Sprafka

H E A L T H
ASSESSMENT

H E A L T H
A S S E S S M E N T

Lois Malasanos, R.N., Ph.D.

Professor and Dean, College of Nursing
University of Florida
Gainesville, Florida

Violet Barkauskas, R.N., C.N.M., M.P.H., Ph.D.

Associate Dean for Administration, School of Nursing
The University of Michigan
Ann Arbor, Michigan

Kathryn Stoltenberg-Allen, R.N., M.S.N.

Formerly Assistant Professor, Department of
Public Health Nursing, College of Nursing,
University of Illinois at the Medical Center,
Chicago, Illinois

Fourth Edition

with **977** illustrations and **6** color plates

The C. V. Mosby Company

ST. LOUIS • BALTIMORE • PHILADELPHIA • TORONTO 1990

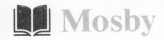

Editor: William Brottmiller
Senior Development Editor: Sally Adkisson
Project Manager: Suzanne Seeley
Production Editor: Jolynn Gower
Designer: Rey Umali
Production: CRACOM Corporation

Fourth Edition

The C.V. Mosby Company
11830 Westline Industrial Drive, St. Louis, Missouri 63146

Library of Congress Cataloging in Publication Data

Malasanos, Lois
  Health assessment/Lois Malasanos, Violet Barkauskas, Kathryn Stoltenberg-Allen. —4th ed.
    p. cm.
  Rev. ed. of: Health assessment/Lois Malasanos . . . [et al.]. 3rd ed. 1986.
  Includes bibliographical references.
  ISBN (invalid) 0-8016-3229-9
  1. Nursing assessment. 2. Medical history taking. 3. Physical diagnosis. I. Barkauskas, Violet. II. Stoltenberg-Allen, Kathryn. III. Health assessment. IV. Title.
  [DNLM: 1. Medical History Taking. 2. Physical Examination. WB 205 M238h]
RT48.M25 1990
616.07′5—dc20
DNLM/DLC
for Library of Congress   89-13173
                                                                CIP

GW/VH/VH 9 8 7 6 5 4 3 2 1

To our family and friends—
who encouraged and sustained us, and

To the students
who have used this book and have gone on
to use assessment skills in their practice,
and to those whose future practice will
benefit from the assessment skills and
good sense presented in these pages.

Contributors

Margaret Fitzgerald, RN,C, MS
(The Interview; Assessment of the Ears, Nose and Throat)

Assistant Professor
Simmons College
Graduate Program in Primary Health Care Nursing
Boston, Massachusetts;
Family Nurse Practitioner
The Family Health Center
Lawrence, Massachusetts

Katharine M. Fortinash, RN, MSN
(Assessment of Mental Status)

Associate Professor Psychiatric Nursing
Grossmont College
San Diego, California

Christina Bergh Jackson, RN, MSN, CPNP
(Assessment of the Pediatric Client)

Faculty
School of Nursing
Eastern College
St. Davids, Pennsylvania;
Pediatric Nurse Practitioner
Private Practice
Paoli, Pennsylvania

Jacqueline L. Kartman, RN,C, MS, CCRN
(Assessment of Sleep-Wakefulness Patterns)

Cardiopulmonary Critical Care Clinical Nurse Specialist
Lutheran Hospital-LaCrosse
LaCrosse, Wisconsin

Linda J. Kerley, RN, MSN
(Assessment of the Musculoskeletal System)

Assistant Professor
East Tennessee State University
Johnson City, Tennessee

Frances K. Lopez-Bushnell, RN,C, EdD, MPH, MSN
(Cultural Considerations in Health Assessment)

Assistant Professor
University of Lowell
College of Health Professions
Family and Community Health Nursing
Lowell, Massachusetts

Mary Meyers-Marquardt, RN, BSN, CCRN
(Assessment of the Neurological System)

Formerly Critical Care Coordinator
Olin E. Teague Veterans' Center
Temple, Texas

Mindi Miller, RN, PhD

Faculty, Department of Human Performance and
Health Sciences
Rice University
Houston, Texas

Carolyn Morris, RN, MSN
(Assessment of the Aging Client)

Clinical Nurse Specialist in Gerontology,
Lecturer in Gerontology
The University of Michigan
School of Nursing
Ann Arbor, Michigan

Linda A. Prinkey, RN, MSN, CCRN
(Decision Making)

Director of Nursing Care
Cardiac Surgical Unit
Alexandria Hospital
Alexandria, Virgina

Ann Herrstrom Skelly, MS, ANP-C
(Assessment of the Skin, Hair, and Nails)

Assistant Professor
Director of Undergraduate Program
University at Buffalo-State University of New York
Buffalo, New York

Denise D. Strathdee, RD, LD
(Nutritional Assessment)

Consultant Dietitian in Private Practice
Total Nutrition Systems
Moline, Illinois

Laura A.M. Talbot, RN, MS
(Assessment Techniques; General Assessment, Including Vital Signs; Assessment of the Abdomen)

Assistant Professor
Texas Christian University
Harris College of Nursing
Fort Worth, Texas;
Doctoral Student
Texas Women's University
Denton, Texas

Preface

Reorganized, redesigned, and considerably rewritten, the fourth edition of *Health Assessment* has been reconceived to reflect recent changes in the practice of health assessment by nurses. Like its previous editions, this book continues to reflect the authors' belief in holistic health assessment, taking into account the client's environment, health practices and beliefs, and physical status. In this edition, assessment is placed into its larger decision-making context. Health assessment is presented as the systematic collection of data that health professionals can use to begin making decisions about how they will intervene to restore or promote health.

The text is designed for students and beginning practitioners. It contains the theory and skills necessary to collect a comprehensive health history and to perform a complete physical examination. These skills can be most effectively mastered when the text is used in conjunction with a structured learning environment, such as a skills lab or a clinical setting in which learners can practice techniques on one another or on properly informed clients. Because the book contains a great deal of substantive detail on examination techniques and findings, the student is not expected to outgrow the text but utilize it as a valuable reference in clinical practice.

A new system of units elucidates the organization of the book. Unit I consists of a series of short chapters on the elements of the health history, capped by an overview chapter that pulls the disparate elements together in a cogent format. The health history, often neglected, is arguably the most important aspect of health assessment, since it alerts the examiner to potential problems and directs the focus of the examination itself. A sensitively gathered health history requires astute communication and observation skills, which are given careful attention in this text. We believe it is the most comprehensive discussion of the health history available to health professionals.

The bulk of the book consists of a body systems approach to the physical examination, Unit II. After short introductory chapters on equipment and techniques and taking vital signs, the physical examination is presented by body systems, a time-honored organizational method conducive to learning. To the extent possible, these chapters follow a consistent format. After a brief review of relevant anatomy and physiology, the examination techniques are presented in depth and carefully illustrated, emphasizing normal findings in the well adult. Then, common abnormal findings are presented that alert the learner to the types of pathology. Finally, by way of summary, the relevant health history, including suggested questions, is reviewed in a boxed format. To facilitate the student's laboratory or clinical experience, perforated cards are bound into the back of the book summarizing the physical examination in both a body systems and a head-to-toe format. These cards are designed to be torn out and carried into the structured practice area to reinforce the habit of an orderly examination. An orderly approach to the examination is indispensible to good technique.

Although the book focuses on the general care of the healthy adult client, no comprehensive text on health assessment can ignore the special assessment techniques required by clients of other age groups. Thus Unit III includes chapters that present assessment techniques unique to pregnant women, children, and older adults.

Other techniques are presented in Unit IV on special populations. Sensitivity to the cultural dimensions of clients has always been a hallmark of this book, and cultural considerations continue to be interwoven throughout the text where appropriate. Nonetheless, because of the multicultural society in the United States and Canada, we have developed a separate chapter that brings cultural considerations into a unified presentation. A functional assessment chapter has been added. Although any client can benefit from a functional assessment, the degree of adaptation to one's environment is especially important for the frail elderly and for disabled clients.

The purpose of performing an assessment is to use the data in clinical decision making. Unit V discusses the use of assessment data. It includes a new chapter on decision making that places assessment in its nursing process context. Emphasis is placed on how the information derived from the assessment is organized. There is little value in obtaining information that is unclear to the practitioner or other members of the health team at a future time when it may be of critical importance as part of an overall data base from which problems are identified and actions planned.

Throughout this text, the consumer of health care is referred to as the *client* because the term implies the ability of a person, whether well or sick, to contract for health care as a responsible participant, with the providers, in the health care process. Health-care providers can no longer expect consumers of health care to accept advice or treatment unless they have been included in the decision-making process. The term *client* also connotes the wide variety of settings in which health care is provided.

The authors are grateful for the wide acceptance of this book over its first three editions. We recognize the obligations that accompany the book's acceptance. It is our goal, once again, to offer a new edition of *Health Assessment* and to provide an innovative product, one which reflects and anticipates the ways in which health care is delivered. The many comments made by students and educators have been instrumental to the revision process and the realization of our goal.

It is also our pleasure to express gratitude to a number of individuals who helped us prepare this edition. Without their support and assistance it would not have been possible. Carrie Schopf, M.D., was our reviewer, supporter, and teacher for the first edition. We are also grateful for the assistance provided by Betsy Perry, R.N., M.P.H., and Lawrence Allen, M.D. The excellent photography of Patricia Urbanus, R.N., M.S.N., C.N.M., continues to serve this book well. Our thanks are also extended to Scott Thorn Barrows, William R. Schwarz, Robert Parshall, Christo Popoff, Marion Howard, and Mary Ann Olson for their outstanding artwork.

Contents

Unit III

Health assessment across the life span

Unit IV

Health assessment of special populations

Unit V

Using health assessment data

Appendixes

Glossary, 796

HEALTH
ASSESSMENT

Color plates

Plate 1
Some common dermatoses and cutaneous manifestations of systemic disorders.

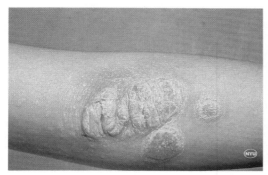

Psoriasis

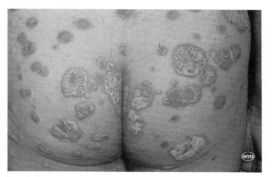

Psoriasis

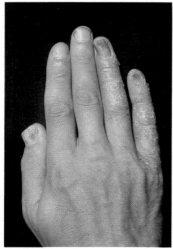

Psoriasis

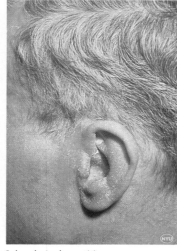

Seborrheic dermatitis

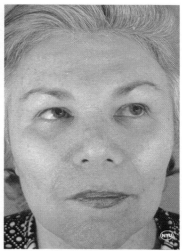

Seborrheic dermatitis

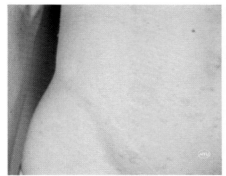

Pityriasis rosea

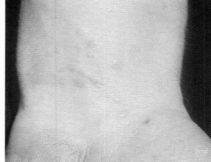

Lichen planus

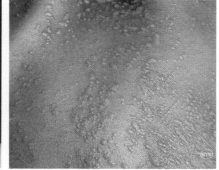

Lichen planus

Continued.

Plate 1, cont'd
Some common dermatoses and cutaneous manifestations of systemic disorders.

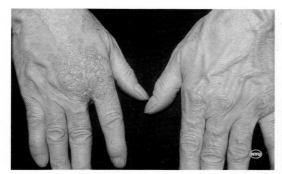

Nummular eczema

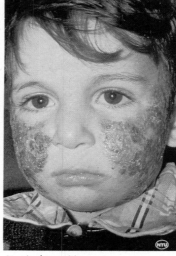

Atopic dermatitis

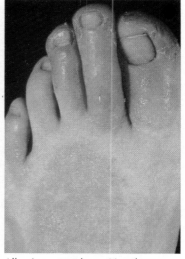

Allergic contact dermatitis—shoe

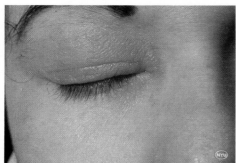

Allergic contact dermatitis—shampoo

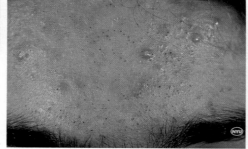

Acne

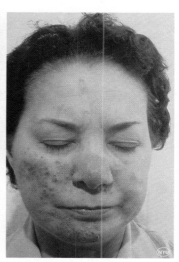

Rosacea

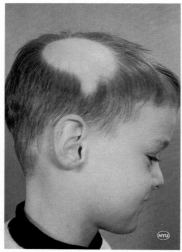

Alopecia areata

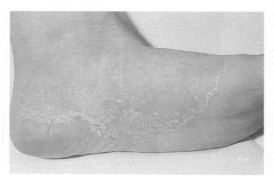

Tinea pedis

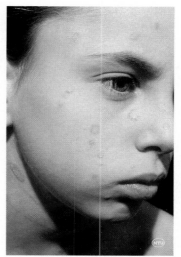

Tinea faciale

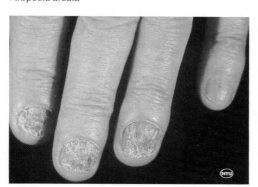

Tinea unguium

Plate 1, cont'd
Some common dermatoses and cutaneous manifestations of systemic disorders.

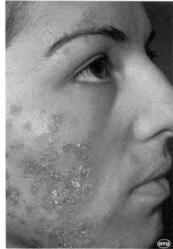

Impetigo contagiosa

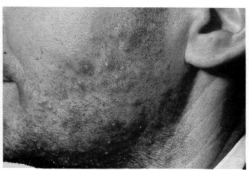

Folliculitis

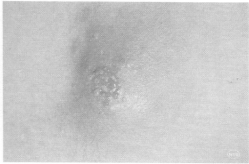

Carbuncle

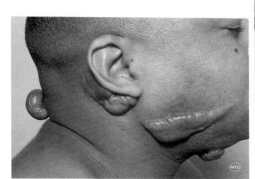

Keloids

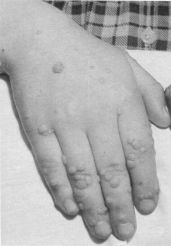

Verruca vulgaris

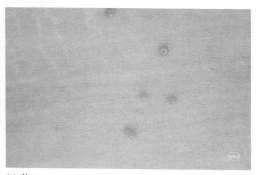

Molluscum contagiosum

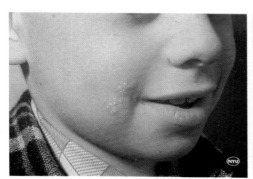

Herpes simplex

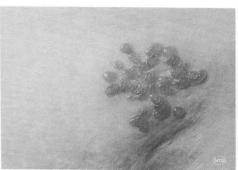

Herpes zoster

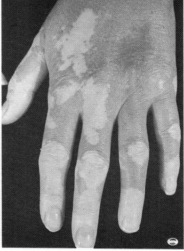

Vitiligo

Continued.

Plate 1, cont'd
Some common dermatoses and cutaneous manifestations of systemic disorders.

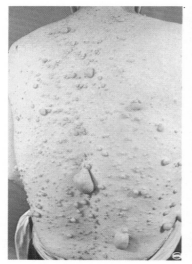

Neurofibromatosis

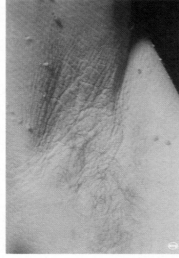

Acanthosis nigricans

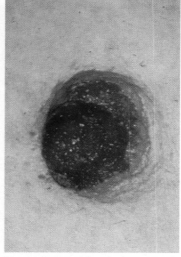

Paget's disease of the nipple
(Courtesy of Stewart, W.D., et. al.:
Dermatology, 1978, The C.V. Mosby Co.)

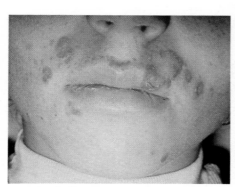

Impetigo (bullous)

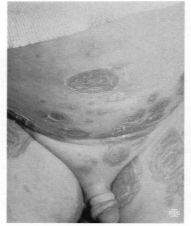

Impetigo (bullous)

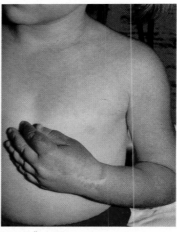

Nevus flammeus

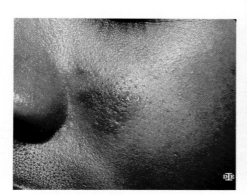

Discoid lupus erythematosus

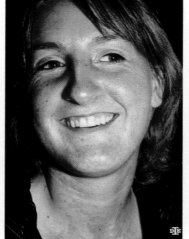

Systemic lupus erythematosus

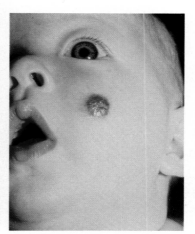

Hemangioma

Plate 1. Courtesy American Academy of Dermatology and Institute for Dermatologic Communication and Education, Evanston, Illinois.

Plate 2
Ear.

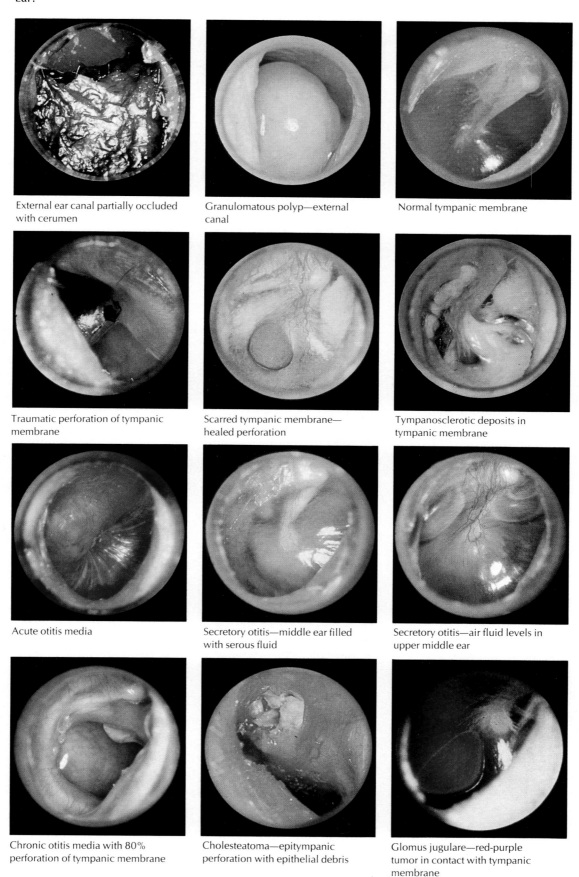

External ear canal partially occluded with cerumen

Granulomatous polyp—external canal

Normal tympanic membrane

Traumatic perforation of tympanic membrane

Scarred tympanic membrane—healed perforation

Tympanosclerotic deposits in tympanic membrane

Acute otitis media

Secretory otitis—middle ear filled with serous fluid

Secretory otitis—air fluid levels in upper middle ear

Chronic otitis media with 80% perforation of tympanic membrane

Cholesteatoma—epitympanic perforation with epithelial debris

Glomus jugulare—red-purple tumor in contact with tympanic membrane

Plate 2. Courtesy Dr. Richard A. Buckingham, Clinical Professor, Otolaryngology, Abraham Lincoln School of Medicine, University of Illinois, Chicago, Illinois.

Plate 3
Nose.

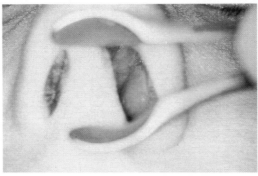

Allergic rhinitis

Plate 4
Mouth.

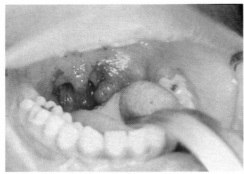

Acute viral pharyngitis

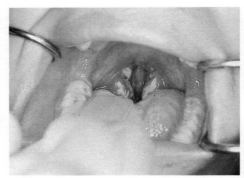

Tonsillitis, pharyngitis

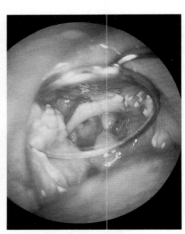

Yeast infection, lingual tonsil, hypopharynx

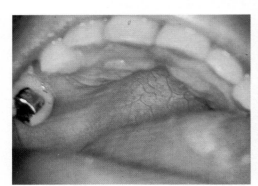

Leukoplakia

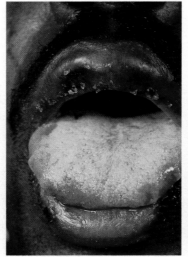

Acute bacterial stomatitis

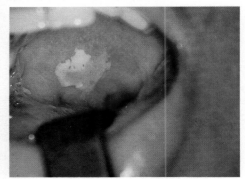

Vincent's angina

Continued.

Plate 4, cont'd
Mouth.

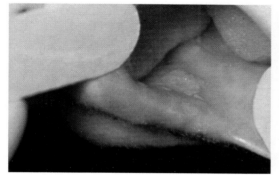

Herpes zoster

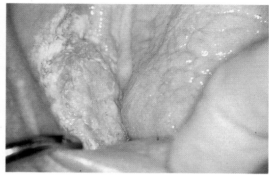

Squamous cell carcinoma

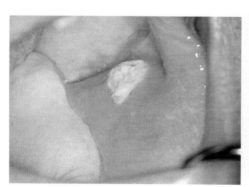

Carcinoma of oral mucosa

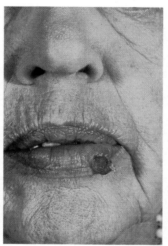

Senile keratosis—lip

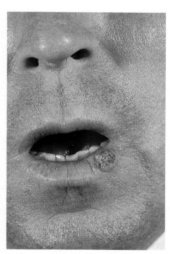

Epidermal carcinoma—lip

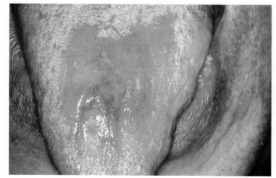

Drug reaction—tongue

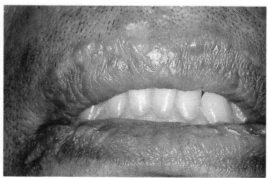

Drug reaction—lip

Plate 4. Courtesy Dr. Edward L. Applebaum, Head, Department of Otolaryngology, University of Illinois Medical Center, Chicago, Illinois.

Plate 5

Eyes.

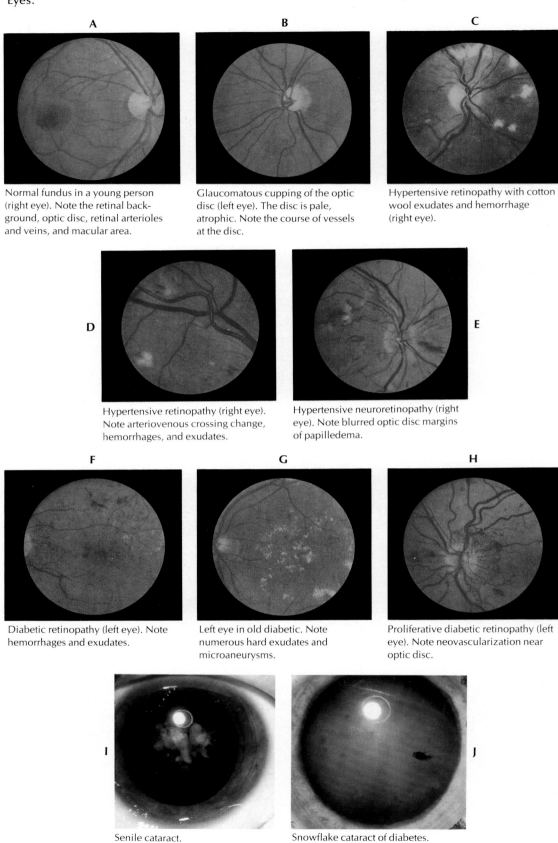

A

Normal fundus in a young person (right eye). Note the retinal background, optic disc, retinal arterioles and veins, and macular area.

B

Glaucomatous cupping of the optic disc (left eye). The disc is pale, atrophic. Note the course of vessels at the disc.

C

Hypertensive retinopathy with cotton wool exudates and hemorrhage (right eye).

D

Hypertensive retinopathy (right eye). Note arteriovenous crossing change, hemorrhages, and exudates.

E

Hypertensive neuroretinopathy (right eye). Note blurred optic disc margins of papilledema.

F

Diabetic retinopathy (left eye). Note hemorrhages and exudates.

G

Left eye in old diabetic. Note numerous hard exudates and microaneurysms.

H

Proliferative diabetic retinopathy (left eye). Note neovascularization near optic disc.

I

Senile cataract.

J

Snowflake cataract of diabetes.

Plate 5. **A** to **H** from Larsen, H.W.: The ocular fundus, Copenhagen, 1976, Munksgaard International Publishers, Ltd. **I** and **J** from Donaldson, D.D.: Atlas of diseases of the eye. The crystalline lens, vol. V, St. Louis, 1976, The C.V. Mosby Co.

Plate 6
Skin changes in the elderly client.

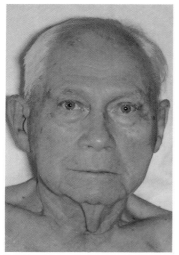

Full face view of 84-year-old man.

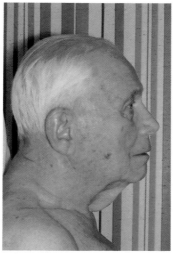

Side view of same subject.

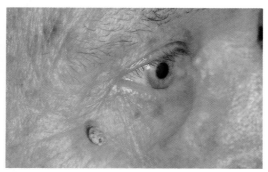

Close-up to emphasize skin wrinkling, sagging, and a prominent seborrheic keratosis.

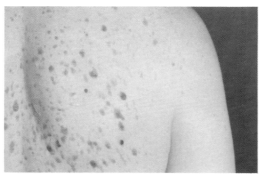

Actinic keratoses.

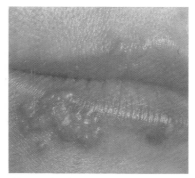

Herpes simplex.

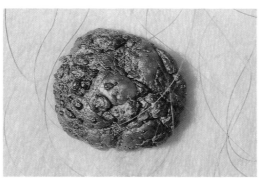

Seborrheic keratosis.

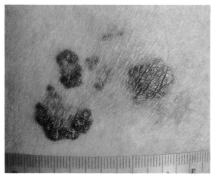

Lentigines malignant.

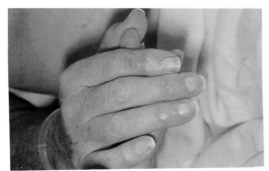

Heberdon's nodules.

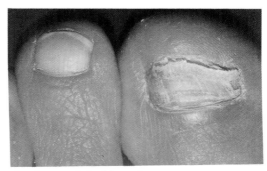

Onychomycosis (nail fungus).

The Health History:

a holistic approach

1

The interview

OBJECTIVES

Upon successful review of this chapter, learners will be able to identify:

- Communication techniques that help fulfill interview purposes

- Purposes and components of a contract between a client and a practitioner

- Methods for facilitating an interview

- Methods of questioning that affect the interview process

- Methods for assuring understanding between client and practitioner

- Nonverbal patterns that communicate data

- Appropriate use of intimate distance, personal, social, and public spaces

- Use of empathy and acceptance in a therapeutic relationship

- Guidelines for obtaining a complete description of a symptom

- Common problems that occur during interviews

The major purpose of the interview conducted before the physical examination is to obtain a health history and to elicit symptoms and the time course of their development. The goal of an effective interview is to obtain a complete and accurate database. However, although assessment may be the main emphasis of a given exchange, the health care provider must use skillful communication techniques to establish the rapport necessary for a full sharing of the client's relevant life experiences. A climate of trust must be established that will allow a full expression of the client's needs. Furthermore, an analysis of the client's reactions during the interview will allow the examiner to predict the client's ability and willingness to comprehend and therefore carry out the directions given as part of the therapeutic plan.

The students of the health care professions have had many years of interacting with fellow human beings and have practiced establishing relationships in many settings. Therefore, the practitioner performs the examination within the context of a professional experience. Most students have learned which communication techniques work well for them, particularly in social settings. The focus of this discussion will be the characteristics of information exchange that will allow the client and health care professional to work toward the mutual goal of establishing a database.

As the interview begins with introductions, a mutual assessment of client and interviewer takes place. The interviewer generally has the advantage of knowing the client's name and may greet him or her warmly, respectfully, and by name. A handshake is appropriate if the examiner is comfortable in reaching out in the initial encounter and the client appears receptive to this.

The interview process is enhanced and facilitated by the client's communication skills and sensitivity to the examiner. To this end, the practitioner must develop a flexible framework for obtaining the information or behavior needed in the assessment that will also facilitate the interaction necessary for a therapeutic relationship.

The most effective place to learn how to interview is at the bedside and in the clinic while dealing with actual clients. Initial interviews should be supervised by a skilled professional who will provide support and suggestions for modification during and after the client session.

It is helpful to have videotapes of practice sessions made so that students may more objectively analyze their own interviewing skills and maximize those special talents made evident by direct viewing. The goal of the effective communicator is to demonstrate concern and sincere desire to engage in tasks necessary to meet the client's health care needs.

The use of a written record of the interview, called a process recording, may be helpful in identifying communication problems. However, a tape recording (with the client's consent) of a verbal interchange between the client and the practitioner may serve the same end. Yet, tape recording may sometimes inhibit the client's willingness to communicate.

Particularly at the first interview, the client should be allowed to talk freely, describing his or her health condition. One frequently observed error is the monopoly of the interview by the practitioner. Frequently clients report that they did not mention symptoms because they did not have an opportunity or were not encouraged to do so—"He asked so many questions that I didn't get a chance to say anything." When one of the participants does most of the talking during the interview, the other may be silent for long periods. The practitioner should bear in mind that clients' perception of what is being said in conversation is often decreased when they are listening to a long presentation. The most effective communication exists when the client takes an active role in the interview. The interview might begin with a general invitation to the client to speak freely, such as "Tell me how do you feel," or " What health concern brings you here?"

CONTRACT

The interview is a verbal and nonverbal exchange that provides for the beginning and development of a relationship. Initially, the participants are strangers, each presenting a particular style of relating and adapting. Defining the terms of the relationship early in the interview allows for reduction of unnecessary stressors and provides goals for the participants. Common symbols (gestures and facial expressions) used between examiner and client should have the same meaning to both partic-

ipants, since the quality of the communication will determine the value of the relationship. Unlike many other associations, the association between the health care professional and the client has a mutual concern, the client's well-being. This commonality of interest will facilitate progress toward the sharing of information, ideas, and emotions. A mutually understandable language and an understanding of the significance of body language, such as gestures and facial expressions, will increase the exchange of information between the client and the practitioner and enrich the data obtained.

Facial expressions are the most widely used nonverbal communication and the message most frequently observed by the client. Eye contact is frequently used. In most ethnic groups, people invite communication with others by looking directly at them. The person who looks another in the eye while talking is generally considered open and honest. However, should the person being gazed on decline the invitation, he or she generally does so by averting eye contact, most often looking downward. Although a short gaze may be interpreted as accessibility and interest on the examiner's part, it is important to avoid long periods of looking directly at the client because this may be interpreted as an invitation to an uncomfortably revealing relationship by the client or as a threatening behavior.

The contract or basic operating agreement between the client and the practitioner is usually a verbal commitment presented by the practitioner. This contract should include:
1. Time and place that the interview and subsequent examinations will occur
2. Duration of time involved in the present and future examinations
3. Number of sessions required
4. Expectations for participation by the client in the assessment process
5. Confidentiality of shared information and findings—responsibilities of each member
6. Rules regarding the presence of other professionals or of the client's relatives or other advocates
7. Cost to the client where applicable
8. Therapeutic goals subsequent to the assessment process

The advantage of the contract to the practitioner is that the client is relieved of misconceptions, fears, or fantasies concerning what might happen during the interview and examination. Thus, the contract establishes norms and role behavior. The practitioner and the client have expectations of each other, and confusion over roles threatens the relationship.

The expectation that there will be shared decision

making in the management of health care should be made very clear to the client. To this end, clients are encouraged to learn more about themselves to identify health needs and to recognize that they have an option in determining if and how health care needs are met.

In traditional health care relationships the health care professional is the authority figure whereas the client is, at least to some degree, the dependent. The client has initiated the interview by seeking help for a problem. In this effort to obtain aid from the professional, the client must determine the kind of information and behavior expected. The professional is obligated to analyze the client's communication pattern to explain to the client what is required for the professional to give the help that is needed. The interaction provides a kind of negotiation for the terms on which the relationship can continue, that is, a contract defining the participants' roles. The verbal and nonverbal dialogue that occurs in the first few minutes of this social exchange may well determine not only the reliability and amount of information the client will furnish to the interviewer but also the character of the relationship that follows.

SETTING

To promote the most effective attention to communication and therefore to build rapport, the practitioner should carefully construct the interview environment to avoid interruption, distraction, or discomfort as shown in the box opposite.

At the outset it should be determined if the time scheduled for the interview is mutually convenient to the client and interviewer. Although geographic privacy may not be obtainable in emergency rooms, large clinics, or multiple bed units in the hospital, psychological protection may be provided. Some of the assurances important to the client are that (1) the client is not being heard by other clients or personnel not concerned in care, (2) the practitioner is giving a high level of attention to the client, and (3) the information the client is sharing will be regarded as confidential or that the conditions of sharing will be defined.

In an ideal setting, the privacy of the client's thoughts and comfort can be guaranteed by conducting the interview in a private room where optimum temperature and lighting can be controlled. Indirect lighting is preferred so the client is not looking into a bright light or exposed to glare from a window.

The practitioner's physical position as related to the client can have implications in the control process. To suggest that the client has the option to control some of the interview, arrange the chairs or other furniture so

---

The Setting

1. Assure a comfortable temperature for both you and your client.
2. Do not seat yourself so the light source is behind you. This forces the client to look into the light. You will then be in a shadow, with your face and gestures difficult to see.
3. An elderly client may feel frightened sitting on an examination table due to altered perceptions of height and space. A child may feel similarly frightened by being up so high and separated from the parent.

---

that a face-to-face alignment to ensure eye contact is possible. The commonly used position of standing over and looking down at the client suggests that the practitioner has assumed leadership for the interchange. Leaning forward appropriately conveys alert attention. However, relaxed body posture should be maintained.

Excessively long interviews are tiring to the client. More than one session may be needed to complete the database, particularly if the health history is complex or the client is critically ill or debilitated.

The client should obtain a sense of the interviewer's full involvement in the process. It is important to be aware of body language that could convey boredom or restlessness, such as shifting from one foot to another, sighing, or edging toward the door.

COMMUNICATION PROCESS

Anxiety may be an anticipated element in an initial interview for both the health care professional and the client. Some of the indications of acute anxiety that may be observed include a furrowed brow, squinting, dilated pupils, tensed facial muscles, distended neck vessels, rapid talk, a dry mouth, frequent hand gestures, a tense posture, an increased heart rate and blood pressure, sweaty palms and axillae, and a sweaty pubic area. Shuffling of feet may indicate the client's desire to escape the interview. The client's anxieties may be associated with the symptoms of illness, with the practitioner's reaction, with fees, or with expectations of future appointments. These anxieties may also be evidence of problems external to the interview. Clues that interview items are producing anxiety include long pauses, nervous laughter, dry coughing, and sighing.

Practitioners are concerned with clients' responses to the interview, with their ability to obtain appropriate information, and with their ability to synthesize the data provided so that the problems can be correctly defined.

To facilitate the development of rapport, health care professionals must use communication skills to project to clients that they are interested and concerned with providing necessary support. A practitioner might convey support by assuring a client, "I want to work with you to find out what is making you feel this way." To demonstrate interest and the willingness to listen, the practitioner must also be aware of the message conveyed nonverbally.

Particular attention is given the remarks made as the client is entering or leaving the room, since these comments frequently have special significance. The client may reveal the chief complaint at these times and avoid mentioning it during the formal interview.

The amount of structure that is brought to bear in the interview depends on the level of organization of ego functioning the client exhibits. In general, the client with the lesser degree of organization needs more structure in the interview to increase the amount of data obtained in a given time and to decrease anxiety.

The communication process involves feedback in that each message sent involves a response. This response affects the next message sent and its reaction. With practice, the examiner will settle in the communication mode that is most effective for the individual client. This is particularly important in the choice of the type of questions used to obtain the health history.

A common communication error that occurs in industrialized nations is that of thinking of the next remark, thereby not fully perceiving what is being said. This is a particular hazard for the student who is not yet fully comfortable with the interview pattern. Such an individual may perceive little of valuable data being given by the client, since that individual must concentrate on the format of questioning and on how best to word the next query.

Types of Questions

Multiple answer questions

Questions should be carefully designed to deal with one issue at a time. Questions should not demand two or more rejoinders, particularly conflicting answers.

Examples of questions to avoid are "Did you have measles, mumps, or whooping cough?" or "Did you have pain in your shoulder or in your chest?"

Open-ended questions

Although the interview is aimed at getting specific answers concerning the events surrounding the client's signs and symptoms, each point should be developed by the client in his or her own words. An open-ended question or suggestion is one aimed at eliciting a response that is more than one or two words long. This type of question is effective in stimulating descriptive or comparative responses. Observation of the client who is describing a symptom may give valuable information concerning attitudes and beliefs. In addition, it allows the client to provide information at a self-determined pace rather than feel forced to divulge information when sharing it may be troublesome. This description may also provide clues to the client's alertness, or level of mental abilities, and to the organization of ego functioning, revealed through the organization of thoughts and vocabulary. Furthermore, rapport is strengthened through the demonstration that the practitioner wants to invest time in hearing the client's thoughts. Examples of open-ended questions or suggestions are "How have you been feeling lately?" and "Tell me about your problem."

The disadvantage of this type of question is that it may result in responses that are not relevant to a specific point being assessed. The client may use the opportunity provided by an open-ended question to digress to avoid discussing relevant data because it is distressing. Although this technique might yield important information, there are times when the examiner needs data quickly and must sacrifice to get it. This is particularly true in emergency care. When the drug overdose victim rouses, the only piece of important data may be elicited by a closed question ("What did you take?")

Closed questions

The closed question is a type of inquiry that requires no more than a one- or two-word answer. This might be agreement or disagreement. The response may be a yes or no and may be answered nonverbally by a nod of the head. This is the kind of question most appropriate for eliciting age, sex, marital status, and other forced-choice responses. Examples of closed questions are "What did you eat for dinner last night?" and "What medication did you take?"

The educationally impoverished or those who lack culturally enriching experiences are often more comfortable with this type of question because they know what is expected. The open-ended question may pose anxiety to the client with poor articulation, who may fear that a display of lack of verbal skill will be a disadvantage with the practitioner. On the other hand, the closed question by its nature limits the amount of information that is obtained in the health history and may convey to the client that the practitioner is too busy or disinterested to listen. It has been observed that practitioners use more closed questions in initial interviews and when the process is stressful, as well as when time is limited.

Directive questions

Questions that lead the client to focus on one set of thoughts are called directive questions. This type of questioning is most often used in reviewing systems or in evaluating client functional levels. Although they are very effective for obtaining information, directive questions should be used with caution. If used in rapid succession, the client may feel rushed into giving information and may not develop a thought fully. The provider should allow the client time for reflection during the use of directive questions.

Leading questions

Questions that carry a suggestion of the kind of information that should be included in the response are called leading questions. The client is presented with an expectation by the practitioner. This kind of question may seriously limit the value of the health history. For example, the question "You haven't ever had venereal disease, have you?" implies that the possibility that the client *has had* venereal disease would be outside the limits of acceptability for the practitioner. The client who has experienced the disease may not say so to avoid disappointing the questioner.

The presence of emotionally charged words in a given question may make the question a biased one. For example, there is one in the question, "You haven't been masturbating, have you?" Since the Judeo-Christian ethic defines masturbating as "bad," bias has been inflicted. In this case the practitioner has suggested that the answer should be no. The client may well avoid all matters dealing with sexuality to avoid losing the practitioner's approval.

The practitioner must balance the goals of efficiency and effectiveness in the interviews. In obtaining a historical database, the practitioner asks the client many questions to obtain thorough, relevant information. However, a comprehensive interview is time-consuming, and practitioners often attempt to save time by asking closed questions. More information is gained by open-ended questions that may supply much relevant and extraneous data. Therefore, the interviewer must consider the relative importance of the interview questions in the gathering of the database to obtain the most useful information within a reasonable time.

Use of Silence

Periods of silence during the interview are helpful in making observations, such as: Is the client comfortable? Angry? Confused? Silence provides an opportunity to assess the level of anxiety in both the practitioner and the client. Also, the client is provided with sufficient time to carefully organize thoughts for a coherent explanation in response to questions. The rapid presentation of questions may not allow the client sufficient time for thought or reflection. Silence is also useful as an indicator of the amount of anxiety the client is experiencing. The client's silence may indicate absorbing thought, boredom. or grief. Silence by the practitioner usually encourages communication by the client.

Facilitation

Facilitation is the act that stimulates the client to continue talking, no matter what the topic. Silence may be facilitative, as are encouraging words such as "Go on", "Mm-hm", and "Yes, I see." The provider who uses facilitation effectively will convey a feeling of caring and empathy to the client.

Methods for Ensuring Understanding

The practitioner must use maneuvers to determine if both participants understand what has been said. A clear understanding of what the client is trying to say is essential to establishing an accurate database. The health history should not contain assumptions of what the client meant but a clear accounting of exactly what was said. Many techniques provide for encouragement of the client to expand on a description or to clarify the explanation that has been given. A workable example might be "Tell me more about it."

Use of a common language

The practitioner must carefully plan questions and give particular care in selecting the vocabulary to be used so that the client perceives the question in the same sense that it is intended by the practitioner. The practitioner is aided in processing the client's language and behavior for what is usual or "normal" by having an understanding of cultural and ethnic differences. Medical terminology or *jargon* should not be used excessively. When medical diagnoses are employed, the meaning should be explained to the client when the words are first used.

Use of jargon or terminology by the provider may serve to build barriers between the two participants. Indeed, the provider may purposely use these terms to avoid communication or to terminate conversations. This practice should be avoided.

If the client uses jargon or terminology, the provider must determine the client's understanding of the word(s). The provider and the client should then agree on the use of the word(s). For example, many lay people use the terms coronary, heart attack, and angina interchangeably.

Planning the questions

The client is asked one question at a time. For the client to give the information needed for the health history, the questions must be phrased so that the client knows what kind of answers are expected. When the client's response is not appropriate, a reordering of the question or a more explicit choice of vocabulary may be indicated. It may be helpful to emphasize the key words in the question. In designing questions, one should avoid the use of ambiguous terms, medical language, or words with more than one meaning.

Use of an example

Comparison with a common experience, that is, a concrete happening, may help to clarify an abstract concept or hazy terminology. The practitioner may use an example as part of the questioning process when the meaning is not clear. For example, the practitioner may ask the client, "Was it as large as a cherry?"

Restatement

Restatement is the formulation of what the client has said in words that are more specific; it provides an opportunity to validate the practitioner's conception. The client is cued to give attention to the thought by phrases such as "Do you mean . . . ," "In other words . . . ," or "If I understand you correctly. . . ."

Reflection

Reflection means repeating a phrase or a sentence the client has just said. The suggestion to the client that the practitioner is still involved in that part of the communication may focus further attention or rumination on that thought. The strategy is aimed toward further elaboration in the form of the recall of facts or feelings that surrounded the circumstance. The technique should allow clarification or expansion of the information just given by the client. Examples are as follows:

Client: My mother has been drinking a fifth a day for 6 years. She's an alcoholic.

Interviewer response: You say your mother is an alcoholic?

Client: The spot on my arm is painful, you know.

Interviewer response: Painful?

Clarification

Questions designed to obtain information to more clearly understand conflicting, abstract, vague, or ambiguous statements are requests for clarification.

You say you felt depressed? Tell me what you mean.
You had constant headaches? Tell me what you remember about them.

Summary

Summary is a technique that allows for the condensation of facts into a well-ordered review. It is particularly useful following a rambling, detailed description. The summary further signals the client that this particular segment of the interview is terminating and suggests that further input is required immediately, since closure is imminent.

Confrontation

Telling clients something about themselves is known as confrontation. This may be a helpful technique to use when inconsistencies are noticed, for example, "When you tell me how painful your arm is, I notice that you are smiling. Why is this?" Confrontation may also be of use in helping the client to discuss emotions, for example, "You say you are not uncomfortable, but you are frowning and your muscles appear very tense." Confrontation is also used to seek further information when the client has presented unrealistic ideas.

Interpretation

The examiner may arrive at a conclusion from the data the client has given. Sharing the interpretation with the client allows the individual to confirm, deny, or offer an interpretation. Making an interpretation involves the risk of being wrong, and the examiner should be prepared to deal with this eventuality. The interpretation may also constitute an act of empathy or confrontation.

Filling in Omitted Data

Clinical impressions reached by the practitioner must be regarded as fluid because in further conversation with the client, new information may be provided. The client may withhold information through fear that sensitive information may be shared indiscriminately or through distrust of the practitioner. Furthermore, the client may regard certain facts as unimportant or irrelevant to the focus of the interview. In many instances when clients are so eager to comply with questions that they give a hurried accounting and leave out significant data. In ordering the data the practitioner may note that information is missing or that there are inconsistencies. Further interviews should be scheduled. The client may simply need to be given a summary of the previous conversation to detect the areas where more information is needed. These gaps may be filled by direct questioning. Another method of asking for the missing facts may be to suggest to the client that the practitioner is confused and must again be told a particular sequence of events. A remark such as the following would invite this input: "Now, tell me again all that you remember from the time you first vomited until you came here."

In addition, the possibility of past evaluation and treatment of symptoms should be investigated. The important facts are those obtained by asking when, where, and by whom. Were laboratory or other diagnostic tests performed? Are results available? What diagnosis was made? Was a treatment instituted? Was the treatment helpful?

Obaining Data from People Other than the Client

The client who is critically ill, confused, or intellectually impaired may be unable to give the information necessary to an adequate history. A close relative or a person who knows the client well may be able to provide the information necessary to understand the presence or nature of problems of the individual being examined. If attempts to obtain the history from the client have been ineffective, it may be prudent to ask permission to go over the details again with the second person. Such comments as "I want to be sure that I have what has happened to you correctly in my mind," or "I'd like to go over this one more time to make sure I've got the facts right and in the correct order," may help to gain the client's permission to interview relatives or friends. The parents may be the only reliable source of information for the young child.

Nonverbal Communication

Nonverbal communication is the use of (1) *body movements,* (2) *touch,* (3) *space or territoriality,* (4) *voice tone,* (5) *time,* (6) *appearance,* (7) *acceptance,* (8) *empathy,* and (9) *termination* to convey emotion or feeling, to state messages, and to impart instruction or direction.

Communication through body movement

Some of the gestures to be observed are movements of the body, limbs, hands, or feet; facial expressions, particularly smiling and frowning; and eye behavior such as blinking, the direction of gaze, and the length of time of gaze. Posture is particularly expressive.

Extension of large muscles is associated with relaxation, whereas contraction of large muscles is associated with anxiety and fear. The individual who sits stretched out and gestures away from the body gives an appearance of assurance.

The posture or movement of the client's body may provide valuable clues to health status. The messages given by the client through body language may provide additional and sometimes more reliable information than words, since many persons employ less conscious control over this aspect of behavior. Thus, by actions clients may convey thoughts that they cannot or refuse to commit to words. Interpretation of the full meaning of the gestures and action of the client must be performed against a comparison of their sociocultural meanings. For instance, the downcast eyes of the Muhammadan woman could be interpreted as the usual or normal response to the practitioner, whereas in the United States one might become alert to other indications of fear, withdrawal, depression, or lack of attentiveness. The use of eye contact assumes a good deal of meaning among Greek and Indian cultures.

Posture. A closed body posture is one in which the limbs are held in defensive positions, that is, close to the body, flexed, with muscles tense. The arms may be held very close to the body as though hugging oneself. The position is most often interpreted as distrustful or anxious. An open body posture is one that is more relaxed, that is, limbs extended, arms hanging loosely at sides.

Facial expression. Clenched teeth and contracted pupils provide a message of tension and may represent an effort to avoid saying something unpleasant to the listener. This expression is generally interpreted as one of anger or hostility.

An individual who smiles constantly may be using this expression as a mask to cover feelings of fear or depression. On the other hand, this may simply be the trademark of an individual with a strong desire to please. The person who covers the mouth with the hands may be expressing a desire to avoid talking.

Eye movement. The practitioner may detect signals of disagreement, aversion, or disgust in the client through subtle eye movements. Dilation of the pupils of the eyes generally accompanies pleasurable experiences, whereas offensive or unpleasant circumstances generally result in contracted pupils.

Touch

The act of touching is one of the most intimate forms of nonverbal communication. It precedes speech in every

---

The Use of Touch

1. Warm your hands and any equipment that may touch the client. A cold touch can convey the feeling that you do not care about the person's comfort.
2. Warn a client of the area you may be touching, particularly if you are approaching from out of the line of vision.
3. Be aware of acceptable behavior for your client's ethnic group. People from some cultures welcome close physical contact, while others consider it highly offensive.

---

person's life. Cultural traditions prescribe the ritual of touch or define the taboos. Touch is regulated by social distancing techniques and is apparent in all living groups, as shown in the box above.

Manners and mores involving touch are given to the developing child through the actions of the family and other close persons. In North America, there is a taboo against touching without permission. In general, when one person touches another, it is in the context of a relationship where touching is appropriate and acceptable to both parties.

Touch has a special meaning among health care professionals. When used properly, it conveys a message of closeness, encouragement, and caring. It plays a prominent role in the provider-client relationship. However, confusion may arise when the client attempts to touch the provider. The provider must be aware of what boundaries feel most comfortable. Negotiation with the client is needed to arrange mutually acceptable limits.

Effect of space or territoriality

A good deal of symbolism has been attributed to one's position in a group. Definition of a cultural group's concern or rejection is provided by distancing. The distance between the practitioner and the client may determine the relationships developed.

Hall has coined the word "proxemics" to describe the use of space by Americans as zones he calls intimate, personal, social, and public.

Intimate distance.   Intimate distance is defined as the distance up to 18 inches from the body. When two people are within this distance, there is awareness of body odor and warmth. Visual detail is sharpened, and the eyes pull inward in accommodation. The voice may automatically lower. The range of vision is such that the individuals are able to focus on one body part only, rather than viewing each other as a whole.

The presence of another body at this close distance is usually associated with activities such as lovemaking, intense verbal interchange, physical punishment, and exchanges of affection. The presence of another body at this close distance intrudes on the senses and is sometimes overwhelming to the client. Although this proximity is needed for the physical examination, it is seldom appropriate to conduct the interview within this space.

Personal distance.   Personal distance limits physical contact and is defined as a distance of 1½ to 4 feet. Although holding and grasping are possible at the near point, touching is the form of physical contact most frequently used. Visual perception is less distorted, and there is a three-dimensional impression of the person involved. As the distance between participants lengthens, the gaze may encompass the entire face rather than a single part of it, such as the eye or the chin. Vocal volume is moderate, and body odors and heat are less intruding. This is the ideal distance for viewing nonverbal behaviors and is the distance most frequently used for the interview. Trust is best developed from this distance.

Social distance.   Social distance provides protection from others without one's having to declare or demand it and is defined as a distance of 4 to 12 feet. The visual image includes more of the total person, and the fine detail of the body is lost. Eye contact becomes more important. Body heat and odor are lost. Vocalization is louder and loses its aura of privacy because it can be overheard. Interaction becomes more ritualized or formal. The threat of domination is less from this distance. This distance allows a limited view of the client's physical aspects, and revelation of attitudes and feelings in general is censored from this distance.

Public distance.   Public distance is defined as separation of communicants by more than 12 feet. Gait and general coordination may be analyzed at this distance while watching the client enter the examining room. Children may be more effectively observed at play when the distance between the child and examiner is increased.

Effect of appearance

Many people in North American society are more generous and outgoing toward physically attractive individuals. Therefore, most adults aim toward an image that is youthful, handsome and well-groomed. In all age levels, clients will present in various states of hygiene and commonly with a physically unattractive appearance. Often the reason the client is seeking health care is due to an illness that alters normal appearance, such as a draining wound, skin rash, or tumor.

As a member of society, the practitioner may come to the interview with preconceived notions about how a person should look and dress. The practitioner must evaluate his or her own value system and not allow these notions to taint the therapeutic relationship. The practitioner must work through attitudes and emotions to interact and touch the less attractive client. Physical signs of limited interaction and touch include restraint of movement, tight musculature, frowning, or touching the person with fingertips only.

Conversely, the client may come to the interview with preconceived notions about how a health care provider should look and dress. Although providers should not stifle a personal sense of style, they should be aware that credibility with the public is usually increased by exhibiting good grooming and attire within commonly accepted standards. This is particularly true when the provider is significantly younger than the client.

Control of space

The hospital room or clinic setting seriously threatens the client's ability to control space. The client is told where and how to sit and how to cooperate with threatening and possibly uncomfortable procedures. Privacy is invaded by multiple members of the health care team.

The client needs time to adjust to the surroundings of the interview and physical examination. Client comfort should be ensured before any questioning or examining is initiated. The client should be allowed to order the disposition of personal belongings. Any questions by the client about uses of the space should be seriously considered and attended to before the interview or examination.

The role of the health care professional is endowed with technical skill, authority, and confidentiality, which helps protect the client from embarrassment when exposing the body or submitting to treatment. To this end, the provider must maintain a professional appearance and attitude and adhere to proper behavior to ensure credibility.

Use of time

The provider is generally perceived by the client to be the person with the superior status in the health care visit. Clients in general realize that providers have many demands on their time. Therefore, most clients will usually tolerate a reasonable delay in the appointment time. However, the provider who is consistently tardy may give the client the impression that the client's time is not valuable. Undue delays should be explained to the client, who should be given the opportunity to reschedule an appointment.

In using the time allotted to the interview, the provider should make every effort to ensure that the process is not interrupted. Potential interruptions include telephone calls and in-person requests from co-workers and other clients. When the provider repeatedly allows the interview to be interrupted, the client may feel that the session is unimportant to the provider. Additionally, these intrusions disrupt the provider's thought processes and may bring about the need to repeat questions. If an interruption is not avoidable, a brief explanation of the nature of the emergency should be provided to the client.

The person with the perceived superior status in a relationship is usually allowed to talk longer. Therefore, the provider will probably speak in longer, uninterrupted lengths than the client. The provider should be aware of the client's reaction to this. For example, if the client interrupts the provider with an unrelated thought during an explanation of treatment requirements, the client may be demonstrating that this information is not of value.

Acceptance

Clients have been shown to be more cooperative when they feel accepted and respected by the health care worker. Gestures that convey acceptability include smiling and moving toward the client without being within the intimate space range (see the discussion on p. 10). Nonverbal messages expressing unfriendliness or tension in the provider include limited eye contact, rushed movements, a lowered voice, and frowning. If the client feels unaccepted by the provider, the relationship may be inhibited and limited in therapeutic value.

Effective communication is best accomplished in a climate of warmth, empathy, and genuineness. The conveyance of a feeling of positive attitude toward the client may be initiated with a hospitable greeting and one's full attention. Clients most frequently interpret warmth from the behavior of health care personnel that includes direct attention and appropriate eye contact by the examiner. Thus, it is important to read or write in the chart minimally while with the client. Other behaviors that have been shown to convey warmth include a relaxed posture while leaning slightly forward in an open arm position and appropriate smiling and nodding. Positive regard may be demonstrated by complimenting aspects of health care that the client is practicing appropriately.

The examiner should guard against communicating haste to the client because the client may believe the examiner has low regard for the interview. Some behaviors that convey impatience are frequent checking of the time, walking to the door, or standing with the hand on the doorknob.

Sincerity or genuineness on the examiner's part may be conveyed by ensuring that there is congruence between the remarks made to the client and the nonverbal cues accompanying the messages. Body language that does not correspond with what is being said may confuse or frighten the client. Facial and body movements should correspond with what is said. The interviewer may have to spend some time learning to be aware of facial, body, and voice behaviors to use them effectively in communicating with clients. Although the practitioner may be frowning because of worry unrelated to the interview, the client in the process of revealing sensitive information may conclude that the information is unacceptable to the interviewer.

Body movements that may convey that the client is uncomfortable include avoidance of eye contact, stiff posture, nervous or inappropriate laughter, and tapping the foot against the floor. The examiner would do well to query the client when these behaviors are observed.

Empathy

Role taking has been suggested to be synonymous with empathy. More simply, it is voluntarily putting oneself in another person's place in one's imagination. The four phases of empathic experience include:

1. Identification—investing oneself in thinking about the person and what is happening to him or her
2. Incorporation—being aware and receptive of the person rather than projecting one's own feelings and thoughts
3. Reverberation—an interaction between the feelings and experiences of the client and the examiner
4. Detachment—return to one's own identity

The insight that is a result of the experience is helpful in understanding and meeting the client's needs. Empathy has been described by some as active listening; it is understanding and acceptance of the client's feelings. Empathic responses may be verbal, for example, "That must have made you feel very frightened" or "That must have been very painful to you." Understanding and acceptance may also be conveyed nonverbally, for example, a hand placed on the client's shoulder.

The interviewer must be correct in responding to the client. Classic errors have been described, such as sympathizing in the assumed painful loss the client felt on the death of his father when in fact the father had been a considerable financial and emotional burden to the client.

Empathy is necessary to the therapeutic relationship. It helps to establish rapport to show understanding and support.

Termination

The interviewer allows the client to terminate the session when the interviewer determines that there are no further questions that would produce productive information in the session. The interviewer signals the client that the interview is in its final phase by saying something such as, "I have no more questions; is there anything more you would like to share with me?" or, "Is there anything we may have omitted?"

HEALTH HISTORY

The first step in health assessment is the interview in which the information of the health history is obtained. This is a structured interview aimed at collecting specific information. This type of interview may present some difficulty for the individual who has been accustomed to less structured methods, that is, more nondirective techniques. Although the client may give a good deal of the history—at least the description of the problem for which help is sought—without the benefit of direct questioning, the complete information of the health history may not be obtained. In that case the practitioner must ask direct questions that will provide the necessary information. In an emergency, the examiner may be forced to use only closed questions.

Encouraging a Complete Description of the Symptom

The descriptions by the client of any changes perceived in the structure of the body or its functions are called *symptoms*. The interview should provide the most accurate and constructive picture of the symptom that can be obtained, since this is the base from which the client's problems can be defined. The practitioner carefully avoids devaluing the client's symptoms by such remarks as, "You have nothing to be nervous about," or, "That's nothing; now, last week we had a really bad case."

Eight criteria can be used to provide this delineation: anatomic location, quality of the symptom, quantity of the symptom, time sequence of the symptom, geographic or environmental locale in which the symptom occurs, precipitating conditions that cause the symptom to be more severe, circumstances that alleviate the symptom, and other symptoms that occur in conjunction with the symptom.

Guideline	*Interview items to elicit symptom description*
1. Anatomic location	"Tell me where it hurts."
Radiation of the symptom	"Show me where it hurts."
2. Quality or character	"What does it feel like?"
	"Can you compare this with something you have felt in the past?"

3. Quantity	"How bad (intense) is the pain?" "How much does the pain immobilize you?" "What effect does the pain have on normal daily activites?"
4. Time sequence	"When did you first notice the pain?" "How long does it last" "How often have you had it since that time?"
5. Geographic or environmental factors	"Where were you when the pain occurred?"
6. Precipitating conditions	"Do you find that the pain occurs at a certain time of day?" "Does heat or cold seem to affect the pain" "What causes the pain?"
Conditions making the symptom more severe	"Have you noticed anything that makes the pain worse?"
7. Alleviating condition	"What seems to help you when you have the pain?"
8. Concomitant symptoms	"Have you noticed any other changes that are present when you have the pain?"

To clarify the use of these guidelines in the interview setting, consider a client who comes for treatment with a chief complaint of pain (see above column). The accuracy of the diagnostic process depends on exploring the ramification of these eight areas for data collection.

Common Problems in Interviewing

McGuire determined that six problem areas were common in the interviewing procedures of senior medical students:

1. Omission of questions aimed to promote discussion of personal or affective matters
2. Failure to explain the purpose of the interviews
3. Inability to keep the patient focused on interview items
4. Emphasis on one or a few problems while failing to explore additional problem areas
5. Failure to seek clarification
6. Failure to be precise in reporting dates and times or chronologic developments of illness or symptoms

Careful attention to these potential trouble spots in the interviewing process may obviate similar difficulties for the learner of interviewing skills.

BIBLIOGRAPHY

Benjamin A: The helping interview, ed 4, Boston, 1985, Houghton Mifflin Co.

Bernstein L and Bernstein RS: Interviewing: a guide for health professionals, ed 3, New York, 1980, Appleton-Century-Crofts.

Bowers A and Thompson J: Clinical manual of health assessment, ed 3, St. Louis, 1987, The CV Mosby Co.

Cormier L, Cormier W, and Weiser R Jr: Interviewing and helping skills for health professionals, Monterey, Calif, 1984, Wadsworth Health Sciences.

DiMatteo MR: A social-psychological analysis of physician-patient rapport toward a science of the art of medicine, J Soc Issues 35:12, 1979.

Enelow AJ and Swisher SN: Interviewing and patient care, New York, 1979, Oxford University Press.

Engel GL and Morgan WL Jr: Interviewing the patient, Philadelphia, 1973, WB Saunders Co.

Foley Rand Sharf B: The five interviewing techniques most frequently overlooked by primary care physicians, Behav Med 26:31, 1981.

Friedman M: Family nursing: theory and assessment, Norwalk, Conn, 1981, Appleton-Century-Crofts.

McGuire P: Teaching essential interviewing skills to medical students. In Osborne PJ, Gruneberg MM, and Eiser JR, editors: Research in psychology and medicine, London, 1979, Academic Press, Inc.

Okun B: Effective helping: interviewing and counseling techniques, Monterey, Calif, 1982, Brooks/Cole Publishing Co.

Potter PA: Pocket nurse guide to physical assessment, ed 2, St Louis, 1990, The CV Mosby Co.

Reiser D and Schoder A: Patient interviewing: the human dimension, Baltimore, 1980, Williams & Wilkins.

Seidel HM and others: Mosby's guide to physical examination, St Louis, 1987, The CV Mosby Co.

Thompson JM: Health assessment: an illustrated pocket guide, ed 2, St Louis, 1988, The CV Mosby Co.

Ware JE Jr, Davies AA, and Stewart AL: The measurement and meaning of patient satisfaction, Health Med Care Serv Rev 1:1, 1978.

2

Psychosocial assessment

OBJECTIVES

Upon successful review of this chapter, learners will be able to recognize:

- Psychosocial theories related to developmental assessment

- Developmental assessment techniques and expected findings during
  Infancy
  Early childhood
  Middle childhood
  Preadolescence
  Adolescence
  Young adulthood
  Middle adulthood
  Late adulthood
  Uses of life change and life experience tools

While learning to perform the health assessment of a client, the beginning practitioner places much emphasis on the physical aspects of that assessment, often being preoccupied with assimilating new skills, handling new tools, performing new techniques, remembering lists of questions for the health history, and performing the components of the physical examination in the correct order. However, from the onset of this learning process it is important to include a perspective on the individual client's whole personhood. This involves taking into account that person's life developmental processes and the phases of growth and maturing through which that individual progresses. This necessitates taking time to observe the client as a person and to discuss and discover the client's world—the interaction and growth within the self, with significant others, and with society at large.

Discussing developmental phases, stages, or crises with the client can provide both practitioner and client with a perspective of greater breadth and depth on the client's life situation and its relationship to health or illness. An openness in discussing the life tasks of individuals can help them appreciate the appropriateness and normalcy of their growth patterns, changes, behaviors, and feelings; it may also assist those who are blocked in their growth in some area to understand and deal with the problem area more effectively.

It is useful to help clients review their past, compare it with the present, look at progressive phases and intervals, and plan for the future in whatever ways are appropriate and necessary. Perhaps most important, it may serve to assist an individual to appreciate both one's similarities to others and one's own unique qualities and to gain assurance in one's efforts to be most fully and healthily one's own person.

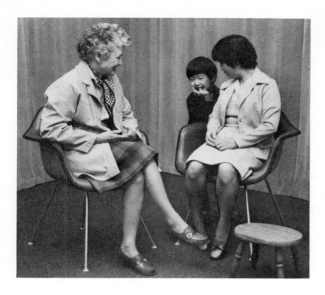

A basic premise to the approach used here is that growth and development are continuous throughout the life cycle. In the past it was often assumed that growth and development occurred during the early years of life but that by adulthood life was stable for a time and then gradually declined. Now it is recognized that human development occurs across the life cycle, with emphasis on various aspects at various times. From birth until death, some aspect of the complex human being is growing or changing in some way. This process of growth and development is both universal and unique and includes physical, emotional, psychological, social, and cognitive components. It ranges from changes that are slow, subtle, and often elusive to those that occur with astonishing rapidity. Another premise basic to this approach is that of change: life has the remarkable property of changing with time while maintaining a core of individuality.

Although developmental phases and categories are used here for purposes of organization, in life such phases are not totally distinct or mutually exclusive. During particular phases, certain aspects of growth may be more prominent, but many overlap across phases and defy neat categorization. Some of the early work done on the development of children by Jean Piaget and of children and adults by Erik Erikson was based on a "stage" approach. One stage and its accomplishments was followed by another, and moving from one to the other was premised on the completion of tasks at the earlier level. Piaget asserted that biologic growth combines with children's interaction with the environment to take them up a development staircase, step by step, each step signaling an increase in complexity of the child's thinking. He believed that changes in memory, perceptual skills, learning

ability, and other aspects of mental development all occurred in this fashion. More recently it has been argued that more variations in children's growth can be observed and that some children develop in one area much more quickly than in others.

Currently, there has been a move away from the stage approach to a more complex view of development wherein an individual may move ahead in certain areas whether or not all tasks are accomplished in other areas. Different areas of development such as cognition and socialization are being studied separately. Each of these areas has a flexible schedule for growth and change; not only age, but also environmental factors, affect this pattern. Still, the contributions of Piaget and Erikson are fundamental to the growth that has occurred in this field and will be used in this chapter.

Development is cyclic: for example, children tend to grow in spurts, then level off for periods, and adolescents tend to have cycles of outward activity and then inner reflection. Adults also experience periods of greater outward involvement and inner orientation. Gesell, Ilg, and Ames suggest that "growth gains are consolidated during recurring periods of relative equilibrium. There is a tendency for stages of increased equilibrium to be followed by stages of lessened equilibrium when the organism makes new inner or outer thrusts into the inner or outer unknown" (1956, p. 20). Also, some aspects of an individual's earlier experiences are probably always a part of him or her. "Childhood does not end nor adulthood begin around adolescence. Rather, the adult is anticipated in the child and the child persists in the adult" (Katchdourian, 1978, p. 51).

The developmental aspects of infancy and childhood have received much attention and study since the late 1800s: there is an abundance of literature on these phases, although much still remains to be studied and understood. Of more recent vintage are the studies and theories advanced on adolescence and on old age. Latest to surface in the literature on human development is material on the age span between youth and old age: middle adulthood.

Erikson is one of the theorists who suggested a developmental framework for the entire life span (1963): his framework is outlined here and will be incorporated into the discussion at the various stages of growth used in this chapter. He suggested eight developmental stages and for each stage identifies a central task and threat to the accomplishment of that task. These central tasks are called developmental "crises," although not in the sense of an emergency but rather "as a term designating a necessary turning point, a crucial moment, when development must move one way or another, marshaling re-

Table 2-1

Erikson's eight stages of development

Stage	Developmental crisis
Infancy	Trust vs mistrust
Childhood	
Early childhood	Autonomy vs shame
Play age	Initiative vs guilt
School age	Industry vs inferiority
Adolescence	
Adolescence	Identity vs identity confusion
Young adulthood	Intimacy vs isolation
Adulthood	
Maturity	Generativity vs self-absorption
Old age	Integrity vs despair

sources of growth, recovery, and further differentiation" (1968, p. 16). Each crisis is marked by a pair of opposite qualities that must be resolved and integrated to allow the person to proceed with ego development. As each challenge is faced, a new strength emerges that contributes to further development. It is "a period of increased vulnerability and heightened potential" (1975, p. 5). Erikson describes the life cycle as the "tendency of individual life to 'round itself out' as a coherent experience and to form a link in the chain of generations from which it receives and to which it contributes both strength and fateful discord" (1975, p. 5). These stages and tasks are shown in Table 2-1.

As a result of studies in recent years that have focused on either men's or women's development across the life span, there has been controversy over the applicability of all the levels of this framework to both sexes. The work of Carol Gilligan, in particular, will be discussed in the adult section of this chapter.

The approach used here is to organize developmental assessment around eight major life phases based on age: infancy, early childhood, middle childhood, preadolescence, adolescence, early adulthood, middle adulthood, and old age. Characteristics of each stage, including developmental tasks, will be described. The length of the chronologic divisions will increase with each division, ranging from months for infants to decades for adults.

A notation on the clinician's impression of a client's developmental tasks and accomplishments can be placed in the health history after the psychological system review. See examples on pp. 129 and 134.

Regarding the tools and tests available to assess different developmental levels, as with the pattern of research mentioned earlier, there are numerous tools devised to assess early childhood stages, but fewer to assess school-age children and adults. Several of the infancy and early childhood assessment tools will be presented, as will two tools used to assist with adult assessment. With adolescents and adults, much developmental assessment is accomplished by talking with the client in an accepting, unrushed manner. Nonthreatening questions about thoughts and feelings, work, family, and other activities and an attitude of active listening will encourage these clients to share significant information about themselves.

The practitioner should not expect to learn everything about a client's developmental accomplishments in one or even in several interviews. It is a personal story that takes time and trust to be told. And again, developmental assessment for a client of any age is a continuous, ongoing process. Life is more like a moving film than a snapshot; it is changing and dynamic and should be regularly reassessed.

INFANCY AND CHILDHOOD

The assessment of a child's development is carried out formally or informally by the practitioner during each examination. The opportunity to observe the development of many children enhances the ability to define the parameters of normal development, and the experienced examiner often responds to subtle behavioral cues with a hunch that all is or is not well with the child. However, it is usually difficult to verify this initial impression and determine the presence or absence of a developmental deficit while examining a child in a busy clinical setting. The practitioner may need to plan additional time to focus attention on assessing the child's development or may need to seek the assistance of experts in child development.

The information obtained from the developmental assessment has many uses. It will aid the practitioner in providing assistance to the parents when they have questions about their child's behavior. Most parents will be interested in learning that their child is developing normally, and with anticipatory guidance they can gain a greater appreciation of ways to support their child's normal development. The developmental assessment also provides information that can be useful at a future time. For instance, the child who has been developing in a normal fashion and then demonstrates a developmental lag presents a different problem than the child who has been consistently slower in development. Finally, the developmental assessment is helpful in screening for some of the more obvious deficits in development that deserve further investigation.

It is most important to keep in mind that the developmental assessment is not a test of the child's intelligence and does not allow the practitioner to make a diagnosis. It does allow the practitioner to collect data that indicate whether the development of the individual child is within the normal range.

Although there are many theories of development that can provide a framework for observing and assessing the development of children, the discussion in this chapter is limited. However, it is reasonable to expect that each practitioner with an interest in children will be challenged to increase understanding of the behavior presented by children of different ages.

The discussion in this section includes a conceptual framework for organizing the developmental assessment; approaches to the developmental assessment of the child, which can be incorporated into the plan for the health history and examination; and a brief discussion of selected screening tests that can be helpful to the practitioner.

A systematic appraisal of the child's development can be organized in different ways. Although each behavior of the child is part of an indivisible whole, it is clinically useful to separate behaviors into several categories whether the assessment is carried out as a part of the health examination or as a more formal procedure. Different categories of behavior are used, but many of the screening tests commonly focus on three categories: fine and gross motor development, language and communication, and personal-social behavior. These categories are especially useful in the assessment of the infant and preschool child, when observable changes occur most rapidly. When the development of the older child is being assessed, it is important to include questions about the child's adjustment to school and the grade level achieved and about his relationships with peers, siblings, and significant adults.

The stages of motor development have been documented and are well known, as is the relationship of motor skills to neuromotor organization. The practitioner will find information about the expected norms for achieving specific motor skills in most standard textbooks of pediatrics or child development. What is not usually discussed in regard to developing motor abilities is the way the child uses these skills. Is the child active and using his skills in a variety of ways? Or is the child quiet, showing little apparent interest or pleasure in walking, running, and climbing? Information on the amount of activity may lead to questions about the environment. Does it offer too much stimulation or too little? Differ-

ences in the use of skills may also be related to organic problems, which are sometimes demonstrated by the hyperactive, impulse-ridden child.

The normal age range for the sequential development of language and communication skills is also well documented, as well as the relationship of speech development to intellectual functioning. The assessment of the child's language and communication skills should provide information about the size of the child's vocabulary, understanding of language, clarity of articulation, and use of phrases and sentences. The speech of the young child is easily disturbed when there are physical problems or problems with the people in the environment. Speech disturbances may be transitory, may indicate an impairment of the hearing or speech apparatus, or may indicate the presence of a mental disability. Although a delay in speech development may be a temporary problem, it is a concern that deserves further investigation even when the child is very young.

Appraisal of the child's personal-social behavior provides information about the child's developing awareness of personhood, ability to interact with people, and adaptive behaviors. These abilities can also be described as the child's intellectual, emotional, and social skills. Erik Erikson's "conceptual itinerary" of the psychosocial stages of life provides a plan, or a guided overview, of the child's changes and adaptive behaviors in each of the sequential stages of childhood.

The practitioner with limited time would be well served to find ways to incorporate aspects of the developmental assessment into the routine health examination of every child. A good deal of information can be gained by including questions about the child's development in the history. Also, since it is traditional to include observations of the child's behavior as part of the general inspection of the physical examination, it is relatively easy to pay special attention to particular aspects of behavior to obtain data about the child's level of functioning. However, it is also well to keep in mind that the behavior demonstrated may not be typical because of the stress from the unfamiliar environment or the particular problems of the illness that the child is experiencing.

Because there are limited opportunities to observe the child's behavior in the clinical setting, the history becomes the major tool for obtaining information about the child's development. First, the history allows the practitioner to obtain data about the factors that will increase the chances of the child's being at risk for problems that may interfere with his development. Una Haynes outlines many of the factors that contribute to the "at risk" status of the child. This information can be elicited from the history of the child in the prenatal, natal, and postnatal periods; from the family history; from the sociologic assessment; from the developmental data; and from the history of illnesses and injuries. The history that reveals problems such as prematurity, precipitate delivery, or hyperbilirubinemia in the first 48 hours of life will alert the practitioner that the child is at greater risk than most children for developmental problems. However, this information should not bias the practitioner's perception of the child's development but should encourage a sense of "benign suspicion," a term used by Sally Provence (1968a) to describe the attitude of the examiner.

The pediatric history as outlined in Chapter 24 includes a developmental history that provides information about the age at which the child achieved certain developmental milestones. This information can be used to determine whether the early development was within average or normal limits. The history of the present health or present illness should include a description of the child's current level of functioning. The practitioner can review the achievements expected of the child at a specific chronologic age as outlined in many texts on child development. The box on p. 19 provides such an outline. Questions about these expected achievements will provide information about the child's current level of development; this information can then be included in the description of the child's present health.

Provence (1968a) mentions two questions that are helpful for the examiner to keep in mind when judging the development of a child: (1) What has the child achieved in the various sectors of development that one can observe, describe, or measure? (2) How does the child make use of the skills and functions available? The first question requires the practitioner to find out about the developmental progress of the infant or child from helplessness at birth to the current level of development. The second question requires the practitioner to find out about the adaptation the child is making to life. The second question is usually more difficult to answer because it is not based on standardized developmental schedules. However, information about the child's adaptation can be obtained by asking the parent(s) to describe the child. This description can be broadened by asking whether the child is quiet or active, happy or sad, and mischievous or very good.

Ronald Illingworth (1975) stresses that purely objective tests result in obtaining information about scorable items in the area of sensorimotor skills and that it is of great importance to also determine the child's alertness, responsiveness, and interest in surroundings, which cannot be scored. Arnold Gessell (1947) calls these latter behaviors "insurance factors." If the child demonstrates these behaviors but has delays in some of the sensori-

motor behaviors, an opinion should be reserved and the child followed over a longer period before the developmental skills are judged.

If questions or concerns about a child's development are identified as the result of the routine appraisal, it is wise to set aside time for a complete developmental assessment that would include a careful review of the history of the developmental milestones and an appraisal of the child's current level of function. It would be appropriate to use one of the more structured screening tests.

Developmental Screening Tests

There are several screening tests that the practitioner may find useful in assessing the development of an infant or young child. Most of them require some training for validity of the test to be ensured.

The clinical assessment of gestational age helps the practitioner to determine that the newborn's gestational age is accurate and to anticipate problems that are related to the infant's maturity or immaturity. Several tools designed for use during the first few days of life assess the physical and neuromuscular maturity of the infant. Included in each of the two major categories are selected items that can be scored and the total score obtained allows the practitioner to make a determination of gestational age. One such tool was designed by Dubowitz (see Appendix) and co-workers (1970). A chart to estimate gestational age was developed by Brazie and Lubchenco and can be found in *Current Pediatric Diagnosis and Treatment* (Kempe, Silver, and O'Brien, 1978). Skill in administering these examinations requires practice with the supervision of an experienced clinician.

The Neonatal Behavioral Assessment Scale (see Appendix) developed by Dr. T. Berry Brazelton and associates is designed to assess the infant's interactive behavior during the neonatal period. "It is an attempt to score the infant's available responses to his environment, and so, indirectly his effect on the environment" (Brazelton, 1973, p. 4). The test includes 27 behavioral items, and repeated assessments are suggested rather than just one assessment. Findings suggest that this tool can be useful in predicting developmental outcomes. It can be used to discriminate between the abnormal and the normal baby. It is also very useful in helping parents understand their infant's behavior when parents are included in the testing process. Training in the proper administration of the test is required.*

---

*A list of trained examiners who can provide training can be obtained by writing to the principal investigator, Dr. T. Berry Brazelton. There are also training films available for use with the published manual. These can be obtained by writing to Educational Development Corporations, 8 Mifflin Place, Cambridge, Mass. 02138.

Child Development from 1 Month to 5 Years

1 Month

Motor

1. Moro reflex present.
2. Vigorous sucking reflex present.
3. Lying prone (face down): lifts head briefly so chin is off table.
4. Lying prone: makes crawling movements with legs.
5. Held in sitting position: back is rounded, head held up momentarily only.
6. Hands tightly fisted.
7. Reflex grasp of object with palm.

Language

8. Startled by sound; quieted by voice.
9. Small throaty noises or vocalizations.

Personal-social-adaptive

10. Ringing bell produces decrease of activity.
11. May follow dangling object with eyes to midline.
12. Lying on back: will briefly look at examiner or change activity.
13. Reacts with generalized body movements when tissue paper is placed on face.

2 Months

Motor

1. Kicks vigorously.
2. Energetic arm movements.
3. Vigorous head turning.
4. Held in ventral suspension (prone): no head droop.
5. Lying prone: lifts head so face makes an approximate 45° angle with table.
6. Held in sitting position: head erect but bobs.
7. Hand goes to mouth.
8. Hands often open (not clenched).

Language

9. Is cooing.
10. Vocalizes single vowel sounds, such as: ah-eh-uh.

Personal-social-adaptive

11. Head and eyes search for sound.
12. Listens to bell ringing.
13. Follows dangling object past midline.
14. Alert expression.
15. Follows moving person with eyes.
16. Smiles back when talked to.

3 Months

Motor

1. Lying prone: lifts head to 90° angle.
2. Lifts head when lying on back (supine).
3. Moro reflex begins to disappear.
4. Grasp reflex nearly gone.
5. Rolls side to back (3–4 months).

Language

6. Chuckling, squealing, grunting, especially when talked to.
7. Listens to music.
8. Vocalizes with two different syllables, such as: a-a, la-la (not distinct), oo-oo.

Personal-social-adaptive

9. Reaches for but misses objects.
10. Holds toy with active grasp when put into hand.
11. Sucks and inspects fingers.
12. Pulls at clothes.
13. Follows object (toy) side to side (and 180°).
14. Looks predominately at examiner.
15. Glances at toy when put into hand.
16. Recognizes mother and bottle.
17. Smiles spontaneously.

4 Months

Motor

1. Sits when well supported.
2. No head lag when pulled to sitting position.
3. Turns head at sound of voice.
4. Lifts head (in supine position) in effort to sit.
5. Lifts head and chest when prone, using hands and forearms.
6. Held erect: pushes feet against table.

Language

7. Laughs aloud (4–5 months).
8. Uses sounds, such as: m-p-b.
9. Repeats series of same sounds.

Personal-social-adaptive

10. Grasps rattle.
11. Plays with own fingers.
12. Reaches for object in front with both hands.
13. Transfers object from hand to hand.
14. Pulls dress over face.
15. Smiles spontaneously at people.
16. Regards raisin (or pellet).

5 Months

Motor

1. Moro reflex gone.
2. Rolls side to side.
3. Rolls back to front.
4. Full head control when pulled to or held in sitting position.
5. Briefly supports most of weight on legs.
6. Scratches on tabletop.

Language

7. Squeals with high voice.
8. Recognizes familiar voices.
9. Coos or stops crying on hearing music.

Personal-social-adaptive

10. Grasps dangling object.
11. Reaches for toy with both hands.
12. Smiles at mirror image.
13. Turns head deliberately to bell.
14. Obviously enjoys being played with.

Continued

Child Development from 1 Month to 5 Years—cont'd

6 Months
Motor

1. Supine: lifts head spontaneously.
2. Bounces on feet when held standing.
3. Sits briefly (tripod fashion).
4. Rolls front to back (6–7 months).
5. Grasps foot and plays with toes.
6. Grasps cube with palm.

Language

7. Vocalizes at mirror image.
8. Makes four or more different sounds.
9. Localizes source of sound (bell, voice).
10. Vague, formless babble (especially with family members).

Personal-social-adaptive

11. Holds one cube in each hand.
12. Puts cube into mouth.
13. Resecures dropped cube.
14. Transfers cube from hand to hand.
15. Conscious of strange sights and persons.
16. Consistent regard of object or person (6–7 months).
17. Uses raking movement to secure raisin or pellet.
18. Resists having toy taken away.
19. Stretches out arms to be taken up (6–8 months).

8 Months
Motor

1. Sits alone (6–8 months).
2. Early stepping movements.
3. Tries to crawl.
4. Stands few seconds, holding on to object.
5. Leans forward to get an object.

Language

6. Two-syllable babble, such as: a-la, ba-ba, oo-goo, a-ma, mama, dada (8–10 months).
7. Listens to conversation (8–10 months).
8. "Shouts" for attention (8–10 months).

Personal-social-adaptive

9. Works to get toy out of reach.
10. Scoops pellet.
11. Rings bell purposely (8–10 months).
12. Drinks from cup.
13. Plays peek-a-boo.
14. Looks for dropped object.
15. Bites and chews toys.
16. Pats mirror image.
17. Bangs spoon on table.
18. Manipulates paper or string.
19. Secures ring by pulling on the string.
20. Feeds self crackers.

10 Months
Motor

1. Gets self into sitting position.
2. Sits steadily (long time).
3. Pulls self to standing position (on bed railing).
4. Crawls on hands and knees.
5. Walks when held or around furniture.
6. Turns around when left on floor.

Language

7. Imitates speech sounds.
8. Shakes head for "no."
9. Waves "bye-bye."
10. Responds to name.
11. Vocalizes in varied jargon-patterns (10–12 months).

Personal-social-adaptive

12. Plays "pat-a-cake."
13. Picks up pellet with finger and thumb.
14. Bangs toys together.
15. Extends toy to a person.
16. Holds own bottle.
17. Removes cube from cup.
18. Drops one cube to get another.
19. Uses handle to lift cup.
20. Initially shy with strangers.

1 Year
Motor

1. Walks with one hand held.
2. Stands alone (or with support).
3. Secures small object with good pincer grasp.
4. Pivots in sitting position.
5. Grasps two cubes in one hand.

Language

6. Uses "mama" or "dada" with specific meaning.
7. "Talks" to toys and people, using fairly long verbal patterns.
8. Has vocabulary of two words besides "mama" and "dada."
9. Babbles to self when alone.
10. Obeys simple requests, such as: "Give me the cup."
11. Reacts to music.

Personal-social-adaptive

12. Cooperates with dressing.
13. Plays with cup, spoon, saucer.
14. Points with index finger.
15. Pokes finger (into stethoscope) to explore.
16. Releases toy into your hand.
17. Tries to take cube out of box.
18. Upwraps a cube.
19. Holds cup to drink.
20. Holds crayon.
21. Tries to imitate scribble.
22. Imitates beating two cubes together.
23. Gives affection.

Continued

Child Development from 1 Month to 5 Years—cont'd

15 Months

Motor

1. Stands alone.
2. Creeps upstairs.
3. Kneels on floor or chair.
4. Gets off floor and walks alone with good balance.
5. Bends over to pick up toy without holding on to furniture.

Language

6. May speak four to six words (15–18 months).
7. Uses jargon.
8. Indicates wants by vocalizing.
9. Knows own name.
10. Enjoys rhymes or jingles.

Personal-social-adaptive

11. Tilts cup to drink.
12. Uses spoon but spills.
13. Builds tower of two cubes.
14. Drops cubes into cup.
15. Helps turn page in book, pats picture.
16. Shows or offers toy.
17. Helps pull off clothes.
18. Puts pellet into bottle without demonstration.
19. Opens lid of box.
20. Likes to push wheeled toys.

18 Months

Motor

1. Runs (stiffly).
2. Walks upstairs—one hand held.
3. Walks backwards.
4. Climbs into chair.
5. Hurls ball.

Language

6. May say six to ten words (18–21 months).
7. Points to at least one body part.
8. Can say "hello" and "thank you."
9. Carries out two directions (one at a time), for instance: "Get ball from table."—"Give ball to mother."
10. Identifies two objects by pointing (or picking up), such as: cup, spoon, dog, car, chair.

Personal-social-adaptive

11. Turns pages.
12. Builds tower of three to four cubes.
13. Puts 10 cubes into cup.
14. Carries or hugs a doll.
15. Takes off shoes and socks.
16. Pulls string toy.
17. Scribbles spontaneously.
18. Dumps raisin from bottle after demonstration.
19. Uses spoon with little spilling.

21 Months

Motor

1. Runs well.
2. Walks downstairs—one hand held.
3. Walks upstairs alone or holding on to rail.
4. Kicks large ball (when demonstrated).

Language

5. May speak fifteen to twenty words (21–24 months).
6. May combine two to three words.
7. Asks for food, drink.
8. Echoes two or more words.
9. Takes three directions (one at a time), for instance: "Take ball from table."—"Give ball to Mommy."—"Put ball on floor."
10. Points to three or more body parts.

Personal-social-adaptive

11. Builds tower of five to six cubes.
12. Folds paper once when shown.
13. Helps with simple household tasks (21–24 months).
14. Removes some clothing purposefully (besides hat or socks).
15. Pulls person to show something.

2 Years

Motor

1. Runs without falling.
2. Walks up and down stairs.
3. Kicks large ball (without demonstration).
4. Throws ball overhand.
5. Claps hands.
6. Opens door.
7. Turns pages in book, singly.

Language

8. Says simple phrases.
9. Says at least one sentence or phrase of four or more syllables.
10. Can repeat four to five syllables.
11. May reproduce about five to six consonant sounds. (Typically: m-p-b-h-w.)
12. Points to four parts of body on command.
13. Asks for things at table by name.
14. Refers to self by name.
15. May use personal pronouns, such as: I-me-you (2–2½ years).

Personal-social-adaptive

16. Builds five- to seven-cube tower.
17. May cut with scissors.
18. Spontaneously dumps raisin from bottle (without demonstration).
19. Throws ball into box.
20. Imitates drawing vertical line from demonstration.
21. Parallel play predominant.

Continued

Child Development from 1 Month to 5 Years—*cont'd*

2½ Years

Motor

1. Jumps in place with both feet.
2. Tries standing on one foot (may not be successful).
3. Holds crayon by fingers.
4. Imitates walking on tiptoe.

Language

5. Refers to self by pronoun (rather than name).
6. Names common objects when asked (key, penny, shoe, box, book).
7. Repeats two digits (one of three trials).
8. Answers simple questions, such as: "What is this?"— "What does the kitty say?"

Personal-social-adaptive

9. Builds tower of eight cubes.
10. Pushes toy with good steering.
11. Helps put things away.
12. Can carry breakable objects.
13. Puts on clothing.
14. Washes and dries hands.
15. Eats with fork.
16. Imitates drawing a horizontal line from demonstration.
17. May imitate drawing a circle from demonstration.

3 Years

Motor

1. Stands on one foot for at least 1 second.
2. Jumps from bottom stair.
3. Alternates feet going upstairs.
4. Pours from a pitcher.
5. Can undo two buttons.
6. Pedals a tricycle.

Language

7. Repeats six syllables, for instance: "I have a little dog."
8. Names three or more objects in a picture.
9. Gives sex. ("Are you a boy or a girl?")
10. Gives full name.
11. Repeats three digits (one of three trials).
12. Knows a few rhymes.
13. Gives appropriate answers to: "What: swims-flies-shoots-boils-bites-melts?"
14. Uses plurals.
15. Knows at least one color.
16. Can reply to questions in at least three word sentences.
17. May have vocabulary of 750 to 1,000 words (3–3½ years).

Personal-social-adaptive

18. Understands taking turns.
19. Copies a circle (from model, without demonstration).
20. Builds three-block pyramid (⬠).
21. Dresses with supervision.
22. Puts 10 pellets into bottle in 30 seconds.
23. Separates easily from mother.
24. Feeds self well.
25. Plays interactive games, such as "tag."

There are few tools designed to assess infant temperament beyond the first month of life. Therefore, the tool developed by William B. Carey and Sean C. McDevitt is useful. They developed the Carey Infant Temperament Questionnaire for detecting the temperament of infants between 4 and 8 months of age. The questionnaire consists of 95 questions relating to behaviors seen during feeding, sleep, elimination, and other activities, and the parent is asked to respond according to a scale from "almost never" to "almost always." Determination of the infant's temperament or behavior is important in understanding how he or she interacts with the environment. The identification of the infant's temperament profile makes it possible to individualize the help offered to parents in handling and caring for their infant. The questionnaire is available from Dr. Carey.*

The Denver Developmental Screening Test (DDST) developed by W.K. Frankenburg and J.B. Dodds is a tool to detect developmental delays during infancy and the preschool years up to 6 years of age (see Appendix). It is not an intelligence quotient (IQ) test, but the results help in estimating the child's current developmental level. It is a valuable tool in determining the child's developmental needs and provides a basis for planning anticipatory guidance. Items were selected from twelve developmental and preschool IQ tests on the basis of (1) ease of administration and interpretation and (2) a relatively short time from the point at which a few children could perform an item to the point at which most children could perform the item. The items are organized to give an overall developmental profile with emphasis on gross motor, language, fine motor-adaptive, and personal-social skills. Both professionals and paraprofessionals can learn to administer the DDST with training. Self-instructional units are available so that each indi-

---

*William B. Carey, M.D., 319 W. Front St., Media, Pa. 19063.

Child Development from 1 Month to 5 Years—*cont'd*

4 Years

Motor

1. Stands on one foot for at least 5 seconds (two of three trials).
2. Hops at least twice on one foot.
3. Can walk heel-to-toe four or more steps (with heel 1 inch or less in front of toe).
4. Can button coat or dress; may lace shoes.

Language

5. Repeats ten-word sentences without errors.
6. Counts three objects, pointing correctly.
7. Repeats three to four digits (4–5 years).
8. Comprehends: "What do you do if: you are hungry, sleepy, cold?"
9. Spontaneous sentences, four to five words long.
10. Likes to ask questions.
11. Understands prepositions, such as: on-under-behind, etc. ("Put the block *on* the table.")
12. Can point to three out of four colors (red, blue, green, yellow).
13. Speech is now an effective communication tool.

Personal-social-adaptive

14. Copies cross (+) without demonstration.
15. Imitates oblique cross (×).
16. Draws a man with four parts.
17. Cooperates with other children in play.
18. Dresses and undresses self (mostly without supervision).
19. Brushes teeth, washes face.
20. Compares lines: "Which is longer?"
21. Folds paper two to three times.
22. Can select heavier from lighter object.
23. Cares for self at toilet.

5 Years

Motor

1. Balances on one foot for 8 to 10 seconds.
2. Skips, using feet alternately.
3. May be able to tie a knot.
4. Catches bounced ball with hands (not arms) in two of three trials.

Language

5. Knows age ("How old are you?")
6. Performs three tasks (with one command), for instance: "Put pen on table—close door—bring me the ball."
7. Knows four colors.
8. Defines use for: fork-horse-key-pencil, etc.
9. Identifies by name: nickel-dime-penny.
10. Asks meaning of words.
11. Asks many "why" questions.
12. Relatively few speech errors remain—90% of consonant sounds are made correctly.
13. Counts number of fingers correctly.
14. Counts by rote to 10.
15. Comments on pictures (descriptions and interpretations).

Personal-social-adaptive

16. Copies a square.
17. Copies oblique cross (×) without demonstration.
18. May print a few letters (5–5½ years).
19. Draws man with at least six identifiable parts.
20. Builds a six-block pyramid from demonstration.
21. Transports things in a wagon.
22. Plays with coloring set, construction toys, puzzles.
23. Participates well in group play.

---

vidual can learn to use a standardized method of test administration. An instructional unit is also available with a manual, workbook, and film for class instruction and a proficiency evaluation. Requests for information about the availability of materials for training should be addressed to LADOCA.*

The Denver Articulation Screening Examination (see Appendix) was developed by Amelia F. Drumwright, a speech pathologist, with the purpose of devising a screening test of articulation skill that would "1.) reliably detect disorders in preschool children aged 2½ to 6 years and 2.) be useful and acceptable to speech pathologists, yet readily understandable to other child workers (doctors, nurses, teachers and subprofessionals)" (Drumwright and others, 1973). The examination requires the child to repeat 22 words that represent 30 speech sounds. The examiner evaluates sound production and makes an overall judgment about the intelligibility of the child's speech. The norms are presented for children between the ages of 2½ and 6 years. The manuals, test materials, and information about training should be requested from LADOCA.

Infancy

During the brief period of infancy, from birth to 18 months, the infant develops from a dependent, helpless newborn into a person who walks, talks, and relates to different people in terms of their importance to the infant's life. Infants enter the world with all sensory systems functioning in at least a rudimentary fashion and begin to interact with and influence their environment from the moment of birth. Very soon they can display a wide range of primary, nonself-conscious emotions: interest, distress, disgust, joy, anger, surprise, sadness, and

---

*LADOCA Project and Publishing Co., East 51st Ave. and Lincoln St., Denver, Colo. 80216.

fear. They are responsive to the caregiver's mood: sadness or happiness affects their behavior. The beginning of a memory function is observed when the infant exhibits differential responsiveness to a novel stimulus and a repeated stimulus. A rudimentary ego identity or sense of self evolves as the infant gradually learns to see himself as separate from the environment and gains feelings of faith and optimism. This relates to Erikson's first stage of trust vs mistrust.

The velocity of growth during the first few months and years of life is greater than at any other time. Infants develop intellectual and motor skills that enable them to move from total dependency at birth to aggressive exploration by 18 months. The newborn weighs an average of 7 to 7½ pounds at birth, loses up to 10% of that weight during the first few days of life, typically regains that weight by the tenth day, and then continues to gain steadily. Birth weight is usually doubled during the first 4 months and tripled by 1 year. During the second year the average weight gain is 6 to 7 pounds. The average length of the newborn is 20 inches, which will increase by 50% during the first year but will not double again until 4 years of age.

Marked changes occur in body contour during infancy. The head grows at a fairly rapid rate during the first year, and the head circumference is greater than the chest circumference. Then the growth of the head slows and the chest circumference becomes greater during the second year. The thickness of the subcutaneous fat increases during the first year, reaching a peak around 9 months, and then decreases during the second year. The plump infant becomes leaner.

The newborn makes many rapid adjustments necessary to sustain life outside the uterus that are actually a continuum of the development during fetal life. At birth, respirations are initiated and changes in the circulatory system occur, the digestive system begins to assimilate the food obtained from an external source, body wastes are excreted, and maintenance of body heat depends on the infant's own resources. Behavior includes many reflex actions that reflect the immaturity of the newborn's nervous system but also assist in adaptation with the new environment. (These reflexes are discussed in Chapter 24, "Assessment of the Pediatric Client.") One of the most striking physiologic changes is the continuing maturation and increasing function of the nervous system. Myelination continues at a rapid rate during the first months of life but is not completed until several years later. The functional development of various body structures probably corresponds to the order of myelination and occurs in a cephalocaudal direction. The development of head control precedes sitting, standing, and walking

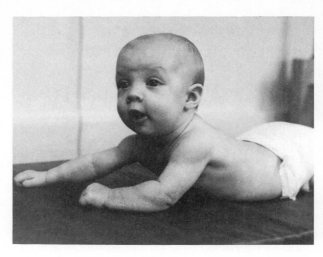

An infant can raise his chest off the table at 3 months of age.

the box on pp. 19-23. As the brain and central nervous system (CNS) continue to develop, there also follows an increasingly sophisticated range of cognitive and behavioral skills.

The first 3 months of life can be called a period of adjustment. Reflexes become more regularized during the first month, and the infant learns how to search and suck and let needs be known. Sleeping and feeding patterns become more regular. The tonic neck reflex becomes more prominent at the end of the first month. During the second and third months new behaviors appear that are not reflexes. The infant begins to follow objects with the eyes, allowing exploration of the environment. There is coordination of movements of hand and mouth, such as sucking the thumb at will. The grasp reflex gradually lessens as more purposeful movements begin. The infant begins to prolong interesting events that occur more or less by accident. The little wails that precede crying may be continued for their own sake. The squeals of the 2 to 3 month old baby are loud, repeated, and joyful. The infant begins to smile in response to environmental stimuli and to vocalize. Most responses are generalized and frequently involve movements of the whole body. The infant during this period has social responses but does not discriminate; any person who can satisfy those needs will be accepted.

In recent years more has been learned about the very young (0 to 6 months) infant's unique adaptive and precocious perception of social stimuli (such as human faces and voices), infant peer recognition and interaction, and the link between early visual recognition memory and later intelligence. The infant is now viewed as more sophisticated perceptually, cognitively, and socially than had been thought even a decade ago (Field, 1982).

By 3 months of age the baby becomes more discriminating and begins to differentiate mother from others and produces special types of smiles and crying for her, which is the beginning of attachment behavior and the development of awareness of the self as separate from her. Between 3 and 6 months, or even earlier, the infant repeats some actions that are interesting as well as prolongs those that occur accidentally, for instance, repeatedly hitting at toys suspended in the crib to produce movement. There is more imitation of facial movements and beginning imitation of sounds. There will be a kind of looking for a displaced object, but not a true search. Infantile reflexes are replaced by purposeful movements, especially those seen in the development of eye-hand coordination. The infant begins to reach for and grasp objects with a raking motion. The tonic neck reflex and Moro reflex disappear during the fifth or sixth month. At 3 months the infant can, while prone, raise the head and chest from a surface with arms extended, and at 4 months the head can be held steadily while the infant is supported in the sitting position. At 6 months the infant can sit without support.

The period between 6 and 12 months is dominated by the social modality of "taking and holding on" as described by Erikson. It is also described by Bowlby (1969) as being a period of active attachment behavior. The infant at 8 to 9 months of age has a beginning permanence concept and becomes fearful that the mother or other primary caregiver will disappear. The infant actively initiates contact with the caregiver and seeks to maintain that contact. There is true searching for a vanished object, although the search may be in several inappropriate places. Behavior becomes more complex and aggressive. There is coordination of earlier repetitive actions into behaviors with a purposeful aim. Now objects are explored more fully by rubbing, banging, and chewing and by discovering the correct procedures for manipulating them. Motor development is dramatic as coordination increases. The pincer grasp, using thumb and forefinger, develops. There is more vocalizing, and the use of pseudowords develops at about 10 to 12 months of age.

Between about 12 and 18 months the infant becomes a toddler. The infant assumes an upright position, and previously acquired motor skills are improved and expanded. Attachment behavior continues to be intense, and the primary caregiver's presence is needed to explore new places or to cope with threatening situations. Most strangers will be treated with caution. The child thoroughly enjoys newly acquired abilities and is enthusiastically persistent and uninhibited in attempts to manipulate objects. The child at this age exhibits repetitive play

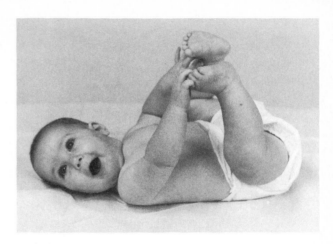

Learning is focused on body actions the first 7 to 9 months of age.

with objects and enjoys putting things in and taking them out of a box as the experimentation with objects and object permanence continues.

Piaget defined the infancy period of cognitive development as the sensorimotor period, "the period of mental development which begins with the capacity for a few reflexes, and ends when language and other symbolic ways of representing the world first appear" (Beard, 1969, p. 33). The infant is egocentric, and sensorimotor learning is related to the self. Recent work has indicated that even the very young infant is a cognitive being capable of rather sophisticated mental operations. For example, infants are more responsive to a new stimulus than to one that has been repeated several times, showing discrimination known as habituation. Their skill at associative learning is demonstrated by showing that infants can learn to turn the head one way or another to earn a reward, for example, a taste of sugar water, and that they have some memory function. They are also able to imitate certain facial gestures, such as sticking out the tongue or opening the mouth, which are indications of early cognitive abilities and integrative function with implications for social development, learning, and communication.

During the first 7 to 9 months of life the infant's learning is focused on body actions. Around 8 to 9 months the concept of what Piaget called "object permanence" can be observed: the infant learns that objects and people continue to exist even when the infant cannot see them. The 5-month-old infant will not reach for an object after it is hidden beneath a piece of cloth, but the 8-month-old infant will. Through this sequence of mental and physical actions and the gradual development of memory, the child begins to have a sense of self as separate from and yet a part of the environment. It is the beginning of the child's construction of reality. During the last months of this period, cognitive development is such that the

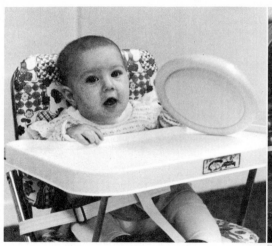
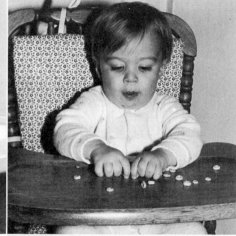
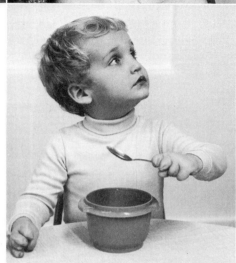

The development of competency is rapid during the first years of life.

infant begins to replace the earlier sensorimotor mental images that are nonverbal and have a highly personal meaning with mental symbols that are the beginning of language: approximately 20 words besides "mama" and "dada" are acquired.

There is a critical period of personality development when the child develops a sense of trust. Successful growth during this period means that the child comes to trust both the self and the people in the environment. According to Erikson (1963), a sense of trust develops when there is a mutual regulation of the baby's pattern of accepting things and the mother's way of giving them that changes as the baby develops. The social modality of the baby's development during the first 6 months is to satisfy needs by getting, receiving, and accepting. This is not passive behavior, since the infant influences people in the environment from birth. The first reflexive behaviors of looking, rooting, sucking, and crying elicit responses in the mother or other caretaking adults that cause them to act in ways that will meet the infant's needs. Parental bonding is influenced by these behaviors. The infant's social modality during the second half of the first year is taking and holding on, which begins with the eruption of teeth and the ability to sit upright and voluntarily reach out. The infant begins to be aware of being separate from the mother. The infant may become more demanding of the mother and is faced with the frustrations that result when the pleasure experienced in biting or grasping and holding on to things is met with interference. The infant displays helpless rage when strong desires are thwarted. When this behavior is understood and the infant continues to receive loving attention, trust in self and others can be maintained and strengthened.

Some of the infant's early emotional expressions, such as timidity and shyness vs expressions of boldness and sociability, may indicate enduring personality characteristics, giving rise to the idea that variables of temperament (e.g., shyness or sociability) are inborn.

Early Childhood

The infant moves into the early childhood years well equipped to continue learning about the self and the world. The ability to see self as separate from the environment, the sense of hope and trust, and the developing intellectual and motor skills allow autonomy to blossom. A basic competence develops with the expansion of language, memory, and self-control. The core problems as described by Erikson are "autonomy vs shame" during the toddler years (from 1 to 3) and "initiative vs guilt" during the preschool years (from 3 to 6).

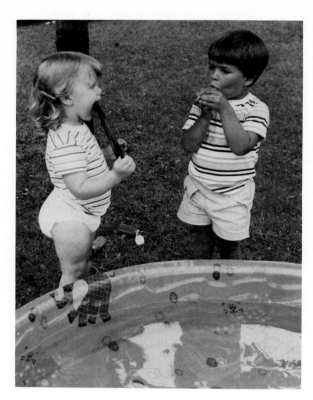

Differences in body contour and posture at 1 year of age and 3 years of age.

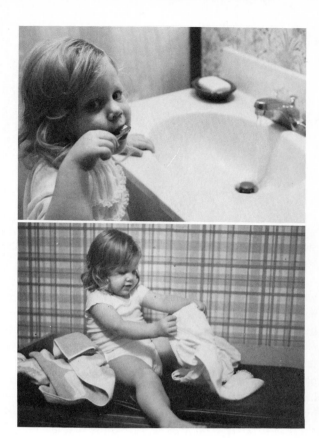

The 3½-year-old takes more responsibility for daily care.

Ego growth is rapid during the second and third years of life as the child continues exploration and learning about objects in the environment and gains increasing mastery of impulses and body functions. A burst of vocabulary occurs toward the end of the second year, as does an emergence of self-awareness and self-conscious emotions such as pride, sympathy, jealousy, guilt, and shame.

Physical growth continues, although at a slower rate. At 2 years the child will have added about 75% of the birth length. Weight increments also continue, although at a slower rate between 2 and 4 years of age, followed by a very gradual acceleration between 4 and 6 years. As the rate of growth in height and weight decreases, it also becomes less consistent month by month.

The changes in the child's physical appearance are dramatic. The toddler beginning to walk looks top-heavy with short legs and a potbelly. Fat pads obliterate the arch of the foot, and most young children appear to be flat-footed until 3 or 4 years of age. There is also a tendency for the legs to bow inward and for lordosis to be apparent. The posture and body proportions change as the chest becomes larger in proportion to the head and the abdomen. After 2 years of age, the extremities continue to grow faster than the trunk, and the jaw and lower face grow more rapidly than the cranium. The subcuta-

neous fat decreases rapidly in thickness during the second year and continues to decrease at a slower rate until 5 or 6 years, while muscle tissue continues to grow. Because of these changes the child becomes less chubby, the potbelly gradually becomes flatter, and the face loses its babyish look. The child age 5 or 6 looks more like an older child than an infant or a toddler.

Other changes that occur include improvement in visual acuity. The infant and young child are farsighted, and visual acuity at 2 years is estimated to be 20/40, compared with 20/20 between 4 and 5 years. The brain reaches 75% of its adult weight by 3 years and approximately 90% by 7 years. The skin changes after the first year, becoming firmer with less water content. The primary teeth continue to erupt, and the child will have the full complement of 20 primary teeth early during the third year, when the second molars erupt.

During the second and third years of life, when neuromuscular coordination and intellectual development make it possible for the child to explore and experiment actively, the toddler strives to establish a sense of autonomy. The child is motivated to assert the self and is uninhibited in pursuing personal goals. However, this wish to assert the self can cause conflict with the parents

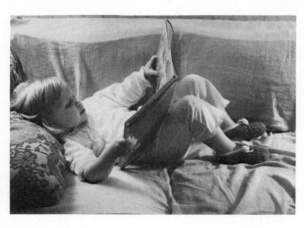

She has learned that she can lie on the couch to read a book like her mother does (3½ years).

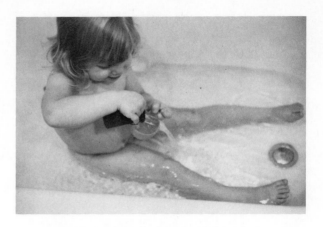

The 3½-year-old enjoys creative water play.

when the child is confronted with the restrictions that are necessary to help the child adapt to society's standards by learning to control the more primitive impulses. This is frustrating, and tantrums are common. It can also be fear-provoking because the child needs and wants the parent's love and approval: despite the independent behavior, the child still wants to please. Therefore, it is important to structure an environment that allows the child to make free choices within limits that are protective. The child gradually learns to accept that there is some safety and comfort in these limitations. Attachment behaviors continue, and although the child becomes increasingly able to play alone for longer periods, there is periodical seeking of the mother or other caregiver and a return to that person if there is any perceived threat. The young child who is faced with a new situation will venture forward with much more assurance if the parent or other caregiver is present and will turn to that person for comfort when things get too difficult. The child during these years is sensitive to changes in the environment because thinking is organized in a global way, such that if there is one alteration in the child's world, everything changes and becomes strange and unmanageable. Therefore, a consistent routine for daily activities is helpful, allowing the child to anticipate what will happen, to learn the behaviors that are expected, and to gain a feeling of controlling the self and performing well. For the 2- to 3-year-old child, rituals can be very important, particularly around bedtime when the child must deal with separation. If everything is done the same way each night, there is reassurance that the world will not change while the child sleeps.

Play during the toddler years begins with exploration and discovery, but as the child grows and gains ability to form mental images, play becomes imaginative and imitative. The toddler enjoys the company of other children and may play with them directly or beside them in parallel play. The younger child may treat others as if they were objects and poke or push them because there is not yet an inner sense that this is hurtful. The pleasure in learning about things by touching and manipulating is also seen in the early attempts at feeding, drinking, washing, brushing teeth, and dressing. The child is initially rather messy, but by about 3 years has gained a fair amount of competence in these areas.

Play during the preschool years becomes increasingly more social, imaginative, and complex. While playing together, children develop concepts, imagination, neuromuscular coordination, and language. "Let's pretend" is a favorite phrase and activity. Erikson describes this as the play age when the child is offered a micro-reality in which to use toys to work out problems and anticipate future roles (1977, p. 99). Through imaginative and creative play the child tries out the roles of different people and also alleviates some of the guilt that occurs as the result of a developing conscience. In play, the child can take on any role and master fears. There can be feelings of strength and adequacy instead of smallness and vulnerability.

Cognitive development is reflected in the child's development of language. Early in the second year of life, the child acquires personal, nonverbal mental images of objects and events; the first words and gestures are also invested with unique personal meanings. Beginning near the end of the second year, vocabulary increases rapidly, which signals the appearance of thought with internal language that allows the child to think about objects and people not present and to anticipate future events. Initially, language does not take the place of action thinking; the young child cannot think through a series of actions but must actually perform them. Thinking is characterized by "centering," meaning that only one attribute of an object or event stands out in the child's perception; for example, the child can sort objects by color or by shape but not by both characteristics.

The child's thinking between the ages of 2 and 7 is limited by egocentrism. There is only one point of view—the child's own, and a belief that everyone else thinks the same way. Children feel no need to justify their own conclusions and take little notice of how other people think. When communicating with other people, there is little attempt to relate to what the other person is saying.

The ages between 3 and 6 are marked by social, emotional, and intellectual development. The child is developing a sense of self as a social person in relation to other people and is also learning a great deal about the physical world. The child identifies with the parents and is motivated to try to be what they want, as well as to be like them. The child is becoming more socially responsive and able to give love and affection. The development of initiative is characterized by the wish to "become," a wish to find out what kind of person the child can be. During the earlier years there was a growth of the sense of self as a separate person with some power to influence the environment and to control impulses and one's own body. These accomplishments make it possible to approach new tasks with wonderful feelings of confidence and an abundance of energy. The child becomes intrusive in a desire to attack new situations. Erikson says the child at this age intrudes into everyone's space with locomotion and into everyone's ears with aggressive talking. Children are noisy, active, and on the move. They thrust themselves into each situation, driven by curiosity and imagination. Love and admiration for the parents and other significant adults intensifies, although it may be mixed with defiance at times; identification with the parents increases. Sexual identification began at an earlier age when the child learned that he was a boy or that she was a girl, but during the preschool years it is heightened. It becomes evident as the child begins to model after the parent of the same sex, learning more of a sex role identity, and becomes acutely aware of sexual differences. The interest in the parent of the opposite sex is somewhat romantic, which results in conflict when the child learns that he or she cannot replace the parent of the same sex, whom the child also loves. These feelings of intense love and the wish to be rid of one parent can cause anxiety and fear because the child believes that wishes are as real as the actual deed. Parents and other significant adults greatly influence early sex role development.

By internalizing the parents' standards and ideals, the child gradually develops a sense of moral responsibility and a conscience, which makes it possible to resist temptation even though the parents are not present. There are feelings of guilt for misbehavior, and at about 5 years of age there will even be some feelings of guilt for wanting to misbehave. This early conscience will be modified throughout the years of childhood as intellectual abilities increase and the ability to identify reasons for moral action becomes more mature.

Creativity develops rapidly in early childhood, often reaching a peak at about age 7. As children begin school, they are often more reluctant to take creative leaps; this probably has much to do with the behavior and responses of adults, who may be more set on "right" answers and the "right" way of doing things, an attitude that can suppress creative growth.

Middle Childhood

During the middle years of childhood, from 6 to 10, the child moves from the close ties of family and home to the larger world of peers, school, and neighborhood. The family "romance" is less intense, and the child is able to go out into the world. It is during this period of latency that the child is free from earlier concentration on sexuality and strong basic drives. Energy can now be directed toward learning the skills and competencies of the mind and body that lead to practical achievements and accomplishments in the world. There is tremendous intellectual growth during this lull before the "storm" of adolescence, and the child is introduced to experiences that help in learning the fundamentals of society and culture.

Physical growth during the middle years of childhood is relatively slow and smooth. The characteristic body type for the individual child has emerged during the middle years; the short child remains short, and the tall child remains tall. The increments in weight are less regular than seen in the young infant and child and may remain stationary for weeks at a time. The approximate annual increase in weight is about 5 to 7 pounds. The average annual increase in height is approximately 2 to 3 inches. Boys on the average are taller and heavier than girls until the adolescent growth spurt, which occurs earlier in girls. Although the growth spurt will be discussed in the section on the preadolescent, it is important to recognize that some elementary-school-age children will already have begun the growth spurt as early as age 8 or 9.

The physical changes that occur make school-age children more agile and graceful. They become slimmer, with longer legs and a lower center of gravity than the younger child. They are stronger and better coordinated and are able to fit into the adult physical environment more easily. There is only a slight increase in the size of

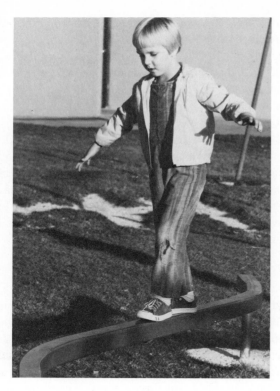

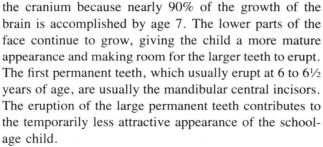

The 6-year-old has good neuromuscular coordination.

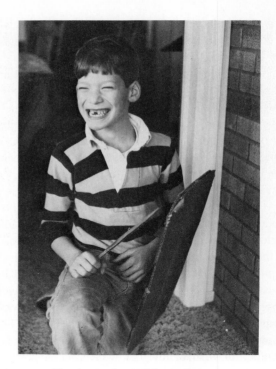

Play is creative and fun at 7 years.

the cranium because nearly 90% of the growth of the brain is accomplished by age 7. The lower parts of the face continue to grow, giving the child a more mature appearance and making room for the larger teeth to erupt. The first permanent teeth, which usually erupt at 6 to 6½ years of age, are usually the mandibular central incisors. The eruption of the large permanent teeth contributes to the temporarily less attractive appearance of the school-age child.

The eyeball continues to grow until 10 or 12 years of age. Visual acuity is usually 20/20 between 4 and 5 years of age, but depth perception is not very accurate until 6 to 7 years of age. Hearing is well-established at a much earlier age. Lymphoid tissue increases steadily until puberty and then decreases. This accounts for the abundance of lymphoid tissues such as adenoids and tonsils. The skeleton continues to ossify, with cartilage being replaced by bone. The child has acquired the basic neuromuscular mechanisms by age 6 or 7 and will spend the school years refining physical skills, resulting in an increase in motor skills and coordination. Thus, the school-age child engages in repetitive practice in all areas of neuromuscular activities from the fine motor skills of writing to the large motor skills used in baseball, bicycle riding, and swimming, depending on individual interests.

By 6 years of age the child's personality has become structured. Through accomplishment of earlier developmental tasks, the child has achieved a concept of

the self, acquired a sense of trust, developed autonomy with some power over impulses and the environment, and incorporated standards of the culture as interpreted by the parents. According to psychoanalytical theory the child has an ego, id, superego, and ego ideal and can deal with the next core problem described by Erikson—industry vs inferiority.

During this period, Erikson says the child becomes a worker, one who is required to develop intellectual, physical, and social skills that contribute to a sense of adequacy. The child is sent to school, and play is transformed into work, games into competition and cooperation, and the freedom of imagination into the duty to perform (Erikson, 1977, pp. 103-104). The child's attainments in interpersonal and social development are important. The child is now able to see a higher organization of behavior in which to participate. The child wants to operate in socially accepted ways of thinking and behaving, can take another person's point of view, and is able to take what is heard and seen and compare it with what the child already knows of reality. The child can reason and act according to rules, which allows for benefit from the school experience and for participation in organized sports or other activities.

As these children move into the larger world of school and peers, they continue to need their parents. Demands for conformity are placed on them by people outside the family, such as teachers, scout leaders, and

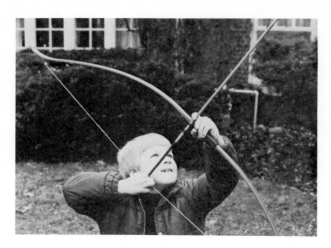

The 8-year-old concentrates on achieving a skill.

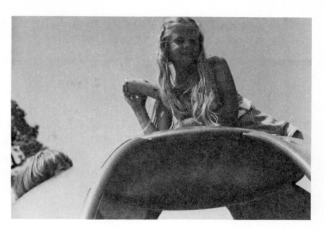

The 10-year-old enjoys her physical skills.

peers. They continue to need parental support and the approval of teachers and other important adults, but they also need to find a place in a group of peers. They are ready to be involved in the private world of children, where adults are not always welcome. This becomes more apparent toward the end of latency, when the child withdraws more into the privacy of the peer group, which is an important socializing agent. Feelings of group solidarity and belongingness are promoted by secret languages and codes as well as a common culture. Together children explore ideas and values as well as their environment.

The cognitive development of the school-age child, according to Piaget, is characterized by the ability to begin to do mentally what the child would have had to do with real action at an earlier age. "Piaget illustrated this by presenting 5-, 6-, and 7-year-old children with six sticks in a row and asking them to take the same number from a pile on the table. The younger children solved the problem by placing the sticks beneath the sample and matching the sticks one by one. The older children merely picked up six sticks and held them in their hands. The older children had counted the sticks mentally" (Elkind, 1974, p. 23). The school-age child also sees the multiple characteristics of objects rather than centering on any one aspect. For instance, in one study Piaget placed 20 white and 7 brown wooden beads in a box and asked individual 5-, 6-, and 7-year-old children if there were more white beads or more wooden beads. The young children could only respond that there were more white beads than brown beads. The older children could determine that there were more wooden beads than white beads because all of the beads were wooden (Elkind, 1974, p. 28). The older children were able to see the whole without losing sight of the uniqueness of the individual parts.

Piaget also found that it is during these years that

the child masters the concept of conservation. The child begins to differentiate between the appearances of things and how they really are. Piaget's classic test is to give the child two jars of equal size containing equal amounts of liquid. The contents of one jar are then poured into two smaller containers of equal size, and the child is asked whether the amount of liquid poured into the two smaller jars is still the same as that remaining in the other container. The younger children cannot comprehend that the liquid has been conserved when placed in smaller containers. The older children can because they can now make mental comparisons rather than actually manipulating objects, can see the whole as well as the parts, and have mastered the concept of conservation. They are ready for the cognitive task of mastering classes, relationships, and quantities of objects.

However, this new ability to reason and to carry out mental operations in solving problems is limited in a very important respect. School-age children can reason about concrete things but not about verbal propositions. They cannot differentiate between their own assumptions and the facts. In other words, they treat their own hypotheses as if they were facts and reject facts that do not agree with that position. Elkind has defined this as "cognitive conceit" (1974, p. 80). For instance, when the child learns that parents are not always right, there are two prevalent assumptions. One of these is that the adults are not too bright, and the other is that the child knows more than the adults. Elkind points out that this behavior is often demonstrated in a spirit of fun or teasing as though the children are aware that they are using a convenient fiction.

Cognitive conceit is also useful in understanding the moral behavior of latency-age children. Children of this age have internalized rules and know what is right and wrong. However, they continue throughout latency to break the rules they see as being made by adults.

Children take the rules as a challenge to their intellectual superiority and attempt to break them without being caught. School-age children continue to operate with this kind of external conscience until the end of childhood, when they start to formulate their own rules that will internally regulate their behavior.

Children experience success during this stage of industry as they participate in many productive activities. They experience a sense of accomplishment that leads to the feelings of adequacy and worth vs the feelings of inferiority that come with repeated failure. School-age children's great desire to win at games and willingness to work to achieve a variety of skills demonstrate their need to be adequate in their own eyes as well as in the eyes of others.

Preadolescence

The precise parameters of age and developmental levels begin to blend and overlap with the late childhood years. From that point on, a range of years, rather than a precise number, describes each developmental level. Some consider the "late childhood" and "early teen" years as a separate and important category known as "preadolescence." It may be helpful to think in terms of this group as youngsters from ages 9 to 12 in the fifth to eighth grades with tasks, characteristics, and behaviors that differentiate them from children and also from adolescents. Youngsters in this group are at an in-between age; they are no longer cuddly children, nor are they quite yet into the dramatic changes that mark the adolescent's world. It might be said that the tasks of preadolescence have to do with preparation for those adolescent changes that lie only a few years ahead. It is a continuation of the change in primary affiliation with the adult society and the codes of parents to an affiliation with those of their peers. Some of the patterns of the child's personality begin to loosen up and alter in some disorganization preparatory to further growth.

Preadolescents characteristically have great physical restlessness. Running is more natural than walking. Sitting still, even through a meal, may seem nearly impossible. Signs of earlier childhood problems, such as nervous habits or antics or bed-wetting, may reappear temporarily before they are discarded. Muscular strength, skill, and agility are very important. In their quiet moments, which may be rather rare, preadolescents may have imaginative daydreams or may sit and stare blankly into space with apparently little on their minds. Although they may well have fears, worries, or concerns, they are not very interested in talking about them, but they may instead symbolically protect themselves from these problems by possessing toy guns, knives, or flashlights.

These years are often very trying times for parents

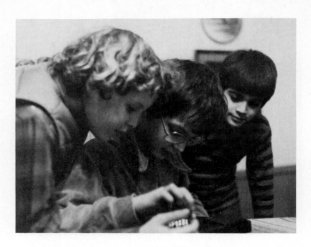

Preadolescence—establishing relationships.

because the parent-child bonds seem to be loosening and breaking. Although preadolescents do love and feel loyalty toward their parents, they may quite frequently treat them with surprising suspicion, distrust, and irritability. They are easily offended and respond to seemingly minor incidents with the ready accusation that adults do not understand them and, furthermore, treat them wrongly. At the same time, they are seemingly unaware of the effect of any of their own inconsiderateness or the feelings of others and are more or less surprised when it is pointed out to them that their behavior has caused some hurt. Other adults in the neighborhood may receive more admiration than the parents receive. Parental recommendations regarding use of language and matters of appearance and cleanliness are often met with a response of indignation and frequent conflict. They are increasingly sensitive about having a parent see their bodies and about public display of affection.

At this stage, some boys and girls have little to do with each other socially, although girls may move through this phase more quickly than boys. Clique and gang formation is a prominent characteristic as they establish strong identification with their peer groups. Often their pals and their peer codes do not meet with parental approval, which serves to make them all the more desirable to the preadolescent.

These changes of preadolescence are not easy for the parents, but neither are they easy for the preadolescent. There are often conflicting and painful choices, but the preadolescent must experience these to move on in the establishment of an individual identity.

ADOLESCENCE

The terms *adolescence* and *adult* are both derived from the Latin word *adolescere* meaning "to grow up." Both stages of life are, indeed, times of growth; however, the

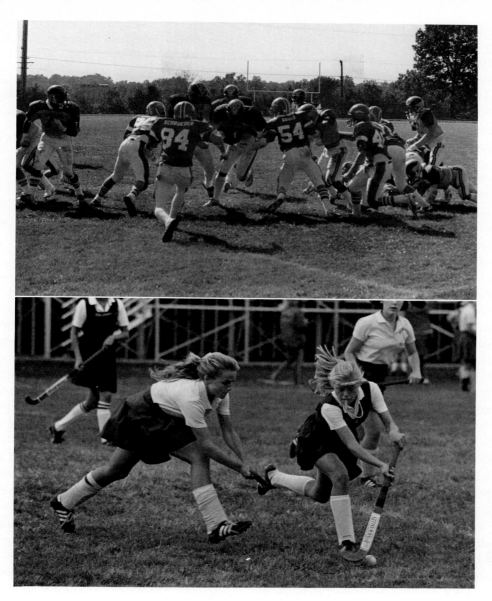

Adolescence—competition.

outward manifestations of growth during adolescence are the most dramatic. The age boundaries of adolescence are variable, although generally the teenage years (13 to 19) are used.

Adolescence is eminently a period of rapid and intense physical growth accompanied by profound changes that affect the entire organism. A physiologic revolution occurs within and great concern develops over what the adolescent appears to be in the eyes of others compared with how the self is viewed. According to Erikson (1963, 1968) the task of adolescence is the development of "ego identity" and the danger of the stage is "role confusion." The social world broadens in adolescence, and the individual develops a growing sensitivity to the perceived judgments of others; one looks at oneself in comparison with others.

The word *conflict* is often associated with the words teenager and adolescent, and adolescence is truly a stage of conflict and turmoil, as well as one of high growth potential in the physical, sexual, and social areas. The adolescent must learn to cope with increasingly intense impulses, now vested in a maturing genital apparatus, an altering body formation, and a powerful muscle system. There is an increased muscular energy and strength, and spurts of physical growth.

Breast development is often the earliest visible sign of puberty in girls, beginning normally between the ages of 8 and 13 and ending between 13 and 18. Girls' pubic hair appears at about age 11 and axillary hair about a year later; the adult pattern of hair distribution is established by about age 14. Most girls begin to menstruate at age 12 to 13 but may normally start as early as 9 or as late as 18; the early cycles tend to be irregular and are often anovulatory.

    In boys, testicular enlargement is usually the first pubescent change, starting between 10 and 13 and ending between 13 and 17. The voice begins to deepen at 13 to 14. The growth of pubic hair occurs between ages 12 and 16; the growth of the beard and chest hair is usually somewhat later, around age 16. The first ejaculation usually occurs at 11 to 13 years, but the sperm are immature.

    The ages of 10 to 12 mark a spurt in height in girls, and by 14 to 15 their height growth is nearly complete. Boys of 12 to 13 have their rapid growth spurt. For some, this is preceded at about age 11 by a "stocky" or "chubby" period, which begins to decline as the spurt in height begins. By age 16, their height growth is nearly complete.

    By the fourteenth year, the body of a girl is more often that of a young woman than that of a child, and for boys that year may mark a transition from boyhood to young manhood.

    The behavioral traits of the adolescent years can also be described. The patterns of behavior during adolescence tend to fluctuate between outer- and inner-directedness as though the learnings of one phase must be tested or reflected on in the next. The adolescent needs periods for readjustment between the changing organism and the expanding environment. Growth is not a uniform, steady process but may show elements of "grown-up" helpfulness or childish lapses. It is an emotional period; the emotions should be considered symptoms of many forces—fears, struggles, and creative construction. Emotional growth requires creative struggle.

    The inner life of the adolescent consists of a mix of emotional peaks and valleys ranging from exhilarating highs to depressing lows. Much of the conflict and growth during these years results from the effort to experience and sort through the meanings of this shifting complex of feelings. Many adolescents also participate in a variety of roles in rapid succession, such as student, teammate, friend, worker, child, outcast, artist, and rebel. The rapid role changes experienced during a day may contribute to the shifting moods so many adolescents experience.

    Adolescents gain satisfaction from meeting challenges that fit their developing skills and interests and that provide them with meaningful rewards. Their growing involvement with many activities and the ability to accomplish tasks takes them beyond the more impulsive and egocentric activities of the childhood years toward the adult world of more widely shared actions, rules, symbols, and communication.

    Without some inner-directedness and an environment that nurtures this kind of growth, the teenage years

---

Major Physical Changes of Adolescence

Female	Male
Breast development	Testicular enlargement
Growth of axillary and pubic hair	Deepening of voice
Onset of menses	Perceptible growth of thyroid cartilage
	Growth of facial, chest, and pubic hair

Both sexes

Spurts of growth in height
Facial and body contours change
Complexion may change with appearance of acne
Increased food intake
Increased muscular strength

---

can be far less productive, maturing, and satisfying. The paths of least resistance to short-term pleasure may lead adolescents to rely on escapes through sexual activities, drugs, or alcohol instead of developing skills that will serve them better in life. Unhealthy and self-defeating behaviors that lead to involvement with addictive activities or to adolescent pregnancy are of great concern at this stage.

    Even reasonably well-integrated adolescents will, from time to time, feel ambivalent about adults who "don't understand me," break-ups in relationships, and the perceived invasion of their privacy and have great concerns about their appearance and popularity.

    A shift in perspective develops gradually with the passing of time. It is a challenge to develop an increasingly complex view of life with a sense of balance, to learn to see another's point of view while clarifying one's own, and to integrate what can be learned from mistakes.

    These fluctuations continue to some degree for several years in the direction of greater maturation. The task of finding an acceptable career, one that is personally and potentially economically adequate, assumes a more central position during the later high school and college years. Sheehy (1974) describes the ages of 18 to 20 as a time of "pulling up roots." College, military service, and short-term trips all provide ways of leaving the family base; peers temporarily become substitutes for family, although rebounds to the family occur from time to time. "The tasks of this passage are to locate ourselves in a peer group role, a sex role, an anticipated occupation, an ideology or world view. As a result, we gather the impetus to leave home physically and the identity to begin leaving home emotionally" (Sheehy, 1974, p. 39). She notes that a stormy progression through this phase prob-

---

> ### *Developmental Tasks of Adolescence*
>
> 1. Continue to expand the sense of individual identity
> 2. Cope with increasingly intense impulses—physical, emotional, and sexual
> 3. Cope with fluctuations between inner- and outer-directedness
> 4. Develop a changing sense of one's body and new capabilities
> 5. Begin to develop self-reliance with decision making
> 6. Develop peer relationships
> 7. Continue formal learning experiences

ably facilitates the normal progression of the adult life cycle.

Friedenberg notes the difficulty of adolescent passage in our Western society and emphasizes the importance of conflict to the individual and to society:

This process (of establishing a clear and stable self-identification) may be frustrated and emptied of meaning in a society which, like our own, is hostile to clarity and vividness. Our culture impedes the clear definition of any faithful self-image. . . . We do not break images . . . we blur and soften them. The resulting pliability gives life in our society its familiar plastic texture. It also makes adolescence more difficult, more dangerous and more troublesome to the adolescent and to society itself. And it makes adolescence rarer. Fewer youngsters really dare to go through with it; they merely undergo puberty and simulate maturity (p.17). . . .

Adolescent conflict is the instrument by which an individual learns the complex, subtle and precious difference between himself and his environment . . . and leads, as a high synthesis to the youth's own adulthood and to critical participation in society as an adult (Friedenberg, 1959, p. 34).

ADULTHOOD

In the past, the phases or stages of adulthood and the accompanying expectations were typically closely related to chronologic age. This is far less the case today: younger people are delaying marriage and children; women are entering the work force in increasing numbers; divorce and remarriage are common, as is the choice to remain single; and older adults are increasing dramatically in number and entering "old" age with better health and the ability to participate actively in numerous aspects of life, including the extended family, travel, politics, and education. The traditional rhythms of the life course are changing, and flexibility is required in adjusting to these shifting social realities. It is more difficult to distinguish the young, middle-aged, and old in terms of major life changes or the ages at which those events occur. Chronologic age is an increasingly unreliable indicator; it is more important to know what life task or challenge a person is currently involved in than to have a particular set of expectations based on age.

The physical changes of adulthood are usually gradual and are less salient than the psychological changes that are occurring. The adult years are marked by a shifting perspective on the self and the world—identity, dreams and expectations, and the levels of satisfaction with various accomplishments are matters that occupy the adult developmental picture. During youth and middle age, people are affected by their experiences and the timing of those experiences, not primarily by biological factors.

Carl Jung focused his extensive psychoanalytic work on the adult years of life. Jung's first developmental stage, extending from about 18 to 35 or 40, was called "youth." He saw this stage as marked by individual development, involvement in the outside world, and investment in a family. During this period the individual's task is to give up the world of childhood while broadening one's horizons and engaging in the task- and achievement-oriented work of the world. Jung saw the second half of life beginning at age 35 or 40, with the change in orientation occurring slowly, developing largely through the unconscious. During this time there is an increased orientation to the inner life through introversion and self-reflection. Throughout life there is a drive toward individuation of the self, but, more markedly during this phase, there is an effort to balance opposing life forces, such as masculine and feminine qualities, while working toward the goal of self-actualization.

Erik Erikson's three stages dealing with adulthood involve for the young adult, ages 20 to 40, the struggle between intimacy and isolation with the capacity for love as the desired result. Middle adulthood, ages 40 to 65, is marked by the struggle between generativity and stagnation. This phase involves the ability to experience pride and pleasure in accomplishments and to guide future generations vs a nonproductive and egocentric life characterized by self-indulgence and personal impoverishment. Old age, from 65 on, involves the struggle between integrity and despair as an individual evaluates life and its accomplishments, seeking to understand, appreciate, and accept life as having had meaning, leading to a sense of integrity, vs the despair generated from a sense that one's life has been meaningless and wasted. Both Jung and Erikson integrated death as the final aspect of the life cycle and as a reality that should be faced and accepted as a part of life.

Carol Gilligan, in her study of the psychosocial processes by which women develop differently than men, takes the position that women's development does not fit

Erikson's model because women's identity formation takes place in a context of ongoing relationship. The female child experiences attachment to the mother that does not require separation for self and sexual identity that the male child requires. Masculine identity becomes defined through separation and is threatened by intimacy, while feminine identity is defined through attachment and is threatened by separation. This leads to life experiences where males tend to have greater difficulty with relationships and females with individuation. She is concerned that when maturity is equated with personal autonomy, a focus on relationships appears to be a weakness rather than a human strength, and she suggests that both forces must be in balance as the person moves toward maturity.

Transitions and changes occur throughout the life cycle, altering in sometimes obvious and sometimes subtle ways: adult roles, relationships, routines, and assumptions (Schlossberg). Certain anticipated transitions are expected to be part of the adult experience, such as working and choosing whether to marry, remain single, or live an alternative life-style. There are also unanticipated transitions, such as losing a job, the unexpected death of someone close, accidents, and major surgery. Nonevent transitions, or events that are expected but fail to occur, include not finding the desired job, not getting married, or not having a family.

Young Adulthood

During the decade of ages 20 to 30, the major task is to achieve relative independence from parental figures and a sense of emotional, social, and economic responsibility for one's own life. Stevenson (1977) suggests the following developmental tasks:

1. Advancing self-development and the enactment of appropriate roles and positions in society
2. Initiating the development of a personal style of life
3. Adjusting to a heterosexual marital relationship or to another companionship style
4. Developing parenting behaviors for biologic offspring or in the broader framework of social parenting
5. Integrating personal values with career development and socioeconomic constraints

Erikson (1963), focusing more narrowly on marriage, describes the task of young adulthood as the development of affiliation or intimacy expressed as mutuality with a loved partner of the opposite sex with whom one is willing and able to regulate the cycles of work, procreation, and recreation. This involves the capacity to commit onself "to concrete affiliations and partnerships and to develop the ethical strength to abide by such commitments, even though they may call for significant sac-

rifices and compromises" (p. 263). The danger of this stage is isolation or an avoidance of those persons and settings that promote and provide intimacy. A young adult whose identity work is not well underway may settle for sets of stereotyped interpersonal relationships that lead to a deep sense of isolation. This false "intimacy" bypasses the accomplishment of improved understanding of one's own inner resources and those of others.

Young adults may move out of the parental home or establish a more equal role with their parents if they stay in it. They begin to establish a style of single living, a marriage relationship, or another companionship style and adapt to the changes and compromises in expectations that their choice requires. Parenting tasks may be initiated by bearing children, adopting, becoming a foster parent, or reaching out in other ways, such as coaching children's teams or participating in child development–oriented organizations. It should also be noted that with divorce and remarriage, a frequent occurrence in American society, stepparenting and single parenting are fairly common situations. As children develop, parenting roles also develop in a reciprocal manner.

The young adult also chooses an area of study, a career, or a vocation and may begin to consider how one's belief about self and humankind affect that choice. Usually leisure activities are selected, and some young adults include participation in local community and organizational activities in addition to career and family development. Sheehy suggests that the focus of the 20s shifts from the interior struggles of late adolescence ("Who am I?" "What is truth?") to a preoccupation with working out external situations ("Where do I go?" "How can I get there?" "How do I put my dreams into effect?"). The tasks revolve around erecting the test structure around the chosen life-style. Becoming caught up in the expectations of others is a pervasive theme, and the impulse to do what one should struggles with the impulses to be experimental and to explore alternative options.

Maturational crises of the 20s occur around these central themes: (1) attempts to increase independence from parents and parental dominance; (2) the choice of a post–secondary education course—school, a job, or the military; and (3) moving into the job or career world and establishing skills.

Middle Adulthood

The middle years of adulthood may be thought of as an intermediate stage of life when growth is strongest in the areas of social and emotional development. By this time, individuals have generally chosen a life-style, a family or single pattern of living, and an occupation and are involved in implementing those choices. The span of time

---

Developmental Tasks of Middlescence

Developmental tasks of middlescence I, the core of the middle years (30–50)	**Developmental tasks of middlescence II, the new middle years (50–70)**
1. Developing socioeconomic consolidation	1. Maintaining flexible views in occupational, civic, political, religious, and social positions
2. Evaluating one's occupation or career in light of a personal value system	2. Keeping current on relevant scientific, political, and cultural changes
3. Helping younger persons (eg., biologic offspring) to become integrated human beings	3. Developing mutually supportive (interdependent) relationships with grown offspring and other members of the younger generation
4. Enhancing or redeveloping intimacy with spouse or most significant other	4. Reevaluating and enhancing the relationship with spouse or most significant other or adjusting to their loss
5. Developing a few deep friendships	5. Helping aged parents or other relatives progress through the last stage of life
6. Helping aging persons (eg., parents or in-laws) progress through the later years of life	6. Deriving satisfaction from increased availability of leisure time
7. Assuming responsible positions in occupational, social, and civic activities, organizations, and communities	7. Preparing for retirement and planning another career when feasible
8. Maintaining and improving the home or other forms of property	8. Adapting self and behavior to signals of accelerated aging processes
9. Using leisure time in satisfying and creative ways	
10. Adjusting to biologic or personal system changes that occur	

From Stevenson JS: Issues and crises during middlescence, New York, 1977, Appleton-Century-Crofts.

---

considered to cover the middle years is variable; some consider ages 40 to 65 and others, ages 30 to 70 as "middle age." However the boundaries are marked, it is probably the longest stage of an individual's life. The boundaries of this stage of life must be considered tentative and flexible. In this text the framework of 30 to 70 years of age, as described by Stevenson (1977), is used. Stevenson uses the term *middlescence* to describe this age span and further subdivides it into two categories: (1) the core middle years, or middlescence I, ages 30 to 50, and (2) the new middle years, or middlescence II, ages 50 to 70. The developmental tasks that she assigns to those subcategories of the middle years are presented in the boxed material above.

Between ages 30 and 50, major goals and activities are in the areas of self-development, assistance to both the younger and older generations, and organizational endeavors. Individuals feel a need to come to terms with their own and with society's value orientations and with the similarities and discrepancies therein. One's own value orientation may undergo a major change or numerous minor changes during these years when patterns are beginning to seem quite set but may not seem comfortably so. Individuals move into various roles and stations in a variety of settings: in the family, at work, in religious organizations, and in community and civic affairs. In Western society, much of the implementation of the goals of major institutions, including business, industry, government, education, religion, and charitable

agencies, is performed by the middle-aged population. Work is a major activity and motivating force. For some the work itself is rewarding and gratifying; for others, the only rewards are the paycheck and the fringe benefits.

Much time during these years goes into promoting the growth of significant others, including one's children, parents, spouse, and friends. Erikson's seventh stage of life, generativity vs stagnation, addresses this issue of producing either another generation or something that may be passed on to the next generation. For some this means parenthood, for others this means generativity through creative acts of expression of altruism. Failure to advance to this stage or develop this task can result, according to Erikson, in a stagnation of self or narcissistic self-indulgence. It should be noted that much of the economic effort and gain of the employed middle-aged population goes toward the support of the younger and older generations. It is important that, while providing these various forms of support and assistance, the middle-aged avoid a need for complete control of these other age groups.

As leisure time increases in the society, the activities that fill that larger portion are worthy of thoughtful consideration. People may choose to develop skills and talents that will serve them well in the present and during retirement. Part of self-knowledge and self-acceptance is an acknowledgment of the changes at the physical, emotional, and intellectual levels that accompany the aging process. The physical alterations may be the most difficult

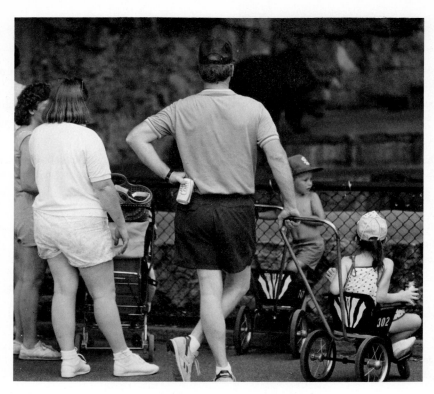

Middle adulthood—the development of a family.

to accept in a culture where the signs of youthfulness are most highly acclaimed. It is most helpful to find some balance between accepting the inevitable changes in appearance while striving to maintain a high level of health with positive approaches toward exercise, diet, and the socioemotional environment. The changes of added years can also be appreciated in terms of emotional and intellectual benefits that can accrue.

During the decades of the 30s and 40s there are several maturational crises that do occur and various situational crises that can occur. Maturational crises are developmental transitions; they are stresses that occur periodically in the life cycle. Situational crises are events that occur with less frequency and predictability and only for certain individuals. Some of the predictable maturational crises in the core middle years occur in the early 30s and again in the early to mid-40s and have to do with the direction one's life seems to be taking. "Why am I doing this and not something else?" "Why am I with this person and not someone else?" "Why this career or talent or role and not another?" "Have I defined myself too narrowly?" are some of the common questions. Much soul-searching about priorities occurs and may lead to changes in residence, job, career, or spouse or to a re-evaluation and acceptance of things as they are. Individuals may approach the 30s realizing that they have expended both time and energy in doing the things their

family and society indicated they "should" do. They may begin to feel too restricted by the career and personal choices made earlier and to realize that other aspects of themselves are struggling to surface and find expression. New choices and alternatives, as well as the old ones, are reconsidered and commitments may be altered or deepened. This may involve an uprooting of the life that seemed to be so well grounded and striking out after a new vision. A job or career change may be sought, single people may renew the search for a partner, and married people may feel discontent leading to a serious review of the marriage and perhaps to separation or divorce. Childless couples reconsider having children, while those who have spent a number of years raising young children may move toward involvement outside the home.

Once these struggles are decided in some way, the following few years may be characterized by a more settled situation during which people put down roots, invest in property, and work earnestly on climbing some particular career or social ladder. Much time and energy are involved in work and child-rearing; satisfaction with a marriage may change.

For many individuals, the mid-30s mark a significant milestone. An awareness of life being at its halfway mark emerges. Time's passage may be felt as never before. There may be a diminishing acceptance of stereotyped roles and acknowledgment that few answers are absolute. Sheehy (1974) refers to the years of 35 to 45 as the "Deadline Decade," a time of reevaluating choices, purposes, and the expenditure of resources. It is a period of uncertainty and opportunity, a chance to restructure a narrower, earlier identity. Individuals may stumble on new aspects of themselves if they give themselves permission to do so.

Davitz and Davitz (1976) have focused on the decade of 40 to 50 and found some similarities as well as a number of differences in the way men and women handle those years. There seems to be a generally increased awareness of one's own mortality as age-group acquaintances begin to develop illnesses and to die, often as a result of a heart attack. People in their 40s become aware, perhaps for the first time, that younger people view them as being in an older age group. Identity questions surface again, as they do with some frequency throughout the adult years, and individuals wonder: "What have I done?" "What have I become?" "Am I doing what is most fulfilling, rewarding, and satisfying for me?" "What am I now?" Occasionally, they wonder what things might be like if they could begin again, but there is also the realization that although one might still make changes, one cannot go back to the beginning.

Parenting may be difficult, especially if the children are adolescents and working out identity problems of their own. Some parenting behaviors may be resented, although the parents may believe they are merely trying to prevent a repeat of their own mistakes. Parents may be attemping to relive their own lives through their maturing children and this is often understandably met with resentment from offspring who are seeking to lead their own lives. Concerns about aging parents also become more prominent.

During the early 40s, men may be enjoying success and promotions at work or may harbor a concern that this is the last chance to make it. Some experience tension from a fear of being passed by and are very sensitive to any indications that peers or superiors are losing confidence. While much energy goes into work or much frustration is experienced there, a sense of boredom with marriage and family life may emerge. Fears regarding sexual drive and loss of potency and masculinity may be experienced. Frustrations may be acted out at home, which tends to be the safest setting, producing more strain on the marriage and family relationship. Extramarital affairs are not uncommon. The emotions are fluctuating, moving from anger to affection and warmth and reflecting some of the internal conflicts about identity at work and at home. These conflicts occur in a context of responsibilities from which the person usually feels he or she cannot escape.

During the mid-40s, the attitude toward work may change from one of total involvement to one of lesser interest with a growing interest in developing a sport or hobby. The meaningfulness of activities is a frequent theme, as daily routines at work and home are rethought and belief in religion, politics, and relationships are reevaluated. This situation offers potential for psychological growth and a reintegration and stabilization of identity. Toward the second half of the 40s, some of the conflicts may be resolved. The stress on the marriage may promote a change in the relationship with greater acceptance of interdependency, or it may lead to a divorce and possibly to remarriage. Greater sexual maturity can provide an enhanced capacity to give and receive pleasure. Work may become more acceptable and viewed more in terms of its responsibilities than in terms of power. During these years aspects of the personality and talents that have been latent may begin to emerge. Physical changes are moderate; weight may increase and recovery time after exertion may be longer.

In our Western society, a woman approaches the age of 40 with a complex mixture of feelings: a sense of greater self-assurance and poise may be counterbalanced with a sense of apprehension. A woman of 40 is frequently thought of as middle-aged, settled, and mature. This set of role expectations may frustrate her, especially if she does not see herself conforming to that model. Involvement in a career may be a source of strength for a woman, since work brings its own rewards and sense of personal accomplishment and her identity is not entirely tied up with her family. It may also be a source of strain, since demands from both work and family may be very high. Women in the work world who may already have experienced some discrimination can find promotions increasingly rare and even resented by a husband who has not been similarly recognized. A woman who has devoted years to home and family may be eager to get into the outside world of school, business, or involvement in community activities.

Weight may become an eminent concern: a battle against weight gain may also be a battle against aging, the loss of physical attractiveness, and all that that implies in our culture. Difficulties in this area may well depend on the amount of self-esteem that has been previously derived from physical attractiveness. Gray hair is yet another manifestation of a physical change accompanying aging and may be a source of distress.

A woman confronted with her own concerns about aging might find these reinforced by her husband's behavior if he appears to be dissatisfied with the marriage. If divorce results, new friends and a new life-style must be developed. If the marital storms are weathered, a closer bond may be forged. Expectations of each spouse for the other may become more based in the facts than the fantasies of the relationship, and mutual dependence is accepted, as well as individual strengths and differences.

Single persons may experience a change in their relationships with married couples; aloneness may become a more prominent theme, despite the positive aspects of independence. The previous choice of career over marriage may be reconsidered, particularly if the parents have died.

Menopause, which normally occurs during the 40s or early 50s, involves both physiologic and psychological changes. The hormonal imbalance may result in episodes of emotional instability, rapid mood shifts, nervousness, irritability, insomnia, and fatigue. Some depression may be involved, but many women react with equanimity. The reaction to menopause may depend on how other developmental crises have been handled. Menopause may be followed by a heightened sexual drive and enjoyment of sex because concerns about pregnancy are absent.

During the "new" middle years, generally ages 50 to 70, individuals have an opportunity to define and integrate the emotional and intellectual growth that has occurred during the earlier adulthood years. It may be a time of changes within the outside of the family resulting in the time and energy to develop new areas of interest. In the work world, many have attained much or most of what they can, although for a few, advancement is still possible. In certain arenas, such as in legislative, business, governmental, religious, and community service areas, these years may be the prime years of activity. Many of the highest positions in these areas are occupied by people in the new middle years. Within the family setting, spouses may be back to the couple stage, or fast approaching it, and must readjust to the contracted nuclear family or to life alone if a spouse should die. Grandparenting is a new role often acquired during this stage. Parents must reassess their relationships with their children and move from the adult-child type of interactions to adult-adult interactions with their offspring who have reached adulthood. Men may become more aware of, less fearful of, and more accepting of their tendencies to provide care and nurturance, while women may accept and develop more fully their assertiveness through an interest in business, politics, or other organizations and activities outside the home. The aging parents of 50- to 70-year-olds often require assistance emotionally, physically, or financially. It continues to be important to help both the older and younger generations continue their own development and not to stifle either with overwhelming controls.

People in this age group, as in any age group, are confronted with rapid changes in technology and in the social environment. However, they often prefer to advise some caution and restraint in the type and rate of change. Life experiences have, one hopes, brought some sense of wisdom and judgment to the middle-aged; although some younger people may view the middle-aged as overly cautious and nonprogressive, the balance between the two views is important. At the same time, openness and flexibility continue to be important characteristics to health and well-being. Those who stay current with ideas and trends will have a more positive approach to life and less need to maintain a defensive posture and will probably communicate more effectively with younger individuals.

Preparation for retirement is a crucial task, perhaps especially for people who have been employed outside the home, but also for those who have maintained the housework. Both must readjust to more shared time. Preparation through adult education or development of new or latent skills can pave the way for a refocusing of talent. In a way, preparation for retirement is lifelong in that people bring to retirement all that they have become throughout the years. Specific planning for retirement should not be delayed until retirement is imminent.

Later Adulthood

As is the case with other stages of adulthood, the parameters of later adulthood and old age are not easy to define. Almost everyone is acquainted with someone who seems "old" at 40 and with someone else who seems "young" at 65. Some gerontologists have attempted to deal with this situation by setting apart the years from 60 to 75 as early old age and the years from 75 on as later old age.

Later adulthood has become a subject of increasing interest to more people over the past several years. Factors influencing this increased interest include the longer life span and the decline in death rates in Western society, leading to increased numbers of the elderly in the population. However, changes in the social and family structure of this society, along with attitudes toward aging and the aged, have created many problems for these ever-larger numbers of old people. Institutional forms of care have been developed but have often proved unsatisfactory; major pieces of legislation have been passed on behalf of the elderly, but often this has not eased the passage of time and the financial, social, and emotional problems that develop. The emphasis on youth and their culture, behavior, and attitudes is accompanied by a negative attitude toward those on the other end of the age spectrum. It is often said that in this culture, all wish to live long but no one wishes to grow old. This is in marked contrast to other cultures, where old age is respected and even revered.

Later adulthood is similar to all other developmental stages in that certain adaptations are necessary and certain developmental tasks must be achieved. Yet these developmental tasks are different from earlier ones in that these are the final ones in life.

Among the most significant developmental and adjustive tasks in later adulthood are:

1. Maintaining or developing activities that enhance self-image, contribute to a sense of worth in society, and help to retain functional capacity
2. Developing new roles as in-laws or grandparents
3. Adapting to numerous losses—economically, socially, emotionally (such as job, friends, spouse)
4. Adapting to physical changes
5. Performing a life review
6. Preparing for one's own death

As both demands from work and family and living arrangements change somewhat with the onset of retirement, time to do other things becomes more available. It is very important that preparation be made for the use of time far in advance of the retirement years. Failure to do so can make the change in time use and availability come as a shock, and the hours may seem empty, heavy, or endless. If, on the other hand, preparation has been made, time can be used to advantage in the development

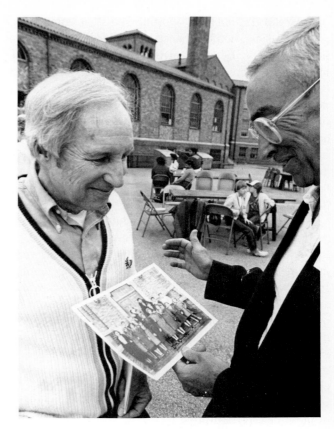

Later adulthood—the life review.

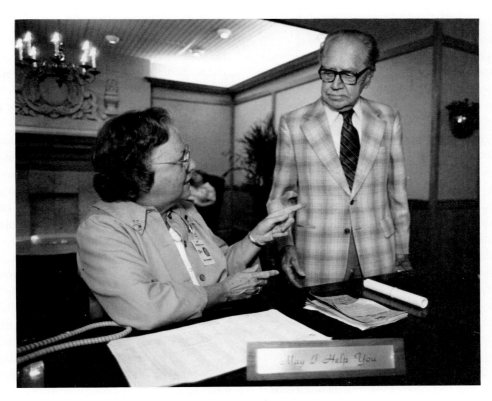

Later adulthood—volunteer work enhances self-worth.

of new careers, hobbies, sporting skills, or community activities. This should enhance both self-worth and functional capacity. Educational opportunities for adults of all ages are increasing. For the older adult, continuing education can provide an opportunity to learn again simply for the pleasure of learning or to develop another set of skills or an avocation. It is important to both physical and mental well-being that individuals continue to be involved in and contribute to society. If one or both elderly spouses have been employed, they must also learn to adjust to having more time together and to meshing their lives effectively.

New roles emerge for older adults as their children marry and have children of their own. Acceptance of their children's spouses into the family network is very instrumental in the ongoing interaction of the family. Interaction with grandchildren can be a very pleasant aspect of aging if it does not become too time-consuming or burdensome. Grandparents should be able to enjoy their grandchildren without having to be overly responsible for them. Another family role that may continue or may begin in early later adulthood is the caretaking of elderly parents who may be ill or at least more dependent. Individuals need to reevaluate personal identity in light of these new roles in life.

It is abundantly evident that numerous losses do accompany the later years of life. Retirement and its consequences must be dealt with. The loss of a job after many years of employment may be one of the greatest developmental and situational crises in an individual's life. As stated earlier, it is crucial to plan far in advance for postretirement activities that enhance self-respect. The loss of a job often includes the loss of the social relationships that were a part of that setting. It may also mean the loss of opportunities for certain kinds of recognition and achievement.

Couples or individuals must learn to adapt their life-style to a retirement income. As retirement incomes become relatively smaller in an inflationary era, this lowered income becomes more of a loss. Homes, entertainment styles, and lifelong travel plans may have to be given up or diminished in scope to meet the costs of food, housing, and health care.

Other losses may include the deaths of friends, a spouse, or other family members. These losses are among the most difficult aspects of later adulthood. Coping with bereavement for one with whom one has shared life experiences, memories, and plans leaves a great personal void. It is important to experience the profound emotions that accompany the loss and then to go on living one's own life and fostering the development of new relationships.

Adaptation to physical changes may also be viewed as a series of losses. Physical strength and vigor do tend to decline gradually over the years. In the 60s and 70s this change is often accompanied by diminishing sensory acuity of the eyes, ears, and taste. The emergence of one or several chronic illnesses may also impinge on strength, self-image, and independent status. The older population does become more dependent on the health care system for more frequent intermittent care and, for a small percentage of them, for full institutional care in various types of nursing homes. The majority of the elderly do continue to live at home and to receive some care from family or significant others; however, their more independent status is decreased. Major tasks are to accept physical changes and their limitations and to conserve strength and resources as necessary.

The process of performing a life review is an important developmental task of later adulthood. Most older persons do spend some time reflecting on their accomplishments and failures, satisfactions, and disappointments in an effort to integrate and evaluate the diverse elements of a life lived so that a reasonably positive view of their life's worth can be reached. Failure to accomplish this task may lead to serious psychological problems. The life review process is far more than useless reminiscence. It allows for some gratification and also for the revision in understanding and clarification of experiences that may have been poorly understood or accepted when they occured. It is an inventory that helps put past successes and failures into some perspective. It is often important for the older person to share some of this material with others, particularly with the younger generation. This can be mutually beneficial because it gives the older person a sense of usefulness and some credit for age and wisdom and can provide the younger person with a sense of history. Today's older Americans have lived through more changes than any other single group in human history. This life developmental task is well described by Erikson (1963) as the eighth cycle of the person: ego integrity vs despair. "It is the acceptance of one's one and only life cycle as something that had to be and that, by necessity, permitted of no substitutions" (p. 268).

Preparation for one's own death, views on death, and the possibility of an afterlife may very likely evolve from the life review process. For many, if not all, it is important to consider the issue of one's own death and to prepare for it in terms of finishing one's business or setting one's affairs in order. This takes many forms: finalizing a will, achieving some goal, resolving some or many interpersonal relationships, and saying one's farewells to significant family members and friends. If the dying process is prolonged because of some chronic illness, the individual will go through several phases of dealing with eventual death. Both popular and professional literature are making available knowledge and information about the process of dying as the final phase of life. To die in a way as close as possible to what the individual desires may be thought of as life's final developmental task.

Adult Assessment Tools

Although there are few tools to assess life changes and their effects on adults, two that have been developed are the Recent Life Changes Questionnaire and the Life Experiences Survey. Both of these are an attempt to assess life stresses and to indicate a possible relationship between life stresses and susceptibility to physical and psychological problems or illnesses.

The Recent Life Changes Questionnaire (Rahe, 1975) is a self-administered questionnaire containing a list of events that subjects respond to by checking those events that they have experienced in the previous 6 months to 1 year (Table 2-2). To determine the scores for these events the researchers had a large group of subjects rate each of the items, with "marriage" assigned to an arbitrary value, with regard to the amount of social readjustment each event required. Mean values for each item were taken to represent the average amount of social readjustment required. The values, called Life Change Units, were added to yield a life stress score. Studies using this tool have shown correlations between high recent life change scores and the development of health problems. This tool does combine a life stress score based on both desirable and undesirable events, and it may be important to take these differences into account in the assessment of an individual's life change and its impact on health. It is also important to consider an individual client's own assessment of both the intensity of the life changes and the strength of his or her coping abilities.

Table 2-2

Recent life changes questionnaire

Scoring weight	
	Health
	Within the time periods listed, have you experienced:
53	1. An illness or injury that:
	(a) Kept you in bed a week or more, or took you to the hospital?
	(b) Was less serious than described above?
15	2. A major change in eating habits?
16	3. A major change in sleeping habits?
19	4. A change in your usual type or amount of recreation?
	*5. Major dental work?
	Work
	Within the time periods listed, have you:
36	6. Changed to a new type of work?
20	7. Changed your work hours or conditions?
29	8. Had a change in your responsibilities at work:
	(a) More responsibilities?
	(b) Less responsibilities?
	(c) Promotion?
	(d) Demotion?
	(e) Transfer?
23	9. Experienced troubles at work:
	(a) With your boss?
	(b) With co-workers?
	(c) With persons under your supervision?
	(d) Other work troubles?

From Rahe RH: Epidemiological studies of life change and illness, Int J Psychiatry Med 6(1-2):133-146, 1975. © Baywood Publishing Co, Inc.
*New questions.
[ ] Scaling weight derived from an earlier (military) scaling study.   *Continued*

Table 2-2

Recent life changes questionnaire—*cont'd*

Scoring weight	
	Work—cont'd
39	10. Experienced a major business readjustment?
45	11. Retired?
47	12. Experienced being:
	(a) Fired from work?
	(b) Laid off from work?
	*13. Taken courses by mail or studied at home to help you in your work?
	Home and family
	Within the time periods listed, have you experienced:
20	14. A change in residence:
	(a) A move within the same town or city?
	(b) A move to a different town, city, or state?
15	15. A change in family "get-togethers"?
44	16. A major change in the health or behavior of a family member (illness, accidents, drug, or disciplinary problems, etc.)?
25	17. Major change in your living conditions (home improvements or a decline in your home or neighborhood)?
100	18. The death of a spouse?
63	19. The death of a:
	(a) Child?
	(b) Brother or sister?
	(c) Parent?
	(d) Other close family member?
37	20. The death of a close friend?
	*21. A change in the marital status of your parents:
	(a) Divorce?
	(b) Remarriage?
50	22. Marriage?
	(**NOTE:** Questions 23-33 concern marriage. For persons never married go to item 34.)
35	23. A change in arguments with your spouse?
29	24. In-law problems?
	25. A separation from spouse:
[45]	(a) Due to work?
65	(b) Due to marital problems?
45	26. A reconciliation with spouse?
73	27. A divorce?
39	28. A gain of a new family member?
	(a) Birth of a child?
	(b) Adoption of a child?
	(c) A relative moving in with you?
26	29. Wife beginning or ceasing work outside the home?
40	30. Wife becoming pregnant?
29	31. A child leaving home:
	(a) Due to marriage?
	(b) To attend college?
	(c) For other reasons?
	*32. Wife having a miscarriage or abortion?
	*33. Birth of a grandchild?

Table 2-2
Recent life changes questionnaire—*cont'd*

Scoring weight	
	Personal and social
	Within the time periods listed, have you experienced:
28	34. A major personal achievement?
24	35. A change in your personal habits (your dress, friends, life-style, etc.)?
39	36. Sexual difficulties?
26	37. Beginning or ceasing school or college?
20	38. A change of school or college?
13	39. A vacation?
19	40. A change in your religious beliefs?
18	41. A change in your social activities (clubs, movies, visiting)?
11	42. A minor violation of the law?
63	43. Legal troubles resulting in your being held in jail?
	*44. A change in your political beliefs?
	*45. A new, close, personal relationship?
	*46. An engagement to marry?
	*47. A "falling out" of a close personal relationship?
	*48. Girlfriend (or boyfriend) problems?
	*49. A loss or damage of personal property?
	*50. An accident?
	*51. A major decision regarding your immediate future?
	Financial
	Within the time periods listed, have you:
17	52. Taken on a moderate purchase, such as a television, car, freezer, etc.?
31	53. Taken on a major purchase or a mortgage loan, such as a home, business, property, etc.?
30	54. Experienced a foreclosure on a mortgage or loan?
38	55. Experienced a major change in finances:
	(a) Increased income?
	(b) Decreased income?
	(c) Credit rating difficulties?

Subjective life change unit (SLCU) instructions
Instructions for scoring your adjustment to your recent life changes

Persons adapt to their recent life changes in different ways. Some people find the adjustment to a residential move, for example, to be enormous, while others find very little life adjustment necessary. You are now requested to "score" each of the recent life changes that you marked with an "X" as to the amount of adjustment you needed to handle the event.

Your scores can range from 1 to 100 "points." If, for example, you experienced a recent residential move but felt it required very little life adjustment, you would choose a low number and place it in the blank to the right of the question boxes. On the other hand, if you recently changed residence and felt it required a near maximal life adjustment, you would place a high number, toward 100, in the blank to the right of that question's boxes. For immediate life adjustment scores you would choose intermediate numbers between 1 and 100.

Please go back through your questionnaire and for each recent life change you indicated with an "X", choose your personal life adjustment score (between 1 and 100) which reflects what you saw to be the amount of life adjustment necessary to cope with or handle the event. Use both your estimates of the intensity of the life change and its duration to arrive at your scores.

The Life Experiences Survey (Sarason, Johnson, and Siegel, 1978) is a self-report tool that allows respondents to indicate events they have experienced over the past year (Table 2-3). It includes events that occur fairly frequently and allows respondents to weigh the desirability or undesirability of events. Ratings are on a seven-point scale from extremely negative (-3) to extremely positive ($+3$). A positive change score is obtained by adding those events rated as positive, the negative change score is obtained by adding the negatively rated events, and a total change score is obtained by adding those two values. Studies by Sarason and others

Table 2-3

The life experiences survey

Listed below are a number of events which sometimes bring about change in the lives of those who experience them and which necessitate social readjustment. *Please check those events which you have experienced in the recent past and indicate the time period during which you have experienced each event.* Be sure that all check marks are directly across from the items they correspond to.

Also, for each item checked below, *please indicate the extent to which you viewed the event as having either a positive or negative impact on your life* at the time the event occurred. That is, *indicate the type and extent of impact that the event had.* A rating of -3 would indicate an extremely negative impact. A rating of 0 suggests no impact either positive or negative. A rating $+3$ would indicate an extremely positive impact.

	0 to 6 mo	7 mo to 1 yr	Extremely negative	Moderately negative	Somewhat negative	No impact	Slightly positive	Moderately positive	Extremely positive
1. Marriage			-3	-2	-1	0	$+1$	$+2$	$+3$
2. Detention in jail or comparable institution			-3	-2	-1	0	$+1$	$+2$	$+3$
3. Death of spouse			-3	-2	-1	0	$+1$	$+2$	$+3$
4. Major change in sleeping habits (much more or much less sleep)			-3	-2	-1	0	$+1$	$+2$	$+3$
5. Death of close family member:									
a. Mother			-3	-2	-1	0	$+1$	$+2$	$+3$
b. Father			-3	-2	-1	0	$+1$	$+2$	$+3$
c. Brother			-3	-2	-1	0	$+1$	$+2$	$+3$
d. Sister			-3	-2	-1	0	$+1$	$+2$	$+3$
e. Grandmother			-3	-2	-1	0	$+1$	$+2$	$+3$
f. Grandfather			-3	-2	-1	0	$+1$	$+2$	$+3$
g. Other (specify)			-3	-2	-1	0	$+1$	$+2$	$+3$
6. Major change in eating habits (much more or much less food intake)			-3	-2	-1	0	$+1$	$+2$	$+3$
7. Foreclosure on mortgage or loan			-3	-2	-1	0	$+1$	$+2$	$+3$
8. Death of close friend			-3	-2	-1	0	$+1$	$+2$	$+3$
9. Outstanding personal achievement			-3	-2	-1	0	$+1$	$+2$	$+3$
10. Minor law violations (traffic tickets, disturbing the peace, etc.)			-3	-2	-1	0	$+1$	$+2$	$+3$
11. *Male:* Wife/girlfriend's pregnancy			-3	-2	-1	0	$+1$	$+2$	$+3$
12. *Female:* Pregnancy			-3	-2	-1	0	$+1$	$+2$	$+3$
13. Changed work situation (different work responsibility, major change in working conditions, working hours, etc.)			-3	-2	-1	0	$+1$	$+2$	$+3$
14. New job			-3	-2	-1	0	$+1$	$+2$	$+3$
15. Serious illness or injury of close family member:									
a. Father			-3	-2	-1	0	$+1$	$+2$	$+3$
b. Mother			-3	-2	-1	0	$+1$	$+2$	$+3$
c. Sister			-3	-2	-1	0	$+1$	$+2$	$+3$
d. Brother			-3	-2	-1	0	$+1$	$+2$	$+3$
e. Grandmother			-3	-2	-1	0	$+1$	$+2$	$+3$
f. Grandfather			-3	-2	-1	0	$+1$	$+2$	$+3$
g. Spouse			-3	-2	-1	0	$+1$	$+2$	$+3$
h. Other (specify)			-3	-2	-1	0	$+1$	$+2$	$+3$

From Sarason IG, Johnson JH, and Siegal JM: Assessing the impact of life changes: development of life experiences survey, J Consult Clin Psychol 46(5):932-946, 1978.

Table 2-3

The life experiences survey—*cont'd*

	0 to 6 mo	7 mo to 1 yr	Extremely negative	Moderately negative	Somewhat negative	No impact	Slightly positive	Moderately positive	Extremely positive
16. Sexual difficulties			−3	−2	−1	0	+1	+2	+3
17. Trouble with employer (in danger of losing job, being suspended, demoted, etc.)			−3	−2	−1	0	+1	+2	+3
18. Trouble with in-laws			−3	−2	−1	0	+1	+2	+3
19. Major change in financial status (a lot better off or a lot worse off)			−3	−2	−1	0	+1	+2	+3
20. Major change in closeness of family members (increased or decreased closeness)			−3	−2	−1	0	+1	+2	+3
21. Gaining a new family member (through birth, adoption, family member moving in, etc.)			−3	−2	−1	0	+1	+2	+3
22. Change of residence			−3	−2	−1	0	+1	+2	+3
23. Marital separation from mate (due to conflict)			−3	−2	−1	0	+1	+2	+3
24. Major change in church activities (increased or decreased attendance)			−3	−2	−1	0	+1	+2	+3
25. Marital reconciliation with mate			−3	−2	−1	0	+1	+2	+3
26. Major change in number of arguments with spouse (a lot more or a lot less arguments)			−3	−2	−1	0	+1	+2	+3
27. *Married male:* Change in wife's work outside the home (beginning work, ceasing work, changing to a new job, etc.)			−3	−2	−1	0	+1	+2	+3
28. *Married female:* Change in husband's work (loss of job, beginning new job, retirement, etc.)			−3	−2	−1	0	+1	+2	+3
29. Major change in usual type and/or amount of recreation			−3	−2	−1	0	+1	+2	+3
30. Borrowing more than $10,000 (buying home, business, etc.)			−3	−2	−1	0	+1	+2	+3
31. Borrowing less than $10,000 (buying car, TV, getting school loan, etc.)			−3	−2	−1	0	+1	+2	+3
32. Being fired from job			−3	−2	−1	0	+1	+2	+3
33. *Male:* Wife/girlfriend having abortion			−3	−2	−1	0	+1	+2	+3
34. *Female:* Having abortion			−3	−2	−1	0	+1	+2	+3
35. Major personal illness or injury			−3	−2	−1	0	+1	+2	+3
36. Major change in social activities, e.g., parties, movies, visiting (increased or decreased participation)			−3	−2	−1	0	+1	+2	+3
37. Major change in living conditions of family (building new home, remodeling, deterioration of home, neighborhood, etc.)			−3	−2	−1	0	+1	+2	+3

Continued

Table 2-3

The life experiences survey—*cont'd*

	0 to 6 mo	7 mo to 1 yr	Extremely negative	Moderately negative	Somewhat negative	No impact	Slightly positive	Moderately positive	Extremely positive
38. Divorce			−3	−2	−1	0	+1	+2	+3
39. Serious injury or illness of close friend			−3	−2	−1	0	+1	+2	+3
40. Retirement from work			−3	−2	−1	0	+1	+2	+3
41. Son or daughter leaving home (due to marriage, college, etc.)			−3	−2	−1	0	+1	+2	+3
42. Ending of formal schooling			−3	−2	−1	0	+1	+2	+3
43. Separation from spouse (due to work, travel, etc.)			−3	−2	−1	0	+1	+2	+3
44. Engagement			−3	−2	−1	0	+1	+2	+3
45. Breaking up with boyfriend/ girlfriend			−3	−2	−1	0	+1	+2	+3
46. Leaving home for the first time			−3	−2	−1	0	+1	+2	+3
47. Reconciliation with boyfriend/ girlfriend			−3	−2	−1	0	+1	+2	+3
Other recent experiences that have had an impact on your life. *List and rate.*									
48. _____			−3	−2	−1	0	+1	+2	+3
49. _____			−3	−2	−1	0	+1	+2	+3
50. _____			−3	−2	−1	0	+1	+2	+3

(1978) suggest that there is a relationship between negative life change as measured by the Life Experiences Survey and problems of a psychological nature. Although the cause-effect relationship is often unclear between life changes and health status, and the effect of life changes or stresses differs from person to person depending on unique characteristics, including the degree of perceived control over events and the degree of psychosocial assets, these tools may be useful to the clinician in obtaining some assessment of the active and recent change factors, some of which may be considered developmental tasks, and their importance in a client's life.

BIBLIOGRAPHY

Baruch GK and others: Lifeprints: new patterns of love and work for today's women, New York, 1983, McGraw-Hill Book Co.

Beard RM: Piaget's developmental outline, New York, 1969, New American Library.

Bier WC: Aging: its challenge to the individual and to society, New York, 1974, Fordham University Press.

Billingham KA: Developmental psychology for the health care professions. Part I. Prenatal through adolescent development, Boulder, Colo, 1982, Westview Press.

Birchenall J and Streight ME: Care of the older adult, Philadelphia, 1973, JB Lippincott Co.

Birren JE and Schaie K Warner, editors: Handbook of the psychology of aging, ed 2, New York, 1985, Van Nostrand Reinhold.

Bowlby J: Attachment and loss, vol 1, Attachment, New York, 1969, Basic Books, Inc.

Brantl VM and Brown ML, editors: Readings in gerontology, St Louis, 1973, The CV Mosby Co.

Brazelton TB: The noenatal behavioral assessment scale, Philadelphia, 1973, JB Lippincott Co.

Bronfenbrenner U: The ecology of human development, Cambridge, 1979, Harvard University Press.

Burnside IM, editor: Nursing and the aged, New York, 1976, McGraw-Hill Book Co.

Butler RN and Lewis MI: Aging and mental health, ed 2, St Louis, 1977, The CV Mosby Co.

Carey WB and McDevitt SC: Revision of the Infant Temperament Questionnaire, Pediatrics 61:735, 1978.

Csikszentmihalyi M and Larson R: Being adolescent: conflict and growth in the teenage years, New York, 1984, Basic Books, Inc, Publishers.

Datan N, Greene AL, and Reese HW, editors: Life-span developmental psychology: intergenerational relations, Hillsdale, NJ, 1986, Lawrence Erlbaum Associates, Inc, Publishers.

Davitz J and Davitz L: Making it from 40 to 50, New York, 1976, Random House, Inc.

DeAngelis C: Basic pediatrics for the primary care providers, Boston, 1976, Little, Brown & Co, Inc.

Drumwright A and others: The Denver Articulation Screening Examination, J Speech Hear Disord 38:3, 1973.

Dubowitz L, Dubowitz V, and Goldberg C: Clinical assessement of gestational age in the newborn infant, J Pediatr 77:1, 1970.

Elkind D: Children and adolescents, ed 2, New York, 1974, Oxford University Press.

Elkind D: The hurried child: growing up too fast too soon, New York, 1981, Addison-Wesley Publishing Co, Inc.

Ellison J: Life's second half: the pleasures of aging, Old Greenwich, Conn, 1978, Devin-Adair Publishers, Inc.

Erickson ML: Assessment and management of developmental changes in children, St Louis, 1976, The CV Mosby Co.

Erikson EH: Childhood and society, ed 2, New York, 1963, WW Norton & Co.

Erikson EH: Identity: youth and crisis, New York, 1968, WW Norton & Co, Inc.

Erikson EH: Life history and the historical moment, New York, 1975, WW Norton & Co, Inc.

Erikson EH: Toys and reason, New York, 1977, WW Norton & Co, Inc.

Erikson EH, editor: Adulthood, New York, 1978, WW Norton & Co, Inc.

Feldman HS and Lopez MA: Developmental psychology for the health care professions. II. Adulthood and aging, Boulder, Colo, 1982, Westview Press, Inc.

Field TM and others, editors: Review of human development, New York, 1982, John Wiley & Sons, Inc.

Frankenburg WK and Camp BW, editors: Pediatric screening tests, Springfield, Ill, 1975, Charles C Thomas, Publisher.

Frankenburg WK and Dodds JB: The Denver Developmental Screening Test, J Pediatr 71:181, 1967.

Friedenberg EZ: The vanishing adolescent, Boston, 1959, Beacon Press.

Gardner JE: The turbulent teens, San Diego, 1982, Oak Tree Publications, Inc.

Gesell A and Amatruda C: Developmental diagnosis, ed 2, New York, 1947, Paul B Hoeber, Inc.

Gesell A, Ilg FL, and Ames LB: Youth: the years from ten to sixteen, New York, 1956, Harper & Row, Publishers, Inc.

Gilligan C: In a different voice: psychological theory and women's development, Cambridge, Mass, 1982, Harvard University Press.

Gould RL: Transformations: growth and change in adult life, New York, 1978, Simon & Schuster, Inc.

Hall CS and Nordby VJ: A primer of Jungian psychology, New York, 1973, New American Library.

Hall E: Growing and changing: what the experts say, New York, 1987, Random House, Inc.

Havighurst R: Developmental task and education, New York, 1952, David McKay Co, Inc.

Havighurst R: Human development and education, St Louis, 1953, Warren H Green, Inc.

Haynes U: A developmental approach to case finding with special reference to cerebral palsy, mental retardation and related disorders, Washington, DC, 1969, US Department of Health, Education, and Welfare, Bureau of Community Health Service.

Holmes TH and Rahe RH: The social readjustment rating scale, J Psychosom Res 11:213-218, 1967.

Illingworth RS: The normal child, ed 5, Baltimore, 1972, Williams & Wilkins.

Illingworth RS: The development of the infant and young child: normal and abnormal, ed 6, Edinburgh, 1975, Churchill Livingstone.

Kagan J: The nature of the child, New York, 1984, Basic Books, Inc, Publishers.

Kaluger G and Kaluger MF: Human development: the span of life, ed 3, St Louis, 1984, The CV Mosby Co.

Kastenbaum R: Humans developing: a life-span perspective, Boston, 1979, Allyn & Bacon, Inc.

Katchdourian HA: Medical perspectives on adulthood. In Erikson EH, editor: Adulthood, New York, 1978, WW Norton & Co, Inc.

Kemp CH, Silver HK, and O'Brien D: Current pediatric diagnosis and treatment, ed 5, Los Altos, Calif, 1978, Lange Medical Publications.

Lerner RM, editor: Developmental psychology: historical and philosophical perspectives, Hillsdale NJ, 1983, Lawrence Erlbaum Associates, Inc, Publishers.

Lerner RM and Spanier GB: Adolescent development: a life-span perspective, New York, 1980, McGraw-Hill Book Co.

Levinson DJ and others: The seasons of a man's life, New York, 1978, Ballantine.

Lipsitt LP: Learning in infancy: cognitive development in babies, J Pediatr 109:172-182, 1984.

Lowenthal ME and others: Four stages of life: a comparative study of women and men facing transitions, San Francisco, 1975, Jossey-Bass Inc, Publishers.

McCluskey KA and Reese HW, editors: Life-span developmental psychology: historical and generational effects, New York, 1984, Academic Press, Inc.

Meltzoff AN: Immediate and deferred imitation in 14- and 24-month-old infants, Child Dev 56:62-72, 1985.

Moos RH, editor: Coping with life crises: an integrated approach, New York, 1986, Plenum Publishing Corp.

Neugarten BL and others: Personality in middle and late life, New York, 1964, Atherton Press.

Neugarten BL: Time, age and the life cycle, Am J Psychiatry 136:887-894, 1979.

Neugarten BL and Datan N: Sociological perspectives on the life cycle. In Baltes PB and Schaie KW, editors: Life-span developmental psychology: personality and socialization, New York, 1973, Academic Press, Inc.

Newman BM and Newman PR: Development through life, Homewood, Ill, 1975, The Dorsey Press.

Osherson S: Finding our fathers: how a man's life is shaped by his relationship with his father, New York, 1986, Ballantine.

Perlmutter M and Hall E: Adult development and aging, New York, 1985, John Wiley & Sons, Inc.

Pfeiffer E: Successful aging: a conference report, Durham, NC, 1973, Duke University Press.

Piaget J: The construction of reality in the child, New York, 1954, Basic Books Inc, Publishers.

Piaget J: Piaget's theory. In Mussen PH, editor: Carmichael's manual of child psychology, New York, 1970, John Wiley & Sons, Inc.

Pikunas J: Human development: an emergent science, New York, 1976, McGraw-Hill Book Co.

Provence S: Developmental assessment. In Green M and Haggerty RJ, editors: Ambulatory pediatrics, Philadelphia, 1968a, WB Saunders Co.

Provence S: Developmental history. In Cooke R, editor: Biological basis of pediatric practice, New York, 1968b, McGraw-Hill Book Co.

Rahe RH: Life changes and near-future illness reports. In Levi L, editor: Emotions: their parameters and measurement, New York, 1975, Raven Press.

Rahe RH: Epidemiological studies of life changes and illness, Int J Psychiatry Med 6:133-146, 1975.

Redl F: When we deal with children: selected writings, New York, 1966, The Free Press.

Riley MW, editor: Aging from birth to death. Washington, DC, 1979, American Association for the Advancement of Science.

Sarason IG, Johnson JH, and Siegel JM: Assessing the impact of life changes: development of the life experiences survey, J Consult Clin Psychol 46:932-946, 1978.

Schlossberg NK: Counseling adults in transition: linking practice with theory, New York, 1984, Springer Publishing Co.

Sheehy G: Passages, New York, 1974, EP Dutton.

Spencer MG and Dorr CJ, editors: Understanding aging: a multidisciplinary approach, New York, 1975, Appleton-Century-Crofts.

Standards of child health care, ed 3, Evanston, Ill, 1977, American Academy of Pediatrics.

Stein M: In midlife: a Jungian perspective, Dallas, 1983, Spring Publications, Inc.

Stevenson JS: Issues and crises during middlescence, New York, 1977, Appleton-Century-Crofts.

Thomas A and Chess S: Temperament and development, New York, 1977, Brunner/Mazel, Inc.

Turner JS and Helms DB: Life span development, Philadelphia, 1979, WB Saunders Co.

Turner R and Reese HW, edtiors: Life-span developmental psychology: intervention, New York, 1980, Academic Press, Inc.

Whitbourne SK, editor: Adult development, ed 2, New York, 1986, Praeger Publishers.

Wolman BB, editor: Handbook of developmental psychology, Englewood Cliffs, NJ, 1982, Prentice-Hall.

3

Nutritional assessment

OBJECTIVES

Upon successful review of this chapter, learners will be able to describe:

- Three major goals for assessing nutritional status
- Primary and secondary deficiency diseases
- Three classifications of malnutrition
- Nutritional deficiencies associated with diseases or conditions
- Procedures and usual findings of
  Anthropometric measurement
  Biochemical measurement
  Clinical examination
  Dietary analysis
- Physical signs suggesting malnutrition
- Recommend dietary allowances and guidelines for good nutrition
- Effects of chronic disease on nutritional status
- Effects of age and activity on nutritional status
- Signs and symptoms of eating disorders
- Roles of registered dietitians

The importance of nutritional assessment in the evaluation of health status cannot be overlooked. Nutrition plays a major role in the way an individual looks, feels, and behaves. The body's ability to fight disease and the effectiveness of any type of therapy in illness greatly depend on the individual's nutritional status.

Three major goals in the assessment of nutritional status include:
1. Identification of malnutrition, and its effects on an individual's health status.
2. Identification of patterns of overconsumption, and their link with the development of obesity, diabetes, hypertension, cardiovascular disease, and cancer
3. Identification of nutritional parameters for optimal health and fitness

Malnutrition has been long recognized and well documented in developing countries. Television commercials and magazine advertisements portraying malnourished children in developing countries describe pictorially its devastating effect on human growth and development. Malnutrition in affluent countries, however, such as the United States, has been identified and revealed in a variety of settings and population groups only within the past 20 years. The existence of *subclinical* nutrient deficiencies is more often seen in developed countries, but overt malnutrition also exists in affluent societies.

The problem of malnutrition in hospitalized patients was brought into focus in the early 1970s (Butterworth, 1974). Another study of hospital patients in a major midwestern city in the mid-1980s revealed a large percentage of patients who had subnormal values for the nutritional assessment parameters studied, and a large number of patients were considered to be at nutritional risk (Kamath and others, 1986.) Nutritional assessment has become recognized as an integral component of health

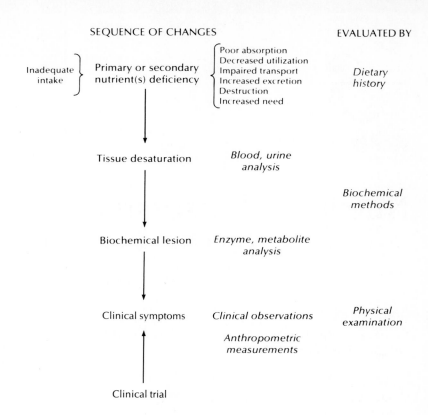

SEQUENCE OF CHANGES   EVALUATED BY

Inadequate intake } Primary or secondary nutrient(s) deficiency { Poor absorption / Decreased utilization / Impaired transport / Increased excretion / Destruction / Increased need   *Dietary history*

Tissue desaturation   *Blood, urine analysis*

Biochemical methods

Biochemical lesion   *Enzyme, metabolite analysis*

Clinical symptoms   *Clinical observations*   *Physical examination*

Anthropometric measurements

Clinical trial

Figure 3-1

Sequence of body changes in the development of malnutrition.

care in terms of preserving patient health and decreasing length and cost of patient hospitalization.

The emphasis in recent years in the United States and Canada has been on a holistic approach to health, going beyond prevention of disease to attainment of high-level wellness (Ardell, 1982). Various aspects of life-style, including food consumption and physical activity patterns, are major components of holistic health. Several chronic disease states can be linked to overconsumption of various nutrients alone or combined with a sedentary life-style. Knowledge of the parameters for optimal health and fitness allows the health care professional to assess an individual's health and fitness status. Assessment of current status and identification of existing patterns are the first steps in helping an individual to make any necessary changes toward optimal health and fitness. As recommendations for optimal nutrient intake and physical activity are modified based on ongoing research and study of population groups, health care professionals have a major responsibility to educate individuals on how to live more healthfully.

MALNUTRITION

Malnutrition is most basically defined as a lack of essential nutrients at the cellular level resulting from psychological, personal, social, educational, economic,

cultural, or political factors in the individual's environment. Malnutrition may exist in the form of a *primary deficiency disease,* which occurs when a specific essential nutrient is lacking in the diet. Malnutrition may also exist as a *secondary deficiency disease* due to the body's inability to digest, absorb, metabolize, or use a specific nutrient properly or because the body has an increased requirement for or increased excretion of a specific nutrient. Malnutrition may be *acute,* a result of temporary conditions and reversible without long-term side effects, or it may be *chronic,* existing over a long period with possible irreversible consequences (Williams, 1985). Although the effects of various forms of malnutrition may be manifested in similar ways, it is important to isolate the cause for successful treatment.

Several steps occur in the development of malnutrition. A primary or secondary nutrient deficiency appears, as noted above. In an attempt to maintain necessary nutrients at the cellular level, the body mobilizes tissue reserves, leading to measurably reduced levels of the nutrients in the tissues. As tissue reserves are depleted and cellular supplies of essential nutrients decrease, biochemical alterations appear, as measured by enzyme and metabolite levels. With further progression, clinical symptoms are manifested. Identification of malnutrition can occur at any of these stages (Figure 3-1).

Table 3-1

Nutrients possibly deficient in specific diseases or conditions

Nutrient*	Disease
Protein	AIDS,† alcoholism, anorexia nervosa, burns, cancer, chronic obstructive pulmonary disease, cystic fibrosis, nephrosis, protein-losing enteropathy, surgical procedures
Fat	Blind loop syndrome, gastrectomy, gluten-induced enteropathy, ileal resection, pancreatic insufficiency, tropical sprue
Thiamin	AIDS,† alcoholism, beriberi, burns, fever, renal failure, thyrotoxicosis, Wernicke's encephalopathy
Riboflavin	AIDS,† alcoholism, burns, fever, renal failure
Niacin	Alcoholism, burns, renal failure
Pyridoxine	AIDS,† alcoholism, burns, renal failure, thyrotoxicosis
Vitamin B_{12}	AIDS,† alcoholism, blind loop syndrome, burns, Crohn's disease, gastrectomy, ileal resection, pernicious anemia, regional enteritis, renal failure
Folate	AIDS,† alcoholism, burns, Crohn's disease, fever, gastrectomy, leukemia, liver disease, macrocytic anemia, psoriasis, renal failure, rheumatoid arthritis, sickle cell anemia
Pantothenic acid	Renal failure, AIDS†
Biotin	Burns
Vitamin C	AIDS,† alcoholism, burns, congestive heart failure, Crohn's disease, drug addiction, fever, peptic ulcer, renal failure, rheumatoid arthritis
Vitamin A	AIDS,† alcoholism, chronic obstructive pulmonary disease, congestive heart failure, Crohn's disease, fever, pancreatic insufficiency, thyrotoxicosis
Vitamin D	AIDS,† cirrhosis of the liver, Crohn's disease, gastrectomy, pancreatic insufficiency
Vitamin E	AIDS,† pancreatic insufficiency, renal failure
Vitamin K	Hemorrhage, pancreatic insufficiency
Calcium	Alcoholism, gastrectomy, intestinal bypass, renal failure
Magnesium	AIDS,† alcoholism, Crohn's disease, intestinal bypass, surgical procedure
Potassium	Alcoholism, cystic fibrosis, intestinal bypass, surgical procedure
Iron	AIDS,† Crohn's disease, gastrectomy, hemorrhage, renal failure
Copper	AIDS,† Crohn's disease, renal failure
Zinc	AIDS,† alcoholism, anorexia nervosa, burns, Crohn's disease, renal failure
Chromium	Renal failure
Selenium	AIDS,† alcoholism
Manganese	Renal failure

*Potential nutrient deficiencies may vary, depending on the extent of a disease, as in anorexia nervosa, or with the particular location in the body and treatment of a disease, as in cancer.

†Vitamins and minerals other than those noted may be deficient in clients with AIDS, but the nutrients noted are particularly important to immune function. AIDS, acquired immunodeficiency syndrome.

Malnutrition can be classified as follows:

1. *Marasmus*—protein calorie malnutrition, evidenced by a client who exhibits weight loss, fat loss, and muscle wasting due to overall calorie-protein deprivation.
2. *Kwashiorkor*—protein malnutrition, evidenced by a client who has adequate fat reserves but, on testing, reveals significant deficits in protein status. The client suffering from kwashiorkor may appear well-nourished, even obese.
3. *Kwashiorkor-marasmus mix*—elements of both states of malnutrition evident in a single client (Kaminski and Winborn, 1978).

Specific nutrient deficiencies may be present in an individual due to lack of adequate intake of the nutrients, or may be associated with various disease states or induced through the use of certain medications, particularly if dietary intake of essential nutrients is marginal. The health care practitioner should use a drug-nutrient interaction handbook to determine possible drug-nutrient interactions a client may be experiencing.

Table 3-1 lists some nutrients that may be deficient in specific diseases or conditions. The existence of a particular disease should alert the health care practitioner to possible nutrient deficiencies.

COMPONENTS OF NUTRITIONAL ASSESSMENT

Nutritional assessment of an individual involves various parameters:

- *Anthropometric measurement*
- *Biochemical measurement*
- *Clinical examination*
- *Dietary analysis*

Anthropometric Measurement

Athropometric measurement is the measurement of size, weight, and proportions of the human body. Most common measurements taken inlcude height, weight, skinfold thickness, and circumference of various body parts, including the head chest, and arm. Measurements taken are compared with appropriate reference standards based on the individual or population being assessed. Standardization of equipment and procedure is essential, so that results are accurate and can be interpreted meaningfully. Results that deviate from standards may indicate malnutrition or overconsumption of various nutrients.

The client should be informed before the physical assessment what areas of the body will be measured, and for what purpose.

For tricep skinfold (TSF) measurement, the client's arm must be exposed (Table 3-2). Clothing should permit easy access to the shoulder area as well as to the upper arm. If other skinfold measurements are being taken, clothing should permit easy access to the particular area while covering private parts of the body to avoid embarrassing the client. Measurements should be taken on the bare skin. Client privacy and assurance of confidentiality are important.

Height

Height is measured in adults and older children by having the client stand erect, without shoes, against a flat vertical measuring surface with a right-angle headboard. Height is measured on the line where the crown of the head intersects the height scale (Fig. 3-2). For small children, height is measured using a wooden length board with the child lying flat on the back (Fig. 3-3). For the nonambulatory elderly and elderly persons who are not able to stand erect due to spinal curvature, specific recumbent measurements have been developed to determine stature.

Height may be recorded in centimeters or in inches. Standards for height exist for children and adolescents and will be discussed in depth in the part of this chapter dealing with pediatric assessment. For adults, the only standard for comparison of measured height is the Mean Height and Weight Table, from the Recommended Dietary Allowances, revised 1980, Food and Nutrition Board (Table 3-3).

Weight

Several types of instruments are commonly used for measuring weight, but the preferred instrument appears to be a balance beam scale with nondetachable weights. Digital electronic platform scales have become increasingly popular and can be modified to weigh individuals in a compromised condition (e.g., in a wheelchair). The client

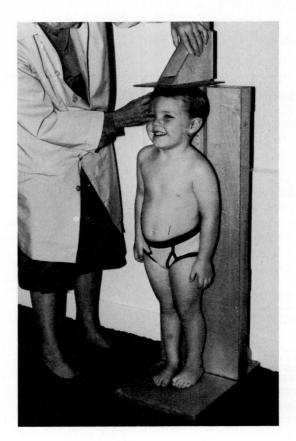

Figure 3-2

Measurement of standing height.

Table 3-2

Anthropometric measurement

Anthropometric measurement	Equipment needed
Weight	Scale, accurate in measuring pounds or kilograms, as well as fractions of these units of measure
Height	Wall scale or rigid freestanding measuring device with a right-angle headboard, or wooden length board, accurate in measuring centimeters or inches, as well as fractions of these units of measure
Midpoint of arm and mid-arm circumference	Nonstretchable cloth tape measure marked in centimeters or special tape designed for use in nutritional assessment that has been developed by companies supplying nutritional products (Inser-tape, Ross Laboratories)
Skinfold thickness	Skinfold calipers

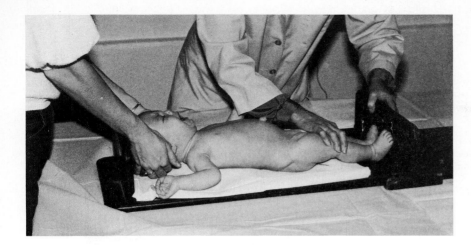

Figure 3-3

Measurement of recumbent length.

Table 3-3

Mean heights and weights and recommended energy intake

Age (yr) and sex group	Weight		Height		Energy		
					Needs		Range in kcal
	kg	lb	cm	in	MJ	kcal	
Infants							
0.0-0.5	6	13	60	24	kg × 0.48	kg × 115	95-145
0.5-1.0	9	20	71	28	kg × 0.44	kg × 105	80-135
Children							
1-3	13	29	90	35	5.5	1300	900-1800
4-6	20	44	112	44	7.1	1700	1300-2300
7-10	28	62	132	52	10.1	2400	1650-3300
Males							
11-14	45	99	157	62	11.3	2700	2000-3700
15-18	66	145	176	69	11.8	2800	2100-3900
19-22	70	154	177	70	12.2	2900	2500-3300
23-50	70	154	178	70	11.3	2700	2300-3100
51-75	70	154	178	70	10.1	2400	2000-2800
76+	70	154	178	70	8.6	2050	1650-2450
Females							
11-14	46	101	157	62	9.2	2200	1500-3000
15-18	55	120	163	64	8.8	2100	1200-3000
19-22	55	120	163	64	8.8	2100	1700-2500
23-50	55	120	163	64	8.4	2000	1600-2400
51-75	55	120	163	64	7.6	1800	1400-2200
76+	55	120	163	64	6.7	1600	1200-2000
Pregnancy						+300	
Lactation						+500	

From Recommended Dietary Allowances, revised 1980, Food and Nutrition Board, Academy of Sciences–National Research Council, Washington, DC. The data in this table have been assembled from the observed median heights and weights of children, together with desirable weights for adults for heights of men (70 in) and women (64 in) between the ages of 18 and 34 years as surveyed in the U.S. population (DHEW/NCHS data).

Energy allowances for the young adults are for men and women doing light work. The allowances for the two older groups represent mean energy needs over these age spans, allowing for a 2% decrease in basal (resting) metabolic rate per decade and a reduction in activity of 200 kcal per day for men and women between 51 and 75 years; 500 kcal for men over 75 years; and 400 kcal for women over 75. The customary range of daily energy output is shown for adults in the range column and is based on a variation in energy needs of ±400 kcal at any one age, emphasizing the wide range of energy intakes appropriate for any group of people.

Energy allowances for children through age 18 are based on median energy intakes of children of these ages followed in longitudinal growth studies. Ranges are the 10th and 90th percentiles of energy intake, to indicate range of energy consumption among children of these ages.

Table 3-4

1959 Metropolitan Life height and weight table*

Men					Women				
Height		Small frame	Medium frame	Large frame	Height		Small frame	Medium frame	Large frame
Feet	Inches				Feet	Inches			
5	2	112-120	118-129	126-141	4	10	92-98	96-107	104-119
5	3	115-123	121-133	129-144	4	11	94-101	98-110	106-122
5	4	118-126	124-136	132-148	5	0	96-104	101-113	109-125
5	5	121-129	127-139	135-152	5	1	99-107	104-116	112-128
5	6	124-133	130-143	138-156	5	2	102-110	107-119	115-131
5	7	128-137	134-147	142-161	5	3	105-113	110-122	118-134
5	8	132-141	138-152	147-166	5	4	108-116	113-126	121-138
5	9	136-145	142-156	151-170	5	5	111-119	116-130	125-142
5	10	140-150	146-160	155-174	5	6	114-123	120-135	129-146
5	11	144-154	150-165	159-179	5	7	118-127	124-139	133-150
6	0	148-158	154-170	164-184	5	8	122-131	128-143	137-154
6	1	152-162	158-175	168-189	5	9	126-135	132-147	141-158
6	2	156-167	162-180	173-194	5	10	130-140	136-151	145-163
6	3	160-171	167-185	178-199	5	11	134-144	140-155	149-168
6	4	164-175	172-190	182-204	6	0	138-148	144-159	153-173

Courtesy Statistical Bulletin, Metropolitan Life Insurance Company, New York.
*Desirable weights for adults ages 25 and over. Weight in pounds according to frame size in indoor clothing wearing shoes with 1-inch (men) or 2-inch (women) heels. For women between 18 and 25, subtract 1 lb for each year under 25.

stands, lies, or sits on the platform, ideally nude or with minimal clothing and without shoes, while weight is recorded in kilograms or pounds. When serial weights are taken, it is important that the client be weighed on the same scale, at approximately the same time of day, and with the same amount of clothing for accurate comparison.

Several standards for weight exist, and the proper standard for the individual being measured must be used. The Mean Height and Weight Table (see Table 3-3) is one standard. Another standard used is the Metropolitan Height and Weight Tables, published first in 1959 (Table 3-4) and revised in 1983 (Table 3-5). The 1983 tables reflect higher desirable weight ranges for all categories than do the 1959 tables. The National Institutes of Health Consensus Development Conference on the Health Implications of Obesity, held in February 1985 (Burton and Foster, 1985), suggested less reliance on these tables alone for a variety of reasons:

They may not be applicable to the entire population, particularly lower socioeconomic groups and some ethnic groups; they ignore other risk factors, such as smoking; they do not measure degree of obesity or regional distribution of fat; and they have relied on an ill-defined concept of "frame size."

If the Metropolitan Life Insurance Tables are used for a standard, the use of the 1959 tables is advised when there is family history of or current indication of disease or risk factors complicated by obesity—particularly high blood pressure, increased serum cholesterol or triglycerides, atherosclerosis, and elevated blood sugar. If such complicating risk factors are not present, the more liberal 1983 tables may be preferred (Burton and Foster, 1985).

The panel recommended the use of the body mass index (BMI) as a reference for comparing weight for adults 20 years and older:

BMI shows a direct and continuous relationship to morbidity and mortality in studies of large populations. The regional distribution of body fat (abdomen in contrast with hips and thighs) was described repeatedly as an important predictor of the health hazards of obesity. High ratios of waist to hip circumference (easily measured with a tape) are associated with a higher risk for illness and decreased life span (Burton and Foster, 1985).

BMI is calculated according to the following formula (Burton and Foster, 1985):

$$BMI = \frac{\text{Weight in kilograms}}{(\text{Height in meters})^2}$$

Nomograms, or graphic representations of the variables used to calculate BMI, were developed to aid in calcu-

Table 3-5

1983 Metropolitan Life table*

Men					Women				
Height		Small frame	Medium frame	Large frame	Height		Small frame	Medium frame	Large frame
Feet	Inches				Feet	Inches			
5	2	128-134	131-141	138-150	4	10	102-111	109-121	118-131
5	3	130-136	133-143	140-153	4	11	103-113	111-123	120-134
5	4	132-138	135-145	142-156	5	0	104-115	113-126	122-137
5	5	134-140	137-148	144-160	5	1	106-118	115-129	125-140
5	6	136-142	139-151	146-164	5	2	108-121	118-132	128-143
5	7	138-145	142-154	149-168	5	3	111-124	121-135	131-147
5	8	140-148	145-157	152-172	5	4	114-127	124-138	134-151
5	9	142-151	148-160	155-176	5	5	117-130	127-141	137-155
5	10	144-154	151-163	158-180	5	6	120-133	130-144	140-159
5	11	146-157	154-166	161-184	5	7	123-136	133-147	143-163
6	0	149-160	157-170	164-188	5	8	126-139	133-150	146-167
6	1	152-164	160-174	168-192	5	9	129-142	139-153	149-170
6	2	155-168	164-178	172-197	5	10	132-145	142-156	152-173
6	3	158-172	167-182	176-202	5	11	135-148	145-159	155-176
6	4	162-176	171-187	181-207	6	0	138-151	148-162	158-179

From Society of Actuaries, Build Study, 1979, Chicago, 1980, Society of Actuaries and Association of Life Insurance Medical Directors of America, Metropolitan Life Insurance Co., New York, 1983. Courtesy Statistical Bulletin, Metropolitan Life Insurance Company, New York.
*Weight in pounds at ages 29 to 59 years according to build. In shoes and 3 lb of indoor clothing for women and 5 lb for men.

lation and interpretation of BMI. Two nomograms are given, based on the 1959 and 1983 Metropolitan Life Insurance Company Tables (Figs. 3-4 and 3-5). The values provided by these nomograms indicate (1) desirable weight, (2) the 20% overweight level, and (3) the 40% overweight level for an individual (Burton and Foster, 1985). The implications of degree of obesity are discussed later in this chapter. From these nomograms, weight values less than desirable are also evident.

The following example is presented:

Female client
Ht = 5 ft 6 in without shoes
Wt = 182 lb without clothes

Health history includes hypertension and elevated triglycerides. Using the nomogram for BMI based on 1959 Metropolitan Life Insurance data, the client's current height and weight are plotted, and a line is drawn intersecting the two points on the scale (Fig. 3-6, *A*). This line intersects the central scale (BMI value) at 29.0. Referring to BMI values for women, we can see that the client is between numbers 2 and 3, which represent 20% and 40% overweight, respectively.

To determine a weight goal for this client, the same nomogram is used, this time plotting the client's current height and point 1 on the BMI scale, correspond-

ing to 21.5 (Fig. 3-6, *B*). A line is drawn intersecting the two points and continued to where it intersects the weight scale. By reading the corresponding number on the weight scale, the weight goal for this client is 133 lb.

Measured weight can also be compared with reference norms listed by percentile, specific for height, sex, and age (Tables 3-6 and 3-7). A formula for calculating desirable body weight, which takes into account frame size, is given in Table 3-8.

Frame size may be determined easily by measuring wrist circumference or elbow breadth (see the box on p. 62). An example using the above is given. An adult male, 6 ft 0 in tall, has a measured elbow breadth of 3¼ in. From the box on p. ?, it is determined that this man has a large frame size. His desirable body weight is calculated:

6 ft = 72 in
5 ft = 60 in
72 in − 60 in = 12 in
106 lb for the first 5 ft, or 60 in
12 × 6 = 72 lb tor 12 in over 5 ft
106 + 72 = 178 lb
Large frame, add 10%, or 18 lb
178 lb + 18 lb = <u>196 lb</u> desirable body weight for this man

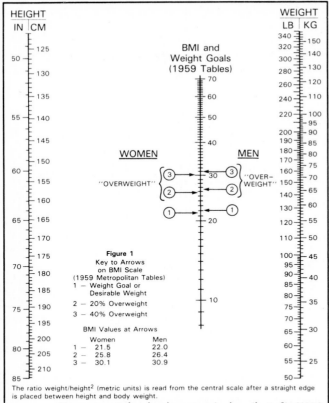

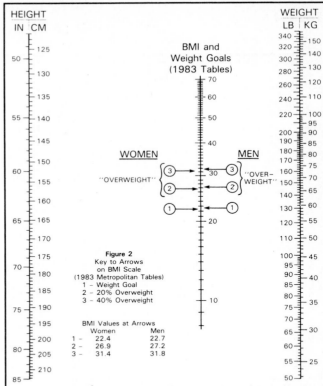

Figure 3-4

Nomogram for body mass index (kg/m²) (1959 Metropolitan Insurance Co. tables. Weights and heights are without clothing. With clothes, add 5 lb (2.3 kg) for men or 3 lb (1.4 kg) for women and 1 in (2.5 cm) in height for shoes.
(From Burton BT and Foster WR: Health implications of obesity: an NIH consensus development conference, J Am Diet Assoc 85(9): 1117-1121, 1985.)

Figure 3-5

Nomogram for body mass index (kg/m²) (1983 Metropolitan Life Insurance Co. tables. Weights and heights are without clothing. With clothes add 5 lb (2.3 kg) for men or 3 lb (1.4 kg) for women and 1 in (2.5 cm) in height for shoes.
(From Burton BT and Foster WR: Health implications of obesity: an NIH consensus development conference, J Am Diet Assoc 85(9):1117-1121, 1985.)

When calculating an individual's desirable weight, it is important to consider the individual's personal weight goal as well as any numbers calculated from a formula. Looking at the person's past weight pattern and ascertaining his idea of a comfortable weight is important if a realistic goal is to be established.

Measured weight can be compared with desirable weight according to the following (Blackburn and others, 1977):

$$\% \text{ Ideal body weight} = \frac{\text{Actual weight}}{\text{Ideal body weight}} \times 100$$

Weight equal to or greater than 20% above or equal to or more than 10% below ideal warrants further investigation.

Determining the percentage of weight change a client has experienced over a specific recent period is important in evaluating nutritional status. The following formula may be used (Blackburn and others, 1977):

$$\% \text{ Weight change} = \frac{\text{Usual weight} - \text{Actual weight}}{\text{Usual weight}} \times 100$$

A change in weight of greater than 10% over 6 months is significant and warrants further investigation.

Circumstances that make the measurement of weight alone an unreliable measure of nutritional status include the body's degree of hydration and increases in muscle mass. For instance, a person who is retaining fluid may appear to be at an appropriate weight for height

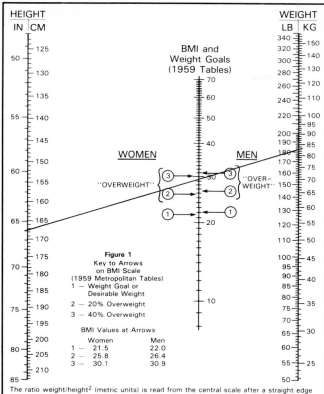

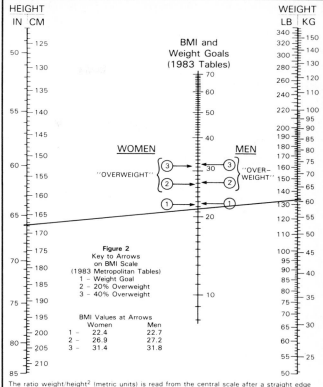

Figure 3-6

Nomograms with examples.
(From Burton BT and Foster WR: Health implications of obesity: an NIH consensus development conference,
J Am Diet Assoc 85(9):1117-1121, 1985.)

but may actually have decreased fat stores and muscle mass. The excess water hides this fact when weight alone is used to assess nutritional status. Another way a weight measurement may be interpreted incorrectly is in an athlete, whose increased muscle mass is reflected in greater total body weight, yet whose fat stores may be low.

Weight standards for children are based on the National Center for Health Statistics Growth Charts, published by Ross Laboratories (see sample on p. 617) and will be discussed in the portion of this chapter dealing with pediatric assessment. Children at either extreme of the scale may require further assessment.

Skinfold thickness

Measuring skinfold thickness is a practical way of determining body fat. Skinfold measurements indicate subcutaneous fat and caloric status. Their accuracy and use-

fulness are greater in assessing clients who are malnourished, normal, or moderately fat as opposed to those who are extremely obese (Kamath, 1986).

Skinfold thickness can be measured at a variety of body sites. The TSF is commonly used for evaluation. Calipers, such as those produced by Cambridge Scientific Industries or Ross Laboratories are used for this measurement, which is made in millimeters (Fig. 3-7). The technique for measurement involves observation and practice for the most accuracy.

In measuring the TSF, the nondominant arm is preferred for measurement. The TSF is measured on the back of the arm midway between the acromion and olecranon process (Fig. 3-8). After the midpoint is assessed and with the arm relaxed, a fold of bare skin above the midpoint and parallel to the long axis is firmly grasped between the clinician's left thumb and forefinger and pulled away from underlying muscle. The contact sur-

Table 3-6

Weight (lb) for height (in), males

Height (in)	Percentile	Age group in years					
		18-24	25-34	35-44	45-54	55-64	65-74
62	50	130	141	143	147	143	143
	15	102	109	115	118	113	116
	5	85	91	98	100	96	100
63	50	135	145	148	152	147	147
	15	107	113	120	123	117	120
	5	90	95	103	105	100	104
64	50	140	150	153	156	153	151
	15	112	118	125	127	123	124
	5	95	100	108	109	106	108
65	50	145	156	158	160	158	156
	15	117	124	130	131	128	129
	5	100	106	113	113	111	113
66	50	150	160	163	164	163	160
	15	122	128	135	135	133	133
	5	105	110	118	117	116	117
67	50	154	165	169	169	168	164
	15	126	133	141	140	138	137
	5	109	115	124	122	121	121
68	50	159	170	174	173	173	169
	15	131	138	146	144	143	142
	5	114	120	129	126	126	126
69	50	164	174	179	177	178	173
	15	136	142	151	148	148	146
	5	119	124	134	130	131	130
70	50	168	179	184	182	183	177
	15	140	147	156	153	153	150
	5	123	129	139	135	136	134
71	50	173	184	190	187	189	182
	15	145	152	162	158	159	155
	5	128	134	145	140	142	139
72	50	178	189	194	191	193	186
	15	150	157	166	162	163	159
	5	133	139	149	144	146	143
73	50	183	194	200	196	197	190
	15	155	162	172	167	167	163
	5	138	144	155	149	150	147
74	50	188	199	205	200	203	194
	15	160	167	177	171	173	167
	5	143	149	160	153	156	151

From Abraham S, Johnson CL, and Najjar MF: Weight by height and age of adults 18-74 years; United States, 1971-74, Advancedata 14:7-8, 1977. Reprinted with permission of Ross Laboratories, Columbus, OH 43216, from Nutritional Assessment Summary Sheet G636, © 1987, Ross Laboratories. 15th Percentile values computed from reference 1 data by Ross Laboratories.

Table 3-7

Weight (lb) for height (in), females

Height (in)	Percentile	Age group in years					
		18-24	25-34	35-44	45-54	55-64	65-74
57	50	114	118	125	129	132	130
	15	85	85	89	94	97	100
	5	68	65	67	73	77	82
58	50	117	121	129	133	136	134
	15	88	88	93	98	101	104
	5	71	68	71	77	81	86
59	50	120	125	133	136	140	137
	15	91	92	97	101	105	107
	5	74	72	75	80	85	89
60	50	123	128	137	140	143	140
	15	94	95	101	105	108	110
	5	77	75	79	84	88	92
61	50	126	132	141	143	147	144
	15	97	99	105	108	112	114
	5	80	79	83	87	92	96
62	50	129	136	144	147	150	147
	15	100	103	108	112	115	117
	5	83	83	86	91	95	99
63	50	132	139	148	150	153	151
	15	103	106	112	115	118	121
	5	86	86	90	94	98	103
64	50	135	142	152	154	157	154
	15	106	109	116	119	122	124
	5	89	89	94	98	102	106
65	50	138	146	156	158	160	158
	15	109	113	120	123	125	128
	5	92	93	98	102	105	110
66	50	141	150	159	161	164	161
	15	112	117	123	126	129	131
	5	95	97	101	105	109	113
67	50	144	153	163	165	167	165
	15	115	120	127	130	132	135
	5	98	100	105	109	112	117
68	50	147	157	167	168	171	169
	15	118	124	131	133	136	139
	5	101	104	109	112	116	121

From Abraham S, Johnson CL, and Najjar MF: Weight by height and age of adults 18-74 years: United States, 1971-74, Advancedata 14:7-8, 1977. Reprinted with permission of Ross Laboratories, Columbus, OH 43216, from Nutritional Assessment Summary Sheet G636, © 1987, Ross Laboratories. 15th Percentile values computed from reference 1 data by Ross Laboratories.

Formula for Calculating Elbow Breadth

Method 1*

Height is recorded without shoes on.
Wrist circumference is measured just distal to the styloid process at the wrist crease on the right arm using a tape measure.
The following formula is used:

$$r = \frac{\text{Height (cm)}}{\text{Wrist circumference (cm)}}$$

Frame size can be determined as follows:

	Males	Females
Small	r > 10.4	r > 11.0
Medium	r = 9.6-10.4	r = 10.1-11.0
Large	r < 9.6	r < 10.1

Method 2†

The patient's right arm is extended forward perpendicular to the body, with the arm bent so the angle at the elbow forms 90° with the fingers pointing up and the palm turned away from the body. The greatest breadth across the elbow joint is measured with a sliding caliper along the axis of the upper arm, on the two prominent bones on either side of the elbow. This is recorded as the elbow breadth. The following data give the elbow breadth measurements for medium-framed men and women of various heights. Measurements lower than those listed indicate a small frame size; higher measurements indicate a large frame size.

	Height in 1″ heels	Elbow breadth
Men	5 ft 2 in-5 ft 3 in	2½ in-2⅞ in
	5 ft 4 in-5 ft 7 in	2⅝ in-2⅞ in
	5 ft 8 in-5 ft 11 in	2¾ in-3 in
	6 ft 0 in-6 ft 3 in	2¾ in-3⅛ in
	6 ft 4 in	2⅞ in-3¼ in
Women	4 ft 10 in-4 ft 11 in	2¼ in-2½ in
	5 ft 0 in-5 ft 3 in	2¼ in-2½ in
	5 ft 4 in-5 ft 7 in	2⅜ in-2⅝ in
	5 ft 8 in-5 ft 11 in	2⅜ in-2⅝ in
	6 ft 0 in	2½ in-2¾ in

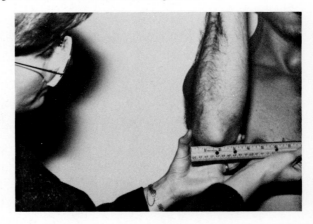

*Data from Grant JP: Handbook of total parenteral nutrition, Philadelphia, 1980, WB Saunders Co.
†Data from the Metropolitan Life Insurance Co, New York, 1983.

Table 3-8

Calculating desirable body weight

Frame size	Adult females	Adult males
Medium	Count 100 lb for the first 5 ft of height, plus 5 lb for each additional inch over 5 ft	Count 106 lb for the first 5 ft of height, plus 6 lb for each additional inch over 5 ft
Small	Subtract 10%	Subtract 10%
Large	Add 10%	Add 10%

From The American Dietetic Association: Handbook of clinical dietetics, New Haven, 1981, Yale University Press.

faces of the caliper are placed on either side of the skinfold directly at the midpoint (Fig. 3-9). When the initial movement of the caliper stops, the measurement is read to the nearest 0.5 mm.

The measurement should be repeated one or two times for reliability. Measurements should be within 1 to 2 mm of each other. If trials yield similar values, record the last value. Tables 3-9 and 3-10 present TSF norms for comparison.

When total body fat is being determined in assessment of physical fitness, various sites on the body are measured and the sum of the skinfold thicknesses is added and compared with norms based on age and sex.

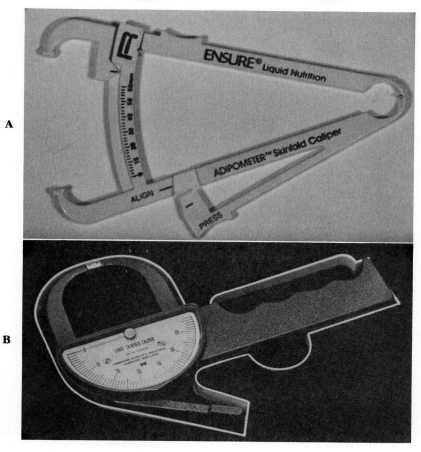

Figure 3-7

A, Ross Adipometer.™ **B,** Lange caliper.
(**A,** Courtesy Ross Laboratories, Columbus OH 43216. **B,** Courtesy Cambridge Scientific Industries, Moose Lodge Road, PO Box 265, Cambridge, MD 21613.)

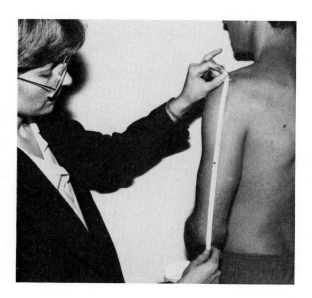

Figure 3-8

Assessing mid-point of upper arm.

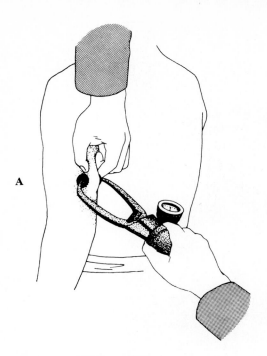

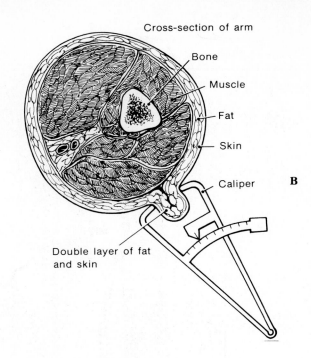

Cross-section of arm
Bone
Muscle
Fat
Skin
Caliper
Double layer of fat
and skin

Figure 3-9

A, Measuring triceps skinfold with calipers. **B,** Cross-section of arm.
(From Guthrie HA: Introductory nutrition, ed 7, St Louis, 1989, The CV Mosby Co. **B,** From Jones DA, Kolassa M, and Baker BA: Health Assessment across the life span, New York, 1984, McGraw-Hill.)

Determining the percentage of body fat gives a better perspective on overall fitness as opposed to weight alone. A discussion of optimal body fat is presented in the portion of this chapter dealing with obesity.

Circumference

Common circumferences measured are the head, chest, mid-arm, and mid-arm muscle. Chest and head circumference are used in assessing infants' growth and brain development and will be discussed in the section on pediatric assessment.

Mid-arm and mid-arm muscle circumference (MAC and MAMC, respectively) are useful in evaluating somatic protein stores and are most commonly used in assessing malnutrition. The MAC is measured in centimeters using a cloth tape around the midpoint of the nondominant arm (Fig. 3-10). The MAMC is calculated from the following formula (Blackburn and others, 1977):

$$MAMC_{(cm)} = MAC_{(cm)} - [3.14 \times TSF_{(cm)}]$$

Values for both the MAC and MAMC can be compared with norms listed in Tables 3-11 through 3-14.

• • •

Anthropometry is of great value as a part of overall assessment, but standardization of instruments and consis-

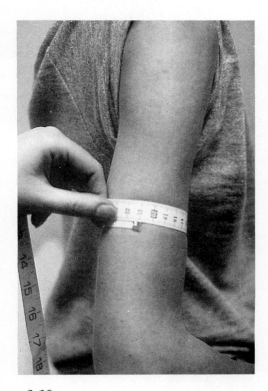

Figure 3-10

Measurement of mid upper arm circumference.
(From Seidel HM and others: Mosby's guide to physical examination, St Louis, 1987, The CV Mosby Co.)

Table 3-9

Triceps skinfold (mm), males

Age (yr)	Percentile		
	50th	**15th**	**5th**
18-19	8.5	6.0	4.5
20-24	10.0	6.0	4.0
25-34	12.0	6.0	4.5
35-44	12.0	7.0	5.0
45-54	11.0	7.0	5.0
55-64	11.0	6.5	5.0
65-74	11.0	6.5	4.5

Basic data on anthropometric measurements and angular measurements of the hip and knee joints for selected age groups 1-74 years of age, United States, 1971-1975. National Health Survey, Vital and Health Statistics Series No. 219, US Dept of Health and Human Services, Public Health Service, 1981, pp 20, 26. Reprinted with permission of Ross Laboratories, Columbus, OH 43216, from Nutritional Assessment Summary Sheet G636, © 1987, Ross Laboratories.

Table 3-10

Triceps skinfold (mm) females

Age (yr)	Percentile		
	50th	**15th**	**5th**
18-19	17.5	12.0	9.0
20-24	18.0	12.0	10.0
25-34	21.0	13.5	10.5
35-44	23.0	16.0	12.0
45-54	25.0	17.0	13.0
55-64	25.0	16.0	11.0
65-74	23.0	16.0	11.5

Basic data on anthropometric measurements and angular measurements of the hip and knee joints for selected age groups 1-74 years of age, United States, 1971-1975. National Health Survey, Vital and Health Statistics Series No. 219, US Dept of Health and Human Services, Public Health Service, 1981, pp 20, 26. Reprinted with permission of Ross Laboratories, Columbus, OH 43216, from Nutritional Assessment Summary Sheet G636, © 1987, Ross Laboratories.

Table 3-11

Mid-arm circumference (cm), males

Age (yr)	Percentile		
	50th	**15th**	**5th**
18-19	30.1	27.4	25.3
20-24	31.0	27.7	26.1
25-34	32.0	28.9	27.0
35-44	32.7	29.6	27.8
45-54	32.1	28.9	26.7
55-64	31.7	28.1	25.6
65-74	30.7	27.3	25.3

Basic data on anthropometric measurements and angular measurements of the hip and knee joints for selected age groups 1-74 years of age, United States, 1971-1975. National Health Survey, Vital and Health Statistics Series No. 219, US Dept of Health and Human Services, Public Health Service, 1981, pp 20, 26. Reprinted with permission of Ross Laboratories, Columbus, OH 43216, from Nutritional Assessment Summary Sheet G636, © 1987, Ross Laboratories.

Table 3-12

Mid-arm circumference (cm), females

Age (yr)	Percentile		
	50th	**15th**	**5th**
18-19	26.2	23.2	22.1
20-24	26.5	23.6	22.2
25-34	27.8	24.8	23.3
35-44	29.2	25.8	24.1
45-54	30.3	26.6	24.3
55-64	30.2	26.1	23.9
65-74	29.9	26.2	23.8

Basic data on anthropometric measurements and angular measurements of the hip and knee joints for selected age groups 1-74 years of age, United States, 1971-1975. National Health Survey, Vital and Health Statistics Series No. 219, US Dept of Health and Human Services, Public Health Service, 1981, pp 20, 26. Reprinted with permission of Ross Laboratories, Columbus, OH 43216, from Nutritional Assessment Summary Sheet G636, © 1987, Ross Laboratories.

tency in technique are critical for reliable measurements. In interpreting anthropometric data, all parameters must be considered together for accurate assessment and serial measurements must be taken to document *changes* in anthropometric status. Measurements at either extreme above or below the 50th percentile warrant further investigation. Measurements significantly lower than the 50th percentile may be considered evidence of depletion;

measurements significantly above the 50th percentile, particularly weight and TSF, may be associated with increased risk of obesity.

Biochemical Measurement

Biochemical measures are useful in indicating malnutrition or the development of diseases as a result of over-

Table 3-13

Mid-arm muscle circumference (cm), males*

Age (yr)	Percentile		
	50th	**15th**	**5th**
18-19	27.4	25.5	23.9
20-24	27.9	25.8	24.8
25-34	28.2	27.0	25.6
35-44	28.9	27.4	26.2
45-54	28.7	26.7	25.1
55-64	28.3	26.2	24.0
65-74	27.2	25.3	23.9

Reprinted with permission of Ross Laboratories, Columbus, OH 43216, from Nutritional Assessment Summary Sheet G636, © 1987, Ross Laboratories.

*Values computed using MAMC (cm) = MAC (cm) − [3.14 × TSF (cm)] from data in Tables 3-8 and 3-10.

Table 3-14

Mid-arm muscle circumference (cm), females*

Age (yr)	Percentile		
	50th	**15th**	**5th**
18-19	20.7	19.4	19.3
20-24	20.8	19.8	19.1
25-34	21.2	20.6	20.0
35-44	22.0	20.8	20.3
45-54	22.5	21.3	20.2
55-64	22.4	21.1	20.5
65-74	22.7	21.2	20.2

Reprinted with permission of Ross Laboratories, Columbus, OH 43216, from Nutritional Assessment Summary Sheet G636, © 1987, Ross Laboratories.

*Values computed using MAMC (cm) = MAC (cm) − [3.14 × TSF (cm)] from data in Tables 3-9 and 3-11.

consumption of nutrients. Serum and urine are commonly used for biochemical assessment.

In assessment of malnutrition, commonly used values include total lymphocyte count (TLC), serum albumin, total iron binding capacity (TIBC), serum transferrin, creatinine height index (CHI), hemoglobin, hematocrit, nitrogen balance, and skin antigen tests. These values, taken with anthropometric measurements, give a good overall picture of an individual's skeletal and visceral protein status as well as fat reserves and immunologic response.

Total lymphocyte count

Depressed TLC has been associated with increased morbidity and mortality. Since 25% of the circulating lymphocytes are B lymphocytes, the TLC partially reflects humoral immunity (acquired immunity in which the role of immunoglobins is prevalent) as well as cell-mediated immunity (acquired immunity in which the role of the small lymphocytes of thymic origin prevail). Because TLC is closely associated with hypoalbuminemia, it is thought to be related to protein deficiency and amenable to correction with appropriate nutritional repletion (Jensen and colleagues, 1981). TLC is expressed in cells/mm³, and Table 3-15 lists normal values for this parameter. The measured value is expressed as percentage of standard, with 60% to 90% of standard indicating moderate depletion and less than 60% of standard indicating severe depletion.

Conditions that may alter the accuracy and meaningfulness of TLC measurement include conditions where leukocytosis is present, such as bacterial infection, severe

Table 3-15

Selected normal values for adults

Hematocrit (vol % red cells)
Male 40%-54%
Female 37%-47%
Hemoglobin
Male 14-17 g/dl
Female 12-15 g/dl
Lymphocytes, total count 1500-3000/mm³
Albumin, serum 4.0-5.5 g/dl
Iron-binding capacity
Total, serum 250-410 µg/dl
Percent saturation 20%-50%
Transferrin 170-250 mg/dl
Creatinine 1.0-1.5 g/24 hr

From Lagua RT, Claudio VS, and Thiele VF: Nutrition and diet therapy reference dictionary, ed 2, St Louis, 1974, The CV Mosby Co. Reprinted with permission of Ross Laboratories, Columbus, OH 43216, from Nutritional Assessment Summary Sheet G636, © 1987, Ross Laboratories.

sepsis, tuberculosis, and chronic leukemia. In these situations, a normal or elevated TLC could be calculated despite overt malnutrition. Relative lymphocytosis is a normal occurrence in children between the ages of 4 months and 4 years (Jensen and associates, 1981).

Leukopenia may also distort the reliability of TLC in evaluation of malnutrition. Leukopenia may be associated with aberrations in white blood cells; it may be induced by certain medications or be a manifestation of viral infection. TLC is not a valid indicator of nutritional status in clients with acquired immunodeficiency syndrome (AIDS).

Serum albumin

Serum albumin is an important parameter in the evaluation of visceral protein stores. A below-normal serum albumin level represents a late manifestation of protein deficiency, which is virtually always associated with clinical signs of malnutrition. Table 3-15 lists normal values for serum albumin. A concentration under 3.4 g/dl warrants further investigation, and a concentration under 2.5 g/dl is associated with severe protein depletion (Jensen and colleagues, 1981). The degree of hydration may have a significant effect on the reliability of serum albumin values.

Total iron binding capacity and serum transferrin

Serum transferrin concentration is another parameter useful in assessing visceral protein status. Serum transferrin is calculated using TIBC according to the following formula (Blackburn and colleagues, 1977):

$$\text{Serum transferrin} = (.8 \times \text{TIBC}) - 43$$

and is assessed in milligrams per deciliter. Normal values are represented in Table 3-15, with results expressed as percentage of standard; values between 60% and 90% of standard indicate moderate depletion, and values under 60% of standard indicate severe depletion.

Creatinine height index

The CHI provides an estimate of skeletal muscle mass, because urinary levels of creatinine depend primarily on the extent of skeletal muscle catabolism, especially during protein depletion. With chronic wasting, creatinine excretion and CHI decrease because muscle protein is catabolized for energy. CHI is expressed as a percentage and calculated as milligrams of creatinine excreted per 24 hours by the client divided by milligrams of creatinine excreted by a normal subject of the same height and sex. (See Table 3-16 for standard urinary creatinine values.) A CHI of 60% to 90% of standard can be interpreted as moderate depletion; under 60% of standard is interpreted as severe depletion. CHI values may be invalid in some cases of renal disease. Accurate collection of urine is crucial in the reliability of this test.

Nitrogen balance

Nitrogen balance indicates if an individual is catabolizing protein stores for energy, as in a malnourished state, and is also useful in assessing the effectiveness of nutritional

Table 3-16

Ideal urinary creatinine value (mg), adults

Male*		Female**	
Height (cm)	Ideal creatinine (mg)	Height (cm)	Ideal creatinine (mg)
157.5	1288	147.3	830
160.0	1325	149.9	851
162.6	1359	152.4	875
165.1	1386	154.9	900
167.6	1426	157.5	925
170.2	1467	160.0	949
172.7	1513	162.6	977
175.3	1555	165.1	1006
177.8	1596	167.6	1044
180.3	1642	170.2	1076
182.9	1691	172.7	1109
185.4	1739	175.3	1141
188.0	1785	177.8	1174
190.5	1831	180.3	1206
193.0	1891	182.9	1240

From Bistrian BR, Blackburn GL, Sherman M, and Scrimshaw NS: Therapeutic index of nutritional depletion in hospitalized patients, Surg Gynecol Obstet 141:512-516, 1975. Reprinted with permission of Ross Laboratories, Columbus, OH 43216, from Nutritional Assessment Summary Sheet G636, © 1987, Ross Laboratories.
*Creatinine coefficient (males) = 23 mg/kg of ideal body weight.
**Creatinine coefficient (females) = 18 mg/kg of ideal body weight.

therapy. Nitrogen balance studies involve calculating protein intake through dietary or intravenous means as well as measuring urine losses. The formula

$$N_2 \text{ balance} = \frac{\text{Protein intake}}{6.25} - (\text{Urinary urea nitrogen} + 4)$$

is used, indicating either a positive or negative value (Blackburn and colleagues, 1977). The degree to which the number is either negative or positive may document the severity of catabolism or the benefit of therapy, respectively.

Nitrogen balance calculated by this formula is unreliable in patients with renal disease and in those in whom urine collection is impaired and may underestimate nitrogen excretion in those patients with burns, diarrhea, vomiting, fistula drainage, and other abnormal nitrogen losses (Jensen and colleagues, 1981).

Hemoglobin and hematocrit

Hemoglobin and hematocrit are measurements that may indicate many nutritional deficiencies. With severe protein malnutrition, the hemoglobin level may reflect protein status. Hemoglobin is expressed in grams per deciliters; hematrocrit is expressed as a percentage. (See Table 3-14 for normal values.) Decreased values may be seen (1) in iron, B_{12}, folate, and pyridoxine (B_6) deficiencies, (2) with chronic blood loss, (3) with overhydration, and (4) with genetic defects. Increased values may be seen in (1) dehydration, (2) chronic anoxia, (3) polycythemia, and (4) the presence of some tumors.

Skin antigen tests

Protein malnutrition is associated with impaired cell-mediated immunity, as manifested by skin antigen testing. Failure of a delayed cutaneous response is termed *anergy* and is a well-documented feature of malnutrition.

Four antigens are commonly used together in skin testing:
- Mumps
- Candida albicans
- Streptokinase/streptodornase
- Purified protein derivative (PPD)

The antigens are injected intradermally, and the area of induration is read after 24 hours and 48 hours. A patient with a response over 15 mm on any *one* test is considered immune competent. The following values indicate a deficit in immune response (Kaminski and Winborn, 1978):

Severe	*Moderate*	*Mild*
<5-0 mm	<10-5 mm	<15-10 mm

Surgery or severe thermal injury will obliterate the immune response; therefore, antigen testing should probably not be done during the first 48 hours following such stresses. Immune response is also diminished in iron-deficiency states but is usually restored once the deficiency is corrected. Skin antigen testing is not valid in clients with AIDS.

Protocol for evaluating therapy

Once malnutrition has been documented and therapy begun, a suggested protocol (Blackburn and others, 1977) for evaluating therapy and the client's nutritional status involves the following:
1. Daily—body weight
2. Twice weekly—nitrogen balance
3. Weekly—TLC
4. Every three weeks—anthropometrics, serum transferrin, skin tests

In assessing the development of diseases that may be due to overconsumption of nutrients, several biochemical values are useful:
- Serum cholesterol, high-density lipoprotein (HDL), low-density lipoprotein (LDL)
- Serum triglyceride
- Serum glucose

One of the primary risk factors in the development of coronary heart disease (CHD) is elevated blood lipid levels. The National Institutes of Health in 1984 made recommendations regarding serum cholesterol levels and relative risk of coronary heart disease (Table 3-17).

Beyond measuring serum cholesterol value, measurement of the high-density fraction and the low-density fraction of the cholesterol molecule gives more insight into the relative risk of heart disease, particularly after age 50. The HDL fraction appears to act as a scavenger molecule in the bloodstream, facilitating removal of cholesterol from the body. Elevated LDL cholesterol is associated with increased CHD risk (American Heart Association, 1980). An optimal LDL:HDL ratio appears to be less than 3:1, with total LDL cholesterol less than 130 mg/dl. An HDL level lower than 35 mg/dl indicates some degree of CHD risk. Diet, exercise, and drug therapy can be used to manipulate unacceptable lipid levels to more desirable levels.

Normal serum triglyceride levels range from 40 to 150 mg/dl. An elevated serum triglyceride level may also be associated with increased risk of CHD, particularly in individuals with other characteristics of increased risk. Individuals with an elevated serum triglyceride level should also be assessed for levels of total cholesterol, HDL, and blood glucose; degree of obesity; alcohol intake; and estrogen-containing medication (American Heart Association, 1980).

Serum glucose

Hyperglycemia is associated with diabetes mellitus, obesity, hypertriglyceridemia, hypertension, and elevated LDL and depressed HDL levels. All are associated with increased risk of CHD. A normal fasting serum glucose value is 80 to 120 mg/dl, but it may vary by 10 mg on either end of the range based on the specific laboratory used for testing.

Table 3-17

Cholesterol recommendations

Age	Blood cholesterol levels (mg/dl)		
	Recommended	Moderate risk	High risk
20-29	under 180	200-220	220+
30-39	under 200	220-240	240+
40+	under 200	240-260	260+

From National Institutes of Health: Cholesterol counts, Bethesda Md, 1985, Public Health Service, US Department of Health and Human Services.

Clinical Examination

Clinical examination of a client involves close physical evaluation and may reveal signs suggesting malnutrition or overconsumption of nutrients. Although clinical examination alone does not permit definitive diagnosis of a nutritional problem, it should not be overlooked in nutritional assessment. Table 3-18 lists physical signs suggesting malnutrition.

Dietary Analysis

Assessment of dietary intake and patterns involves eliciting information regarding usual foods consumed and habits of food purchasing, preparation, and consumption. Individuals rely on food for much more than physical nourishment. Food may represent cultural and ethnic background and socioeconomic status and have many emotional or psychological meanings. It is important to

Table 3-18

Physical signs suggesting malnutrition

Body area	Signs associated with malnutrition	Possible causes
Hair	Lack of natural shine; hair dull, dry, thin, and sparse; color changes (flag sign); can be easily plucked	Protein-calorie (P-C) deficiency; may be deficiency of other nutrients
Face	Skin color loss; skin dark over cheeks and eyes	P-C deficiency; deficiency of B complex vitamins
	Moon face; enlarged parotid glands	P-C deficiency
	Scaling of skin around nostrils	Niacin, riboflavin, pyridoxine deficiency
Eyes	Small, yellowish lumps around eyes (xanthelasma); white rings around both eyes (corneal arcus)	Hyperlipidemia
	Eye membranes pale (pale conjunctivae)	Vitamin B_{12}, folic acid, or iron-deficiency anemia
	Xerophthalmia: (1) night blindness, (2) dryness of eye membranes (conjunctival xerosis), and (3) dull-appearing or soft cornea (corneal xerosis)	Vitamin A deficiency
	Redness of membranes (conjunctival injection); ring of fine blood vessels around cornea (circumcorneal injection); Bitot's spots	General poor nutrition
	Redness and fissuring of eyelid corners (angular palpebritis)	Niacin and riboflavin deficiency
Lips	Redness and swelling of mouth or lips (cheilosis), especially corners of mouth (angular fissures and scars)	Niacin, riboflavin, iron, or vitamin B_6 deficiency
Tongue	Swelling; scarlet and raw tongue; smooth tongue; swollen sores; hyperemic and hypertrophic papillae; atrophic papillae	Folic acid, niacin, riboflavin, vitamin B_{12}, pyridoxine, iron or zinc deficiency
	Magenta (purplish) tongue	Riboflavin deficiency
Gums	Spongy and bleeding	Vitamin C deficiency
Teeth	Teeth may be missing or erupting abnormally	General poor nutrition
	Caries	Excessive intake of highly refined carbohydrates; general poor nutrition
	Gray or white spots (fluorosis)	Excessive fluoride intake
Glands	Thyroid enlargement	Iodine deficiency or toxicity
	Parotid enlargement (cheeks become swollen)	General poor nutrition
	Hypogonadism	Zinc deficiency
Skin	Small or large tumors around joints of hands, legs, or skin (xanthoma)	Hyperlipidemia
	Dryness of skin (xerosis); sandpaper feel of skin (follicular hyperkeratosis); flakiness of skin	Vitamin A deficiency or excess; essential fatty acid deficiency; P-C deficiency

From Roberts SLW: Nutrition assessment manual, Iowa City, 1977. University of Iowa Hospitals and Clinics. Reprinted with permission.

Continued

Table 3-18

Physical signs suggesting malnutrition—*cont'd*

Body area	Signs associated with malnutrition	Possible causes
	Black and blue marks due to skin bleeding (petechiae)	Vitamin C or K deficiency
	Skin swollen and dark; red swollen pigmentation of exposed areas (pellagrous dermatosis)	Niacin deficiency
	Lack of fat under skin	P-C deficiency
	Yellow skin	Carotene toxicity
	Hyperpigmentation	Multiple vitamin deficiencies
	Cutaneous flushing	Niacin toxicity
Nails	Nails spoon shaped (koilonychial)	Iron deficiency
Cardiovascular system	Tachycardia (heart beat greater than 100); enlarged heart	Thiamine deficiency
	Elevated blood pressure	Excessive sodium intake
	CHD	Excessive cholesterol, fat, or caloric intake
Nervous system	Listlessness	P-C deficiency
	Loss of position and vibratory sense; decrease and loss of ankle and knee reflexes	Vitamin B_{12} and thiamine deficiency
Muscular and skeletal systems	Muscle weakness	Phosphorus deficiency
	Muscles have "wasted" appearance	P-C deficiency
	Baby's skull bones are thin and soft; round swelling of front and side of head (frontal and parietal bossing); baby's soft spot on head does not harden (persistently open anterior fontanelle); small bumps on both sides of chest wall (ribs); bowed legs; swelling of ends of bones (epiphyseal swelling)	Vitamin D and calcium deficiency
	Musculoskeletal hemorrhages	Vitamin C deficiency
	Pseudoparalysis	
	Calf tenderness	Thiamine deficiency
	Bilateral edema of lower extremities	Protein deficiency
	Demineralization of bone (osteoporosis)	Calcium deficiency
Gastrointestinal system	Liver enlargement	Protein deficiency
	Liver and spleen enlargement	Hyperlipidemia
	Gastritis	Niacin toxicity
	Anorexia, nausea	Magnesium deficiency
	Nausea and vomiting	Vitamin A toxicity
General	Growth failure	P-C or zinc deficiency

gain as much background information into daily food habits as possible to aid in client assessment and identification of any nutritional problems, therapy, and education.

In assessment of actual food intake, a 24 hour recall method may be used. In this method, the client is asked to recall everything consumed within the past 24 hours including all foods, fluids, and any vitamins, minerals, or other supplements. The interviewer should not be biased about the client's responses to questions based on personal habits or knowledge of recommended food consumption.

Another method of ascertaining food intake involves the client's keeping food records for 1 to 3 days.

A detailed food record sheet, an example of which is given in the box on p. 71, supplies a wide variety of information regarding habits of consumption and behaviors linked with food consumption. Because an individual's weekends or days away from work or school may differ from the usual "routine," clients are asked to provide at least one weekend day in their records.

Using food records as above, it is possible to use one of many popular computer programs to analyze the client's actual intake according to the Recommended Dietary Allowances (RDAs) based on age and sex (Table 3-19) and the Estimated Safe and Adequate Daily Dietary Intakes of Additional Selected Vitamins and Minerals (Table 3-20 on p. 74). Intakes of two thirds or greater

\multicolumn{6}{c}{*Sample Food Record Sheet*}					

Sample Food Record Sheet

Name: Height:
Date: Weight:
Age: Sex:

Foods and fluids consumed	Amount	Time of day	Place	Alone or with whom	Mood while eating
Note: Include water and any vitamins, minerals, and nutritional supplements. Specify brand name whenever possible.	*Be as specific as possible: oz., cups, etc.*				

of the RDA are considered adequate, although individuals may require greater amounts of a specific nutrient in particular situations.

Without computer analysis, the records can be quickly assessed using the "Guide to Good Eating," developed by the National Dairy Council, as shown in Table 3-21 on p. 75. A more detailed but very time-consuming analysis can be performed using food analysis reference books.

Further information may be elicited in a detailed dietary history by asking the client to answer the following:

1. Do you eat away from home?
2. What restaurants do you frequent?
3. Who cooks at home?
4. What methods of food preparation are normally used—e.g., baking, broiling, frying?
5. What are your particular food likes and dislikes?
6. What are your food allergies or intolerances?
7. What medications do you take, including vitamins, minerals, or other nutritional supplements?
8. Do you have drug allergies?
9. What are your significant medical problems, past and present?
10. Have you any difficulty chewing or swallowing?
11. Have you any problems with nausea, vomiting, diarrhea, or constipation?
12. What is your occupation? (Note the amount of time sedentary vs physically active.)
13. What are your hobbies or relaxation activities?
14. Do you exercise—type, frequency, intensity, and duration?
15. What is your target weight, if different than current weight?
16. What is your pattern of weight throughout life?
17. Have you had any significant change in weight within the last 6 months?
18. Have you ever followed dietary restrictions?
19. Have you ever received nutritional counseling? By whom?
20. Have you any episodes of food bingeing and purging?
21. Have you consumed nonfood substances (pica)?
22. Are there any religious restrictions regarding your food preparation or consumption?
23. Do you participate in special food programs?
24. How many people are in your household?

Table 3-19

Recommended dietary allowances

Age (yr) and sex group	Weight		Height		Protein (g)	Fat-soluble vitamins			
						Vitamin A (µg R.E.†)	Vitamin D (µg‡)	Vitamin E (mg α-TE§)	Vitamin C (mg)
	kg	lb	cm	in					
Infants									
0.0-0.5	6	13	60	24	kg × 2.2	420	10	3	35
0.5-1.0	9	20	71	28	kg × 2.0	400	10	4	35
Children									
1-3	13	29	90	35	23	400	10	5	45
4-6	20	44	112	44	30	500	10	6	45
7-10	28	62	132	52	34	700	10	7	45
Males									
11-14	45	99	157	62	45	1,000	10	8	50
15-18	66	145	176	69	56	1,000	10	10	60
19-22	70	154	177	70	56	1,000	7.5	10	60
23-50	70	154	178	70	56	1,000	5	10	60
51+	70	154	178	70	56	1,000	5	10	60
Females									
11-14	46	101	157	62	46	800	10	8	50
15-18	55	120	163	64	46	800	10	8	60
19-22	55	120	163	64	44	800	7.5	8	60
23-50	55	120	163	64	44	800	5	8	60
51+	55	120	163	64	44	800	5	8	60
Pregnancy					+30	+200	+5	+2	+20
Lactation					+20	+400	+5	+3	+40

From Recommended Dietary Allowances, Revised 1980, Food and Nutrition Board, National Academy of Sciences—National Research Council, Washington, DC.

*The allowances are intended to provide for individual variations among most normal persons as they live in the United States under usual environmental stresses. Diets should be based on a variety of common foods to provide other nutrients for which human requirements have been less well defined.

†Retinol equivalents: 1 retinol equivalent = 1 µg retinol or 6 µg β-carotene.

‡As cholecaciferol: 10 µg cholecalciferol = 400 IU of vitamin D.

§α-tocopherol equivalents: 1 mg d-α-tocopherol = 1 α TE.

It may be necessary to rephrase a question or statement in various ways during an interview to ascertain the reliability of information given.

Estimated calorie needs

Table 3-3 lists mean heights and weights and mean values as well as ranges for recommended caloric intake. An individual's needs may vary considerably due to present nutritional status, activity, or compromising medical conditions.

Table 3-22 on p. 76 gives formulas for calculating estimated caloric expenditure in various types of injury or trauma.

Estimated protein needs

Table 3-20 lists suggested daily protein intakes for maintaining good health. As with caloric needs, an individual's protein needs may vary due to present nutritional status, activity, or compromising medical condition.

The information gathered in the four parameters of nutritional assessment—anthropometric measurement, biochemical measurement, clinical examination, and dietary analysis—must be integrated thoroughly to present a detailed, clear analysis of the client's current state of health and well-being. A sample nutritional assessment form is given on pp. 78-79.

	Water-soluble vitamins					Minerals					
Thiamine (mg)	Ribo-flavin (mg)	Niacin (mg NE‖)	Vitamin B_6 (mg)	Folacin¶ (µg)	Vitamin B_{12} (µg)	Calcium (mg)	Phosphorus (mg)	Magnesium (mg)	Iron (mg)	Zinc (mg)	Iodine (mg)
0.3	0.4	6	0.3	30	0.5#	360	240	50	10	3	40
0.5	0.6	8	0.6	45	1.5	540	360	70	15	5	50
0.7	0.8	9	0.9	100	2.0	800	800	150	15	10	70
0.9	1.0	11	1.3	200	2.5	800	800	200	10	10	90
1.2	1.4	16	1.6	300	3.0	800	800	250	10	10	120
1.4	1.6	18	1.8	400	3.0	1,200	1,200	350	18	15	150
1.4	1.7	18	2.0	400	3.0	1,200	1,200	400	18	15	150
1.5	1.7	19	2.2	400	3.0	800	800	350	10	15	150
1.4	1.6	18	2.2	400	3.0	800	800	350	10	15	150
1.2	1.4	16	2.2	400	3.0	800	800	350	10	15	150
1.1	1.3	15	1.8	400	3.0	1,200	1,200	300	18	15	150
1.1	1.3	14	2.0	400	3.0	1,200	1,200	300	18	15	150
1.1	1.3	14	2.0	400	3.0	800	800	300	18	15	150
1.0	1.2	13	2.0	400	3.0	800	800	300	18	15	150
1.0	1.2	13	2.0	400	3.0	800	800	300	10	15	150
+0.4	+0.3	+2	+0.6	+400	+1.0	+400	+400	+150	**	+5	+25
+0.5	+0.5	+5	+0.5	+100	+1.0	+400	+400	+150	**	+10	+50

‖1 NE (niacin equivalent) = 1 mg niacin or 60 mg dietary tryptophan.

¶The folacin allowances refer to dietary sources as determined by *Lactobacillus casei* assay after treatment with enzymes ("conjugases") to make polyglutamyl forms of the vitamin available to the test organism.

#The RDA for vitamin B_{12} in infants is based on average concentration of the vitamin in human milk. The allowances after weaning are based on energy intake (as recommended by the American Academy of Pediatrics) and consideration of other factors, such as intestinal absorption.

**The increased requirement during pregnancy cannot be met by the iron content of habitual American diets nor by the existing iron stores of many women; therefore, the use of 30-60 mg of supplemental iron is recommended. Iron needs during lactation are not substantially different from those of nonpregnant women, but continued supplementation of the mother for 2-3 months after parturition is advisable to replenish stores depleted by pregnancy.

CHRONIC DISEASES

Diet and physical activity have an effect on various chronic diseases, as discussed below.

Obesity

Overweight is defined as an excess of body weight compared with predetermined standards. *Obesity* is defined as an excess of body fat. A body fat greater than 25% of total body weight for men and greater than 30% of total body weight for women indicates obesity. Obesity threatens health as follows:

1. Obesity may aggravate existing health conditions such as high blood pressure, cardiovascular problems, liver disorders, and arthritis and may pose increased risk for development of these diseases.
2. Obesity is often found with diabetes, particularly type II.
3. Obesity can increase the risk of developing gall bladder disease.
4. Obesity can increase surgical risks.
5. Obestiy restricts mobility, which can lower one's general level of fitness.
6. Obesity can decrease life expectancy. The morbidly obese have the highest rate of premature death.

Table 3-20

Estimated safe and adequate daily dietary intakes of additional selected vitamins and minerals

Age group (yr)	Vitamins			Trace elements*						Electrolytes		
	Vitamin K (µg)	Biotin (µg)	Pantothenic acid (mg)	Copper (mg)	Manganese (mg)	Fluoride (mg)	Chromium (mg)	Selenium (mg)	Molybdenum (mg)	Sodium (mg)	Potassium (mg)	Chloride (mg)
Infants												
0.0-0.5	12	35	2	0.5-0.7	0.5-0.7	0.1-0.5	0.01-0.04	0.01-0.04	0.03-0.06	115-350	350-925	275-700
0.5-1.0	10-20	50	3	0.7-1.0	0.7-1.0	0.2-1.0	0.02-0.06	0.02-0.06	0.04-0.08	250-750	425-1275	400-1200
Children and adolescents												
1-3	15-30	65	3	1.0-1.5	1.0-1.5	0.5-1.5	0.02-0.08	0.02-0.08	0.05-0.1	325-975	550-1650	500-1500
4-6	20-40	85	3-4	1.5-2.0	1.5-2.0	1.0-2.5	0.03-0.12	0.03-0.12	0.06-0.15	450-1350	775-2325	700-2100
7-10	30-60	120	4-5	2.0-2.5	2.0-3.0	1.5-2.5	0.05-0.2	0.05-0.2	0.1-0.3	600-1800	1000-3000	925-2775
11+	50-100	100-200	4-7	2.0-3.0	2.5-5.0	1.5-2.5	0.05-0.2	0.05-0.2	0.15-0.5	900-2700	1525-4575	1400-4200
Adults	70-140	100-200	4-7	2.0-3.0	2.5-5.0	1.5-4.0	0.05-0.2	0.05-0.2	0.15-0.5	1100-3300	1875-5625	1700-5100

From Recommended Dietary Allowances, Revised 1980. Food and Nutrition Board, National Academy of Sciences–National Research Council. Because there is less information on which to base allowances, these figures are not given in the main table of the RDAS and are provided here in the form of ranges of recommended intakes.

* Since the toxic levels for many trace elements may be only several times usual intakes, the upper levels for the trace elements given in this table should not be habitually exceeded.

Table 3-21

Guide to good eating: A recommended daily pattern

The recommended daily pattern provides the foundation for a nutritious, healthful diet.
The recommended servings from the four food groups for adults supply about 1200 calories. The chart below gives recommendations
for the number and size of servings for several categories of people.

Food group	Recommended number of servings					Food group	Recommended number of servings				
	Child	Teen-ager	Adult	Pregnant woman	Lactating woman		Child	Teen-ager	Adult	Pregnant woman	Lactating woman
Milk	3	4	2	4	4	**Fruit-vegetable**	4	4	4	4	4
1 cup milk, yogurt, OR						½ cup cooked or juice 1 cup raw Portion commonly served such as a medium-size apple or banana					
Calcium equivalent:											
1½ slices (1½ oz) cheddar cheese* 1 cup pudding 1¾ cups ice cream 2 cups cottage cheese*						**Grain,** whole grain, fortified enriched					
						1 slice bread 1 cup ready-to-eat cereal ½ cup cooked cereal, pasta, grits					
Meat	2	2	2	3	2						
2 ounces cooked, lean meat, fish, poultry, OR											
Protein equivalent:											
2 eggs 2 slices (2 oz) cheddar cheese* ½ cup cottage cheese* 1 cup dried beans, peas 4 tbsp peanut butter											

*Count cheese as serving of milk OR meat, not both simultaneously.
"Others" complement but do not replace foods from the four food groups. Amounts should be determined by individual caloric needs.
Courtesy National Dairy Council, 1977.

In addition, obese individuals often suffer emotional and psychological difficulties (National Dairy Council, 1985).

Assessment of the obese individual involves a close look at

1. Current height and weight
2. BMI—degree of overweight
3. Percentage of body fat (may not be reliable with the severely obese client)
4. Abnormalities that may be present in blood pressure, serum lipids, and serum glucose
5. Food consumption and habits
6. Physical activity patterns

Height, weight, BMI, and degree of obesity can be determined by methods previously described in this chapter. Body composition can be measured using skinfold calipers. A variety of sites on the body are usually measured, and the estimated total body fat is determined by comparing measured values to tables based on age and sex. A range of *optimal* total body fat for healthy adult females is estimated to be 16% to 23%; for healthy adult males, it is estimated to be 7% to 16%. ·

Table 3-22

Estimated caloric expenditure (ECE)

$ECE \text{ (men)} = (66.47 + 13.75W + 5.0H - 6.76A) \times \text{(activity factor)} \times \text{(injury factor)}$
$ECE \text{ (women)} = (655.10 + 9.56W + 1.85H - 4.68A) \times \text{(activity factor)} \times \text{(injury factor)}$

	Activity factor	Injury factor	Trauma: Skeletal use 1.35	Burns: Body Surface Area
W = weight in kg	Confined to bed,	Surgery: Minor, use 1.10	Head injury with	(BSA)
H = height in cm	use 1.20	Major, use 1.20	steroid therapy,	40% BSA, use
A = age in yr	Out of bed, use	Infection: Mild, use 1.20	use 1.60	1.50
	1.30	Moderate, use	Blunt, use 1.35	100% BSA, use
		1.40		1.95
		Severe, use 1.80		

From Long CL, Schaffel N, Geiger JW et al: Metabolic response to injury and illness: Estimation of energy and protein needs from indirect calorimetry and nitrogen balance, JPEN 3:452-456, 1979, and Long CL: Energy and protein requirements in stress and trauma. In Critical Care Nursing Currents, vol 2, no 2, Columbus, OH, 1984, Ross Laboratories, pp. 7-12. Reprinted with permission of Ross Laboratories, Columbus, OH 43216, from Nutritional Assessment Summary Sheet G636, © 1987, Ross Laboratories.

Weight reduction is recommended in the following circumstances:

1. Excess body weight of 20% or more. This corresponds to a BMI above 26.4 for men and 25.8 for women (see Table 3-4 and Fig. 3-4) or above 27.2 for men and 26.9 for women (see Table 3-5 and Fig. 3-5).
2. Family history or risk factors for maturity-onset (type II) diabetes.
3. High blood pressure.
4. Hypertriglyceridemia or hypercholesterolemia.
5. CHD (or atherosclerosis).
6. Gout.
7. Functional impairment due to heart disease, chronic obstructive pulmonary disease, or osteoarthritis of the spine, hips, and knees (which bear weight).
8. History of childhood obesity (Burton and Foster, 1985).

A team approach is suggested in the diagnosis and treatment of obesity. In many cases, when elevations of blood sugar, blood pressure, or serum lipids coexist with obesity, a loss of body fat and achievement of desirable weight will reduce these elevations. Psychological factors important in assessment and treatment of obesity are discussed in the section on assessment of eating disorders later in this chapter.

Diabetes

Diabetes, although not caused by dietary or activity factors alone, may be aggravated by obesity, poor food choices, and a sedentary life-style. The diabetic client is at increased risk of developing microvascular complications. In assessing the diabetic client, the practitioner must pay close attention to the following:

1. Current height and weight versus desirable weight for height
2. Regularity of physical activity patterns
3. Daily food consumption patterns:
   a. Calories consumed
   b. Percentages of carbohydrate, protein, and fat in the diet
   c. Types of dietary fat consumed
   d. Amount of dietary fiber consumed
   e. Regularity of meal schedule
   f. Methods of food preparation
4. Monitoring of blood and/or urine glucose

Dietary and activity recommendations should be based on maintaining desirable weight, controlling blood sugar and serum lipid levels, and promoting a generalized state of fitness.

Hypertension

Predisposing factors that increase a person's risk of developing hypertension include heredity, sex, age, race, obesity, and sensitivity to sodium. Related factors that appear to have some effect on hypertension include heavy alcohol consumption, use of oral contraceptives, and a sedentary life-style. Nutritional assessment of the client with hypertension or of the client who is at increased risk for developing hypertension involves assessment of weight and dietary factors, with particular attention to the amount of sodium and calories consumed as well as the overall balance of nutrients in the diet. Assessment of physical activity patterns is important. BMI has been related to hypertension, and it is estimated that 25% to 35% of hypertensive individuals are overweight. It has been shown that moderate weight loss can produce decreases in blood pressure similar to those produced with initial doses of diuretics (Elmer, 1985).

Assessment of needs is based on

1. Achieving and maintaining desirable weight
2. Reducing sodium intake, if elevated, to suggested levels based on the severity of hypertension and the client's past response to diet or drug modifications
3. Ensuring a balance of all essential nutrients in the diet
4. Promoting regular physical activity according to individual tolerance

Coronary Heart Disease

The three major risk factors in the development of CHD are high blood cholesterol, hypertension, and cigarette smoking. Other risk factors in the development of CHD include

- Emotional stress
- Sedentary life-style
- Overweight
- Diabetes
- Heart abnormalities
- Family history of heart disease
- Age
- Sex
- Race

The American Heart Association's (1986) current recommendations for healthy adult Americans include the following:

1. Saturated fat intake should be less than 10% of calories.
2. Total fat intake should be less than 30% of calories.
3. Cholesterol intake should be less than 100 mg/1000 calories, not to exceed 300 mg daily.
4. Protein intake should be approximately 15% of calories.
5. Carbohydrate intake should make up 50% to 55% or more of calories, with emphasis on increasing sources of complex carbohydrates.
6. Sodium intake should be reduced to approximately 1 g/1000 calories, not to exceed 3 g daily.
7. If alcoholic beverages are consumed, the limit should be 15% of total calories, not to exceed 50 ml of ethanol daily.
8. Total calories should be sufficient to maintain the individual's body weight (see Table 3-3).
9. A wide variety of foods should be consumed.

Modification of the diet in individuals whose lipid levels are elevated involves individualization. It appears that HDL levels may be positively affected by regular physical activity and by modifying specific types of fat consumed. LDL levels may be lowered by modifying

dietary saturated fat and cholesterol intake and by regulating body weight combined with exercise training.

Cancer

Scientific research has demonstrated an association between the amount of dietary fat consumed and the incidence of cancer, especially of the breast, large bowel, and prostate. Certain nutrients and other food constituents, such as vitamins A, C, and E, selenium, and dietary fiber, may be potential anticancer substances when consumed at levels found in a balanced diet. In certain geographic areas, it has been shown that excess consumption of smoked or salt-cured foods may elevate the risk of stomach and esophageal cancer. There is little or no evidence that many Americans fall into this category. In addition, although alcoholic beverages are low in most nutrients, they are high in calories. A high intake of such "empty" calories reduces the intake of other nutrient-rich foods needed in a balanced diet. When excessive alcohol consumption is combined with cigarette smoking, cancers of the mouth, esophagus, and larynx are increased. Also, excessive alcohol consumption may be a factor in the development of liver cancer.

The American Institute for Cancer Research has produced the following dietary guidelines to lower cancer risk:

1. Reduce daily intake of dietary fat—both saturated and unsaturated—from the current average of approximately 40% to a level of 30% of total calories.
2. Increase consumption of fruits, vegetables, and whole grain cereals.
3. Consume salt-cured, smoked, and charcoal-broiled foods in moderation.
4. Drink alcoholic beverages in moderation.

These guidelines to lower cancer risks are consistent with and extend the *Dietary Guidelines for Americans* published by the U.S. Departments of Agriculture and Health and Human Services. Nutritional assessment involves dietary analysis with the above guidelines in mind.

SPECIALTY POPULATIONS AND CONCERNS

Pediatric Assessment

Pediatric assessment involves evaluating growth and activity patterns as well as foods consumed and eating behavior. Height, weight, head circumference, and growth pattern can be evaluated using the National Center for Health Statistics growth charts, (see sample on p. 617). Table 3-23 lists standards for height and weight for children 4 to 18 years of age. Specific attention should be

Nutritional Assessment

Name: _____ Age: _____ Gender: _____

Date: _____

Address: _____

Telephone: _____

Present Health Condition or Health Problem: _____

Parameter	Value	Percentile	Degree of depletion or elevation
0 + Weight/height	_____ kg _____ cm	_____	_____
0 + Usual weight	_____ kg	_____	_____
0 + % Weight change	_____ %	NVA*	NVA*
0 + Desirable weight	_____ kg	NVA*	NVA*
0 + Tricep skinfold	_____ mm	_____	_____
+ Mid-arm circumference	_____ cm	_____	_____
+ Mid-arm muscle circumference	_____ cm	_____	_____
0 Body fat	_____ %	NVA*	_____

Parameter	Value	% Of standard	Degree of depletion or elevation
+ Total lymphocyte count	_____ mm³	_____	_____
0 + Serum albumin	_____ g/dl	_____	_____
+ Total iron binding capacity	_____ μg/dl	NVA*	NVA*
+ Serum transferrin	_____ mg/dl	_____	_____
+ Urinary creatinine	_____ mg	NVA*	NVA*
+ Creatinine height index	_____ %	_____	_____
0 + Hemoglobin	_____ mg/dl	NVA*	_____
0 + Hematocrit	_____ %	NVA*	_____
0 Serum cholesterol	_____ mg/dl	NVA*	_____
0 LDL:HDL ratio	_____	NVA*	_____
0 Serum triglyceride	_____ mg/dl	NVA*	_____
+ Nitrogen balance	_____ pos. or neg. number	NVA*	_____
+ Cellular immunity	_____ pos. or neg.	NVA*	_____
0 Serum glucose	_____ mg/dl	NVA*	_____

+ indicates parameters which may be used to assess malnutrition.

0 indicates parameters which may be used to assess physical fitness or determine existence or risk of various chronic diseases, such as CHD, diabetes, and so on.

*NVA means no value appropriate.

Clinical: Unusual physical signs _____

_____

_____

_____

Dietary: Approximate number of calories consumed per 24 hours _____

Approximate grams of protein consumed per 24 hours _____

Estimated caloric needs per 24 hours _____

Estimated protein needs per 24 hours _____

Adequacy of basic food groups _____

Nutrient deficiencies _____

_____

Nutrient excesses _____

_____

Daily fluid intake _____

Other dietary information pertinent to current health status _____

_____

_____

Problem identification: _____

_____

Action plan: _____

_____

_____

_____

_____

_____

_____

_____

Table 3-23

Height and weight of children 4 to 18 years of age

Ages (yr)	Height (in)			Weight (lb)		
	5th P*	50th P	95th P	5th P	50th P	95th P
Boys						
4	38.3	40.8	43.3	30.0	36.1	42.2
5	40.3	43.4	46.4	33.0	40.3	47.6
6	42.8	45.9	49.0	36.0	44.7	53.4
7	44.8	48.1	51.4	40.3	50.9	61.5
8	46.9	50.5	54.1	44.4	57.4	70.4
9	48.8	52.8	56.8	48.0	64.4	80.4
10	50.6	54.9	59.2	51.4	71.4	91.4
11	51.9	56.4	60.9	53.3	78.9	102.5
12	53.5	58.6	63.7	60.0	86.0	113.5
13	55.2	61.3	67.4	65.3	98.6	131.9
14	57.5	64.1	70.7	75.5	111.8	148.1
15	61.0	66.9	72.8	88.0	124.3	160.6
16	63.8	68.9	74.0	97.8	133.8	169.8
17	65.2	69.8	74.4	106.5	139.8	174.0
18	65.9	70.2	74.5	110.3	144.8	179.3
Girls						
4	38.1	40.7	43.3	28.8	36.1	43.4
5	40.6	43.4	46.2	32.2	40.9	49.6
6	42.8	45.9	49.0	35.5	45.7	55.9
7	44.5	47.8	51.1	38.3	51.0	63.7
8	46.4	50.0	53.6	42.0	57.2	72.4
9	48.2	52.2	56.2	45.1	63.6	82.1
10	49.9	54.5	59.1	48.2	71.0	95.0
11	51.9	57.0	62.1	55.4	82.0	108.6
12	54.1	59.5	64.9	63.9	94.4	124.9
13	57.1	62.2	66.8	72.8	105.5	138.2
14	58.5	63.1	67.7	83.0	113.0	144.0
15	59.5	63.8	68.1	89.5	120.0	150.5
16	59.8	64.1	68.4	95.1	123.0	150.1
17	60.1	64.2	68.3	97.9	125.8	153.7
18	60.1	64.4	68.7	96.0	126.2	156.4

From Falkner F: Some physical growth standards for white North American children, Pediatrics 29:448, 1962.
*P, percentile.

paid to *individuality* and *consistency* in the growth pattern, recognizing that trends and variations may occur. Height indicates long-term nutritional status, while weight signals a change in nutritional status. Measurements in children and adolescents below the 15th percentile may indicate some type of disorder and warrant closer investigation of the condition. Children and adolescents whose weight is at the 85th percentile or greater may warrant closer investigation of food habits and activity patterns, especially if rapid changes are seen. The development of eating disorders can begin in early childhood, and early intervention is critical if the individual is to mature with a healthy view of food and the eating experience.

The assessment of food intake and eating behavior begins with the infant. The information contained under Nutritional Data in Chapter 24, Assessment of the Pediatric Client, details important aspects of infant feeding that should be included in pediatric assessment. Determining the appropriateness of the formula used, if the child is not breast-fed, is important, along with ensuring that the child is growing at a consistent rate. Developmental patterns and the introduction of solid foods may be assessed according to the schedules shown in Tables 3-24 through 3-26. The child who is growing normally will experience changes in appetite and food intake as growth trends occur. Refer to Table 3-21 for recommended daily servings from the four basic food groups for children and teens.

Along with the basics, an evaluation of types of foods consumed, method of preparation (e.g., fresh, convenience, fried, baked), and snacking habits will indicate other aspects of nutritional quality such as the level of fat, sodium, sugar, and so on.

Evaluation of a child's or adolescent's intake of iron, calcium, and vitamins A and C may indicate a less than desirable intake. The RDAs for these nutrients, along with other essential nutrients, are found in Table 3-19. Inclusion of recommended servings from the basic food groups every day ensures that the average healthy child's nutrient needs will be met.

Nutritional assessment of the pediatric client involves assessment of family attitudes toward food, family knowledge of proper nutrition, and family food budget.

Maternal Assessment

Assessment of maternal nutrition would begin, ideally, once a woman has decided to conceive but before conception. A health evaluation including assessment of the woman's current height and weight status, dietary intake, and any preexisting health concerns allows the health care practitioner to determine if the client is in optimal health or if changes in health habits (e.g., diet and exercise) would serve to make pregnancy healthier and safer for the mother and baby.

Because the majority of women are seen for evaluation once conception has occurred, the pregnant woman should be assessed early in the pregnancy.

Prepregnancy weight and maternal weight gain have both been positively associated with infant birth

Table 3-24

Developmental patterns and feeding style in the first 6 months

	Birth	1 mo	2 mo	3 mo	4 mo	5 mo	6 mo
Mouth pattern:	Sucking, "extrusion" pattern.				Beginning swallow pattern; can transfer food from front of tongue to back. Beginning of drooling		
Hand coordination:	Random motion of hands				Hands beginning to go to mouth		Palmar grasp
Body control:	Prone on back; can raise head when on stomach				Sits supported; loses balance when reaches		Sits unsupported; can balance while manipulating with hands
Digestive ability:	Can digest appropriate milk				Intestinal amylase begins to increase to allow starch digestion		
Homeostatic ability:	Low; needs carefully adapted formula						
Nutritional requirements:	Relatively high nutrient requirement for rapid growth		Iron stores depleted in premature infants			Iron stores begin to be depleted in term babies	
Feeding style:	Nipple-feeding by breast or bottle					Beginning spoon feeding	
Food selection:	Breast milk or formula					Beginning solids: iron source	

From Satter E: Child of mine—feeding with love and good sense, Palo Alto, Calif, Bull Publishing Company 1983, 1986. Reprinted with permission.

weight (Committee on Maternal Nutrition, 1970). Table 3-27 gives values for optimum weight gain during pregnancy, based on the results of two studies performed in the United States. In the two studies, overweight was defined at different levels (20% and 35% or more above normal, according to the Table of Standard Weight for Height suggested for use by the American College of Obstetricians and Gynecologists, which is based on the 1959 Metropolitan Life Insurance Company Actuarial Tables), but it appeared that a 15 lb weight gain during pregnancy for the overweight woman was the *minimum* amount required to produce a healthy fetus in terms of birthweight and infant mortality.

The pattern of weight gain is important, with about 2 to 4 lb as an average gain during the first trimester and an average weight gain of about 1 lb per week during the second and third trimesters.

The recommended number of servings from the basic food groups for pregnant and lactating women can be found in Table 3-21. Supplementation of the pregnant woman's diet with 30 to 60 mg of iron daily during the second and third trimesters, as well as a daily supplement of 0.2 to 0.4 mg of folate, is commonly advised. Other nutritional considerations involve the mother's use of caffeine, artificial sweeteners, and alcohol during pregnancy. The safest strategy, in terms of protecting the baby

Table 3-25

Development patterns and feeding recommendations

	6 mo	7 mo	8 mo	9 mo	10 mo	11 mo	12 mo	13 mo	14 mo	15 mo	16 mo
Mouth pattern:	Beginning swallow pattern; can transfer food from front of tongue to back		Beginning chewing pattern; side-to-side motion of tongue and mashing food with jaws				Continuing maturation of biting, chewing, swallowing				
Hand coordination:	Palmar grasp	Pincer grasp beginning	Grabs spoon		Can get spoon in mouth but generally turns it over		Beginning mastery of spoon—still spilling most times			Spoon to mouth—with load intact	
	Urge to put anything in mouth continues until about three; increased risk for poisoning throughout this time										
Body control:	Sits unsupported; can balance while manipulating with hands		Continuing improvement in balance while sitting								
		Begins to stand; can pull self to feet and move around					Beginning and increasing mastery of walking				
Digestive:		Gastric acid volume begins to increase			Can handle balanced amounts of all reasonably soft, moderately-seasoned family food						
Homeostatic ability:		Increasing ability to maintain hydration and chemical balance									
Nutritional requirements:	Iron stores begin to be depleted in term babies		Gradually increasing proportion of adequate diet offered by foods other than milk feeding							All daily nutritional requirements provided by a mixed table food diet: primary source of nutrients and calories in table food and cup	
Feeding style:	Spoon feeding	Introduce cup at meals		Begin self-feeding with cup; beginning proficiency with spoon						Reasonably adept with spoon and cup. Can feed self with spoon, drink from cup. Weaned from bottle. Continuance of breastfeeding up to baby and parents	
Food selection:	Semisolid foods	Increase texture, stiffness of solids				Pieces of soft, cooked foods					

From Satter, E.: Child of mine—feeding with love and good sense, Palo Alto, Calif, 1983, 1986, Bull Publishing Company. Reprinted with permission.
Ages overlap and are given as ranges because of variations in rate of infant development.

Table 3-26

Feeding schedule: Six to twelve months

	4-7 months*	6-8 months	7-10 months	10-12 months
Milk feeding	Breast milk or formula	Breast milk or formula	Breast milk or formula	Breast milk or formula Evaporated milk diluted 1:1 with water Whole pasteurized milk or combination
Cereal and bread	Begin iron—fortified baby cereal mixed with milk feeding	Continue baby cereal; begin other breads and cereals	Continue baby cereal Other breads and cereals from table	Continue baby cereal until 18 months Total of four servings bread and cereal from table
Fruit and vegetables (including juice)	None	Begin juice from cup: 3 oz vitamin C source Begin fork-mashed, soft fruits and vegetables	3 oz juice Pieces of soft and cooked fruits and vegetables from table	Table-food diet to allow 4 servings a day, including juice
Meat and other protein sources	None	None	Gradually begin milled or finely cut meat. Casseroles, ground beef, eggs, fish, peanut butter, legumes, cheese	Two servings daily; one ounce total, meat or equivalent

From Satter, E.: Child of mine—feeding with love and good sense, Palo Alto, Calif, 1983, 1986, Bull Publishing Company. Reprinted with permission.
Ages overlap and are given as ranges because of variations in rate of infant development.

Table 3-27

Optimal weight gain in pregnancy

Weight status at conception	Weight gain (lb) for lowest infant mortality
Normal weight	27
Underweight	30
Overweight	15

From Satter, E.: Child of mine—feeding with love and good sense, Palo Alto, Calif, 1983, 1986, Bull Publishing Company. Reprinted with permission.

from possible side effects, is to abstain from using these substances in the diet. Amounts of these substances consumed by the pregnant woman must be evaluated. Assessment of the mother's intake of dietary fiber, found in whole grains, fruits and vegetables (especially raw), and legumes, as well as assessment of fluid intake is helpful in preventing constipation.

Assessment of the mother's diet while breast-feeding is important, following the recommendations listed in Table 3-21, as well as ensuring that the mother is drinking enough fluids to quench her thirst, thereby supporting milk production. It is important during this time that the mother not omit basic foods—and thus essential nutrients—from her diet in an attempt to lose weight rapidly. Alcohol, caffeine, and artificial sweeteners should be used with caution, as in the pregnant woman.

Geriatric Assessment

Assessment of the older individual involves recognizing changes that occur during the aging process. In the process of aging, some lean body mass is lost as the weight of vital organs decreases, while increased fat deposition occurs, mainly around internal organs, with some deposition in the blood. Total body water decreases slightly. A decrease in bone mass is experienced, more so in women than in men.

Because of bodily changes that occur during aging and the difficulty of obtaining certain measurements, anthropometric measurement is not entirely appropriate for the geriatric population. The particular measurements that may be difficult to obtain in some elderly clients include height, weight, skinfold thickness, and MAC. Various recumbent measurements can be used to assess nutritional status when standard methods are not possible.

Reference data have been established for anthropometric assessment of the elderly. The appropriate data must be used for accurate assessment and interpretation of nutritional status. Taking into account a decrease in basal metabolic rate and generally decreasing physical activity with aging, recommended energy intake decreases with age, as listed in Table 3-3. Because a decreased number of calories is needed to maintain weight at an appropriate level, the foods consumed must be of high nutrient density. Physiologic changes occurring during aging may interfere with the body's ability to digest, absorb, and use food consumed. In addition, many elderly persons are taking one or more drugs, which may interfere with the body's use of nutrients consumed.

Other common characteristics in the geriatric client that are important in nutritional assessment include (1) tooth loss, (2) loss of perception of taste and smell, (3) changes in vision, (4) specific physical and psychological disorders, and (5) social isolation. All these factors affect the food choices a person might make. Causes and any possible corrections should be evaluated thoroughly so that the feeding environment is as pleasant and as positive an experience as possible, ensuring consumption of a nutritious diet. Alterations in the composition and consistency of the diet and the timing and size of meals and snacks may be necessary. An evaluation of activity habits is important, considering that moderate activity is thought to have a positive effect on health and well-being.

The following laboratory values may be altered in the elderly:

May be increased

Serum glucose
Serum cholesterol
Serum triglycerides
Blood urea nitrogen

May be decreased

Hemoglobin
Hematocrit
Serum albumin
Creatinine clearance
Adrenocorticotropic hormone

Assessment of the Physically Active

Assessment of the physically active client involves evaluating physical status, including such factors as body composition, flexibility, muscular strength, and cardiovascular endurance. For a healthy individual, suggested laboratory analysis could include serum cholesterol, serum glucose, hemoglobin, and hematocrit determina-

tions. The measurement of blood pressure is of further value in assessing health status.

Nutritional assessment involves a close look at energy expended during various activities as well as evaluation of the client's current dietary patterns regarding calories consumed; percentages of carbohydrate, protein, and fat in the diet; balance and variety of food consumption; appropriate amounts of vitamins and minerals in the diet; and fluid consumption.

Table 3-28 lists caloric expenditure for various recreational activities based on body weight. Endurance athletes may require as many as 5000 to 6000 calories daily to supply sufficient energy for performance. *Where* these calories are obtained, in terms of food sources, can have a tremendous impact on the athlete's health and performance.

Table 3-21 is used as a guideline for consumption by physically active individuals. Although endurance athletes appear to require slightly more protein than nonathletic and moderately active adults (1.2 g of protein/kg body weight daily vs 0.8 g of protein/kg body weight daily, respectively), these needs are usually met without any problem if the endurance athlete consumes 15% of total calories daily in the form of protein. The recommended amounts of carbohydrate, protein, and fat in the diet of the nontraining adult are as follows:

• 55% to 60% of calories in the form of carbohydrate
• 12% to 15% of calories in the form of protein
• Up to 30% of calories in the form of fat

Endurance training athletes are advised to increase the carbohydrate content of their diet slightly, up to about 65% of total calories, to increase muscle glycogen stores and ensure available energy to the body during the training process. The food groups that supply the major amounts of carbohydrate in the diet are the grain group and the fruit and vegetable group. Foods in the milk group also supply some carbohydrate but may supply unwanted fat if not chosen carefully.

It is important to assess if an individual is consuming adequate fluid to meet metabolic needs. A sedentary individual needs approximately 1 l of water daily per 1000 calories consumed, and large, very active athletes may require two or three times this amount. Inadequate fluid intake hampers performance and can cause serious heat-related problems.

Specific concerns related to nutritional health of athletes involve the misuse of dietary supplements (vitamins, minerals, and protein) and the development of eating disorders in an attempt to achieve an unrealistic body size or shape. Although athletes require a few vitamins and minerals in increased amounts, these needs can be easily met through a diet that is varied and bal-

Table 3-28

Calories used per minute in popular recreational activities

Activity	Weight (lb)					
	110	130	150	170	190	209
Lying at ease	1.1	1.3	1.5	1.7	1.9	2.1
Sitting quietly	1.1	1.2	1.4	1.6	1.8	2.0
Knitting, sewing	1.2	1.4	1.6	1.8	2.0	2.2
Card playing	1.3	1.5	1.7	1.9	2.2	2.4
Piano playing	2.0	2.4	2.7	3.1	3.4	3.8
Horse riding, walking	2.1	2.4	2.8	3.2	3.5	3.9
Canoeing	2.2	2.6	3.0	3.4	3.8	4.2
Volleyball	2.5	3.0	3.4	3.9	4.3	4.8
Ballroom dancing	2.6	3.0	3.5	3.9	4.4	4.8
Fishing	3.1	3.7	4.2	4.8	5.3	5.9
Cleaning	3.1	3.7	4.2	4.8	5.3	5.9
Walking, normal pace	4.0	4.7	5.4	6.2	6.9	7.6
Golf	4.3	5.0	5.8	6.5	7.3	8.1
Badminton	4.9	5.7	6.6	7.5	8.3	9.2
Downhill skiing	4.9	5.8	6.7	7.5	8.4	9.3
Bicycling, 9.4 mph	5.0	5.9	6.8	7.7	8.6	9.5
Aerobic or disco dancing	5.2	6.1	7.0	7.9	8.9	9.8
Tennis	5.5	6.4	7.4	8.4	9.4	10.4
Swimming, crawl	6.4	7.6	8.7	9.9	11.0	12.2
Jogging, 11½ minute miles	6.8	8.0	9.2	10.5	11.7	12.9
Basketball	6.9	8.1	9.4	10.6	11.9	13.1
Cross-country skiing	7.2	8.4	9.7	11.0	12.3	13.6

Modified from McArdle WD, Katch FI, and Katch VL: Exercise Physiology: Energy, Nutrition, and Human Performance, Philadelphia, 1981, Lea & Febiger. Data from Bannister EW and Brown SR: The relative energy requirements of physical activity. In Falls HB, editor: Exercise Physiology, New York, 1968, Academic Press, Howley ET and Glover ME: The caloric costs of running and walking one mile for men and women, Med Sci Sports 6:235, 1974, and Passmore R and Durnin IVGA: Human energy expenditure, Physiol Rev 35:801:1955, Courtesy National Dairy Council.

anced and that supplies enough calories to meet energy needs. The athlete who consumes megadoses of vitamins, minerals, or protein in an attempt to increase muscle mass or improve performance may cause serious toxicities or risk developing such problems as renal disease from long-term overload of protein. According to O'Neil and colleagues (1986), "Athletes at high risk for developing iron deficiency include male and female long-distance runners, menstruating girls and women, children, vegetar-

ians, and other individuals who do not meet iron needs through diet."

Although athletes do not generally require more calcium than nonathletes, the athlete's diet should be assessed for adequate calcium consumption, providing at least the RDA. The amenorrheic athlete's calcium needs may be increased, resembling the needs of postmenopausal women.

Athletes, because they may be told to lose a few pounds to make weight, wish to be a certain body size or shape for a specific sport, or are striving toward perfectionism, may be prone to consume inadequate diets to meet nutritional needs as well as to develop eating disorders. Assessment of eating disorders is discussed in the next section.

Because of the positive effects of regular physical activity in controlling weight, increasing cardiovascular fitness, reducing stress, and contributing to an overall sense of health and well-being, an assessment of current activity patterns is important in determining health status and providing recommendations to the client.

Assessment of Eating Disorders

An eating disorder is an aberration of the function and process of eating, indicating a complexity of psychological, emotional, and social problems or maladaptation. Assessment of eating disorders involves identification of

1. The signs and symptoms associated with particular disorders
2. Medical, psychological, and social complications or consequences resulting from particular disorders
3. A client's present nutritional status, dietary habits, activity patterns, and psychological background

Two major categories of eating disorders will be discussed, anorexia nervosa and bulimia nervosa. Psychological aspects of obesity are also mentioned in this section, although obesity is technically classified as a physical disorder.

Anorexia nervosa

Anorexia nervosa is "characterized by persistent, intentional loss of weight and maintenance of weight at an abnormally low level" (Huse and Lucas, 1983). Discriminating features in identifying the disorder include those listed in the box on p. 86.

Onset of the disorder typically occurs in early to late adolescence but may range from prepubescence to, rarely, the early thirties. Anorexia nervosa occurs predominantly in females. The symptoms and signs associated with anorexia nervosa are listed in Table 3-29. Common laboratory abnormalities are shown in the box on p. 86, and clinical features of anorexia nervosa in-

---

Discriminating Features in Identifying Anorexia Nervosa

1. Self-inflicted weight loss accompanied thereafter by a sustained avoidance of mature body shape, which cannot be directly ascribed to other identifiable psychiatric causes, cachexia-inducing diseases, or externally imposed demands for reduced food intake.
2. A morbid and persistent dread of fat.
3. The manipulation of body weight through dietary restraint, self-induced vomiting, abuse of purgatives, or excessive exercise.
4. Disturbances in body image manifest in the misrepresentation of actual body dimensions or extreme loathing of bodily functions.
5. Amenorrhea and the development of other behavioral-physiologic sequelae of starvation.

From Brownell KD and Foreyt JP, editors: Handbook of eating disorders: physiology, psychology, and treatment of obesity, anorexia, and bulimia, New York, 1986, Basic Books.

---

opposite, and clinical features of anorexia nervosa include those listed in Table 3-30. Medical complications resulting from anorexia nervosa involve various organ systems (see the box on p. 87).

Nutritional assessment involves the following:
1. Anthropometric measurement to assess current physical status
2. Biochemical evaluation for nutrient deficiencies
3. Clinical examination
4. Detailed dietary history, determining
   a. Development of the disorder
   b. Current food consumption—calories, protein, other nutrients
   c. *Patterns* of food intake and eating behavior
   d. Psychological and social influences on eating behavior
   e. Use of any drugs, including vitamins, minerals, laxatives, and diuretics
   f. Exercise habits

From assessment data, a treatment plan involving medical, nutritional, and psychological intervention can be determined.

Bulimia nervosa

Bulimia nervosa is typically characterized by episodes of binge eating, or rapid consumption of large amounts of food within a given time, alternating with episodes of vomiting, use of laxatives or diuretics, strict dieting, or exercise to prevent weight gain. Bulimia nervosa usually begins during adolescence or early adulthood and occurs

---

Table 3-29

Symptoms and signs of anorexia nervosa

Symptoms	Prevalence of symptoms (%)	Signs	Prevalence of signs (%)
Amenorrhea	100	Hypotension	20-85
Constipation	20	Hypothermia	15-85
Bloating	30	Dry skin	25-85
Abdominal pain	20	Bradycardia	25-90
Cold intolerance	20	Lanugo	20-80
Lethargy	20	Edema	20-25
Excess energy	35	Petechiae	10

From Brownell KD and Foreyt JP, editors: Handbook of eating disorders: physiology, psychology, and treatment of obesity, anorexia, and bulimia, New York, 1986, Basic Books.

Common Laboratory Abnormalities Seen in Patients With Anorexia Nervosa

Metabolic abnormalities

Hypercholesterolemia
Hypercarotenemia
Hypozincemia
Abnormal liver functions
Abnormal glucose tolerance
Fasting hypoglycemia
Hypocalcemia

Gastrointestinal abnormalities

Elevated amylase

Cardiovascular abnormalities

Electrocardiogram abnormalities

Renal abnormalities

Elevated blood urea nitrogen
Decreased glomerular filtration rate
Urinary concentrating defect

Central nervous system abnormalities

Electroencephalogram abnormality

Computed tomography scan abnormality

Fluid and electrolyte abnormalities

Hypochloremia
Hypokalemia
Metabolic alkalosis
Metabolic acidosis

Hematological abnormalities

Pancytopenia
Relative lymphocytosis
Bone marrow hypocellularity
Thrombocytopenia

Endocrine abnormalities

Low luteinizing hormone, follicle-stimulating hormone
Low urinary gonadotropins
Low urinary estrogen
Low triiodothyronine
Elevated growth hormone
Elevated cortisol
Dexamethasone suppression test nonsuppression

From Brownell KD and Foreyt JP, editors: Handbook of eating disorders: physiology, psychology, and treatment of obesity, anorexia, and bulimia, New York, 1986, Basic Books.

Table 3-30

Clinical features of anorexia nervosa

Feature	Anorexia nervosa
Intense drive for thinness	Marked
Self-imposed starvation	Marked (due to fear of body size)
Disturbance in body image	Present (lack of awareness of change in body size and lack of satisfaction or pleasure in the body)
Appetite	Maintained (but with fear of giving in to impulse)
Satiety	Usually bloating, nausea, early satiety
Avoidance of specific foods	Present (for carbohydrates or foods presumed to be high in "calories")
Bulimia	Present in 30% to 50%
Vomiting	Present (to prevent weight gain)
Laxative abuse	Present (to prevent weight gain)
Activity level	Increased
Amenorrhea	Present

From: Garfinkel PE and others, Can Med Assoc 129:940, 1983.

Medical Complications of Anorexia Nervosa

Metabolic complications

Yellowing of skin
Impaired taste
Hypoglycemia

Gastrointestinal complications

Altered gastric emptying
Salivary gland swelling
Superior mesenteric artery syndrome
Gastric dilatation
Constipation

Cardiovascular complications

Bradycardia
Arrhythmias
Pericardial effusion
Edema
Heart failure

Renal complications

Water concentration defect
Kaliopenic nephropathy

Fluid and electrolyte complications

Dehydration
Weakness
Tetany

Hematologic complications

Bleeding diathesis
Anemia

Dental problems

Decalcification
Caries

Endocrine complications

Amenorrhea
Lack of sexual interest
Impotence

General complications

Weakness
Hypothermia

From Brownell KD and Foreyt JP, editors: Handbook of eating disorders: physiology, psychology, and treatment of obesity, anorexia, and bulimia, New York, 1986, Basic Books.

---

predominantly in females. The disorder occurs in individuals of normal weight as well as in obese persons and persons with anorexic behavior (Kirkley, 1986). Diagnostic criteria for bulimia nervosa are outlined in the box opposite.

Laboratory and medical complications can be extensive and, as with anorexia nervosa, involve various organ systems (see box on p. 88).

The bulimic individual may show no outward signs of the disorder. Physical complaints may bring the client in for medical treatment. Bulimic behavior is secretive, and, as with anorexics, denial may exist.

Dietary analysis should detail the following:
1. Weight history
2. Dieting history and behavior
3. History of the bulimic behavior
4. Patterns of bingeing and purging
5. Foods consumed during a binge—"trigger" foods
6. Food likes and dislikes
7. Eating behavior and pattern when not bingeing
8. Feelings regarding food and self
9. Exercise habits

As with anorexia nervosa, psychological assessment by a qualified professional is critical for treatment to be individualized and successful.

Diagnostic Criteria for 307.51 Bulimia Nervosa

1. Recurrent episodes of binge eating (rapid consumption of a large amount of food in a discrete time).
2. A feeling of lack of control over eating behavior during the eating binges.
3. The person regularly engages in either self-induced vomiting, use of laxatives or diuretics, strict dieting or fasting, or vigorous exercise to prevent weight gain.
4. A minimum average of two binge eating episodes a week for at least 3 months.
5. Persistent overconcern with body shape and weight.

From the *Diagnostic and Statistical Manual of Mental Disorders*, ed 3, rev. Washington DC, 1987, American Psychiatric Association. Reprinted with permission.

Laboratory Abnormalities and Medical Complications of Bulimia

Renal complications

Dehydration
Hypokalemic nephropathy

Gastrointestinal complications

Gastric dilatation
Sialodenosis
Amylase elevations
Pancreatitis

Electrolyte abnormalities

Hyperuricemia
Hypokalemia
Alkalosis
Acidosis

Laxative abuse complications

Hyperuremia
Hypocalcemia
Tetany
Osteomalacia
Clubbing
Skin pigmentation
Hypomagnesemia
Fluid retention
Malabsorption syndromes
Protein-losing enteropathy
Cathartic colon

Hematologic abnormalities

Bleeding tendency

Neurologic abnormalities

Electroencephalogram abnormalities

Endocrine abnormalities

Blunted thyroid-stimulating hormone response to thyroid-releasing hormone
Pathologic growth hormone response to thyroid-releasing hormone glucose
Prolactin elevations
Dexamethasone suppression test nonsuppression

Dental problems

Caries
Enamel erosion

From Brownell KD and Foreyt JP, editors: Handbook of eating disorders: physiology, psychology, and treatment of obesity, anorexia, and bulimia, New York, 1986, Basic Books.

Obesity

Obesity may result from a complexity of factors, and several theories regarding the development of obesity exist. In terms of psychological aspects of obesity, the use of food to handle other problems in life results in overconsumption, weight gain, and possibly other health risks. The obese individual often knows *what* to eat, but the control of eating behavior is elusive. An overweight individual may consume much less than a thin individual in terms of total calories, but a decreased metabolic rate, often due to repeated strict dieting and low activity levels,

may aid the body's storage of fat. Being overweight may be a predisposing factor in some cases of anorexia nervosa; adolescent obesity may be a predisposing factor in the development of bulimia nervosa in adult life. Important in planning a holistic therapy program is a detailed diet history, including

1. Weight history
2. History and patterns of dieting
3. Present food consumption
4. Eating behavior patterns
5. Exercise habits
6. Feelings about food—psychological meanings

THE REGISTERED DIETITIAN

The registered dietitian is the health care professional best qualified to work as a member of the health care team in assessing an individual's nutritional needs, planning appropriate nutritional intervention, and educating the individual on a healthy life-style. Registered dietitians can be found in a variety of settings, including hospitals and clinics, community health care, extended care facilities, private practice, business and industry, the armed forces, and educational settings. A client with a suspected or diagnosed nutritional problem or concern can be referred to the registered dietitian for further assessment, counseling, and follow-up regarding the problem or concern. As people strive toward high-level wellness, registered dietitians do much preventive counseling in the area of health and fitness. National, state, and local dietetic associations exist to serve the public and act as a resource to the community and other professionals.

SUMMARY

Because food is basic to life, assessment of nutritional status is an essential component of health assessment. The parameters of nutritional assessment, including

- *A*nthropometric measurement
- *B*iochemical measurement
- *C*linical examination
- *D*ietary analysis

can be applied to any client, noting particular features that may be of value in assessing a specific condition or disorder. Integration of all these components, along with other health assessment data obtained, is important in evaluating health status accurately and in recommending any treatment or client education.

BIBLIOGRAPHY

Ardell DB: Fourteen days to a wellness lifestyle, San Rafael, Calif, 1982, Whatever Publishing.

American Dietetic Association: Handbook of clinical dietetics, New Haven, Conn, 1981, Yale University Press.

American Heart Association: About high blood pressure, 1986, Dallas, American Heart Association.

American Heart Association: Dietary guidelines for healthy American adults, Dallas, 1986, American Heart Association.

American Heart Association: Risk factors and coronary disease: a statement for physicians, Dallas, 1980, American Heart Association.

The American Institute for Cancer Research: Dietary guidelines to lower cancer risk, Washington DC, 1988, The American Institute for Cancer Research.

Blackburn GL, and others: Nutritional and metabolic assessment of the hospitalized patient, JPEN 1:11-22, 1977.

Burton BT and Foster WR: Health implications of obesity: an NIH consensus development conference, J Am Diet Assoc 85:1117-1121, 1985.

Butterworth CE Jr: The skeleton in the hospital closet, Nutrition Today 9:4-8, 1974.

Chumlea WC, Roche AF, and Mukherjee, D: Nutritional assessment of the elderly through anthropometry, Columbus, Ohio, 1987, Ross Laboratories.

Committee on Maternal Nutrition, Food and Nutrition Board, National Research Council, National Academy of Sciences: Maternal nutrition and the course of pregnancy: summer report, Bethesda, Md, 1970, Department of Health and Human Services.

Elmer PJ: "Dietary intervention in hypertension: current status, weight and sodium, and new directions," Iowa City, 1985. Presented at Diet Therapy USA.

Huse DM and Lucas AR: Dietary treatment of anorexia nervosa, J Am Diet Assoc 83:687-690, 1983.

Jensen TG, Englert DM, and Dudrick SJ: Interpretation of nutritional assessment data, Nutr Support Serv 1:14-20, 1981.

Kamath SK, and others: Hospital malnutrition: a 33-hospital screening study, J Am Diet Assoc 86:203-206, 1986.

Kaminski MV Jr and Winborn AL: Nutritional assessment guide, Chicago, 1978, Midwest Nutrition, Education, and Research Foundation.

Kirkley BG: Bulimia: clinical characteristics, development, and etiology, J Am Diet Assoc 86:468-472, 1986.

National Dairy Council: LIFESTEPS®, Rosemont, IL, 1985, The Council.

O'Neil FT, Hynak-Hankinson MT, and Gorman J: Research and application of current topics in sports nutrition, J Am Diet Assoc 86:1007-1012, 1986.

Satter E: Child of mine—feeding with love and good sense, Palo Alto, Calif, 1983, 1986, Bull Publishing Co.

National Institutes of Health: Cholesterol counts, Bethesda, Md, 1985, Public Health Service, U.S. Department of Health and Human Services.

Williams SR: Nutrition and diet therapy, ed: St Louis, 1985, The CV Mosby Co.

4

Assessment of sleep-wakefulness patterns

OBJECTIVES

Upon successful review of this chapter, learners will be able to describe:

- Circadian rhythms, biologic functions and peaks

- Effects of environmental time and age on circadian rhythmicity

- Factors that influence sleep-wakefulness patterns

- Usual physiologic and affective findings associated with the four stages of sleep

- Differences in sleep patterns of children and adults

- Neurologic changes that occur with sleep deprivation

- Causes and conditions of primary sleep disorders and possible treatments

- Causes and conditions of secondary sleep disorders and possible treatments

- Causes and conditions of parasomnias and possible treatments

- Effects of chronic illness on sleep patterns

- Assessment techniques that help elicit sleep pattern data

HUMAN CIRCADIAN RHYTHMS

Normal human beings are characterized as organisms that adapt bodily functions in such a way as to have a different physiochemical and psychological makeup for each hour of the day. Yet each of these changes is carefully regulated for the given hour, and the variations of one day closely resemble those of each other day. The ability to maintain a relative internal constancy has been termed *homeostasis* or, more precisely, *homeokinesis*. Thus, healthy individuals represent the integration of a myriad of cyclic alterations of psychophysiologic functions.

Biologic rhythms have been described for all levels of biologic functions. The external stimuli that are most likely to affect the human are those who periods most closely correspond to endogenous rhythms. Considerable evidence has supported the possibility of endogenous timekeeping. The most prevalent rhythms, when freed from the effects of the environment, are periods of 23 to 25 hours called circadian. *Circadian rhythms* (L. *circa*, about; and *dies*, day) are defined as those functions with a period of 20 to 28 hours. The normal sleep-wakefulness pattern in humans follows the circadian rhythm. Circadian rhythms persist even when an organism is isolated from time cues (free-running cycles). Humans who have been placed in a chamber where the levels of light, temperature, food, and sounds are kept constant have circadian rhythms that more directly reflect the behavior of the human clock(s).

There is a wide range of biologic rhythms, with periods of less than a second to more than a year (Table 4-1). *Ultradian rhythms* are those periods less than 24 hours. Ultradian rhythms in the human being include the electrical activity of the brain as recorded by electroencephalogram (EEG), heartbeat, and breathing. *Infradian*

Table 4-1

Types of biologic rhythms

Rhythm	Time period	Example
Ultradian	<24 hours	Electrical activity of brain (EEG)
		Heartbeat
		Respiratory rate
		Sleep cycles
Circadian	20-28 hours	Most human rhythms
		Vital signs
		Serum electrolyte values
		Urine electrolyte values
		Hormones of the pituitary gland
Infradian	>28 hours	Menstrual cycle
		Sexual hormones

rhythms are characterized by periods longer than 28 hours, an example of which is the menstrual cycle.

The suprachiasmatic nuclei of the hypothalamus have been demonstrated to be the anatomic structures necessary to the control of many circadian rhythms, including the sleep-wakefulness cycle. There are felt to be two types of circadian oscillators. Type X oscillators have a periodicity of 24.5 hours and control rapid eye movement (REM) sleep and cortisol secretion. Type Y oscillators have a periodicity of 33 hours and control the cycles of slow wave (non-rapid eye movement [NREM]) sleep and growth hormone (GH). These oscillators interact with each other, giving an overall circadian rhythm in humans of approximately 25.3 hours. Because the circadian rhythm in humans is slightly longer than the 24-hour light-dark cycle, entraining stimuli are necessary to adapt the sleep-wake cycle to the environmental cycle. It is known that relatively few chemical compounds interfere with circadian rhythms. One class of chemicals that is known to reset the timing of circadian clocks is methylxanthines, an example of which is caffeine.

Since the cyclic nature of human function has been defined, a good deal of experimentation has been focused on determining whether one or more factors in the environment cause the rhythms. Further work has been devoted to locating receptors in humans that sense these external factors and are responsible for establishing the rhythms.

Human beings adapt to environmental cues of an immediate nature as well as to external sequences or cycles of regularly changing conditions. Examples of regular external periodicities that are thought to be in-

corporated into organisms' adaptive behavior are the tides, the light-dark cycle, the lunar cycle, and the seasons. This adaptive process involves establishing an endogenous rhythm that approximately corresponds to the environmental stimulus. These rhythms are known as the biologic clocks that allow the organisms to adjust to the changes occurring outside. Once the internal rhythm is established, the environmental cue that caused the change becomes a synchronizing stimulus and is called a *Zeitgeber* (Ger. *Zeit,* time; and *Geber,* giver). Examples of these stimuli include light and darkness, waking time, meal time, and other less well-defined factors.

The influence most frequently observed in plants and animals is the day-night, or light-dark cycle. Such circadian rhythms have been identified for all cells and functions of the human body from enzyme levels to complex neural events. Because most human rhythms are 23 to 25 hours long, they are termed circadian. However, although most human functions are entrained by a period approximating 24 hours, the peaks (high-function point) and troughs (low-function point) of daily rhythms for various functions can occur at different times; and although these functional records show phase relationships to each other, it is not known if all the rhythms for the various functions are entrained by *Zeitgeber* stimuli or by other rhythms internal to the person.

It has been shown that cells may be influenced directly by gravity and electrostatic magnetic fields. The nervous system seems important to the control of rhythms in higher organisms, particularly as related to photoperiodicity. At least one researcher has hypothesized different levels of rhythm organizations: neural, endocrine, and cellular. In this system, the neural system is thought to be entrained by dominant synchronizers and the cellular elements by weaker synchronizers. In human beings, it is necessary to include a fourth level, psychosocial organization, which may serve to modify rhythmic trends.

In the human, social cues are considered to be important *Zeitgebers.* An experiment comparing groups of subjects isolated from time cues exhibited free-running periods different from each other. When a subject was moved from one group to another, a progressive phase shift occurred to resynchronize that person with the new group.

It has been hypothesized that functions such as the sleep-wakefulness cycle are weakly entrained, whereas functions such as urinary output, body temperature, adrenocortical secretion, enzyme production, and cellular division are more strongly incorporated. Data to support this hypothesis are those from experiments wherein subjects are placed in lightproof and soundproof enclosures for weeks to months. As many stimuli as possible are removed, and this is termed the *free-running condition*, which means that cyclic events occur in the absence of their respective *Zeitgeber*. The sleep-wakefulness cycle becomes desynchronized to 30 to 33 hours. The more deeply entrained cycles, the vegetative functions, retain a 25-hour cycle. Thus, many endogenous cycles may be in new phase relationships.

The 24-hour temperature rhythm was defined soon after the development of the clinical thermometer in the 18th century. However, a refined experimental approach to the study of biologic rhythms in human physiology had its origin in the 1920s, when it was shown that rhythms occur even in metabolism. Table 4-2 reflects some of the data useful to the health care professional in this still relatively unknown field.

The measures of physiologic function that have been used as diagnostic indicators have been shown to exhibit a circadian rhythm. The human body has been shown to have a diurnal rhythm of peaks and troughs for nearly every laboratory value and physiologic measurement. The variation from high (peak) to low (trough) for some values may be minor, as little as 10% of plasma potassium concentration, but the changes over a 24-hour period may be markedly variable, as in the case of plasma cortisol, which is quite low before sleep and reaches a daily peak just before awakening. It is now considered good practice to take into account the time of day at which the plasma cortisol was obtained.

It has been shown that the sensitivity to many pharmacologic agents (such as morphine and ethanol) to bacteria, and to carcinogens varies over the 24-hour period. Thus, the time the client takes a given medication may influence the effectiveness of the drug. In addition, the body is more sensitive to toxic effects of some drugs at specific times of the day.

Some cycles appear to be significantly related to one another; for instance, the pulse rate and respiratory rate in the normal adult demonstrate a 4:1 ratio, and any long-term deviation from this ratio may be the diagnostic feature of abnormal function. Moreover, it has been shown that clients with respiratory failure resulting from bronchial asthma have a greatly exaggerated rhythm of bronchial constriction around 6 AM. This observation led to increased vigilance in observance of clients at this time, as well as focusing treatment at this phase of the rhythm.

Nocturnal diuresis has been given as an example of a phase change (180 degrees) in a biologic rhythm; the change in time for this function was recognized as abnormal and given diagnostic significance long before circadian rhythms were well defined.

Table 4-2

Time of maximum amplitude of physiologic rhythms in a person whose sleep cycle is 11 PM to 7 AM

Physiologic rhythms	Peak of cycle*
Vital signs	
Temperature (rectal)	4-6 PM
Heart rate	4 PM
Respiratory rate	2-3 PM
Blood pressure	7-10 PM
Cardiac output	Midnight
Venous pressure	Midnight
Oxygen consumption	Midnight
Physical vigor	3-4 PM
Optical reaction time	3 AM
Grip strength	2-8 PM
Blood	
Sodium	4-5 PM
Calcium	9-10 PM
17-Hydroxycorticosteroid	7-8 AM
Hematocrit	9-10 PM
Polymorphonuclear cells	12-1 PM
Lymphocytes and monocytes	11-3 AM
Urine	
Sodium	12-1 PM
Potassium	12-1 PM
Calcium	3-4 PM
Magnesium	1 AM
Dopamine	3 PM
Catecholamines	5-7 PM
Vanillylmandelic acid	5-7 PM
17-Hydroxycorticosteroid	9-10 AM
Rate of excretion	8-9 AM
Mitosis—epidermal	11-12 PM
Body weight	6-7 PM

*The valley or low period for these values occurs approximately 12 hours later.

Periodic mood changes are described in both normal mental states and in emotional illnesses. Dramatic changes in affect occur in manic-depressive illness. One group has reported that some hormonal functions may free run whereas other rhythms adhere to the 24-hour cycle and has correlated depression with the times when hormonal functions are out of phase.

FACTORS INFLUENCING CIRCADIAN RHYTHMICITY

The human being, like most other species on earth, evolved in a regular 24-hour light-dark cycle. Yet many changes have occurred in human life-style that have an effect on circadian rhythmicity. The invention of the light bulb caused an interference with light-dark cycles.

Persons who have experienced unconventional sleep-wake schedules, such as persons working evening and night shifts and persons traveling across time zones, may have disruption of circadian rhythms. That is, the rhythm of such individuals may be out of phase with persons sleeping in the nighttime hours and with the majority of persons in that time zone.

The hospital environment may disrupt the circadian rhythms of patients subjected to relatively constant levels of noise, light, and activity around the clock, such as occurs in intensive care units.

A good deal of work has been devoted to determining whether interference with circadian rhythms results in disorders in the affected individual. Two particularly fruitful areas for this study have been work situations requiring a change in the sleep-wakefulness pattern and rapid travel across time zones.

Shift Work

Industrial shift workers demonstrate changes in accuracy and accident proneness. Some 16% of workers in the United States and about 60 million persons worldwide are known to rotate between day and night shifts or to be assigned permanently to evening or night work. Workers who change shifts give an indication of some imbalance in rhythms.

The major health disruptions associated with shift work are disruptions of sleep and digestive disorders. It is not feasible for shift workers to sleep at the normal phase of the circadian cycle. Sleep may occur at the phase of maximum arousal of the endogenous rhythm. Other persons in their lives may be awake and making noise as the shift worker tries to sleep. Food may be available only at times of days when the hormones and enzymes of the gastrointestinal tract are at low ebb. As many as 80% of persons who rotate shifts report sleep disruption, including insomnia and sleepiness at work. Disruptions of the circadian cycle have been associated with emotional disturbance and impaired coordination. Temperature changes over the 24-hour period are reduced in amplitude. The work schedules of health care professionals, particularly house officers and nurses, often disrupt circadian synchrony.

Long-distance Travel

Long-distance travel across time zones results in a derangement of rhythms so that several days are required to adapt to local time. A 5-hour flight westward results in a readjustment period of 2 days for the sleep-wakefulness cycle, 5 days for body temperature, and 8 days for cortisol secretion.

Travel by airplane produces rapid shifts in environmental light-dark cycles. At one time travel in an easterly or westerly direction was sufficiently slow that the time zones below the Arctic Circle (500 to 1000 miles wide) could not be traversed in a single day, and the light-dark cycle rarely deviated more than a few minutes from 24 hours, which is well within the range of entrainment. Since the advent of widespread commercial jet travel, increasing numbers of people fly on trips that cross more than one time zone. The symptoms developed by persons who travel across time zones have been labeled *jet lag* and include disruption of sleep, gastrointestinal disturbances, decreased attention span, diminished alertness, and a general feeling of malaise. Although most persons can cope with a phase shift across a single time zone, the symptomatology is increasingly severe as the number of zones traveled is increased. Persons with the lowest amplitude of rhythms shifted most readily. Circadian resynchronization occurs more rapidly for most people after westbound travel (phase delay) than for eastbound (phase advance) flights.

The advice given to the traveler who will stay in a new time zone for several weeks for rhythm adjustment is to maximize the strength of external *Zeitgebers*, particularly social cues. Adjustment to the new time zone is facilitated by being active in the new daytime and sleeping during the new night, eating meals at local times, and seeking out social contact of persons adjusted to the new time schedule. Short visits to a new time zone may best be accommodated with the least stress by maintaining home schedules for activities, eating, and social contact.

Age

It is known that the age of an animal determines the strength of entrainment by a *Zeitgeber*. The newborn may require several weeks of neural maturation for accurate entrainment to occur. Entrainment to local time takes much longer at 3½ months of age compared with 16½ months.

Circadian clocks have been shown to run faster with advancing age. That is, the free-running period gradually shortens. The change may not be caused by a change in the master clock regulating the timing of the organism. Hormonal changes that occur with aging may alter the clock function.

The coupling to environmental cues appears weaker with aging. For instance, the sleep-wake cycle appears to be less precisely synchronized to environmental time with age. The amplitude of circadian rhythms also diminishes with age.

SLEEP-WAKEFULNESS PATTERNS

Sleep has been identified as a basic human need. The phenomenon of sleep can relieve the individual of stress and responsibility when a break is needed to recharge the person's spirit, mind, and body; or it can remain maddeningly aloof when it is needed most. The inability to sleep and rest is one of the causes as well as one of the accompaniments of disease.

Sleep is defined as a normal, physiologic condition that can be regarded as a state of consciousness generally occurring at the low phase of the circadian rhythm, from which one can be aroused by stimuli of sufficient magnitude. Sleep is a complex physiologic phenomenon influenced by pathophysiologic, physical, psychological, environmental, and maturational factors. Sleep patterns are highly individual. The cyclic pattern of sleep stages for REM and non-REM sleep and the circadian rhythmic synchronization of sleep are influenced, for example, by chronic and acute illness, stress, age, pain, medication, hospitalization, sensory overload and deprivation, and life-style disruptions. Although the precise function of sleep is not clear, most persons agree that the act of sleep is refreshing and that it is a time of physiologic and psychosocial reintegration.

Clients may complain of sleep-pattern disturbance as a primary problem or one due to another condition. It has been recorded that one fifth to one third of clients who seek health care complain of a difficulty related to sleep. It has been estimated that 20% to 40% of the U.S. population has some type of sleep disturbance. Thus, the magnitude of sleep problems can be appreciated both in the number of individuals involved and in the degree to which a client may be incapacitated.

Factors identified as influencing the length of time an individual will spend sleeping and the quality of that sleep are (1) anxiety related to the need to meet a task, such as waking at an early hour for work; (2) the promise of pleasurable activity, such as starting a vacation; (3) the conditioned patterns of sleeping; (4) physiologic makeup; (5) age; and (6) physiologic alteration, such as disease. Whether the individual had a "good night's sleep" has been found to depend on the number of awakenings and on the total number of hours of sleep.

The primary care provider is the most appropriate person to evaluate the client with sleep-pattern disturbance. The practitioner must be aware of the individual's unique rest and sleep needs.

Sleep Research

Sleep research has been systematically conducted for only the past 40 years. Before this time sleep was thought to be a relatively simple, uniform state. It is now recognized that sleep is a complex cyclic progression of stages with changes in neurochemistry and skeletal muscle activity. The reported findings of research have shown the diagnostic value of having the client report the sleep-wakefulness pattern as part of the history. These data will indicate the need for further intervention. The EEG tracings of subjects who are asleep have been analyzed by many researchers. The findings have been correlated with physiologic alterations that accompany various EEG sleep patterns as well as with affective phenomena reported by the subjects when they awaken naturally or are awakened by the observers. These studies have indicated that clients' complaints of inability to sleep well may have their basis in organic diseases.

Furthermore, observation for signs of sleep disturbance may yield valuable data for the ongoing assessment and management of the hospitalized client. It has been shown that sleep consists of cyclic patterns of physiologic signs that recur periodically throughout the night.

The physiologic measurements most valuable to defining the sleep pattern are (1) the recordings of electrical potential made from electrodes placed on the surface of the head (EEG), (2) the tracing made from sensors (electro-oculogram [EOG]) of ocular movement made from both eyes, and (3) the record derived from sensors for skeletal muscle tone (electromyogram [EMG]); these sensors are generally placed beneath the client's jaw.

The differentiation of sleep stages from the EEG tracing is based on alterations in the frequency and amplitude of the brain wave tracings recorded from subjects who are asleep (Fig. 4-1). Waves of 8 to 12 cycles per second (cps) are called alpha activity and are the typical waveforms of a person at rest. Sleep spindles are defined as bursts of waves of 12 to 16 cps, and those greater than 12 (mean 20 cps) cps are called beta activity. Slower waves of 4 to 7 cps are called theta activity, and those of 1 to 3 cps are described as delta activity (Table 4-3).

Table 4-3

Differentiation of brain wave tracings

EEG pattern	CPS	Sleep-wakefulness cycle
Beta	>12 (average 20)	Alert wakefulness; REM sleep
Sleep spindles	12-16	Stage 2
Alpha	8-12	Relaxed wakefulness; stage 1
Theta	4-7	
Delta	1-3	Stages 3 and 4

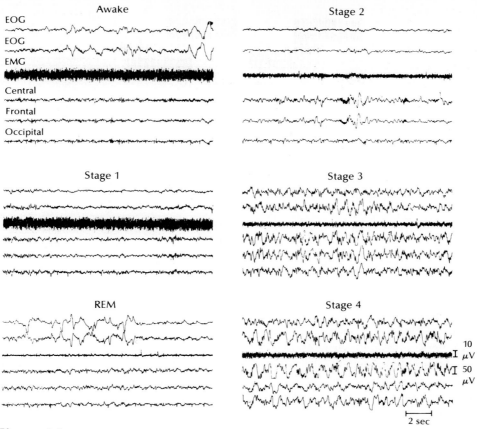

Figure 4-1

Sleep stages. The same six channels are used throughout, as labeled in the *awake* record. *EOG,* Eye movements; *EMG,* muscle tonus from beneath the chin. Note the high EMG and eye movements in the awake state, the absence of REMs in stage 1 (NREM), and REMs with decreased muscle tonus during REM sleep. Stages 2, 3, and 4 show progressive slowing of frequency and an increase in amplitude of the EEG.

(From Kales A and others: Ann Intern Med 68:1078, 1968.)

The normal adult has low-amplitude, fast-frequency activity in the waking state. Alpha activity is the most frequent type of activity recorded during what the subject believed was a period of rest.

Some authorities refer to the awake and resting states as stage 0 of the sleep cycle. During sleep, four characteristic tracings of NREM sleep can be isolated, making up the stages of sleep called NREM stages 1, 2, 3, and 4 and a fifth stage of REM. These five stages constitute the sleep cycle (Table 4-4).

The Sleep Cycle

In the critical stage of falling asleep, alpha waves decrease in the EEG record. Sleep spindle waveforms appear within 1 to 2 minutes and herald the beginning of NREM stage 2. Stage 2 lasts 5 to 10 minutes, and its termination marks the end of light sleep. NREM stage 3 is identified on the EEG record as the appearance of delta

Table 4-4

Principal levels of human activity

Level of activity	EEG pattern	Skeletal muscle
Awake (or arousal)		
Stage 0	Beta-aroused	Corticospinal control
	Alpha-relaxed	Modified by basal ganglia and cerebellum
NREM sleep		
Stage 1	Beta to theta	Turning occurs
Stage 2	Sleep spindles	Movements in response to stimuli
Stage 3	Delta	
Stage 4	Delta	
REM sleep	Beta	Atonia

Table 4-5

The initial sleep cycle

Stages of sleep	EEG brainwaves	Time span	Approximate percentage of total night's sleep	Affective aspects	Physiologic alterations
NREM (slow wave) sleep					
Stage 1	Alpha activity (may be beta to theta)	1-7 min	5%-10%	Fleeting thoughts; may be unaware of being asleep	Light sleep, easily awakened; pulse rate decreased 10-30 beats per min; basal metabolism rate (BMR) decreased 10%-15%; temperature and respiration decreased; muscle tone minimal; knee jerks abolished; slight decrease in blood pressure
Stage 2	Sleep spindles	5-10 min	50%		
Stage 3	Delta activity appears (20% to 50%)	10 min	10%-20%		Transition sleep
Stage 4	Delta activity predominates (75%)	5-15 min			Deep sleep; difficult to awaken
REM sleep	Desynchronized pattern of low-voltage beta activity—similar to waking EEG	10 min, first cycle; 10-12 min, second cycle; 20-30 min as length of total sleep increases	20%-25%	Dreams believed to occur	Physiologically active; paradoxical muscle movements, that is, rapid eye movements; increase in cerebral blood flow, brain temperature, and body oxygen consumption (most skeletal muscle tone depressed; tendon reflexes depressed)

The sleeper, on falling asleep, goes through NREM stages 1 through 4 and then returns to stage 3 and then to stage 2, followed by a period of REM sleep. This pattern is considered a sleep cycle and usually takes 90 minutes (see Fig. 4-2). Further sleep involves stages 2, 3, and sometimes 4, returning to stage 3 and then to stage 2, with another slightly longer REM period.

activity. These slow waves make up 20% to 50% of the EEG sleep record. This transition stage between light and deep sleep may last about 10 minutes. As stage 4 sleep is entered, sleep spindles disappear and high-voltage slow waves occupy 50% or more of the EEG record. This stage lasts from 5 to 15 minutes.

During these four stages of sleep, eye movements are not observed and skeletal muscle tone is only slightly less in amplitude than during the waking state. Calling these four stages NREM allows for categorization of sleep into two categories: NREM and REM (Table 4-5).

During a normal sleeping period, the client experiences NREM stage 1 sleep followed by NREM stages 2, 3, and 4 sleep. Then there is a reverse from NREM stage 4 sleep to NREM stages 3 and 2. After about 60 to 90 minutes of this pattern of sleep, the first period of REM sleep occurs. The EEG is characterized by lower voltage and by the absence of big, slow waves and sleep spindles.

Gross eye movements can be seen and recorded (EOG). The first REM period of sleep lasts approximatey 10 minutes and is characterized by a lack of body movement. This period is thought to be the time that most dreaming occurs. The client may recall the dream only if awakened during the REM stage. Dreaming associated with REM sleep is not easily correlated with waking activities and is therefore less realistic. The remembered ideation occurring in NREM sleep seems more like the thinking that surrounds daily life activities.

At the end of the initial REM period, the sleeper returns to NREM stages 2, 3, and sometimes 4, returning again to stage 3 and then to stage 2. This second period of NREM sleep lasts about 60 to 90 minutes. This is followed by another, slightly longer REM period (10 to 12 minutes). The transition from stage to stage is accompanied by body movement. A healthy adult probably turns 30 to 40 times during a night's sleep. The mobility of sleep protects the sleeper from the hazards of remaining motionless, that is, pressure changes in the micro-circulation, thrombus formation, or diminished respiration, which might possibly lead to pneumonia.

Sleep stages are regulated by an ultradian rhythm of approximately 90 minutes (70- to 110-minute cycles) throughout the night. The pattern of the cycles changes over the course of a normal night's sleep. As the night progresses, there are decreasing periods of delta sleep and more frequent and longer periods of REM, and later in the sleep period more REMs are observed per minute.

As the sleep period continues, the length of the NREM sleep periods decreases and the length of the REM periods increases. In addition, the depth of sleep, usually that of stages 2 and 3, decreases. Thus, the client achieves the greatest amount of stages 3 and 4 sleep early in the sleep period, whereas most of the REM sleep occurs in the later cycles of the sleep period (see Fig. 4-1).

The total number of cycles in a normal sleep period ranges from four to six, depending on the total length of the sleep period.

REM sleep

Phasic activity that occurs during REM sleep may be considered that of an arousal state generated by bursts of central nervous system (CNS) activity, resulting in muscle twitches, eye movements, phasic changes in pupil size and cardiopulmonary irregularities. REM sleep has been described as a physiologically active period. The forebrain appears to be aroused. Animal studies have demonstrated that there is an increase in cerebral blood flow as well as in brain temperature. Lability of cardiopulmonary parameters is the rule with REM sleep; there is a marked variation in heart and respiratory rate as well as in blood pressure.

Tonic inhibition of skeletal muscles occurs during REM sleep. The absence of EMG activity, particularly as recorded from the digastric or neck muscles, has been cited to support the statement that there is generalized, skeletal motor inhibition. This large muscle paralysis has been conjectured to be a mechanism for preventing the dreamer from acting out dreams. Tendon reflexes are also suppressed.

Phasically occurring conjugated eye movements or REMs provided the title for this phase of the sleep cycle. Some muscle twitches that affect the jaw and distal muscles of the limbs have been observed. These movements are produced by short-lasting but powerful excitatory volleys. Although some movement is observed, the volleys cannot overcome the postural atonia.

On the other hand, some muscles are not suppressed. These are the diaphragm, the extraocular, middle ear, and intercostal muscles, some facial muscles, and the muscles of the pharynx and larynx. Penile erection

may occur in REM sleep, an observation used clinically to evaluate impotence. The presence of an erection during sleep rules out pathophysiologic etiology from psychogenic causes of impotence.

Peripheral resistance is decreased and an associated reduction in mean blood pressure results. Arterial blood pressure values are lower during the first hours of sleep and gradually increase toward the second part of the night.

Heart rate decreases during REM sleep compared with wakefulness have been reported. Increased variability of heart rate compared with NREM sleep has been consistently reported, made up of phasically occurring tachycardia. Respiratory rate has been shown to be slightly increased during REM sleep, but, like heart rate, can be highly variable. Respiratory irregularities often include short-lasting central apneas. Blood gases are similar in REM and NREM sleep. Penile erection has been consistently observed in REM sleep; the response is more marked during the late night. Endocrine decreases in prolactin secretion have been observed during REM sleep.

This stage is also referred to as paradoxical rhombencephalic, emergent, dream, or desynchronized sleep. Although data show that most REM sleep occurs during the last half of the sleep period, REM can occur during naps if the nap is long enough. For the night sleeper, morning naps contain largely REM sleep, whereas afternoon naps are largely made up of NREM stage 4 sleep. Several investigators have posited that REM sleep serves to reprogram the brain, particularly through the assimilation of new experiences into the existing personality structure. Some theorists contend that the function of REM sleep is to keep disturbing or threatening information from reaching the waking consciousness. Another theory is that the REM arousal periods are the mechanism for vigilance during the rest period that may have contributed to our distant ancestors' survival.

NREM stages 3 and 4 (slow wave) sleep

NREM sleep represents 80% of the total sleeping time and is also called slow wave sleep. Slow wave sleep is characterized by a decrease in tempo of the body's physiologic processes. The basal metabolism rate (BMR) is decreased 10% to 15%, resulting in a decrease in body temperature of approximately 1° F. The pulse rate is decreased 10 to 30 beats, and the respiratory rate shows compensatory slowing. The blood pressure is slightly decreased. Muscle tone is minimal and knee jerks are abolished. All these characteristics represent an acute inhibitory process. Reflexes are weaker and slower to appear. The pupils of the eye are constricted in sleep and, with relaxation of the extraocular muscles, appear to "roll," that is, are not aligned. Growth hormone is known to be secreted in NREM stage 4.

Significance of the sleep stages in health assessment

The clinical significance of the presence or absence of the sleep stages in humans is still not clearly understood. Furthermore, it is difficult to make a judgment from the client's explanations of sleep patterns whether there is more REM or NREM sleep deprivation. Some investigators have reported, however, that loss of REM sleep is more likely to cause agitation and irritability or, in some persons, apathy and depression. Most clients report malaise or tiredness when the REM sleep period is shortened.

The EEG pattern may provide support to other data in differentiating such conditions as depression, narcolepsy, endocrine abnormality, or drug dependency.

Sleep Patterns Throughout the Life Cycle

Over the life cycle, decrements are noted in the time spent in total sleep, in NREM stage 4 sleep, and in REM sleep.

Sleep patterns in the young adult. The young, physically active, healthy adult spends 20% to 25% of sleep time in REM sleep, 50% in stage 2 sleep, and 5% to 10% in stage 1 sleep. The remaining 10% to 20% of sleep time is spent in a combination of stages 3 and 4 sleep (Fig. 4-2). Although most adults sleep 7 to 9 hours a day, many normal individuals sleep more than 9 hours, and another group of normal individuals sleep 6 hours or less in a 24-hour period. One study showed that the long sleepers had a high incidence of mild to moderate anxiety, depression, and social introversion, whereas the short sleepers were predominantly healthy, efficient, and energetic persons who tended to work hard or otherwise keep busy and who were satisfied with themselves and their lives.

Sleep patterns in the infant and child. The newborn spends 50% of sleep time in REM sleep. By the age of 1 year, this is reduced to 20% to 30%, which approximates the adult value. Stage 4 sleep is greater in amount during childhood. Sleep cycles in the neonate are 45 to 60 minutes long and increase as the individual matures. The total sleep time for the normal newborn may be 14 to 18 hours a day. The child develops normal sleep cycles between 2 and 5 years of age.

Sleep patterns in the aged. "Can't sleep at night" is a frequent description of the sleep of the elderly client. Stage 4 sleep is markedly decreased and sometimes absent in the aged adult. The total sleeping time is diminished as a result of frequent and prolonged wak-

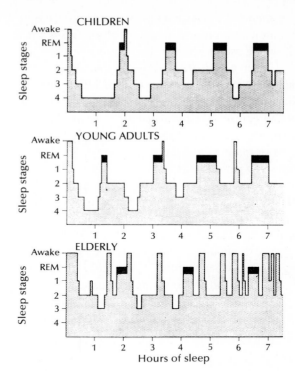

Figure 4-2

Sleep cycles of normal subjects. The sleep of children and young adults shows early preponderance of stages 3 and 4, progressive lengthening of the first three REM periods, and infrequent awakenings. In elderly adults there is little or no stage 4 sleep, REM periods are fairly uniform in length, and awakenings are frequent and often lengthy.
(From Kales A and others: Ann Intern Med 68:1078, 1968.)

ing periods. This is distinguished from the early morning awakening in clinical depression.

Although REM sleep continues to occupy 20% to 25% of the total sleep time, REM latency at every period (the time from the onset of sleep to the first REM activity) is decreased, and the first REM period is longer. The EEG record may show poorly formed spindles that occur at a lower frequency. Insomniacs who are less than 50 years of age generally have difficulty in falling asleep; those over 50 complain of difficulty in staying asleep or in awakening early in the morning. It has been shown that these age-related sleep changes may begin at age 30 in men and age 50 in women.

The sleep-deprived elderly client shows deficits in stages 3 and 4 and REM activity. A question to elicit a description of sleep pattern changes relevant to the aging process might be "Is your sleep the same as it has always been?"

Average sleep times

The average sleep time is 16 hours in neonates, 8 hours at age 12, 7 hours for ages 25 to 45, and 6½ hours for the elderly. It has been shown that older persons stay in bed longer but sleep less than younger individuals.

BEHAVIORS OR DISORDERS RELATED TO SLEEP

Effects of Sleep Deprivation

A disruption in sleeping affects family life, employment, and general social adjustment. Sleep laboratory experiments have been conducted to determine the effects of sleep loss in human beings. The loss of 60 to 200 hours of sleep resulted in the following observations: feelings of fatigue, irritability, difficulty in concentrating, difficulty in maintaining orientation, illusions, hallucinations—particularly visual and tactile, decreased psychomotor ability, decreased incentive to work, mild nystagmus, tremor of hands, and increase in glucocorticoid and adrenergic hormone secretion.

The affective description associated with sleep loss includes tiredness or fatigue, increased anxiety, irritability, and sleepiness. Neurologic changes associated with sleep loss have included decreased reflexes, muscle tremor, particularly of the hands; skeletal muscle weakness, such as neck flexion; lack of coordination of motor movements; dysarthria and decreased facial expressive movements; and decreased attention span. Prolonged sleep deprivation has been accompanied by delusions, hallucinations, visual distortions, and paranoid and psychotic behavior. The sleep-deprived individual may appear apathetic or hyperactive and agitated. The poorest performance of the sleep-deprived individual occurs in monotonous and prolonged tasks. Accurate assessment of functioning on short-term tasks is difficult because these individuals appear capable of concentrating effectively for short periods.

Anterior pituitary hormone secretion (GH, adreno-corticotropic hormone [ACTH], and thyroid-stimulating hormone [TSH]) follows a circadian rhythm with maximum secretion rates occurring in the early morning during the later period of sleep. It is known that growth is delayed when insufficient sleep is obtained.

Laboratory tests performed on sleep-deprived individuals show an increase in creatinine phosphokinase (CPK), glucose, and cortisol but a decrease in plasma iron and cholesterol.

The individual has an increased total sleep time following total sleep deprivation, with the increment reflected to stages 3 and 4. Although total REM sleep is increased in the first recovery night, the percentage of REM activity shows little actual change. The second night REM sleep is in greater proportion than that of the subject before the sleep loss; this is REM rebound. An-

---

Sleep Disorders

Conditions associated with excessive daytime sleepiness	Conditions associated with chronic insomnia
Sleep apnea	Pain
Narcolepsy	Sleep apnea
Stimulant dependency	Restless legs syndrome
Shift change ⎱ Circadian	Nocturnal myoclonus
Change of ⎰ rhythm	Alpha sleep
time zone ⎰ disruption	Depression—nonpsychotic, i.e., loss of a loved one
Resulting from:	Exercise just before sleep
Hypothyroidism	Caffeine
Brain tumor	Coffee > 4 cups
	Tea
	Colas
	Resulting from:
	Aging
	Hyperthyroidism
	Anorexia nervosa
	Psychoses:
	Depression
	Manic-depressive illness
	Schizophrenia
	Change of ⎱ Circadian
	time zone ⎰ rhythm
	Shift change ⎰ disruption
	Environmental discomfort
	Noise
	Cold
	Drug dependency and drug withdrawal
	Steroid administration
	Alcoholism

---

imals that are selectively deprived of REM sleep for several nights are hyperactive and have excessive appetite for food and sexual activity. Those deprived of NREM sleep are less responsive than normal.

Most sleeping pills decrease REM sleep and, therefore, dreaming. Withdrawal of the medication is followed by an increase in REM sleep and dreaming.

Psychotropic drugs (or those that alter the function of the CNS), sedatives or tranquilizers, hypnotic antidepressants, and stimulants have been observed to alter the course of sleep.

The box above lists various sleep disorders.

Primary Sleep Disorders

Primary sleep disorders are those in which disordered sleep is the only symptom or sign of a problem. These disorders include sleeping periods in excess or less than what is considered a normal sleeping period. Insomnia is the general term for a shortened sleeping period. Hypersomnia and narcolepsy are examples of conditions wherein the client sleeps longer than the normal individual.

Disorders of initiating and maintaining sleep (DIMS)

Insomnia. The term *insomnia,* which literally means a complete lack of sleep in common usage, includes the inability to fall asleep, frequent or prolonged awakening, or shortened sleep periods (early morning awakening).

EEG studies of insomniacs have shown the affected individual to have varying sleep spindle production, longer sleep latencies, shorter sleep periods, and less efficient sleep. These individuals are believed to have greater levels of REM sleep than other persons.

General causes of insomnia. Transient insomnia may occur with changes of shift at work or with travel across time zones. Insomnia often accompanies health problems, for example, pain, physical discomfort, fear, or depression. Poor sleep may accompany stressful periods such as the loss of a loved one or pressures from school or job. Environmental factors such as noise or cold can interrupt sleep. Drugs have been shown to be a cause of insomnia, for example, amphetamines, steroid preparations, central adrenergic blockers, and bronchodilating drugs. Insomnia may follow the withdrawal of short-acting benzodiazepine hypnotics. An excess of caffeine in coffee, tea, or colas may interfere with sleep. Insomnia is known to occur more commonly in those over 30 years of age than in younger individuals and is most likely to occur in women older than 50.

Individuals with insomnia have been shown to have higher levels of physiologic arousal before and during the sleep period. The poorer sleeper has more body movements during sleep. Both heart rate and temperature are increased before and during sleep.

Several subgroups of insomniacs have been cited based on the pattern of sleep loss. They are described as follows:

1. *Initial insomnia:* Inability to fall asleep, usually as a result of rumination on situational stress, sleep phobia, or anxiety. Autonomic activity is higher during sleep in these persons compared with the normal sleeper. The normal individual falls asleep in 10 to 15 minutes.

   The cause of sleep latency may be apparent from the history. Examples of questions that might reveal situational stress or anxiety as the cause of initial insomnia include: "How are things going at work?" "Have you had a lot of worries lately?" or "How are you getting along with your spouse?" Initial insomnia is the most common type of sleep loss in young adults.

2. *Delayed sleep phase insomnia:* Difficulty in falling asleep at night followed by difficulty awakening in the morning. Sleep time is relatively constant, and sleep pattern is essentially normal. The disorder affects approximately 10% of clients reporting difficulty in sleeping. The disorder can be tolerated by adjustments in activity schedules, and therefore it is probable that many more persons do not report this disorder.

3. *Maintenance or intermittent insomnia.* Disruption of sleep occurring during midcycle as a result of a startle reaction from internal or external stimuli. This is the most common type of insomnia.

4. *Terminal insomnia:* Early awakening. This may be a result of aging or may be an important sign of depression. It could also mean the person is napping during the day or retiring early.

5. *Imaginary insomnia:* Subjective insomnia. The person appears to have slept but claims to have had no sleep.

   Both the shift worker who has incurred a change in working hours and the traveler who has crossed a time zone have disrupted circadian rhythms and may suffer insomnia. These individuals complain of daytime sleepiness, anxiety, or depression and have somatic symptoms and impaired psychomotor ability.

   Insomniacs often show an improved sleeping pattern following a judicious increase in activity and exercise during the waking period. However, activity just before bedtime has an excitatory effect in most instances. A thorough assessment of a client who reports insomnia includes a description of activities of daily living. It is important, particularly, to determine the amount and vigorousness of exercise subscribed to by the client who has difficulty sleeping.

   Some investigators have suggested that most insomniacs have problems in sexual adjustment or functioning. The client's description of sexual activity is therefore assessed.

   Sleep has been shown to be improved by:

1. A regular time to go to bed and time to rise (Explanation: A regular schedule strengthens the sleep-wake cycle.)
2. Regular daily exercise (Explanation: Exercise may increase levels of endogenous opioids.)
3. Soundproof room or ear plugs (Explanation: Loud noises are known to disrupt sleep; eliminating anti-sleep stimuli should improve sleep.)

4. A light bedtime snack such as milk or tuna fish (Explanation: Tryptophan, a precursor of serotonin, and perhaps other amino acids have sleep-inducing effects. Foods rich in tryptophan, such as milk and tuna fish, might be soporific.)
5. Avoidance of alcohol (Explanation: Alcohol reduces sleep latency and increases slow wave sleep but is associated with increased wakefulness after sleep onset as a result of REM breakthrough.)
6. Avoidance of caffeine (Explanation: Caffeine is a stimulant and is known to modify circadian rhythms.)
7. Avoidance of smoking (Explanation: Both nicotine and the resultant increased carbon monoxide blood levels may cause arousal.)

Persons with insomnia should not stay in bed tossing and turning but should get up and find an absorbing and satisfying activity until they feel tired again.

Nocturnal myoclonus. Chronic insomnia may be symptomatic of nocturnal myoclonus. Clients complain of frequent arousals and aching leg muscles at night and in the morning. Nocturnal myoclonus is a condition characterized by marked muscle contraction resulting in jerking of one or both legs. The jerking has a periodicity of approximately 28 seconds and occurs in NREM sleep. When the contractions are pronounced, EEG arousal is noted and the client may be aroused to consciousness (one of ten cases). Nocturnal myoclonus has been observed in 10% to 20% of chronic insomniacs. The client's sleeping partner may complain of being kicked at night. Treatment may include clonazepam or benzodiazepines. Measures to reduce stress in the patient's life may decrease exacerbations.

Restless legs syndrome. Restless legs syndrome (RLS) is a problem incurred during the waking state; the affected individual is unable to keep the body, particularly the legs, at rest for the time necessary for falling asleep. The client complains of discomfort when the legs are immobile or when lying down for more than 15 to 20 seconds. Deep paresthesias are also common. These symptoms may prevent the client from falling asleep. Opioids such as oxycodone are used to treat patients with RLS. Increased anxiety should be addressed in any treatment plan.

Sleep apnea

Sleep apnea is a periodic cessation of breathing that occurs during sleep. Sleep apneas are further classified by nature into central, obstructive, and mixed forms of sleep apnea. The central apneas are those in which there is failure of neural output initiating respiration. Obstructive apneas are those in which there is a drive to breathe; however, airflow is obstructed, usually at the level of the posterior pharynx. Mixed apnea syndromes are a combination of central and obstructive components, usually with the central component followed by airflow obstruction.

Sleep apnea is diagnosed in the sleep laboratory with polysomnography, monitoring of muscle movements, an ear oximeter, a nasal or oral thermistor, and a chest wall motion monitor or strain gauge. In obstructive sleep apnea, there is a pause in nasal and oral airflow, although respiratory efforts continue as evidenced by thoracic strain gauge recordings. Desaturation is associated with the pause in respiration. Central sleep apnea is documented again with a pause in nasal and oral airflow coinciding with lack of respiratory movements on the thoracic strain gauge. There is desaturation to a lesser degree, however. Mixed sleep apnea is a combination of both types, with the central component preceding the obstructive component.

Obstructive sleep apnea. The client diagnosed as having obstructive sleep apnea is typically a middle-aged overweight man with a history of hypertension who complains of excessive daytime sleepiness. Periods of heavy snoring and morning headache are frequent complaints. Enlarged adenoids or tonsils predispose to this disorder, which results from relaxation of the muscles of the nasopharynx, hypopharynx, and pharynx during sleep. The period of apnea leads to progressive hypercapnia, hypoxemia, increased pulmonary arterial pressures, and possibly life-threatening cardiac arrhythmias. Treatment modalities include avoidance of alcohol and respiratory suppressants such as benzodiazepines, weight loss, medroxyprogesterone acetate, protriptyline, and theophylline. Nasal continuous positive airway pressure (CPAP) has been helpful to many patients, making the need for tracheostomy less common. The surgical removal of redundant tissue in the pharynx, called uvulopalatopharyngoplasty (UPPP), is another option.

Central sleep apnea. In general, persons with central sleep apnea tend to be older than those with obstructive apnea, although central apnea occurs in infants and may be involved in the apnea of prematurity and in sudden infant death syndrome (SIDS). Patients complain of daytime sleepiness, fatigue, loss of libido, or impotence. Persons with central sleep apnea have responded to treatment with protriptyline, diaphragmatic pacing, and nasal CPAP.

Disorders of excessive somnolence (DOES)

Hypersomnia. *Hypersomnia* is the term used to describe the condition wherein an individual tends to sleep for excessive periods. In some clients the sleep period may be extended to 16 to 18 hours a day. The episodes of hypersomnia may be acute or chronic. The EEG sleep patterning is normal. Victims of hypersomnia are found to have higher pulse and respiratory rates than normal individuals during both sleep and wakefulness.

Perihypersomnia is a condition that is described as an increased need for sleep (18 to 20 hours a day) that lasts for only a few days, following which the client is fine.

Hypersomnia has been correlated with uremia, increased intracranial pressure, and diabetic acidosis. The hypothyroid client may report longer hours spent in sleep and sleepiness when awake.

In some cases hypersomnia may be a conversion symptom. The severely anxious client may be escaping discomfort in sleep. The hysterical personality and the depressed individual are predisposed to conversion symptoms. This mechanism should be looked for particularly when the need to sleep occurs repeatedly in conjunction with potentially troublesome experiences, such as "Whenever my in-laws come for a visit."

Narcolepsy.   Narcolepsy ("sleep attacks") is the term used to describe the excessive daytime drowsiness or uncontrolled onset of sleep. Although the pathophysiology of narcolepsy is not clearly understood, it is safe to say that the condition is a disorder in the sleep regulatory mechanism. The episode of sleep occurs when the client is engaged in what are considered to be wake-time activities. Some 10% of diagnosed narcoleptics have described situations of falling asleep while driving and causing accidents. Others have fallen asleep in such unusual activities as standing at attention while in the military service or while eating. It is particularly important to be alert to the evidence that will establish the diagnosis so that treatment may be instituted, since the untreated narcoleptic is dangerous to the self and to others. The annual incidence is thought to be at least 0.07% in the United States.

The episodes of involuntary sleep may begin just before puberty, that is, at approximately 12 years of age in girls and 14 years of age in boys. The range of age for the first attack may occur any time between 10 and 40, however. The familial involvement should be explored, since family members show an incidence of narcolepsy 20 times that of the general population.

Clinical records indicate that affected individuals may have the condition for as long as 15 years before it is diagnosed. This is particularly unfortunate, since the attacks can be eliminated by amphetamines or methylphenidate (Ritalin) hydrochloride.

Because most normal people feel sleepy from time to time during the day, particularly at quiet times, such as during a dull lecture or television broadcast, a careful history is necessary to differentiate this dozing phenomenon from narcolepsy.

Automatism is sometimes reported by the narcoleptic victim's relatives. The person appears to be awake but may act irrationally. The client does not remember the episode.

Diagnosed narcoleptics are observed to sleep fewer hours than their normal counterparts, and the sleep they do obtain is interrupted and restless. They fall asleep remarkably quickly, sometimes within 15 seconds after lying down, and complain of difficulty in waking up.

Narcolepsy has been described as a tetrad of four symptoms: sleep attacks, cataplexy, hypnagogic hallucinations, and sleep paralysis. The final two symptoms occur in the transition period between sleep and wakefulness and indicate narcolepsy only when accompanied by the preceding symptoms.

Sleep attacks.   The uncontrolled sleep in the early stages of the disorder occurs infrequently and under conditions that are described by normal people as sleep inducing. The episodes increase in number and occur in increasingly bizarre circumstances. Eventually the episodes occur 3 to 5 times a day, lasting 5 to 15 minutes. Some of these victims fall asleep without warning, whereas others feel sleepy for minutes or hours before succumbing to sleep.

Cataplexy.   Approximately 4 to 5 years after the disorder is initiated, the client may experience cataplexy, an abrupt weakness or paralysis of voluntary muscles seen predominantly in the arms, legs, and face. There are many gradations of the loss of voluntary skeletal contraction. The episode may be experienced as only a fleeting weakness or as the inability to move quickly. On the other hand, all the skeletal muscles may be paralyzed. The intraocular muscles are a frequent exception. The client may still be capable of perceiving the external environment and may describe the attacks as "My knees buckled," "My jaws sagged," "I couldn't speak," "The muscles of my neck were twitching," or "I couldn't walk."

The cataplectic attack may last from a half second to 10 minutes, and the client may experience them only once or twice a year or as often as 100 times a day. The attacks appear to be triggered by strong emotion, loud noise, a startle reaction, or sudden fright. Hearty laughter has frequently been implicated as a stimulus to the episodes.

Hypnagogic hallucinations.   These attacks may be described as dream episodes. They are generally disturbing or frightening dreams that occur as the client is falling asleep. The client describes the dream as very real— "As if I were right there"—and the feeling as one of being awake. This can occur in the normal individual.

Sleep paralysis.   The phenomenon of sleep paralysis is a skeletal muscle paralysis of varying degrees that occurs when the client awakes or is falling asleep. The client describes the arousal as one of waking and being aware of external conditions but unable to move or speak. If undisturbed, the client recovers gradually. However, if stimulated, as by touching, paralysis ameliorates quickly. Sleep paralysis may occur in as many as 2% to 3% of the normal population.

Relation to REM sleep. Although nacrolepsy has been linked to epilepsy in the past because of similar EEG patterning, it is not the same, nor can narcolepsy be logically attributed to depression or schizophrenia. More acceptable in the light of research findings is that narcolepsy is related to REM sleep. REM activity can be recorded during sleep attacks. The victim has a REM period at the beginning of the long sleep period. Some individuals with cataplexy experience REM sleep before recovery. Both hypnagogic hallucinations and sleep paralysis in normal individuals have been associated with REM activity.

Treatment. Treatment of narcolepsy includes good sleep hygiene and the use of stimulants such as dextroamphetamine, methylphenidate, and pemoline. Cataplectic attacks are treated with imipramine, clomipramine, or protriptyline (antidepressants). Support groups have been sponsored by the American Narcolepsy Association.

Parasomnias (Disorders of Partial Arousal)

Parasomnia is the term used for those patterns of waking behavior that appear during sleep. Some of those most common behaviors are night terrors, somnambulism (sleepwalking), sleep talking, bruxism (teeth grinding), and enuresis (bed-wetting).

Night terrors and dream anxiety attacks (nightmares). Night terrors occur during slow wave sleep (stages 3 and 4). Children who experience night terrors generally do not display daytime anxiety, whereas adults are likely to have anxiety symptoms.

Night terror–sleep terror. The individual with night or sleep terror has repeated episodes of abrupt awakening with symptoms of anxiety that last about 1 to 10 minutes. The episodes generally occur between 30 and 200 minutes after onset of sleep during sleep stages 3 and 4. Anxiety symptoms include tachycardia, rapid breathing, dilated pupils, sweating, and piloerection, indicating sympathetic arousal. Efforts to comfort the victim of night terrors are generally unsuccessful.

Dream anxiety attacks. Dream anxiety attacks are the most common and are considered to be milder than night terrors. They occur in the middle of sleep or later. Autonomic anxiety signs may accompany these episodes. Mental confusion frequently occurs, particularly if the sleeper is awakened suddenly.

Somnambulism. Sleepwalking is common (1% to 6%) in children between the ages of 5 and 12 years. It occurs more often in children than in adults. Boys are affected more frequently than girls. Sleepwalking has familial relationships; it is more common among family members than among the general population. Both sleepwalking and night terrors occur during stages 3 and 4 of sleep, usually between 30 and 200 minutes after onset of sleep. The sleepwalker may not awaken during the episode if active for fewer than 3 to 4 minutes but will show an awakening pattern if up longer. During ambulation the sleeper functions at a low level of awareness and critical skill.

The essential feature of sleepwalking is repeated episodes of a sequence of complex behaviors, including leaving the bed and walking. The walking periods may last from a few minutes to half an hour. The sleepwalker does not appear to be conscious and is amnesic for the episode. The face of the sleepwalker is expressionless, and efforts to communicate with the somnambulist produce little response. Although the sleepwalker appears able to see and does walk around objects, coordination is poor and stumbling and falling are hazards, particularly in going down stairs. Some sleepwalkers have walked through windows.

It is important to teach the family to protect the sleepwalker from injury by installing safety rails or guards, locks on windows, and having the somnambulist's bedroom on the ground floor.

Sleep talking. Articulation during sleep appears to be a frequent occurrence. Talking during sleep generally occurs during NREM sleep and body movement.

Bruxism. Grinding of the teeth during the sleep period, called bruxism, may occur in as many as 15% of the population. Evidence of the practice may be seen in damaged teeth or supporting structures. EEG studies demonstrate that bruxism generally is seen during stage 2 sleep.

Enuresis. The problem of enuresis has long been considered a genitourinary problem, although a pathologic condition of this system is seldom found. Primary enuresis is bed-wetting during sleep. It persists from birth to at least age 6. Secondary enuresis refers to bed-wetting during sleep by an individual who has physiologic control of micturition. This is primarily a disorder of childhood that is identified in 5% to 15% of all preadolescent children, and it may have a familial pattern. However, enuresis has been observed to exist in some sample adult groups at a rate of 1% to 2%.

Enuresis occurs more frequently in boys than in girls. Researchers have demonstrated more frequent bladder contractions and greater heart rate during the entire sleep period of those individuals affected, although the act of urination occurs in stage 2. The episode of bed-wetting occurs during slow wave sleep. Children with enuresis are generally described as deep sleepers, that is, difficult to rouse from sleep. Whereas primary enuresis may be the result of a pathophysiologic defect, secondary enuresis may be reflected to psychological factors.

In assessing the enuretic child, one should explore the affective state surrounding this condition with both the child and parents. Although data from sleep laboratories demonstrate that 90% of enuretic children are asleep when bed-wetting occurs, in most cases studied the parents believed that the child had control over the occurrence. The parents punished the child, producing shame, embarrassment, guilt, or anxiety. To investigate how the episodes have been dealt with, the following questions might be used.

To the parents: "How have you felt about your child's wetting the bed?" If this question is nonproductive, more specific information might be gained by asking, "Do you feel he (she) could prevent the bed-wetting?" or "Do you punish him (her) when he (she) wets the bed?"

To the child: "How do you feel when you wake up after wetting the bed?"

Secondary Sleep Disorders

Secondary sleep disorders are those sleep disturbances associated with other clinical disorders. Those clinical entities often accompanied by sleep disorders are alterations in thyroid hormone secretion, chronic renal insufficiency, depression, schizophrenia, alcoholism, and anorexia nervosa.

Alterations in thyroid hormone secretion. Individuals with both hyposecretion and hypersecretion of the thyroid have derangements of stage 3 and 4 sleep. Individuals with hyperthyroid conditions have decreased stages 3 and 4 sleep time, whereas persons with hypothyroid conditions show increases. Sleep patterns return to normal with adequate treatment to bring the client into the euthyroid range.

Chronic renal insufficiency. The client who undergoes dialysis treatments for chronic renal insufficiency has been observed to have sleep disturbances that occur with greatest frequency just before dialysis and are improved after the dialysis. Investigation has shown that sleep disturbances correlate with the uremic condition.

Depression. Depression is both a mental illness and a symptom. Depression is seen in the grieving process over significant loss of a loved one or possession. The depressed client has prolonged latency in achieving

sleep, more rapid transition from stage to stage, more frequent awakening, less slow wave sleep, less total sleep time, and more REM activity.

Depression as a mental illness is that which is incurred without significant loss. A subgroup of depressives is made up of those individuals who alternate between periods of depression and mania. The classical clinical description of the sleep pattern in depression is that of early morning awakening. Stage 4 sleep decreases in both manic and depressive clients. During the manic phase the client is observed to have decreased total sleep time and decreased REM activity. Depressed periods are associated with normal sleep time.

Schizophrenia. Some investigators have reported anorexia and a reduction in REM sleep in the early phases of schizophrenia. Stages 3 and 4 sleep are also significantly reduced in the schizophrenic. Greater eye movement has been reported in hallucinating schizophrenics than in nonhallucinating individuals.

Alcoholism. Studies have shown that the subject who has drunk 6 oz of 95% alcohol before sleep shows REM deprivation during the sleep period, whereas the person who drinks small amounts of alcohol may not show changes in the sleep pattern. Because alcohol is a CNS depressant, it may help the client get to sleep; but because it is a short-acting drug, it does not affect sleep maintenance. Furthermore, it may diminish REM sleep in the early hours of the sleep period and therefore contribute to a rebound increase of REM activity in the latter hours of sleep. Withdrawal studies of chronic alcoholics showed that sleep periods were made up almost entirely of REM sleep. These alcoholics frequently awakened from REM to experience hallucinations.

Both slow wave and REM sleep appear to be decreased in acute alcoholic psychosis. Initially, slow wave activity appears to increase, whereas REM sleep is suppressed. As the condition progresses both may disappear. As mentioned above, REM rebound has been employed to explain the hallucinations that occur on withdrawal of alcohol. The rebound of slow wave sleep has been cited as the harbinger of recovery from the psychosis.

Anorexia nervosa. The individual experiencing anorexia nervosa has a protein-calorie deficiency that is accompanied by a patterned sleep disturbance. There is a reduction of the deeper sleep stages, 3 and 4, as well as of REM sleep. Although stage 1 sleep is increased, there is a reduction in total sleep time.

Sleep-Provoked Disorders: Sleep Patterns in Chronic Illness

The sleep-provoked disorders include symptoms and signs of chronic clinical diseases that are elicited during sleep (Table 4-6).

Table 4-6

Clinical observations associated with stages of sleep

Stage of sleep	Associated clinical condition
NREM sleep	
Stage 1	Myoclonic jerks
	Bruxism
Stage 2	Bruxism
	Enuresis most likely to occur
Stage 3	Night terrors
	Sleepwalking
	Sleep talking
	Hypothyroidism—metabolic rate most depressed
All stages	Enuresis
	Bronchial asthma—except stage 4 in childhood
REM sleep	Nocturnal erection or emission
	Migraine headaches
	Gastric acid secretion increased
	Duodenal ulcer—incidence of epigastric pain
	Coronary atherosclerosis
	ECG changes
	Anginal attacks
	Bronchial asthma in children

Pain. Clients who experience chronic pain may complain of sleeplessness. These clients awaken frequently and stay awake for long periods. Pain due to rheumatoid arthritis may disrupt sleep. Early morning stiffness is a frequent symptom in persons with rheumatoid arthritis. Individuals with angina pectoris tend to underestimate their actual number of movements. Clients with angina may experience pain during REM sleep. On awakening they may report an upsetting dream. A direct cause-and-effect relationship has not been established.

Duodenal ulcer. Clients with duodenal ulcer often awaken in the night and complain of epigastric pain, which is relieved by food or antacid. It has been shown that these incidents are correlated with an increased secretion of gastric hydrochloric acid (three to 20 times greater than normal), particularly related to REM sleep; normal subjects studied did not demonstrate this increase in secretion.

Cardiovascular symptoms. The pain of myocardial ischemia frequently accompanies REM sleep. Observations of patients with myocardial infarctions have shown that premature ventricular contractions (PVCs) are increased during or immediately following REM sleep. The horizontal position generally assumed during sleep results in an increased plasma volume as gravity effects on the fluid compartments are obviated. The increased

cardiac input may lead to left ventricular failure, resulting in pulmonary edema and dyspnea. Because many of the manifestations of heart disease do occur during the sleep period, many clients express a fear of going to sleep. This fear of falling asleep is particularly true of the client with angina pectoris or cardiac arrhythmia.

Respiratory alterations. Clients with emphysema have increased carbon dixoide tension and decreased oxygen saturation during sleep.

Children with asthma have been shown to have a decreased amount of stage 4 sleep compared with normal children. In children asthmatic attacks originate in the late part of the sleep period, when the child is not in stage 4 sleep. In adults they may occur in any sleep stage. There is a decrease in total sleep time and frequent awakenings.

Asthmatics frequently have bronchial spasm during REM sleep periods.

Metabolic disorders. Individuals with diabetes mellitus have been shown to have variable levels of blood glucose during the sleep period. Thus, diabetic individuals who are being regulated for the first time or who are out of control may need special surveillance during sleep.

Migraine headaches. Individuals with migraine headaches and with cluster headaches who suffered severe headache on awakening were monitored by EEG, which showed that the headache began during REM sleep.

ASSESSMENT OF SLEEP HABITS

The sleep-wake cycle is an obvious function of temporal organization. If the client cannot sleep at night or falls asleep during the daytime, it is likely that help will be sought to correct these subjective symptoms. Sleep disruptions may be debilitating and interfere with daytime activities.

The simplest and probably most accurate way, outside a sleep laboratory, to evaluate sleep-wake disorders is to have the client record the times of going to sleep and awakening for sleep periods, including naps, for a week. In most cases the health care provider sees the client for the first time in an ambulatory setting and must interview the client to obtain the information that will help to define the characteristics of the disorder and the 24-hour sleep-wakefulness pattern. Additional information may be obtained from the client's bed partner.

In most cases it is more productive to allow clients to describe their sleep habits in their own words. An open-ended question may provide the stimulus to the client to give all the information pertinent to assessment. Examples of such questions are as follows:

Table 4-7

Effects of pharmaceutical agents on the sleep cycle

Decrease time		Increase time		Allow normal time	
Drug	**Dosage**	**Drug**	**Dosage**	**Drug**	**Dosage**
REM sleep					
Placidyl	500 mg	Reserpine	1-2 mg	Chloral hydrate	0.5 g
Doriden	500 mg	LSD	30 μg		1.0 g
Seconal	100 mg				1.5 g
Phenobarbital	200 mg				
Nembutal	100 mg			Dalmane	15-30 mg
Quaalude	300 mg			Quaalude	150 mg
Benadryl	50 mg			Librium	50-100 mg
Scopolamine	0.006 mg/kg			Valium	5-10 mg
Morphine				Triazolam	0.125-0.25 mg
Heroin					
Alcohol	1 g/kg				
Tofranil	50 mg				
Elavil	50-75 mg				
Miltown	1200 mg				
Amphetamine	15 mg				
Stage 4 sleep					
Doriden	500 mg	Antidepressants in the presence of depression			
Nembutal	100 mg				
Valium	10 mg				
Librium	50 mg				
Reserpine	0.14 mg/kg				
Chloral hydrate	1.5 g				

"How have you been sleeping?"
"Can you tell me about your sleeping habits?"
"Are you getting enough rest?"
"Tell me about your sleep problem."

An adequate history includes a general sleep history, a psychological history, and a drug history. The description obtained of the sleep problem should include the 24-hour pattern of sleep and wakefulness.

There are times when the practitioner must ask more specific questions to understand the client's sleep habits. The suggested questions (see p. 107) may serve as a guide for this assessment. Only those questions need be used that will elicit the information not given by the more general query.

A technique that might more clearly define the sleep-activity cycle is to provide the client with a graph form on which to record the hours of sleep. The client should be encouraged to keep a record over a long enough period that the pattern is well demonstrated on the graph.

Clients might be taught to color code various activities to give the examiner, as well as themselves, a clearer picture of circadian rhythm. Even a simple written daily record of the sleep-activity cycle may prove helpful. At any rate, a diary of several days' sleep-activity cycles will allow the examiner a broader database from which to advise the client.

The medication the client has been taking must be assessed. Cases of insomnia resulting from drug interaction have been recorded, and many drugs currently prescribed for induction of sleep may change the EEG activity pattern. Some of these changes are summarized in Table 4-7. The drugs listed in this table should be given particular attention in assessing the client's sleep pattern.

Aspects of sleep pattern	Questions to elicit sleep pattern
Time retired	What time do you usually go to bed?
Initial insomnia	Do you fall asleep right away?
	How long does it take you to fall asleep?
	How often do you have trouble falling asleep? Does it occur every night? Every other night? Just the weekend? Every Monday?
	How do you feel before you fall asleep?
Maintenance insomnia	Do you wake up in the night? How often does this occur?
	What wakes you up once you have fallen asleep? Is there something that helps you get back to sleep?
Arousal-terminal insomnia	What time do you wake up? How often do you get up this early? What wakes you up at this early hour?
	What do you do once you wake up?
Quality of sleep (affective response)	How do you feel when you get up?
	Do you feel rested after a night's sleep?
Naps	Do you nap during the day?
Dreams, night terrors	Do you dream at night?
	Are your dreams ever frightening?
	Do your dreams ever wake you?
	How do you feel when you wake up from a bad dream?
Bruxism	Has anyone ever told you that you grind your teeth in your sleep?
Somnabulism	Has anyone ever told you that you walk in your sleep?
	Have you ever awakened in some place different than the one in which you went to sleep?
	Have you ever awakened to find furniture or other objects moved around in your home?
Daytime activity work pattern	What kind of work do you do?
Shift change	What hours do you work?
Recreation, exercise	What kind of activity is involved in your work?
	What do you do for fun?
	Are you engaged in any exercise?
Home responsibilities	Do you work at home? What kind of work do you do at home?
Sleep environment	
Bedding (mattress, pillows, blankets)	Do you need any special bedding to help you sleep?
	How many pillows do you use?
Light	Do you sleep with the lights off?
	Does having a light on at night bother you?
Noise	Do you have to have it very quiet to sleep?
	Do noises keep you awake at night? Wake you up?

Aspects of sleep pattern	Questions to elicit sleep pattern
Ventilation	Do you open the window at night?
Temperature	Do you need the bedroom to be cold [warm] to sleep well?
Special activities associated with sleep	
Bath, massage	What do you do just before going to bed?
Food	Do you eat before you go to bed?
	Do you like to have a snack before bed?
Drink (warm milk, water)	Do you like a drink before going to bed?
	What do you prefer as your bedtime beverage?
Medication	Do you take any medicine to help you sleep?
	Are you taking anything to keep you awake in the daytime?
	Are you taking any medicine at all?
Personal beliefs about sleep	How much sleep do you think you should have to stay healthy?
	What will happen if you don't get enough sleep?
Internal stimuli	How does the way you sleep affect your family?
Psychiatric disorders (anxiety, depression, schizophrenia)	How have your spirits been?
	Have you had a lot of worries lately?
Alteration as a result of physical condition (stimulus, electrolyte imbalance)	How have you been sleeping?

BIBLIOGRAPHY

Aschoff J: Circadian systems in man and their implications, Hosp Pract 11:51, 1976.

Aschoff J and others: Reentrainment of circadian rhythms after phase-shifts of the zeitgeber, Chronobiologica 2:22, 1975.

Bale P and White M: The effects of smoking on the health and sleep of sports women, Br J Sports Med 16:149, 1982.

Dement WC: Some must watch while some must sleep, San Francisco, 1976, San Francisco Book Co., Inc.

Folk GE: Biological rhythms. In Folk, GE, editor: Textbook of environmental physiology, ed 4, Philadelphia, 1986, Lea & Febiger.

Ganten D and Pfaff D, editors: Sleep: clinical and experimental aspects, New York, 1982, Springer-Verlag New York, Inc.

Guilleminault C, Tilkin A, and Dement WC: The sleep apnea syndromes, Ann Rev Med 27:465, 1976.

Guilleminault C and Dement W, editors: Sleep apnea syndromes, New York, 1978, Alan R. Liss, Inc.

Hudgel D: Diagnosis and therapy of sleep apnea, J Fam Pract 12:1001, 1981.

Kales A and Kales J: Sleep disorders, N Engl J Med 290:487, 1974.

Kales A, Soldatos C, and Kales J: Taking a sleep history, Am Fam Physician 22:101, 1980.

Kales JD: Aging and sleep. In Goldmann R and Rockstein M, editors: Physiology and pathology of human aging, New York, 1975, Academic Press, Inc.

Kales JD and others: Resource for managing sleep disorders, JAMA 241:2413, 1979.

Kiester E Jr: I keep falling asleep: what's wrong with me? Today's Health 54:40, 1976.

Kupfer D and Reynolds C III: Sleep disorders, Hosp Pract 18:101, 1983.

Luce GC: Biological rhythms in psychiatry and medicine, U.S. Department of Health, Education, and Welfare, National Institute of Mental Health, Public Health Service pub no 2088, 1970, U.S. Government Printing Office.

Mendelson W: Sleep and its disorders, New York, 1977, Plenum Publishing Corp.

Miles LE and Dement WC: Sleep and aging, Sleep 3:119, 1980.

Moore-Ede M, Sulzman F, and Fuller C: The clocks that time us, Cambridge, Mass, 1982, Harvard University Press.

Orem J and Bames C, editors: Physiology in sleep, New York, 1980, Academic Press, Inc.

Orr W, Altshuler K, and Stahl M: Managing sleep complaints, Chicago, 1982, Year Book Medical Publishers, Inc.

Rechtschaffen A and Kales A: A manual of standardized terminology, techniques and scoring for sleep stages in human subjects, National Institute of Health publ no 204, Washington DC, 1968, U.S. Government Printing Office.

Soldatos CR, Kales A, and Kales JD: Management of insomnia, Ann Rev Med 30:301, 1979.

Webb W, editor: Biological rhythms, sleep and performance, New York, 1982, John Wiley & Sons, Inc.

5

The health history

OBJECTIVES

Upon successful review of this chapter, learners will be able to explain:

- Guidelines used for taking a health history

- Three types of health histories

- Information appropriate for a health history format
  Biographical data
  Chief complaint or request
  Present illness or health status
  Past history
  Current health information
  Family history
  Review of physical, sociologic and psychologic systems
  Developmental data
  Nutritional data

- Purposes of a recorded health history

The health history is an extremely important part of the health assessment. Its performance is the primary vehicle by which rapport is established between the practitioner and the client. The information derived from the history-taking interview assists the practitioner in assessing and diagnosing the client's health problems and in obtaining knowledge of the client's problems and needs within the context of that particular client's life. The health history not only records the client's problems but also describes the client as a whole and in relation to the social and physical environment. Thus, it records not only weaknesses and abnormalities but also the strengths that will support therapy and care.

Other important components of the history database are the client's perceptions regarding health, illness, and experiences with health delivery systems. These perceptions must be known if future care is to be relevant and, consequently, effective. Guidelines for taking the health history are shown in the box on p. 110.

In practice, the taking of the health history is implemented in two phases: (1) the client interview phase, which elicits the information, and (2) the recording of data phase. The information for taking a history, as presented in this chapter, is organized according to a systematic method for recording the history. The client interview (Fig. 5-1) may not proceed in the same sequence. Each portion of the health history discussed contains descriptions of processes for both eliciting and summarizing data. Examples of two recorded health histories are included at the end of this chapter.

The health history usually occurs in the examiner's office or the client's home or hospital room. If the interview is in the examiner's space, the examiner has developed mechanisms of controlling the environment to

---

Guidelines for Taking the Health History

1. Establish an environment conducive to effective communication; that is, one that is private, comfortable, and quiet.
2. Allow the client to state problems and expectations for the encounter.
3. Provide the client with an orientation to the structure, purposes, and expectations of the health history.
4. Make some judgment early in the interview about the priorities for the encounter given the constraints of the interviewer and the client. Communicate and negotiate priorities with the client.
5. If the client has already encountered a provider within the health care system, review pertinent recorded information before the interview.
6. Make a judgment about the balance between allowing a patient to talk in an unstructured manner and the need to structure requested information.
7. Clarify the client's definitions of all key terms and descriptors.
8. Avoid questions that can be answered as yes or no if detailed information is desired.
9. Keep notes adequate enough for future recording. Specific quantitative data is especially subject to faulty recall.
10. Record the health history as soon as possible after the interview.

---

facilitate privacy, comfort, and quiet. However, if the interview is in the client's space, the examiner must assess the environment and, in some cases, alter it to facilitate an adequate interview by, for example, closing the curtains in a multibed hospital room or requesting that the television be turned off in the home.

Regardless if the examiner or the client initiates the encounter, clients will have various perceptions regarding the encounter's purpose and content. Clarification of the client's purpose and expectations, and orientation of the client early in the encounter to the examiner's goals and needs, will minimize potential for misunderstanding and frustration. Often the client's purposes and priorities are different from the examiner's, or the examiner may have an inaccurate perception of the client's purposes. Discrepancies must be clarified and negotiated.

There are various types of health histories:

1. A *complete health history* as described in this chapter. This type of health history is taken on initial visits to health care facilities when the providers within the facilities will be providing comprehensive or continuous care.

2. An *interval health history* is used to collect information in visits following the one in which an initial database is collected. Depending on the time since the last entry to the history and the purpose of the encounter, selected information about current problems and updates of historical information are obtained.

3. A *problem-focused health history* is used to collect data about a specific problem system or region.

A balance between allowing clients to talk and tell their story in their own way and efficient use of time must be achieved. Clients must be able to provide information they consider relevant; however, examiners must probe, clarify, and quantify in structured ways. Since the examiner is the "expert" in history taking, the examiner must take the lead in managing the interview to obtain appropriate information as efficiently as possible. Also, time is not an infinite resource: often other clients are waiting for services, and the costs of encounters must be controlled.

The interviewer should take notes during data collection; however, it is usually not possible to write the entire health history during the interview. Forms are useful in structuring note taking and are very appropriate for many data components. The interviewer should record as much of the health history during the interview as possible and the remainder soon after the interview.

FORMAT

The health history, as described in this chapter, is an extremely complete one. In many actual client care situations, it may not be possible, or even appropriate, to obtain the complete history at the first encounter or at all. For clients receiving continuous care, the history can be obtained in portions during several encounters.

For clients requiring episodic care, decisions regarding the data essential for immediate therapy guide the content of the history.

However, the beginning historian should practice obtaining the complete health history to develop skill in interviewing and in recording data and to establish priorities for focused interviews. During this practice process the learner will develop an appreciation for the client management implications of each portion of the health history.

The format used in this text for the complete health history is as follows (see the box on p. 111):

A. Biographical information
B. Chief complaint or client's request for care
C. Present illness or present health status
D. Past history
E. Current health information

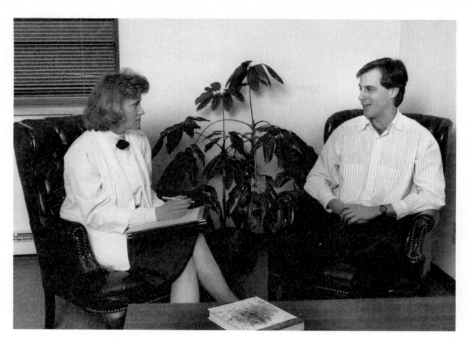

Figure 5-1

A comfortable arrangement for a health history.

Suggested Script for Introducing Components of the Health History

Biographical information

"I will start the history by asking you some general questions about yourself. First, could you please give me the correct spelling of your full name."

Chief complaint

"Please tell me why you came to see me today."

Client history

"Because some of the health problems you had in the past may have some implications for what we do today, I will now be asking you about your past illnesses, health problems, and immunizations."

Current health information

"Because my advice must take into account your current health habits and practices, I will now ask you about various questions about your current habits and medications."

Family history

Ill client: Because others in your family may have health problems that relate to your problems or affect your treatment, I will ask you some questions about their health.

Well client: Because others in your family may have health problems that relate to your current health risks and future health, I will ask you some questions about their health.

Review of systems
Physical systems

Up to now in the interview, we have concentrated on only several parts of your body. To have a complete picture of your physical health, I will now ask you a number of questions about the other parts of your body.

Sociological systems and psychological systems

Because I want to know more about you as a total person, I will now ask you some questions about you, your family, and your relationships with others.

Developmental data

[Usually the interview up to this point in the history will provide information for this section.]

Nutritional data

Because nutrition is important to health, I will next ask you some questions about your diet.

F. Family history
G. Review of systems
   1. Physical
   2. Sociologic
   3. Psychological
H. Developmental data
I. Nutritional data

Biographical Information

At the beginning of any health record, there should be a place to record commonly used and sometimes critical biographical information. This information should be obtained early during the client's first visit or admission; otherwise, it may be omitted, only to be needed in an emergency or at a time when the client is unavailable or unable to respond.

The following information should be recorded in the introductory, biographical section of the history:
A. Full name
B. Address and telephone numbers
   1. Client's permanent
   2. Contact of client
C. Birthdate
D. Sex
E. Race
F. Religion
G. Marital status
H. Social Security number
I. Occupation
   1. Usual
   2. Present
J. Birthplace
K. Source of referral
L. Usual source of health care
M. Source and reliability of information
N. Date of interview

First, the client's name is recorded. Persons in an ethnically homogenous geographic area often have similar names. Precise identification, using first, middle, and last names, assists in ensuring accurate information retrieval and coordination. If additional identifying information is needed, parents' names, including the mother's maiden name, can be recorded.

Next, the client's full mailing address and telephone number are recorded. Also recorded are the name, address, and telephone number of one of the client's friends or relatives, someone with whom the client is in frequent contact and who would be willing and able to relay a message to the client in an emergency or if the client could not be located.

Birthplace, sex, race, marital status, and religion information are self-explanatory. Many health problems

and needs are related to age, sex, race, or social situation. This information might be correlated with problems discovered later in the history.

There are justifiable reasons for including the client's Social Security number, including the precise identification of each client and a potential access to a large pool of health-related information. Potential violations of confidentiality are a disadvantage.

A significant difference may exist between the client's current and usual occupations. The nature of the difference may indicate the severity of the client's health problems and the level of disability resulting from them. In addition, knowledge of past occupations might provide clues to past or present environmental hazards contributing to the present illness. A mine worker with a respiratory system complaint is an example.

Knowledge of the client's birthplace provides geographic implications for the origin of problems and cultural implications for therapy and health maintenance.

If the current caregiver is not the usual and primary source of the client's care, the name and address of the individual or institution so identified should be recorded. In addition, the practitioner should record the reason for the client's entering a new health care system. The client may be in crisis, he may be dissatisfied with past care, or he may be "shopping." If the past source of care possesses significant data about the client's health and if the client intends to continue in the current health care system, the client should be asked to sign a permission for the transfer of information. Later in the health history, the practitioner will have the opportunity to record, in some detail, past patterns of health care.

The source of client payment for care is usually information included on administrative records. However, information here might be useful in guiding the choice of intervention.

Next, the practitioner makes a statement about the source of the information to follow. In most cases the source is the client, but this cannot be assumed unless the information is specifically identified. If the information is given by someone other than the client, the degree of the informant's contact with the client should be described. For example, in the case of a child, the practitioner would use the history given by a grandmother who resides with the child differently from one given by a grandmother who visits the child once a week.

Along with the statement of the informant, an evaluation of reliability is made. For example, one of the following may be stated: "inconsistent," "unclear about recent events," "evasive," or "cooperative and reliable." These statements serve as simple criteria by which the remainder of the information in the history is judged by other health care providers and may indicate a need to retake or supplement the history at a future date or to consult with other informants to determine the accuracy of the data.

The history is dated. In a situation where the client's condition changes rapidly, events can be correlated only if their temporal relationships are known.

Chief Complaint or Client's Request for Care

The chief complaint (CC) statement is a short statement, in the client's own words and recorded in quotation marks, that indicates the client's purpose for requesting health care at this time. In the case of a client who is ill, the CC statement is of the acute or chronic problem(s) that is the client's priority for treatment. The CC statement, whenever relevant, includes a notation of the problem's duration. The duration, as stated by the client, may not be the actual duration of the symptoms. However, it is an indication of the time during which the complaint has become intolerable enough to motivate the client to seek help.

In the case of a well client, the CC statement may be a statement of the client's request for a health examination for health screening, health promotion, or disease case-finding purposes.

The CC statement is not a diagnostic statement. Actually, it is very hazardous to state a chief complaint in diagnostic terms. For example, a client who has frequent asthmatic attacks appears for treatment with respiratory system complaints and states that he is having an "asthmatic attack." This may not be the case. In this early portion of the history, client and interviewer bias must be avoided; otherwise the interview and the problem solving may be set in one, potentially wrong direction.

The following are examples of adequately stated chief complaints.

> Chest pain for 3 days.
> Swollen ankles for 2 weeks.
> Fever and headache for 24 hours.
> Pap smear needed. Last Pap 9/8/83.
> Physical examination needed for camp.

The following are examples of inadequately stated chief complaints:

> Thinks she might be pregnant.
> Sick.
> Nausea and vomiting.
> Hypertension.

The CC statement may seem superfluous, especially since the next section on the present illness describes the symptoms in detail. However, this is one of the few places in the recorded history of an encounter with the health care system where clients have the opportunity to have recorded, in their own words, their needs. Too often, the practitioner loses sight of the client's priorities for care. The consistent recording of a chief complaint or reason for the visit will assist in keeping the system responsive to the client's perceived needs.

In some instances the client may present several complaints. No more than three should be stated in this portion of the history, and the client's stated priorities should be noted first. There is the opportunity to discuss all problems in the present illness portion of the health history.

Present Illness or Present Health Status

The present illness (PI) section describes the information relevant to the chief complaint. In the case of a client with a health problem, this portion of the health history challenges the practitioner's interviewing, clinical knowledge, and written communication skills. The practitioner must learn the minute details of the chief complaint and its associated phenomena. Information must be comprehensive, recorded concisely and comprehensively, and provide the practitioner with enough information to initiate additional assessment and the intervention measures.

The interviewing and recording for the present illness portion of the health history is especially difficult for beginning practitioners because the processes require skill in interviewing and history taking as well as clinical knowledge. Outlining the progression of the present illness before writing the narrative discussion is sometimes helpful. Although the student learning health assessment has probably not yet learned client care management, the student may find the referral to clinical management references for the system(s) discussed with the patient will often alert him or her to the most valuable pieces of data and highlight important omissions, which can be incorporated in future interviews.

In the case of a well client, the interviewer usually describes the client's usual health and briefly summarizes the health maintenance needs and activities.

The following are the components of the PI section:

I. Introduction
   A. Client's summary
   B. Usual health
II. Investigation of symptoms: chronological story
   A. Onset
   B. Date
   C. Manner (gradual or sudden)
   D. Duration
   E. Precipitating factors

F. Course since onset
   1. Incidence (frequency)
   2. Manner
   3. Duration (longest, shortest, and average times)
   4. Patterns of remissions and exacerbations
G. Location
H. Quality
 I. Quantity
 J. Setting
K. Associated phenomena
L. Alleviating or aggravating factors
III. Negative information
IV. Relevant family information
V. Disability assessment

Introduction.   The introduction to the PI section should be succinct; its major purpose is to provide the reader with a general orientation to the client.

The introduction indicates the client's previous admissions or visits, if any, to the institution or service. Next, there is a short summary of the client's biographical data. Age, race, marital status, employment status, and occupation are the items of information usually recorded. If the client is being hospitalized and has been hospitalized in the past, the client's total number of hospitalizations and the number of hospitalizations for complaints related to the current illness are noted.

The practitioner next describes the client's usual health and records any significant past diagnoses or past or current health problems.

Investigation of symptoms: chronologic story.   The practitioner usually initiates the PI description by asking the client: "Tell me about it [the problem mentioned in the CC statement]," or "How did it start and what has happened since it started?" The client will usually respond to this inquiry with a long but usually diagnostically incomplete discourse about health problems and needs. The practitioner exercises skill in determining when to interrupt the client and more specifically direct the responses by asking additional, clarifying questions and when to allow the client to continue the narration of significant events.

The practitioner needs a mental or actual list of the areas of symptom investigation as an aid in attaining comprehensive information. Regardless of the nature of a problem, each of the areas of investigation is relevant, and any health problem analysis would be incomplete without the description of all areas.

The practitioner also attempts to determine the chronologic sequence of the client's problem. The client is apt to best remember the most recent episode of illness

and, in the case of prolonged illness, will need direction in tracing the problem back to its first symptomatic event. Once this first event is identified, it is investigated in detail and its date, manner of onset, duration, and precipitating factors are described in the recording.

Each symptom's course since onset is described. Frequency in a specific time interval is determined. Clients may state vaguely that they have a symptom "all the time." This may mean once a month to one client or ten times a day to another. To obtain specific information, the practitioner might ask, "How many times a day (or a week, or a month) does it occur?" Although the practitioner avoids suggesting answers with his questions, occasionally it may be necessary to pursue frequency with leading questions, for example, "Does it occur more often than five times a day?"

The practitioner determines the usual manner of onset for the illness episodes. Any change in onset is specifically mentioned. In the case of many episodes, the longest, shortest, and average durations of the episodes are noted. If there have been only several episodes, the length of each is identified.

In prolonged illnesses, the patterns of remission and exacerbation are described according to their duration and frequency. The practitioner must be watchful for environmental or other clues that might be precipitating factors for the illness events.

In recording, several suggested methods can be used in assisting readers to identify temporal relationships easily. The practitioner describes the initial event first and then the subsequent events. The chronologic story may be indexed in the lefthand column of the history sheet, using the reference base *prior to admission* (PTA). For example, the index might be listed as follows: "6 years PTA," "3 years PTA," "6 months PTA," "1 day PTA," and so on, with the corresponding narrative alongside and below the temporal index heading.

A method of demonstrating the progression of illness is accomplished by the use of a diagram illustrating the disease process (Fig. 5-2). A diagram is especially helpful in the case of multisymptomatic illnesses.

As the chronologic story evolves, the other areas of symptom investigation are integrated into the text of the narrative. Whenever appropriate, the sign's or symptom's location, quality, quantity, setting, associated phenomena, and alleviating and aggravating factors are described, especially whenever there is a change in any of them.

Location.   The exact site of the sign or symptom is determined. Subjective events, such as pain, pose some problem. Having a client point to the exact point of pain

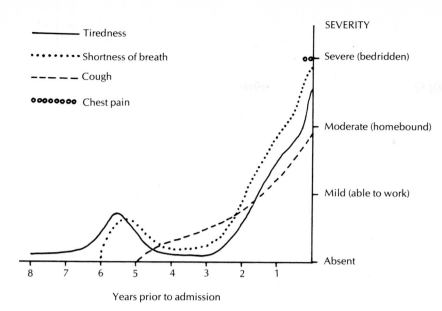

Figure 5-2

Use of a graph to illustrate symptomatic progress of an illness.

and trace its radiation with a finger assists in location. In recording location, one uses body hemispheres and landmarks.

Quality. Quality refers to the unique properties of the complaint. Signs, such as discharge, are described according to their color, texture, composition, appearance, and odor. Sound and temperature may be descriptive attributes of other phenomena.

Subjective events, such as pain, challenge the creativity of the practitioner. The quality of pain is frequently characterized as dull, aching, sharp, nagging, throbbing, stabbing, or squeezing.

Whenever appropriate, the client's descriptions are used with quotation marks.

Quantity. Quantity refers to the size, extent, number, or amount, for example, of the pain, rash, discharge, or lesion. With objective signs, the practitioner can use commonly understood measures, such as centimeters, cups, or tablespoons. In describing subjective events, pain, for example, one should note that evaluations such as "a little" or "a lot" have different meanings among persons. The quality of such phenomena can be more accurately understood by describing the client's response to the symptom. For example, does the client stop and sit or continue on with an activity?

Setting. Whenever something occurs, the client is somewhere and is either with someone or alone. Physically or psychologically the setting may have an effect on the client, and knowledge of this information may provide the practitioner with clues of the cause of the problem and implications for treatment.

Associated phenomena. Associated phenomena are those symptoms that occur with the chief complaint. They may be related to the chief complaint or may be a part of a totally different syndrome. Often the client will spontaneously identify these events. In addition, the practitioner may ask if there is anything else occurring with the chief complaint or ask about the presence or absence of certain specific events. A complete review of the implicated problem system or systems is indicated. Positive responses are recorded with a complete description of all reported symptoms. Negative responses are recorded in the negative information section.

Alleviating or aggravating factors. When an illness occurs, people often accommodate to it or treat themselves. They may decrease activity, eat more or less, wait, or actively medicate and treat themselves. The practitioner should nonpunitively probe into the client's actions in response to the problem and into the effect of these actions. If there has been professional intervention, the nature, source, and effect of each intervention are recorded. The client, through treatment or through accommodation, may have discovered something that alleviates the symptom. The client is asked what makes the problem better. The client's solution may provide valuable therapeutic data and may reflect the nature of the adaptation to illness.

The client is asked about that which makes the chief complaint worse. Usually clients have noticed aggravating factors but may need assistance in recalling them. The practitioner may ask about the effect of movement, positioning, or eating, for example. Again, valuable therapeutic data may be obtained.

Negative information.   In analyzing a problem, one may find negative information as significant as positive information in determining the diagnosis.

Each system implicated in the PI section is thoroughly reviewed. All the client's positive replies are recorded in the text of the chronologic story. All the negative information is recorded in this separate category of the PI section.

Relevant family history.   The client is queried about any problem similar to the chief complaint in blood relatives. Positive replies are recorded, identifying specifically the relative and the problem. A negative reply is recorded generally, for example, "None of the client's blood relatives has diabetes."

Disability assessment.   The practitioner determines the extent to which the symptoms identified in the PI section have affected the client's total life. Not only are the physiological effects determined, but also the sociological, psychological, and financial impacts of the problem.

Past History

The purpose of the past history (PH) section of the health history is to identify all major past health problems of the client.

The following indicates the information to be obtained and recorded in the PH section of the health history:

The recording of childhood illnesses is probably more relevant to and more easily obtained for a child's history than for an adult's history. However, all adults should be asked minimally if they have had rheumatic fever. Whenever there is a positive reply, the age of the client at occurrence, the fact or absence of a medical diagnosis, and the sequelae of the disease are determined.

The client is asked to recall accidents and disabling injuries, regardless of whether he was hospitalized for them or was treated on an outpatient basis. The precipitating event, the extent of injry, the fact or absence of medical care, the names of the practitioner and institution, and the sequelae are determined and recorded. The practitioner investigates for patterns of injuries or for the presence of consistent environmental hazards.

Descriptions of hospitalizations include all the times the client was admitted to an inpatient unit. Dates of stay, the primary practitioner, the name and address of the hospital, the admitting complaint, the discharge diagnosis, and the follow-up care and sequelae should all be recorded.

Obstetric hospitalizations are recorded in the review of systems portion of the health history under the review of the female genital system.

Operations are recorded together, under this specific category. The history should include as complete a description of the nature of the repair or removal as is possible. However, clients are generally and unnecessarily unaware of the nature of their operations. Past records may need to be consulted for accurate and complete information.

Clients may have had major, acute illnesses or chronic illnesses that have not required hospitalization. The course of treatment, the person making the diagnosis, and the follow-up care and sequelae are noted.

Information under the categories of hospitalizations, operations, and other major illnesses may, in some cases, be redundant. Information is not recorded more than once, but the presence of a past problem is stated, and the reader is referred to the section where the original notation was made.

Immunizations are recorded as to type and date. Good immunization records are often kept for children but not usually for adults. For adults, it is advisable to obtain the exact or approximate date of the last tetanus immunization.

Current Health Information

The purpose of the current health information section is to record major, current, health-related information. A recommended outline for the information is as follows:
A. Allergies
   1. Environmental
   2. Ingestion
   3. Drug
   4. Other
B. Habits
   1. Alcohol
   2. Tobacco
   3. Drugs
   4. Caffeine
C. Medications taken regularly
   1. By health care provider prescription
   2. By self-prescription
D. Exercise patterns
E. Sleep patterns

The practitioner specifically asks about allergies to food, environmental factors, animals, and drugs. (The practitioner should particularly ask about past administrations and reactions are noted in the record.) If the client has an allergy, specific information is obtained about the causative factor, the reaction, the diagnosis of causative factor, the therapy, and the sequelae. Caution must be exercised in assessing drug allergies. A drug reaction may not always be an allergic response; it may be an interaction with a concurrently administered drug, a misdose, or a side effect.

Habits that may have relevance to the health of an individual are excessive alcohol, coffee, or tea ingestion; smoking; and the addictive use of legal or illegal mood-altering substances. In the case of habits, the number of cigarettes, ounces, tablets, and so on per day are noted along with the duration of the habit.

If therapy is to be logically planned by informed practitioners, all medications currently being used by the client must be known and recorded. Clients usually admit to vague patterns, such as "a white pill once a day for water," but forget to tell the practitioner about the aspirin or antacid they take several times a day unless they are specifically asked about nonprescription items. Here, the health practitioner has the opportunity to educate clients about the names, doses, and uses of their medications and about the necessity of knowing such information.

The pattern of sedentary and active activities in the client's usual routine is explored. A weekly pattern of activity is recorded.

The client's sleep pattern is explored. The usual daily routine is recorded.

Family History

The purpose of the famiy history (FH) section is to learn about the general health of the client's blood relatives, spouse, and children and to identify any illnesses of environmental, genetic, or familial nature that might have implications for the client's current or future health problems and needs or to their solution or resolution.

The health status of the client's family is significant for several reasons. First, the client's health status affects and is affected by health conditions in other family members. Communicable diseases are an example. Second, heredity and constitutional factors are associated with the causation of many diseases. A strong family history of certain problems might be important clues in assessment and diagnosis.

The practitioner inquires about the health of the client's consanguineous family members, including maternal and paternal grandparents, parents, siblings, aunts, uncles, spouse, and children. For certain situations, information regarding roommates, sexual partners, and significant others might be relevant to a family history. Information is obtained about the current health status, presence of disease, and current age or age at death of each family member. If a member is deceased, the cause of death is recorded.

If the nature of the client's established or possible illnesses have known or suspected familial tendencies, the client is again questioned about similar problems of family members.

Inquiries about the presence of the following dis-

eases are made because of their genetic, familial, or environmental tendencies: alcoholism, allergies, epilepsy, diabetes, hematologic disorders (such as hemophilia, sickle cell anemia, thalassemia, hemolytic jaundice, and s evere anemia), Huntington's chorea, cancer, hypertension, arteriosclerosis, gout, obesity, coronary artery disease, tuberculosis, and kidney disease. Often printed history forms list these diseases, and the interviewer can check if the client or a family member has the diagnosis. The interviewer may inquire about additional diseases because of the client's family history, occupation, socioeconomic status, ethnic origins, or environment.

The information in the FH section may be outlined in the record or put in the form of a family tree chart. Fig. 5-3 is an example of such a chart. This type of chart is especially useful in situations where genetically transmitted diseases are present or suspected or if the understanding of family composition is an important factor in management. The box on p. 119 includes the traditionally used symbols for genogram notations.

Review of Systems

The review of systems (ROS) portion of the history includes a collection of data about the past and present health of each of the client's systems. This review of the client's physical, sociologic, and psychological health status may identify problems not uncovered previously in the history and provides an opportunity to indicate client strengths and liabilities.

Generally, the ROS portion of the history is organized from cephalad to caudad, from physical to psychosocial. Clients are instructed that they will be asked a number of questions. Both beginning and experienced interviewers normally need a checklist or written reminder of the questions usually asked each client.

Physical systems

In the review of physical systems section, the practitioner asks about symptoms or asks a specific question and then pauses, allowing the client to think and respond. If the client responds positively, the examiner analyzes the symptoms according to the characteristics of symptoms discussed in the PI section of the history. The practitioner asks questions quickly enough to be efficient, yet slowly enough to allow the client time to think. Questions generally emphasize the presence of past or current common anatomic or functional problems of the system and the health functioning and maintenance of the system.

Obviously, the signs and symptoms must be creatively translated into questions and terms that the client can understand. For example, questions concerning a

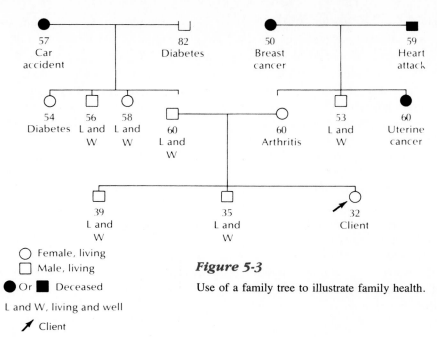

Female, living
Male, living
Or ■ Deceased
L and W, living and well
Client

Figure 5-3

Use of a family tree to illustrate family health.

symptom such as intermittent claudication would need to be presented in lay, descriptive terms.

The presence or absence of all signs or symptoms regarding which inquiry has been made is stated in the record. The general term *negative* for a total system is meaningless; the reader, if not the recorder, does not know which questions were asked and consequently does not know the context of *negative;* if the reader is also the recorder, he or she probably will not, after time, remember which specific questions were asked. An exception might exist in a health care system where the review of physical systems section is routinized and where *negative* indicates an inquiry into and a negative response to predetermined, universally known, and always-reviewed items of exploration.

In the PI section the practitioner has already reviewed the problem system thoroughly. The practitioner can, under that system in the review of physical systems section, advise the reader to refer to the PI section for information about that system.

Systems and body regions for review and exploration of health status, functional and anatomic problems, and health maintenance in the review of physical systems section are as follows:

General

Usual state of health
Episodes of chills
Episodes of weakness or malaise
Fatigue
Fever
Recent and significant gain or loss of weight (if present, amount, time interval, and possible causes are recorded)
Sweats
Usual, maximum, and minimum weight

Skin

Usual state of health
Previously diagnosed and treated disease
Color changes
Dryness
Ecchymoses
Lesions

Masses
Odors
Petechiae
Pruritus
Temperature changes
Texture changes
Care habits

Hair

Usual state of health
Alopecia or hair loss
Excessive growth or change in distribution
Texture changes

Use of dyes

Nails

Usual state of health
Changes in appearance
Texture changes

Head and face

Usual state of health
Dizziness
History of trauma
Injuries
Pain

Syncope
Unusual or frequent headache

Eyes

Usual state of health
Visual acuity, without and with corrective lenses, if applicable
Cataracts
Changes in visual fields or vision

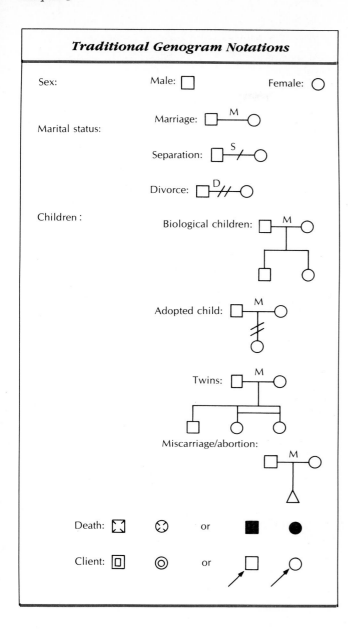

Diplopia
Excessive tearing
Glaucoma
Date of last ophthalmologic examination
Visual disturbances, such as rainbows around lights, flashing
 lights, or blind spots
Infections
Pain
Pattern of eye examinations
Photophobia
Pruritus
Redness
Unusual discharge or sensations

Ears

Usual state of health	Tinnitus, buzzing, ringing
Use of prosthetic devices	Otalgia
Discharge	Vertigo (subjective or objective)

Hearing ability	Care habits, especially ear cleaning
Infections	
Presence of excessive environmental noise	

Nose and sinuses

Usual state of health	Pain in infraorbital or sinus areas
Olfactory ability	Postnasal drip
Discharge (seasonal associations)	Sinus infection
Epistaxis	Sneezing (frequent or prolonged)
Frequency of colds	
Obstruction	

Mouth and throat

Usual state of health	Hoarseness
Use of prosthetic devices	Lesions
Abscesses	Odors
Bleeding or swelling of gums	Pain
Change in taste	Sore throats
Dysphagia	Voice changes
Dryness	Pattern of dental care
Excessive salivation	Pattern of dental hygiene

Neck and nodes

Usual state of health	Swelling
Masses	Tenderness
Node enlargement	
Pain with movement or palpation	

Breasts

Usual state of health	Tenderness
Dimples	Self-examination pattern
Discharge	
Masses	
Pain	

Respiratory and cardiovascular systems

Usual state of health
Past diagnosis of respiratory or cardiovascular system disease
Cough
Cyanosis
Dyspnea (if present, amount of exertion precipitating it is recorded)
Edema
Hemoptysis
High blood pressure
Orthopnea (number of pillows needed to sleep comfortably is recorded)
Pain (exact location and radiation and effect of respiration are recorded)
Palpitations
Sputum
Stridor
Wheezing
Paroxysmal nocturnal dyspnea
Date of last roentgenogram and electrocardiogram

Gastrointestinal system

Usual state of health
Appetite
Bowel habits
Previously diagnosed problems
Abdominal pain
Ascites
Change in stool color
Constipation
Diarrhea
Dyschezia
Dysphagia
Flatulence
Food idiosyncrasies

Hematemesis
Hemorrhoids
Hernia
Indigestion
Infections
Jaundice
Nausea
Pyrosis
Rectal bleeding
Rectal discomfort
Recent changes in habits
Thirst
Vomiting
Previous roentgenograms

Urinary system

Usual state of health
Past diagnosed problems
Usual patterns of urination
Anuria
Change in stream
Dysuria
Enuresis
Flank pain
Frequency
Hematuria
Hesitancy of stream

Incontinence
Nocturia
Oliguria
Polyruia
Pyuria
Retention
Stress incontinence
Suprapubic pain
Urgency
Urine color change
Urine odor change

Genital system

Male
Usual state of health
Lesions
Impotence
Masses

Pain
Prostate problems
Swelling

Female
Usual state of health
Diagnosed problems
Lesions
Pruritus
Vaginal discharge
Frequency of Pap smear
Menstrual history
  Age at menarche
  Frequency of menses
  Duration of flow
  Amount of flow
  Date of last menstrual period (LMP)
  Dysmenorrhea
  Menorrhagia
  Metorrhagia
  Polymenorrhea
  Amenorrhea
Dyspareunia

Obstetric history (for each pregnancy)
  Prenatal course
  Complications of pregnancy
  Duration of pregnancy
  Description of labor
  Date of delivery
  Type of delivery (vaginal, cesarean section)
  Condition, sex, and weight of baby
  Postpartum course
  Place of prenatal care and hospitalization

Both sexes
Ability to perform and enjoy satisfactory sexual intercourse

Infertility
Sterility
Veneral disease

Extremities and musculoskeletal system

Usual state of health
Past diagnosis of disease
Extremities
  Coldness
  Deformities
  Discoloration
  Edema
  Intermittent claudication
  Pain
  Thrombophlebitis

Muscles
  Cramping
  Pain
  Weakness
Bones and joints
  Stiffness
  Swelling
  Redness
  Heat
  Limitation of movement
  Fractures
  Back pain

Central nervous system

Usual state of health
Past diagnosis of disease
Anxiety
General behavior change
Loss of consciousness
Mood change
Nervousness
Seizures
Speech
  Aphasia
  Dysarthria
Cognitive ability
  Changes in memory
  Disorientation
  Hallucinations

Motor
  Ataxia
  Imbalance
  Paralysis
  Paresis
  Tic
  Tremor
  Spasm
Sensory
  Pain
  Paresthesia (hyperesthesia, anesthesia)

Endocrine system

History of physical growth and development
Adult changes in size of head, hands, or feet
Diagnosis of diabetes or thyroid disease
Presence of secondary sex characteristics
Dryness of skin or hair
Exophthalmos
Goiter
Hair distribution
Hormone therapy
Hypoglycemia
Intolerance of heat or cold
Polydipsia
Polyuria
Polyphagia
Postural hypotension
Weakness

Hematopoietic system

Past diagnosis of disease
Anemia
Bleeding tendencies
Blood transfusion

Blood type
Bruising
Exposure to radiation
Lymphadenopathy

Sociologic system

The practitioner cannot effectively diagnose a disorder or treat a client by knowing the client's physical status only. The client is a unique and whole person. For therapy to be effective, the problem must be assessed and treated within the context of that person. The practitioner should, in some organized way, gather information about the client's sociologic, psychological, developmental, and nutritional status.

The following is a suggested organization of sociologic data:

A. Relationships with family and significant others
   1. Client's position in the family
   2. Persons with whom client lives
   3. Persons with whom client relates
   4. Recent family crisis or changes
B. Environment
   1. Home
   2. Community
   3. Work
   4. Recent changes in environment
C. Occupational history
   1. Jobs held
   2. Satisfaction with present and past employment
   3. Current place of employment
D. Economic status and resources
   1. Source of income
   2. Perception of adequacy or inadequacy of income
   3. Effect of illness on economic status
E. Educational level
   1. Highest degree or grade attained
   2. Judgment of intellect relative to age
F. Daily profile
   1. Rest-activity patterns
   2. Social activities
   3. Special weekend activities
   4. Recent changes in daily activities
G. Patterns of health care
   1. Private and public primary care agencies
   2. Dental care
   3. Preventive care
   4. Emergency care

This outline is recommended for gathering the sociologic data of the majority of adult clients; obviously, adaptations are needed for some individuals. Many clients may be unaccustomed to extensive questioning about nonphysical matters during the taking of a health history. The practitioner may need to explain the use of such data by stating to the client, for example, "To treat you most effectively, it is important that I know something about you as a person."

First, the practitioner asks about the client's role or roles in the family and household. A member may have a societally assigned role, relating to birth, for example, that of son, father, or grandfather, as well as a circumstantially defined role, for example, that of pro-

vider, "black sheep," child, and so on. Both should be identified.

Next, the practitioner inquires about the people with whom the client lives and relates on a regular basis. Information can be used to hypothesize, for example, the effect on the family of a long illness of the provider. Also, the practitioner could identify strengths in the presence of strong family or friend relationships. The client should also be asked about the closeness and compatibility of the relationships. Sometimes unsatisfactory social relationships produce stress, which can be a factor in exacerbating or causing illness.

Each client should be asked if any recent event has had a significant impact. Resultant positive data might provide clues of causation or implications for prevention of illness.

Physical and psychological environments can have a profound effect on an individual's health status and potential. The practitioner asks about the client's satisfaction with the appearance and general comfort of house, community, and work situation. The practitioner might ask if the client considers the environment healthy or unhealthy. The pursuit of "why" in the case of negative responses will provide the practitioner some insight into the client's value system, possible information regarding significant health hazards, clues to the cause of the present illness, and a validation of the negative response. The practitioner again asks about recent change or loss. Positive responses are recorded.

Occupational history information can be used to identify past environmental hazards, to determine the fit between personal ability and productivity, and to plan rehabilitation. The practitioner asks about jobs held, satisfaction with those jobs, and the place of current employment.

The practitioner does not, in many cases, need to know the exact annual income but should know the source of income and the client's assessment of its adequacy. Clients whose resources are too insufficient to enable them to follow therapy must be identified early and appropriate referral for financial assistance made. In the case of probable prolonged illness, financial reserves are discussed and recorded. If the client is covered by any health insurance, the type of insurance, the name of the insurer, and the policy number are recorded.

The educational level of the client is determined, and the highest degree or grade completed is recorded. The practitioner must also wish to judge intellectual ability relative to age. Interviewing up to this point in the history has provided the opportunity for extensive observation of the client's understanding, response, and judgment.

Knowledge of the client's daily pattern helps the practitioner know the client as a person, with habits that encourage or impede health. The practitioner asks the client to describe a typical 24-hour day and to indicate weekend differences. Work, activity, sleep, rest, and recreational pursuits are specifically identified in the recording.

Part of the client's past social interaction has been with the health care system, and past responses may predict future patterns. The client is asked about health agencies used for acute, preventive, and maintenance health care. It can be determined whether the client is a health facility "shopper" or whether care has had continuity.

Psychological system

The following is an outline of the information obtained and recorded in the psychological assessment of the client.

A. Cognitive abilities
  1. Comprehension
  2. Learning patterns
  3. Memory
B. Responses to illness and health
  1. Reaction to illness
  2. Coping patterns
  3. Value of health
C. Response to care
  1. Perceptions of the caregivers
  2. Compliance
D. Cultural implications for care
  1. Patterns of therapy
  2. Patterns of illness response

In the assessment of cognitive abilities, the practitioner determines the client's comprehension ability. Usually this assessment is accomplished more indirectly than directly. Up to this point in the history-taking process, the client has demonstrated the ability to respond to some rather complex questions. The recording is the practitioner's judgment summary regarding the client's general comprehension ability.

Since education should be an essential component of all therapy, it is useful to determine the client's health-learning patterns. Some clients need personal instructions; others learn best through reading or group discussion. Knowledge of the client's preference can enable efficient use of provider effort and also involve the client in decision making concerning the process of therapy.

A discussion of the client's behavior in past illnesses and in health will probably predict future responses. The practitioner asks: "What does health mean to you, and what do you do to keep yourself healthy?" "How do you feel, and what do you do when you become slightly ill? When you become very ill?" "Who do you go to for help if you are ill?" Most clients will be able to answer these questions easily. A summary of the client's responses is recorded concisely. Information can alert the practitioner about strengths, weaknesses, and possible problems in therapy.

Skill may be required in learning the client's real responses to care, since people are often placed in a position of subjugation by the health care system. The practitioner might ask the client how comfortable he or she feels in asking questions of health care providers and if he or she feels like a partner in care with them. Answers may be recorded verbatim or summarized.

The practitioner asks about the client's amount of compliance to past courses of therapy. If compliance has been minimal, reasons should be determined for noncompliance. Problems resulting from lack of understanding and financial constraints are more easily solved than problems relating to distrust, indifference, or denial.

If the client is of a cultural group different from that of the practitioner and the majority of the care providers, it would be useful to ask the client what he or she expects of care and therapy, and what general things are done in that culture for persons with similar needs. If the chief complaint is of an illness, the practitioner asks about the feelings and responses of the client and significant others to the fact of the illness. Responses may guide the care provider into more efficient and fewer unacceptable routes of intervention.

Developmental Data

A detailed description of the developmental assessment is presented in Chapter 2, Psychosocial Assessment. The recording of this data minimally includes a summary of the client's development to date and a statement of current developmental functioning.

Nutritional Data

A detailed description of nutritional assessment is presented in Chapter 3, Nutritional Assessment. The recording of data minimally includes a description of an average day's food intake; an assessment of adequacy, inadequacy, or excess of the components of the Basic Four food groups; and the presence of any past nutritional problems.

COMPUTER-ASSISTED HISTORIES

Computer science is becoming an important and permanent component of health care technology, and the computer can assist in obtaining the client health history. Studies have demonstrated that use of the computer in history taking can save practitioner time; can yield a reliable, comprehensive, and readable printout; and is acceptable to clients. In personnel-deficient situations, where time allocated to history taking has been inadequate, the computer-assisted history can be superior to verbal histories.

Computer systems for history taking can be either practitioner- or client-interactive. The client-interactive systems are more commonly used because they are more likely to save practitioner time. A number of client-interactive, computerized, history-taking systems are available. Wakefield and Yarnell (1975) describe a number of both computer-assisted and other self-administered histories that would be very helpful to those considering the use of client self-administered, data collection techniques.

Self-administered histories involve the client's either completing a paper-and-pencil questionnaire or interacting with a computer. In the paper-and-pencil questionnaire situation, the client's responses are computerized in a variety of ways and the practitioner receives a printout of responses. In the client-interactive systems, the client responds to inquires from a computer terminal. Clients have been generally favorable to computer-assisted interviews, and printouts using such systems have been complete, accurate, and legible.

In any client self-administered system, practitioner time is needed to review the client's history, but usually this review requires only a relatively small amount of time. The amount of time spent by the client in the history-taking process is not shortened by the computer-assisted methods, however. Client age, number of client's problems, and time required by the client to complete the instructional portion of the computer program are positively correlated with overall time needed to give a computer history, and the number of client's years of formal education is negatively correlated with overall time.

The computer-assisted history is more appropriate to the ambulatory client than to the hospitalized client. The ambulatory client can be scheduled for a computer interview or can complete a form for computerization with the printout to be available to the practitioner for an appointment in several days. For hospitalized clients, information is generally immediately needed, and client access to terminals becomes problematic. Also, often the hospitalized client is too ill to complete a questionnaire or to use a computer terminal.

Practitioner-based computer systems for history taking involve either the practitioner's direct interaction with a computer, which is programed for questions relating to the history and into which answers are placed, or the practitioner's completion of a form that is com-puter-processed at a later time. The computer-interactive systems require a terminal for each practitioner, a situation that may not be cost-effective in ambulatory care situations. The use of the questionnaire for computerization has been used more extensively. The advantage of this latter method is that a legible printout is produced, an improvement over most handwritten documents.

The computer-assisted history can be as effective as the verbal history and may be more effective because remembering items for review is not a problem. Any question that can be asked verbally can be programmed into a computer system, and computer technology allows for additional branching questions if certain significant responses are given. Before additional assessment and therapy it is imperative that any client self-administered history be discussed, reviewed, and verified by the practitioner to determine the validity of significant responses: the client may have misunderstood instructions, or there may have been mechanical errors reflected in the information.

As computers become more prevalent in health care systems, especially microcomputers, the use of computer-assisted histories is likely to increase. However, there will always exist situations in which the computer history is not feasible and a verbal history is necessary. Therefore, skill in history taking is, and will continue to be, an important ability of the health care practitioner.

WRITTEN RECORD OF THE HEALTH HISTORY

The written record is the permanent, legal, and working documentation of what was seen, heard, and felt during the examination. It will serve as the baseline by which subsequent changes will be evaluated and therapy advised. It is very often used by a reader who does not have access to the recorder and is consequently subject to interpretation.

It is important that the recorded history be as objective, clear, complete, and concise as possible. The history should be free of recorder bias. The history is not the place for the recorder to bias the reader wtih opinions of diagnoses. Other portions of a client's record allow for the recorder to elaborate on hypotheses and plans.

In addition, the client's responses should be integrated in an accurate but objective way. This can be accomplished in one of two ways: (1) by paraphrasing the client, using, for example, statements such as "States he had the same symptoms 4 years ago" or "Denies chest pain," or (2) by quoting the client directly, for example, "The pain was so severe, I fell back into the chair I had just gotten up from."

Because most health histories are read over time

by multiple health care providers, the clarity of the presentation is very important. A clear presentation is often difficult for the beginning historian, but colleague and instructor feedback about written histories will assist in identifying strengths and deficits in this area. Most beginners must pay specific attention to chronology and the quality and quantity of symptoms.

The record should be a complete history of the practitioner-client encounter. It should be specific enough for the reader to clearly determine what was asked and examined and the result of the interview and examination. An entry such as "Eyes—negative" or "Eyes—normal" does not supply information regarding questions asked about the eyes. The "range of normal" is wide. Change in condition, even within the range of "normal," may be significant for an individual client.

The record, however, should be concise. Regional entries should be easily located and read. An extremely verbose and disorganized record may be less effective than an incomplete one because its appearance may frustrate the busy reader, who simply will not read it. The recording does not need to contain whole sentences. Use of clear phrases can save much time and space.

Two examples of recorded health histories are presented. One is an example of a history taken from an ill client who is being admitted to a hospital. The other is an example of a history taken from a well client. An example of a recorded physical examination is included in Chapter 28, Integration of the Physical Assessment and Documentation.

Example of a Recorded Health History: Ill Client

Client: John Donald Doe
Address: 9037 N. Sheridan St.
　　　　St. Louis, Mo. 63125
Telephone: 735-1946
Contact: Mrs. Clara Doe (mother)
Address: Same address as above; client will move in with mother after discharge from hospital
Telephone: Same telephone number as above
Birthdate: March 3, 1960　　　　**Sex:** Male　　　　**Race:** White
Religion: Presbyterian (inactive)　　　　**Marital status:** Separated
Social Security number: 097-32-7259
Usual occupation: Offset printer
Present occupation: None; on disability for 1 year
Birthplace: New York, N.Y.
Source of referral: Self
Usual source of health care: Dr. Ryan
　　　　　　1346 W. North Ave.
　　　　　　St. Louis, Mo. 63122
Source and reliability of information: Client; attempted to be cooperative; however, was frequently vague about the nature and time of events
Date of interview: Jan. 9, 1989

Chief complaint

"Pain in the left side of stomach for 2 days."

Present illness
Usual health

This is the fifth Healer's Hospital admission for this 29-year-old white, separated, unemployed male who has been drinking an average of 2 to 3 fifths of hard liquor daily. Total past admissions number 8; none of these has been for abdominal complaints. Client is presently on disability income as a result of a diagnosis of tuberculosis (11/88). Also has a history of drug abuse and gastric ulcer.

Example of a Recorded Health History: Ill Client—*cont'd*

Chronological story

14 years PTA*	Began drinking heavily and regularly.
7 years PTA	Diagnosed as having a gastric ulcer by Dr. Ryan. Treated by him on an outpatient basis with Maalox and Valium prn. Had x-rays at that time. Has complained of slight to moderate gastric discomfort and food intolerance intermittently since then. Unable to relate the specific frequency or specific characteristics of episodes of illness. States that they are usually accompanied by "hangovers." Generally experiences left upper quadrant (LUQ) discomfort, feelings of hunger, nausea, and vomiting of mucous material 6 to 8 hours after drinking heavily. Drinks heavily 3 to 4 days a week and states symptoms occur approximately 2 times a week. Appetite generally has been good. Meal patterns are erratic. Takes Valium for sleep each night. Drinks 2 to 3 8-oz bottles of Maalox per week. No pattern of follow-up care with Dr. Ryan. Symptoms relieved somewhat with Maalox. Bowel movements have been regular, formed, and brown.
1 day PTA	Had not been drinking the night before. Awoke at approximately 7:00 AM and took several alcoholic drinks (amount approximately 1 cup). An hour after an attempt to drink orange juice experienced nausea and vomiting.
	At 10:00 AM walked to his mother's home (2 blocks). On arriving, experienced a sharp, continuous, nonradiating pain in his upper left abdominal area. Indicates LUQ. The intensity required him to lie down. Position changes provided no relief. A whole bottle of Maalox did not affect the pain, which built in intensity over the next 2 hours. After 2 hours the pain remained constant but was more nagging than sharp. Tried to take some soup and orange juice but immediately vomited it. At 2:00 PM vomited again, and this time there were red streaks in the vomitus, which was a green, thick material. (Exact amount of vomitus or blood streaks unknown.)
	Throughout the remainder of the afternoon and early evening, took 5 mg Valium for a total of 4 times. Obtained no relief; pain remained nagging and continuous. Was able to walk with no increase in discomfort but felt most comfortable lying down.
	At bedtime took a sleeping pill but states it did not really help him sleep. Spent a fitful night, and the pain persisted with increased intensity. States he took his temperature at midnight and had a fever of 102° F.
Date of admission	Rose at 9:00 AM and was driven to Dr. Ryan's office but found it closed. Then came directly to Healer's outpatient clinic, where he was seen and admitted.

Negative information

Denies unusual weakness, chills, or fever before the onset of symptoms. Denies injury to the abdomen, unusual activity or exercise, pain in other locations, diarrhea, constipation, change in stools, jaundice, ascites, flatulence, hemorrhoids, rectal bleeding, or dysphagia.

Relevant family history

The only significant family history (hx) for a serious, persistent gastrointestinal disorder was a maternal uncle who was a heavy drinker and who died of stomach cancer at age 40.

Disability assessment

Client states that he has not felt really well in the past 7 years. Has not spent a great deal of time in bed but has not worked regularly and has been either drinking or "hung over" most of the time. Was diagnosed as having tuberculosis, 11/88, and was placed on a disability income plan at that time. This insurance will cover medical expenses.

Past history
Childhood illnesses

Exact illnesses or dates unknown. Assumes he had all childhood illnesses, for example, measles, mumps, chickenpox; denies hx of rheumatic fever.

Injuries

Client unable to provide exact dates for any of the following:
1. Age 9 (1969). Hit in the eye by rock. States has had a permanent decrease in vision in that eye. No medical care.
2. Age 14 (1974). In an automobile accident. Was hospitalized in Lakeside Hospital, Chicago, for 1 week. Physician unknown. Discharged from hospital with no follow-up required.
3. Age 15 or 16 (1975 or 1976). Fractured right ankle while playing football. Cast applied at Johnson Hospital, Chicago, and was followed in their orthopedic clinic. Apparently healed.
4. Age 18 (1978). Head injury from blow with blunt object, which was thrown. Was unconscious for approximately 30 minutes. Head sutured in emergency room (ER) of Healer's Hospital, St. Louis. No follow-up except for removal of sutures. No sequelae.
5. Age 21 (1981). Stab wound in left shoulder; was attacked and robbed. Sutured in ER of Lakeside Hospital, Chicago. No follow-up except for removal of sutures. No sequelae.

---

*PTA, prior to admission.

Continued

Example of a Recorded Health History: Ill Client—*cont'd*

Hospitalizations

1. Age 10 (1970). Hernia repair at Lakeside Hospital, Chicago. Dates and events of hospitalization unclear.
2. Age 14 (1974). Automobile accident. See item 2 under Injuries.
3. Age 20 (1980). Pneumonia. Under the care of Dr. Warner at St. Peter's Hospital, Chicago. Hospitalized for 2 weeks during December. No follow-up.
4. Age 23 (1983). Surgery for priapism at Lakeside Hospital. Under the care of Dr. Meyer. Follow-up for 1 year after surgery because was unable to obtain an erection. No other complications or current disability.
5. Age 24 (1984). Drug overdose. Under the care of Dr. Ryan, Healer's Hospital, St. Louis. Hospitalized for 2 weeks; was to start methadone maintenance; did not. Dates of stay not known.
6. Age 26 (1986). Drug overdose. Under the care of Dr. Ryan, Healer's Hospital. In the hospital for 1 week. Discharged against medical advice.
7. Age 28 (1988). Drug overdose. Under the care of Dr. Ryan. Hospitalized at Healer's Hospital for 2 weeks (1/83). Discharged on methadone maintenance.
8. Age 28 (1988). Hemorrhoidectomy. Under the care of Dr. Ryan and Dr. Jones, Healer's Hospital. Hospitalized 1 week. No complications; 1 follow-up visit.

Operations

See Hospitalizations for details.
1. Age 10 (1970). Hernia repair.
2. Age 23 (1983). Correction of priapism.
3. Age 28 (1988). Hemorrhoidectomy.

Other major illnesses

1. Age 23 (1983). Diagnosed as having a gastric ulcer by Dr. Ryan after an outpatient evaluation including x-rays. See Present illness section for follow-up and sequelae.
2. Age 28 (1988). Tuberculosis diagnosed and treated by staff of the St. Louis Health Department as an outpatient. Medications for 1 year. Off medications for the past 3 months. Followed with yearly x-rays and evaluation.

Current health information
Allergies

None known. Denies allergies to penicillin, other drugs, foods, or environmental components; has had at least 3 courses of penicillin.

Immunizations

Unknown.

Habits

Cigarettes—smokes 1 pack a day. Habit regular since age 12.
Hard drugs—all types, including heroin. 1984-1988 had a "$90-a-day habit."
Alcohol—started to drink heavily at age 16. Drinking decreased during period of drug addiction. Has been drinking 2 to 3 fifths of hard liquor a day for the past 2 years.
Coffee—drinks 6 to 7 cups a day.

Medications

Maalox—for ulcer prn with varied dosage since 1983. Prescribed by Dr. Ryan. Client states he uses 2 to 3 8-oz bottles a week.
Valium—10 mg prn for ulcer and nervousness since 1983. Client states he uses at least 1 to 2 tablets a day.
Methadone—40 mg daily for 6 months, 1988. Given through drug abuse program.
Streptomycin—IM daily, dose? For TB, 11/88 to 9/89.
INH—tid for TB, 11/88 to 9/89.
Salve—name unknown, a nonprescription drug; topically every day for scaling skin on soles of feet; since approximately 8/89.
Magnesium citrate—for constipation approximately once (×1) monthly or less frequently; prescribed by self. Uses 1 tbsp prn.
Sleeping pill—prn. Name and dose unknown. Prescribed by Dr. Ryan; 1 every night.

Exercise patterns

Largely sedentary due to life-style and low energy. No regularly scheduled exercise.

Sleep patterns

Sleeps about 7 to 8 hours during a 24-hour period. Often patterns are irregular because of alcohol consumption.

Example of a Recorded Health History: Ill Client—*cont'd*

Family history

Maternal and paternal grandparents deceased. Ages at death and causes of death unknown. Denies family hx of diabetes, blood disorders, arteriosclerosis, gout, obesity, coronary artery disease, tuberculosis, cancer, hypertension, epilepsy, kidney disease, or allergic disorders. Uncertain about health history of aunts and uncles.

Mother—age 52; alive and well.

Father—deceased, age 50, 1975; cause unknown.

Siblings—no maternal miscarriages.

1. ♀ Age 27; alive and well.
2. ♂ Age 20; deceased 1988; drug overdose.
3. ♀ Age 21; alive and well.
4. ♂ Age 18; deceased 1985; gunshot wound.
5. ♀ Age 19; alive and well.

Children

1. ♂ Age 10; alive and well.
2. ♂ Age 7; alive and well.

Wife—age 31; obese, otherwise well.

Review of physical systems
General

Chronically ill, white male adult; usual wt about 176 lb. Reports approximately 10-lb wt loss over the past 3- to 4-month period. Feels this is a result of not eating when drinking heavily. States he has felt a generalized fatigue and malaise for over 1 year, since onset of TB, but denies requiring daily naps or extra sleep. States he cannot exercise due to fatigue. Denies chills (other than those associated with present illness), sweats, and seizures.

Skin, hair, and nails

Denies lesions, color changes, ecchymoses, petechiae, texture changes, unusual odors, or infections. Pruritus; soles of feet dry and scaling for 6 months; condition stable (using nonprescription salve, name unknown). States he has had small cracks at corners of mouth for 1 month. Denies cold sores. States hair breaks off and falls out but denies patchy alopecia. Denies brittle, cracking, or peeling nails. States bites nails. Has 1 birthmark on upper back but is not aware of any change in size or color.

Head and face

Denies pain, headache, dizziness, or vertigo. Hx of injury with blow to forehead. Reports frequent losses of consciousness after drinking; duration unknown, probably 1 to 8 hours.

Eyes

Has worn corrective lenses since 1970, age 10. States rt eye 20/20, lt eye 20/50. Hx of 1 eye injury, age 9. States visual acuity decreased after injury. Denies pain, infection, watery or itching eyes, diplopia, blurred vision, glaucoma, cataracts, decreased peripheral vision. Last ophthalmological examination 2 years ago.

Ears

Denies hearing loss. Denies discharge, pain, irritation, or ringing in ears. States he was "cut in a fight" on rt auricle. Cleans ears with a toothpick.

Nose and sinuses

Denies sinus pain, postnasal drip, discharge, epistaxis, soreness, excessive sneezing, or obstructed breathing. Denies injuries. States he has approximately 2 colds a year. Olfaction not good; attributes this to smoking.

Oral cavity

Complains of frequent dryness in mouth and cracking of lips and tongue. No false teeth. Gums bleed frequently. Denies hoarseness, pain, odor, frequent sore throats, voice change. Dental care infrequent. Brushes teeth "occasionally."

Neck

Denies pain, stiffness, or limitation of range of motion. Denies masses.

Nodes

Denies enlarged or tender nodes in neck, axillary, or inguinal area.

Continued

Example of a Recorded Health History: Ill Client—cont'd

Breasts

Denies surgery, pain, masses, or discharge.

Chest and respiratory system

Denies pain, wheezing, asthma, or bronchitis. Hx of pneumonia, age 20 (see Hospitalizations). Denies shortness of breath or dyspnea. Sleeps on 2 pillows but is not dependent on them for breathing. Hx of TB, 1988-1989. Last chest x-ray on present admission, negative. States he had 1 episode of hemoptysis, 1983, associated with his ulcer. Details of this unclear. States he has "smoker's cough" (dry cough in the morning) but denies sputum.

Cardiovascular system

Denies chest pain, coronary artery disease, rheumatic fever, or heart murmur. Denies hypertension, palpitations, cyanosis, or diagnosis of cardiac disorder. States he has occasional slight edema in rt ankle.

Gastrointestinal system

See PI. Also see Hospitalizations re hemorrhoidectomy. Appetite good. Denies dysphagia, belching, or hematemesis. Hx of ulcer (see PI) and hernia repair (see Hospitalizations). Denies melena, clay-colored stools, or diarrhea. Takes laxative, magnesium citrate, approximately $\times 1$ monthly or less for constipation. Denies jaundice. Reports decreased appetite with alcohol intake but denies specific intolerance to any food.

Genitourinary system

Denies bladder or kidney infections, urgency, frequency, hesitancy, painful micturition, incontinence, nocturia, or polyuria, hx of VD. Denies testicular pain. Hx of surgery for priapism with inability to have erection for 1 year following (p) surgery. No dysfunction at present. States sex life is "fair." Alcohol decreases "urge."

Extremities

Hx of fractured rt ankle, age 15 or 16. Reports swelling of ankle without pain. Denies varicose veins, thrombophlebitis, joint pain, stiffness, swelling, gout, arthritis, limitation of movement, or color changes.

Back

Denies pain, stiffness, limitation of movement, or disk disease.

Central nervous system

Reports loss of consciousness (1978) following blow to head; duration approximately 30 minutes. Denies clumsiness of movement, weakness, paralysis, tremor, neuralgia, or paresthesia. States he is a "nervous" person but denies hx of nervous breakdown. Hx of drug and alcohol abuse. States he will periodically (every 2 to 3 weeks) have spontaneous jerky movement of legs during rest. There are 4 to 5 movements in each episode. This has never occurred while legs were bearing weight. Denies disorientation or memory disorders. Denies seizures or epilepsy. "Passes out" frequently after heavy alcohol ingestion and sleeps for 5 to 6 hours. Wakes with headache and nausea.

Hematopoietic system

Denies bleeding, bruising, blood transfusion, or exposure to x-rays or toxic agents.

Endocrine system

Denies diabetes, thyroid disease, or intolerance to heat or cold. Growth has been within normal range.

Review of sociologic system
Family relationships

Has been separated from wife for 6 to 7 months and is in the process of being divorced. States his marital problems do not interfere with seeing his children. Plans to move to his mother's home when discharged from hospital. States relationships with his family are good.

Occupational history

Offset printer since 1986. Presently unemployed. Was advised not to work for 6 months when tuberculosis was diagnosed and has not been "able to get back to work." States he liked that occupation but expresses no urgency to return to work.

Example of a Recorded Health History: Ill Client—*cont'd*

Economic status

On disability income, because of tuberculosis and need to rest. States he does not have trouble making ends meet on present income.

Daily profile

Lives alone in a room. States he spends time during the day at home or with friends, drinking. Has no special hobbies or activities to occupy time. Has habit of heavy daily drinking. States "I just hang around all day." Does do some spur-of-the-moment traveling. Weekdays are no different than weekends. States he dropped out of college because of disinterest.

Educational level

States he is "smart enough." Dropped out of college after 2 years because of disinterest. States he has no aspiration except to "get by in life."

Patterns of health care

Has maintained relationship with same physician for the episodic care for the last 10 years. Does return for periodic examinations and follow-up when symptoms "scare him."

Environmental data

Birthplace—New York, N.Y. No travel outside of USA; no armed forces duty.
Home—Plans to move to his mother's home. Will share the 5-bedroom residence with his mother and 2 siblings. Neighborhood is residential; describes it as "beautiful."

Review of psychological system
Cognitive abilities

Oriented to present events. Has fairly adequate vocabulary. Has a fair to poor memory. Cannot recall details of some important events. No history of psychiatric treatment.

Response to illness

States he "quit" drinking when he entered the hospital and plans to abstain in the future. Verbalizes that his health problems are his own fault and that he will die soon if he does not resolve them. States illness does not bother him except when "it gets out of control." Definition of health entails being able to play baseball again.

Response to care

States he has sometimes not followed medical advice, because of fear or because drugs or alcohol did not allow him to think "straight." "People have been nice to me." States all care has been "OK."

Cultural implications

Inactive Presbyterian at present but is concerned about conflict with religious beliefs and life-style. Fourth-generation American.

Developmental data

Adult male who has had problems with interpersonal relationships in his marriage. Has demonstrated drug and alcohol abuse since entering adulthood. Does not express concern regarding his inability to work; has abandoned his college attendance. Immediate plans for the future involve moving in with his mother and trying to stop drinking. Speaks of his children as playmates; expresses few fathering needs or activities.

Nutritional data

States he does not eat or has erratic meal patterns when drinking heavily and must build his tolerance to food by taking liquids such as soup or juices after drinking. States he does eat 3 complete meals daily when not drinking. Includes foods from the four basic food groups.

Continued

Example of a Recorded Health History: Well Client

Client: Mary Rose Doe
Address: 1056 N. East St.
            St. Louis, Mo. 63047
Telephone: 278-9274
Contact: Mrs. Elsa Smith (mother)
Address: 3496 Oak St.
            St. Louis, Mo. 63047
Telephone: 926-8711
Birthdate: Feb. 6, 1959   **Sex:** Female   **Race:** Black
Religion: Methodist (active)   **Marital status:** Married
Social Security number: 396-47-8911
Usual occupation: Grade school teacher
Present occupation: Same—Greenwich School
Birthplace: Greenwood, Mississippi
Source of referral: Self
Usual source of health care: St. Louis Health Maintenance Organization
                                 4693 C. Division St.
                                 St. Louis, Mo. 63044
Source and reliability of information: Client; cooperative, apparently reliable
Date of interview: Dec. 12, 1989.

Reason for visit

Annual physical examination; last exam, 1/88.

Present health status
Usual health

This is the third St. Louis Health Maintenance Organization (HMO) visit for this 30-year-old black, married, female school teacher who has been in good health for all of her life. Client has been hospitalized twice for the purposes of normal childbirth only. Has no major chronic diseases.

Summary

Client is presently well and requests a physical examination for health maintenance and screening purposes. Is concerned about a strong family history of hypertension and believes that monitoring of her blood pressure status is important.

   Also requests a Pap smear and evaluation for continuance of oral contraceptives. Has been taking Ortho-Novum 1 + 50 since the birth of her last child in 1983. Client enrolled in the health plan a year ago.

Past history
Childhood illnesses

Had rubella, chickenpox—not diagnosed by a physician. Has not had rheumatic fever.

Injuries

None.

Hospitalizations

See obstetrical data in Review of physical systems.
1. Age 20 (1979). Childbirth.
2. Age 24 (1983). Childbirth.

Operations

None.

Major illnesses

None.

Current health information
Allergies

None known. Denies allergy to penicillin, other drugs, foods, or environmental components. Has had a course of penicillin (10 d, oral).

Example of a Recorded Health History: Well Client—*cont'd*

Immunizations

Had full series of diphtheria-pertussis-tetanus (DPT) when a preschooler. Had oral polio when an adolescent. No others.

Habits

Cigarettes—smoked 15 cigarettes a day for 5 years (age 20-25).
Hard drugs—none.
Alcohol—drinks 3 to 4 mixed drinks during a weekend.
Coffee, tea—drinks approximately 10 cups of coffee a day. Drinks tea rarely.

Medications

Ortho-Novum 1 + 50 oral contraceptive since 1983.
Aspirin (ASA) for headache—takes approximately × 10 gr twice a month.
Milk of magnesia for constipation—takes 1 tablespoon about once a month.
One-a-Day multiple vitamins—takes 1 a day.

Exercise patterns

Attends aerobics classes 2 to 3 times a week during the winter. In summer, walks 3 to 4 times a week.

Sleep patterns

Sleeps 7 to 8 hours a night regularly with occasional naps on weekends.

Family history

Denies family history of diabetes, blood disorder, gout, obesity, tuberculosis, epilepsy, kidney disease, or gastrointestinal disease.

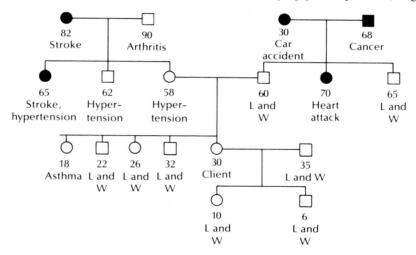

Review of physical systems
General

Usually well. Usual-minimum-maximum weight: 135-125-160 lb. No recent increase or decrease in weight. Denies fatigue, malaise, chills, sweats, fever, seizures, or fainting. Reports height as 5 ft 6 in.

Skin, hair, and nails

Denies lesions, color change, ecchymoses, masses, petechiae, texture changes, pruritus, sweating, or unusual odors. No alopecia or brittle hair. Denies brittle, cracking, or peeling nails. No birthmarks. Washes hair once a week; does not use dyes.

Head ad face

Denies pain, dizziness, vertigo, or history of injury or loss of consciousness.

Eyes

Has worn corrective lenses since age 7; currently wears contact lenses all day. Denies recent change in visual acuity, pain, infection, watery or itching eyes, diplopia, blurred vision, glaucoma, cataracts, or decreased peripheral vision. Last ophthalmoscopic examination, 2 years ago.

Continued

Example of a Recorded Health History: Well Client—*cont'd*

Ears

Denies hearing loss, discharge, pain, irritation, or ringing in the ears. Cleans ears with cotton-tipped applicator.

Nose and sinuses

States she has sinus pain, congestion, and subsequent nasal discharge several times each winter. Takes Contact prn (approximately 1 q 12 hours × 3 d) for each episode of rhinitis; gets relief. Denies epistaxis, soreness, excessive sneezing, obstructed breathing, or injuries. States olfaction is good.

Oral cavity

Visits a dentist every 6 months for cleaning and examination. Brushes teeth twice a day. Denies toothache, lesions, soreness, bleeding of gums, coated tongue, disturbance of taste, hoarseness, or frequent sore throat.

Neck

Denies pain, stiffness, limitation of movement, or masses.

Nodes

Denies enlarged or tender nodes in neck, axillary, or inguinal area.

Breasts

Denies masses, pain, tenderness, or discharge. Examines breasts monthly, right after menses.

Chest and respiratory system

Denies pain, wheezing, shortness of breath, dyspnea, hemoptysis, or cough. Denies hx of asthma, pneumonia, or bronchitis. Has yearly chest x-ray, required for work in the schools.

Cardiovascular system

Denies precordial pain, palpitations, cyanosis, edema, or intermittent claudication. Frequently bicycles in summer and downhill skis in winter. Walks 2 miles a day. Denies diagnosis of heart murmur, hypertension, coronary artery disease, or rheumatic fever.

Gastrointestinal system

Denies history of gastrointestinal (GI) disease. Appetite good. Bowels active daily, stools are always brown. Denies pain, constipation, diarrhea, flatulence, vomiting, hemorrhoids, hernias, jaundice, pyrosis, or bleeding. Has never had GI x-rays.

Genitourinary system

Denies hx of bladder or kidney infections, hematuria, urgency, frequency, dysuria, incontinence, nocturia, polyuria, or VD. Menses— onset 13 years; frequency, every 26 to 30 days; duration, 5 days; flow, heavy for 3 days, light for 2 days; last menstrual period (LMP), 12/1/89. Denies dysmenorrhea, menorrhagia, metrorrhagic discharge, or pruritus. Last Pap smear, 12/88.

Obstetric history

1. Sept. 12, 1979. Girl, 6 lb, 8 oz. Vaginal delivery at St. Francis Hospital, St. Louis. Prenatal, intrapartum, and postpartum course normal for mother and baby.
2. Oct. 9, 1983. Boy 7 lb, 2 oz. Vaginal delivery at St. Francis Hospital, St. Louis. Prenatal, intrapartum, and postpartum course normal for mother and baby.

Sexual history

Age at first intercourse was 17 years. Enjoys intercourse with husband—no dyspareunia and able to achieve satisfactory orgasm most of the time. Using oral birth control medication. Not sure yet if she will have another child. Will consider sterilization when family is complete.

Extremities

No past problems. Denies deformities, varicose veins, thrombophlebitis, joint pain, stiffness, swelling, gout, arthritis, limitation of movement, color changes, or temperature changes.

Back

No past problems. Denies pain, stiffness, or limitation of movement; no history of disk disease.

Example of a Recorded Health History: Well Client—*cont'd*

Central nervous system

No past problems. Denies loss of consciousness, clumsiness of movement, difficulty with balance, weakness, paralysis, tremor, neuralgia, paresthesia, history of emotional disorders, drug or alcohol dependency, disorientation, memory lapses, or seizures. Speech articulate.

Hematopoietic system

No past problems. Denies excessive bleeding and bruising, blood transfusions, or excessive exposure to x-rays or toxic agents. Blood type A, Rh positive.

Endocrine system

Denies history of diabetes or thyroid disease, polyuria, polydipsia, polydysplasia, intolerance to heat or cold, or hirsutism.

Review of sociologic system
Family relationships

Lives in own home with husband and 2 children. Husband is a school teacher also; couple shares finances, child-rearing, and housekeeping responsibilities. Client's parents live ½ mile away, and relationships are described as "good." Couple has several close friends; also, siblings are in frequent contact. No recent family crisis or change.

Occupational history

Has been a grade school teacher for 5 years. No other jobs. Holds bachelor's and master's degrees and feels secure that she can retain her job as long as she wants it. Enjoys children and states job is very satisfying.

Economic status

Client and husband achieve a combined gross income of over $60,000 a year. Feels this is very adequate. Has hospitalization insurance.

Daily profile

During the week, works 8 AM to 3 PM. Returns home around 3:30 and works until 5 PM on school work. Then cooks dinner and interacts with family. Has meetings 1 or 2 evenings a week. Weekends, client and husband usually have 1 evening out with friends, to movie or concert. Family attends church each Sunday. Client is involved with photography as a hobby.

Education level

Highest degree attained is the master's degree. Obtains most of health knowledge by reading.

Patterns of health care

Has always had a primary care provider. Cared for by Dr. Richard Smith, a family practitioner until first pregnancy. Then seen regularly by Dr. Janice Lawson for obstetric and gynecologic care. Family enrolled in HMO a year ago; all family members are being seen here. Dental care regular and at the HMO.

Environmental data

Birthplace—Greenwood, Miss. Grew up in Trenton, N.J.
Home—family lives in their own 8-room home in a residential St. Louis neighborhood. Client describes home as comfortable.
  Has lived there for 10 years.
Community—community is middle income, integrated, consisting primarily of young professional families.
Work—teaches fourth grade in a community school. States that the work situation is fairly good. School is in good condition, and
  classes are small. A recent stress is a new assistant principal with whom client does not get along. May consider transfer to
  another school.

Review of psychological system
Cognitive abilities

Oriented to time, place, and person ($\times 3$). Is articulate, asks questions, has a good memory. Able to understand directions.

Response to illness

States she has never been seriously ill, so does not know what personal response would be. Feels she is "too busy" to be ill for any length of time. Uses the resources of HMO for preventive and therapeutic needs of self and family.

Continued

---

*Example of a Recorded Health History: Ill Client—*cont'd

Response to care

States she enjoys encounters with health care providers. States she usually follows through on the advice that is given. Feels that the services of the HMO are adequate to meet her family care needs and she has been very satisfied with the care to date.

Cultural implications

Client states she and her family are involved in a racially integrated community. She grew up in a predominantly black northern community. Cannot identify any way in which her black culture would especially affect her response to illness or therapy in the case of illness. Active Methodist; believes that religious concerns would influence her response to illness and treatment.

Developmental data

Adult female; wife, mother, and career teacher.

Nutritional data

Diet adequate; high in fats and carbohydrates. Has no food intolerances.
Usual breakfast—toast with butter, fried egg, orange juice, and coffee with cream.
Usual lunch—eats with school children; consists of meat, 1 vegetable, 1 carbohydrate, dessert, and beverage.
Dinner—meat (beef, chicken, or pork), salad, 1 vegetable, potato or bread, dessert, and coffee with cream.
Snacks—may have cheese and crackers or peanuts in the evening.

BIBLIOGRAPHY

Becker CE: Key elements of the occupational history for the general physician, West J Med 137:581, 1982.

Beitman BD, and others: Steps toward patient acknolwedgement of psychosocial factors, J Fam Pract 15:1119, 1982.

Bernstein L and Bernstein RS: Interviewing: a guide for health professionals, ed 4, Norwalk, CT, 1985, Appleton-Century-Crofts.

Burack RC and Carpenter RR: The predictive value of the presenting complaint, J Fam Pract 16:749, 1983.

Coye MJ and Rosenstock L: The occupational health history in a family practice setting, Am Fam Physician 28:229, 1983.

Crouch MA and Thiedke CC: Documentation of family health history in the outpatient record, J Fam Pract 22:169-174, 1986.

Froelich RE and Bishop FM: Clinical interviewing skills: a programmed manual for data gathering, evaluation, and patient management, ed 3, St. Louis, 1977, The CV Mosby Co.

Gelehrter TD: The family history and genetic counseling: tools for preventing and managing inherited disorders, Postgrad Med 73:119, 1983.

Lilford RJ, Glyn-Evans D, and Chard T: The use of a patient-interactive microcomputer system to obtain histories in an infertility and gynecologic endocrinology clinic, Am J Obstet Gynecol 146:374, 1983.

Mackenzie TB: The initial patient interview: identifying when psychosocial factors are at work, Postgrad Med 74:259, 1983.

Mahoney EA and Verdisco LA: How to collect and record a health history, ed 2, Philadelphia, 1982, JB Lippincott Co.

Minkoff H: The medical significance of the obstetric history, Am Fam Physician 27:164, 1983.

Palchick YS: Obtaining a practical case history and examination, Dent Clin North Am 27:505, 1983.

Romriell GE and Streeper SN: The medical history, Dent Clin North Am 26:3, 1982.

Roter DL and Hall JA: Physicians' interviewing styles and medical information obtained from patients, J Gen Intern Med 2:325-329, 1987.

Schneiderman H: The review of systems: an important part of a comprehensive examination, Postgrad Med 71:151, 1982.

Scully C and Boyle P: Reliability of a self-administered questionnaire for screening for medical problems in dentistry, Community Dent Oral Epidemiol 11:105, 1983.

Skarfors E, Waem U, and Lidell C: Findings at a reexamination of a self-administered questionnaire after two and a half years in a sample of sixty-year-old men, Scand J Soc Med 8:137, 1980.

Stout F and Doering P: The problematic drug history, Dent Clin North Am 27:387, 1983.

Taking the occupational history, Ann Intern Med 99:641, 1983.

Truitt CA, Longe RL, and Taylor AT: The evaluation of a medication history method, Drug Intell Clin Pharm 16:592, 1982.

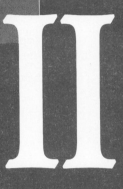

II

Physical Assessment

6

Assessment techniques

OBJECTIVES

Upon successful review of this chapter, learners will be able to state related rationale and to demonstrate:

- Four assessment techniques used during a physical examination

- Differences between subjective and objective data

- Three steps for conducting an efficient examination

- Six possible client positions during an examination

- Hand regions used for palpation

- Immediate and mediate percussion techniques

- Five percussion sounds produced in different body regions

- Differences among sound intensity, pitch, duration, and quality

- Uses of acoustic, magnetic, and electronic stethoscopes

- Equipment preparation for a health assessment

The four assessment techniques in the physical examination are inspection, palpation, percussion, and auscultation. The examiner uses these techniques as an organizing framework to bring the four senses of sight, hearing, touch, and smell into focus. The overall goal of the physical examination is to identify variations from the normal state. The information will then become a part of the client's database.

The database provides subjective and objective information. Subjective information is the client's verbalized perceptions and interpretations. In the interview, the history and review of systems provide subjective information. This information alerts the nurse on what area to focus the examination.

Objective information is obtained through the physical examination. It is data observed or measured by the examiner using all the senses. This information is used to support subjective information given during the interview. Although the major emphasis of this volume is health assessment, certain physiologic functions and perceptions are considered integral to examination of the client, that is, the skills that contribute to physical investigation. Objective data are obtained through these processes. The four techniques of inspection, palpation, percussion, and auscultation are described here. These techniques are further developed in chapters dealing with their application for specific organs and systems.

PREPARATION FOR THE EXAMINATION

To conduct an efficient examination, a consistent pattern of performing the examination is necessary. This will prevent omitting a step and, possibly, vital information. The examiner must be compulsive in the examination routine. A head-to-toe approach is used. The region to be examined must be exposed completely to ensure an accurate finding.

Table 6-1

Positions for examination

Position	Areas assessed	Rationale	Limitations
Sitting	Head and neck, back, posterior thorax and lungs, anterior thorax and lungs, breasts, axilla, heart, vital signs, and upper extremities	Sitting upright provides full expansion of lungs and provides better visualization of symmetry of upper body parts	Client who is physically weakened may be unable to sit. Use supine position with head of bed elevated instead
Supine	Head and neck, anterior thorax and lungs, breasts, axilla, heart, abdomen, extremities, pulses	Most normally relaxed position. Prevents contracture of abdominal muscles. Provides easy access to pulse sites	If client becomes short of breath easily, examiner may need to raise head of bed
Dorsal recumbent	Head and neck, anterior thorax and lungs, breasts, axilla, heart	Certain clients with painful disorders are more comfortable with knees flexed	Not used for abdominal assessment as position promotes contracture of abdominal muscles
Lithotomy	Female genitalia and genital tract	Provides maximal exposure of genitalia and facilitates insertion of vaginal speculum	Embarrassing and uncomfortable position; thus minimize time client spends in this position. Keep client well draped. Patient with severe arthritis or other joint deformity may be unable to assume position
Sims' position	Rectum	Flexion of hip and knee improves exposure of rectal area	Joint deformities may hinder client's ability to bend hip and knee
Prone	Musculoskeletal	Position used only to assess extension of hip joint	Position intolerable for client with respiratory difficulties

From Potter P: Pocket nurse guide to physical assessment, St Louis, 1986, The CV Mosby Co.

The procedure is explained to the client at the beginning of the evaluation and restated as the examination proceeds. Assisting in appropriate positions and warning of uncomfortable maneuvers will be necessary. Table 6-1 summarizes the positions used for assessing different body parts.

EXAMINATION TECHNIQUES

Inspection

Inspection (L. *inspectio,* the act of beholding) is the act of concentrating attention to the thorough and unhurried visualization of the client. Inspection also involves listening to any sounds emanating from the client and being attuned to any odors that may be present.

Lighting must be adequate. Either daylight or artificial light is suitable. The specific cues to which the examiner should be alert are discussed in Chapter 7 on general assessment.

Palpation

By palpation (L. *palpatio,* the act of touching), the examiner's hands may be used to augment the data gathered

through inspection. The skilled examiner will use the most sensitive parts of the hand for each type of palpation (Table 6-2). The examiner may use touch to seek out and determine the extent of tenderness and tremor or spasm of muscle tissues or to elicit crepitus in bones and joints.

HELPFUL HINT: Always palpate areas of tenderness last.

Individual structures within body cavities, particularly the abdomen, may be palpated for position, size, shape, consistency, and mobility. The examining hand may be used to detect masses. Palpation may also serve to evaluate abnormal collections of fluid. Both light and deep palpation may be used in the examination. Light palpation is always performed first. In the case of superficial masses the fingers are moved in a circular motion in the region suspected of containing a mass. The skin and hair are examined for moisture and texture through the use of touch.

Percussion

Percussion (L. *percussio,* the act of striking) involves a cause-and-effect relationship. This summary term in-

Table 6-2

Discriminating areas of the hands used in palpation

Discriminating sense	Sensitive regions of the hands
Fine tactile discrimination	Fingertips
Skin texture	General differences: fingertips
	Fine discrimination: back of the hands and fingers
Position, consistency, and form of a structure or mass	Fingertips using the grasping fingers
Vibration	Palmar aspects of the metacarpophalangeal joints (ball of the hand)
	Alternative method: ulnar side of the hand
Temperature	Dorsa of the hands or fingers (back of the hand)

From Talbot L and Marquardt M: Pocket guide to critical care assessment, St Louis, 1989, The CV Mosby Co.

cludes the act of striking or otherwise producing the impact of one object against another—this is the cause. The result of this rapping is the production of a shock wave that in some cases results in vibration. The vibration may produce sound waves that may reach the ear to be interpreted as sound. In the process of physical diagnosis, percussion means the striking or tapping of a body surface such as the back or the abdomen while listening with the unassisted ear or with the stethoscope.

Auenbrugger, the originator of the technique, described what has been termed *immediate percussion.* Immediate percussion means the striking of a finger or hand directly against the body. The term *mediate percussion* is used to describe the refinement in technique that was developed some time in the 19th century. Instruments called the *pleximeter* and *plexor* were devised. The plexor was a small rubber hammer, much like the reflex hammers used today. It was used to strike a blow against the pleximeter, a small, flat, solid object, often made of ivory, that was held firmly in place against the client's body.

Mediate percussion using the middle finger of one hand as the plexor that strikes against the middle finger (pleximeter) of the other hand is the method in use in current clinical practice.

The passive hand is placed gently against the body surface while the distal portion of the middle finger is placed firmly against the skin. The middle finger is dealt a blow at or immediately distal to the distal interphalangeal joint with the middle finger of the other hand. The

blow must be delivered crisply and sharply and with the plexor perpendicular to the pleximeter.

The speed and force of a blow by the plexor are made possible by wrist action. The hand is flexed back on the forearm and brought forward with a clean, snapping motion that follows a fast strike and rapid removal of the plexor (Fig. 6-1) without dampening the vibration. Fingernails of the plexor finger should be cut sufficiently short to avoid cutting the skin of the pleximeter. Fatty tissue overlying the tissue to be percussed may dampen the blow. To overcome this, it has been suggested that more force can be brought to bear on the body surface by striking the lateral aspect of the thumb. Rapid pronation of the forearm is used to provide the quick, striking movement.

The vibration produced through percussion involves only the tissue closely adjacent to the pleximeter (approximately 3 to 5 cm). Percussion over bones is affected by lateral transmission of vibration.

The change from resonance to dullness is more easily perceived than the dull-to-resonant transition. Thus, the examiner organizes a percussion protocol to progress from more resonant regions to lesser ones.

Fist percussion is, as the name implies, striking with the hand in a fisted position. The blow is delivered with the lateral aspect of the hand. The purpose of this type of percussion is to elicit sensation by the vibration of the tissue. The most common applications are to stimulate pain or tenderness caused by hepatitis, cholecystitis, or kidney disease.

The sound waves that result from percussion are evaluated with reference to intensity, pitch, quality, and duration (Table 6-3).

Sound is produced by vibrating structures. The vibrations generate a series of compression waves in the medium that is capable of sound transmission. Solids, liquids, and gases that are sufficiently elastic to convert energy to motion may transmit sound. The compression waves initiate vibrations of the tympanic membrane, which moves in and out with the frequency of the sound waves. The mechanical energy of the compression waves is transduced into neural signs by receptor structures of the middle ear. These neural signals are transmitted to the temporal cortex and perceived as sound.

Intensity, loudness. The physical property of sound called *intensity* produces the effect of loudness in the human auditory apparatus. As a sound wave travels through a point in the air, the air molecules are compressed and then expanded in the wake of the compression wave. The difference between maximum pressure and minimum pressure is the amplitude of the sound wave. The greater the displacement of air, the more

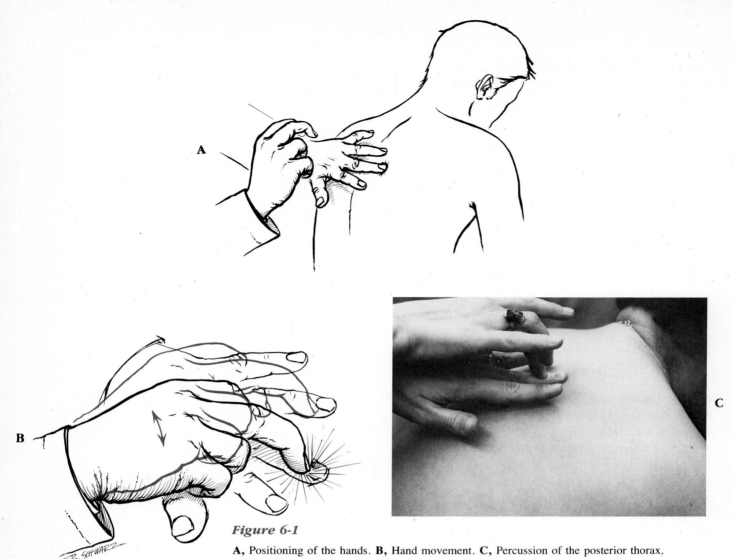

Figure 6-1

A, Positioning of the hands. **B,** Hand movement. **C,** Percussion of the posterior thorax.

movement during vibration of the tympanic membrane and the louder the perception of sound. Loudness is a psychological variable as well. The individual listener may be attentive to or selectively unaware of the many sounds in the environment. Also various alterations in the conduction apparatus of the ear or the sensory neural components of audition may produce alteration in the perception of sound.

Pitch, frequency. The frequency of sound is a physical property that corresponds to the number of vibrations of the sound source per second. *Pitch* is related to the frequency of sound.

The waveform of a sound of single frequency is sinusoidal, ⁓⁓⁓⁓ , with perfectly matched hills (peaks) and valleys (troughs). The distance from one peak to the next is 1 cycle. The recording of frequency is in cycles per second (cps) or hertz (Hz). The human ear can detect sounds in the frequency range of

15 to 30 cps to 20,000 cps. With advancing age, the human ear becomes progressively less sensitive to the higher sound frequencies. The sounds of speech and music (250 to 2,048 cps) are most frequently lost. However, most sounds of importance in physical diagnosis are in the frequency range below 1,000 cps and more particularly in the range of 40 to 500 cps. Thus, the ability to hear sounds that are important to health assessment is not compromised by aging.

Quality, harmonics. *Harmonic,* or *overtone,* refers to the physical property of sound that causes the psychological effect called quality or *timbre.* A sound of single frequency produces a pure tone. The lowest frequency at which a piano wire vibrates is called the *fundamental.* Most objects vibrate at more than one frequency. The piano wire may vibrate as a single unit or in halves or thirds that oscillate at their own frequency. These frequencies will be whole-number multiples of the

Table 6-3

Sounds produced by percussion

Record of finding	Intensity	Pitch	Duration	Quality	Anatomic region where sounds may be encountered
Tympany	Loud	High	Moderate	Drumlike	Air in closed structure vibrates in concert with tissue surrounding it; the gastric air bubble; air in intestine
Hyperresonance	Very loud	Very low	Long	Booming	Air-filled lungs, as in emphysema
Resonance	Moderate to loud	Low	Long	Hollow	Normal lung
Dullness	Soft to moderate	High	Moderate	Thudlike	Liver
Flatness	Soft	High	Short	Flat	Muscle

single frequency. The fundamental and the multiples of the single frequency are the harmonics. Sound quality is produced by the sum of the harmonics present and their intensities. The quality is recorded in descriptive terms such as *humming, buzzing,* or *roaring.* The fundamental is the first harmonic. A musical sound is one wherein the mix of intensity and pitch is pleasing to the ear, whereas *noise* is the term given an unpleasant sensation. Most sounds heard in the course of the physical examination are perceived as noise.

An axiom of the physical examination is that, like the drum, the more air the tissue contains (the less dense the tissue), the deeper, louder, and longer the sound will be. The corollary is that the more compact the tissue, the higher, fainter, and shorter the sound will be. The sounds elicited in percussion are recorded in relation to the density of the tissue being vibrated. The least dense tissues produce tympany, whereas successively more dense tissue results in hyperresonance, resonance, dullness, and flatness.

The percussion hammer (see Fig. 20-48) is used to strike a blow to tendons that serves to stretch the tendon such that a deep tendon reflex is elicited. This will be described in greater detail in the neurologic examination (see Chapter 20).

Auscultation

Auscultation (L. *auscultate,* to listen to) is the process of listening for the sounds produced by the human body. The sounds of particular importance are those produced by (1) the thoracic or abdominal viscera and (2) the movement of blood in the cardiovascular system. *Direct,* or *immediate, auscultation* is accomplished by the unassisted ear, that is, without any amplifying device. This form of auscultation often involves the application of the ear directly to a body surface where the sound is most prominent. The use of a sound augmentation device such

as a stethoscope in the detection of body sounds is called *mediate auscultation.*

Hippocrates described chest sounds in his writings, and Harvey mentioned heart sounds in the early 1600s. Direct, or immediate, auscultation was practiced until 1816, when Laennec devised the first stethoscope, which consisted of a series of rolled up papers held in place with gummed paper. Laennec continued to improve the device and ultimately used a wooden tubing with an earpiece. Later, flexible ear trumpets were modified for use in auscultation. This monaural form of mediate auscultation was succeeded by a binaural instrument in the middle of the 19th century.

The three types of stethoscopes that enjoy clinical popularity today are the acoustic, magnetic, and electronic stethoscopes.

The *acoustic stethoscope* (Fig. 6-2) is essentially a closed cylinder, which serves to inhibit the dissipation of the compression waves produced by the sound source in the column. The diaphragm of the acoustic stethoscope screens out low-frequency sounds and is therefore most effective in assessing high-frequency sounds. The diaphragm is applied firmly to the skin so that it moves synchronously with the body wall.

HELPFUL HINT: A water-soluble jelly applied to the diaphragm will improve the transmission of sound.

The bell-type head is most effective in detecting low-frequency sounds. Care is taken not to flatten the skin by pressing the bell too firmly, since the vibrations of the surface tissues in response to visceral vibration are the source of sound; stretching these tissues inhibits vibration, actually converting the tissue to a diaphragm. The bell chestpiece should be wide enough to span an intercostal space in an adult and deep enough so that it will not fill with tissue.

Several sizes of earpieces are supplied with better

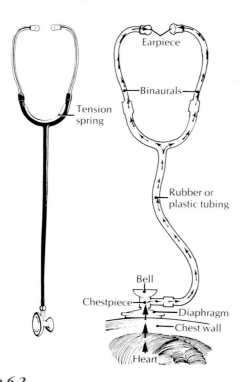

Figure 6-2

Acoustic stethoscope.
(Adapted from Patient Care, March 15, 1974. © Copyright 1974, Miller & Fink Corp., Darien, Conn. All rights reserved.)

stethoscopes. The examiner should determine which size fits the external meatus most snugly. The earpieces should occlude the meatus, thus blocking extraneous sound. However, the earpieces should not cause the examiner pain. Earpieces that are too small will enter the ear canal, causing pain. The binaurals (metal tubing) are angled somewhat toward the nose of the wearer to project the sound onto the tympanic membrane. The direction of the angle may be adjusted by the tension spring. The tubing should not be longer than 12 to 14 in to minimize sound distortion. It is more likely that with longer tubing the sound will be diminished.

An internal bore of ⅛ in has been suggested for best sound transmission. The purpose of the stethoscope is to exclude environmental sound; the system does not magnify sound.

The Harvey stethoscope, a variation of the acoustic type, has three heads: a bell for low frequencies, a corrugated diaphragm for midrange, and a flat diaphragm for high frequencies. This stethoscope also has separate tubes leading to each head.

The *magnetic stethoscope* (Fig. 6-3) has a single head that is a diaphragm. Magnetic attraction is established between an iron disk on the interior surface of the diaphragm and a permanent magnet installed behind it in

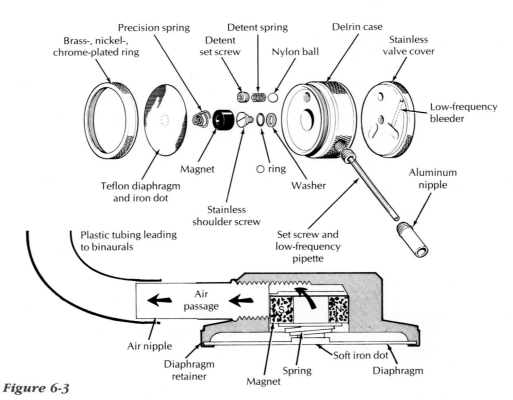

Figure 6-3

Magnetic stethoscope.
(From Patient Care, March 15, 1974. © Copyright 1974, Miller & Fink Corp., Darien, Conn. All rights reserved.)

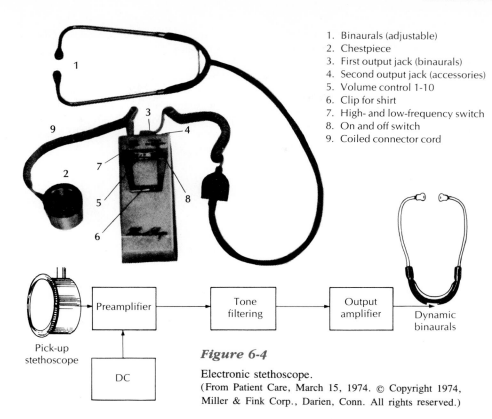

1. Binaurals (adjustable)
2. Chestpiece
3. First output jack (binaurals)
4. Second output jack (accessories)
5. Volume control 1-10
6. Clip for shirt
7. High- and low-frequency switch
8. On and off switch
9. Coiled connector cord

Figure 6-4

Electronic stethoscope.
(From Patient Care, March 15, 1974. © Copyright 1974, Miller & Fink Corp., Darien, Conn. All rights reserved.)

Suggested Equipment for Health Assessment

Sphygmomanometer
Stethoscope
Ophthalmoscope
Otoscope
Percussion hammer
Tuning fork
Cotton balls
Cotton-tipped applicators
Tongue blades
Ruler
Tape measure—metal or nonstretchable plastic
Safety pins
Vaginal speculum
Examination gloves
Flashlight

the head. A strong spring keeps the diaphragm bowed outward when not compressed against a body surface. Application of the diaphragm with the appropriate amount of pressure allows activation of the air column. A dial allows the user to adjust for high-, low-, and full-frequency sounds.

The *electronic stethoscope* (Fig. 6-4) functions when a diaphragm or microphone vibrates due to body surface vibrations. These vibrations are transduced into electrical pulses, which are amplified and converted back to sound at a low speaker.

The use of the stethoscope is described in Chapter 14, Assessment of the Respiratory System, and in Chapter 15, Cardiovascular Assessment: the Heart and the Neck Vessels.

BIBLIOGRAPHY

Andreopoulos S, editor: Primary care: where medicine fails, New York, 1974, John Wiley & Sons, Inc.

Breslow L and Somers AR: The lifetime health monitoring program: a practical approach to preventive medicine, N Engl J Med 296:601, 1977.

Canadian Task Force: Report on the periodic health examination, Can Med Assoc J 121:1193, 1980.

Collen MF: Periodic health examinations, Primary Care 3:197, 1976.

Dales LG, Friedman GD, and Collen MF: Evaluating periodic multiphasic health checkups: a controlled trial, J Chronic Dis 32:385, 1979.

Garfield SR and others: Evaluation of new ambulatory medical care delivery system, N Engl J Med 294:426, 1976.

Hart CR: Screening in general practice, Edinburgh, 1975, Churchill Livingstone.

Javits J: National health care policy for the future, J Politics Policy Law 1:5, 1976.

King C: Refining your assessment techniques, RN 46:42-47, 1983.

Leavell HR and Clark EG: Preventive medicine for the doctor in his community, ed 3, New York, 1965, McGraw-Hill Book Co.

Mushkin SJ, editor: Consumer incentives for health care, New York, 1974, Prodist.

Rappaport MD and Sprague HB: The effects of tubing bore on stethoscope efficiency, Am Heart J 42:605, 1951.

Somers AR: Lifetime health monitoring: preventive care for the child in utero, Patient Care 13:162, 1979.

Somers AR: Lifetime health monitoring: preventive care: age 1 through adolescence, Patient Care 13:201, 1979.

Somers AR: Lifetime health monitoring: a whole-life plan for well patient care, Patient Care 13(11):83, 1979.

Spitzer WO and others: The Burlington randomized trial of the nurse practitioner, N Engl J Med 290:251, 1974.

Talbot L and Marquardt M: Pocket guide to critical care assessment, St Louis, 1989, The CV Mosby Co.

7

General assessment, including vital signs

OBJECTIVES

Upon successful review of this chapter, learners will be able to state related rationale and to demonstrate:

- General inspection techniques and common findings

- Assessment of body morphology:
  Musculoskeletal, posture, and gait
  Skin, hair, and nails
  Face and eyes
  Apparent age and hygiene
  Speech and communication
  Mental status

- Assessment of vital signs:
  Factors influencing temperature
  Temperature measurements with thermometry
  Oral, rectal, and axillary temperatures
  Fever patterns and conditions
  Pulse points
  Usual rate, elasticity, and pulsation findings
  Pulsation irregularities
  Normal systolic and diastolic blood pressure
  Blood pressure measurements by palpation, mercury gravity and aneroid sphygmomanometer, and electronic manometers
  Blood pressure variations
  Hypotension and hypertension

Having concluded the general remarks about health assessment and the discussion of methods of obtaining subjective data from the client, the examiner proceeds to those techniques that allow the *objective* measurements of health assessment—the physical examination. Pathologic phenomena are recognized and localized through the client's and examiner's coordinated efforts. Symptoms can be elicited only in the interview. The client's description allows the examiner to look at the nature of the complaint from the vantage point of the client's perception. The examiner often gains valuable insights from the client's presentation on whether a pathologic condition of tissue or function exists. Furthermore, indications of the client's cooperation, motivation, and objectives may be obtained. However, the examiner's observations are essential to verifying the client's descriptions and identifying signs of which the client was unaware. Furthermore, the tools of physical assessment allow exploration of facets not usually available to the client. Conclusions about an individual's health are drawn from synthesizing information from the client's description and the physical assessment.

SURVEY OR GENERAL INSPECTION

The survey or general inspection begins with those observations made when the client enters the room, during introductions, and as he or she follows instructions for seating before the interview begins. It is the *overall impression of the client's general state of health* and *outstanding characteristics.*

The general observations continue throughout the interview. In some cases this initial impression sets the focus of the interview and of the physical examination. For instance, some feature of the client's appearance may point immediately to the problem; sparse, fine hair, for example, may indicate the need to look further for the edema, slow speech, hoarse voice, and sluggish movement of the hypothyroid individual.

Certain characteristics typically are noted in this section of the physical examination record: *apparent age; sex; race; body type (constitution), stature, and symmetry; weight and nutritional status; posture and motor activity; mental status; speech; general skin condition; apparent state of health and signs of distress or disorder.* These factors are not limited to a single system of the body but are instead parameters for the total or whole person—the general appearance, head to toe.

In general, the survey proceeds in a *cephalocaudal* (head to toe) direction. The examiner observes thoroughly and discerningly. Many professionals experience some difficulty in gazing at the client without doing some task simultaneously. However, total absorption in the process of looking and perceiving must be achieved.

The practitioner perceives only that to which he or she is prepared to attend. Therefore, the practitioner should keep a plan in mind for stimuli to perceive, associate, and respond to. Although the term *inspection* implies restriction to visual stimuli, the examination may include smell, hearing, and touch as well.

Every attempt should be made to concentrate on the person being examined. The complete absorption with the client is learned with practice and careful guarding against distractions from the environment and internally against preoccupations with unrelated thoughts. The purpose of total and focused concentration on the client is to allow the examiner to process information with all sensory circuits.

An example of the record of the general survey might read as follows:

Mr. A. is an alert, loquacious, asthenic 25-year-old white male who appears younger than his stated age and exhibits no indication of distress. He does not appear acutely or chronically ill.

Accurate observations can only be made in good light. This is particularly important in assessing skin color.

Although this initial survey may be considered a scanning procedure, the highlights gathered by the astute practitioner may be used as the basis for planning those portions of the examination deserving special attention and perhaps for establishing the client's problem list.

The Client as a Whole

The general impression of wellness should be assessed. Historically, health and illness have been defined as opposites. For instance, the World Health Organization

---

Screening Examination

1. Working from head to toe, perform a general inspection or survey for an overall impression of the client's general state of health and outstanding characteristics. Note the apparent age, sex, race, body type, stature and symmetry, weight and nutritional status, posture and motor activity, mental status, speech, general skin condition, and apparent state of health and signs of distress.
2. Assess the vital signs. Take the temperature, pulse, respiratory rate, and blood pressure. Use the techniques of inspection, palpation, and auscultation to assess these cardinal signs.
3. The usual range for temperature is 97° to 99.6° F. Note that multiple factors influence body temperature. Take a complete history to ensure the accuracy of the temperature reading.
4. The pulse rate is between 50 to 100 beats per minute based on American Heart Association (AHA) standards. Count the pulse for 1 full minute to obtain a complete evaluation of the rate, rhythm, and volume.
5. The normal systolic blood pressure range is 95 to 140 mm Hg. The normal diastolic pressure range is 60 to 90 mm Hg. When using a sphygmomanometer, be sure to use the appropriate size cuff to ensure an accurate reading.

(WHO) has defined health as "a state of complete physical, mental, and social well-being and not merely the absence of disease." By implication, any other condition is defined as illness. More recently, health and illness have been described in terms of a continuum. This conceptualization expresses the philosophy that the human being is never in a state of absolute wellness, or nonillness; that the person, in fact, varies from conditions of high-level wellness to markedly poor health, close to death. Illness is considered to exist when there is a disturbance or failure in either the biophysical or psychosocial function or development, so that observable (signs) or felt (symptoms) changes in the body are present. Mental or emotional illness is said to exist when the individual demonstrates inappropriate or inadequate behavior in a given social context. Essentially, high-level wellness for an individual means that health is such that the person functions optimally.

Some terse but typical kinds of descriptions that have appeared as survey summaries are as follows:

He appears acutely ill.
He appears chronically ill.
He appears frail.

The supporting documentation for these general terms makes the description more meaningful. For instance, the description of *chronically ill* might include terms such as *cachectic* or *dehydrated* or other, more descriptive terms.

The practitioner should be aware of signs of distress in the patient. Detection of distress may predicate dealing with the underlying problem immediately and curtailing the full interview and physical examination for the present. Some of the signs that might require intervention are (1) anxiety that may be indicated by anxious or tense facies, fidgety movements, cold, moist palms, and an apparent inability to process questions normally; (2) pain that may be indicated by drawn features, moaning, writhing, or guarding of the painful part; (3) cardiopulmonary distress that may be signaled by labored breathing, wheezing, or coughing (Since the color of the skin is determined by the amount of oxygen-carrying hemoglobin and by the constriction or dilatation of the capillary beds, cyanosis and pallor are excellent indications of cardiopulmonary distress); (4) alteration in consciousness; or (5) hemorrhage.

Observation of the Face

The examiner's attention is generally drawn to the face first. The face is observed for *symmetry, contour,* and normal facial expression. Individuals suffering from Parkinson's syndrome tend to have motionless faces. Limited movement of the musculature leads to a paucity of facial expression. In addition, the blinking rate is slowed so that the client appears to stare. The facial changes that occur with acromegaly include a prominent supraorbital ridge, jutting jaw, and enlarged nose and lips. In myxedema (hypothyroidism) the features are flattened because of the swelling occasioned by fluid retention caused by the accumulation of mucopolysaccharides. The face appears heavy and coarse. The individual with Bell's palsy has paralysis of muscles served by the facial nerve and is unable to close the eye; the face appears flaccid, and the mouth droops on the affected side. (See section on nonverbal communication in the interview.)

Body Type and Stature

A concise description of the client's bodily proportions should be included in the written record of the general survey.

Normal Body Types

Although the constitution is to some degree genetically determined in the sense that endocrine control is inherited, the environment may play a significant role in altering the physiognomy. Descriptions of several normal body types (constitutions) by Draper and colleagues

(1944) may help the examiner understand the variation of anatomy seen in groups of normal individuals.

Sthenic type. The sthenic constitution is one of average height, well-developed musculature, wide shoulders with a subcostal angle that is approximately a right angle, and a flat abdomen. The most frequently observed type of face is ovoid, and the dental arch is round and wide.

Hypersthenic type. The hypersthenic body build is short and stocky and the most likely of the body types to be obese. The chest is shorter and broader than is the sthenic build. The costal margin is a wider angle (obtuse). The heart is likely to lie in a transverse position. The abdominal wall is thicker than in the sthenic constitution. Roentgenographic examination reveals the stomach to be higher in the abdomen and more or less in a transverse configuration. The face is more rectangular, as is the dental arch.

Hyposthenic type. The hyposthenic body build is often characterized as tall and willowy. The musculature is poorly developed. The subcostal angle is more acute than in the sthenic type. The chest is long and flat, with the heart in a more midline and vertical position. Since abdominal muscles are not as well developed, the abdominal wall may sag outward. The stomach is observed to be lower in the abdomen and more vertical in position. The neck is long. The face is triangular (narrower and more pointed), as is the dental arch.

Asthenic type. The asthenic body build is an exaggeration of the hyposthenic constitution.

• • •

An essential part of the assessment of children or, for that matter, anyone who has not completed the growth cycle, is the accurate, serial measurement of height and weight. Growth charts (see Chapter 24) assembled from data gathered from large populations allow a comparison of the pattern growth of an individual child with national standards. Children with inherited disorders of growth are known to deviate from the normal standards throughout most of the growth period; for example, children who have genetically determined tall stature grow at a normal rate and thus their growth curves are parallel to the normal curve but higher. An acquired alteration in growth would be deduced from a curve that followed the normal growth curve for some time and subsequently deviated. Chronic diseases of a nonendocrine nature known to cause short stature include diseases of the heart, lungs, kidneys, liver, gastrointestinal tract, bones and cartilage, blood-forming organs, and central nervous system (CNS). Lack of psychosocial stimulation may also lead to growth retardation (failure to thrive). Endocrine diseases known to inhibit the growth processes are hypothyroidism, glucocorticoid excess, and growth hormone (GH) deficiency. Because it is possible to treat those individuals who have a GH deficiency, it is necessary to differentiate this disorder from other growth patterns. Children who were known to have intrauterine growth retardation or who have a family history of less than normal height or a family pattern of delayed growth are generally not referred unless they are three standard deviations below the mean height for their age.

Gross Abnormalities in Body Build

Two rules of thumb that have been suggested in comparing body parts for appropriate development are (1) the distance from fingertip to fingertip of outstretched arms should equal the height; and (2) the distance from the crown to the pubic symphysis should roughly equal the distance from the pubic symphysis to the sole. Normally the ratio of the upper segment measurement to that of the lower segment is about 0.92 in whites and 0.85 in blacks.

Marfan's syndrome. Elongated arms and limbs compared with the trunk may indicate hypogonadism or Marfan's syndrome, a genetic disorder.

In Marfan's syndrome, an inherited generalized disorder of connective tissue, the tubular bones are elongated and the ratio is lower. In addition, the arm span exceeds the height.

Hyposomatotropism.   *Dwarfism* is the general term used to mean an abnormally small person who has normal body proportions. Achondroplastic dwarfism refers to that individual who has abnormally small limbs but a normal-size trunk and head. This is the result of a disorder of cartilaginous growth.

Pituitary hyposomatic dwarfism.   Pituitary dwarfism is the consequence of hyposecretion of GH. That deficiency in GH has little effect over fetal growth is evidenced by the relatively normal size at birth of babies who have no pituitary gland. However, the length at birth of the infant with hyposecretion of GH is less than that of the normal infant. The rate of growth declines in the first months of life and may be noticeable by the sixth month but more frequently is diagnosed between that age and around 3 years, at which time physical growth is half that of normal. However, because the epiphyseal closure is retarded, growth continues into the 40s and 50s, ending at the height of 4 or 5 feet. General health is maintained, and normal immune mechanisms are present. Mental development is usually normal for chronologic age. Men are affected twice as often as women. Many of the children appear obese, with adipose depositions over the iliac crest and lower abdomen. Sec-

ondary teeth erupt late. In adult life these dwarfs often develop wrinkles about the eyes and mouth and appear prematurely old.

Laron dwarfism.   Laron dwarfism is a genetically transmitted (mendelian recessive) form of dwarfism that occurs in Oriental, Jewish, and other Middle Eastern peoples. The condition is characterized by high levels of GH and low levels of somatomedin (SF), although metabolic response to exogenous GH hormones is subnormal.

African pigmy.   The condition known as *African pigmy* is polygenically transmitted and is characterized by resistance to both GH and SF.

• • •

Growth failure can follow any serious illness or nutritional deficiency in childhood. Prolonged corticosteroid therapy has been associated with early epiphyseal closure and growth lag. Some of the diseases associated with growth failure are Laurence-Moon-Biedl syndrome, mongolism, achondroplasia, neurofibromatosis, severe congenital heart disease, congenital hemolytic anemia, and progeria.

Failure to thrive.   Growth failure occurs in some children who suffer parental neglect or are deprived of love and affection. These children are characterized by distortions of appetite-feeding patterns and by the eating of food not considered nourishing or edible (pica). Bloating may be present, and clinical symptoms like those of malabsorption may be present.

Hypothyroidism.   Hypothyroidism, beginning in infancy, is called cretinism and is characterized by retarded bone maturation and multiple abnormal areas of epiphyseal ossification. Juvenile myxedema is also a cause of retarded growth.

Gonadal dysfunction.   Gonadal dysplasia should be suspected in short girls with primary amenorrhea and congenital anomalies such as webbing of the neck, short metacarpal or metatarsal bones, or increased carrying angle of the elbows. (X chromosome defect may be noted on cytologic examination.)

Hypersomatotropism.   Hypersomatotropism is characterized by abnormally enhanced secretion of GH.

Tall stature may be genetic and may be a cause for concern in girls. Treatment with estrogen has been shown to accelerate epiphyseal closure. However, the long-term effects of estrogen therapy are not known, and controversy surrounds the advisability of treatment with this hormone.

Gigantism.   The hypersecretion of GH occurring before puberty and before the ossification of the epiphyseal plates causes overgrowth of the long bones, and gigantism results. The length of time of long bone growth is also lengthened, since the gonadal secretion is depressed. Adrenocorticotropic hormone (ACTH) or thyroid-stimulating hormone (TSH) secretion may be deficient.

Excessive GH in children is caused by an actively secreting pituitary tumor. Because the tumor may be treated by radiation or surgery, these individuals are referred to specialists.

Cerebral gigantism (Soto's syndrome) is a growth disorder wherein the individual is abnormally tall at birth and continues to grow at a more rapid than normal rate until the second or third year, after which growth is normal. The disorder is not thought to be hormonally engendered and may be genetic. The affected children are generally mentally retarded.

Acromegaly. Acromegaly is a disease caused by hypersecretion of GH; it is evidenced clinically in the fourth or fifth decade. In most instances, growth of the acral (small) parts proceeds so slowly that their appreciation may not occur until the changes are well advanced. Bony and soft tissue growth is apparent clinically. Bony changes in the skull are most apparent. The mandible is increased in length and width. Prognathism or overbite of the lower incisors beyond the upper incisors by as much as a half inch is a characteristic of acromegaly. There is little increase in height, since the epiphyseal plates have closed. The teeth become separated as the jaw elongates. The features are exaggerated as a result of the expansion of the facial, molar, and frontal bones. The skull itself, as well as the sinuses, may be markedly enlarged. However, in some individuals only a single feature appears grossly enlarged, such as the jaw or the supraorbital ridge. Arthralgia and arthritis are commonly present in acromegaly.

With the increased total mass of connective tissue that occurs concomitantly with the retention of interstitial fluid, the skin appears coarse and leathery and the pores and markings of the skin appear enlarged. In addition, the hands are large with broad fingers and wide palms, thereby earning the description "spade hand." The tongue is frequently enlarged and furrowed. The body hair is coarse and increased in amount. On physical examination both cardiomegaly and hepatomegaly may be found.

Hyperthyroid conditions are associated with increased mitosis and skeletal growth.

Symmetry

The arrangement of most structures of the human body is symmetric; that is, size and shape of parts correspond. Inspection that reveals obvious areas of lack of symmetry should be noted and investigated later.

Weight

The client should be weighed and the height measured to compare these parameters with actuarial tables prepared by insurance companies of average weights and heights.

HELPFUL HINT: The client may be weighed with or without clothes. The circumstances in which weighing was done should be noted. Height should be measured without the client wearing shoes.

Unexplained weight loss frequently accompanies acute and chronic disease and may be one of the early signs of illness. Weight loss may occur as a result of fever, infection, neoplastic disease, endocrine or metabolic disorders, drug intoxication, disorders of the mouth and pharynx, and psychiatric disorders.

Patterns of adiposity are described here so that the typical fat deposits of obesity may be differentiated from those of disease states.

A sex difference is apparent in adipose deposition. Women are observed to have fat deposits over the shoulders, breasts, buttocks or lateral aspect of the thighs, and pubic symphysis. The fat deposits in men are more evenly dispersed throughout the body.

The fat deposition that is characteristic of Cushing's syndrome (hyperadrenalism) or administration of the glucocorticoid hormone is found in the facial, nuchal, truncal, and girdle areas. This kind of obesity has been termed centripetal "buffalo" obesity.

In addition to fat deposition patterns, there are other differences between simple obesity and Cushing's syndrome that may be helpful in establishing the diagnosis.

Obesity	*Cushing's syndrome*
Thick skin	Thin skin
Pale striae	Purplish striae
Absence of plethora	Plethora
Preservation of muscle strength	Protein wasting resulting in muscle weakness
No evidence of osteoporosis	Evidence of osteoporosis
Uniform distribution of fat—sex related	Redistribution of fat deposits Truncal obesity "Buffalo hump"—cervicodorsal fat "Moon facies" Thin extremities

Growth is arrested in Cushing's syndrome; therefore, the obese child who is growing rapidly probably does not have this disease.

It is well to remember that the increased serum levels of the glucocorticoids may be a result of delayed metabolism of these hormones by the liver or of increased production of estrogen.

Apparent Age

There is great disparity in the apparent age of individuals at the same chronologic age. These differences arise as a result of such influences as heredity, sex, past medical history, and life experiences.

Physical changes that have been associated with the aging process are elevations in blood pressure, decreased cardiac output and stroke volume as well as lessened pulmonary reserve. However, those changes, like the "aches and pains" of old age, may be preventable or at least treatable with judicious exercise and hormone replacement. The kyphosis in women that once indicated the presence of osteoporosis may be prevented with postmenopausal hormones and maintenance of calcium balance through diet and medication.

There are some indications that may help the practitioner in estimating the apparent age. Elastic fibers in the corium of the skin decline in number with advancing age. As the individual ages, the skin loses turgor, that is, its ability to return to its normal contour when released after being picked up between the examiner's fingers. The skin appears dull, moves less readily, sags, and wrinkles. These changes are noticeable in middle age and are first observable in the anterior neck and chin.

Hair begins to decline in amount in the middle years as the sex hormones decrease in amount.

Progeria is the term for premature senility occurring in childhood. The stature is small; the face looks old and wizened; the skin is dry and thin and the hair scanty; and sexual organs are infantile.

Precocious puberty is the term for premature maturation of the gonads accompanied by secondary sexual characteristics.

Posture

"Harmonious movement leads to harmonious thought" (Plato). Posture is a part of body image. It is customary to correlate good body alignment with good health. Good posture depends on a normal sense of balance—muscular coordination as well as conditioned learning. Appropriate posture in any circumstance is that which requires the least investment of energy.

Minimum muscular effort is required to maintain an upright posture when the line of the center of gravity bisects the principal weight-bearing joints and is the same distance from each foot. Upright posture requires the contraction of the antigravity muscles. Specifically, these muscles are erector spinae, gluteals, quadriceps, and calf muscles. Other muscles contributing to upright posture are the abdominal muscles.

Proprioception and Posture

Eye muscles. The extraocular muscles of the eye and the vestibular function are integrated to maintain the upright individual's eyes in a horizontal plane and to maintain fixation of the eye on the selected object. Eye muscles play a role in *proprioception*, whereas the *exteroceptive* impulses are received through the retina. It is important to note that a normal person can balance in the dark when all other neural functions are adequate.

Vestibular organs. Disorders of the vestibular system are known to lead to loss of balance. However, an individual can learn to balance even when all vestibular function is lost. An individual with no vestibular function cannot adjust to rapid postural adjustments or maintain eye fixation in a moving vehicle.

Muscles, tendons, and joints. Proprioceptive impulses from the muscles, tendons, and joints provide information about the body's position in space and major influences in the maintenance of posture. These impulses are integrated in the mid-brain and cerebellum.

Exteroception and Posture

Stimulation of the retina of the eye results in the head's turning and in fixation of the eye.

Posture of the Elderly

Bone and joint changes contribute to the bent posture that has been ascribed to the elderly in the literature of all eras. Joint degeneration and osteoporosis occur with aging. The intervertebral disks decrease in height and osteoporotic changes are noted, particularly in the vertebrae. Thus, changes are correlated with the waning of estrogen levels in women and testosterone in men. Although osteoporosis may be prevented or controlled with appropriate care, aging changes such as widening and flattening of the third cervical vertebrae and drying of the intervertebral disks produce alteration such that any given individual may be as much as 1 in shorter than his or her usual adult height.

Although it is generally observed that all muscles decline in girth and strength with aging, the muscles of the trunk are particularly affected. Thus, weakness of the abdominal muscles also contributes to the slumped posture.

There is some correlative evidence that appropriate exercise may aid the person to maintain erect posture. The Chinese shadow boxing exercises are purported to maintain body awareness and posture despite advancing years. Abnormal posture is most likely to result from pathologic conditions of the muscles, bones, joints, or neurologic system.

Poor posture maintained over a long period results in painful joints, ligaments, and muscles. Occupations requiring positions that deviate from normal alignment may result in chronic pain or deformity, for example, bent shoulders in mine workers and painful shoulders in sewing machine operators. Frequent changes of posture are necessary for comfort.

Bent or disordered body alignment may lead to changes of the surrounding soft tissue. An example of this is the change in lung volume and ventilation, as well as in circulation, that occurs with scoliosis.

Certain pathologic conditions are characterized by specific postures, for example, the deviation of the spine toward the affected side in sciatica and the maintenance of a position that elevates the clavicles, such as leaning forward on extended arms, by the client with chronic obstructive lung disease.

The practitioner should develop a protocol for accurately observing the main postures of the body in all its common acts. Beginning observations are made by watching the client come into the room and sit down and by observing while the client lies on the examining table. It is important to note whether the client sits tensely or slumps in the chair. Rigid positioning of the neck may be the result of a fixated spine. Respiratory distress may result when the patient tries to lie flat. Hyperextension of the neck and muscular rigidity may indicate meningitis. Leaning to one side may be a response to a fractured rib. Carcinoma of the tail of the pancreas may result in complaints of pain over the lower thoracic spine when the client is asked to lie flat. Girdle muscle weakness patterns may be seen when a person rises from a chair or climbs stairs.

Gait

The characteristics of the client's walk often provide clues to the pathophysiology involved in the client's problems. The client with a disorder in *gait* should be observed for natural stance and for the attitude and dominant positions of the trunk, legs, and arms. The patient may be asked to walk a straight line. The rapidity or slowness of step may be noteworthy, as well as the style of movement. Table 7-1 presents various types of gait that are readily recognized.

The phases of normal gait are stance and swing. The components of stance are described in reference to the pressure exerted by the part of the foot contacting the surface beneath it: (1) heel strike, (2) full foot, (3) midstance of the foot, and (4) metatarsal pushoff.

The normal heel strike is quiet and smoothly coordinated. The knee is in extension during the heel strike. The movement to full contact of the foot with the floor should be complete and proceed smoothly. The midstance of the foot is the shift of weight onto the foot. The weight should be supported evenly by all aspects of the foot. The hip will be displaced 2 to 5 cm over the weight-bearing foot. The knee is slightly flexed during weight bearing. During metatarsal pushoff, a smoothly coordinated lift off the floor is observed. The metatarsal joint is extended. In the swing phase following the contact of the foot with the floor, three components are acceleration, midswing, and deceleration. The acceleration component is the contraction of the quadriceps muscle to initiate extension of the leg and forward swing of the leg. Knee flexion results in elevation of the foot, which is accompanied by dorsiflexion of the foot to allow ground clearance. The foot remains in dorsiflexion in midswing. Deceleration involves a contraction of the hamstring muscles to inhibit forward swing of the leg in preparation for the subsequent heel strike.

In normal gait the shoulders rotate 180 degrees out of phase with the pelvis. This is seen as an equal and symmetric arm swing.

Body Movements

Body movements are observed to detect lack of coordination and tremor occurring at rest or stimulated by voluntary movement. The amplitude of tremor or involuntary movement may be fine or coarse and may be confined to a single muscle or be generalized to the entire body. Examples of generalized involvement of skeletal muscles in involuntary contraction include the convulsive movements of epilepsy and the choreiform movements of Huntington's chorea. Asymmetry of body movement frequently occurs with damage to the CNS or with peripheral nerve damage.

Hair and Hair Growth Patterns

Inspection for hair growth is made on the following body regions: scalp, beard, mustache, ears, hypogastric area, thoracic area, lower limbs, genital area, lumbosacral area, upper back, midphalangeal area, pubis, and axillae.

The hair is assessed for growth characteristics, distribution, density of growth, appearance, and hygiene.

In the present evolutionary state of *Homo sapiens,* hair growth patterns have a great deal of social value. Whereas in lower animals the skin covering of hair may afford warmth and protection of exposed body parts from friction during motion, in human beings hair serves a decorative function.

Hair growth is influenced by hereditary and racial factors. Excessive hairiness is thought to be a dominant

Table 7-1

Diagnostic patterns of gait

Form	Description	Associated disorders
Spastic	Leg held stiffly—does not flex freely; jerking movements; poorly coordinated; short steps dragging all of foot over floor	Multiple sclerosis; syringomyelia; cerebral spastic diplegia
Scissors	Spasticity of adductor muscles of legs with legs held close together adducted; one knee may cross over the other; feet further separated	Spastic paraplegia; paresis; cerebral palsy (choreoathetosis)
Atactic (cerebellar gait)	Staggering, reeling, lurching; steps uncertain; some shorter or longer than intended; may lurch to one side	Acute disease of cerebellum, cerebellar tracts of brain; severe alcohol and barbiturate intoxication
Sensory atactic	Uncertainty, irregularity, and stamping of feet Depends on vision for clues	Interruption of afferent fibers for proprioception—tabes dorsalis Pernicious anemia
Slapping (steppage); weak muscles of dorsiflexion (footdrop)	Walks on broad base with feet wide apart; raises foot abnormally high to be certain of clearing the floor with the toes (steppage)—slapping noises as foot strikes floor; eyes on floor to observe where to place foot	Peripheral nerve disease; paralysis of pretibial and peroneal muscles; posterior column disease; tertiary syphilis
Foot dragging (hemiplegic gait)	Affected foot dragged in semicircle with toes outward; arms on affected side held rigidly against chest wall	Hemiplegia and paraplegia
Festinating (parkinsonian gait)	Body rigid, trunk bent forward—flexion of hips, knees; short, mincing steps barely clear ground—shuffling; arms carried ahead of body in abduction; wrists extended, fingers flexed at metacarpal joints—do not swing; may make sudden hastening forward movement (propulsion) or backward movement (retropulsion)	Parkinsonism
Waddling or rolling (dystrophic gait)	Proximal muscle weakness Steps regular, but uncertain; often lumbar lordosis; exaggerated elevation of one hip, depression of other	Muscular dystrophy

hereditary trait in the presence of androgens, whereas thinning or absence of hair is a recessive trait.

Although hair growth is continuous in some animals, in most animals, including humans, hair growth is cyclic. Hair growth occurs in what is known as an anagen phase; it then enters a telogen, or resting, phase before it is pushed out and new hair grows in the follicle.

The anagen phase may continue for years in areas such as the scalp. This long phase of growth contributes to longer hairs. Pubic hair, on the other hand, grows for only a few months.

Hair growth can be described in terms of cycle, rate of growth, size, and density.

Hair grows at various rates. The most rapid rate of growth is that of the beard, followed by that of the scalp, axillae, thighs, and eyebrows. Long hairs regenerate most rapidly. More rapid regrowth is noted in scalp hair in men than in women, but in men regrowth is slower in the axillae and on the thighs. The normal rate of head hair growth is 0.35 mm per day or 10 to 12 mm per

month in adults. Hair grows more rapidly in children. The rate of hair growth is affected by environmental temperature and by the general state of health. Extremely cold temperatures such as those experienced in the Antarctic, impede hair growth, whereas hot climates appear to promote increased length.

General protein production is inhibited in starvation, and this is reflected in reduced hair growth and dullness in appearance. Chemotherapeutic drugs inhibit cell division and thereby inhibit hair growth. X-ray radiation causes hair to switch to the telogen phase and causes atrophy of perifollicular structures, resulting in hair loss.

White persons have more abundant and coarser body hair growth than do Asians. Facial hirsutism has been described for more than 40% of white women. Japanese women, on the other hand, do not develop excessive facial hair growth, and Japanese men have sparser beards than do white men. Blacks have kinky hair, whereas whites have straight or wavy to curly hair. Mongolians and American Indians have straight hair.

A heavier distribution of hair is correlated with darker skin pigmentation; that is, the brunette individual is more likely to have more hair than the blonde person.

Some male hair growth characteristics may be normal for women of certain ethnic or familial groups and could include hair growth on the upper lip; sideburns; and hair growth on the intermammary periareolar area, abdomen, and lower limbs.

Because of the variations in hair growth patterns among individuals, it is more important to note marked changes in hair growth characteristics. Hair growth increases in normal sites have been associated with adrenal tumors.

Hair has been classified into three categories: primary, secondary, and terminal hair. Primary hair is the very fine, thinly pigmented short hair of the fetus. Secondary hair resembles primary hair structurally but appears postnatally. This secondary hair is generally distributed over the body and is the hair type involved in hypertrichosis. This hair is often termed *lanuginous* or *vellus* and is not hormonally influenced. Terminal hair is a coarser and more heavily pigmented growth that appears at the time of puberty. Axillary and pubic terminal hair is called *ambosexual* hair. Adrenal hormones initiate the growth of this coarse hair, which is also influenced by ovarian and testicular hormones. True sexual hair is that which grows on the face, chest, abdomen, back and extremities.

The hair may also be classified by the types of hormonal influences the growth receives:
1. Hair dependent on GH is that which grows on the head, eyelashes, eyebrows, midphalangeal area, and distal portions of limbs and, to some extent, on the lumbosacral area.
2. Hair dependent on female hormones is that which grows on the pubic area, axillary limbs, and hypogastric area. The male hypogastric or pubic hair configuration is that of a diamond with its superior angle at the umbilicus, whereas the female pubic hair pattern is triangular with the base over the mons.
3. Hair dependent on male hormones is that of the beard, mustache, nasal tip, and ear, and body hair (particularly on the back).

Morphologic characteristics of the hair found in various anatomic sites are described in Table 7-2.

Hirsutism, the appearance of excessive hair in normal and abnormal sites, can be most disturbing to the affected female client. The degree of overgrowth need not be marked to pose a threat to the client's feelings of femininity.

On noting hirsutism in the female client, the ex-

Table 7-2

Morphologic hair types in humans

Growth site	Description	Length (mm)
Head	Relatively small root; tapered tip; many variations	1000
Eyebrow and eyelash	Curved; smooth; coarse; punctate tip	10
Beard and mustache	Relatively longer root than scalp hair; blunt tip	300
Body	Fine; long tip	Up to 60
Pubic	Coarse; irregular; asymmetric; usually curved but may be spiral tufted	Up to 60
Axillary	Coarse; straighter than pubic hair; may be spiral tufted in blacks	Up to 50

aminer is alerted to note the presence of other virilizing signs, which include a deepening of the voice, clitoral enlargement, and changes in fat distribution.

Hirsutism has been observed in the following pathophysiologic conditions: bilateral polycystic ovary, Cushing's syndrome, and ovarian tumor.

Because of the identity confusion that may exist in the presence of hirsutism, the examiner approaches the investigation of the problem with sensitively phrased queries.

Description of the hirsute condition may be facilitated by Table 7-3.

Hair Loss

Balding. Balding *(alopecia)* is more frequently noted in those individuals with abundant growth of coarse, or terminal, hair on the body and is thought to be related to androgen production. Male pattern baldness is recession of the hairline and baldness of the crown.

Generally, the man with a hairline that is low on the forehead does not bald. As a rule, women do not bald unless androgens are present in relatively increased amounts or the baldness occurs as a result of another disease.

Alopecia areata. Alopecia areata is an autoimmune disorder thought to be genetic in cause. The persons affected with alopecia areata frequently have other autoimmune disorders such as vitiligo, Hashimoto's thyroiditis, or diabetes mellitus. Some 35% of clients with alopecia areata have an endocrine disease.

Table 7-3

Classification of hirsutism

Stage	Site	Symbols for recording quantity, quality*
1	Lanuginous hair Not in virilizing sites	D_1Q_1
2	Coarser hair as in men Distribution sites: Upper lips Sideburns Intermammary area Periareolar area Midabdomen	D_1Q_2
3	Same sites as stage 2, as well as: Upper back Shoulders Inner thighs Ears, nose Supragluteal and gluteal areas Temporal recession	D_2Q_2 to D_3Q_3
4	Same sites as stage 3; in addition shows other signs of virilization	D_3Q_3

*D, Quantity: D_1, mild; D_2, moderate; D_3 profuse. Q, Quality: Q_1, fine; Q_2, coarse; Q_3, very coarse.

Fungal infections. Fungal infections may cause hair loss. The fungal contamination is frequently acquired from pets and contaminated cosmetics.

Pohl's sign. Pohl's sign is a constriction of the hair shaft that occurs as a result of systemic illness or malnutrition. Illnesses associated with constriction of the shaft and hair loss are hypopituitarism, hypothyroidism, hyperthyroidism, and uncontrolled diabetes.

Chemical, thermal, and physically abusive treatment of the hair causes damage to the surface characterized by breaking and splitting.

Odors

The odor of the body and breath should be noted. The smell of alcohol on the client's breath alerts one to look for other effects of this CNS depressant. The fruity odor of acetone indicates that diabetes and starvation must be ruled out, whereas a fetid breath points to the possibility of an oral or pulmonary infection or may simply be the result of poor oral hygiene but may indicate infection or foreign body with infection. The odor of ammonia may be detectable in the patient with uremia. Body odor may be related to the activities of the sweat and sebaceous glands and to the general cleanliness of the body.

The odors emanating from the client may provide clues helpful in defining the client's condition. Some diseases are characterized by particular odors emanating from the mouth. The odors known to have diagnostic importance are listed in the boxed material on p. 155.

Nails

The nails may indicate the level of concern and care the person has for appearance. The nails are inspected as to length, cleanliness, neatness of filing, and, if the client is a woman, the presence and condition of polish. The examiner further notes the texture, recording thickness and ridging when present (see Chapter 8 for inspection of the nails).

Personal Hygiene

General cleanliness of the body is an important indication of the individual's self-esteem and of the availability of necessary supplies to maintain good body care. Again, this is a socioculturally flavored value. It is important to note that deodorants are not used in all cultures. Although shaving of the legs is a norm in some groups of women in the United States, it is not practiced by other women.

Manner of Dress

The fit of the clothing should be noted, as well as the attendance to current style. In addition, the general cleanliness and neatness of clothing may provide further clues to the client's cultural or socioeconomic status as well as ego strength. The unshaven or unwashed signs of neglect by relatives or others for the dependent client or of self-neglect should be carefully noted.

Speech

The manner of speech* is the cornerstone to diagnosis of both emotional and physical illness. The characteristics that should be noted include the following:
1. *Pace:* A fast or rapid-fire manner of delivery may indicate hyperthyroidism, whereas slow speech and a thick, hoarse voice are typical of hypothyroidism.
2. *Clarity:* The ability to enunciate clearly may be lost in motor nerve disease of the tongue, jaws, or lips. Slurred speech can result from CNS damage.
3. *Vocabulary:* The choice of words may indicate the client's level of education, and an accent may indicate socioeconomic class or a particular region of the country.
4. *Sentence structure:* The client's sentences may give some indication of cortical associative abilities.

*See Chapter 2 on assessment of mental status.

Association of Breath Smells to Disease

Breath odor	Description	Condition associated with odor
Halitosis, fetid	Odor of necrotic tissue	Pyorrhea
		Poor dental hygiene
		Tonsillitis
		Sinusitis
		Lung abscess
		Bronchiectasis
Feculent	Odor of feces	Bowel obstruction
Fetor hepaticus	Described as "fishy," "mousy" odor	Hepatic failure
Acid	Acrid, acid smell	Peptic disease
Uriniferous, ammoniacal	Azotemia, odor of urine	Renal failure
Acetone	Odor of acetone, described as smell of fruit, rotting apples	Diabetic ketoacidosis
Bitter almonds	Odor of the bitter almond	Cyanide poisoning

5. *Tone of voice:* The voice should be observed for hoarseness, whining, or squeaky characteristics.
6. *Strength of voice:* Voice strength is evaluated in terms of loudness or softness in delivery of speech.

Some typical observations might be as follows:

1. *Aphasia:* Inability to express onself through speech (motor or expressive) or loss of verbal comprehension (receptive or sensory).
2. *Anarthria, dysarthria:* Loss of motor power to speak distinctly (stammering or stuttering).
3. *Aphonia, dysphonia:* Inability to produce sounds from the larynx. This is not the result of a brain lesion. A possible cause might be laryngitis or malignancy.

In addition to observing the client's speech, one may find it useful to assess a sample of the client's writing for intactness of structures coordinating this complex act and for the client's ability to express thoughts in this medium.

Construction of a simple drawing may provide clues to cerebellar function and may help to unmask dementia.

Mental Status*

The focus in this survey is to determine the client's problems in living and the psychodynamics underlying them. It is important that the client's own words be used in describing the problems.

The kind of information that is relevant will include the client's state of awareness from alertness to dullness to unconsciousness or coma. The client's ability to comprehend what he or she is told is described, as well as level of education. The speed of responses to questions and reaction time in following instructions for

*See Chapter 2 on assessment of mental status.

motor activity may provide valuable clues. The length of attention span should be recorded. The facial expression should be observed at rest and during the early verbal interaction with the client for indications of anxiety, depression, apathy, and pain.

The client who slumps slowly into the chair should be observed for further indications of depression, such as carelessness in grooming and in dress or a short attention span.

The levels of cooperation can be described on a continuum from passive acceptance to rigid resistance. The level of aggressiveness may be described by descriptive terms relative to the client's relationship to the environment.

Mood has been described by such terms as hostility, resentment, depression, fearfulness, distrustfulness, elation, and euphoria. The difficulty in using these terms is that they may mean different things to the people who use them and to those who read the history. For instance, the client who looks down while being interviewed might be described as "depressed," "withdrawn," "serious," or "thoughtful" by different observers. To obviate this confusion, it is best to describe the behavior observed.

The client's use of vocabulary and the complexity of sentence structure should be recorded, as well as use of medical or other professional terminology.

Awareness is recorded in descriptive terms, relating the client's apparent perception of external stimuli and response to physiologic stimuli.

The client's orientation for person, place, and time is assessed. Bear in mind that orientation usually is initially lost in the sphere of time, followed by place, and finally by person. Deviation from this order should be reported.

ASSESSMENT OF VITAL SIGNS

The clinical assessment of temperature, pulse, respiratory rate, and blood pressure is the most frequent clinical measurement made by the health practitioner. These measures of neural and circulatory function provide valuable data in the diagnosis of disease states. Irregularity of these parameters warrants further investigation. Because of the importance of these indicators in predicting the effectiveness of bodily function, they have been termed the *vital* or *cardinal* signs. Vital signs are assessed as the initial maneuver in any examination.

The history should be carefully attended for symptoms that would indicate alterations in the vital signs. These might include "pounding" of the heart, faintness, or dizziness.

The techniques used in the assessment of vital signs include inspection, palpation, and auscultation.

Inspection may reveal changes in color such as the flush of fever, the pallor in response to cold, or the dusky blueness of cyanosis. The bluish color observed as cyanosis results from an increased amount of reduced hemoglobin in superficial blood vessels. It is most readily identified in the vessels beneath the tongue or in the buccal mucosa. The examiner observes the chest for morphologic changes that may indicate a pathologic condition. For instance, in those individuals with chronic obstructive pulmonary disease, the anteroposterior diameter is often as great as the transverse diameter, and the ribs are observed to flare in the horizontal plane rather than downward. This structural change is thought to be the result of the long period of overinflation of the lungs.

The chest is also observed for defects of the thoracic cage that might change the nature of respiration. Some of these are pigeon or chicken breast (the sternum is markedly protuberant, as in a bird), funnel chest or *pectus excavatum* (sternal retraction), and scoliosis.

Symmetry of thoracic expansion is noted. Bulging or retraction of the interspaces is recorded.

In addition to the assessment of pulsations, *palpation* may be used to determine temperature. Since the dorsal aspect of the hand is more sensitive to temperature variation, it is recommended that the backs of the fingers be used in this rough measure of temperature. Palpation may also reveal moisture and texture variations as well as the vibration of shivering.

Auscultation of the precordial area is employed to further evaluate the irregular pulse. Listening over the heart while simultaneously palpating a peripheral pulse is helpful in detecting a pulse deficit. Auscultation is the technique used to evaluate the sounds produced as a result of sphygmomanometer (Gr. *sphygmos,* pulse) manipulation.

The examiner must bear in mind that the assessment of vital signs is done in the interest of establishing a database so that on future occasions the client may be compared to baseline values—in essence, serves as a control.

Measurements of clinical significance are those that reveal variation from the client's basal value or from the last measurement. This is important in view of the considerable variability noted among individuals. The ranges of normal for temperature, for example, are 97° to 99.6° F (36.1° to 37.6° C).

The examiner must bear in mind the fact that the manner of approach to the client may alter the vital signs should the client react emotionally to the examiner's actions. For instance, a brusque, impatient, rude interaction or awkward handling of the instruments may upset the client, increasing pulse rate, respiration, blood pressure, and even temperature if the interaction is prolonged.

Temperature

The optimum temperature for metabolic function of all cells of the human body is considered to be 98.6° F (37° C) for most individuals, and the core temperature of the human body is maintained at this level within very narrow limits. Although some individuals have a normal core temperature of 97° F and the range of normal extends to 99.6° F, the temperature of the individual shows little variation. Nichols (1972) found afebrile oral temperatures from 96.9° to 99.6° F among individuals.

Temperature regulation is an excellent example of both homeostasis and biologic rhythms. The accomplishment of the reasonably steady core temperature is a function of the hypothalamus, which serves as the thermostat. Two hypothalamic centers trigger heat-dissipating or heat-conserving mechanisms. The delivery of overwarmed blood to thermoreceptors in an anterior hypothalamic site results in sweating and redistribution of blood, so that surface capillaries are dilated (flushing). The loss of temperature from the skin is related to the delivery of blood flow to the skin and to the evaporation of sweat. This loss of heat is related to the difference in temperature between the skin and the external environment.

Conduction, convection, radiation, and evaporation are the physical phenomena involved. Heat is lost from the object of higher temperature to the object of lower temperature by *conduction. Convection* is the loss of heat to the molecules of air. Warm air rises, carrying the heat away. Conduction and convection cannot occur when external objects and ambient temperature are greater than that of the body.

Radiation is the loss of heat by electromagnetic

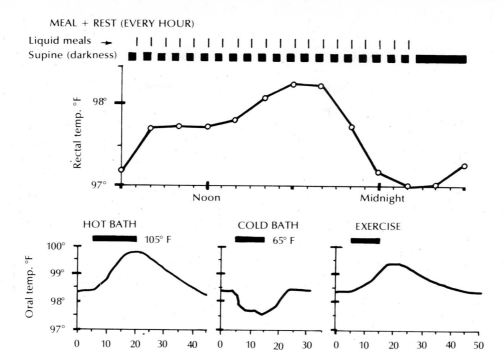

Figure 7-1

Factors influencing the body temperature of human beings. The body temperature is nicely regulated, but exact maintenance is altered by many factors, such as hot baths, cold water, and exercise. Also, there is a daily resetting of temperature regulation that persists in a resting individual if the influence of exercise or meals is removed. If standardized exercise is carried out at noon and at midnight, the day-night regulation is still apparent in the exercise body temperature.
(From Folk GE, editor: Textbook of environmental physiology, ed 2, Philadelphia, 1974, Lea & Febiger; in part from Green JH: An introduction to human physiology, ed 4, Oxford, 1976, Oxford University Press.)

infrared waves. The radiation does not heat the air through which it passes.

Evaporation is the conversion of liquid to gaseous form. The liquid involved is sweat. Perspiration in humans is the insensible, thermal sweat from the eccrine glands and the autonomic, or emotional, sweat arising from the palms and soles. Insensible perspiration is moisture of diffusion principally noted from the corneum, from the sweat glands of the skin, and from the lungs. Insensible perspiration and thermal sweat are the most important in terms of heat loss. Evaporation of thermal sweat from the body requires 0.58 calorie per 1 ml of sweat. Vaporization of perspiration depends on ambient humidity and does not occur when air is highly saturated with water.

When overcooled blood is delivered to thermoreceptors in a posterior hypothalamic site, heat-conserving mechanisms are instituted. These functions include reduction of blood flow to the distal extremities as a result of shunting through venae comitantes from large arteries to similar veins and constriction of peripheral capillary beds (blanching). Compensatory heat production is en-

hanced both at the metabolic level (nonshivering thermogenesis) and through voluntary muscle contraction and shivering. Shivering occurs when vasoconstriction is ineffective in preventing heat loss.

Thermoreceptors in the skin sense ambient temperature and transmit neural signals to the spinal cord at all levels for relay through the spinothalamic tracts to the thalamus. These neural messages are thought to act as stimuli to the hypothalamic centers.

Factors influencing temperature

Biologic rhythms are reflected in temperature assessment (Fig. 7-1). Diurnal variations of 1.0° to 1.5° F are observed; the trough occurs in the hours before waking and the peak in the late afternoon or early evening.

Secretion of hormones affects the body temperature. Increased secretion of thyroid hormones is associated with increased heat production. Progesterone secretion at the time of ovulation is correlated with temperature increases of 0.5° to 1.0° F, which continue until the menses. Both estrogen and testosterone may increase the rate of cellular metabolism.

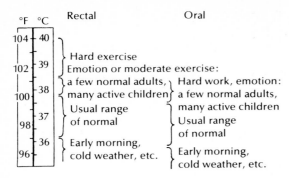

Figure 7-2

Estimate of ranges in rectal and oral temperatures found in healthy persons. This suggests that it would be wise to replace the red arrow on the clinical thermometer with a red band covering the space between 96.5° and 99.3° F (35.9° to 37.8° C).

(From DuBois EF: Fever and the regulation of body temperature, American Lecture Series, pub no 13, 1948. Courtesy Charles C Thomas, Publisher, Springfield, Ill.)

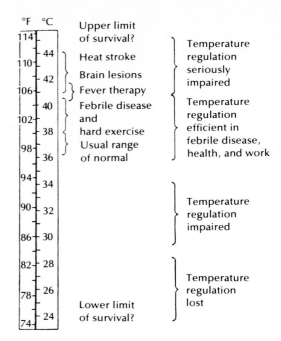

Figure 7-3

Extremes of human body temperatures with an attempt to define the zones of temperature regulation.

(From DuBois EF: Fever and the regulation of body temperature, American Lecture Series, pub no 13, 1948. Courtesy Charles C Thomas, Publisher, Springfield, Ill.)

There are some *environmental effects* on temperature. Although body temperature may be little altered by seasonal changes in environmental temperature, hot and cold baths are known to produce temporary changes in temperature, as shown in Fig. 7-1.

The physiologic changes incurred in *exercise* are also known to increase body temperature (Fig. 7-2). The temperature rise associated with the *eating of food* is said to be a result of the specific dynamic activity (SDA) of the food.

Drugs that alter circulation or metabolism will also affect body temperature.

Age is a factor in temperature assessment. Because heat control mechanisms are not as well established in the child as in the adult, considerable variation in temperature may occur.

HELPFUL HINT: Because multiple factors can affect the body's temperature, it is advisable to obtain a thorough nursing history to account for these multiple variables.

Temperature recording

Body temperature is recorded in degrees centigrade (°C) or in degrees Fahrenheit (°F) according to the protocol of the agency. Because the United States is committed to the future adoption of the metric system, the practitioner would do well to think of temperature in degrees centigrade. Scales may be readily converted through the use of the following formulas:

$$°C = \frac{5}{9} (°F - 32)$$
$$°F = \frac{9}{5} °C + 32$$

Table 7-4 equates Fahrenheit and centigrade temperatures in the range compatible with survival in the human being.

Table 7-4

Metric-Fahrenheit equivalents for possible range of human temperature

Fahrenheit (degrees)	Centigrade (degrees)
93.2	34.0
95.0	35.0
96.8	36.0
98.6	37.0
100.4	38.0
102.2	39.0
104.0	40.0
105.8	41.0
107.6	42.0
109.4	43.0

Temperature regulation

Temperature control may be altered so that the mechanisms of control may be effective at a higher or lower level. An example of this might be seen in the individual exposed to marked exercise. During the first few days the core temperature may reach values of 102° F (38.9° C), but with adaptation the individual may undergo

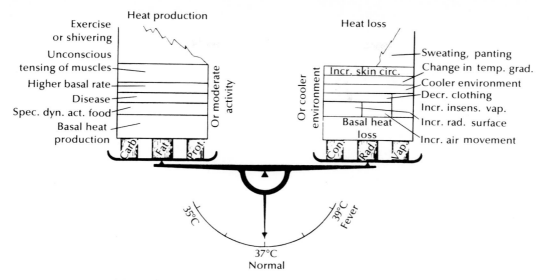

Figure 7-4

Balance between factors increasing heat production and heat loss.
(From DuBois EF: Bull NY Acad Med 15:143, 1939.)

a decrease to 100° F (37.8° C), which will be maintained as long as the exercise is carried on.

Fever, or elevation of temperature because of the effect of pyrogens on the hypothalamus, also affects this type of core temperature resetting.

Temperature regulation becomes impaired or lost when extreme variations of temperature occur (Fig. 7-3). It results from the balance of heat loss and heat conservation functions. These are summarized in Fig. 7-4.

Temperature Acclimatization

Clients who have spent a good deal of time in very cold climates show an increased ability to tolerate cold. Changes that have been measured in these individuals are (1) increased metabolic rate with increased rates of secretion of thyroid hormones, (2) reduction in shivering, and (3) growth of hair.

Adaptation to heat involves changes in the secretion of sweat. The amount of sweat produced declines from the profuse, dripping early response to a quantity that will evaporate on reaching the air.

Thermometry

Glass thermometry. The clinical glass thermometer has been in use since the 15th century. The thermometer reflects heat changes through the expansion of mercury. The accuracy of the instrument is determined by the amount and quality of the mercury and by the calibrations identified on the glass tube.

Recent studies have shown the glass thermometer to be subject to inaccuracy. Furthermore, in most subjects the oral thermometer must be left in place for 8 minutes for women and 9 minutes for men to obtain full registration of the instrument at room temperatures of 65° to 75° F (18.3° to 23.9° C). Thus, the readings obtained for shorter registration periods must be considered to be approximations of the actual temperature of the client.

Other disadvantages in the use of the glass thermometer are frequent breakage and danger to the client through the use of rigid glass rod. In several instances the rectal wall was perforated due to inappropriate placement of a glass thermometer.

The examiner may also build in error through improper reading of the thermometer. The eyes must be at a 90-degree angle to the meniscus of the mercury to avoid parallax error.

Electronic thermometry. The electronic thermometer has been in use over the past decade. The advantages to be realized with the fully charged, correctly calibrated instrument are speed and accuracy of measurement. The probes used in these thermometers are unbreakable, thus obviating damage from broken glass and mercury ingestion, which are hazards with the traditional clinical thermometer.

The electronic thermometers are claimed to provide increased accuracy over glass thermometers by providing correct readings within 0.2° F. Thirty seconds is required for registration without lip closure. Less examiner time is required in the use of these thermometers.

Oral, rectal, and axillary temperature assessment

Differences in temperatures recorded from the mouth, rectum, or axilla have been shown to reflect the length of time the thermometer is allowed to register rather than actual variation in temperature from one site to another.

Oral temperature. The oral temperature registration is the most convenient method for the client. This site for temperature determination is the one used unless the client is an infant, unconscious, confused, or has shown erratic behavior.

A 5- to 15-minute wait is recommended before temperature assessment if the client has ingested hot or iced liquids, to allow the temperature to stabilize. Small temperature increases will occur if the client has smoked in the 2 minutes preceding the temperature assessment. The oral thermometer may take as long as 8 to 9 minutes to reach maximum registration. Other assessment procedures may be done at this time.

Rectal temperature. The rectal site for temperature registration is preferable for the confused or comatose client, the individual who is unable to close the mouth, the client who is receiving oxygen, or the client who may bite the thermometer for other reasons.

The rectal temperature is routinely ordered as the general mode of temperature registration in some agencies.

The thermometer placed in the rectum will register adequately within a 2-minute time span in adults and within 3 minutes in premature infants.

Axillary temperature. Eleven minutes has been shown to be the maximum length of time necessary for the full registration of axillary temperature. This method has been shown to be safe and accurate for infants and small children.

Correlation of pulse and temperature

Marked increases in temperature are accompanied by increments in pulse and respiratory rates because oxygen requirements are known to increase 7% for every 1° F (10% for every 1° C) rise in temperature. Since reducing cellular temperatures results in a decreased rate of cell metabolism, oxygen consumption is lessened in hypothermia; therefore, pulse and respiratory rates also decline.

Fever

Fever, or *pyrexia,* is the elevation of body temperature above normal limits compared with a given individual's basal data. Fever may be a valid diagnosis when the temperature is found to be 98.6° F (37° C) for a specific client if normal temperature ranges about 97° F (36.1° C).

Not all causes of fever are related to disease. Exercise may cause a temporary elevation of temperature, which subsides when the activity is stopped.

It has been suggested that a temperature above 97° F in a client who has been lying in bed (whose metabolism is basal) indicates the presence of disease. The association of an elevated temperature with disease is called a fever.

Fever is caused by those conditions that contribute to heat production, that prevent heat loss, or that affect the heat-regulating centers of the CNS.

Fevers are described according to the chronologic pattern of occurrence and amplitude. Frequently, recognition of the pattern may help to establish the diagnosis. The following paragraphs present descriptions of fever.

A *continuous* or *sustained fever* is one in which there is a persistent elevation of temperature without a return to normal values for that individual. This pattern is typical of typhoid or typhus fever.

An *intermittent fever* is one in which there are major diurnal variations, so that there is a daily elevation of temperature with a drop to subnormal or normal values in the same 24-hour period. When there is a marked difference between the peaks and the troughs of the temperature the fever is called *hectic* or *septic.* This type of fever is seen in pyrogenic infection.

Remittent fever is characterized by a temperature elevation that does not return to normal level but shows marked spikes of even further increased temperature on the febrile baseline. This appears in sustained or continuous fever, in which there are only slight variations from the elevated set point.

Relapsing fever is one in which febrile periods alternate with periods of normal temperature. This pattern of fever is seen in malaria, relapsing fever, and the Pel-Ebstein fever of Hodgkin's disease.

Fever may also be described by the rate pattern of dissolution. *Lysis* is the gradual disappearance of fever, whereas *crisis* is the rapid (less than 36 hours) decrease of temperature to normal.

The development of the febrile condition and its abatement have been described in three stages, called cold, hot, and defervescence.

The period of a developing increase in core temperature is characterized by heat conservation reactions. The affected individual has diminished cutaneous circulation, and the skin looks blanched and feels cold. Heat production is attested to by shivering and piloerection ("goose pimples"). Chills and rigor are the extremes of shivering that produce rapid increases in temperature.

The hot stage is the period after the fever has peaked (regulated at the new set point). During this stage blood flow to the periphery is increased. The affected individual's body radiates excess heat, feels hot, and is flushed.

The stage of defervescence is the period of fever abatement and is characterized by heat-loss mechanisms; particularly prominent is vasodilation and sweating. Diaphoresis is diffuse perspiration, which may accompany fever abatement.

Respiratory Pattern

The assessment of the respiratory pattern is discussed in Chapter 14, Assessment of the Respiratory System.

Pulsation

The assessment of central pulses discussed in Chapter 15, Assessment of the Cardiovascular System, should be read before this section.

Assessment of the peripheral arterial pulse has been a part of the health care professional's routine procedure throughout recorded medical history. The peripheral arterial pulse is a pressure wave transmitted from the left ventricle to the root of the aorta to the peripheral vessels.

Examination of the peripheral (radial) arterial pulsation gives less information concerning left ventricular ejection or aortic valvular function than does the assessment of the more central (carotid) arteries because the normal arterial pulse expands normal peripheral arteries only slightly. The information obtained is a necessary part of the database, however, because the nature of the peripheral pulse gives an indication of cardiac function and of perfusion of the peripheral tissues. These peripheral pulsations are evaluated in terms of rate, amplitude (indicating volume), rhythm, and symmetry regularity. They may also be auscultated for the presence of bruits.

Arterial pulses are most accurately examined while the client is reclining with the trunk of the body elevated about 15 to 30 degrees.

Parameters of arterial pulsation

Visual and palpable pulsations result from diameter changes incurred through vessel filling and through straightening of the vessel. These pulsations are referred to as arterial pulse waves.

Pressure changes in the wall of the artery are felt through the overlying skin and subcutaneous tissue. The arterial pressure pulse wave is sensed through the pressure receptors in the pads of the examiner's fingers, which are superimposed on the vessel wall, as in pressure of

Table 7-5

Chronologic variations in pulse rate

Age	Pulse rate (beats/min)
Birth	70-170
Neonate	120-140
1 year	80-140
2 years	80-130
3 years	80-120
4 years	70-115
Adult	60-100
Conditioned athlete	$\cong 50$

paired arterial pulses exerted against the wall. The pulse is best palpated over arteries that are close to the surface of the body and that lie over a bony surface. The arteries that are palpated during the health examination include the superficial temporal, carotid, brachial, ulnar, radial, femoral, popliteal, dorsal pedal (dorsalis pedis), and posterior tibial.

Rate. As defined by the AHA, the heart rate is normal when it is between 50 and 100 beats per minute.

The pulse rate is counted for 1 full minute to evaluate rate, rhythm, and volume accurately. Some authorities recommend counting for 15 to 30 seconds for those pulses that are normal on palpation and to extend the period of evaluation only when irregularities are detected.

A diurnal rhythm is noted for pulse rate. The lowest rate is seen in the early morning hours, and the most rapid rates are observed in the late afternoon and evening.

Chronologically the pulse rate decreases from infancy through the middle years; it tends to increase in the older client (Table 7-5).

A sex difference is noted in that women have demonstrated a rate 5 to 10 beats per minute faster than men.

Volume. Pulse volume is estimated from the feel of the vessel as blood flows through it with each heartbeat. *Bounding* is the descriptive term used to describe the full pulse that is difficult to depress with the fingertips. The normal pulse is easily palpable, does not fade in and out, and is not easily obliterated. Weak, feeble, and thready are descriptive words for the pulse of a vessel that has low volume. The artery in this case is readily compressed. The absent pulse is not palpable.

Amplitude. The strength of the left ventricular contraction is reflected in the amplitude of the pulsation.

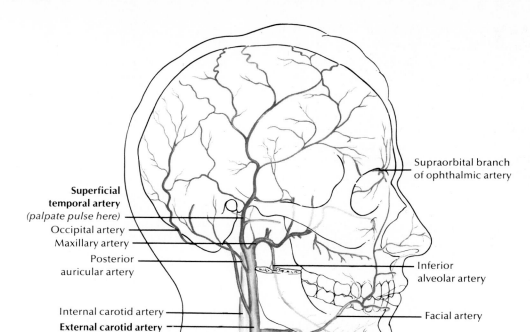

Figure 7-5

Arteries of the head and neck.
(Modified from Francis CC and Martin AH: Introduction to human anatomy, ed 7, St Louis, 1975, The CV Mosby Co.)

This may be recorded as follows:

3 + Bounding, hyperkinetic
2 + Normal
1 + Weak, thready, hypokinetic
0   Absent

Elasticity of the arterial wall

Elasticity of the arterial wall is reflected by the expansibility or deformability of the artery as it is palpated by the examiner's fingers. The normal artery is soft and pliable, whereas the sclerotic vessel may be more resistant to occlusion, even hard and cordlike. The artery may feel beaded and tortuous to touch in the individual with arteriosclerosis.

Palpation of arterial pulses— pulse points

Superficial temporal pulse.   The superficial temporal artery is accessible to palpation anterior to the tragus of the ear and upward to the temple and is frequently used in the clinical evaluation of pulsation (Figs. 7-5 and 7-6).

Carotid pulse.   Examination of the carotid and jugular pulse is described in Chapter 15. Fig. 7-7 shows one method of palpation of the carotid artery.

The carotid pulse is easily accessible and is frequently the pulse evaluated in emergency situations.

The easiest method of locating the carotid is by placing the fingers lightly over the trachea and allowing them to slide into the trough between the trachea and the sternocleidomastoid muscle. The carotid will be felt immediately below the examining fingers. The pulse is palpated in the lower half of the artery to avoid pressure on the carotid sinus. Care should be taken to avoid undue pressure on the carotids to avoid stimulation of the baroreceptors of the carotid sinus and a resultant slowing of the heart and a decrease in blood pressure. All symmetric pulses except the carotid may be measured simultaneously. The carotid pulses should not be measured simultaneously. Excessive biarterial pressure may dangerously occlude the blood supply to the brain.

Radial pulse.   The radial pulse is the one most frequently used as an initial indication of the rate and rhythm of pulsation, the pattern of pulsation, and the

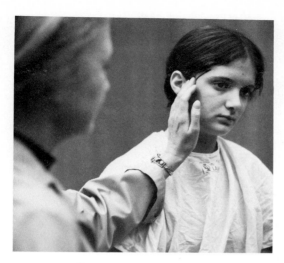

Figure 7-6

Palpation of the superficial temporal artery.

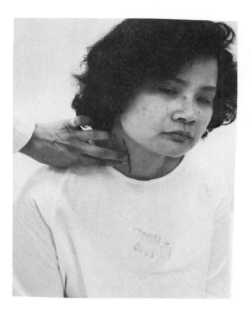

Figure 7-7

Palpation of the carotid artery.

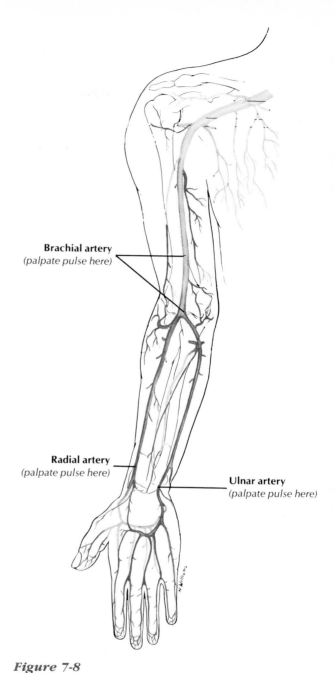

Brachial artery
(palpate pulse here)

Radial artery
(palpate pulse here)

Ulnar artery
(palpate pulse here)

Figure 7-8

Arteries of the upper extremity.
(Adapted from Francis CC and Martin AH: Introduction to human anatomy, ed 7, St Louis, 1975, The CV Mosby Co.)

shape (consistency) of the arterial wall. This pulse is easily accessible to the examiner, and its evaluation causes little inconvenience to the client. Other pulses easily evaluated in the upper extremity are the ulnar and brachial pulses (Fig. 7-8).

The radial pulse is readily assessed by placing the pads of the examiner's second and third (or first, second, and third) fingers on the palmar surface of the relaxed and slightly flexed wrist medial to the radial styloid process (Fig. 7-9). Occasionally the arteries run a deeper and more lateral course. Both radial pulses should be felt simultaneously for an assessment of symmetry. The fingers should exert sufficient pressure to occlude the artery during diastole, yet allow the vessel to return to normal contour during systole.

Ulnar pulse. The ulnar artery may be compressed against the ulna on the palmar surface of the wrist. It is not used as frequently as the radial artery in evaluation.

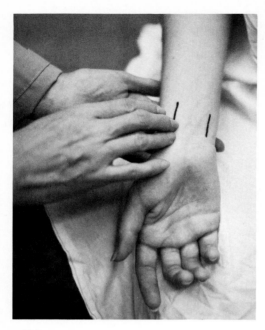

Figure 7-9

Palpation of the radial pulse. The site for palpation of the ulnar artery is also marked.

Brachial pulse. Brachial pulse assessment by auscultation is a part of the blood pressure evaluation. The pulse is palpated as it passes through the upper half of the cubital fossa at the midline (anterior surface of the elbow joint) because halfway through the fossa it bifurcates into the radial and ulnar arteries. The brachial artery is palpated medial to the biceps tendon. The brachial artery may be used to determine the arterial waveform, as can the carotid artery. The waveform of more peripheral arteries may be distorted and therefore provide less valuable data.

Femoral pulse. The pads of the examiner's fingers explore the groin in the area just inferior to the midpoint of the inguinal ligament. This is also approximately midway between the anterior superior iliac spine and the symphysis pubis (Figs. 7-10 and 7-11).

Popliteal pulse. Since the popliteal artery is situated relatively deeply in the soft tissues behind the knee, the knee should be flexed for examination of the pulsation in this artery. The pulse may be readily examined with the client in either the dorsal recumbent (Fig. 7-12) or prone position (Fig. 7-13). The fingertips are pressed deeply into the popliteal fossa.

Dorsal pedal pulse. The pads of the examining fingers examine the dorsum of the foot. The foot should be dorsiflexed to obviate traction on the artery, preferably to 90 degrees (Fig. 7-14).

When the dorsal pedal pulse is congenitally ab-

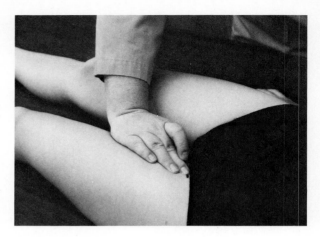

Figure 7-10

Palpation of the femoral pulse.

sent, pulsation may sometimes be discerned in the lateral tarsal artery, located in the proximal dorsum of the foot, or in the peroneal artery, anterior to the lateral malleolus.

Although only one pedal pulse can occasionally be palpated, this need not necessarily indicate arterial insufficiency; it may be a result of clinically insignificant congenital variation in the arteries to the foot.

One or both dorsal pedal pulses have been noted to be absent in 12% of children and in 17% of adults. Whereas whites seldom show an absence of the posterior tibial pulse, a 9% incidence of absence has been found in black adults.

Posterior tibial pulse. The pads of the examining fingers palpate posterior or inferior to the tibial medial malleolus while the client's foot is dorsiflexed, preferably to 90 degrees (Fig. 7-15).

The examination of the pulses of an extremity begins with the most distal pulse point. Normal pulses in the dorsal pedal and posterior tibial arteries indicate that there is no disruption of flow to the extremity, whereas a weak or absent pulse is expected to be found distal to an obstruction. However, the observation of an indication that an individual has a disease known to produce a peripheral vascular change, such as circulatory impairment or diabetes, dictates the examination of all the superficial pulse points. A thorough assessment includes assessment of all pulse points.

Irregularities in pulsation (Fig. 7-16)

Tachycardia. Rates persistently over 100 beats per minute *(tachycardia)* suggest some abnormality (Table 7-6). However, hyperkinetic heart action can be the result of exercise, anger, anxiety, or fear in the normal client. Heart rates are increased during fever, anemia, hypoxia, and low volume states (shock).

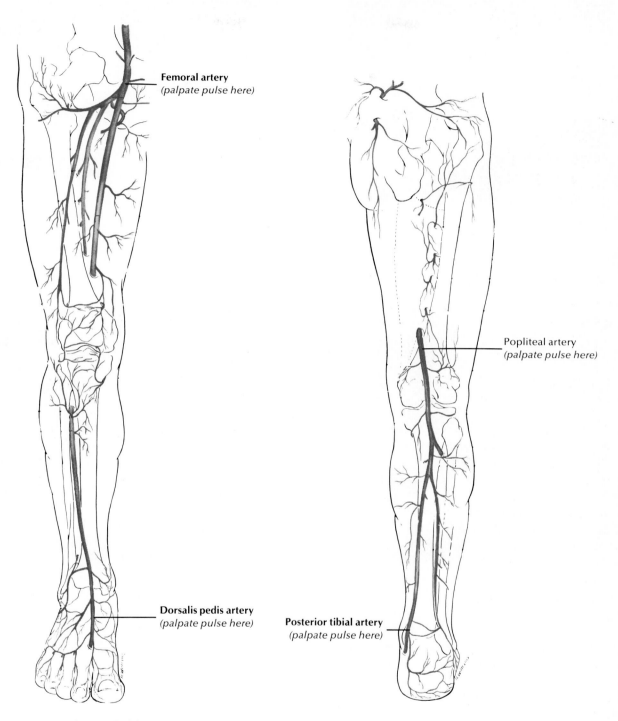

Femoral artery
(palpate pulse here)

Popliteal artery
(palpate pulse here)

Dorsalis pedis artery
(palpate pulse here)

Posterior tibial artery
(palpate pulse here)

Figure 7-11

Arteries of the lower extremity.
(Adapted from Francis CC and Martin AH: Introduction to human anatomy, ed 7, St Louis, 1975, The CV Mosby Co.)

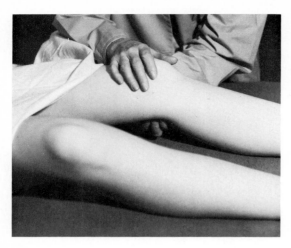

Figure 7-12

Palpation of the popliteal pulse with client in the dorsal recumbent position.

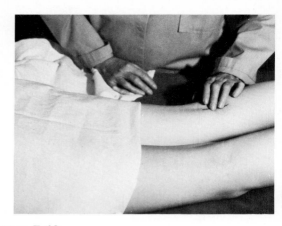

Figure 7-13

Palpation of the popliteal pulse with client in the prone position.

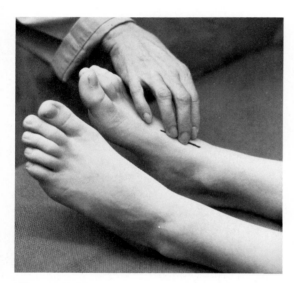

Figure 7-14

Palpation of the dorsal pedal pulse.

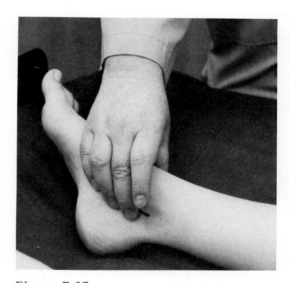

Figure 7-15

Palpation of posterior tibial pulse.

Bradycardia. A slow heart rate less than 50 beats per minute is known as *bradycardia* (Table 7-7). These slow rates may indicate stimulation of the parasympathetic system or failure in the electrical conduction system of the heart. Bradycardia may be iatrogenically produced through overdoses of digitalis.

The well-trained athlete may have cardiac rates less than 50 beats per minute.

Irregular rhythm—pulse deficit. Cardiac arrhythmias, that is, atrial fibrillation, atrial flutter with block, and second degree heart block resulting in dropped beats, irregular sinus depolarization, and premature complexes result in an irregular rhythm of the pulse.

Pulse deficit means that the number of pressure waves palpable at the peripheral pulse point is less than the actual number of muscular contractions of the heart. Pressure waves initiated by weak, premature ventricular contractions may not be transmitted to the periphery. Simultaneous measurement at the precordium and peripheral pulse point reveals this deficit.

Bigeminal pulse. A pulse that alternates in amplitude from beat to beat may be produced by a small,

Table 7-6

Characteristics of common forms of tachycardia

Type	Rhythm, amplitude	Most common ventricular rate (beats/min)	Onset	Termination	Effect of carotid sinus massage
Sinus tachycardia	Regular; constant amplitude	Usually 170	Gradual	Gradual	Gradual slowing and return to previous state
Paroxysmal atrial tachycardia (PAT)	Regular; constant amplitude	170	Abrupt	Abrupt	Sudden slowing of heart rate or no change
Paroxysmal atrial flutter	Flutter, regular; uniform amplitude	170	Abrupt		Sudden diminution of rate or temporarily irregular rhythm
Ventricular tachycardia	Irregular; variable amplitude	140	Sudden		No effect

Table 7-7

Characteristics of common forms of bradycardia

Type	Rhythm, amplitude	Most common ventricular rate (beats/min)	Effect of exercise
Sinus bradycardia	Regular; constant amplitude	40	Rate increases appropriately through varying degrees of exercise
Incomplete heart block	Constant amplitude	40	May double or become irregular in response to exercise
Complete heart block		40	Increases only slightly in response to exercise

premature ventricular beat after a strong beat, resulting from normal electrical cardiac conduction. The strong pulse occurs after a long diastolic filling phase following the premature beat. The pulse is irregular. This condition is called bigeminal pulse and can be identified by simultaneously palpating the radial pulse and listening at the precordium.

Pulsus alternans. *Pulsus alternans* is a pulse that alternates between strong and weak beats while the rhythm is regular. When the variation is marked, the alternation from weak to strong beats is palpable. However, it may be necessary to use the sphygmomanometer and stethoscope to determine minor changes. The examiner will hear the alternation of loud and soft sounds in pulsus alternans. (See assessment of pulsus alternans in the section on blood pressure in this chapter.)

Pulsus paradoxus. Arterial pressure is known to fluctuate physiologically with the respiratory cycle, falling with inspiration and rising with expiration. This variation is detectable at normal respiratory amplitude but is more marked during forced respiratory volumes. Two mechanisms appear to explain this effect. First, the changes in pleural pressure during respiration appear to affect the arteries and veins as they enter or leave the thoracic cage, altering the gradients whereby blood enters or leaves the thorax. Second, the relationship between the ventricles of the heart is such that distention of one results in alteration of the filling characteristics (distensibility or compliance) of the other. Reduction in pleural pressure during inspiration increases the return of systemic venous blood to the right ventricle. The increase in right ventricular filling pressure results in a shift of the interventricular septum leftward, thus reducing the amount of blood that is accepted by the left ventricle. The resultant decrease in left ventricular end diastolic pressure decreases the stroke work of the subsequent left

NORMAL PULSE

POSSIBLE CAUSE

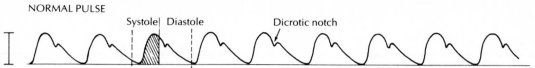

mm Hg

Graphic recording of pulse pressure as obtained from electrical transducer. The normal pulse is easily palpable but may be obliterated by pressure. The wave of a single pulsation rises in systole, reaches a summit, and descends more slowly in diastole. The secondary rise in pressure, noted in diastole, is associated with closure of the aortic valve. The point at which the increase in pressure changes the downward slope is known as the dicrotic notch. This may not be palpable. The difference in pressure from the endpoint of diastole to the summit is the amplitude. Normal amplitude (30-40 mm Hg) is recorded as 2 +. A pulse of greater amplitude is called strong, and one of lesser amplitude is weak or faint.

Partial arterial occlusion
Myocardial infarction
Myocarditis
Pericardial effusion shock
Stenosis of valves: aortic,
    mitral, pulmonic, tricuspid

SMALL, WEAK PULSE

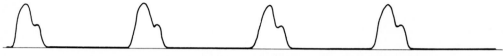

A weak pulse may be difficult to feel, and the vessel may be obliterated easily by the fingers. The pulse may "fade out" (be impalpable). This pulse is recorded as 1 +. The pulsation is slower to rise, has a sustained summit, and falls more slowly than the normal. A pulse that is weak and variable in amplitude is called thready.

Hypovolemia
Physical obstruction to
    left ventricular output,
    e.g., aortic stenosis

LARGE, BOUNDING PULSE

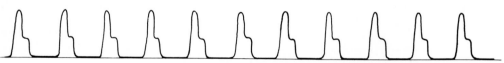

The large, bounding (also called hyperkinetic or strong) pulse is readily palpable. It does not "fade out" and is not easily obliterated by the examining fingers. This pulse is recorded as 3 +.

Exercise
Anxiety
Fever
Hyperthyroidism
Aortic rigidity or
    atherosclerosis

WATER-HAMMER PULSE

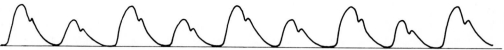

The water-hammer pulse (also known as collapsing) has a greater amplitude than the normal pulse, a rapid rise to a narrow summit, and a sudden descent.

Patent ductus arteriosus
Aortic regurgitation

PULSUS ALTERNANS

Pulsus alternans is characterized by alternation of a pulsation of small amplitude with the pulsation of large amplitude while the rhythm is normal.

Left ventricular failure
More significant if pulse
    slow

Figure 7-16

Table of pulses.

ventricular systole. Thus, although there is an increase in right ventricular output, left ventricular output is decreased. In conditions characterized by distention of the venous system, for example, right ventricular failure as a result of severe obstructive lung disease or pericardial tamponade, a greater fall in pleural pressure and, thus, arterial pressure occurs. This is called pulsus paradoxus.

The variation in arterial pressure may be objectively measured only through the use of a stethoscope and sphygmomanometer. Following detection of systolic

BIGEMINAL PULSE   POSSIBLE CAUSE

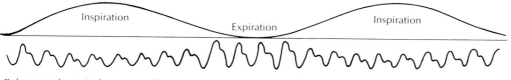

Disorder of rhythm

Bigeminal pulsations result from a normal pulsation followed by a premature contraction. The amplitude of the pulsation of the premature contraction is less than that of the normal pulsation.

PULSUS PARADOXUS

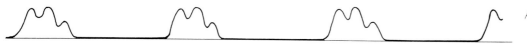

Premature cardiac contraction

Tracheobronchial obstruction
Bronchial asthma
Emphysema
Pericardial effusion
Constrictive pericarditis

Pulsus paradoxus is characterized by an exaggerated decrease (>10 mm Hg) in the amplitude of pulsation during inspiration and increased amplitude during expiration. (See text for measurement with sphygmomanometer.)

PULSUS BISFERIENS

Aortic stenosis combined
   with aortic insufficiency

Pulsus bisferiens is best detected by palpation of the carotid artery. This pulsation is characterized by two main peaks. The first is termed percussion wave and the second, tidal wave. Although the mechanism is not clear, the first peak is believed to be the pulse pressure and the second, reverberation from the periphery.

IRREGULAR PULSE RHYTHM

Pulse deficit means that the number of pressure waves palpable at the peripheral vessel is less than the cardiac contractions.

Cardiac arrhythmia
Atrial fibrillation
Atrial flutter with block
Second-degree heart block
Irregular sinus depolarization
Premature complexes
Weak, premature ventric-
   ular contractions

Figure 7-16 cont'd

Table of pulses.

pressure, the first noted Korotkoff sound, the pressure is allowed to decrease very slowly until sounds can be heard throughout the respiratory cycle. The decrease in arterial pressure during inspiration in the normal individual may be 10 ± 5 mm Hg. A difference greater than 15 mm Hg indicates pulsus paradoxus.

Palpitations.   In the resting state the normal individual is unaware of the beating of the heart. *Palpitation* is the term used to record a description given by the client of the perception of the feeling of the heartbeat (Table 7-8). Such expression as "pounding," "thudding," "fluttering," "flopping," and "skipping" are common descriptive terms used by clients to describe this phenomenon. Palpitation is more common just before falling asleep or during sleep.

Physiologic palpitations may be experienced by the normal individual following strenuous exercise or when aroused emotionally or sexually. In this case the cardiac contraction is of greater rate and amplitude. Several pathophysiologic states are also associated with a hyperkinetic heart (anemia, fever, hypoglycemia, and thyrotoxicosis). Irregularities in cardiac rhythm have also been associated with palpitations, particularly extra systoles and ectopic tachycardia. The chief complaint of palpitations is frequently correlated with psychopathology.

A common feature of the anxiety state, palpitations may be related to the increased adrenergic activity that is present in this arousal state. This relationship creates some problem for the examiner; since the presence

Table 7-8

Guide to causes of palpitations

Possible cause	Signs and symptoms
Menopausal symptom	Associated with heat "flashes" or perspiration
Drugs known to produce a hyperkinetic heart	History of ingestion of mono-amine oxidase inhibitors, thyroid replacement or stimulatory drugs, adrenergic drugs, alcohol, tea, coffee
Hemorrhage, hypoglycemia, pheochromocytoma	Sudden occurrence of palpitation not related to exercise or emotional arousal
Hypervolemia	Blood pressure is elevated
Psychopathology	Clinical examination reveals no evidence of hyperkinetic heart or irregularity of rate
Postural hypotension	Palpitations occur when individual stands
Anemia, fever, atrial fibrillation, thyrotoxicosis, exposure to environmental heat	Clinical examination reveals hyperkinetic heart
Extra systoles	Irregular "skips"

of palpitations frequently creates anxiety, careful questions will be necessary to minimize this effect.

Arterial insufficiency

Assessment of the arterial pulsation is particularly important in those individuals suspected of or diagnosed as having diseases known to compromise the arterial circulation. Some of these pathophysiologic conditions are diabetes, atherosclerosis, Buerger's disease, Raynaud's disease, and arterial aneurysm.

Signs and symptoms of arterial insufficiency include intermittent claudication, increased pallor on elevation of the extremity, a prolonged venous filling time following elevation of the extremity, flush incurred by gravitational effect if the extremity is below the level of the heart, and tissue death (gangrene). Symptoms may also include easy fatigability. Ischemic pain may be incurred by simple resistance exercises. Intermittent claudication is the transient ischemic pain encountered by the client in the arms when they are being used or in the legs during walking.

The impaired flow of arterial insufficiency may be adequate to serve the metabolic activities of the muscle at rest but does not maintain the circulation necessary to the increased metabolic rates of exercise. The pain is theorized to be the result of the buildup of metabolic acids that stimulate the sensory nerves. It is described as cramping or "tightness" and sometimes likened to being in a vise. Many clients, however, do not recognize the discomfort as pain but describe aching, cramping, burning, tiredness, numbness, or weakness of the calf muscles.

Intermittent claudication in the arms may be confused with the pain of angina pectoris. The examiner must carefully define the fact that the pain occurred with work and disappeared with rest. Subclavian arterial insufficiency may result in dizziness and faintness.

In both arterial insufficiency and venous stasis, calf pain is experienced that is relieved during sleep (see comparison in boxed material on p. 171).

Physical examination of the client thought to have arterial insufficiency includes auscultation of the arteries, palpation of the pulses, and observations of cutaneous color; examination should be done before and after exercise.

Absence of pulsation in the femoral artery and at least one peripheral vessel is a criterion for the diagnosis of arterial insufficiency.

Arterial insufficiency in the arm, although generally thought to be less frequent than that of the leg, may frequently be demonstrated through changes in murmurs, pulses, and skin color after exercise.

Importance of exercise testing in determining arterial insufficiency of the extremities. Exercise testing of the poorly perfused limb is based on the inability of the occluded vessel to increase blood flow to meet the increased demands for oxygen. Bruits that were present only in systole continue into diastole, since there is a relatively decreased diastolic pressure distal to the obstruction, which promotes forward flow (Fig. 7-17, see also Fig. 15-31).

In clients with intermittent claudication the pulses diminish in amplitude following exercise. Cutaneous ischemia may be apparent.

The amount of the exercise needed to produce these vascular changes is usually not more than that which is part of daily living. Flexion-extension exercises of the arms and legs (deep knee bends) or walking may produce these changes.

Homans' sign. Thrombosis of the deep veins of the calf muscles may be detected by forced dorsiflexion of the foot. This maneuver compresses the veins and causes pain. The complaint of pain by the client when this maneuver is performed indicates *Homans' sign.* It is important to remember that deep venous thrombosis may be silent, that is, not give rise to pain.

Differentiation of Arterial Insufficiency from Venous Stasis

	Client's response	
Interview	**Arterial insufficiency (intermittent claudication)**	**Venous stasis**
When does the pain occur?	Walking	Standing
What makes the pain worse?	Cold	
What helps to get rid of the pain?	Standing	Elevation
	Stopping to rest	
Do you notice swelling in your feet or legs?	No	Yes
Inspection of involved extremity		
Pulses	Decreased amplitude or absent	
Skin	Cool to touch	Brownish pigmentation
	Pallor, rubor on elevation	
	Shiny	
	Hair loss	
	Nails thickened, ridged	
If ulcer present	Irregular edges	Shallow exudate covering
	Pale, boggy, granulation tissue	Located on side of ankle
	Eschar covering	
	Gangrene possible	No gangrene
	Located on toes or sites of trauma	

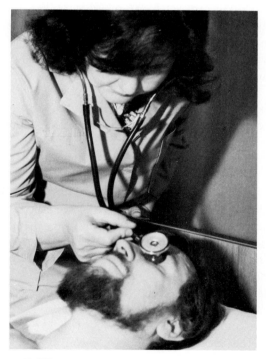

Figure 7-17

Listening for an ocular bruit. The bell of the stethoscope is applied to form a right seal around the orbit.
(From Burnside JW: Physical diagnosis: an introduction to clinical medicine, ed 16, Baltimore, 1981, Williams & Wilkins.)

Auscultation for arterial murmurs

All accessible arteries should be ausculated in the client suspected of arteriovascular disease. Murmurs are not present over major arteries in the normal adult, and only faint ones are heard in the healthy child.

Arterial murmurs (bruits) may result from hyperdynamic cardiac states or from irregularity of arterial walls.

The bell of the stethoscope is used to detect bruits over major vessels. The instrument is held lightly to avoid occluding the underlying vessel. Should the examiner detect a murmur, the limb is exercised if no contraindication exists, and the auscultation is repeated. The auscultation of a systolic murmur that extends into diastole in the postexercise state connotes some degree of arterial obstruction.

Sphygmomanometer detection of arterial flow

Failure to palpate pedal pulsation may require the use of the sphygmomanometer to detect arterial flow. The pneumatic cuff is inflated to a pressure between the systolic and diastolic blood pressure. Oscillation of the needle (aneroid) or mercury column (mercury) in synchrony with the ventricular contraction indicates blood flow to the extremity. A disadvantage of this method is that it does not indicate the adequacy of the flow volume.

Blood pressure

Arterial blood pressure is the force exerted by the blood against the wall of the artery as the heart contracts and relaxes. *Systolic arterial blood pressure* is the force exerted against the wall of the artery when the ventricles are contracted, and *diastolic arterial blood pressure* is the force when the heart is in the filling or relaxed phase. *Pulse pressure* is the difference between the *systolic* and *diastolic* blood pressures. The usual pulse pressure is between 30 and 40 mm Hg.

The blood pressure is determined by the cardiac output and peripheral resistance. Thus, the blood pressure reflects the volume of fluid in the cardiovascular system and elasticity of the arterial walls.

The screening examination is especially important to recognize the client who has a disorder in blood pressure, particularly hypertension (persistently elevated blood pressure). Because hypertension may be present without symptoms, it is known as the silent disease. The client who does not feel ill does not usually come to a clinic or hospital for health care. Thus, this examination may be instrumental in getting the hypertensive client into the therapeutic milieu in time to prevent some of the sequelae of hypertension.

A measure of the functions of the cardiovascular system may be accomplished through assessment of peripheral arterial blood pressure. The peripheral blood pressure is the force exerted against the walls of the vessels and the force responsible for the flow of blood through the arteries, capillaries, and veins. The pressure is the result of the interaction of cardiac output and peripheral resistance and is dependent on the velocity of the arterial blood, the intravascular volume, and the elasticity of the arterial walls.

Stephen Hales made the first recorded direct measurement of blood pressure in 1733 when he cannulated the artery of a horse, allowing the blood to rise in a glass tube. He was also able to demonstrate the changes in blood pressure that occur in systole and diastole as he watched the blood rise and fall in the tube with each heartbeat. Almost a century later (1828), Poiseuille attached a mercury-filled tube to a cannulated artery. Since mercury is 13.6 times heavier than blood or water, the column in the tube was much shorter. Several instruments for the indirect method of blood pressure measurement were devised in the late 1800s.

The systemic arterial blood pressure may be assessed either by direct or indirect methods. The direct method requires cannulation of the artery but is the trusted method of measurement. Routine, direct arterial blood pressures are not measured, because of the potential sequelae, though the risks are small. Indirect blood pressure measurement can be made without opening the artery. The valid methods of indirect measurement are those that are closest in values to those made from direct techniques. Direct blood pressure standards are used to calibrate indirect pressure instruments.

Indirect measurement

Indirect methods of blood pressure measurement involve the following three physiologic facts: (1) the arterial wall may be occluded by direct pressure, resulting in obliteration of the pulse distal to the compression; (2) oscillations that vary directly with the amount of pressure being applied may be measured from the compressed artery; and (3) the normal extremity blanches (pales) when its arterial blood supply is occluded by pressure, and there is flushing or return of color when the pressure is removed.

The most commonly used method of indirect assessment of blood pressure is the auscultatory technique. For the procedure a sphygmomanometer and a stethoscope are used.

The two types of sphygmomanometers commonly used to assess arterial blood pressure are the mercury gravity and the aneroid instruments. Each instrument includes a pressure manometer, an inflatable rubber bladder encased in a cloth cuff, and a rubber hand bulb with a pressure control valve.

The air distensible bladder encased in the cloth cuff is used to occlude an artery. The cuff is long enough to encircle the extremity and be fastened securely in place. The covering cuff must be made of elastic material so pressure is applied evenly to the limb.

The mercury gravity manometer (Fig. 7-18) is made up of a straight glass tube connected to a reservoir of mercury. The reservoir in turn is connected to the pressure bulb, so that pressure created on the bulb causes the mercury to rise in the tube. Because the weight of mercury depends on gravity, a given amount of pressure will always support a column of mercury of the same height if the tube is straight and of uniform diameter. The mercury manometer does not need further calibration after the initial setting.

The aneroid sphygmomanometer (Fig. 7-19) is made up of a metal bellows connected to the compression cuff. Changes in pressure within the apparatus cause the bellows to expand and collapse. The movement of the bellows rotates a gear that moves a pointer across the calibrated dial. The aneroid sphygmomanometer is calibrated against a mercury manometer, since the more

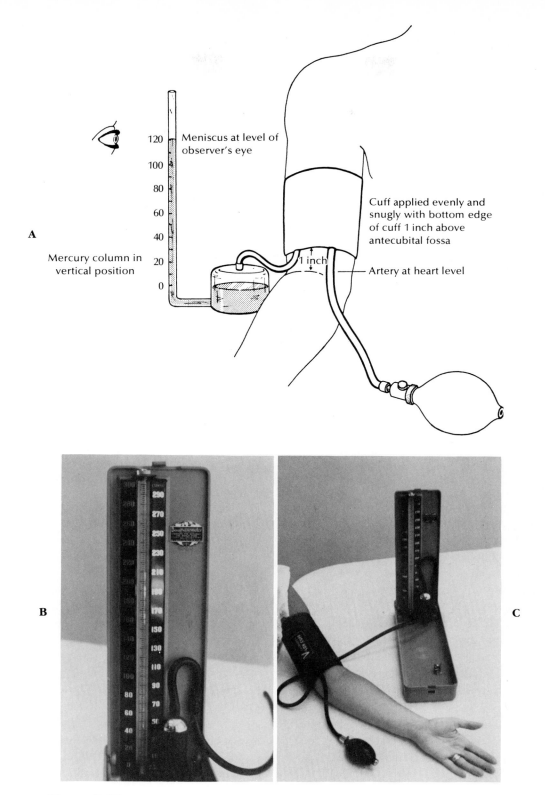

Figure 7-18

A, Mercury gravity manometer (diagrammatic). **B,** Mercury manometer. **C,** Mercury sphygmo-manometer applied to client.

(**A** from Burch GE and DePasquale NP: Primer of clinical measurement of blood pressure, St Louis, 1962, The CV Mosby Co. **B** and **C** reproduced with permission from Chicago Heart Association: Blood pressure measurement: a handbook for instructors, © 1979, The Association.)

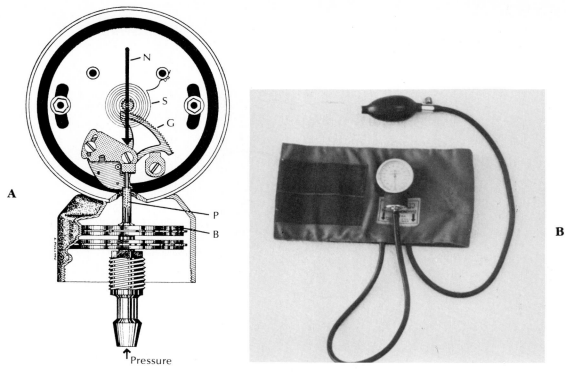

Figure 7-19

A, Aneroid sphygmomanometer (diagrammatic). Variations within the bellow *(B)* activate a pin *(P)*, which sets a gear *(G)* into motion. The gear, in turn, operates the spring *(S)*, which causes the needle *(N)* to move across the face of a calibrated dial. **B,** Aneroid sphygmomanometer.
(**A** from Burch GE and DePasquale NP: Primer of clinical measurement of blood pressure, St Louis, 1962, The CV Mosby Co. **B** reproduced with permission from Chicago Heart Association: Blood pressure measurement: a handbook for instructors, © 1979, The Association.)

complex mechanisms have been shown to need frequent adjustment. This is simply done by using a connecting Y tube between the manometers.

Electronic blood pressure measurement. Electronic cuff manometer consoles are available. They are easier to manipulate, since no stethoscope is required. This type of equipment is especially advantageous for hearing-impaired health care professionals and for clients who are hearing impaired and who monitor their own blood pressure. Some models have error indicators.

The electronic models are more expensive than the aneroid or mercury manometers. The opportunity for error is greater, since the electronic units are less accurate and use batteries. Another disadvantage is that calibration may be performed only by the manufacturer.

Taking blood pressure*
1. Assist the client to a comfortable sitting position, with arm slightly flexed, forearm supported at heart level, and palm turned up. Expose the upper arm fully.
2. Palpate the brachial artery. Position the cuff 2.5 cm (1 in) above the site of brachial artery pulsation (antecubital space). Center the arrows marked on the cuff over the brachial artery.
3. Be sure the cuff is fully deflated. Wrap the cuff evenly and snugly around the upper arm. Be sure the manometer is positioned at eye level.
4. If you do not know the client's normal systolic pressure, palpate the radial artery and inflate the cuff to a pressure 30 mm Hg above the point at which radial pulsation disappears. Deflate the cuff and wait 30 seconds.
5. Place the stethoscope earpieces in the ears and be sure sounds are clear, not muffled.
6. Relocate the brachial artery and place the diaphragm (or the bell) of the stethoscope over it.
7. Close the valve of the pressure bulb clockwise until tight.
8. Inflate the cuff to 30 mm Hg above the client's normal systolic level.

*Modified from Potter PA and Perry AG: Fundamentals of nursing: concepts, process, and practice, St Louis, 1985, The CV Mosby Co.

9. Slowly release the valve, allowing the mercury to fall at a rate of 2 to 3 mm Hg per second. Note the point on the manometer at which the first clear sound is heard. Continue to deflate the cuff gradually, noting the point at which a muffled or dampened sound appears. Continue cuff deflation, noting the point on the manometer at which sound disappears.

10. Deflate the cuff rapidly and remove it from the client's arm unless you need to repeat the measurement. If repeating the procedure, wait 30 seconds.

HELPFUL HINT: An alternative method to auscultation of the blood pressure is palpation of the diastolic pressure. It is usually used when Korotkoff sounds are inaudible or require verification.

Measurement of blood pressure by palpation. The brachial artery is palpated below the cuff, and the cuff is inflated to 30 mm Hg beyond the point at which the pulse is obliterated. The air pressure in the bladder is released at a rate of 2 to 3 mm Hg per heartbeat, and systolic blood pressure is recorded at the point at which pulsations first become palpable. The diastolic pressure is said to coincide with the cessation of vibrations in the artery. The diastolic value is difficult to obtain. However, in a test situation, more than 79% of the values obtained were within ± 4 mm Hg of those obtained by auscultatory procedures.

Auscultatory method of arterial blood pressure assessment. When the cuff is properly placed on the limb, the arterial blood can flow past the cuff only when arterial pressure exceeds that in the cuff. Partial obstruction of arterial blood flow disturbs the laminar flow pattern, creating turbulence. This turbulence produces sounds called *Korotkoff sounds* and can be heard over arteries distal to the cuff through a stethoscope (Fig. 7-20).

The bell of the stethoscope is more effective than the diaphragm in transmitting the low-frequency Korotkoff sounds. The bell is applied snugly over the artery; care is taken not to press hard enough to close the artery.

The deflated cuff is applied, without wrinkles, snugly around the upper arm so that the edge of the cuff is 2 to 3 cm above the site at which the bell of the stethoscope is to be placed. The artery is palpated, and the cuff is inflated at a rate of 12 to 20 mm Hg per second to a peak of 30 mm Hg higher than the point at which the pulse was obliterated. The cuff is then deflated at a rate of 2 to 3 mm Hg per heartbeat. The level of the meniscus of the mercury column at which the Korotkoff sounds are changed is noted.

The *systolic blood pressure* is recorded for that point at which the Korotkoff sounds are initially heard.

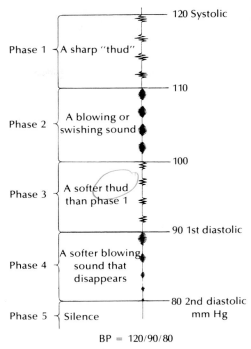

Figure 7-20

Phases of the Korotkoff sounds.
(From Burch GE and DePasquale NP: Primer of clinical measurement of blood pressure, St Louis, 1962, The CV Mosby Co.)

This is also the beginning of *phase 1,* which starts with faint, clear, and rhythmic tapping or thumping noises that gradually increase in intensity. At this point the intraluminal pressure is the same as the cuff pressure but not great enough to produce a radial pulse.

Phase 2 is characterized by a murmur or swishing sound heard as the vessel distends with blood, creating eddies and producing vibration of the vessel wall. *Phase 3* is the period during which the sounds are crisper and more intense. In this phase the vessel remains open in systole but obliterated in diastole.

The *muffling* of the Korotkoff sounds is the guidepost for the beginning of *phase 4,* and the pressure at this point is believed by many authorities to be the closest to the *diastolic arterial pressure* measured by a direct method. At this point the cuff pressure falls below the intraluminal pressure. It is frequently called the first diastolic pressure. The second diastolic pressure and *phase 5* are said to be present when the Korotkoff sounds are no longer heard. Phase 5 marks the period wherein the vessel remains open during the entire cycle.

If muffling of the Korotkoff sounds is established as indicating diastolic level, the value will be about 8 mm Hg greater than that obtained by the direct method.

Disappearance of the Korotkoff sounds is a risky criterion for diastolic pressure, since the sounds do not abate in some individuals until a pressure well below the diastolic value is reached.

Thus, three values are recorded: the systolic pressure, the point of muffling of the Korotkoff sounds, and the disappearance of the sounds. An example of the record might be 120/78/54. This method has the approval of WHO and AHA.

Korotkoff sounds may be heard all the way to zero on the sphygmomanometer scale. This occurs frequently in healthy children and in certain hyperdynamic states such as the aftermath to vigorous exercise, in thyrotoxicosis, or in severe anemia. In this case the pressure at the beginning of phase 4 is noted and recorded, as well as a description of sound heard to 0 mm Hg.

Cuff size. If the cuff is too narrow, the blood pressure reading will be erroneously high. A wide cuff increases the risk of an erroneously low reading.

The sphygmomanometer cuff should be 20% to 25% wider than the diameter of the extremity in which the blood pressure is being taken. Another recommendation is that the bladder width be equal to two fifths the circumference of the limb. A more liberal approximation suggests that the cuff should cover two thirds of the upper arm. Ideally, the bladder should completely encircle the extremity and should be snugly applied. Cuffs may be obtained in several sizes (Table 7-9).

CAUTION: The cuff size is determined by the diameter of the limb, not the client's age.

The examiner's eye must be at a direct line with the level of the meniscus of the mercury column to avoid parallax error, and the mercury column must be kept in a vertical position.

The cuff should be deflated completely (0 mm Hg) between successive readings. At least a 15-second interval is allowed between readings, with the cuff completely deflated, to avoid spurious readings as a result of venous congestion.

The bladder and the pressure bulbs should be monitored for leaks. Erratic inflation or deflation usually indicates a leak.

Measurement of blood pressure in the leg. The blood pressure in the leg may be measured with the client in either the supine or prone position. The Korotkoff sounds are evaluated over the popliteal artery.

In the popliteal artery, the systolic arterial blood pressure is higher (10 ± 5 mm Hg) than in the brachial artery, whereas the diastolic pressure is generally lower. This difference is magnified in aortic insufficiency and in some hyperdynamic states such as after exercise.

Increasing audibility of the Korotkoff sounds in infants and the flush test. Occasionally the Korotkoff sounds are not heard over the brachial artery

Table 7-9

Dimensions for appropriate size cuff

	Range of dimensions of bladder (cm)	
	Width	**Length**
Newborn	2.5-4.0	5.0-10.0
Infant	6.0-8.0	12.0-13.5
Child	9.0-10.0	17.0-22.5
Adult	12.0-13.0	22.0-23.5
Large adult arm	15.5	30.0
Adult thigh	18.0	36.0

From The National Heart, Lung, and Blood Institute's Task Force on Blood Pressure Control in Children: Report of the Task Force on Blood Pressure Control in Children, Pediatrics Supplement 59 (suppl 5):797, 1977. Copyright American Academy of Pediatrics 1977.

in infants. A suggestion for making the sounds audible is to hold the infant's arm upright for 1 to 2 minutes with the cuff in place. The pressure is measured immediately on lowering the arm.

If the Korotkoff sounds cannot be obtained, a flush pressure that approximates the mean blood pressure may be measured in the upper or lower extremity. The procedure for this test is as follows: The properly sized cuff is placed around the infant's wrist or ankle. An elasticized bandage is placed around the extremity distal to the cuff to promote vascular emptying. The bladder pressure of the sphygmomanometer is raised to approximately 150 mm Hg. The bandage is removed, and the cuff pressure is decreased at a rate of 2 to 3 mm Hg per heartbeat until a vascular flush (rubor) is observed. The appearance of the flush is correlated with the sphygmomanometer reading.

Auscultatory gap. Occasionally, as the pneumatic cuff is being deflated, the Korotkoff sounds disappear and then are heard 10 to 15 mm Hg later. This is called auscultatory gap. The examiner records systolic blood pressure at the onset of the first sound. Thus, the auscultatory gap will not be cause for error if the cuff was inflated to 20 mm Hg above the point at which the artery was occluded as determined by palpation.

Normal systolic and diastolic pressure. In adults the systolic blood pressure has a normal range of 95 to 140 mm Hg; 120 mm Hg is cited as average (when measured in the brachial artery). Normal diastolic pressure ranges from 60 to 90 mm Hg; 80 mm Hg is average.

The systolic blood pressure in the neonatal period may range about 60 mm Hg. It has been recommended that a systolic blood pressure less than 55 mm Hg be considered hypotension. Blood pressure gradually increases until adolescence, when an accelerated rise is incurred. Thus, at about 17 or 18 years, blood pressure reaches adult levels.

The proper application of the auscultatory method yields values that are within 4 ± 5 mm Hg of the direct method of measurement.

Normal variations in blood pressure recordings. The blood pressure in a normal individual varies continually with respiration, autonomic state, emotional levels, and biologic rhythms. Furthermore, successive readings of indirect measures of blood pressure by the same or different observers may differ by as much as 10 mm Hg.

In the normal individual, the *change from a supine to an erect position* causes a slight decrease in systolic blood pressure (less than 15 mm Hg) and in diastolic pressure (less than 5 mm Hg). Marked drops in pressure (greater than 30 mm Hg) incurred when the individual stands may indicate a vasopressor defect or hypovolemia.

The blood pressure also shows a *24-hour,* or *circadian, pattern.* Consistent with the other vital signs, the blood pressure has higher values in the afternoon and evening hours and lower values in the late hours of sleep.

Because blood pressure is readily altered by *stressful events,* an effort should be made to relax the client as much as possible before taking the blood pressure.

Food and exercise also affect the blood pressure. It is recommended that the individual should not eat or exercise in the 30 minutes before the determination is made. The extremity should be at heart level for a period of approximately 5 minutes.

Differences in blood pressure indicating disease. The initial examination of blood pressure should include a measurement in both arms and one from the leg. Differences in blood pressure between the two arms may be caused by congenital aortic obstruction (coarctation), by acquired conditions such as aortic dissection, or by obstruction of the arteries of the upper arm.

Constriction or obstruction of the aorta may be suspected when the pressure assessed in the client's arms exceeds that in the legs, particularly when the differences are great.

Coarctation of the aorta must be suspected when the brachial pressure markedly exceeds that of the popliteal artery. This reversal of gradient may also accompany other obstructive lesions of the aorta or obstructive lesions in proximal arteries of the leg.

Assessment of pulsus paradoxus. Arterial blood pressure in healthy human beings is known to vary as much as 10 mm Hg during relaxed respiration. The decrease with inspiration may be 10 ± 5 mm Hg,

whereas on exhalation proportionate increase is noted. A difference greater than 15 mm Hg indicates pulsus paradoxus. These fluctuations may be more accurately assessed by raising the cuff pressure to a level greater than systolic pressure and by allowing the cuff to deflate very slowly while the client breathes normally.

Assessment of pulsus alternans. Pulsus alternans is pulse beat to pulse beat variation in systolic pressure. Although the presence of pulsus alternans may be readily determined from palpation of the pulse, when it is marked, it may be accurately assessed through the use of the sphygmomanometer.

The cuff is inflated to 20 mm Hg above the systolic pressure as determined by palpation. On deflation to phase 1, only alternate beats are heard. Later all beats are audible and palpable. After still further deflation all beats are of equal intensity. The difference between this point and the peak systolic level is often used in determining the degree of pulsus alternans.

Pulse pressure. The pulse pressure is the difference between systolic and diastolic pressure. The normal value is generally 30 to 40 mm Hg. The heart rate may influence the pulse pressure. With a slowly beating heart the period of flow or "runoff" from the aorta to the periphery is lengthened, lowering the diastolic pressure, thus increasing the pulse pressure.

A wide pulse pressure accompanied by bradycardia frequently indicates increased intracranial pressure, aortic insufficiency, patent ductus arteriosus, and arteriovenous fistula. The pulse pressure is also increased in hyperkinetic states such as hyperthyroidism or after vigorous exercise. Although the stroke volume may be greater, rapid runoff may result in low diastolic recordings.

With increased peripheral resistance, runoff to the peripheral circulation is less; thus, more blood accumulates in the aorta, and both systolic and diastolic blood pressure increase.

A small stroke volume will tend to decrease the pulse pressure.

Hypertension and hypotension

Hypertension. WHO defines hypertension as a persistent elevation of blood pressure greater than 140/90. AHA recommends that 160/95 be the defining point for hypertension in the client over 40 years of age. Elevation of either systolic or diastolic blood pressure is an indication for further diagnostic tests.

If the definition of hypertension in the adult is accepted as a diastolic pressure in excess of 90 mm Hg, then about 15% of whites and 30% of blacks in the United

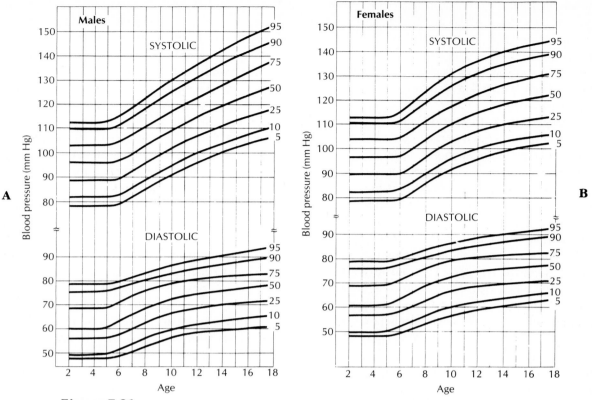

Figure 7-21

Percentiles of blood pressure measurement (right arm, seated). **A,** Men. **B,** Women.
(From the National Heart, Lung, and Blood Institute's Task Force on Blood Pressure Control in Children: Pediatrics 59 [suppl 5]:797, 1977. Copyright American Academy of Pediatrics 1977.)

States have hypertension. One study estimated that one half of hypertensive persons have not been identified.

The structures most frequently observed to suffer damage as peripheral resistance is increased are the heart, the kidneys, and the brain. Vessel changes are best observed in the retina. Sclerosis, hemorrhage, and exudates typify the alterations seen in hypertension.

The incidence of cerebrovascular accident (CVA) is increased by high pressure in the vessels in the brain.

An exaggerated pulsus paradoxus is observed in persons with pericardial effusion, constrictive pericarditis, severe chronic obstructive pulmonary disease, and hypovolemia.

Increased cardiac work is required to pump the blood against the increased peripheral resistance. Thus, congestive heart failure, left ventricular hypertrophy, or angina pectoris may result from hypertension.

The examiner must bear in mind other signs and symptoms that accompany hypertension. These might include severe headache, blurred vision, and signs of renal disease.

Pulsus alternans may be detected in tachypnea if the respiratory rate is half the heart rate, immediately

following ventricular ectopic contractions, in myocardial failure resulting from severe organic heart disease, and in bigeminal rhythm.

Although it is accepted that the routine measurement of blood pressure in all children from newborn through adolescence is imperative to the diagnosis of hypertension, this practice is frequently neglected. The screening examination may yield an incidence of hypertension of approximately 2.3% in children 4 to 15 years of age. Early detection of these hypertensive children may mean that diagnosis and treatment may be initiated in time to prevent the sequelae of the underlying disease process. It has been shown that 90% of adults are subject to essential or idiopathic hypertension, whereas this is true only for 20% of children. The blood pressure is recorded each time the child is seen and is considered with other developmental data.

Hypertension is said to exist in children with either the systolic or diastolic blood pressure is greater than the 95th percentile for age, that is, two standard deviations above the mean. Fig. 7-21 shows the range of blood pressures obtained in children.

The blood pressure as measured by Doppler technique has demonstrated that blood pressure rises rapidly from between 4 days and 6 weeks and then remains reasonably stable until the first year. The 95th percentile for blood pressure between 6 weeks and 6 years is about 115 mm Hg. Note the progressive increase in blood pressure that is incurred from 1 year to age 15.

The observation of a brachial blood pressure of 150 mm Hg or more may indicate secondary hypertension resulting from renal or endocrine disease or coarctation of the aorta. Coarctation of the aorta is also suspected when the blood pressure in the arms exceeds that in the legs by 30 mm Hg. The normal difference in the infant is that the brachial blood pressure is 17 ± 10 mm Hg greater than in the legs.

The findings of an elevated blood pressure in the pediatric client alert the examiner to look for indications of hypertensive encephalopathy (hyperactivity, excitability, and fundal changes).

The Task Force on Blood Pressure in Children (1987) recommended that nondrug therapies such as diet, exercise, and behavior modification be pursued aggressively in treating the mildest cases of high blood pressure. The recommendations were made in response to research data indicating toxicity and side effects of antihypertensive drugs.

Weight reduction was recommended with the justification that weight loss often results in a substantial decrease in blood pressure even when ideal weight is not achieved. The report advised that high blood cholesterol levels be reduced even though definitive information of the effect on blood pressure is not available. Restriction of dietary sodium to an amount equal to 2 g was also recommended. Alcohol consumption was advised to be less than 4 oz of hard liquor, 16 oz of wine, or 48 oz of beer a day.

A regular program of exercise was recommended, as well as behavior modification therapies such as relaxation and biofeedback. The committee said a diastolic pressure less than 85 mm Hg can be considered normal, but a reading of 85 to 89 mm Hg is high normal and should be watched.

Hypotension. Hypotension has been defined as a persistent blood pressure less than 95/60.

Hypotension in the absence of other signs or symptoms is generally innocent. In fact, lower blood pressures may be considered beneficial because the heart does not have to pump as hard to circulate the blood. The blood pressure must be high enough to ensure an adequate blood supply to the kidneys, brain, and other body tissues.

However, sudden changes in blood pressure may produce changes in body function. Sudden drops in nor-

mal blood pressure may result in fainting. This is observed in orthostatic hypotension. In this case, the blood pressure may be normal when the individual is reclining but drops when the individual rises to a sitting or standing position, particularly when the position change is a rapid one. Faintness and dizziness from orthostatic hypotension is common in individuals who have been confined to bed or have diseases of the nervous system.

A drop in blood pressure may also follow severe injury, hemorrhage, and endotoxin-producing infections. In hypovolemic or endotoxic shock, the Korotkoff sounds will be less audible or absent. Since the peripheral blood pressure is an important parameter for determining the method of treatment, ultrasonic direct or invasive techniques of blood pressure assessment may be used. Some other signs of shock might include increased pulse and respiratory rates, dizziness, confusion, blurred vision diaphoresis, and cold and clammy skin.

Respiratory rate, volume, and rhythm assessment are described in Chapter 14 on assessment of the respiratory system.

BIBLIOGRAPHY

Adelman EM: When patient's blood pressure falls, what does it mean? What should you do? Nurs 80 10:26, 1980.

American Heart Association: Recommendations for human blood pressure determination by sphygmomanometers, Dallas, 1980, The Association.

Atkins E: Fever: a new perspective on an old phenomenon, N Engl J Med 308:958, 1983.

Centers for Disease Control: Recommendations for prevention of HIV transmission in health-care settings, MMWR (suppl) 36:SS, Aug. 21, 1987.

Eoff M and Joyce B: Temperature measurements in children, Am J Nurs 81:1010, 1981.

Bernheim HA and others: Fever: pathogenesis, pathophysiology, and purpose, Ann Intern Med 91:261, 1979.

Birdsall C: How accurate are your blood pressures? Am J Nurs 84:1414, 1984.

Birdsall C: How do you interpret pulses? Am J Nurs 85:785, 1985.

Donaldson JF: Therapy of acute fever: a comparative approach, Hosp Pract [Off] 9:125, 1981.

Draper G, Dupertuis C, and Caughey J, Jr: Human constitution in clinical medicine, New York, 1944, PB Hoeber, Inc.

Dressler DK and others: A comparison of oral and rectal temperature measurement on patients receiving oxygen by mask, Nurs Res 32:373, 1983.

Electronic thermometers: the better alternative? Health Devices 12:18, 1982.

Griffin JP: Fever: when to leave it alone, Nurs 86 16:58, 1986.

Guerevich I: Fever: when to worry about it, RN 48:14, 1985.

Guyton AC: Textbook of medical physiology, ed 6, Philadelphia, 1986, WB Saunders Co.

Joint National Committee on Detection, Evaluation, and Treatment of High Blood Pressure: The 1984 report of the Joint National Committee on Detection, Evaluation and Treatment of High Blood Pressure, Arch Intern Med 144:1045, May 1984.

Lim-Levy F: The effect of oxygen inhalation on oral temperature, Nurs Res 31:150, 1982.

McCarron K: Fever: the cardinal vital sign, CCQ, 15, July 1986.

Mountcastle VB: Medical physiology, vol 2, ed 14, St Louis, 1980, The CV Mosby Co.

Nichols GA: Time analysis of afebrile and febrile temperature reading, Nurs Res 21:463, 1972.

Nichols GA and others: Oral, axillary, and rectal temperature determinations and relationships, Nurs Res 15:307, 1966.

Nichols GA and others: Taking oral temperature of febrile patients, Nurs Res 18:448, 1969.

Nichols GA and others: Measuring oral and rectal temperatures of febrile children, Nurs Res 21:261, 1972.

Petersdorf RC: Disturbances of heat regulation. In Isselbacher KJ and others, editors: Harrison's principles of internal medicine, ed 9, New York, 1980, McGraw-Hill Book Co.

Task Force on Blood Pressure Control in Children: Report of Second Task Force on Blood Pressure Control in Children—1987, Pediatrics, 79:1-15, 1987.

Thibodeau GA: Anatomy and physiology, St Louis, 1987, The CV Mosby Co.

Whaley LF and Wong DL: Nursing care of infants and children, ed 3, St Louis, 1987, The CV Mosby Co.

8

Assessment of skin, hair, and nails

OBJECTIVES

Upon successful review of this chapter, learners will be able to:

- Describe anatomy and physiology of the integumentary system

- State related rationale and demonstrate assessment of
  Skin and sebaceous gland characteristics
  Hair characteristics
  Nail and finger characteristics

- Recognize stages of dermatitis

- Distinguish between primary and secondary skin lesions

- Recognize conditions and locations of common skin lesions

- Describe how to assess a skin lesion

The skin, or integumentary system, is an organ system readily accessible to examination. As a membrane barrier between the individual and the external environment, the skin responds to changes in the external environment and also reflects changes in the internal environment. A careful examination of the skin may yield valuable information about the client's general health, along with specific information that will aid in identifying a systemic disease or a specific problem of the skin. It is important to describe the skin of the healthy client, as well as the skin of the client with a health problem, paying special attention to any deviation from normal. (The examination of the sclera and conjunctiva is discussed in Chapter 10, and the examination of the oral mucosa is discussed in Chapter 9.)

The examination of the skin requires some understanding of the structure and function of the system and familiarity with the appearance of the skin, hair, nails, and mucous membranes in health and disease. This chapter includes a brief discussion of the anatomy and function of the skin, methods for conducting a systematic examination of the skin and appendages, and an approach to the description and classification of skin lesions.

ANATOMY AND FUNCTION

The skin has many important functions, including (1) assisting in maintaining an internal environment by providing a barrier to loss of water and electrolytes; (2) providing protection from external agents injurious to the internal environment; (3) regulating body heat; (4) functioning as a sense organ for touch, temperature, and pain; (5) providing self-maintenance and wound repair; (6) maintaining buffered protective skin film by eccrine and sebaceous glands; (7) participating in production of vitamin D; and (8) delaying hypersensitivity reaction to foreign substances.

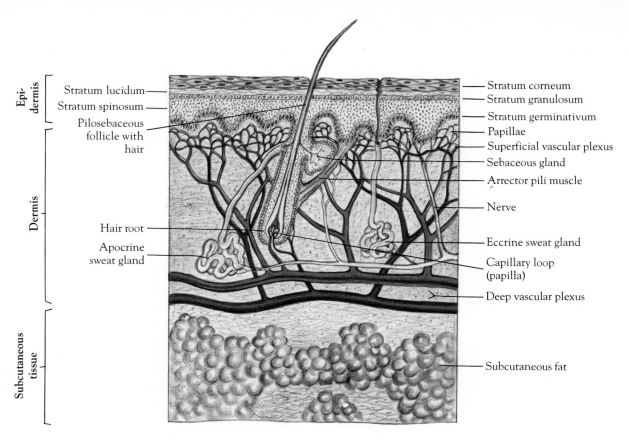

Figure 8-1

Structures of skin.
(From Thompson JM and others: Clinical nursing, ed 1, St Louis, 1987, The CV Mosby Co.)

The skin is divided into three layers: the epidermis, the dermis, and the subcutaneous tissues (Fig. 8-1).

The epidermis is an avascular, cornified cellular structure. The epidermis, or external epithelial layer, is continuous with the mucous membranes and lining of the ear canals. It is stratified into several layers and is composed chiefly of keratinocytes, cells that produce keratin. Keratin makes up much of the horny material in the outermost epidermal layer of dead cells and is the principal constituent of the harder, keratinized structures of nails and hair. The innermost layer of the epidermis contains melanocytes, the source of melanin, the pigment that gives color to the skin and hair. This outer layer is constantly shed in an inconspicuous way and replenished by mitosis of the underlying cells, so there is almost a complete turnover every 3 to 4 weeks.

Epidermal appendages include the hair, nails, eccrine sweat glands, apocrine sweat glands, and sebaceous glands. These are formed by invagination of the epidermis into the underlying dermis. The hair and nails are keratinized appendages and have no significant function in human beings. The eccrine, sebaceous, and apocrine appendages are glandular. The sebaceous glands usually arise from the hair follicles and produce sebum, which has a lubricating effect on the horny outer layer of the epidermis. The eccrine sweat glands are widely distributed and have an important function in the dissipation of body heat as sweat is produced and evaporated. The apocrine sweat glands are found in the axillary and genital areas and usually open into the hair follicles. The sweat produced by the apocrine glands decomposes when contaminated by bacteria, resulting in the characteristic body odor.

The dermis underlying the epidermis constitutes the bulk of the skin. It is often referred to as the "true skin." A tough connective tissue that contains lymphatics and nerves and is highly vascular, it supports and nourishes the epidermis.

The subcutaneous layer immediately under the dermis is distinguished by the storage of fat and is important in temperature insulation.

Tips for Assessing Dark Skin

1. Skin color should be observed in the sclera, conjunctiva, buccal mucosa, tongue, lips, nail beds, palms, and soles.
2. Inspection should be accompanied by palpation, especially if inflammation or edema is suspected.
3. Findings should always be correlated with the patient's history to arrive at a nursing diagnosis.
4. *Pallor* in brown-skinned patients may present as a yellowish brown tinge to the skin. In a black-skinned patient the skin will appear "ashen-gray." It can be difficult to determine. Pallor in dark-skinned individuals is characterized by absence of the underlying red tones in the skin.
5. *Jaundice* may be observed in the sclera but should not be confused with the normal yellow pigmentation of the dark-skinned black patient. The best place to inspect is in that portion of the sclera that is observable when the eye is open. If jaundice is suspected, the posterior portion of the hard palate should also be observed for a yellowish cast. This is most effective when done in bright daylight.
6. The *oral mucosa* of dark-skinned individuals may have a normal freckling of pigmentation that may also be evident in the gums, the borders of the tongue, and the lining of the cheeks.
7. The *gingiva* normally may have a dark blue color that may appear blotchy or be evenly distributed.
8. *Petechiae* are best observed over areas of lighter pigmentation—the abdomen, gluteal areas, and volar aspect of the forearm. They may also be seen in the palpebral conjunctiva and buccal mucosa.
9. To differentiate petechiae and ecchymosis from erythema, remember that pressure over the area will cause erythema to blanch but will not affect either petechiae or ecchymosis.
10. *Erythema* usually is associated with increased skin temperature, so palpation should also be used if an inflammatory condition is suspected.
11. *Edema* may reduce the intensity of the color of an area of skin because of the increased distance between the external epithelium and the pigmented layers. Therefore, darker skin would appear lighter. On palpation the skin may feel "tight."
12. *Cyanosis* can often be difficult to determine in dark-skinned individuals. Familiarity with the precyanotic color is often helpful. However, if this is not possible, close inspection of the nail beds, lips, palpebral conjunctiva, palms, and soles should show evidence of cyanosis.
13. *Skin rashes* may be assessed by palpating for changes in skin texture.

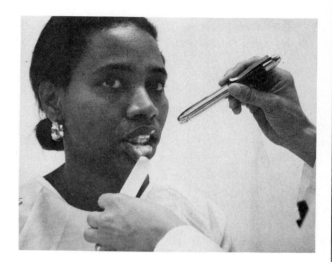

In black individuals pallor and cyanosis are best detected by examining the mucosa of the mouth (above) and the palpebral conjunctiva of the eye.

From Roach B: Color changes in dark skin, Nursing '77, January, 1977.

EXAMINATION

The examination of the skin and appendages begins with a general inspection, followed by a detailed examination. A good source of illumination is necessary; indirect natural daylight is preferred. A small magnifying glass will aid in the examination of individual lesions of the skin. A clear flexible measure is helpful in assessing the size of the lesions.

The examination may begin with an observation of the entire integument with the client disrobed or a more simple approach may be taken: the skin that is exposed may be surveyed, followed by inspection of the skin, mucous membranes, and epidermal appendages of each body part as it is examined. Comparison of symmetric anatomic areas is made throughout the examination. The two major techniques used are inspection and palpation.

The skin is inspected for color and vascularity and for evidence of perspiration, edema, injuries, or skin lesions. During the examination the practitioner should think about the underlying structures and the particular kind of exposure of a body part. It is also helpful to note those changes in the skin that indicate past injuries and habits, such as calluses, stains, scars, needle marks, and insect bites, and to note the grooming of hair and nails. See the box above for tips on assessing dark skin.

Skin Color

Skin color varies from person to person and from one part of the body to another but is normally a whitish pink

---

Tips for Evaluating Skin Color Changes

If you notice a color change in the client's skin, consider:
- The lighting in the examination room
- The position of the patient or the extremity
- The room temperature
- The patient's emotional condition
- The cleanliness of the integument
- The presence of edema

---

or a brown shade, depending on race. The exposed areas of the body, including the face, ears, back of neck, and backs of hands and arms, are noticeably different and may be more damaged after long exposure to the sun and weather. The vascular flush areas are the cheeks, the bridge of the nose, the neck, the upper chest, the flexor surfaces of the extremities, and the genital area. These areas may be involved in a vascular disturbance or may demonstrate increased color caused by blushing or temperature elevation. They should be compared with areas of less vascularity. The pigment labile areas are the face, the backs of the hands, the flexors of the wrists, the axillae, the mammary areolae, the midline of the abdomen, and the genital area. These areas may demonstrate normal systemic pigmentary changes, such as occur during pregnancy. See box above.

Other changes in skin color should be noted as evidence of systemic disease. Cyanosis, a dusky blue color, may be observed in the nail beds and in the lips and the oral mucosa. It results from decreased oxyhemoglobin binding, or decreased oxygenation of the blood, and can be caused by pulmonary or heart disease, by abnormalities of hemoglobin, or by cold. The yellow or green hue of jaundice occurs when tissue bilirubin is increased and may be noted first in the sclerae and then in the mucous membranes and the skin. Pallor, or decreased color in the skin, results from decreased blood flow to the superficial vessels or from decreased amounts of hemoglobin in the blood; it is most evident in the face, the palpebral conjunctiva, the mouth, and the nails. Generalized redness of the skin may be caused by fever, whereas defined areas of redness may be the result of a localized infection or sunburn. Other localized changes in color may indicate a problem such as edema, which tends to blanch skin color. Alterations in the normal pattern of pigmentation result from changes in the distribution of melanin or in the function of the melanocytes in the epidermis; hyperpigmentation or depigmentation can occur. The nevus, or birthmark, is an example of a defined area of hyperpigmentation that may be an innocent manifestation, such as the mongolian spots found

on infants, or may be a more serious finding, such as the numerous café au lait spots of neurofibromatosis. Depigmentation of the skin, which is seen in vitiligo, may involve only one or few areas or be more generalized. Common sites of vitiligo are the face, neck, axillae, groin, anogenital area, eyelids, hands, and wrists. Table 8-1 lists other conditions causing variations in pigmentation.

Skin Palpation

Palpation of the skin is used to amplify the findings observed on inspection and is usually carried out simultaneously as each body part is examined. Changes in temperature, moisture, texture, and turgor are detected by palpation.

Temperature of the skin is increased when blood flow through the dermis is increased. Localized areas of skin hyperthermia are noted in the presence of a burn or a localized infection. Generalized skin hyperthermia involving all the integument may occur when there is fever associated with a localized or systemic disease. Temperature of the skin is reduced when there is a decrease in blood flow in the dermis. Generalized skin hypothermia occurs when the client is in shock, whereas localized hypothermia occurs in conditions such as arteriosclerosis.

The moisture found on the skin will vary from one body area to another. It is normal to find the soles of the feet, the palms of the hands, and the intertriginous areas—where two surfaces are close together—containing more moisture than other parts. The amount of moisture found over the entire integument also varies with changes in the environmental temperature, with muscular activity, and with body temperature. The skin functions in the regulation of body temperature and produces perspiration that evaporates, thus cooling the body when the temperature is increased. The skin is normally drier during the winter months, when environmental temperatures and humidity are decreased, and as the individual ages. Abnormal dryness of the skin occurs with dehydration; the skin will feel dry even when the temperature is increased. Dryness of the skin is also found in conditions such as myxedema and chronic nephritis.

Texture refers to the fineness or coarseness of the skin, and changes may indicate local irritation or trauma to defined skin areas or may be associated with problems of other systems. The skin becomes soft and smooth in hyperthyroidism and rough and dry in hypothyroidism.

Turgor refers to the elasticity of the skin and is most easily determined by picking up a fold of skin over the abdomen and observing how quickly it returns to its normal shape. There is a loss of turgor associated with dehydration, and the skin demonstrates a laxness and a

Table 8-1

Variation in pigmentation

Condition	Characteristic color	Location
Diffuse hyperpigmentation		
Addison's disease, ACTH-producing tumors*	Tan to brown, "bronzing"	Generalized, more marked on exposed areas, flexures, mucous membrane of mouth
Arsenic toxicity	Dusky, diffuse, paler spots	Trunk, extremities
Chloasma (mask of pregnancy), phenytoin ingestion	Tan to brown	Forehead—adjacent to hair line, malar prominence, upper lip, chin
Hemochromatosis	Bronze to grayish brown, deposits of hemosiderin	Generalized
Ichthyosis	Tan, fine to coarse scales	Generalized
Malabsorption syndrome (sprue)	Tan to brown patches	Any area of body
Scleroderma	Yellow to tan (may also have depigmentation)	Generalized
Uremia (chronic renal failure)	Yellow-brown, retention of urinary chromogens	Generalized
Lack of pigmentation		
Vitiligo	Circumscribed lack of pigmentation	
Albinism—hereditary	Complete or partial lack of melanin	Generalized (universal albinism), skin, hair, eyes

*ACTH, adrenocorticotropic hormone.

loss of normal mobility, returning to place slowly. Loss of turgor is also associated with aging; the skin becomes wrinkled and lax. Increased turgor is associated with an increase in tension, which causes the skin to return to place quickly when pinched. Increased turgor is seen in progressive systemic sclerosis (PSS), a connective tissue disorder.

Hair

The hair over the entire body is examined to determine the distribution, quantity, and quality. There is a normal male or female hair pattern that evolves after puberty, and a deviation may indicate an endocrine problem. The pattern of hair distribution in the male genital area is diamond-shaped, while the pattern of hair distribution in the female genital area is triangular. Changes in the quantity of the hair are also important. Hirsutism, increased hair growth, is found in conditions such as Cushing's syndrome and acromegaly. Decreased hair growth or loss of hair may be associated with hypopituitarism or a pyogenic infection. Types of alopecia, or hair loss, are listed in Table 8-2. The quality of the hair is determined by the color and texture. Changes in color such as graying occur normally with aging, but patchy gray hair may develop following nerve injuries. Changes in texture of hair associated with hypothyroidism include dryness and coarseness, and changes associated with hyperthyroidism include increased silkiness and fineness.

Table 8-2

Alopecia—hair loss

Type of alopecia	Description
Androgen (in female)	Thinning of scalp hair; male pattern hirsutism on body
Areata	Circumscribed bald areas; sudden onset, usually reversible.
Chemical	Hair brittle, breaks off
Cicatricial	Permanent localized loss of hair associated with scarring
Drug or radiation	Generalized loss of hair caused by antineoplastic agents, such as gold, thallium, and arsenic, or by radiation
Male pattern	Receding of anterior hairline, temples, and vertex; hereditary
Mucinosis	Erythmatous papules or plaques without hair
Syphilitic	Generalized thinning of hair or baldness; mucous patches without hair

Nails

The assessment of the nails is important to determine not only their condition but also possible evidence of systemic diseases. The nails are examined for shape, normal dorsal curvature, adhesion to the nail bed, regularity of the nail surface, color, and thickness. The skin folds around the

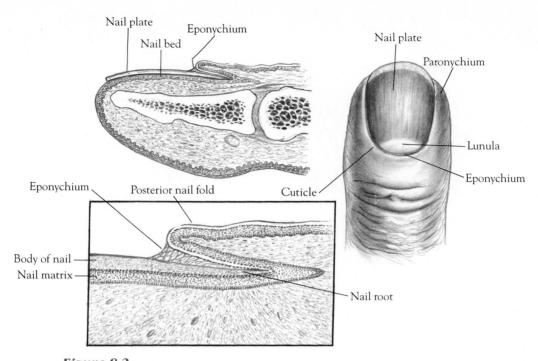

Figure 8-2

Structures of nail.
(From Thompson JM and others: Clinical nursing, ed 1, St Louis, 1987, The CV Mosby Co.)

nails are examined for any color changes, swelling, increased temperature, and tenderness (Fig. 8-2).

The nails are keratinized appendages of the epidermis, as are hairs. The nails consist of (1) the nail matrix (root), wherein the nail plate is developed; (2) the nail plate; (3) the nail bed, which is attached to the nail plate; and (4) the periungual tissue, including the eponychium and the perionychium.

The nail matrix is not visible. The lunula, located at the base of the visible nail, has the shape of a half moon. The whiter color of the lunula compared with the more distal nail is caused by the uptake of keratolytic granules and by the lunula's looser connection to the underlying vascularized derma. A bluish hue can be observed in the nails of more darkly pigmented subjects. The size of the lunula is variable and may not be visible in older subjects.

The nail plate is a horny, semitransparent structure with a dorsal convexity. The nail bed lies distal to the lunula and is not known to participate in nail formation. The visible nail has a roughly rectangular shape. Normal thickness of the nail is 0.3 to 0.65 mm, being somewhat thicker in men.

The free edge of the nail fold is continuous with the cuticle, which is an extension of the stratum corneum of the dorsum of the finger. The eponychium lies below this and is the anterior extension of the roof of the nail fold on the nail plate. The hyponychium is the portion of the fingertip underlying the free portion of the nail. The perionychium is the epidermis bordering the nail.

Nail growth

The nail plate is formed continuously and uniformly at all points in the matrix. The plate is pushed forward by cells of the germinative layer of the matrix. The fingernail growth rate in the normal adult has been reported variously as 0.1 to 1 mm per day. The rate varies with nutrition, age, and activity level.

Nail growth also has a circadian and seasonal rhythm. It is greater in the morning, lessening progressively in the afternoon and the night. Nail growth is greater in warm seasons than in cold, and accelerated growth has been observed in warm climates. The growth rate slows with aging. The total time required for reaching the free margin of the nail from the lunula is called the migration time and is normally 130 days. The time required for complete renewal of the fingernail (regeneration time) is 170 days, while that of the toenail is 1 to 1½ years.

Nail absence

Anonychia is the complete absence of the nail. This condition is usually congenital.

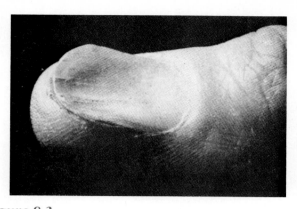

Figure 8-3

Koilonychia.
(From Samman PD: The nails in disease, London, 1978, William Heinemann Medical Books, Ltd.)

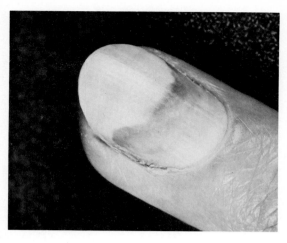

Figure 8-4

Onycholysis.
(From Samman PD: The nails in disease, London, 1978, William Heinemann Medical Books, Ltd.)

Changes in nail curvature

Platyonychia is flattening of the nails, although color, consistency, and thickness are not altered. This may be hereditary or may be the forerunner of koilonychia.

Koilonychia describes a nail that has the general shape of a spoon. The color is generally white, and the nail is opaque. The concave portion of the nail is particularly fragile. When all the nails are not involved, the cause may be chronic eczema or a tumor of the nail bed. Systemic diseases associated with koilonychia are hypochromic anemias, chronic infections, malnutrition, pellagra, and Raynaud's disease (Fig. 8-3).

Racket nail is a flattened and expanded nail, usually the thumb. It has been considered a sign of secondary syphilis.

Changes in nail adhesion

Onycholysis is separation of the nail from the nail bed, originating at the free edge and progressing proximally. Although the condition may be congenital, it has also been associated with disorders of the thyroid—both hypothyroidism and hyperthyroidism—repeated trauma, peripheral arteriospasm (as in Raynaud's disease), hypochromic anemias, syphilis, eczema, and acrocyanosis (Fig. 8-4).

Onychomadesis is the separation of the nail starting at the roof of the nail and progressing to the free margin. This condition is the result of a lesion of the matrix and the hyponychium. The separation may be the result of peripheral neuritis, amyotrophy, hemiplegias, thrombosis, vascular disease, frostbite, exanthemas (scarlet fever, measles), or hypocalcemia.

Paronychia is an inflammation of the folds of tissue surrounding the nails leading to erythema, with inflammation, swelling, and induration of the nail fold accompanied by pain and tenderness. It is the most common complaint related to the nails. Drops of pus may be extruded from beneath the nail fold ulceration. The ulceration tends to involve surrounding tissues. The lesion generally involves the distal third of the nail, which may be broken or destroyed as necrosis progresses. This condition is common in diabetic persons. *Candida albicans,* staphylococci, and streptococci are most frequently involved. Third-stage syphilis and leprosy may lead to paronychia (Fig. 8-5).

Changes in the nail surface

Beau's lines (Beau's striations, transverse sulci) are striations approximately 1 mm deep and 0.1 to 0.5 mm wide running across the entire nail perpendicular to the longitudinal axis. The color is the same as the remainder of the nail. Beau's lines are thought to be caused by an arrest of nail growth at the matrix. If the retardation of growth is repeated, another line may result. Because the nail grows at a rate of approximately 0.1 mm per day and the eponychium is about 3 mm long, it is possible to calculate the point in time at which the hiatus in nail production occurred. Beau's lines have been associated with the acute phase of infectious diseases, malnutrition, and anemia (Fig. 8-6).

Pitting deformities of the nail may vary from pinpoint to pinhead size and may be linear or irregular in distribution. These depressions have been observed in psoriasis, peripheral vascular disease, diabetes, and infectious diseases such as syphilis and tuberculosis (Fig. 8-7).

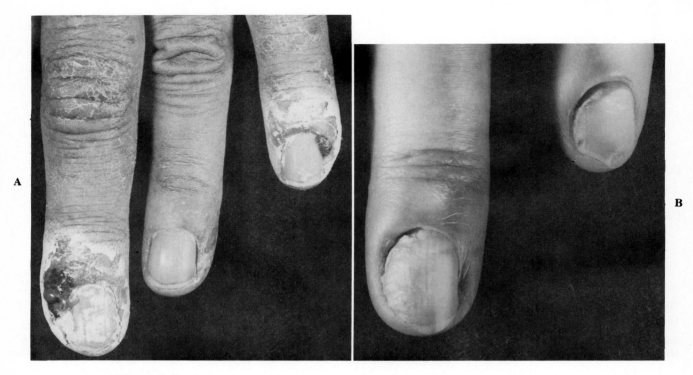

Figure 8-5

A, Acute paronychia. **B,** Chronic paronychia—early stage. Note loss of cuticle and bolstering of posterior nail fold.

(From Samman PD: The nails in disease, London, 1978, William Heinemann Medical Books, Ltd.)

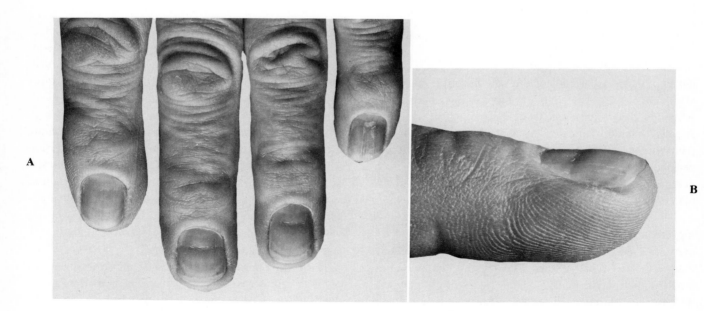

Figure 8-6

A, Beau's lines. **B,** Beau's lines, side view.

(From Samman PD: The nails in disease, London, 1978, William Heinemann Medical Books, Ltd.)

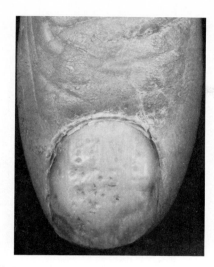

Figure 8-7

Psoriasis—nail pitting.
(From Samman PD: The nails in disease, London, 1978, William
Heinemann Medical Books, Ltd.)

Mees' lines are crescent-shaped transverse lines similar in color to the lunula. They have been observed in arsenic poisoning.

Striated nails are characterized by longitudinal ridges running the length of the nail and are associated with increased fragility. Nail striations have been observed in malnutrition, anemia, defective peripheral circulation, chronic infections, and psoriasis. Nail striations are frequently observed in the elderly.

Changes in nail color

Leukonychia is characterized by white striations or 1- to 2-mm dots that progress to the free edge of the nail as growth proceeds. The white areas may result from trauma, infections, vascular disease, psoriasis, and arsenic poisoning.

Leukonychia totalis (white nails) is a condition in which the entire nail plate is white. Although the white nail may be congenital, this type of nail has been associated with hypocalcemia, severe hypochromic anemia, leprosy, hepatic cirrhosis, and arsenic poisoning. Paired narrow white bands parallel to the lunula have been associated with hypoalbuminemia. These white lines affect the nail bed rather than the nail plate.

Melanonychia is the presence of brown color in the nail plate resulting from a melanin redistribution in the melanophore cells. Normal nails in white persons are not pigmented, but the nails are pigmented in black persons from adolescence. An increase in pigment of the nails may be seen in Addison's disease and malaria.

Pigment band is a single black or brown streak in

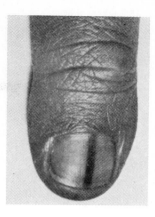

Figure 8-8

Pigment band probably caused by a junctional nevus.
(From Samman PD: The nails in disease, London, 1978, William Heinemann Medical Books, Ltd.)

the nail of a white person. The development of such a line may be caused by junctional nevus in the nail matrix. Brown striations are common in black persons (Fig. 8-8).

Bluish nails are observed in cyanosis and venous stasis. Sulfhydric acid poisoning results in the formation of sulfhemoglobin, which creates a blue tinge as it circulates in the capillary bed beneath the nail. Wilson's disease has been associated with a bluish tint of the lunula. *Pseudomonas aeruginosa* infection is associated with a bluish gray color of the entire nail.

Changes in nail thickness

Thickening or hypertrophy of the nail is generally caused by trauma. The nail of the small toe is often the only one affected; it takes on a clawlike shape. Thickening of the nails has been associated with psoriasis, fungal infection, defective vascular supply, and trauma. Thinning of the nail has been linked to defective peripheral circulation and nutritional anemias.

Brittleness of the nails is a common sign. Systemic diseases associated with brittle nails are nutritional anemias and impaired peripheral circulation. Prolonged exposure to water and alkaline substances has also been associated with brittle nails.

Clubbing of fingers

Clubbing of fingers (drumstick fingers) is associated with a decrease of oxygen supply in general. The resultant changes in the nail have been called *hippocratic* or *watch-glass* nails. The watch-glass nail is longer in the longitudinal axis than in the transverse axis, and the dorsal convexity is increased (Fig. 8-9). The nail is thickened, hard, shiny, and curved at the free end. The matrix atro-

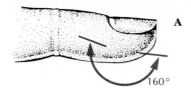

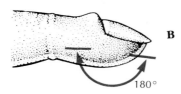

Figure 8-9

A, Normal angle of the nail. **B,** Abnormal angle of the nail seen in late clubbing.

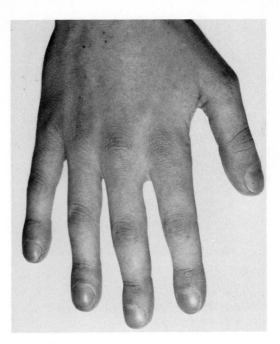

Figure 8-10

Finger clubbing.
(From Samman PD: The nails in disease, London, 1978, William Heinemann Medical Books, Ltd.)

phies. Early in the process the normal angle of the nail to the nail base (160 degrees) is lost. The nails are flatter and may be at a 180-degree angle to the nail base. In advanced cases the entire nail is pushed away from the base at an angle greater than 180 degrees and feels "spongy." (The student may simulate this spongy feel by grasping the distal phalanx on the lateral aspects of a finger at the level of the nail bed of one hand firmly between thumb and middle finger of the opposite hand. After a second or two the lunula will feel spongy when pressed down by the nail of the index finger of the examining hand.) The distal phalanx becomes enlarged as the condition progresses. Clubbing is associated with respiratory (emphysema, chronic obstructive lung disease, carcinoma of the lung) and cardiovascular diseases and cirrhosis. Clubbing occurs in all the digits but is most readily seen in the fingers (Fig. 8-10).

Sebaceous Glands

The sebaceous glands, which are more numerous over the face and scalp areas, normally become more active during adolescence, resulting in increased oiliness of the skin. A sudden increase in the oil of the skin at other ages would not be normal and may suggest an endocrine problem.

SKIN LESIONS: DESCRIPTION AND CLASSIFICATION

The initial examination of any skin lesion should be carried out at a distance of 3 ft or more to determine the general characteristics of the eruption. This first observation should provide the opportunity to determine the location, distribution, and configuration of the lesions. A closer examination is required next to determine the color, size, shape, texture, firmness, and morphologic characteristics of the individual lesions (see boxed material on p. 192).

It is not possible to discuss the particular manifestations of the many skin problems that the examiner may find in practice. This discussion is limited to a few examples that demonstrate some of the different characteristics of skin lesions that will assist the examiner in describing the problem when consulting a dermatologist or a textbook on dermatology.

The distribution of skin lesions is fairly simple to describe according to the location or body region affected and the symmetry or asymmetry of findings in comparable body parts. The examiner must keep in mind the characteristic patterns that provide the major clue in the diagnosis of a specific skin problem. Fig. 8-11 illustrates a few distribution patterns by specific problems.

The configuration of skin lesions is equally important in defining the problem. Configuration refers to the arrangement or position of several lesions in relation to each other. For example, the skin lesions of tinea corporis, ringworm of the body, have an annular configuration that is circular. Some of the terms used to describe the configuration of skin lesions are as follows:

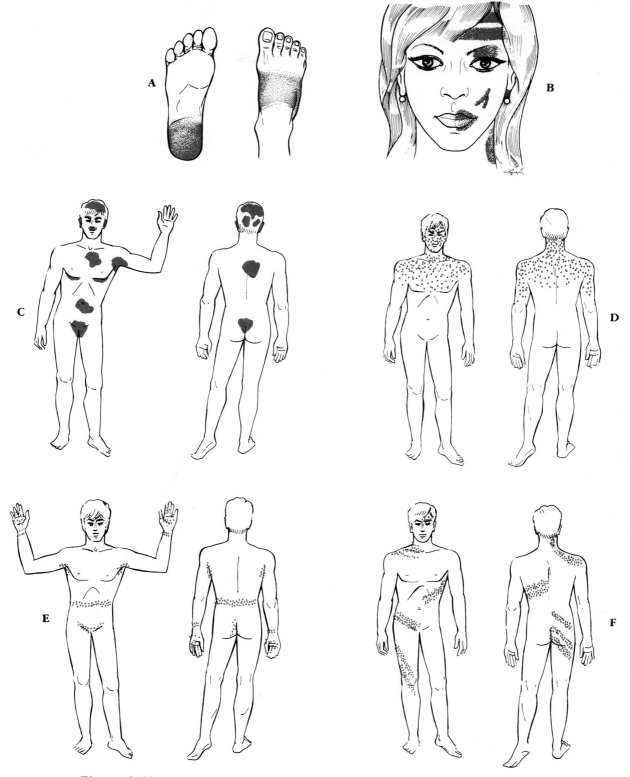

Figure 8-11

Distribution of lesions in selected problems of the skin. **A,** Contact dermatitis (shoes). **B,** Contact dermatitis (cosmetics, perfumes, earrings). **C,** Seborrheic dermatitis. **D,** Acne. **E,** Scabies. **F,** Herpes zoster.

<table>
<tr><td>Grouped</td><td>Lesions clustered together</td></tr>
<tr><td>Herpetiform or zosteriform</td><td>Multiple groups of vesicles erupting unilaterally following the course of cutaneous nerves</td></tr>
<tr><td>Linear</td><td>Lesions arranged in a line</td></tr>
<tr><td>Annular</td><td>Lesions arranged in a circle, ring-shaped</td></tr>
<tr><td>Polycyclic</td><td>Multiple annular arrangements of lesions</td></tr>
<tr><td>Arciform</td><td>Lesions arranged in an arc, bow-shaped</td></tr>
<tr><td>Reticular</td><td>Lesions meshed in the form of a network</td></tr>
<tr><td>Confluent</td><td>Lesions become merged together, not discrete</td></tr>
</table>

Tips for Assessing Skin Lesions

If a lesion is present, consider
- Are there any associated symptoms, for example, pruritus?
- What is the chronology of the appearance of these lesions? Are they changing in morphology? Are they disappearing?
- Are there associated variables or precipitants, such as
  Environmental exposure
  Injuries
  Infection
  Use of medications (prescribed or self-treatment)
  Diet
  Clothing
  Emotions
  Personal care items such as soap and cosmetics

Fig. 8-12 illustrates some of the different configurations that occur.

The color of the individual lesion should be described. There may be no discoloration, or many colors may be seen, as with ecchymosis when the initial dark-red and dark-blue colors are fading and a yellow color

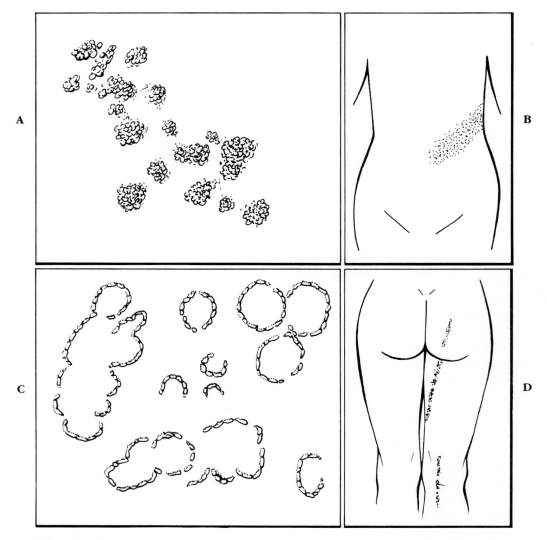

Figure 8-12

Examples of different configurations of skin lesions. **A,** Grouped. **B,** Zosteriform. **C,** Annular (circular) and arciform (arc). **D,** Linear.

is seen. The lesions may be well defined with the color changes limited to the borders of the lesion and are referred to as "circumscribed," or the borders may be undefined with the color changes spread over a large area and described as "diffuse." Diascopy is used to observe for color changes of a lesion when pressure is applied. A transparent slide is pressed against the skin to express blood from the capillaries and superficial venules. Telangiectases will blanch, whereas petechial or purpuric lesions will not.

The lesions are gently palpated to determine the texture and firmness of the individual lesion and in some instances to determine the actual shape of the lesion.

Finally, there is a morphologic classification of skin lesions that classifies lesions in terms of structure. It is important to identify the morphological structure of the individual lesion to identify the specific problem (Table 8-3). Lesions are classified as primary or second-

ary. *Primary lesions* are those that appear initially in response to some change in the external or internal environment of the skin. *Secondary lesions* do not appear initially but result from modifications such as trauma, chronicity, or infection in the primary lesion. For instance, the primary lesion may be a vesicle, which is a small, circumscribed, elevated lesion containing clear fluid. The vesicle will rupture, leaving a small moist area, which is classified as a secondary lesion called an *erosion*. Figs. 8-13 and 8-14 illustrate some of the primary and secondary lesions. Tables 8-4 to 8-6 (pp. 196-201) identify various skin lesions.

The following are examples of the recording of selected abnormal skin findings.
1. *Measles (rubeola):* Skin is hot and dry with an erythematous, confluent, maculopapular rash covering the neck, trunk, arms, and abdomen but fading from the face. Discrete erythematous maculopapular le-

---

Table 8-3

Identification of skin lesions

	Name of lesion	Description	<1 cm	>1 cm
Type of lesion:				
Primary	Macule—patch	Flat, circumscribed discoloration	Macule (Fig. 8-13, *A*)	Patch (Fig. 8-13, *A*)
	Papule—plaque	Solid, elevated lesion	Papule (Fig. 8-13, *B*)	Plaque (Fig. 8-13, *B*)
	Nodule—tumor	Solid, elevated lesion also has depth	Nodule (Fig. 8-13, *C*)	Tumor (Fig. 8-13, *D*)
	Vesicle—bulla	Fluid filled, superficial, elevated	Vesicle (Fig. 8-13, *D*)	Bulla (Fig. 8-13, *E*)
Primary of	Pustule (Fig. 8-13, *F*)	Vesicle or bulla containing pus		
varying	Wheal (Fig. 8-13, *G*)	Lesion caused by cutaneous edema irregular in shape, elevated, transient		
size	Telangiectasia	Dilated capillary, fine red line(s)		
Secondary	Scale (Fig. 8-14, *A*)	Accumulation of loose surface epithelium		
	Crust (Fig. 8-14, *B*)	Dried surface fluids: serum or pus		
	Excoriation	Scratch mark		
	Erosion (Fig. 8-14, *C*)	Superficial denuded lesion		
	Scar (Fig. 8-14, *D*)	First red, then pale smooth hyaline wound repair; may be flat, depressed, elevated, or hypertrophic (keloid)		
	Ulcer	Loss of tissue from a surface caused by destruction of a superficial lesion		
	Atrophy	Thinning of skin, loss of hair and sweat glands		
	Fissure (Fig. 8-14, *E*)	Linear crack in skin that extends to dermis		
	Lichenification	Thickening of skin caused by chronic scratching		

Number of lesions: ☐ Single ☐ Numerous ☐ Actual count
Size of lesion: (Measure)
Shape of lesion: ☐ Round ☐ Oval ☐ Umbilicated ☐ Irregular
Color of lesion: ☐ Red ☐ Brown ☐ Black ☐ Gray-blue ☐ White ☐ Purple ☐ Orange ☐ Yellow
  ☐ Circumscribed? ☐ Diffuse? ☐ Change with diascopy*?
Configuration: ☐ Single ☐ Grouped: ☐ Herpetiform ☐ Linear ☐ Annular ☐ Arciform ☐ Reticular ☐ Scattered
Distribution: ☐ Localized ☐ Generalized ☐ Symmetrical
  Site of predilection _____

---

*Diascopy consists of the application of firm pressure against a microscope slide or clear plastic placed over a skin lesion, allowing identification of capillary dilatation and thus differentiating telangiectasia from purpura. The technique also makes lymphoma, sarcoidosis, and tuberculosis of the skin appear yellow-brown.

Figure 8-13

Descriptions and characteristics of primary skin lesions.
(From Thompson JM and others: Clinical nursing, ed 1, St Louis, 1987,
The CV Mosby Co.)

Macule—flat; nonpal-
pable; circumscribed;
less than 1 cm in di-
ameter; brown, red,
purple, white, or tan
in color
Examples: Freckles;
flat moles; rubella;
rubeola; drug erup-
tions

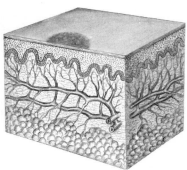

Patch—flat; nonpal-
pable; irregular in
shape; macule greater
than 1 cm in diame-
ter
Examples: Vitiligo;
port-wine marks

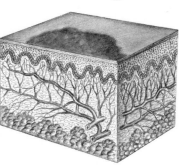

Papule—elevated; pal-
pable; firm; circum-
scribed; less than 1
cm in diameter;
brown, red, pink,
tan, or bluish red in
color
Examples: Warts;
drug-related erup-
tions; pigmented
nevi; eczema

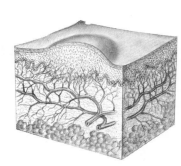

Plaque—elevated; flat
topped; firm; rough;
superficial papule
greater than 1 cm in
diameter; may be co-
alesced papules
Examples: Psoriasis;
seborrheic and ac-
tinic keratoses; ec-
zema

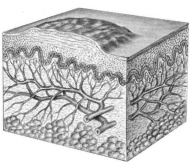

Wheal—elevated, ir-
regular-shaped area
of cutaneous edema;
solid, transient,
changing; variable di-
ameter; pale pink in
color
Examples: Urticaria;
insect bites

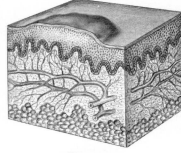

Nodule—elevated; firm;
circumscribed; palpa-
ble; deeper in dermis
than papule; 1 to 2
cm in diameter
Examples: Erythema
nodosum; lipomas

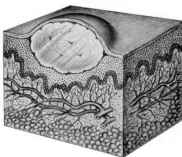

Tumor—elevated; solid;
may or may not be
clearly demarcated;
greater than 2 cm in
diameter; may or
may not vary from
skin color
Example: Neoplasms

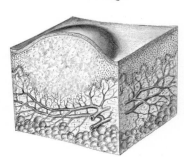

Vesicle—elevated; cir-
cumscribed; superfi-
cial; filled with se-
rous fluid; less than
1 cm in diameter
Examples: Blister;
varicella

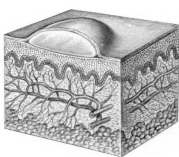

Bulla—vesicle greater
than 1 cm in di-
ameter
Examples: Blister;
pemphigus vulgaris

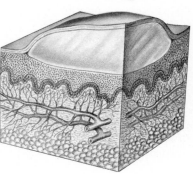

Pustule—elevated; superficial; similar to vesicle but filled with purulent fluid
Examples: Impetigo; acne; variola; herpes zoster

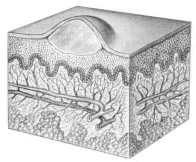

Cyst—elevated; circumscribed; palpable; encapsulated; filled with liquid or semi-solid material
Example: Sebaceous cyst

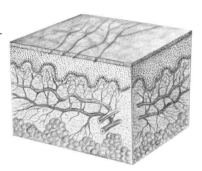

Telangiectasia—fine, irregular red line produced by dilation of capillary
Example: Telangiectasia in rosacea

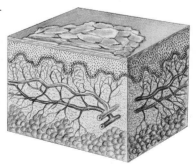

Figure 8-13, cont'd

Crust—dried serum, blood, or purulent exudate; slightly elevated; size varies; brown, red, black, tan, or straw in color
Examples: Scab on abrasion; eczema; impetigo

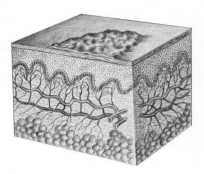

Lichenification—rough, thickened epidermis; accentuated skin markings due to rubbing or irritation; often involves flexor aspect of extremity
Example: Chronic dermatitis

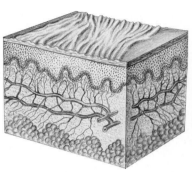

Scar—thin to thick fibrous tissue replacing injured dermis; irregular; pink, red, or white in color; may be atrophic or hypertrophic
Examples: Healed wound or surgical incision

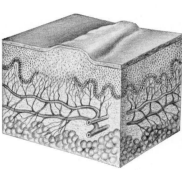

Keloid—irregularly shaped, elevated, progressively enlarging scar; grows beyond boundaries of wound; due to excessive collagen formation during healing
Examples: Keloid from ear piercing or burn scar

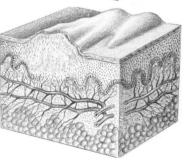

Figure 8-14

Description and characteristics of secondary skin lesions.
(From Thompson JM and others: Clinical nursing, ed 1, St Louis, 1987, The CV Mosby Co.)

Scale—heaped-up keratinized cells; flaky exfoliation; irregular; thick or thin; dry or oily; varied size; silver, white, or tan in color
Examples: Psoriasis; exfoliative dermatitis

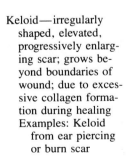

Excoriation—loss of epidermis; linear or hollowed-out crusted area; dermis exposed
Examples: Abrasion; scratch

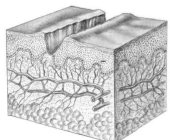

Continued

Fissure—linear crack
or break from epidermis to dermis; small;
deep; red
Examples: Athlete's
foot; cheilosis

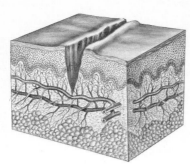

Erosion—loss of all or
part of epidermis; depressed; moist; glistening; follows rupture of vesicle or
bulla; larger than
fissure
Examples: Varicella;
variola following
rupture

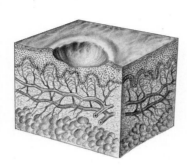

Ulcer—loss of epidermis and dermis; concave; varies in size;
exudative; red or reddish blue
Examples: Decubiti;
stasis ulcers

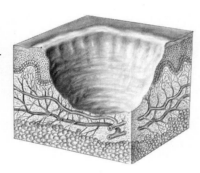

Atrophy—thinning of
skin surface and loss
of skin markings;
skin translucent and
paperlike
Examples: Striae;
aged skin

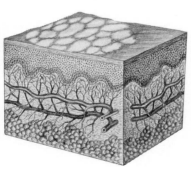

Figure 8-14, cont'd

Table 8-4

Stages of dermatitis

Stage	Lesions
Acute	Erythema, edema, vesicles, exudate, crusting
Subacute	Erythema, residual crusting, scaling
Chronic	Scaling, hyperpigmentation, lichenification, fissuring

sions are densely scattered over the lower extremities.
2. *Impetigo:* Skin is dark brown, warm, moist, elastic, and smooth, except for four irregularly grouped, moist, honey-colored crusted pustular lesions, 1 to 2 cm in diameter, inferior to the right lower lip.
3. *Vitiligo:* Skin is light brown, warm, moist, elastic, and smooth, with several nontender, macular, depigmented, roughly oval-shaped areas varying in size from 1 by 2 cm to 3 by 4 cm and scattered over dorsal surfaces of both hands.
4. *Ecchymosis:* Skin is light pink, warm, elastic, and smooth with a tender, 8- by 10-cm, irregularly shaped, dark purple to green-yellow macular area over extensor surface of the left shoulder.

Table 8-5

Common lesions of the skin

Condition	Lesion	Location
Actinic keratosis	Macule; scaling; red	Areas exposed to sunlight; scalp; ears
Atopic dermatitis	Dry, scaling inflammation; pruritus; excoriated lichenification; abnormally sensitive to environmental irritants	Forehead; cheeks; flexure regions; may be generalized
Contact dermatitis	Erythema; pruritus resulting from environmental irritant	Area of contact
Discoid lupus erythematosus	Discrete with hyperkeratotic plugs; scaling; central atrophy; scarring, red	Paranasal area; eyebrows; upper midback
Eczema		
Allergic	Erythema to exudate	Scalp; nose; forehead; eyelids; neck (from shampoo or hair dye); feet (from shoes); ears (from hearing aids or glasses); hands (from rubber gloves)
Chronic hereditary	Laminated silvery scales, tiny bleeding spots if scale pulled off	Points of trauma; genitalia
Nummular	Round lesions; moist surface; crusting; excoriation	Extensor surfaces of arms and legs
Intertrigo	Moist patches or erosions; borders well demarcated; red; associated with friction; macerated	Skin folds (warm and moist); breasts; axilla; inguinal regions, between toes, marked in obesity
Pityriasis rosea (unknown cause)	Macules; scaling, oval shape; long axis follows lines of cleavage; red	Herald patch; then generalized
Psoriasis	Early lesion discrete; deep red patches; scaling; later discrete or confluent patches; plaques; gray-white thick scale; scale may appear shiny (disorder of keratin synthesis, hereditary)	May arise in one skin area or may appear as generalized skin involvement
Rosacea	Papules; pustules; oiliness; erythema; telangiectasia may be present	Face
Seborrhea	Noninflammatory dryness and scaling "dandruff" or oiliness	Scalp; face
Seborrheic dermatitis	Inflammation; dryness; scaling (loose, flaky); oiliness; pruritus; may be crushed; eczematous	Scalp; ears; face (nasolabial fold, temples, eyelids); shoulders; navel; perianal region
Seborrheic keratosis	Early lesion—tan macule; progresses to papules, plaques; surface brown, rough	Any area; common on trunk
Scleroderma	Indurated; atrophic; shiny; skin appears tight, fastened down; hyperpigmentation or depigmentation	Generalized; tight facies; claw fingers
Systemic lupus erythematosus	Purpuric lesions; erythema; telangiectasia	Malar prominence over joints
Vascular		
Nevus flammeus (port wine stain)	Plaque; plexus of capillaries may have rough surface; red or purple	Present at birth; 50% on nuchal area
Nevus vasculosus	Capillary hemangioma; single tumor; rough surface; bright or dark red	75% in head region; appear in first or second month; most disappear by age 7
Spider nevus (arteriolar spider or spider angioma)	Small branching; arteriole, red; blanches on pressure	Any area; most common on face, neck, arms, and upper trunk
Telangiectasia	Capillary dilatation; red; blanches on pressure	Lips, tongue, nose, palms, and fingers

Continued

Table 8-5

Common lesions of the skin—*cont'd*

Condition	Lesion	Location
Extravasation of blood		
Senile purpura	Ecchymoses; large areas blue-black, then green-yellow, then yellow; lesions do not blanch	Usually occurs on the dorsum of the hand or forearm
Neoplasia		
Paget's disease	Crusted dermatitis; moist verrucous surface; pruritus	Nipple and areola (manifestation of deeper intraductal malignancy)
Kaposi's sarcoma (associated with AIDS*)	Reddish brown plaques and nodules often associated with lymphedema	Most commonly seen on lower extremities
Scar		
Striae	Linear; depressed; red-blue first, then silvery white	Abdomen, buttocks, or breasts; less often on thighs, upper arms, and back
Bacterial infection		
Erysipelas	Acute; edematous; red; tender	Face; limbs; abdomen
Impetigo	Yellow crusts; erythematous base; rapid spreading	Facial area; may be localized or may spread
Leprosy	Macules—tan to pink; nodules—yellowish; may ulcerate; incubation about 3 years	
Scarlet fever	Confluent, diffuse, blanching dermatitis; erythematous 1-7 days after—sore throat, fever	Generalized
Syphilis (secondary)	Macules; papules; lymphadenopathy; malaise, myalgia; low-grade fever	Mucous membranes; palms; soles
Syphilitic chancre	Small, round, red macule; erodes to indurated ulcer (1-2 cm); regional lymphadenopathy	Breast; vulva; penis
Trichomonas infection		
Trichomoniasis	Granular vaginal mucosa; bright red; petechiae may be present; discharge "foamy"	Vaginal; labia
***Candida* infection**		
Candida	Patch borders well demarcated; flaccid pustules; patches creamy white; erythematous base; curdlike white discharge, pruritus patches; erythema	Inguinal region; vagina; glans penis
Viral infection		
Rubella, rubeola, roseola	Macules; discrete; erythematous; fever; lymphadenopathy (rubella); Koplik's spots (rubeola); 2- to 3-week incubation (rubella); then malaise, fever	Appear on trunk first; spread peripherally
Varicella (chickenpox)	Papule; vesicle; erythematous base; first clear fluid, then turbid; crusting on fourth day; 2-week incubation; 24-hour fever; malaise	First on chest and back; then face, arms, and legs
Variola (smallpox)	Macules; erythematous; progress to umbilicated lesions; then pustules, firm, round; then crusting; 2- to 3-week incubation; 5-day prodromal; toxic myalgia; fever	More lesions on face, extremities

*AIDS, acquired immunodeficiency syndrome
†HIV, human immunodeficiency virus. HIV has been implicated as the cause of AIDS.

Table 8-5

Common lesions of the skin—*cont'd*

Condition	Lesion	Location
HIV† infection		
	Variety of dermatoses (macules, papules, nodules, plaques): bacterial, fungal, parasitic, viral; worsening of psoriasis, seborrheic dermatitis; herpes simplex, herpes zoster, oral candidiasis	Anywhere on body, including all mucosal surfaces
Fungal infection		
Tinea corporis (ringworm)	Scaling; red with pale center; vesicular border; pruritic	Face; neck; extremities
Tinea cruris	Scaling; crescentic; red-brown	Axilla; inguinal region
Tinea pedis (fungal infection of foot)	Scaling; circular; vesicular border; red; chronic-hyperkeratotic	Feet
Infestations		
Pediculosis capitis	Pruritus; white concretions on hair—nits	Hair of scalp
Variation in pigmentation		
Hyperpigmentation		
Café au lait spots	Patches; light tan (six or more larger than 1.5 cm indicative of neurofibromatosis)	Anywhere on the skin
Freckle (ephelis)	Discrete; macule; tan to brown	Pigmenting increased in areas exposed to sun
Lentigo		
Juvenile	Discrete macule; brown	Not affected by sun exposure
Senile	Single-macule; scaling; yellowish brown; may be dark brown	Exposed surfaces, forehead, cheeks, extensor surfaces of limbs
Malignant	Mottled; irregular macule; enlarging; tan-brown, black-white; may ulcerate—then red	Face, also eyelids, conjunctiva, lips, penis, axilla
Mongolian spots	Patch; irregular; dark blue or purple (chromophobe like cell in skin)	Sacrum; present at birth; more common with darker pigmented individuals; disappear spontaneously by age 4
Nevus	Macule; pigmented or nonpigmented; may be present at birth or arise later	
Peutz-Jeghers syndrome	Brown spots; abdominal pain	Lips; fingers, toes
Depigmentation		
Vitiligo		
Addison's disease	Circumscribed patch(es) of depigmentation	Face, neck, axillae, groins, anogenital area, eyelids, hands, and wrist
Pernicious anemia		
Thyrotoxicosis		

Table 8-6

Common raised lesions

Condition	Lesion	Location
Acne vulgaris	Comedones; papules; pustules; cysts; scars	Face; back; shoulders; upper arms
Dermatitis herpetiformis (chronic)	Macules; papules; vesicles; excoriated vesicles; pruritus (intense); residual hyperpigmentation; hereditary	Scalp; interscapular; sacral
Leukoplakia	Plaque; thick; indurated; white	Mucous membrane; mouth; labia; vagina
Lichen planus (unknown cause)	Maculopapular lesion; deep red to purple; pruritus; hyperkeratotic	Flexor surfaces of wrists; palms; soles; ankles; abdomen; sacrum
Lichen simplex (chronic)	Plaque; dry; lichenification; hyperpigmentation	Scalp; labia
Seborrheic keratosis	Single plaque; soft lesion with rough surface; brown	Back, chest, scalp, face, backs of hands, and external surfaces of forearms
Lipid disorder		
Xanthelasma	Papules or plaques; yellow; lipid deposits	Eyelids
Cysts		
Epidermoid and sebaceous cysts	Fluctuant, globular lesions	Scalp, face, back, or scrotum
Milia	Pinhead (1-2 mm) white, sebaceous cyst	Infraorbital skin; nose; chin; common in newborn
Neoplasia		
Acrochordon (skin tag)	Pedunculated skin tag; skin color	Neck; axilla; groin
Basal cell carcinoma	Nodolar—rolled edge; tendency to ulcerate in center	Face, scalp, ears, or neck
Basal cell epithelioma	May follow actinic keratosis; papule or nodule—rolled edge; ulcer—nonhealing	Face, scalp, upper back
Squamous cell carcinoma	Nodule; indurated; ulcer—nonhealing; history of overexposure to sun, x-ray films; often opaque	Often on head (75%); hands (15%)
Dermatofibroma	Tumor; discrete; dome-shaped; brown; less than 1 cm	Usually legs
Lipoma	Fatty tumor; soft	Trunk, nuchal area, arms, and thighs
Malignant melanoma	Arises from pigmented nevus; indurated: may be flat or elevated, eroded or ulcerated	Any area of skin or mucous membrane
Neurofibroma	Pedunculated; soft; flaccid lesion; skin color black, brown, rose, white	Anywhere on the skin, including the palms and soles
Pigmented nevus	Single or multiple dome-shaped lesions; may be hairy; brown to black; present at birth	Anywhere on the skin
Vascular		
Angioma (sometimes called senile angioma)	Papule; vascular; cherry red; pinhead (1-3 mm); most adults after climacteric	Usually on trunk
Hyperkeratosis		
Clavus (corn)	Hyperkeratosis; hard; tender; shape—inverted cone	Dorsum of toes; most common on fifth toe
Cutaneous horn	Horn projection of hyperkeratotic lesion	Face, arms, scalp, and dorsum of the hand

Table 8-6

Common raised lesions—*cont'd*

Condition	Lesion	Location
Wheals		
Dermographism	Wheal in response to scratch or pressure; (histamine easily released)	Anywhere on the skin
Erythema multiforme (varied causes)	Wheal like; round, darker, depressed center (target appearance)	Arms and legs first; then on body
Urticaria	Wheal; pale on erythematous base; pruritus; transient	Usually trunk but may appear anywhere on body
Bullae		
Pemphigus	Bullae; flaccid, moist, fluid-filled rupture easily bleeds; erythematous base; from lack of mucopolysaccharide protein for intercellular cement	Skin—all parts mucous membrane
From bacterial infection		
Chancroid	Vesicopustule; ulcer; ragged, undermined edges; shallow; may be multiple; red; lymphadenopathy	Genitalia—male and female
Folliculitis	Discrete perifollicular papules and pustules; erythematous	Any hairy area
Furuncle	Swelling becomes pustular; red; tender; painful	Any hairy site but most common on neck, buttocks, wrists, and ankles
From viral infection		
Herpes simplex	Vesicles; grouped; may be recurrent	Lips; anywhere on face
Herpes zoster	Tenderness; burning; pruritus; vesicles later crusting; erythematous base; hypersensitivity; localized lymphadenopathy	Pathway of a peripheral nerve, may have postherpetic neuralgia
Molluscum contagiosum	Multiple, discrete globules; waxy depression in center	Trunk
Verruca acuminata	Papillary (cauliflower like); red; soft	Penis; vulva; perianal area
Verruca plantaris (plantar wart)	Circumscribed callus; surrounded by hyperkeratosis; black dots; tender	Plantar surface of foot or toes
Verruca vulgaris (wart)	Single or multiple; tan	Hands
From infestation		
Pediculosis corporis (body lice)	Wheal; central hemorrhagic spot; linear excoriations; later dry, scaly pigmentation	Trunk; can be generalized
Pediculosis pubis (pubic lice)	Papules; discrete; excoriated; gray-white dots at base of hair—nits; lice may be seen at base of hairs	Genital region; lower abdomen; chest; axillae; eyebrows; eyelashes
	Gray-blue macules	May be present on abdomen; thighs; axillae
Scabies	Vesicles; papules; pruritus	Skin folds

Health History
Skin, Nails, and Hair

NOTE: A yes response to any question *must* be further investigated. Use the following indicators throughout the assessment: (1) onset (specific date, sudden or gradual), (2) duration, (3) frequency, (4) precipitating factors, (5) aggravating or alleviating factors, (6) treatment received, and (7) outcome.

Present status

1. Have you had recent changes in scalp or body hair?
   a. Description: location, distribution, quality, quantity, color
   b. Cause: chemical irritants, drugs, irradiation, heredity, disease, fever, medication
3. Do you have prolonged exposure to the sun?
   a. Cause: job-related, sunbathing
4. Do you have a mole(s) that recently changed?
   a. Description: size, shape, color, raised, flat, drainage

Past history

1. Have you had skin reactions, lesions, or rashes?
   a. Location: face, trunk, extremities, skin folds, generalized, mucous membranes
   b. Description: red, raised, flat, crusty, vesicles, itching, draining, scaly, thickening, pustules, wheal
   c. Configuration: symmetrical, asymmetrical, clustered, linear, circular, confluent
   d. Cause: clothing, dentures, jewelry, solvents, soaps, cosmetics, animal hair or dander, acids, emotions, injuries, medications, foods
2. Have your nails changed?
   a. Description: shape, color, texture, nailbed adhesion

3. Have you been exposed to infectious diseases that cause skin reactions?
   a. When
   b. Type: herpes zoster, herpes simplex, measles, scarlet fever, typhoid fever, syphilis, rheumatic fever, impetigo

Associated conditions

1. Have you had unusual emotional stress?
2. Do you have a hormonal imbalance?
3. Do you have heart disease or circulatory impairment?
4. Have you had bacterial or fungal skin conditions?
   a. Type
   b. Location
5. Have you ever had skin tumors or skin cancer?
   a. Type
   b. Location

Family history

1. Do males in your family have male-pattern baldness?
2. Do family members have psoriasis?
3. Has a family member had a skin malignancy?

Sample assessment record

Client states the mole at back waistline has recently changed color and bled slightly yesterday. States waistbands aggravate mole. Denies any change in scalp/body hair and excessive sun exposure. Mole previously was approximately 5 mm in size, round, flat, and brown colored. Denies skin reactions and other lesions. Denies nail changes and exposure to infectious disease. Denies having other health problems, and there is no family history of cancer.

BIBLIOGRAPHY

Binnick SA: Skin diseases: diagnosis and management in clinical practice, Menlo Park, Calif, 1982, Addison-Wesley Publishing Co.

DeNicola P and Morsiani M: Nail diseases in internal medicine, Springfield, Ill, 1974, Charles C Thomas, Publishers.

Fitzpatrick TG and others: Dermatology in general medicine, ed 4, New York, 1987, McGraw-Hill Book Co.

Lazarus GS and Goldsmith LA: Diagnosis of skin disease, Philadelphia, 1980, FA Davis Co.

Roach LB: Assessment color changes in dark skin, Nursing '77, January 1977, pp. 48-51.

Rook A and Wilkerson DS: Textbook of dermatology, ed 3, Oxford, Mass, 1979, Blackwell Scientific Publications.

Samman PD: The nails in disease, London, 1978, William Heinemann Medical Books.

Sauer GC: Manual of skin diseases, ed 6, Philadelphia, 1988, JB Lippincott Co.

Stewart WD, Danto JL, and Maddin S: Dermatology: diagnosis and treatment of cutaneous disorders, ed 6, St. Louis, 1986, The CV Mosby Co.

chapter

9

Assessment of ears, nose, and throat

OBJECTIVES

Upon successful review of this chapter, learners will be able to:

- Describe anatomy and physiology of the ears, nose, mouth, and throat

- Distinguish between conductive and sensorineural hearing loss

- State related rationale and demonstrate
    External and internal ear assessment
    Auditory function assessment
    External and internal nasal assessment
    Mouth, jaw, and oropharynx assessment

- Recognize abnormalities and common problems of the ears, nose, mouth, and throat

The examination of the ears, nose, and throat is an important part of every physical examination because it provides the opportunity to inspect directly or indirectly most parts of the upper respiratory system and the first division of the digestive system. The clinical examination of these body orifices can provide information about the client's general health as well as information about significant local disease. The methods of examination are primarily inspection and palpation.

The client should be seated for the ear, nose, and throat examination with the examiner's head at approximately the same level as that of the client. The necessary equipment includes an otoscope with various sizes of speculums, tongue blades, 4- by 4-in gauze sponges, disposable latex gloves (see Safety First box on p. 206), and a tuning fork (512 cycles per second [cps]). A good light source such as a gooseneck lamp with a 100- to 150-watt bulb is helpful, but if not available, a penlight can be used. A dental mirror and a nasal speculum may also be helpful.

Discussion is focused on each of the three areas: the ears, the nose and paranasal sinuses, and the mouth and oropharynx. The portion of the chapter on each area includes a brief review of the anatomy and physiology, a description of the methods to be used in the examination, and some of the common findings of which the examiner should be aware when examining the particular area.

EARS

Anatomy and Physiology

The ear is a sensory organ that functions both in hearing and in equilibrium. It has three parts: the external ear, the middle ear, and the inner ear. Fig. 9-1 illustrates the structures of the ear.

Figure 9-1

External auditory canal, middle ear, and inner ear.

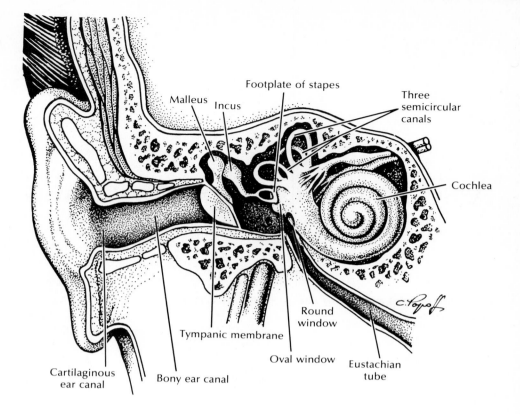

The external ear has two divisions, the flap called the auricle, or *pinna,* and the canal called the external auditory canal, or *meatus.* Stretching across the proximal portion of the canal is the tympanic membrane, which separates the external ear from the middle ear. The auricle is composed of cartilage, closely adherent perichondrium, and skin. The main components of the auricle are the helix, anthelix, crus of helix, lobule, tragus, antitragus, and concha (Fig. 9-2). The *mastoid process* is not part of the external ear but is a bony prominence found posterior to the lower part of the auricle.

The external auditory canal, which is about 1 in long, has a skeleton of cartilage in its outer third and a skeleton of bone in its inner two thirds. It has a slight curve with the outer one third of the canal directed upward and toward the back of the head, whereas the inner two thirds is directed down and forward. The skin of the inner ear is very thin and sensitive.

The tympanic membrane, which covers the proximal end of the auditory canal, is made up of layers of skin, fibrous tissue, and mucous membrane (Fig. 9-3). The membrane is shiny, translucent, and pearl gray. The position of the eardrum is oblique with respect to the ear canal. The anteroinferior quadrant is most distant from the examiner, which accounts for the cone of light or the light reflex. The membrane is slightly concave and is pulled inward at its center by one of the ossicles, the

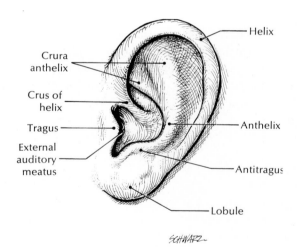

Figure 9-2

Structures of the external ear.

malleus, of the middle ear. The short process of the malleus protrudes into the eardrum superiorly, and the handle of the malleus extends downward from the short process to the umbo, the point of maximum concavity. Most of the membrane is taut and is known as the pars tensa. A small part superiorly is less taut and is known as the pars flaccida. The dense fibrous ring surrounding the tympanic membrane, except for the anterior and posterior malleolar folds superiorly, is the anulus.

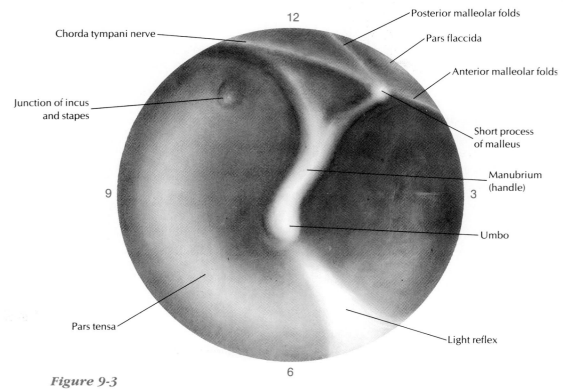

12

Chorda tympani nerve

Posterior malleolar folds

Pars flaccida

Anterior malleolar folds

Junction of incus
and stapes

Short process
of malleus

Manubrium
(handle)

9   3

Umbo

Pars tensa

Light reflex

6

Figure 9-3

Usual landmarks of right tympanic membrane with "clock" superimposed.
(From Whaley LF and Wong DL: Nursing care of infants and children, ed 2, St Louis, 1987, The
CV Mosby Co.)

The middle ear is a small, air-filled cavity located in the temporal bone. It contains three small bones called the *auditory ossicles:* the *malleus,* the *incus,* and the *stapes.* The middle ear cavity contains several openings. One is from the external auditory meatus and is covered by the tympanic membrane. There are two openings into the inner ear, the oval window into which the stapes fits and the round window covered by a membrane. Another opening connects the middle ear with the eustachian tube. The middle ear performs three functions: (1) it transmits sound vibrations across the ossicle chain to the inner ear's oval window, (2) it protects the auditory apparatus from intense vibrations, and (3) it equalizes the air pressure on both sides of the dividing tympanic membrane to prevent the tympanic membrane from being ruptured.

The inner ear is made up of two parts, the bony labyrinth and, inside this structure, a membranous labyrinth. The bony *labyrinth* consists of three parts: the vestibule, the semicircular canals, and the cochlea. The vestibule and the semicircular canals comprise the organs of equilibrium. The cochlea comprises the organ of hearing. The cochlea is a coiled structure that contains the organ of Corti, which transmits stimuli to the cochlear branch of the auditory nerve (cranial nerve [CN] VIII).

Hearing occurs when sound waves enter the external auditory canal and strike the tympanic membrane, causing it to vibrate at the same rate as the sound waves striking it. The auricle does not direct or amplify sound and has little apparent usefulness. The vibrations are transmitted through the auditory ossicles of the middle ear to the oval window. From the oval window the vibrations travel through the fluid of the cochlea, winding up at the round window, where they are dissipated. The vibrations of the membrane cause the delicate hair cells of the organ of Corti to beat against the membrane of Corti, acting as a stimuli setting up impulses in the sensory endings of the cochlear branch of the auditory nerve (CN VIII).

Hearing Loss

There are several types of hearing loss. However, almost every form may be classified under one of three headings: conductive hearing loss, sensorineural or perceptive hearing loss, or mixed hearing loss.

Conductive hearing loss occurs when there are external or middle ear disorders such as impacted cerumen, perforation of the tympanic membrane, serum or pus in the middle ear, or a fusion of the ossicles. The vibrations are not adequately transmitted to the inner ear through the ear canal, tympanic membrane, middle ear, and ossicular chain; a partial loss of hearing occurs.

Sensorineural, or perceptive, hearing loss occurs when there is a disorder in the inner ear, the auditory nerve, or the brain. Vibrations are transmitted to the inner ear, but an impairment of the cochlea or auditory nerve attenuates the nervous impulses from the cochlea to the brain.

Mixed hearing loss is a combination of conductive and sensorineural loss in the same ear.

Examination

The examination of the external ear begins with an inspection of both auricles to determine their position, size, and symmetry. Then the lateral and medial surfaces of each auricle and the surrounding tissues are inspected to determine the skin color and the presence of deformities, lesions, or nodules. The auricles and mastoid areas are palpated for evidence of swelling, tenderness, or nodules.

Manipulation of the auricle can also be helpful. Ordinarily there is no discomfort if the client has an otitis media. If pressure on the tragus or gently pulling on the auricle causes pain, the client may have external otitis. Although fairly simple, this part of the examination is frequently neglected.

Examination of the external auditory canal and tympanic membrane requires additional lighting. The examiner should become acquainted with the use and maintenance of the electric otoscope. For the otoscope to be effective, the batteries should be changed frequently (if using a rechargeable model, recharge frequently) to ensure optimum efficiency. The focus of light should be directed out of the end of the speculum. Some speculum carriers are movable and can be out of alignment with the bulb carrier. Some older models have a bulb carrier that can be bent, causing the light to be deflected to one side of the speculum.

Before inserting the speculum in the client's ear, the practitioner should carefully inspect the opening of the auditory canal for redness, swelling, narrowing of canal, a foreign body, or discharge. Any discharge should be described in terms of appearance and odor. A putrid odor may indicate mastoid disease with bone destruction. After this inspection, the speculum can be inserted. The following points should, however, be remembered:

1. Use the largest speculum that can be inserted in the ear without pain.
2. The client's head should be tipped toward the opposite shoulder for easy examination of the canal and tympanic membrane.

> ### *Safety First*
>
> As the 1990's begin, health care providers are becoming increasingly aware of the need to protect themselves and their clients from the threat of infection. Practitioners must be aware than whenever they come in close physical contact with clients, infection may be transmitted between persons.
>
> The concept of *universal precautions* has thus been developed. Briefly, this concept proposes that the provider avoid contact with all the client's bodily fluids. One of the front-line measures for this avoidance is the use of latex gloves, which should be worn when examining the client's ear, mouth, and throat. Disposable specula and tongue blades must be available. Eye goggles should be considered when dealing with secretions that may be passed through the air, possibly falling into the examiner's eye.

---

3. In adults the ear canal may be straightened by pulling the auricle upward and backward; in young children and infants it may be straightened by pulling the auricle downward (Fig. 9-4).
4. The inner two thirds of the external meatus, which has a bony skeleton, is sensitive to pressure. Insert the speculum gently and not too far to avoid causing pain.
5. The angle at which the speculum is inserted into the meatus must be varied, or only a limited area of the tympanic membrane will be seen.

The auditory canal should be inspected for cerumen, redness, or swelling. The appearance of the normal canal varies in diameter, shape, and growth of hairs. Hair growth is limited to the outer third of the canal, but the hairs may be numerous.

> ### *Approach to the Examination: Little Ears, Special Problems*
>
> Young children (usually under age 4) perceive having their ears examined as a threatening act. It is usually best to leave the ear until the end of the examination, when the practitioner has had more time to build a relationship with the young client.
>
> Once a relationship is established, the practitioner can try to make the ear examination fun. Show the child how to "blow out the candle" by shutting down the otoscope light while the child puffs. Let the child look through the magnifying lens of the otoscope head at a familiar object to see how big it can be. Use your imagination! Sell your examination!

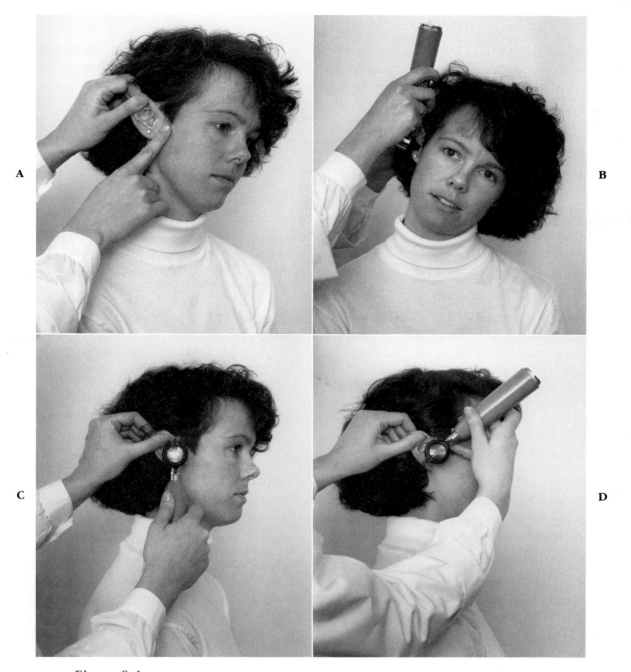

Figure 9-4

Examination of the ear with the otoscope. **A,** Inspection of the meatus. **B,** Client's head is tipped toward the opposite shoulder. **C** and **D,** Two ways of holding the otoscope.

Another aspect of the examination of the auditory canal is the evaluation of *cerumen,* which is produced by the sebaceous glands and the apocrine sweat glands in the canal. There are apparently racial variations in color, and black or brown cerumen will be noted in the client with darker skin coloring. There is also some difference in the color of fresh cerumen compared with older, drier cerumen; the former is lighter yellow or even pink, and the latter is a darker, yellowish brown. A small amount of cerumen will not interfere with the examination; the examiner can look past it and visualize the tympanic membrane. However, if the wax is excessive, it may be necessary to remove it.

Two methods that can be used for removing wax

are curettement and irrigation. *Curettement* is appropriate if the wax is soft or if the tympanic membrane could be perforated. However, it should not be done except by a skilled clinician. The closeness of the blood vessels and nerves to the surface makes it easy to cause bleeding and pain. There is also a risk of perforating the tympanic membrane if the client moves or the curet is used with too much vigor. *Irrigation* may be used when the wax is dry and hard but should not be carried out if there is a possibility that the membrane is perforated. Lukewarm water is used for the irrigation, which is done by repeatedly injecting the water from a syringe toward the posterosuperior canal wall. This procedure may make the client feel dizzy.

The examination of the tympanic membrane (see Fig. 9-3) requires a careful assessment of the color of the membrane and the identification of landmarks. The membrane is usually translucent pearl gray; in disease it may be yellow, white, red, or dull gray. Some membranes have white flecks or dense white plaques that are the result of healed inflammatory disease. The landmarks are identified, beginning with the light reflex, which is a triangular cone of reflected light seen in the anteroinferior quadrant of the membrane. A diffuse or spotty light is not normal. At the top point of the light reflex toward the center of the membrane is the umbo, the inferior point of the handle of the malleus. Anterior and superior to the umbo is the long process of the malleus, which appears as a whitish line extending from the umbo to the juncture of the malleolar folds, where the small white projection of the short process of the malleus can be seen. The malleolar folds and the pars flaccida, the relaxed portion of the membrane, are superior and lateral to the short process. Finally, an attempt should be made to follow the anulus around the periphery of the pars tensa. It is in the areas close to the anulus that perforations are frequently noted.

Normal tympanic membranes vary to some extent in size, shape, and color. It is only by examining many normal, healthy membranes that the ability to recognize the abnormal membrane is acquired.

Fluid in the middle ear may sometimes be identified by air bubbles or a fluid level seen through the tympanic membrane. Also, the membrane may be amber.

Bulging of the tympanic membrane may occur when fluid forms in the middle ear. The pressure increases, and the membrane may bulge outward in one part, or the entire membrane may bulge, obliterating some or all of the landmarks. The light reflex is usually lost, and the membrane appears dull. The cause of this fluid may be pus from otitis media or serum from serous otitis media.

Retraction of the tympanic membrane occurs when pressure is reduced resulting from obstruction of the eustachian tube, usually associated with an upper respiratory system infection. The retraction of the membrane causes the landmarks to be accentuated. The light reflex may appear less prominent.

Testing of auditory function

Clinical testing of auditory function is a process that starts early in the physical examination of the client. Understanding the spoken word is the principal use of hearing, and it may become apparent during the interview that there is an impairment or loss of auditory function. The actual testing of auditory function should be delayed until the end of the examination, after obvious problems related to hearing may have been identified. A precise measurement of hearing requires the use of the audiometer, but a good estimate of hearing can be made during the physical examination with the use of the tests discussed in this section.

Simple assessment of auditory acuity requires that only one ear be tested at a time. Therefore, it is necessary to mask the hearing in the ear not being tested. The examiner may occlude one of the client's ears by gently placing a finger against the opening of the auditory canal.

Voice tests are frequently used in estimating the client's hearing. The testing is begun with a very low whisper; the lips of the examiner should be 1 or 2 ft away from the unoccluded ear. The examiner exhales and softly whispers numbers that the client is to repeat. If necessary, the intensity of the voice is increased to a medium whisper and then to a loud whisper; then to a soft, then medium, then loud voice. To prevent lip-reading during the voice tests, the examiner may stand behind the client. If it is more convenient to be in front of the client, the client should be asked to close the eyes.

The watch tick is useful in testing but should not be used exclusively, because it provides only a high-frequency sound. The ticking watch is moved away from the ear until the client can no longer hear the sound.

Does Your Watch Tick?

Most battery-operated watches do not make a ticking sound; therefore they are of no value in the hearing screening. An alternate method is to rub the tips of the fingers together. Start about 4 ft from the client, approaching from an angle out of the person's range of vision. Move in closer until the client can hear the sound. Normally this will be about one arm's length from the client's ear.

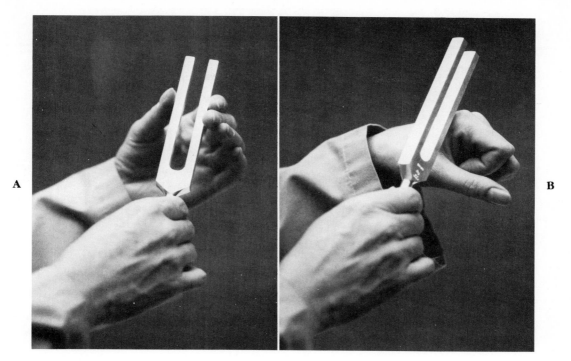

Figure 9-5

Activating the tuning fork. **A,** Stroking the fork. **B,** Tapping the fork on the knuckle.

Tuning fork tests are useful in determining whether the client has a conductive or a perceptive hearing loss. A fork with frequencies of 500 to 1000 cps is used because it can provide an estimate of hearing loss in the speech frequencies of roughly 500 to 2000 cps. The tuning fork is held by the base without the fingers touching either of the two prongs. The sound vibrations are softened or stopped entirely when the prongs of the fork are touched or held. The fork is activated by gently stroking or tapping on the knuckles of the opposite hand (Fig. 9-5). It should be made to ring softly, not harshly.

The terms *bone conduction* and *air conduction* must be clearly understood in the discussion of tuning fork tests. *Air conduction* implies the transmission of sound through the ear canal, tympanic membrane, and ossicular chain to the cochlea and auditory nerve. *Bone conduction* implies that sound is transmitted through the bones of the skull to the cochlea and auditory nerve. The client with normal auditory function will hear sound twice as long by air conduction, when the tuning fork is held opposite the external meatus, as he or she will by bone conduction, when the base of the tuning fork is placed on the mastoid bone.

The Rinne test makes use of air conduction and bone conduction. The tuning fork is used to compare the conduction of sound through the mastoid bone and the conduction of sound through the auditory meatus (Table 9-1). There are two different methods of performing the Rinne test, but the principle remains the same: the sound will be heard twice as long by air conduction as by bone conduction when there is no conductive hearing loss (Fig. 9-6). The most common method is to place the activated tuning fork against the mastoid bone until the client can no longer hear the sound and then move the fork ½ to 1 in from the auditory meatus. The client with no conductive hearing loss will continue to hear the sound by air conduction.

The second method merely reverses the order. The activated tuning fork is held 1 in from the auditory meatus; when the client can no longer hear the sound, the base of the fork is placed immediately on the mastoid bone. If the client cannot hear the sound when the fork is placed on the mastoid bone, the Rinne test is considered positive and the client does not have a conductive hearing loss. If the opposite is true and the client can hear the sound better by bone conduction, his Rinne test is negative and there is a conductive hearing loss. A positive Rinne with *an overall reduction in the time* where the sound is heard and normal ratio of air conduction to bone conduction is maintained results when there is a sensorineural hearing loss. This demonstrates that the client does not hear well by either air conduction or bone conduction.

The *Weber test,* which makes use of bone con-

Table 9-1

Hearing tests using tuning forks

Hearing	Weber (bone conduction)	Rinne (air and bone conduction)
Normal	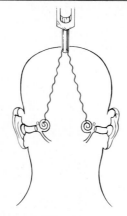**Normal hearing** Sound does not lateralize to either side; heard equally well in both ears	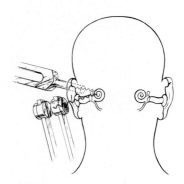**Normal hearing** "Positive Rinne." Sound is heard twice as long by air conduction as by bone conduction
Conduction loss (problem of external or middle ear)	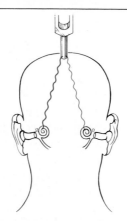**Conductive deafness in right ear** Sound lateralizes to defective ear because few extraneous sounds are carried through external or middle ear	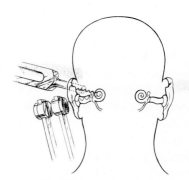**Conductive deafness in right ear** "Negative Rinne." Sound heard longer by bone conduction than by air conduction
Sensorineural loss (perceptive problem of inner ear or nerve)	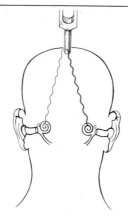**Perceptive deafness of right ear** Sound lateralizes to the better ear	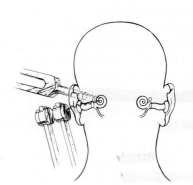**Perceptive deafness of right ear** "Positive Rinne." Sound is heard longer by air conduction than by bone conduction

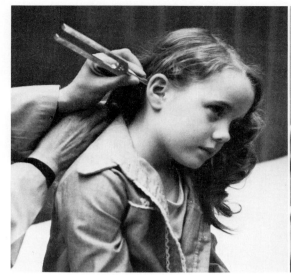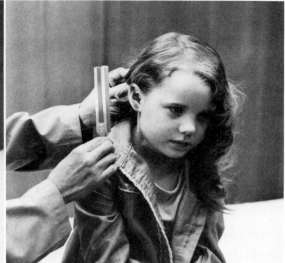

Figure 9-6

Rinne test. **A,** Bone conduction. **B,** Air conduction.

duction, is carried out by placing the base of the vibrating tuning fork on the vertex of the skull, on the forehead, or on the front teeth and asking the client if the sound is clearer in one ear or in the other (Fig. 9-7). In conductive deafness, the sound is referred to the deafer ear. This happens because the cochlea on that side will be undisturbed by extraneous sounds in the environment; these sounds are not transmitted because of a problem or defect in the ear canal or middle ear. In perceptive deafness, the sound is referred to the better ear because the cochlea or auditory nerve is functioning more effectively.

The caloric tests that measure labyrinthine function of the inner ear are discussed in Chapter 20 on neurologic assessment.

NOSE AND PARANASAL SINUSES

Anatomy and Physiology

The nose is the sensory organ for smell. It also warms, moistens, and filters the air inspired into the respiratory system.

The functions of the paranasal sinuses are not definitely known, but they may perform the same functions as the nose—that of warming, moistening, and filtering air. They also aid in voice resonance.

The nose is divided into the external nose and the internal nose or nasal cavity (Fig. 9-8). The upper third of the nose is bone; the remainder of the nose is cartilage. The nasal cavity is divided by the septum into two narrow cavities. The cavities have two openings: the anterior cavity is the vestibule where the naris is located and is thickly lined with small hairs; the posterior opening, or choana, leads to the throat. The nasal septum forms the

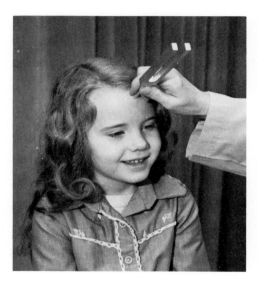

Figure 9-7

Weber test.

medial walls. The lateral walls are divided into the inferior, middle, and superior turbinate bones, which protrude into the nasal cavity. The turbinates are covered by a highly vascular mucous membrane. Below each turbinate is a meatus named according to the turbinate above it. The nasolacrimal duct drains into the inferior meatus, and most of the paranasal sinuses drain into the middle meatus. There is a plexus of blood vessels in the mucosa of the anterior nasal septum, which is a common site for epistaxis.

The receptors for smell are located in the olfactory area in the roof of the nasal cavity and upper third of the

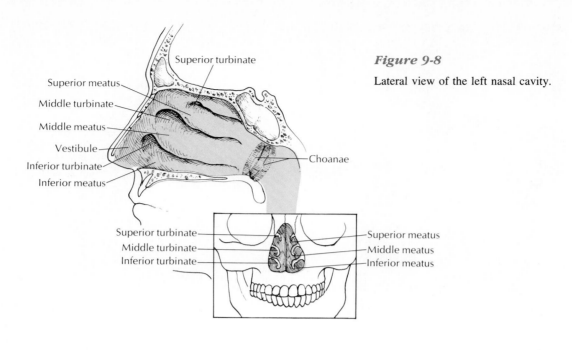

Figure 9-8

Lateral view of the left nasal cavity.

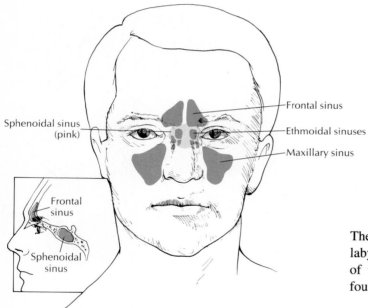

Figure 9-9

Anterior view of the frontal and maxillary sinuses.

The ethmoidal sinuses are small and occupy the ethmoidal labyrinth between the orbit of the eye and the upper part of the cavity of the nose. The sphenoidal sinuses are found in the body of the sphenoid.

Examination

The external portion of the nose is inspected for any deviations in shape, size, or color; the nares are inspected for flaring or discharge (Fig. 9-10). The ridge and soft tissues of the nose are palpated for displacement of the bone and cartilage and for tenderness or masses.

Examination of the nasal function includes determination of the ability to smell and the patency of the nasal cavities. To determine if the nasal cavities are patent, the client is asked to close the mouth, exert pressure on one naris with a finger, and breathe through the opposite naris. The procedure is repeated to determine the potency of the opposite naris. To determine the adequacy of function of the olfactory nerve (CN I), the client is

septum. The receptor cells, grouped as filaments, pass through openings of the cribriform plate, become the olfactory nerve (CN I), and transmit neural impulses for smell to the temporal lobe of the brain.

The paranasal sinuses are air-filled, paired extensions of the nasal cavities within the bones of the skull. They are the frontal, the maxillary, the ethmoidal, and the sphenoidal sinuses (Fig. 9-9). Their openings into the nasal cavity are narrow and easily obstructed. The frontal sinuses are located in the anterior part of the frontal bone. The maxillary sinuses, the largest of the paranasal sinuses, are located in the body of the maxilla.

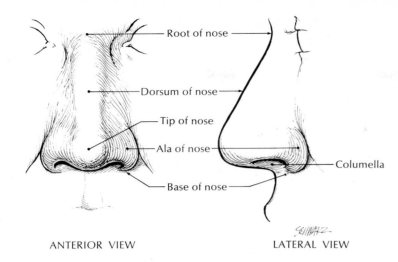

Root of nose

Dorsum of nose

Tip of nose

Ala of nose

Columella

Base of nose

ANTERIOR VIEW   LATERAL VIEW

Figure 9-10

External structure of the nose.

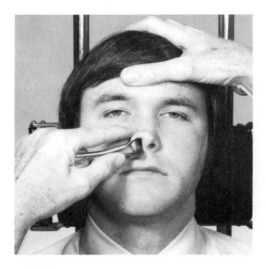

Figure 9-11

Proper position for insertion of nasal speculum.
(From Prior JA, Silberstein JS, and Stang JM: Physical diagnosis: the history and examination of the patient, ed 6, St Louis, 1981, The CV Mosby Co.)

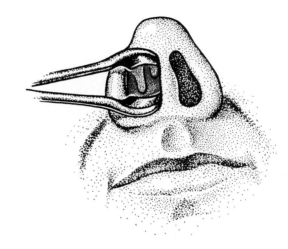

Figure 9-12

Examination of the anterior nasal cavity. View of the inferior and middle turbinates.

asked to close the eyes and occlude one naris again. The examiner places an aromatic substance, such as coffee or alcohol, close to the client's nose and asks the client to identify the odor. Each side is tested separately.

The examination of the nasal cavities may be carried out in several ways. The electric otoscope with the short, broad nasal speculum may be used or the nasal speculum with a penlight. The examination can also be carried out by using the thumb of the left hand to push the tip of the nose upward while shining a light into the naris. The last method is the easiest to perform and the most comfortable for the client. If the otoscope or speculum is used, the instrument is held in the left hand and the index finger is placed on the side of the nose to stabilize the position of the speculum and prevent dis-

placement (Fig. 9-11). The right hand is used to position the head and hold the light. Care must be taken not to apply pressure on the nasal septum because of its great sensitivity; but if a nasal speculum is being used, the blades must be opened as far as possible.

Examination of the nasal cavity through the anterior naris is limited to the vestibule, the anterior portion of the septum, and the inferior and middle turbinates. It is necessary to change the position of the client's head several times during the examination to inspect the various areas. With the client's head tipped back, the inferior and middle turbinates can be seen (Fig. 9-12). The septum is inspected for deviation, exudate, and perforation. The septum is rarely straight. The lateral walls of the nasal cavities and the inferior and middle turbinates are

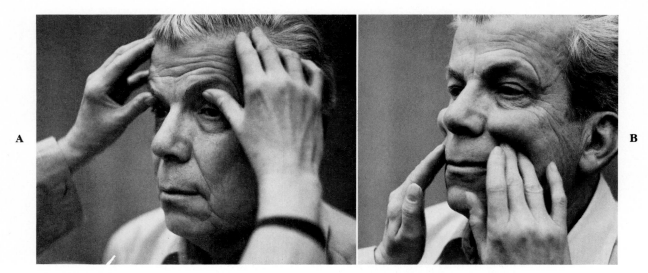

Figure 9-13

Palpation of the frontal **(A)** and maxillary **(B)** sinuses.

examined for polyps, swelling, exudate, and change in color. The nasal mucosa is normally redder than the oral mucosa. Increased redness indicates infection. Pale, boggy turbinates are typical of allergy, while redness with edema may indicate localized irritation. Any drainage from the middle meatus, which drains several of the paranasal sinuses, is important and should be described. The floor of the vestibule should be carefully inspected for evidence of a foreign body.

The secretions should be noted. The normal nasal secretion is mucoid. Watery secretions may indicate an acute upper respiratory infection or an allergic rhinitis. Purulent, crusty, or bloody secretions are abnormal.

Examination of the paranasal sinuses is made indirectly. Information about their condition is gained by inspection and palpation of the overlying tissues or by transillumination. Only the frontal and maxillary sinuses are accessible for examination. Palpation for examination of the maxillary sinuses is performed on the maxillary areas of the cheeks, where tenderness may be elicited. By palpating both cheeks simultaneously, one can determine differences in tenderness. Swelling of the cheek rarely occurs in maxillary sinusitis. The frontal sinuses can be palpated by finger pressure below the eyebrows. Palpation of the sinuses is demonstrated in Fig. 9-13. Both the maxillary and the frontal sinuses may also be percussed by lightly tapping with the index finger to determine if the client feels pain.

Transillumination of the maxillary sinuses is accomplished in a completely darkened room by shining a bright light in the client's mouth. The frontal sinus is transilluminated by shining a light through the medial aspect of the supraorbital rim. Transillumination has lim-

itations as a diagnostic tool, since even normal sinuses will show differences in the amount of transillumination. However, infected sinuses may be opaque.

MOUTH AND OROPHARYNX

Anatomy and Physiology

The mouth is the first division of the digestive tube and an entry site to the respiratory system. The oropharynx conducts air to and from the larynx and food to the esophagus from the mouth. The structures of the mouth and oropharynx are illustrated in Fig. 9-14.

The boundaries of the mouth are the lips anteriorly and the soft palate and uvula posteriorly. The floor is formed by the mandibular bone, which is covered by loose, mobile tissue. The roof of the oral cavity is formed by the hard and soft palates. They are distinctly different in color; the soft palate is pink, and the hard palate is lighter. The uvula is a muscular organ that hangs down from the posterior margin of the soft palate. The muscles of *mastication* are innervated by two main nerves: the trigeminal nerve (CNV) and the facial nerve (CN VII).

The mouth contains the tongue, gums, teeth, and salivary glands. The tongue is composed of a mass of striated muscles interspersed with fat and many glands. The dorsal surface is rough resulting from the presence of papillae. The ventral surface toward the floor of the mouth is smooth and shows large veins. The fold of mucous membrane that joins the tongue to the floor of the mouth is the frenulum. The tongue is innervated by the hypoglossal nerve (CN XII). The sensory receptors for taste are the glossopharyngeal nerve (CN IX) and the facial nerve (CN VII).

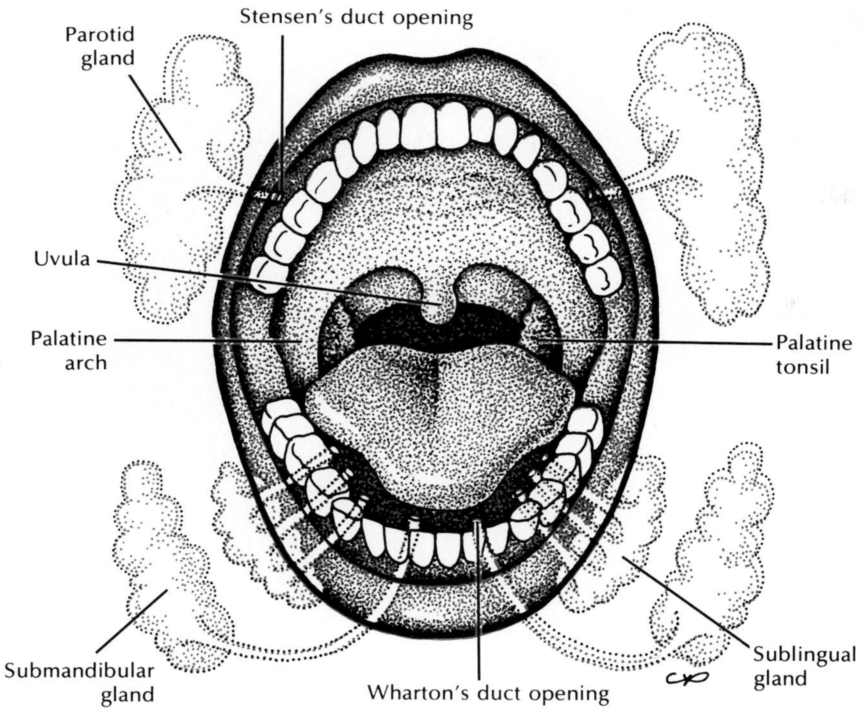

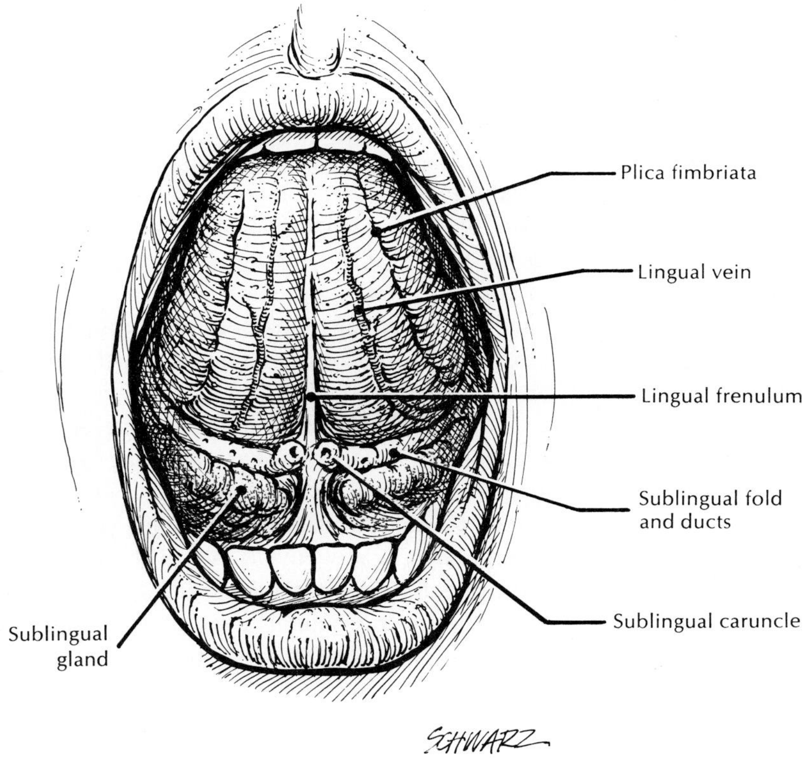

Figure 9-14

Structures of the mouth.

The gums are composed of fibrous tissue covered with a smooth mucous membrane and are attached to the alveolar margins of the jaws and to the necks of the teeth. In the adult there are 32 teeth, 16 in each arch.

Three pairs of salivary glands secrete into the oral cavity. They are the parotid, submandibular, and sublin-gual salivary glands. The largest is the parotid gland, which lies in front of and below the external ear. The parotid (Stensen's) duct opens into the buccal membrane opposite the second molar. The submandibular gland lies below and in front of the parotid gland. The submandib-ular (Wharton's) duct opens at the side of the frenulum on the floor of the mouth. The sublingual gland is the smallest salivary gland and lies in the floor of the mouth. It raises the mucous membrane, covering its superior surface to form the sublingual fold. It has numerous small openings, which open on the sublingual fold.

The oropharynx is the section of the pharynx that is posterior to the oral cavity and most accessible to examination. The nasopharynx lies behind the nasal cavities and is superior to the oropharynx. The laryngopharynx is inferior to the oropharynx. Along both lateral walls of the oropharynx are two palatine arches, and between them are the tonsils. The tonsils are usually the same color as the surrounding tissue and do not normally extend beyond the pillars. Tonsillar tissue in children enlarges until puberty and then shrinks back into the folds of the arches. Consequently, a child's tonsils may normally be larger than an adult's. The posterior pharyngeal wall that is visible during the clinical examination may show many small blood vessels and small areas of pink or red lymphoid tissue.

Examination

The examination is conducted from the anterior to the posterior areas of the mouth and begins with the external components of the mouth and jaw.

The lips are inspected for symmetry, color, edema, or surface abnormalities. The client is asked to open and close the mouth to demonstrate the mobility of the mandible and the occlusion of the teeth. The temporomandibular joint is palpated while the mouth is opened wide and then closed, for any tenderness, crepitus, or deviation (Fig. 9-15). Pressure applied to the joint during closing of the mouth may result in referred pain to the ear; a common cause of the referred pain is malocclusion. The lips are palpated for induration.

The client is asked to remove dentures, if worn, for the rest of the mouth and throat examination. A good source of additional light is essential in examination of the mouth and throat.

The oral mucosal surfaces are normally light pink and are kept moist by saliva. The surfaces are examined

---

Tips on Examining the Throat

When examining the throat, first ask the client to open wide and say "ah" with the tongue extended. With this procedure, most people will be able to lower the tongue and open the pharynx sufficiently to visualize the pharynx properly. Use a tongue blade only if absolutely needed, since many clients will have an involuntary gag response to any object placed in the mouth.

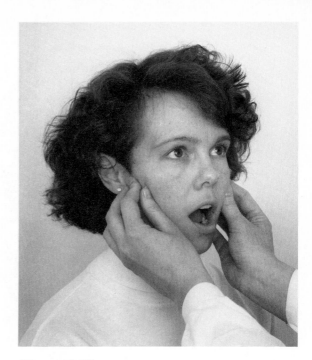

Figure 9-15

Palpatation of the temporomandibular joint.

systematically to ensure that all areas are inspected (Fig. 9-16). The examiner may use two tongue depressors or the fingers as retractors. With the client's mouth partially open, the mucosa in the anteroinferior area between the lower lip and gum is examined. With the mouth wide open, the buccal mucosa and Stensen's duct (the opening to the parotid gland, opposite the upper second molar) of the right cheek are examined. The maxillary mucobuccal fold between the upper lip and gum is examined next; then the mucosa and Stensen's duct of the left cheek are examined.

The examination of the tongue begins with inspection of the dorsum for any swelling, variation in size or color, coating, or ulceration. The client is asked to extend the tongue to demonstrate any deviation, tremor, or limitation of movement; any of these would indicate impairment of the hypoglossal nerve (CN XII). To inspect the posterior and lateral areas of the tongue, a 4- by 4-in piece of gauze is wrapped around the tip of the extended tongue and the examiner's gloved hand is used to hold and position the tongue (Fig. 9-17). The tongue is swung to the left, and the right lateral border is inspected. The position is reversed, and the left lateral border is examined. The tongue is released, and the client is asked to touch the tip of the tongue to the palate. The ventral surface is observed for swelling or varicosities. The floor of the mouth is inspected for abnormalities or swelling; Wharton's ducts (the openings of the subman-

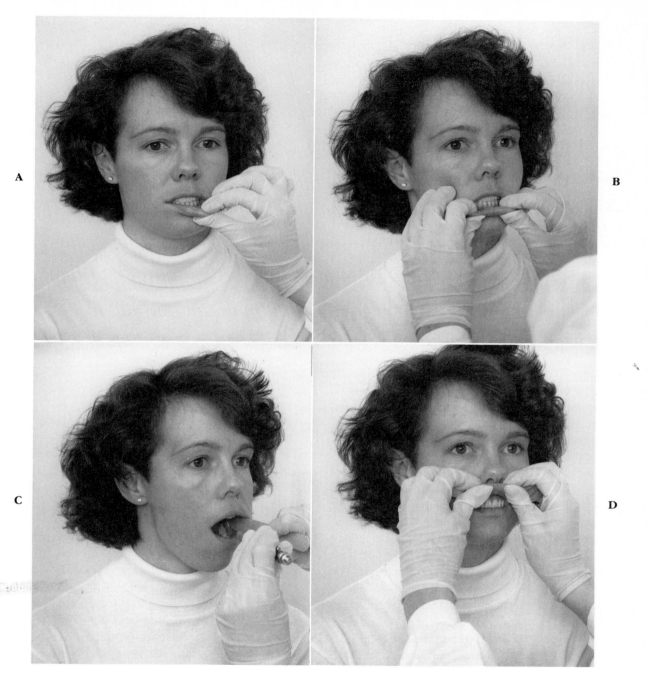

Figure 9-16

Examination of the lips and oral mucosa. **A,** Palpatation of the lips. **B,** Inspection of the mucosa of the lower anterior area. **C,** Inspection of mucosa of each cheek with identification of Stensen's duct opening. **D,** Inspection of mucosa of the upper anterior area.

dibular glands), the frenulum, and the sublingual ridge are identified. The entire tongue and the floor of the mouth are carefully palpated, because some diseases or tumors cause little change in the surface and can only be detected by palpation.

The examination of the teeth and gums is not a substitute for a dental examination but should reveal gross

problems that need attention. A dental mirror can be used productively as a retractor and to reflect some of the surfaces of the teeth and gums that are not readily accessible. The teeth are inspected for caries, missing teeth, and malocclusions. The examination is conducted systematically so that each tooth of one arch is visualized before those of the other arch. Any soft discolorations

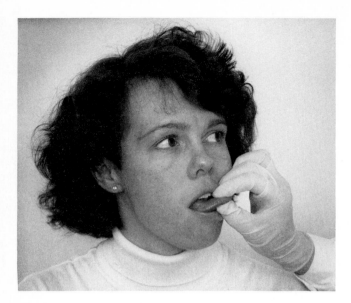

Figure 9-17

Examination of the tongue.

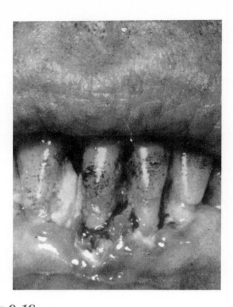

Figure 9-18

Advanced pyorrhea.
(From Prior JA, Silberstein JS, and Stang JM: Physical diagnosis: the history and examination of the patient, ed 6, St Louis, 1981, The CV Mosby Co.)

on the crown of a tooth should be suspected as carious. The teeth are counted, taking into consideration the client's age in determining the number of primary teeth, 20, or permanent teeth, 32, that are present and the number missing.

The dental screening form in Fig. 9-19 illustrates the correct numbering of teeth. The permanent teeth of the adult or older child are counted, beginning at the right third molar of the upper arch to the upper left third molar and then continuing with the left third molar of the lower arch to the lower right third molar. The third molars are the so-called wisdom teeth and may not be visible. The primary teeth of the child are given alphabetical letters, but the sequence for lettering is the same as for numbering. The letters begin with the right second molar, "A," of the upper arch and continue around to the left second molar, "J," and then to the left lower arch.

Malocclusions, such as two teeth in the space for one, overlapping of teeth, and missing teeth with wide spaces should be noted. The palpation of the temporomandibular joint with opening and closing of the mouth, described in the beginning of the oral examination, is helpful in demonstrating normal or abnormal occlusion such as the lower teeth biting outside the upper teeth (underbite) or the upper front teeth protruding and hanging over the lower front teeth (overbite).

The gums are inspected in the same systematic way as the teeth with the completion of one arch and then the other arch. Any signs of inflammation and hemorrhage of the gums (gingivitis) may indicate more se-

rious periodontal disease (pyorrhea) involving the bones and ligaments that anchor the tooth in its socket (Fig. 9-18). Any stains, tartar (calculus), or loose teeth are noted as signs of periodontal disease. Fig. 9-19 is a form that can be used in recording observations made during the examination of the teeth and gums.

With the client's head back, the palate and uvula are inspected. It may be necessary to depress the base of the tongue with a tongue depressor. The difference in color of the hard and soft palate is noted, as is any abnormality of architecture. An exostosis (torus palatinus) is frequently found in the midline of the posterior two thirds of the hard palate (Fig. 9-20). This is a smooth, symmetric bony structure resulting from the downgrowth of the palatal processes. Such bony growths are benign. The uvula may be bifid and part of a submucosal cleft palate. The client is asked to say, "Ah," and the rise of the soft palate and uvula is noted. Any deviation or lack of movement indicates impairment of the vagus nerve (CN X).

The oropharynx is inspected while the client's head is back, and the base of the tongue is gently depressed with a tongue depressor. The anterior palatine arches and the posterior arches are inspected for inflammation or swelling. The size of the tonsils is estimated, and any exudate is noted. A grading system to describe the size of tonsils can be used: grade 1, tonsils behind the pillar; grade 2, between pillar and uvula; grade 3,

DENTAL SCREENING FORM

DENTAL CARIES
1. No apparent caries.
2. Indicate caries on chart.

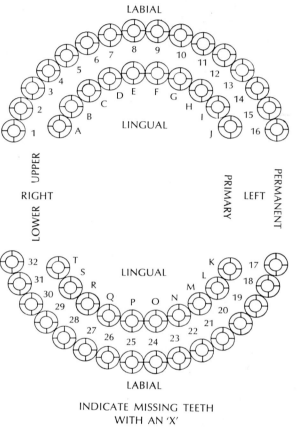

INDICATE MISSING TEETH
WITH AN 'X'

GUMS	NORMAL	GINGIVITIS	PERIODONTITIS
CALCULUS	NONE	LIGHT	HEAVY
ORAL HYGIENE	CLEAN	POOR	VERY POOR
OCCLUSION	NORMAL	OVERBITE	UNDERBITE

RECOMMENDATION

A. Immediate dental care not indicated
B. Dental care indicated ——————— Emergency ——————— Routine ———————

Figure 9-19

Dental screening form.

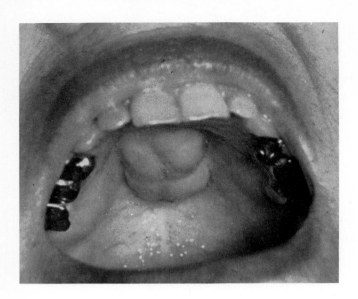

Figure 9-20

Exostosis.
(From Prior JA, Silberstein JS, and Stang JM: Physical diagnosis: the history and examination of the patient, ed 6, St Louis, 1981, The CV Mosby Co.)

Health History

Ears, Nose and Throat

NOTE: A yes response to any question *must* be further investigated. Use the following indicators throughout the assessment: (1) onset (specific date, sudden or gradual), (2) duration, (3) frequency, (4) precipitating factors, (5) aggravating or alleviating factors, (6) treatment received, and (7) outcome.

Present status

1. Have you experienced hearing loss?
   a. Type
   b. Hearing aid: any problems
2. Do you have drainage from your ears?
   a. Description: waxy, purulent, clear
3. Do you have nose bleeds?
   a. Treatment required
4. Do you have sensations in your ears?
   a. Description: fullness, pain, ringing/buzzing
5. Do you have allergies?
   a. Allergin: pollen, chemicals, animals, clothing fibers
6. Do you have any nose discharge?
   a. Description: watery, mucoid, crusty, bloody, purulent
7. Do you have unpleasant mouth taste or odor?
   a. Cause: throat infections, dental caries, dentures, foods, other health conditions
8. Do you have swollen or bleeding gums?
9. Do you wear dentures?
   a. Chewing difficulties
   b. Mouth ulcerations
10. Do you have variations in your tongue character?
    a. Description: swelling, size change, color, coating, ulceration
11. Do you have difficulty swallowing?
    a. Description: pain, tightness, "catching," substernal fullness, vomiting

Past history

1. Have you had any trauma to your nose or ears?
   a. Nature: structural damage, foreign body, sharp blow
2. Have you experienced dizziness?
3. Have you had cerumen build up requiring professional removal?
4. Have you had frequent sore thraots?
5. Have you had ear, nose, throat, mouth, or teeth surgery?
   a. Type
   b. When
   c. Residual effects

Associated conditions

1. Do you have high blood pressure?
2. Do you have any blood dyscrasias?
3. Do you have vitamin K deficiency?

Family history

1. Do you have a family history of hearing loss?
2. Does anyone in your family experience nose bleeds?

Sample assessment record

Client states that nose bleeding following a sneezing episode occurs two to three times weekly lasting 5 to 10 minutes. Client is allergic to wool and mold. Nares has been packed twice in the last 3 months, but bleeding usually stops with ice pack applied across nose. Denies nose trauma, surgery, and hypertension. Father has one to two nose bleeds per week due to vitamin K deficiency.

Findings in Common Problems in the Ear, Nose, and Throat

Sinusitis (infection or inflammation of one or more of the paranasal sinuses). Tenderness to palpation or percussion over one or more sinuses. Swollen, pale, dull red nasal mucosa.

Otitis media (infection of the middle ear). Red, nonmobile tympanic membrane with loss of bony landmarks and light reflex. A positive Weber test lateralizes to affected side.

Serous otitis (filling the middle ear with noninfected fluid). Amber tympanic membrane, loss of light reflex, possible presence of fluid line and air bubbles.

Pharyngitis (inflammation of the mucous membranes of the pharynx, of viral or bacterial origin). Red posterior pharynx, possible white coating (exudate), enlarged tonsils if present.

touching the uvula; and grade 4, to the midline. The posterior wall of the oropharynx is examined for any change in color. The glossopharyngeal nerve (CN IX) and the vagus nerve (CN X) are tested by touching the posterior wall of the pharynx on each side. The normal response is a gag reflex. A unilaterally impaired gag reflex usually indicates impairment of glossopharyngeal and vagal function.

Throughout the examination of the mouth and throat, attention should be given to mouth odors, which may result from systemic or oral disease.

BIBLIOGRAPHY

Ballantyne J and Groves J: Scott-Brown's diseases of the ear, nose, and throat, ed 4, Philadelphia, 1979, JB Lippincott Co.

Cody D and others: Diseases of the ears, nose and throat: a guide to diagnosis and management, Chicago, 1981, Year Book Medical Publishers.

DeWeese DD and Saunders WH: Textbook of otolaryngology, ed 6, St Louis, 1982, The CV Mosby Co.

10

Assessment of the eyes

OBJECTIVES

Upon successful review of this chapter, learners will be able to:

- Describe anatomy and physiology of the eyes
- State related rationale and demonstrate assessment of
  - Visual acuity
  - Extraocular muscle function
  - Color vision
  - Ocular structures
  - Eyes, using ophthalmoscope and tonometer instruments
- Outline history relevant to an eye examination
- Recognize visual acuity, visual field, and extraocular neuromuscular defects

A thorough examination of the eyes can reveal a wealth of information on both local and systemic health and disease processes. Observation of the eyes in conjunction with facial expression and body posture frequently reveals information about the client's emotional status.

The eye examination involves multiple components, and students practicing it should learn a thorough and efficient arrangement of the various components. The ordering of these parts should focus both on completeness of the examination and on positioning the client comfortably.

This examination encompasses measurement of visual acuity, evaluation of visual fields, testing of ocular movements, inspection of ocular structures, testing of nerve reflexes, and the ophthalmoscopic examination. Tonometry should also be included, especially for persons over 40 years of age. Inspection is the principal physical examination technique used.

Anatomy and Physiology

OCULAR STRUCTURES

The structures of the eyelid and the globe of the eye are shown in Figs. 10-1 and 10-2.

Eyelids and Eyelashes

The eyelashes are evenly distributed along the margin of the lids and curve outward. The eyelids serve a protective function, covering the anterior aspect of the eye and lubricating its surface. The lids should be able to close completely, so that the upper and lower lid margins approximate. When the eyes are open, the upper lid normally covers a small portion of the iris and the cornea

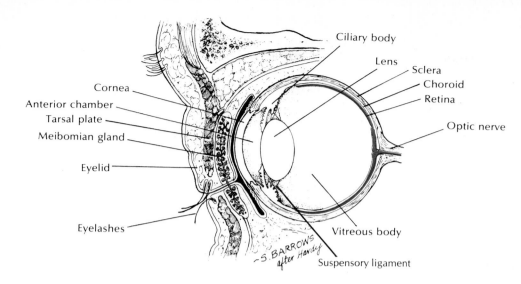

Figure 10-1

Structures of the eyelid and globe.

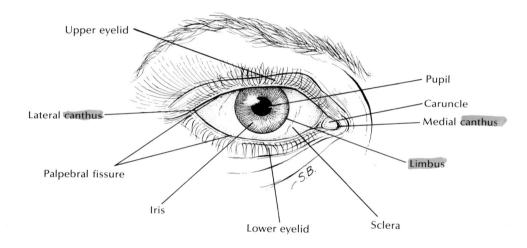

Figure 10-2

Anterior view of the eye.

overlying it, coming about midway between the limbus and the pupil. The margin of the lower lid lies at or just below the limbus. The limbus is the junction line where the cornea and sclera meet. The distance between the lid margins, called the palpebral fissure, should be equal in both eyes. The tarsal plates are thin strips of connective tissue that lie within the lid and give the lid some form and consistency.

Conjunctiva

Lining the lids and covering the anterior portion of the eyeball is the conjunctiva. This continuous, transparent structure is divided into two portions: palpebral and bulbar. The palpebral portion lines the lids and appears shiny pink or red because it overlies the fleshy vascular structures of the lids; the bulbar portion lies over the sclera.

The palpebral conjunctiva recesses into the folds of the lids and is continuous with the bulbar conjunctiva,

which lies loosely over the sclera to the limbus, where it merges with the corneal epithelium. This portion of the conjunctiva is normally clear; the white color comes from the sclera below. The bulbar portion does, however, contain many small blood vessels; these are normally visible and may become dilated, producing varying degrees of redness. A small fleshy elevation, the caruncle, is located in the nasal corner of the conjunctiva. Yellowish, triangular deposits, called pinguecula, may occur in the bulbar conjunctiva near the limbus. These are essentially normal senile changes caused by a hyaline degeneration of fibrous tissue. The meibomian glands, which secrete an oily, lubricating substance, appear as vertical yellow striations on the palpebral conjunctiva.

Sclera

The sclera is the white portion of the eye visible anteriorly. Normally, several small, distinct conjunctival ves-

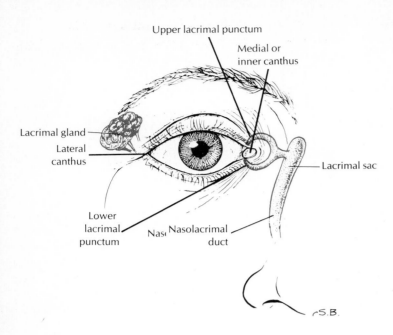

Figure 10-3

Lacrimal apparatus.

Upper lacrimal punctum

Medial or
inner canthus

Lacrimal gland

Lateral
canthus

Lacrimal sac

Lower
lacrimal
punctum

Nas Nasolacrimal
duct

S.B.

sels are visible over the sclera, particularly around the periphery. In some dark-complected persons, small, dark-pigmented dots may be visible on the sclera near the limbus.

The sclera is composed of fibrous tissue. It is supplied with sensory innervation by the ciliary nerve. Inflammation of the sclera is very painful.

Cornea

The cornea, like the bulbar conjunctiva, is a smooth, moist, transparent tissue. It covers the area over the pupil and iris and merges with the conjunctiva at the limbus. It is normally invisible except for the light reflections from its surface. The cornea is quite sensitive to touch; this sensation is transmitted by the ophthalmic branch of the trigeminal nerve (cranial nerve [CN] V). Stimulation of either cornea causes a blinking reflex in both eyes, which is transmitted by the facial nerve (CN VII).

Anterior Chamber

The anterior chamber is bounded anteriorly by the cornea, laterally by the sclera and the ciliary body, and posteriorly by the iris and that portion of the lens within the pupillary opening. It is filled with aqueous, which is constantly produced by the ciliary body. The function of the anterior chamber is very important, because the relation between the rate of aqueous production and the resistance to aqueous outflow at the anterior chamber angle determines the intraocular pressure, which is 15 mm Hg ± 3 mm Hg in normal eyes.

Lacrimal Apparatus

The components of the lacrimal apparatus are illustrated in Fig. 10-3. The lacrimal gland, located above and slightly lateral to the eye, produces tears, which moisten and lubricate the conjunctiva and cornea. The tears are washed across the eye and then drain through the puncta, which are located on the nasal end of both upper and lower lids. The tears then pass into the nasolacrimal sac, located in the medial portion of the orbit, and from there through the nasolacrimal duct to the nose. Of these several components of the lacrimal system, only the puncta are normally visible.

Iris

The iris is a doughnut-shaped pigmented structure containing two involuntary muscles. It is located in front of the lens and behind the anterior chamber. The iris, along with the ciliary body and suspensory ligament, forms the interior portion of the choroid. The iris functions as a diaphragm within the image-forming portion of the eye. The diaphragm has a variable aperture—the pupil. The aperture's size, or pupillary opening, varies with the amount of light striking the retina. The surface of the iris is composed of numerous fibrils that vary in color within a given iris and from person to person. Posterior to the layer of fibrils are the dilator and sphincter muscles. The deepest layer of the iris is the pigment epithelium. The iris attaches to the ciliary body.

Pupils

The pupils are normally round and equal in size. A small percentage of individuals (about 5%) do have a slight but noticeable difference in the size of their pupils. Although this may be normal, the finding should be regarded with some suspicion. The size of the pupils is controlled by the autonomic nervous system. Stimulation of the parasympathetic fibers leads to constriction of the pupils; stimulation of the sympathetic fibers produces dilatation. The amount of ambient light influences the size; normally, increasing illumination causes pupillary constriction, whereas diminishing illumination causes dilatation. The pupils also constrict in response to accommodation, which is the change in focus from a distant to a near object.

The size of the pupils does vary in individuals exposed to the same degree of ambient light. Pupils tend to be smaller in infants and older persons; myopic (nearsighted) persons tend to have larger pupils, whereas hyperopic (farsighted) persons tend to have smaller pupils. The normal pupil is between 2 and 6 mm in diameter. Pupils of less than 2 mm are considered miotic; those greater than 6 mm are considered mydriatic.

The constricting response of the pupils to a bright direct light, a pupillary reflex, consists of both a direct and a consensual reaction. The direct reaction refers to the constriction of the pupil receiving the increased illumination. The constriction of the pupil that is not receiving increased illumination is the consensual reaction. The optic nerve (CN II) mediates the afferent arc of this reflex from each eye, and the oculomotor nerve (CN III) mediates the efferent arc to both eyes; thus the presence of both direct and consensual responses indicates the functioning of these two cranial nerves.

The accommodation response of the pupils consists of convergence of the eyes and constriction of the pupils as the glance is shifted from a distant to a near object.

The rapidity of the responses to both light and accommodation varies in normal persons. What is important is the presence of the responses and the equality of the responses in both eyes.

Lens

Directly behind the iris and at the pupillary opening lies the lens, the center of the refracting system of the eye. It is normally transparent and has no blood vessels, nerves, or connective tissue. It is composed of epithelial cells within an elastic membrane, the lens capsule. The thickness of the lens is controlled by muscles of the ciliary body, and it is the changes in thickness of the lens that enable the eye to focus on objects both far and near. Thus, the coordinated functions of the muscles of the iris and the muscles of the ciliary body acting on the lens

control the amount of light permitted to reach the neurosensory elements of the retina and the focusing of objects on the retina.

Vitreous

The vitreous is a normally transparent material occupying the area posterior to the lens, the posterior chamber. It is surrounded by the retina.

Retina

The eyeball is a spherical structure lined from the inside toward the outside by the retina, the choroid, and the sclera. Within this sphere lies the vitreous body.

The layers of the eyeball accessible to physical examination are the sclera anteriorly and the retina interiorly; the retina is visible with the ophthalmoscope.

The retina is reddish orange because of the deeper vascular supply and the deeper pigmented layers. The pigment present in the posterior layers of the retina also accounts for its slightly stippled appearance. Normally, the color of the retina is quite uniform throughout, with no patches of light or dark discoloration.

Observable on the retina are several important structures, including the optic disc, or nerve head of the optic nerve, with its physiologic cup; the four sets of retinal vessels, which emerge from the optic disc and travel medially and laterally around the retina; the macular area, where central vision is concentrated; and the retinal background itself (Fig. 10-4 and the color plate on the eye).

Optic disc

The optic disc is located on the nasal half of the retina. Important characteristics of the disc include its size, shape, color, the nature of the margins, and the physiologic cup. The optic disc is about 1.5 mm in diameter and is round to vertically oval. It ranges from creamy yellow to pink; it is lighter than the surrounding retina. (See color plate of eye.) The color of both the disc and the retinal background vary from one individual to another; it is somewhat lighter in fair-complected, light-haired people and slightly darker in dark-complected, dark-haired people.

The margins of the disc are usually sharp and are clearly demarcated from the surrounding retina, although several normal variations deserve comment. The nasal outline may normally be somewhat more blurred than the temporal outline. Dense pigment deposits may be situated about the disc margins, particularly in dark-complected people. A whitish to grayish crescent of scleral tissue

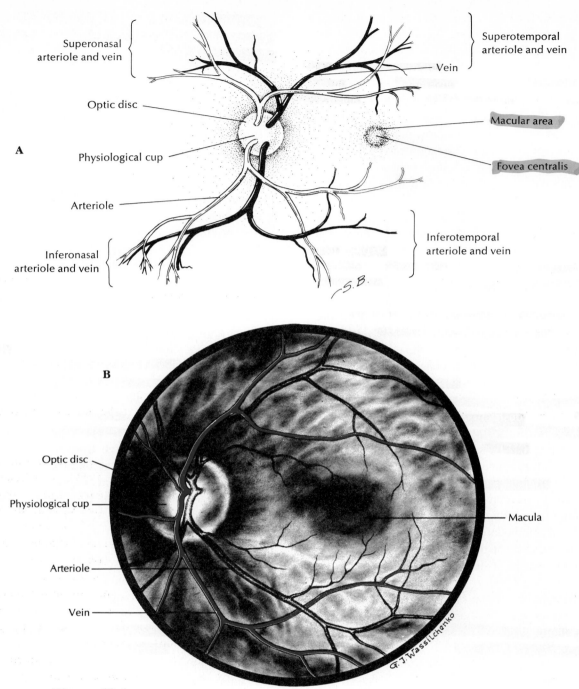

Figure 10-4

A and **B,** Retinal structures of the left eye.
(**B** from Whaley LF and Wong DL: Nursing care of infants and children, ed 2, St Louis, 1983, The CV Mosby Co.)

may be present immediately adjacent to the disc, particularly on the temporal side.

Most discs have a small depression just temporal to the center of the disc; slightly lighter than the rest of the disc, this depression is yellowish white and is called the physiologic cup or physiologic depression. In normal individuals it does not extend completely to the disc margins but may occupy one fourth to one third of the area of the disc.

Retinal vessels

As shown in Fig. 10-4, four sets of retinal vessels emerge from the optic disc and wind outward, becoming smaller at the periphery. Each set includes an arteriole and a vein

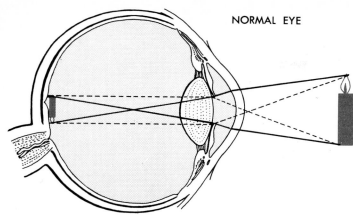

NORMAL EYE

Figure 10-5

In the normal eye, light rays from an object are refracted by the cornea, aqueous humor, lens, and vitreous humor and converge on the fovea of the retina, where an inverted image is clearly formed.
(From Anthony CP and Thibodeau GA: Textbook of anatomy and physiology, ed 12, St Louis, 1987, The CV Mosby Co.)

amaurosis fugax

and is known by the quadrant of the retina that it supplies: superonasal, inferonasal, inferotemporal, or superotemporal. Important characteristics of the vessels include color, size, regularity of caliber, arteriolar light reflex, and the characteristics where one vessel crosses another.

The vessel walls are normally quite transparent, and the "color" of the vessels describes the oxygenated or deoxygenated blood they carry. Thus, the arterioles are a brighter red than the veins, which are dark red. The arterioles are about 25% smaller than the veins; thus, an arteriole-to-vein (A:V) ratio of 2:3 or 4:5 is normal. When observed, arterioles have a narrow light reflex from the centerline of the vessel. Pulsations are sometimes visible in the veins near the optic disc and are caused by the forcing of blood out of the eye through the vein with each systole. Veins do not show a light reflex. Normally, both arterioles and veins show a gradually and regularly diminished diameter as they go from the disc to the periphery. They normally cross and intertwine; but where the vessels cross one another, there should be no change in the course or caliber of either vessel.

Retinal background and macular area

The neurosensory elements, rods and cones, are contained in the retina. At a point temporal to the disc at the posterior pole of the eye, there is a slight depression in the retina, known as the fovea centralis. The cones are most heavily concentrated here, making this the point of central vision and most acute color and daylight vision. The retinal area immediately around this is called the macula. The macular area usually has no visible retinal vessels; it is nourished by choroidal vessels and appears slightly darker than the rest of the retinal background.

PHYSIOLOGY OF VISION

For a clear visual image to be perceived, light reflected from an object must pass through the cornea, anterior chamber, lens, and vitreous fluid, be focused on the retina

where the neural receptors, the rods and cones, are activated, and carry the impulse along the optic nerve and tract to the visual cortex.

Formation of a Retinal Image

To produce a clear image on the retina, four processes must occur:
1. Refraction, or bending, of the light rays
2. Accommodation, or change in curvature, of the lens
3. Constriction of the pupil
4. Convergence of the eyes

Refraction is the bending or deflecting of light rays that occurs when rays of light pass obliquely from one transparent medium into another of different density. In the eye these media are the cornea, aqueous humor in the anterior chamber, lens, and vitreous humor, which, in the normal eye, work in conjunction to bring an object 20 ft or more away into focus on the retina (Fig. 10-5).

Accommodation for near vision enables the eye to focus on near objects by increase in the curvature of the lens, constriction of the pupils, and convergence of the eyes. Light rays from close objects are divergent and must be bent to focus on the retina. The curvature of the lens is increased to accomplish this: Contraction of the ciliary muscle causes the elastic lens to bulge.

The pupils constrict due to contraction of the circular fibers of the iris. This prevents divergent light rays from an object from coming into the eye through the peripheral portions of the cornea and lens. The pupil constricts both for near vision and in the presence of bright light.

Convergence is the movement of eyes inward to bring together the visual axes on the object viewed. Single binocular vision requires that light rays from an object fall on corresponding points of the two retinas so that one object is seen instead of two. The extraocular muscles hold the visual axes of the two eyes parallel.

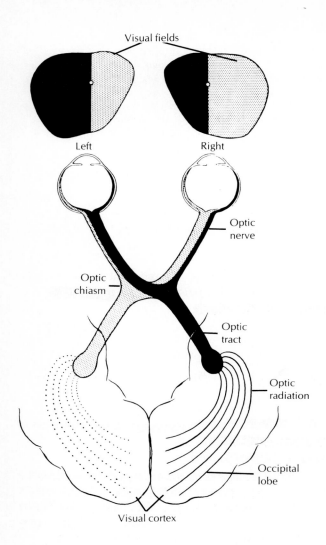

Visual fields

Left   Right

Optic
nerve

Optic
chiasm

Optic
tract

Optic
radiation

Occipital
lobe

Visual cortex

Figure 10-6

Representation of the visual field in the optic pathways.
(From Havener WH: Synopsis of ophthalmology, ed 6, St Louis, 1984,
The CV Mosby Co.)

Visual Pathways and Visual Fields

The images formed on the retina are reversed right to left
and are upside down; thus, an object in the upper nasal
field of vision will be formed on the lower temporal
quadrant of the retina. The light stimulates neuron impulses that are conducted through the retina, the optic
nerve, and the optic tract to the visual cortex of the
occipital lobes.

The layout (spatial arrangement) of the nerve fibers in the retina is maintained in the optic nerve; that
is, temporal (lateral) fibers run along the lateral side of
the nerve, and nasal (medial) fibers run along the medial
portion of the nerve. However, at the optic chiasm, the
nasal or medial fibers cross over and join the temporal
or lateral fibers of the opposite optic tract. Thus, the left
optic tract contains fibers only from the left half of each
retina (the right half of each field of vision), and the right
optic tract contains fibers only from the right half of each
retina (left half of each field of vision). By this sequence

of pathways and events, conscious vision is produced.
The relationship of visual pathways and fields of vision
is illustrated in Fig. 10-6.

Neuromuscular Aspects

Six muscles of each eye, working in a coordinated
"yoked" fashion with the other eye, control eye movement, which normally occurs in conjugate, parallel fashion except during convergence, when a very close object
is visualized. These six muscles include the superior,
inferior, lateral, and medial rectus muscles; the superior
oblique muscle; and the inferior oblique muscle. This
parallelism of the axis of the eye makes possible single-
image, binocular vision. Thus, the yoked muscles are the
muscles in each eye that work together to move the eyes
in parallel motion to any given position of gaze. For
example, the left lateral rectus and the right medial rectus
are yoked muscles working concurrently to move the gaze

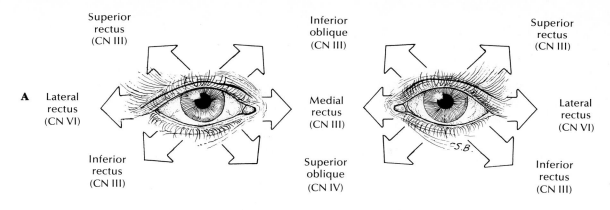

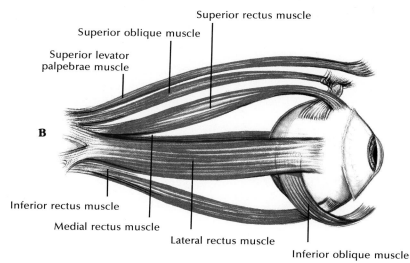

Figure 10-7

A, Movement generated by the six extraocular muscles. **B,** Muscles of the right orbit as viewed from the side.

(**B** from Anthony CP and Kolthoff NJ: Textbook of anatomy and physiology, ed 9, St Louis, 1975, The CV Mosby Co.)

to the left. The attachment of the muscles to the globe of the eye and the direction of their action are illustrated in Fig. 10-7.

These six eye muscles are innervated by three cranial nerves. The oculomotor nerve (CN III) innervates four muscles: the superior, inferior, and medial rectus muscles and the inferior oblique muscle. The trochlear nerve (CN IV) innervates the superior oblique muscle, and the abducens nerve (CN VI) innervates the lateral rectus muscle. A mnemonic device helpful for remembering this innervation is: LR_6SO_4, or lateral rectus—CN VI, superior oblique—CN IV, the four remaining eye muscles all being innervated by CN III.

Six of the 12 cranial nerves and portions of the cerebral hemispheres are involved in the total neurologic innervation of the eye and related structures. Table 10-1 summarizes the relationship of the six cranial nerves to the eye structures.

Table 10-1

Relationship of cranial nerves to eye structures

Cranial nerve		Activity
II	Optic	Mediates vision
III	Oculomotor	Innervates medial, superior, and inferior rectus muscles; inferior oblique muscle; musculature elevating the eyelid (levator palpebrae); and muscles of the iris and ciliary body
IV	Trochlear	Innervates superior oblique muscle
V	Trigeminal, ophthalmic division	Innervates sensory portion of corneal reflex
VI	Abducens	Innervates lateral rectus muscle
VII	Facial	Innervates lacrimal glands and musculature involved in lid closure (orbicularis oculi)

Color Vision

Color vision is a cone function. Deficiency in color perception is inherited in approximately 7% of men and 0.5% of women (Newell, p. 146). Visual acuity is normal, but color perception is depressed to varying degrees. It is disturbed in a variety of diseases of the optic nerve, in fovea centralis, in nutritional disturbances, and after ingestion of toxic drugs.

Examination

RELEVANT HEALTH HISTORY

1. Adequacy of vision in each eye; use of corrective lenses
2. Difficulty with vision
   a. Near or distant
   b. Central, peripheral, or specific area
   c. Constant or intermittent
   d. Presence of floaters, halos around lights
   e. Double vision
   f. Abnormal movements
3. Pain
   a. In or around eye
   b. Superficial or deep
   c. Onset: abrupt or gradual
   d. Associated symptoms: itching, burning, photophobia, or other sensation
4. Abnormal secretions
   a. Color
   b. Consistency
   c. Onset and duration
   d. Excessive or decreased tearing
5. History of trauma to the eyes
   a. History of incident
   b. Structures damaged
   c. Efforts to correct damage and degree of success
6. History of eye surgery
   a. Condition(s) requiring eye surgery
   b. When and where performed
   c. Results
7. History of illnesses affecting the eyes
   a. Hypertension
   b. Diabetes
   c. Glaucoma
   d. Cataract
   e. Eye infections
8. Family history of eye diseases such as retinoblastoma, color blindness, or other conditions, as in No. 7 above.

INTRODUCTION AND PREPARATION FOR THE EXAMINATION

Examination of the functions and the structures of the eyes involves multiple procedures and should be performed in a manner that provides efficient access to physical findings while maintaining the greatest degree of comfort for the client. There are, of course, numerous ways to organize this examination; the method suggested here is to examine initially the functions of visual acuity, both central and peripheral, and ocular motility. This assessment of function is followed by the examination of ocular structures, starting with the outermost structures and working toward the retina. Finally, intraocular tension should be checked as appropriate. The method allows the examiner to perform much of the ocular examination before touching any of the rather sensitive eye structures and reserves the somewhat uncomfortable procedures of ophthalmoscopic examination and tonometry until last.

Several pieces of equipment are required for the eye examination. These should be organized before the examination is begun:

• Visual acuity chart for distant vision
• Rosenbaum chart or newspaper clipping with several sizes of print for assessing near vision
• Opaque card or eye cover for assessing visual acuity, visual fields, and muscle function
• Penlight for assessing pupillary reflexes and external structures
• Cotton-tipped applicator for eversion of the upper lid
• Wisp of cotton for assessing corneal reflex
• Ophthalmoscope for assessing ocular media and for the retinal examination
• Tonometer for assessing ocular pressure

In addition to the equipment needed, a darkened room is necessary to enable the examiner to assess the pupillary reflexes and to perform the funduscopic examination with greater ease.

EXAMINATION TECHNIQUES

In examination of the eye, the range of normal is broad and the variations from normal are numerous. Much time, patience, and practice are required to assess the normal and common abnormal eye patterns.

Visual Acuity

The assessment of visual acuity is a simple and rewarding test of ocular function. Findings in a normal range of visual acuity give the examiner an indication of the clarity of the transparent media (cornea, anterior body, lens, and vitreous body), the adequacy of macular (central) vision,

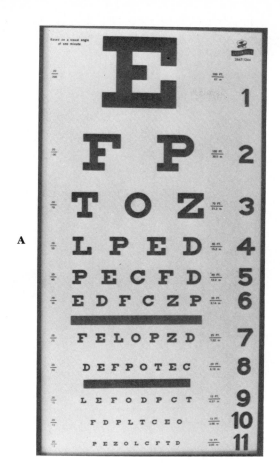

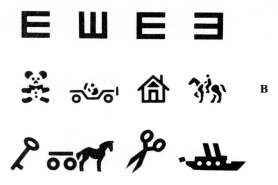

Figure 10-8

A, Snellen's chart. **B,** Test objects used in testing visual acuity. In successive lines are shown the illiterate E, the Henry F. Allen preschool vision test, and the Osterberg chart.
(**A** courtesy Graham-Field Surgical Co., Inc., New Hyde Park, NY; **B** adapted from Newell FW: Ophthalmology: principles and concepts, ed 5, St Louis, 1982, The CV Mosby Co.)

and the functioning of the nerve fibers from the macula to the occipital cortex.

Traditionally, Snellen's chart (Fig. 10-8, *A*) with various sizes of letters is used. For individuals who are illiterate or are unfamiliar with the Western alphabet, the illiterate E chart, in which the letter E faces in different directions, may be used (Fig. 10-8, *B*). A variety of charts have been designed to test children who cannot yet recognize the letters of the alphabet (Fig. 10-8, *B*). The chart has standardized numbers at the end of each line of letters; these numbers indicate the degree of visual acuity when measured from a distance of 20 ft. The numerator is 20, the distance in feet between the chart and the client, or the standard testing distance. The denominator is the distance from which the normal eye can read the lettering; therefore, the larger the denominator, the poorer the vision. It is important to note that although the terms *numerator* and *denominator* are commonly used, the measurement is not a fraction or a percentage of normal vision. Measurement of 20/20 vision in a client indicates a normal eye and optic pathway. Measurement of less than 20/20 vision indicates either a refractive error or some other optic disorder. Only one eye should be

tested at a time; the other may be covered with an opaque card or eye cover, not with the client's fingers. The room used for this test should be well-lighted. A person who wears corrective lenses may be tested with and without them; this allows for an assessment of the adequacy of the correction. Reading glasses, however, do blur distant vision.

Persons who cannot see the largest letter on the chart (20/200) should be checked to see if they can perceive hand movements about 12 in from their eyes or if they can perceive the light of the penlight directed into their eyes.

A gross assessment of near vision is performed in the client who complains of reading difficulty and in persons over 40 years of age. A Rosenbaum chart (Fig. 10-8, *C*) or a newspaper with various sizes of print may be used for this. With advancing age the lens may become less flexible, resulting in difficulty with near vision. This condition is known as presbyopia.

Visual Fields

The assessment of visual acuity indicates the functioning of the macular area, the area of central vision. However,

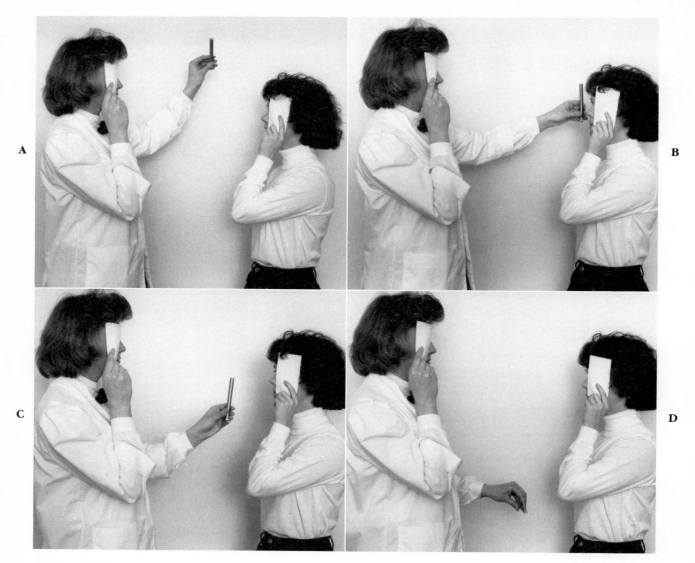

Figure 10-9

To examine the visual fields, the examiner and client cover opposite eyes with an opaque card; the examiner brings in a penlight or other small object from the superior (**A**), temporal (**B**), nasal (**C**), and inferior (**D**) fields of vision.

it does not test the sensitivity of the other areas of the retina, which perceive the more peripheral stimuli. The visual field confrontation test provides a rather gross measurement of peripheral vision.

The performance of this test assumes that the examiner has normal visual fields, since the client's visual fields are compared with the examiner's. The examiner and the client sit or stand opposite each other with their eyes at the same horizontal level at a distance of 1½ to 2 ft apart. The client covers one eye with an opaque card or eye cover, and the examiner covers his or her own eye opposite the client's covered eye; that is, if the client's right eye is covered, then the examiner's left eye

is covered. This leaves the client's and the examiner's same field of vision open for inspection.

The client is asked to stare directly at the examiner's open eye while the examiner stares directly at the client's open eye. Neither looks out at the object approaching from the periphery. The examiner holds a small object, such as a pencil or penlight, in the hand and gradually moves it in from the periphery of both directions horizontally and from above and below. The object should be beyond the limits of the field of vision initially, held equidistant from both persons, and then advanced toward the center. The client and the examiner should be able to visualize the object at the same time. It is often difficult for the examiner to move the test object out far enough so that neither person can see it, especially in the temporal field. It may be necessary for the examiner to hold the object slightly closer to the client in the temporal field, moving it to a line equidistant between them as it is brought in (Fig. 10-9).

This test provides only a crude estimate of visual fields, and although it would pick up larger field defects, such as hemianopsias, quadrantanopsias, or large scotomas, it does not ascertain small lesions or changes. Hemianopsia is blindness for one half the field of vision in one eye or in both eyes. Quadrantanopsia is blindness in one fourth the field of vision in one eye or in both eyes. A scotoma is an islandlike blind area in the visual field. Thus, clinical use of this test is limited to gross screening. Any suspicions of decreasing peripheral vision, such as occurs with glaucoma and some brain lesions, should be referred for the more accurate quantitative measurements that can be performed with a perimeter or tangent screen. These tests are more useful for detecting, evaluating, and following visual pathway damage, whereas the confrontation method may fail to detect early evidence of damage, possibly delaying timely intervention.

Extraocular Muscle Function

There are three aspects to the assessment of extraocular muscle function: the corneal light reflex, the six cardinal positions of gaze, and the cover-uncover test. Basic to each of these is the observation of the parallelism of the eyes and ocular movements.

Corneal light reflex

The parallelism, or alignment, of the anteroposterior axes of the two eyes can be assessed by observing the reflection of a light from the cornea. The client is requested to stare straight ahead while the examiner shines a penlight on the corneas from a distance of 12 to 15 in. The bright dot of light reflected from the shiny surface of the corneas should be located in a symmetric position, for example, at the 1 o'clock position in the right eye and the 11 o'clock position in the left eye. An asymmetric reflex will indicate a deviating eye and a probable muscle imbalance. A weak or paralyzed extraocular muscle is a cause of ocular deviation.

Six cardinal positions of gaze

The second mode of assessing muscle function is movement of the eyes through the six cardinal positions of gaze:

$$
\begin{array}{ccc}
& SR \rightarrow IO & \quad IO \rightarrow SR \\
LR \; {}_{5}\nearrow \quad {}_{6} \qquad {}_{1}\searrow & \quad {}_{6}\nearrow \quad {}_{1}\searrow \\
\quad {}_{5}\swarrow \quad {}_{4} \qquad {}_{3} \; {}_{2}\, MR & {}_{5}\nwarrow \quad {}_{4} \qquad {}_{3} \; {}_{2}\, LR \\
IR \leftarrow SO & \quad SO \leftarrow IR
\end{array}
$$

Right eye   **Left eye**

These six positions are used because the muscle indicated is weak or paralyzed if the eye will not turn to that particular position. As stated earlier, the normal eye muscles work in yoked fashion, so that when the left eye is moved to the upward and outward position, the right eye moves to the upward and inward position.

The client is asked to follow a small object held by the examiner, which is moved to each position in a clockwise fashion. The client holds the head in a fixed position, and only the eyes follow the examiner's object. The examiner asks the client to fix the gaze momentarily in the extreme position of each of the six positions; and while the client is doing so, the examiner notes any jerking movements of the eye, or nystagmus. On extreme lateral gaze, some eyes will develop a rhythmic twitching motion, known as end-position nystagmus. A few beats of nystagmus on extreme lateral gaze are normal, but any other nystagmus is abnormal. Three of the six positions are illustrated in Fig. 10-10.

After examining the extraocular muscles in the six cardinal positions, the examiner observes the relationship of the upper eyelid to the globe while directing the client's eyes from an upward to a downward gaze. The lid should overlap the iris slightly throughout this movement; no sclera should show between the iris and the upper lid.

Cover-uncover test

A third, more delicate method of assessing muscle function is the cover-uncover test. Maintenance of parallel eyes is a result of the fusion reflex, which makes binocular vision possible. If a muscle imbalance is present and the fusion reflex is blocked when one eye is covered, this weakness can be observed.

The examiner asks the client to look at a specific fixation point, such as the examiner's nose, with both eyes. Then the examiner covers one eye with an opaque card or eye cover and while doing so observes the uncovered eye to see if it moves to fix on the object (Fig. 10-11, *A*). If it does move, then it was not straight before the other eye was covered. The examiner then removes the opaque cover from the covered eye and observes for any movement of the eye just uncovered (Fig. 10-11, *B*). When an eye is covered, the appearance of an object on that retina is suppressed. The eye relaxes, and if there is a weak tendency in one of the extraocular muscles, the eye drifts to another resting position. Then, when the

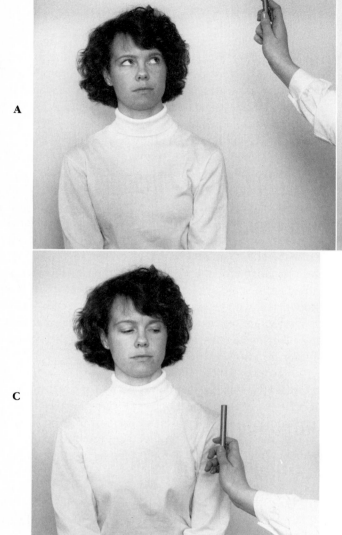

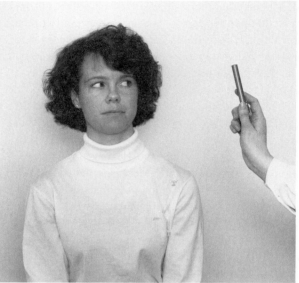

Figure 10-10

To assess extraocular muscle function, the examiner directs the client's gaze into the six cardinal positions. Shown here: upward and left (**A**), left lateral (**B**), and downward and left (**C**). The client's gaze is then directed to the right in these three positions.

Ocular Structures

The ocular structures to be examined include the eyelashes and eyelids, the conjunctiva, the cornea, the anterior chamber, the lacrimal apparatus, the sclera, the iris, the pupil, the lens, the vitreous body, and the retina.

Examination of outermost structures

Eyelids and eyelashes. The functions of the lids are to protect and lubricate the anterior portions of the globe. They are inspected for the ability to close completely, for position and color, and for any lesions, infection, or edema. When the lids do not close properly, drying of the cornea may result in serious damage.

The examiner observes for equality in the height of the palpebral fissures. The margins of the upper lids normally fall between the superior pupil margin and the superior limbus.

Raised yellow plaques, 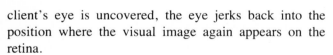 xanthelasma, may appear on the lids near the inner canthi; these grow slowly and may disappear spontaneously.

It is at this time that the position of the globe, whether it is normal, prominent, or sunken, can be most easily observed.

client's eye is uncovered, the eye jerks back into the position where the visual image again appears on the retina.

The examiner then repeats this procedure on the other eye.

Color Vision Testing

Suspected defects in color vision, or screening for certain industrial or vehicle operation jobs, should include testing with color plates. These plates have numbers outlined in one color surrounded by confusion colors that are similar in color or intensity. The individual with a color vision deficiency is unable to see the number (Ichikawa and associates, 1978).

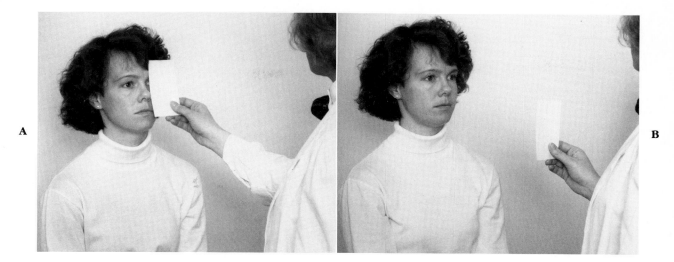

Figure 10-11
Cover-uncover test.

The distribution, condition, and position of the eyelashes are noted. The eyelashes should be evenly distributed and should curve outward.

Conjunctiva.   The bulbar and palpebral portions of the conjunctiva are examined by separating the lids widely and having the client look up, down, and to each side. When separating the lids, the examiner should exert no pressure against the eyeball; rather, the examiner should hold the lids against the ridges of the bony orbit surrounding the eye (Fig. 10-12). The client is then instructed to direct the gaze upward and to each side. Many small blood vessels are normally visible through the clear conjunctiva. The white sclera is, of course, visible through the bulbar portion.

Although eversion of the upper lid is not a necessary part of the normal or screening examination, the beginning examiner should learn a careful technique for performing lid eversion when it is indicated. The entire procedure should be explained to the client before it is begun, and reassurance should be given during the process. In the absence of gentleness, carefulness, and reassurance, the client is very likely to become tense when the sensitive eye structures are manipulated, thereby making the examination much more difficult for all persons involved.

Eversion of the upper eyelid is performed as follows (Fig. 10-13).

1. Ask the client to look down but to keep the eyes slightly open. This relaxes the levator muscle, whereas closing the eyes contracts the orbicularis muscle, preventing lid eversion.
2. Gently grasp the upper eyelashes and pull gently

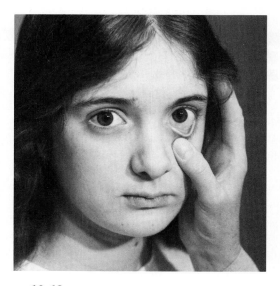

Figure 10-12

The examiner inspects the conjunctiva by moving the lower lid downward over the bony orbit.

downward. Do not pull the lashes outward or upward; this, too, causes muscle contraction.

3. Place a cotton-tipped applicator about 1 cm above the lid margin on the upper tarsal border and push gently downward with the applicator while still holding the lashes. This everts the lid.
4. Hold the lashes of the everted lid against the upper ridge of the bony orbit, just beneath the eyebrow, never pushing against the eyeball.
5. Examine the lid for swelling, infection, or a foreign object.

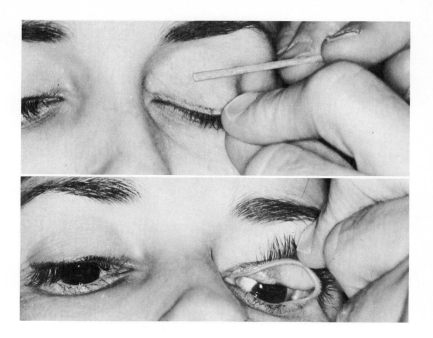

6. To return the lid to its normal position, move the lashes slightly forward and ask the client to look up and then to blink. The lid returns easily to a normal position.

Sclera.   The sclera is easily observed during assessment of the conjunctiva. It is normally white, although some pigmented deposits are within the range of normal.

Cornea.   The cornea is best observed by directing the light of a penlight at it obliquely from several positions. The cornea should be transparent, smooth, shiny, and bright. There should be no irregularities in the surface, and the features of the iris should be fully visible through the cornea. In older persons the appearance of arcus senilis is normal. Arcus senilis is a white ring located around the periphery of the cornea; it is composed of lipid deposits.

Testing of the corneal reflex may be reserved for later in the eye examination, after all external structures are checked, but is discussed here as part of the complete assessment of the cornea. Corneal sensitivity is tested by bringing a wisp of cotton from the lateral side of the eye and brushing it lightly across the corneal surface (Fig. 10-14). The normal response is lid closure of both eyes when either eye is brushed. A different wisp of cotton should be used for each eye.

Anterior chamber.   The anterior chamber is easily observed in conjunction with the cornea. The technique of oblique illumination is also useful in assessing the anterior chamber. This, too, is a transparent structure. Any visible material in it is abnormal. The depth of the

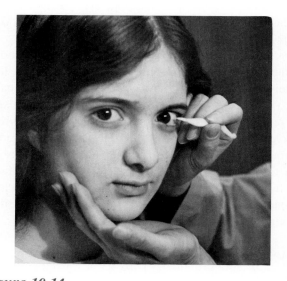

Figure 10-14

Testing for corneal sensitivity, the examiner brings in a wisp of cotton from the side and lightly brushes it over the cornea.

chamber should be noted by looking at the eye from the side instead of from directly in front. The depth is the distance between the cornea and the iris. From a side view, the iris should appear quite flat and should not be bulging forward (see Fig. 10-29, *A*).

Lacrimal apparatus.   Of the various components of the lacrimal apparatus, including the lacrimal gland, the puncta, the lacrimal sac, and the nasolacrimal duct, only the puncta can normally be observed. These

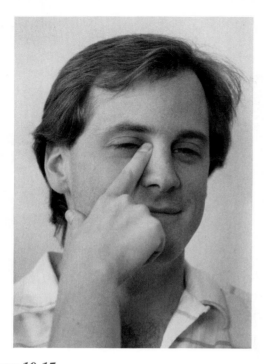

Figure 10-15

To examine the lacrimal sac, the examiner presses with the index finger against the client's lower inner orbital rim, *not* against the nose.

are located on the upper and lower nasal margins of the lids.

Blockage of the nasolacrimal duct can be checked by pressing against the lacrimal sac with the index finger or cotton-tipped applicator inside the lower inner orbital rim, not against the side of the nose (Fig. 10-15). In the presence of blockage, this will cause regurgitation of material through the puncta.

Iris. The iris should be observed for shape and coloration.

Pupils. Examination of the pupils involves several observations, including assessment of their size, shape, reaction to light, and accommodation.

The pupils are normally round and equal in size. The pupillary response to light consists of both a direct and consensual reaction. The beam of a penlight is brought in from the side and directed on one eye at a time. The eye toward which the light is directed is observed for the direct response of constriction. Simultaneously, the other eye is observed for a consensual response of constriction. Each eye is observed for both the direct and consensual response. Normally, both responses are present; however, the rapidity with which the pupils respond does vary. A room that can be darkened to facilitate dilatation is helpful in assessing constriction in

The notation *PERRLA* stands for *pupils equal, round, react to light,* and *accommodate.*

response to light; a sunny, well-lighted room can make assessment of constriction responses very difficult.

The test for pupillary accommodation is the examination for change in pupillary size as the gaze is switched from a distant to a near object. It is performed by asking the client to stare at an object across the room. Visualization of a distant object normally causes pupillary dilatation. The client is then asked to fix the gaze on the examiner's index finger, which is placed 5 to 6 in from the client's nose. The normal response is pupillary constriction and convergence of the eyes. The rapidity of the response varies; the response is slower in older persons.

Ophthalmoscopic examination

Examination of other ocular structures includes observation of the lens, the vitreous body, and the retinal structures and is performed with an ophthalmoscope.

The instrument and its assembly. The head of an ophthalmoscope and the five apertures that may be available are shown in Fig. 10-16. The ophthalmoscope head is seated in the handle by fitting the handle into the ophthalmoscope head. Push the head in the direction of the handle while turning in a clockwise direction until the stop is felt.

The ophthalmoscope is turned on by depressing the button on the rheostat and turning the rheostat clockwise to the appropriate intensity of light. The instrument is turned off after use to prevent shortening the useful life of the bulb and the battery life in battery-operated ophthalmoscopes. The beginner may become familiar with the apertures by projecting them onto a piece of paper. The aperture may be changed by moving the aperture selection lever.

The structure being examined is brought into focus by rotating the lens selector dial until the image becomes clear. The instrument may be held and focused with one hand. On the front of the ophthalmoscope head is an illuminated aperture displaying the number of the lens in position before the viewing aperture. The value of the lens is indicated in diopters. Black numbers are for positive values; red figures are for negative values.

When the lens selector is rotated clockwise beginning with zero (0) the positive numbers ($+1$, $+2$, $+3$, $+4$, $+5$, $+6$, $+8$, $+10$, $+12$, $+15$, $+20$, $+40$) appear, and when the selector is rotated counterclockwise

Figure 10-16

The head and five apertures of an ophthalmoscope. **A,** Hemispot is used for small pupil examinations and to aid in eliminating the corneal light reflex. **B,** Full spot is provided in two different sizes. The small one is used for undilated pupils or to eliminate the corneal reflex in examination of the macula. The large one is used for dilated pupils. The large beam is the one most frequently used because it provides a wide field for the general fundus examination. **C,** Red-free filter is a green beam used for examining the optic disc for pallor and the retina for hemorrhages. Hemorrhages appear black with the red-free filter, whereas melanin deposits appear gray. **D,** Fixation star and polar co-ordinates (grid) are used to determine the fixation pattern and for relating the characteristics, size, and location of fundal lesions. **E,** Slit is used for examining the anterior segment of the eye and for determining the elevation or depression of fundal lesions.

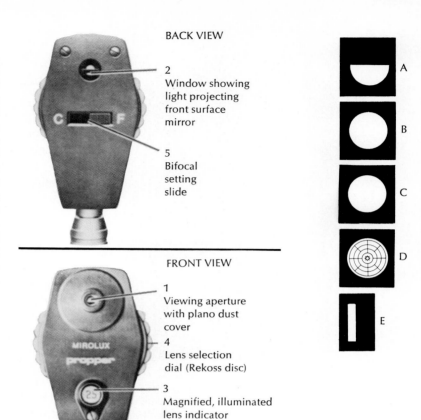

BACK VIEW

2
Window showing
light projecting
front surface
mirror

5
Bifocal
setting
slide

FRONT VIEW

1
Viewing aperture
with plano dust
cover

4
Lens selection
dial (Rekoss disc)

3
Magnified, illuminated
lens indicator

6
Aperture
selection

A
B
C
D
E

from zero (0) the negative numbers (-1, -2, -3, -4, -5, -6, -8, -10, -15, -20, -25) are seen.

The lens system can compensate for hyperopia or myopia. However, there is no correction for astigmatism.

Examination with the ophthalmoscope. The examination with the ophthalmoscope is best accomplished in a semidarkened or darkened room. If darkening the room does not adequately dilate the client's pupils, 10% phenylephrine hydrochloride, 0.5% Mydriacyl, or 1% Cyclogyl drops may be instilled in the client's eyes. Before using dilating drops, however, it is absolutely essential to rule out any suspicion of glaucoma. If the client wears corrective lenses, the examination may be done either with or without them. It is generally easier to perform the examination without the client's glasses on unless there is a high degree of astigmatism. The client's contact lenses may be left in place on the cornea. The examiner may choose to perform the retinal examination wearing or not wearing his or her own corrective lenses. Both ways should be tried to determine which is more satisfactory to the examiner.

Use of the ophthalmoscope (see also Chapter 1). The head of the ophthalmoscope is equipped with a series of lenses that are changed by moving the round, white wheel. The 0 lens is clear glass; the red, or negative, numbers focus farther away; and the black, or positive, numbers focus closer to the ophthalmoscope. Several apertures and filters for the light are built into most ophthalmoscopes; however, the round aperture with white light is best for most examinations. The examiner should read the manual accompanying the ophthalmoscope for information on other apertures and filters. The light should be turned to maximum brightness unless the client cannot tolerate it.

The client's cooperation is essential to the performance of this examination. The client is asked to stare directly ahead at some object across the room, such as the light switch or the corner of a picture. This assists in two ways: staring at a distant point encourages dilatation of the pupils, and staring at one fixed point helps to prevent the eyes from rotating and moving about so much that it is impossible for the examiner to focus on any of the retinal structures.

The client is told to blink from time to time during the examination. If blinking becomes so frequent that it is difficult to visualize the retinal structures, the examiner

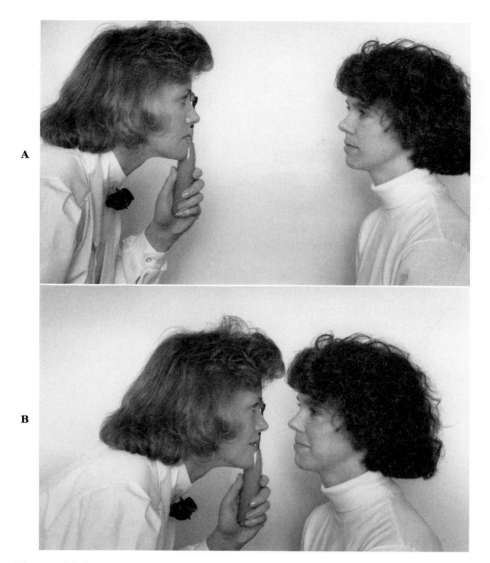

Figure 10-17

A, The examiner uses the ophthalmoscope to inspect the lens and vitreous body from a distance of about 12 inches. The examiner uses the left eye and left hand to examine the client's left eye. **B,** Moving in closer to the client's eye, the examiner studies the retinal structures.

may elevate the upper lid and hold it against the upper orbital rim.

The examiner holds the ophthalmoscope in the right hand and to the right eye to examine the client's right eye, and in the left hand and to the left eye to examine the client's left eye. The examiner initially sets the ophthalmoscope lens at 0, holds the viewing aperture directly in front of the eye with the top of the ophthalmoscope against the forehead, and begins about 12 inches away from the client's eye (Fig. 10-17, *A*). The index finger of the hand holding the ophthalmoscope rests on the lens wheel to permit focusing during the examination.

The bright circle of light is flashed on the eye through the pupil; a red glow, the red reflex, is visible through the pupil of the normal eye. While continuing to focus on the red reflex, the examiner moves close to the eye being examined (Fig. 10-17, *B*). If the examiner loses sight of the red reflex, it is usually because the light is no longer directed through the pupil and is resting instead on the iris or sclera. If this occurs, it is easiest to relocate the red reflex by backing away several inches and redirecting the beam of light. As the examiner moves close to the eye, the lenses are rotated to the positive numbers (+15 to +20), which focus on the near objects. At this setting the anterior chamber and lens are examined for transparency; there should be no clouding or opacities.

Gradually rotating the lens back toward 0, the examiner also observes the vitreous body for transparency. At this setting the examiner begins to look for some retinal structure, such as a vessel or the disc. Once some structure is located, the lens wheel is rotated until it is brought into focus. In a myopic or nearsighted person, whose eyeball is more elongated than normal, the more negative lenses will be needed to focus farther back. In a farsighted client the lens wheel is rotated toward the positive numbers. Focusing is quite individual and does depend on the refractive status of both the client and the examiner.

Often, a vessel is detected first and can be followed in toward the optic disc. If the examiner directs the beam of light through the pupil in a slightly nasalward direction, the beam will fall on or near the optic disc initially.

Retinal structures.   Examination of the various retinal structures should be performed in a consistent and orderly fashion. The following order is recommended: (1) optic disc, (2) retinal vessels, (3) retinal background, and (4) macular area.

The disc is examined for its size, shape, color, the distinctness of its margins, and the physiologic cup. The disc is also used as a standard measurement device. The distance from the disc and the size of other findings are estimated in terms of disc diameters (DD); for example, an alteration slightly larger than the disc situated in the upper portion of the fundus may be described as being 1 × 2 DD in size and 3 DD away from the disc at 1:30 (clock position) in the left eye (Fig. 10-18).

The retinal vessels are examined for their color; the A:V ratio is determined; arteriovenous crossings are examined for indentations; and the arterioles are examined for their light reflex. Each set of vessels should be followed out from the disc to the periphery. The retinal background is examined for its color and regularity of appearance and for any areas of light or dark color alterations. The more peripheral reaches of the vessels and retinal background can be examined by having the client direct the gaze upward, downward, and to each side. Observation of the macular area is reserved for last, because having a bright light directed at the center of acutest vision is very uncomfortable for the client. The macula is about 1 DD in size and is located 2 DD temporal to the optic disc. It appears as an avascular area with the bright spot of light reflected from its center, the fovea. This area can be examined by having the client look directly at the examining light. When the client does so,

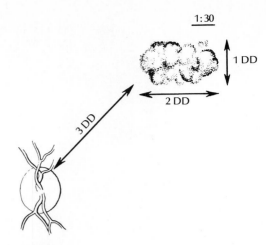

Figure 10-18

Method of giving position and dimensions of a lesion in terms of disc diameters.
(From Havener WH: Synopsis of ophthalmology, ed 6, St Louis, 1984, The CV Mosby Co.)

the examiner is visualizing the macula. (See color plate of eye.)

Intraocular Pressure

Screening for intraocular pressure is best accomplished with the Schiøtz tonometer, which measures the ease with which the cornea may be indented by the plunger of the instrument (Fig. 10-19). A soft eye is easily indented; a hard eye is indented with greater difficulty. Instructions accompanying the instrument on measurement and cleaning should be followed carefully.

For an accurate tonometry reading, the client should be either recumbent or reclining in a chair. A tight collar or tie must be loosened to avoid an artificial increase in intraocular pressure caused by impeded venous return from the jugular system. If contact lenses are worn, they should be removed. Before proceeding, the examiner explains the procedure to the client. The cornea of each eye is then anesthetized by instilling a drop of a topical anesthetic such as proparacaine hydrochloride. Any tearing may be blotted with a tissue, but the eye should not be rubbed. The client is then asked to fix the gaze directly overhead and to breathe regularly. The examiner uses the thumb and index finger of one hand to hold the client's upper and lower lids against the bony orbital rim; with the other hand, the footplate of the vertically held tonometer is placed lightly on the center of the cornea (Fig. 10-20). The reading is taken, and the footplate is lifted, not slid, off the cornea. The lower the reading on the tonometer scale, the greater the pressure. The tonometer should be carefully cleaned after each procedure.

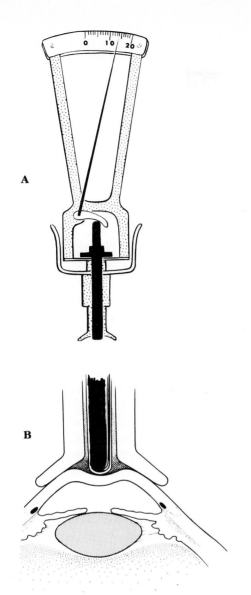

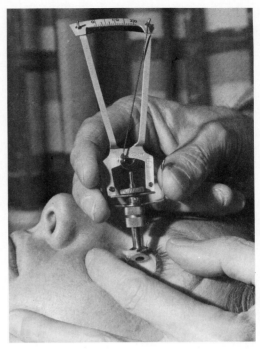

Figure 10-20

Screening for intraocular pressure.
(From Prior JA, Silberstein JS, and Stang JM: Physical diagnosis: the history and examination of the patient, ed 6, St Louis, 1981, The CV Mosby Co.)

Figure 10-19

A, Schiøtz tonometer in which the plunger, in black, measures the ease of indentation of the cornea. **B,** Indentation of the anesthetized cornea by the plunger of the tonometer to measure ocular tension. (From Newell FW: Ophthalmology: principles and concepts, ed 5, St Louis, 1986, The CV Mosby Co.)

It should be remembered that examination of the depth of the anterior chamber, assessment of the visual fields, and examination of the optic nerve head are also components of the examination for increased intraocular pressure, or glaucoma.

All persons over 40 years of age should be checked regularly by tonometry. Glaucoma is a major cause of blindness, and although it cannot be reversed, it can be halted.

Variations from Health

Variations from health in the function and the various structures of the eye will be addressed.

The following conditions are contraindications to performing tonometry:
1. Any ocular infection or discharge
2. Recent ocular injury
3. Herpes on the face or eyelids
4. Corneal edema, distortion, thickening, or scarring
5. Marked nystagmus
6. Uncontrollable coughing
7. Significant apprehension or blepharospasm

DISTURBANCES OF VISUAL FUNCTION

Abnormalities of visual function include numerous variations, among which the following are not uncommon:
1. Diminished visual acuity
2. Decreased central or peripheral vision
3. Defects in color vision
4. Diplopia, or double vision
5. Faulty adaptation to the dark

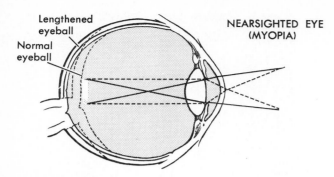

Figure 10-21

Nearsighted, or myopic, eye focuses the image in front of the retina. This may occur when the eyeball is too long or the lens is too thick. Correction is by concave lens.
(From Anthony CP and Thibodeau GA: Textbook of anatomy and physiology, ed 12, St Louis, 1987, The CV Mosby Co.)

6. Visualization of objects within the eye
7. Iridescent vision, "halos"

Diminished Visual Acuity

Error of refraction is a common variation from normal vision. This is an inability to focus rays of light on the retina under the stated conditions. Common errors of refraction include nearsightedness, farsightedness, and astigmatism.

Nearsightedness

In this condition, also known as myopia, the eye focuses the image in front of the retina. This can occur when the eyeball is too long or the lens is too thick (Fig. 10-21).

Farsightedness

In this condition, also known as hyperopia, the eye focuses the image at a hypothetical distance behind the retina. This can occur when the eyeball is too short or the lens is too thin (Fig. 10-22). As people age, they typically become farsighted as the lens becomes more rigid, losing its elasticity. The ciliary muscles become weaker, and the lens cannot bulge to accommodate for near vision. This condition is known as presbyopia.

Astigmatism

This occurs when there is uneven curvature of the cornea or the lens, causing rays to be focused at different points on the retina.

Decreased Central or Peripheral Vision

Defects in the field of vision may be caused by lesions of the retina, lesions along the optic nerve, at the optic chiasm where portions of each nerve cross over to the opposite side, along the optic tract, or in the occipital

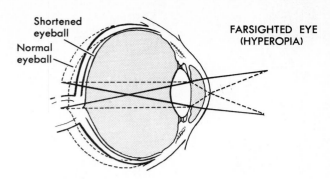

Figure 10-22

The farsighted, or hyperopic, eye could only focus the image at a hypothetical distance behind the retina. This may occur when the eyeball is too short or the lens is too thin. Correction is by convex lens.
(From Anthony CP and Thibodeau GA: Textbook of anatomy and physiology, ed 2, St Louis, 1987, The CV Mosby Co.)

lobes (Fig. 10-23). The resulting defect in vision may be central or peripheral, depending on the lesion's nature and location. Peripheral defects are described as temporal, nasal, superior, or inferior. The visual field reflects the visual function in the opposite areas of the retina involved. Therefore, a temporal visual field defect reflects a defect of the nasal retina, and a superior field defect reflects an inferior retinal defect. Likewise, an inferior nasal retinal defect would cause a defect in the superior temporal field of vision.

If the lesion is in the retina of one eye or along one optic nerve anterior to the chiasm, vision is affected in that eye. Lesions occurring at the optic chiasm, along the optic tract, or in the occipital lobes affect the visual fields of both eyes because of the crossing and mixing of fibers from both eyes at the chiasm. Lesions at the optic chiasm, as from a pituitary tumor, cause a loss of vision from the nasal portion of each retina, resulting in a loss of both temporal fields of vision. This condition is called *bitemporal hemianopsia* (Gk, *hemi*, half; *an*, negative; *opsi*, vision).

Nerve fibers from both eyes mingle behind the chiasm in the optic tracts and in the brain. Lesions along the optic tract or in the temporal, parietal, or occipital lobes will impair the same half of the field of vision in both eyes. For example, a lesion of the right optic tract or right side of the brain will result in visual field defects in the right nasal field and in the left temporal field. This condition is termed *homonymous hemianopsia* and may be caused by occlusion of the middled cerebral artery. The effects of such lesions on the field of vision are illustrated in Fig. 10-24.

The location of disease on the retina determines the type of resultant visual field defects. Macular defects

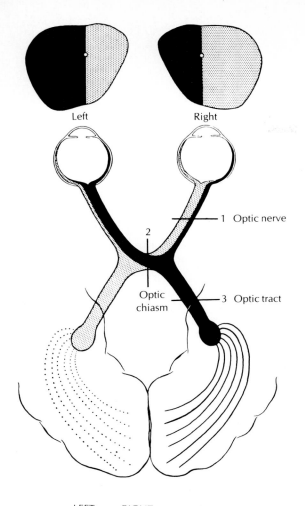

Left

Right

1 Optic nerve

2

Optic chiasm

3 Optic tract

Figure 10-23

Visual field defects. *1*, Blind right eye; *2*, bitemporal hemianopia—no temporal vision; *3*, left homonymous hemianopia—no vision in left field of either eye.

(Adapted from Havener WH: Synopsis of ophthalmology, ed 6, St Louis, 1984, The CV Mosby Co.)

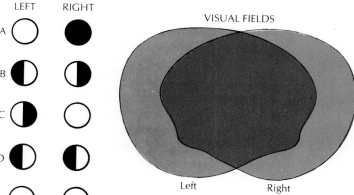

LEFT   RIGHT

A

B

C

D

E

F

A—Total blindness of right eye

B—Bitemporal hemianopsia

C—Left nasal hemianopsia

D—Left homonymous hemianopsia

E—Left homonymous hemianopsia inferior quadrant

F—Left homonymous hemianopsia superior quadrant

VISUAL FIELDS

Left   Right

Figure 10-24

Visual fields showing optic nerve, optic chiasm, optic tracks, and optic radiations. Examples of various visual field defects.

(From Rudy EB: Advanced neurological and neurosurgical nursing, St Louis, 1984, The CV Mosby Co.)

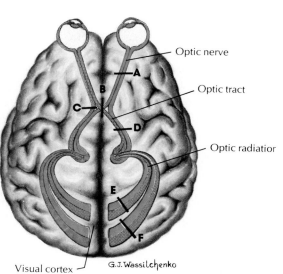

Optic nerve

A

B

Optic tract

C

D

Optic radiation

E

F

Visual cortex   G.J.Wassilchenko

lead to a central blind area. Localized damage in other areas of the retina will cause a loss of vision corresponding to the involved area. A blind spot is known as a scotoma, that is, an area of blindness surrounded by an area of vision. Advanced diabetic retinopathy may cause macular damage, resulting in a loss of central vision. Glaucoma, or increased intraocular pressure, causes decreased peripheral vision because of the damage caused by the elevated pressure. As the disease advances, it may also cause a loss of central vision. A retinal detachment will cause loss of vision from that portion of the retina where the detachment occurs.

Blindness

Generally, a person is considered legally blind when the best visual acuity with corrective lenses in the better eye is 20/200 or less, or when the peripheral visual field is constricted to within 20 degrees. Major causes of blindness in North America are glaucoma, unoperated cataract, and retinal disorders, mainly diabetic retinopathy and macular degeneration.

Defects in Color Vision

A variety of conditions may disturb color vision, including diseases of the optic nerve, the fovea centralis, and macular area where the cones are most highly concentrated and nutritional disturbances. In macular degeneration, the decrease in color vision parallels the loss of visual acuity. The color-deficient person is unable to see the figures on color plates, which are easily recognizable to the person with normal color vision.

Diplopia

Double vision occurs whenever the visual axes are not directed simultaneously to the same object. It is a cardinal sign of weakness of one or more of the extraocular muscles and occurs only if binocular vision has developed.

Faulty Adaptation to Light or Dark

Night blindness is caused by pigmentary degeneration of the retina, optic nerve disease, glaucoma, or vitamin A deficiency occurring because of inadequate nutrition or cirrhosis of the liver. A client may complain of slow recovery of vision experienced during nighttime driving after the headlights of a passing car shine in the eyes.

Visualization of Objects Within the Eye

Translucent specks of various shapes and sizes that float across the visual field and can be seen only when the eye is open are called *floaters*. Small remnants of hyaloid vascular system in the vitreous humor, they can be seen

Table 10-2

Diagnostic clues to dysfunction of extraocular neuromuscular units

Position to which eye will not turn	Muscle	Cranial nerve
Straight nasal	Medial rectus	III
Up and nasal	Interior oblique	III
Down and nasal	Superior oblique	IV
Straight temporal	Lateral rectus	VI
Up and temporal	Superior rectus	III
Down and temporal	Inferior rectus	III

as small dots that dart away as one tries to look at them. Sudden showers of floaters may occur in the periphery of the visual field with vitreous hemorrhage. This may be the initial symptom of hole formation preceding retinal separation. The location of the floaters may be helpful in locating the retinal tear. The sudden appearance of a moderately large floater is the main symptom of vitreous detachment.

Iridescent Vision

This term describes the halos or rainbows that are seen surrounding bright lights when there is corneal edema. This may follow a rapid increase in intraocular pressure with acute glaucoma, after prolonged wearing of hard contact lenses, with corneal abrasion, and with cataracts.

EXTRAOCULAR NEUROMUSCULAR FUNCTION

An asymmetric corneal light reflex, an inability of the eyes to move in parallel fashion to the six cardinal positions of gaze, or an abnormal cover test indicates a weakness or paralysis of one or more of the extraocular muscles or a defect in the nerve supplying it. Table 10-2 indicates the muscle and cranial nerve involved when the eye will not turn to one of these six positions.

Examples of the effects of nerve lesions are as follows:
1. *Oculomotor paralysis (CN III):* the eye turns down and out with drooping of the upper lid.
2. *Abducens paralysis (CN VI):* the eye turns in toward the nose because of unopposed action of the medial rectus.

Carrying the fixation point of the six cardinal positions out to the extremes will exaggerate a defect. A disparity of the anteroposterior axes of the eyes is called strabismus. Deviations in these axes may be detected during the cover test, which blocks the fusion reflex of

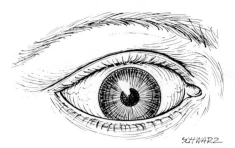

Figure 10-25

Lid lag.

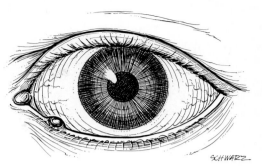

Figure 10-26

Hordeolum or sty.

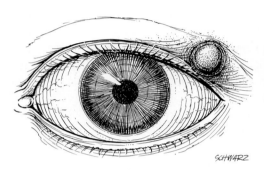

Figure 10-27

Chalazion.

the eyes. A mild weakness of the extraocular muscles is called *phoria*. If there is a weak tendency during the cover test, a definitely perceptible jerk of the eye is noted when the cover is removed. *Tropia* is a more pronounced imbalance producing a permanent disparity in the axes of the eyes. A mild outward deviation of the eye is called *exophoria*; an inward deviation is called *esophoria*. The rhythmic twitching motion of nystagmus may be normal at the end of the lateral position but is abnormal when the eyes are in any other position.

OCULAR STRUCTURES

Eyelids and Eyelashes

Faulty positioning of the eyelids occurs in a variety of ways. The lid margins may fall above or below the middle part of the iris. A drooping lid margin, *ptosis,* that falls at the pupil or below may indicate an oculomotor nerve lesion or a congenital condition. If the lid margin falls above the limbus so that some sclera is visible, thyroid disease may be present. In the presence of thyroid disease the lid may lag behind the limbus as the gaze moves from an upward to a downward position (Fig. 10-25). Another type of faulty positioning of the lids is improper approximation of the lids to the eyeballs. The lids may be loose or lax and roll outward. This condition is called *ectropion*. Because the puncta cannot effectively drain the tears, *epiphora* (tearing) results. The lids may also roll inward because of lid spasm or the contraction of scar tissue. This condition is called *entropion*. Because the lashes are pulled inward, they may produce corneal irritation.

The tissues within the lids are loosely connected and collect excess fluid rather readily. Edema of the lids may be a manifestation of local or systemic disease. Examples of systemic problems that may cause lid edema include allergy, heart failure, nephrosis, and thyroid deficiency.

The glands of the lids may be sites of infection. A localized infection of the small glands around the eye-

lashes in the hair follicle at the lid margin is a hordeolum, or sty (Fig. 10-26). The meibomian glands lying within the posterior portion of the lid may develop an infection or a retention cyst, known as a chalazion (Fig. 10-27); crusting or scaling at the lid margins may occur as a result of staphylococcal infection or seborrheic dermatitis. If a lid infection is present or suspected, the lids may be gently palpated by moving the examining finger across the lid surface. Pressure should never be exerted over the eye in an effort to separate the lids. As mentioned earlier, the bony orbital rims should be used as points over which to slide the lids.

Xanthelasma, the raised yellow plaques that may appear on the lids, may have no pathologic significance, or they may be associated with hypercholesterolemia.

Conjunctiva

Infectious disease of the conjunctiva typically produces engorgement of the conjunctival vessels and a discharge. The infected vessels are usually more pronounced at the fornices. Small subconjunctival hemorrhages may result from more severe involvement, although in some persons these may also result from sneezing, coughing, or lifting.

Sclera

Changes in the color of the sclera may indicate systemic disease. For example, jaundice manifests its presence in the eyes as a yellow discoloration, scleral icterus. Excessive bilirubinemia may be evident as scleral icterus before jaundice of the skin becomes apparent. In the presence of osteogenesis imperfecta the sclera is bluish.

Cornea

The cornea is a very sensitive structure, and pain and photophobia are common manifestations of corneal disease. Any dullness, irregularities, or opacities of the cornea are abnormal. Two of the more frequent abnormalities affecting the cornea are abrasions and opacities. Although an abrasion may cause the surface to look irregular or may cast a shadow on the iris, it may be invisible and detectable only with fluorescein stain. A client suspected

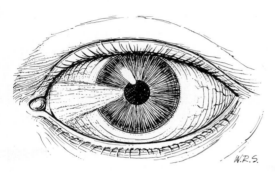

Figure 10-28

Pterygium.

of having corneal abrasion should be referred to an ophthalmologist.

Abnormal growth of bulbar conjunctival tissue from the edge toward the center of the cornea, known as pterygium, may interfere with vision (Fig. 10-28).

Although the presence of arcus senilis is normal in elderly people, in younger individuals it may be associated with abnormal lipid metabolism.

Anterior Chamber

Abnormalities observable in the anterior chamber are a decrease in depth and any foreign material interrupting the normal transparency. A shallow anterior chamber may be a sign of closed-angle glaucoma or may predispose the eye to glaucoma (Fig. 10-29). Symptoms typical of glaucoma include pain, redness, and seeing colored halos around lights. As the increased intraocular pressure causes the iris to become displaced anteriorly, there is less distance between the cornea and the iris. As a result of this anterior displacement, light directed obliquely from the temporal side will illuminate only the temporal side, and the nasal side will appear darker or shadowed. The presence of a shallow anterior chamber is a contraindication to the use of dilating drops for the ophthalmoscopic examination.

Any cloudiness of the aqueous fluid or accumulation of blood (hyphema) or purulent material (hypopyon) is abnormal. Hyphema may be caused by trauma or may result from spontaneous hemorrhage. If the hyphema is mild, the red blood cells settle out inferiorly by gravity to a height of a few millimeters. In severe

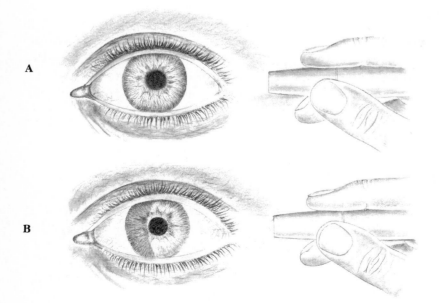

A

B

Figure 10-29

Evaluation of depth of anterior chambers. **A,** Normal anterior chamber. **B,** Shallow anterior chamber. (From Seidel HM and others: Mosby's guide to physical examination, St Louis, 1987, The CV Mosby Co.)

hyphemas, the entire anterior chamber may be filled with blood.

Lacrimal Apparatus

Both the lacrimal gland, which produces tears, and the system that drains the tears are subject to certain abnormalities. The lacrimal gland may be swollen as a result of infection or tumor. Infection with consequent blockage of the lacrimal sac or duct may occur with associated findings of swelling, redness, warmth, pain, and purulent discharge. The swelling tends to occur in the area below the inner canthus. The technique for examining for infection in the lacrimal sac is to press with the examining finger against the *inner* orbital rim (not against the nose), then to gently depress the lower lid over the lower orbital rim to observe for regurgitation of fluid through the puncta.

As mentioned earlier, ectropion may cause tearing because of inadequate drainage. Any unusual markings or growths should be noted. Persistent tearing of an infant's eye suggests either a blocked tear duct or congenital glaucoma.

Iris

Iritis, inflammation of the iris, results in throbbing pain and visual blurring and is associated with the findings of circumcorneal injection, a deep pinkish red flush about the cornea, and a constricted pupil. This is in contrast to conjunctivitis, wherein the infected vessels tend to extend from the periphery toward the center. The iris may become inflamed because of bacterial infections, which may also lead to the production of a purulent exudate, as well as to diffuse congestion around the iris. If the lens has been removed, the normal support of the iris is absent and the iris will, with movements of the eye, have a tremulous, fluttering motion

Pupils

Abnormalities of the pupils include alterations in size and in reflexes. Although a slight but noticeable difference in pupil size does occur in about 5% of the population, this finding should be regarded with suspicion because it can be an indication of central nervous system (CNS) disease. Inequality in the size of the pupils is known as *anisocoria. Dyscoria* is a congenital abnormality in the shape of the pupils.

Mydriasis, enlargement of the pupils, may result from emotional influences, recent or old local trauma, acute glaucoma, systemic reaction to parasympatholytic or sympathomimetic drugs, or the local use of dilating drops. A unilateral fixed enlarged pupil may be caused by local trauma to the eye or head injury. Fixed dilation of both eyes occurs with deep anesthesia, CNS injury, and circulatory arrest.

Miosis, constriction of the pupils, is associated with iritis, use of morphine, and glaucoma treatment by pilocarpine and is seen physiologically with sleep.

Any irregularity in pupil contour is abnormal and may result from iritis, trauma, CNS syphilis, or congenital defects.

Failure of the pupils to react to light with preservation of the accommodation reaction is another characteristic of CNS syphilis. This is known as the *Argyll Robertson pupil*.

In the case of monocular blindness, the blind eye and optic tract will transmit no response to light, and neither pupil will constrict. However, when the unaffected eye receives illumination, both pupils will constrict because the efferent pupil constriction stimuli are distributed evenly to both eyes.

Lens

Opacities in any of the clear portions of the eye (anterior chamber, lens, or vitreous body) will appear as dark shadows on black spots within the red reflex on ophthalmoscopic examination because they prevent light from being reflected back to the examiner's eye. An opacity within the lens is referred to as a cataract. These opacities vary in appearance; some look like pieces of coral, some look like various-shaped crystals, and others have a stellate, or starlike, appearance. Cataract formation may be associated with various systemic disorders, may occur as the complex of findings in various hereditary syndromes, or may result from senescent changes within the lens. In certain endocrine disorders, such as diabetes mellitus, the metabolic disturbance results in abnormal lens fiber formation and cataracts. Such cataracts typically attack young persons more frequently than older persons, are bilateral, progress rapidly, and have a classic snowflake appearance. Senile cataracts occur as a result of various degenerative processes within the lenticular material. Typical symptoms include cloudiness of vision, particularly in bright light, a decrease in the visual field, and occasionally the appearance of black spots with movements of the eyes. Because of the increase in the size of the lens with a maturing cataract, the depth of the anterior chamber may be diminished, thus precipitating glaucoma. (See color plate of eye.)

Retinal Structures

Optic disc

Three of the major conditions causing alterations of the optic disc are papilledema, glaucoma, and optic atrophy. Papilledema, or swelling of the optic nerve head, causes

Blurred disc margin

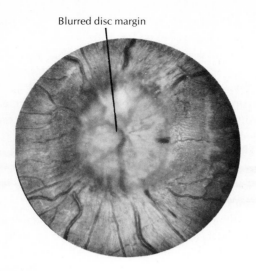

Figure 10-30

Papilledema.
(From Newell FW: Ophthalmology: principles and concepts, ed 5, St Louis, 1982, The CV Mosby Co.)

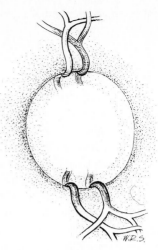

Figure 10-31

Glaucomatous cupping.

the margins of the disc to become blurred and indistinct (Fig. 10-30). The nerve head appears out of focus with the surrounding retina. The degree of elevation can be assessed by focusing first on the disc and then on the surrounding retina and noting the difference in diopters on the ophthalmoscope.

Papilledema is a sign of increased intracranial pressure. This causes decreased venous drainage from the eye, hence venous stasis, or the accumulation and leakage of fluid, leading to edematous appearance of the disc. This condition may be associated with malignant hypertension, eclampsia, brain tumor, and hematoma.

The increased intraocular pressure of glaucoma gradually exerts pressure anteriorly against the iris, as mentioned earlier, and posteriorly against the optic disc, causing increasing cupping (Fig. 10-31). This may be noted by observing the course of vessels as they emerge from the center and over the disc margins, since glaucoma may cause a vessel to seem to disappear from sight at the disc rim and then reappear at a slightly different site just past the rim. The pressure of glaucoma may also eventually cause pallor of the disc, a sign of optic atrophy. Advanced cupping and optic atrophy are late findings of the disease; the early findings are very subtle and are likely to be very difficult to recognize. Thus, the need for careful tonometry as a far more sensitive indicator is reemphasized.

Death of the optic nerve fibers leads to the disappearance of the tiny disc vessels that give the disc its normal pinkish color and results in optic pallor. The disc appears pale and white, either in a section or throughout. NOTE: The scleral crescent, a normal, crescent-shaped

area around the rim of the disc only, should not be mistaken for disc pallor.

Retinal vessels

Changes in caliber and alterations at crossings can occur in the retinal vessels. Changes in these vascular structures often indicate systemic diseases, such as hypertension. Because any vessel caliber changes may not be evenly distributed along the course of the vessel, vessels should be observed from the disc to the periphery. Arterioles, normally about two thirds to three fourths of the diameter of the corresponding veins, are subject to a decrease in diameter as a result of constriction of the vessels or reduced blood flow to the eye. In hypertension, arterioles may become narrowed to a 3:5 or 2:4 or less ratio. More rarely, veins may increase in diameter as a result of conditions causing more blood to circulate to the eye or conditions impeding the exit of blood from the eye.

The condition of the arteriole vessel walls determines their color. Normally, they are transparent and reflect the color of the column of blood within, but they may develop sclerotic or sheathing changes, causing them to become opaque and lighter. The width of the light reflex from the arteriolar wall also increases with arteriosclerosis to one third or more of the width of the vessel. In advanced stages, the vessels may appear as fine, silvery lines.

Changes at arteriolovenous crossings include an apparent narrowing or blocking of the vein where an arteriole crosses over it. This appearance is the result of some degree of concealment of the underlying veins by an abnormally opaque arteriole wall and occurs with longstanding hypertension; it is initially apparent as venous narrowing and later as a more complete interruption of

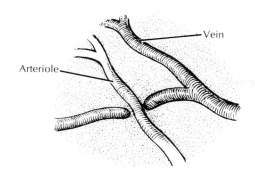

Figure 10-32

Arteriovenous nicking.

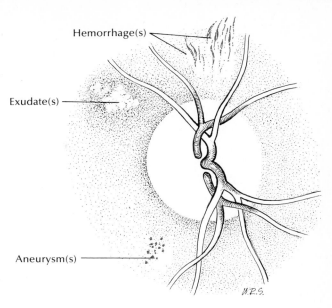

Figure 10-33

Abnormalities of the retinal background: microaneurysms, exudates, and hemorrhages.

the vessel. These changes are referred to as arteriovenous nicking (Fig. 10-32).

Emboli in a retinal vessel cause abrupt narrowing of arterioles and abrupt dilation of a vein as it impedes return flow.

Retinal background

Among the more common abnormalities to appear on the retinal background are microaneurysms, exudates, and hemorrhages (Fig. 10-33). Microaneurysms, outpouchings in the walls of capillaries, appear as tiny bright red dots on the retina. These are frequently associated with diabetes mellitus.

Exudates are whitish yellow infiltrates that may occur alongside vessel walls. They are rather round, appearing somewhat like a small cumulus cloud, and may have hazy or distinct edges. Exudates may be associated with systemic diseases, including diabetes mellitus and hypertension, and may occur with degenerative or inflammatory diseases of the retina. They may be resorbed over time.

Hemorrhages are bright to dark red, may be small and round, as is commonly found with diabetes mellitus, or linear and flame shaped, as occurs in hypertension. Bleeding may occur from retinal or choroidal vessels into the preretinal, retinal, or choroidal areas.

The retina itself may be damaged by the development of a hole, tear, or detachment. Retinal detachment is a serious condition in which the retinal layer pulls away from the choroid.

Problems such as those just described may affect any part of the retinal background, including the macular area. Depending on the area affected, resultant difficulty with central or peripheral vision may occur.

In the case of any retinal abnormality, the color, shape, size, and proximity to the disc or vessels should be described.

Eye pain and discomfort

The sensation of a superficial foreign body may be caused by:
- Lesion in the eyelid
- Foreign body on the cornea or conjunctiva
- Loss of corneal or conjunctival epithelium

Deep severe eye pain within the eye may be present in a variety of disorders requiring immediate attention, such as:
- Inflammation of the ciliary body
- Rapid increase in intraocular pressure, such as occurs with angle closure glaucoma

In these instances, the eye is red and vision is decreased.

Many relatively minor ocular abnormalities may manifest themselves by burning, itching, or uncomfortable eyes. Symptoms may originate from inadequately corrected refractive error, fatigue, and conjunctivitis.

Abnormal eye secretions

The following are some characteristics of the more common abnormal eye secretions.
- Purulent material is found in the conjunctival sac in mucopurulent conjunctivitis. The eyelashes may be stuck together by the dried exudate; it may be difficult to open the eyes in the morning.
- A tenacious, stringy secretion occurs in allergic inflammation of the conjunctiva.
- Foamy secretions at the inner canthus are produced by *Corynebacterium xerosis*.
- A stringy secretion and excoriation of the canthus char-

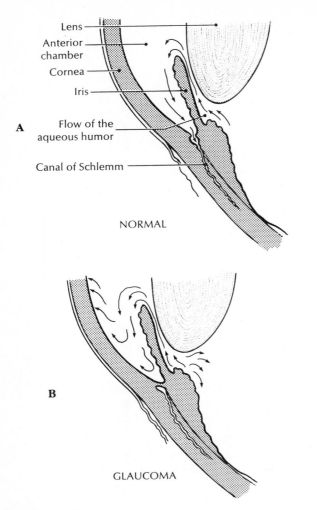

A

Lens
Anterior chamber
Cornea
Iris
Flow of the aqueous humor
Canal of Schlemm

NORMAL

B

GLAUCOMA

Figure 10-34

A, Normal flow of aqueous. **B,** Closed angle glaucoma: the flow of aqueous is blocked.

acterizes inflammation caused by diplobacillus of Morax-Axenfeld.

• Excess tearing may occur because of excessive production of tears or inadequate drainage leading to an overflow of the normal volume of tears. Persistent tearing in one or both eyes of an infant is a cardinal sign of congenital glaucoma. Tearing also occurs with photophobia, in inflammation of the cornea and conjunctiva, and in inflammation of the ciliary body.

INCREASED INTRAOCULAR PRESSURE

Glaucoma is a disease characterized by increased intraocular pressure resulting from an inadequate drainage system for the aqueous fluid. Normal intraocular pressure is 15 mm Hg ± 3 mm Hg. Untreated glaucomatous eyes with field loss have a mean measure of 22 mm Hg ± 5 mm Hg. If not treated, it results in damage to the optic nerve, with subsequent loss of peripheral vision and may

lead eventually to blindness. It is divided into open-angle and closed-angle categories. In the open-angle types the aqueous humor flows into the anterior chamber but has impaired outflow through the canal of Schlemm. In closed-angle glaucoma, the iris is displaced anteriorly so that the anterior chamber is narrowed and drainage of the aqueous humor into the anterior chamber is blocked, leading to accumulation in the posterior chamber. The disease may be chronic or acute, primary, secondary, or congenital, and painless or painful. It is frequently asymptomatic and proceeds so gradually that it may go unnoticed until well advanced. Primary glaucomas include chronic open-angle, chronic and acute closed-angle, and congenital.

Approximately 90% of the primary glaucomas are the mainly asymptomatic chronic open-angle type. Open-angle glaucoma is usually asymptomatic. The intraocular pressure gradually increases over several years and, although it may reach a high level, corneal edema and ocular pain do not occur. In early stages, peripheral vision is not affected. Measurement of visual field by confrontation is of little value until late in the disease.

Closed-angle glaucoma, which may be acute or chronic, occurs in the individual with an abnormally narrow space or angle formed by the iris and the cornea. The adhesions that form decrease or totally inhibit the normal flow of the aqueous (Fig. 10-34). Symptoms including ocular pain and blurred vision are related to sudden intermittent increases in intraocular pressure. There may be repeated attacks of ocular pain and blurred vision occurring after a prolonged time in darkness, after emotional upset, or after situations that cause pupillary dilation.

In congenital glaucoma, certain developmental defects interfere with the flow of aqueous. Symptoms include tearing, photophobia, and blepharospasm or spasm of the orbicularis oculi muscle. Secondary glaucoma may be of the open- or closed-angle type and may result from a number of causes including trauma, drugs, inflammation, and neovascularization.

Persons particularly at risk for glaucoma include those who are diabetic, hypertensive, or black; those who have had eye injuries; large-eyed children; and those with a family history of glaucoma. It is the third major cause of blindness in the United States. It is detectable and treatable and should be a part of a regular screening examination for those at risk and for all persons over age 40.

SCREENING EXAMINATION OF THE EYES

1. Vision when corrected with glasses, if necessary, is normal in each eye for near and far, each eye being measured separately.

Health History
Eyes

NOTE: A yes response to any question *must* be further investigated. Use the following indicators throughout the assessment: (1) onset (specific date, sudden or gradual), (2) duration, (3) frequency, (4) precipitating factors, (5) aggravating or alleviating factors, (6) treatment received, and (7) outcome.

Present status

1. Do you need corrective lenses for vision?
   a. Type: glasses, contact lenses, bifocal, trifocal
   b. Correction required: farsighted, nearsighted, presbyopia, cataract
2. Do you have other vision abnormalities?
   a. Description: halos around lights, nightblindness, central or peripheral only vision, double vision, half-fields vision, floating spots
3. Do you have pain in or around your eyes?
   a. Description: dull, sharp, shooting, throbbing
   b. Associated problems: itching, burning, redness, tearing, photophobia
4. Do you have abnormal secretions from your eye(s)?
   a. Description: purulent, tenacious, stringy, foamy, excessive tearing
5. Do you have swelling around your eyes?

Past history

1. Have you had trauma to your eye(s)?
   a. Type
2. Have you had eye surgery?
   a. Type
   b. When
3. Have you had an eye infection?
   a. Type: conjunctivitis, corneal ulceration or infection, sty
4. Have you had glaucoma or cataracts?

Associated conditions

1. Do you have any other illnesses affecting your eyes?
   a. Hypertension, diabetes, glaucoma, cataract, eye infections, multiple sclerosis, CVA, syphilis

Family history

1. Is there family history of eye disease?
   a. Type: color blindness, cataracts, glaucoma, infection

Sample assessment record

Client states presence of floating spots and flashes of light in right eye. Has seen floating spots for several weeks but began seeing flashes of light today after lifting a heavy box. Wears corrective lenses for myopia since age 8. Denies other vision abnormalities, pain, abnormal eye secretions, and periorbital edema. Denies eye trauma and surgery. Denies glaucoma, diabetes, hypertension, cataracts, and eye infections. Has no history of other systemic problems. Mother had bilateral cataracts removed at age 72.

2. Peripheral visual field of each eye is intact on gross testing.
3. Ocular movements are normal, the axes of the eyes are parallel.
4. Each pupil constricts when the retina of each eye is stimulated by light; pupils are equal.
5. The optic discs are flat and of normal color; they are not swollen or atrophic.

BIBLIOGRAPHY

Albert DM: Jaeger's atlas of diseases of the ocular fundus, Philadelphia, 1972, WB Saunders Co.

Anderson D: Testing the field of vision, St Louis, 1982, The CV Mosby Co.

Anthony CP and Thibodeau GA: Textbook of anatomy and physiology, St Louis, 1987, The CV Mosby Co.

Blodi FC, Allen L, and Frazier O: Stereoscopic manual of the ocular fundus in local and systemic disease, vol II, St Louis, 1970, The CV Mosby Co.

Donaldson DD: Atlas of external diseases of the eye, vol IV, Anterior chamber, iris, and ciliary body, St Louis, 1973, The CV Mosby Co.

Donaldson DD: Atlas of disease of the anterior segment of the eye, vol V, The crystalline lens, St Louis, 1976, The CV Mosby Co.

Harrington DO: The visual fields: a textbook and atlas of clinical perimetry, ed 5, St Louis, 1981, The CV Mosby Co.

Ichikawa H and others: Standard pseudoisochromatic plates, Tokyo, 1978, Igaku-Shoin.

Jackson CRS: The eye in general practice, Baltimore, 1972, Williams & Wilkins.

Mechner F: Patient assessment: examination of the eye, part I, Am J Nurs 74:1, part II, 75:1, 1974.

Medcom: Selected topics in ophthalmology, Medcom Clinical Lecture Guides, Garden Grove, Calif, 1983, Medcom, Inc.

Newell FW: Ophthalmology: principles and concepts, ed 6, St Louis, 1986, The CV Mosby Co.

Potts AM, editor: The assessment of visual function, St Louis, 1972, The CV Mosby Co.

Stein HA and Slatt BJ: The ophthalmic assistant: fundamentals and clinical practice, ed 4, St Louis, 1983, The CV Mosby Co.

Thomas BA, editor: Introduction to ophthalmoscopy, Kalamazoo, Mich, 1976, The Upjohn Co.

Trever-Roper PD and Curran PV: The eye and its disorders, ed 2, Oxford, 1984, Blackwell Scientific Publications.

chapter 111

Assessment of the head, face, and neck

OBJECTIVES

Upon successful review of this chapter, learners will be able to:

- Describe anatomy and physiology of the head, face, and neck

- State related rationale and demonstrate assessment of the
  Head
  Face
  Neck
  Thyroid gland

- Recognize variations of health associated with
  Head pain
  Head injury
  Neck discomfort
  Thyroid dysfunction

- Differentiate effects of hyperthyroidism and hypothyroidism on body structures and systems

Numerous structures of the head, face, and neck are examined during the clinical assessment process. These include

Head	*Face*	*Neck*
Position	Facial expression	Neck muscles
Scalp and hair	Facial skin	Cervical vertebrae
	Bony structures	Trachea
	Eyes (see Chapter 10)	Thyroid gland
	Nose, mouth, and ears (see Chapter 9)	Carotid arteries and jugular veins (see Chapter 15)
		Cervical lymph nodes (see Chapter 12)

As indicated above, the examination of some of these structures is covered in other chapters in this text. The student practitioner should be aware of gradually learning to integrate all these components by regional area.

Anatomy and Physiology

HEAD

The skull is composed of seven bones that, in adulthood, are fused along suture lines. These bones include (Figure 11-1)

- Two frontal
- Two parietal
- Two temporal
- One occipital

The skull protects the sensitive structure of the brain. The movable (nonfused) lower jaw bone, or mandible, and the fused bones of the face, including

- Frontal
- Nasal
- Zygomatic
- Lacrimal

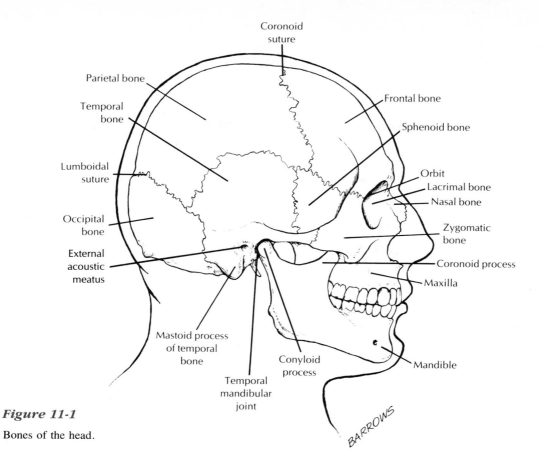

Figure 11-1

Bones of the head.

• Sphenoid

• Maxilla

Bones form the facial contours and provide protection and cavities for the special sense organs. The bones are used to identify regions of the head and overlying structures.

The skin overlying the superior, lateral, and posterior portions of the skull is called the scalp and is normally covered with hair, although there may be a pattern of loss, particularly in the adult male.

FACE

Variations in facial appearance are as numerous as the earth's population, and the face is usually one of an individual's most distinguishing characteristics. Also, the appearance of any one person's face may change considerably from time to time depending on facial expression, emotional condition, nutritional status, and illness states.

The eyes, nose, and mouth are generally symmetric, as are the ears. The palpebral fissures, the distance between the upper and lower lids of the eye, are equal, as are the nasolabial folds, the skin creases extending from the angle of the nose to the corner of the mouth. Within the range of normal, there are many persons with slightly asymmetric characteristic features or expressions.

Sensation of the face is mediated by the trigeminal nerve, cranial nerve (CN) V (Fig. 11-2), which has three sensory branches: (1) the ophthalmic, (2) the maxillary, and (3) the mandibular. The muscles of facial expression are ennervated by the facial nerve, CN VII.

The major artery accessible on the face is the temporal artery, which passes just anterior to the ear over the temporal bone and onto the forehead.

NECK

The major structures of the neck are

• Sternocleidomastoid and trapezius muscles

• Trachea

• Thyroid gland

• Carotid arteries and jugular veins

• Cervical lymph nodes

• Cervical vertebrae

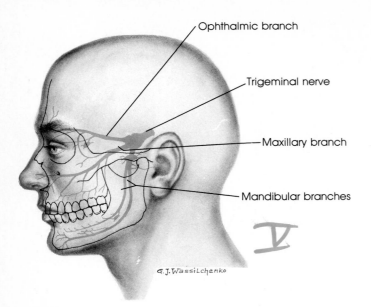

Figure 11-2

Trigeminal nerve with innervation to the face by ophthalmic, maxillary, and mandibular branches.
(From Rudy EB: Advanced neurological and neurosurgical nursing, St Louis, 1984, The CV Mosby Co.)

Neck Muscles

The two major neck muscles, the sternocleidomastoid and the trapezius, provide support and mobility for the neck, enabling the head to flex, extend, rotate, and flex laterally. Each sternocleidomastoid muscle extends from the upper sternum and proximal one third portion of the clavical to the mastoid process of the temporal bone posterior to the ear (Fig. 11-3). This symmetric pair of muscles is involved in turning and lateral flexion of the head. The two trapezius muscles are large, flat, and triangular; together they form a trapezoidal pattern. Each trapezius muscle extends from the seventh cervical vertebra and all the thoracic vertebrae and the spine of the scapula to the occipital bone of the skull (Fig. 11-4). The trapezius muscles are involved in the movements of shrugging the shoulders, pulling the scapulae downward and toward the vertebral column, rotating the head to the side, and extending the head backward. The sternocleidomastoid and trapezius muscles are ennervated by the spinal accessory nerve, CN XI.

Both sets of muscles and their position in relation to other neck structures are used to describe anatomic landmarks and physical findings. These muscles divide each side of the neck into two triangles: anterior and posterior. The parameters of the anterior triangle are the mandible superiorly, the sternocleidomastoid muscle lat-

Figure 11-3

Sternocleidomastoid muscle and the anterior and posterior triangles.

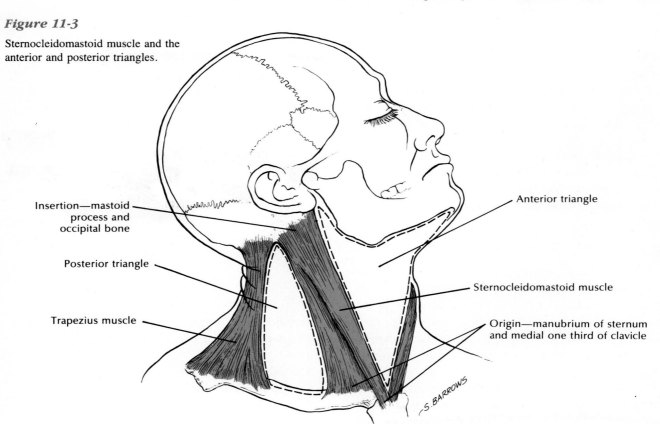

erally, and the midline of the trachea medially (see Fig. 11-3). Within the anterior triangle along the midline of the anterior neck lie the hyoid bone, cricoid cartilage, thyroid cartilage, trachea, and thyroid gland (Fig. 11-5). Also within the anterior triangle are the anterior cervical lymph nodes, the carotid artery, and the internal jugular vein, which run just anterior and parallel to the anterior aspect of the sternocleidomastoid muscle. The external jugular vein crosses the sternocleidomastoid muscle diagonally (see Fig. 15-18). The parameters of the posterior triangle are the sternocleidomastoid muscle laterally, the trapezius muscle posteriorly, and the clavicle inferiorly. Several groups of lymph nodes lie within the posterior triangle including the posterior cervical and spinal nerve chain lymph nodes (see Fig. 12-7).

Midline Neck Structures

Anterior midline neck structures include the following (see Fig. 11-5):

1. The hyoid bone, which lies just below the mandible at the angle of the floor of the mouth.
2. The thyroid cartilage, which is shaped like a shield and is the largest of the cartilaginous structures of the neck. The upper edge is notched, and its level corresponds to the level of the bifurcation of the common carotid artery into the internal and external carotid arteries.
3. The cricoid cartilage, which is the uppermost ring of the trachea. It is palpable just below the thyroid cartilage.
4. The tracheal rings.
5. The isthmus of the thyroid gland, which lies across the trachea below the cricoid cartilage.

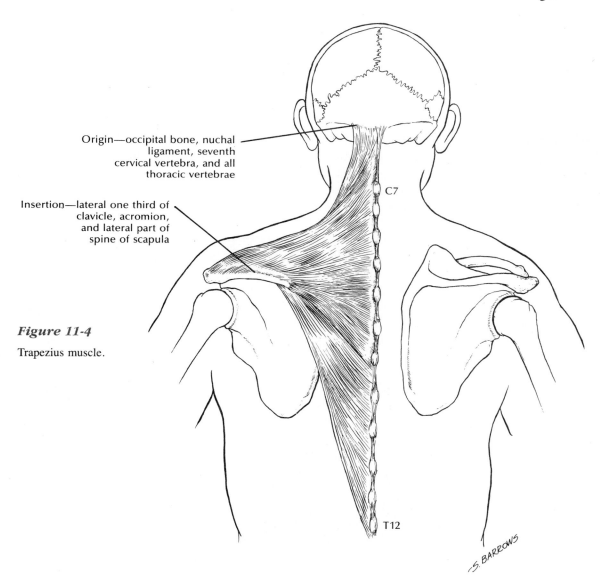

Origin—occipital bone, nuchal ligament, seventh cervical vertebra, and all thoracic vertebrae

Insertion—lateral one third of clavicle, acromion, and lateral part of spine of scapula

C7

T12

—S. BARROWS

Figure 11-4

Trapezius muscle.

Figure 11-5

Midline neck structures.

Midline neck structures.

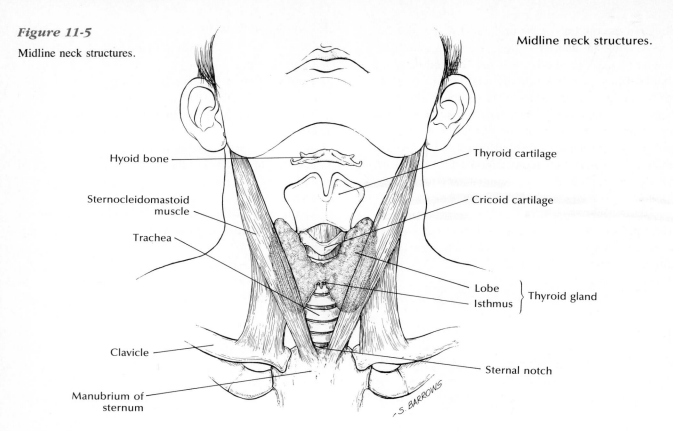

Hyoid bone

Sternocleidomastoid muscle

Trachea

Clavicle

Manubrium of sternum

Thyroid cartilage

Cricoid cartilage

Lobe
Isthmus } Thyroid gland

Sternal notch

~S. BARROWS

Thyroid Gland

The thyroid gland is the largest endocrine gland in the body and the only one accessible to direct physical examination. Its normal functions are essential for normal physical growth and development and for maintenance of metabolic stability. It produces two hormones: thyroxine, T_4, and triiodothyronine, T_3. These hormones influence the concentration and activity of numerous enzymes as well as the metabolism of substrates, vitamins, and minerals. The secretion and degradation rates of all other hormones as well as their target tissue responses are also affected by the thyroid hormones. Thus, thyroid hormones affect virtually all the tissues and organ sysems of the body.

The thyroid gland is butterfly shaped, with two lateral lobes lying on either side of the trachea and a connecting isthmus that joins the lobes in the lower half just inferior to the cricoid cartilage. The lobes curve posteriorly around the cartilage; the lateral portions are covered by the sternocleidomastoid muscles. The normal adult thyroid gland weighs about 15 to 20 g in the male and 20 to 25 g in the female. It is larger in women than in men, particularly during adolescence, pregnancy, and around menopause. The lobes are irregular and cone shaped, each about 5 cm long, 3 cm in diameter, and 2 cm thick (Fig. 11-6). The thyroid arteries supply the highly vascular thyroid tissue. The recurrent laryngeal nerves run behind the lobes of the thyroid gland. The thyroid atrophies somewhat during normal aging.

Examination

RELEVANT HEALTH HISTORY

Headache

1. Location, onset, duration, character of pain, aggravating and alleviating factors
2. Associated symptoms—visual changes including photophobia, hemianopsia, visual distortion of objects, and lacrimation; gastrointestinal changes including nausea, vomiting, and diarrhea
3. Precipitating events and factors such as stressful situations, foods, food additives, alcohol, allergies, menstrual cycle, and oral contraceptives
4. Effects of treatment efforts including sleep, medication, and meditation
5. History of headaches—client's and family's history

A chart or outline (Table 11-1) that helps the client and clinician record the description of the pattern of headaches over time may be helpful in determining the type or types of headache from which the client is suffering.

ANTERIOR   POSTERIOR

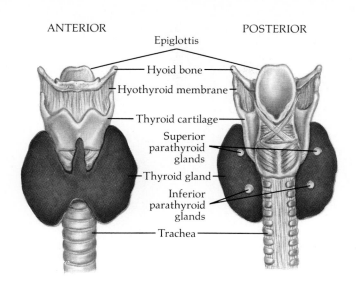

Figure 11-6

Anterior and posterior views of the thyroid gland and nearby structures.
(From Thompson J: Clinical nursing, St Louis, 1986, The CV Mosby Co.

Table 11-1

Sample headache record

Date	Onset	End	Location	Severity 1 = mild 10 = severe	Efforts to relieve	Relief 1 = good relief 10 = no relief	Possible precipitating factors

Head Injury

1. History of trauma, state of consciousness and behaviors after event, and sequelae
2. Predisposing factors such as seizure disorder, visual changes, light-headedness, and fainting
3. Associated symptoms such as pain, change in breathing pattern, visual changes, and gastrointestinal symptoms
4. History of head surgery or other treatments to head such as radiation

Neck Ache or Stiffness

1. History of injury, strain, or bacterial or viral illness
2. Presence of masses, tenderness, or swelling
3. Character of dysfunction
   a. Limitation of motion
   b. Pain or discomfort, radiation patterns to shoulders, arms, or back
4. Effects of treatment efforts: heat, cold, medication, or movement

Thyroid Dysfunction

1. Changes in sleep pattern or energy level: fatigue, drowsiness, lethargy, or insomnia
2. Changes in emotional patterns: mood changes, irritability, nervousness, or emotional lability
3. Hair loss, change in texture of hair or skin, or brittleness of nails
4. Altered sensitivity to cold or heat
5. Cardiorespiratory changes: dyspnea on exertion, tachycardia, or cardiac irregularity

6. Changes in appetite, weight loss, bowel habits, thirst, or frequency of urination
7. Changes in menstrual pattern
8. Hoarseness, difficulty swallowing, swelling, or pain or tenderness in the neck
9. History of radiation to the head or neck
10. Treatments used: surgery or medication
11. Family history of medullary carcinoma of the thyroid

The presence of thyroid disease is usually suspected by signs and symptoms other than in the neck, although with diffuse goiter, thyroiditis, and cancer, signs and symptoms may be referable only to the neck.

PREPARATION FOR THE EXAMINATION

Examination of the head, face, and neck involves the assessment of numerous structures; several organs of special sensation including sight, smell, taste, and hearing; and portions of some body systems, including the cardiovascular, lymphatic, and musculoskeletal. Thus, it is an area of the body where many aspects of the physical examination are concentrated.

Equipment required for the examination includes a stethoscope, a glass of water, and a tape measure. There are no special environmental considerations other than a room warmed or cooled to a comfortable temperature and one that provides privacy for the client. This portion of the physical examination is done with the client in a sitting position. The assessment techniques used are inspection, palpation, and auscultation.

EXAMINATION

Head

The head is examined by observing the position of the head, any unusual movements, the size, shape, and symmetry of the skull, and the condition of the scalp and hair. To inspect the scalp, the hair should be parted in several areas. Wigs or other hairpieces should be removed. The examiner notes the texture and amount of hair and the use of coloring or lubricating agents. The condition of the hair may be a useful indicator of the client's emotional status, social group identification, and personal hygiene. The scalp should be palpated in several areas with a gentle rotary motion; it should move freely over the skull. No depressions, swelling, or tenderness are expected.

Face

The examiner observes the facial expression, the color and condition of the facial skin, and the shape and symmetry of the facial features, including the eyebrows, eyes,

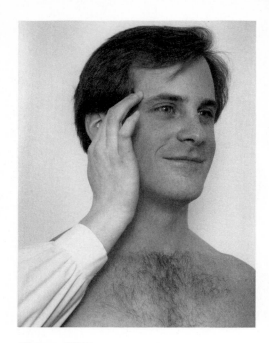

Figure 11-7

Palpatation of temporal artery.

palpebral fissures, mouth, and nasolabial folds. The head should be held upright and still, and the facial features should be symmetric at rest and with a change of expression, although a slight amount of asymmetry is common.

The examiner tests facial muscle function by asking the client to elevate and lower the eyebrows, frown, close the eyes tightly, puff the cheeks, show the teeth, and smile. (See also Chapter 20 on neurologic assessment.)

The temporal artery is palpated just anterior to and, in some cases, slightly above the tragus of the ear (Fig. 11-7). Any thickening, hardness, or tenderness of the vessel is noted. Using the bell of the stethoscope, the temporal artery is auscultated for a bruit, which is a blowing sound of blood in the vessel.

Neck

Midline structures and muscles

A long, slender neck will be easier to inspect and palpate than a short, thick neck. The neck is inspected for symmetry and stability in its usual position. The neck muscles are inspected for symmetry of the musculature, and the areas over and around the muscles are inspected for any abnormal masses or swelling.

Muscle function is assessed by checking for range of motion in slight hyperextension, in lateral rotation to each side, and in flexion with the chin to the chest wall (Fig. 11-8). These motions should be smooth and should not cause pain or dizziness. The midline structures are

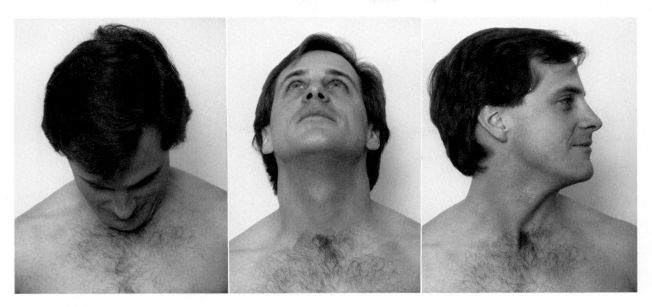

Figure 11-8

Movements of the neck: flexion, extension, and lateral rotation.

inspected for symmetry. The jugular veins and carotid arteries should not be distended or prominent.

The midline cartilages, including the thyroid and cricoid cartilages and the tracheal rings, are palpated for symmetry. The trachea should be centered and equidistant from the sternocleidomastoid muscle. The cartilages should be smooth, nontender, and move easily under the examiner's fingers when the client swallows.

The neck is then palpated for any masses and for area lymph nodes. (See Chapter 12.) Muscle strength is tested against resistance. The sternocleidomastoid is tested by having the client turn the head to one side and then the other against the resistance of the examiner's hand. Trapezius muscle strength is assessed by asking the client to shrug the shoulders against the resistance of the examiner's hands. (See Chapter 18.) On the posterior aspect of the neck, the cervical vertebrae are inspected and palpated for symmetry, tenderness, masses, or swelling.

Thyroid gland

It is easier to estimate the size and shape of the thyroid gland in young or slender individuals, but it becomes more difficult in the presence of kyphosis, a short neck, obesity, or prior neck surgery. The normal gland may be impalpable or easily palpable with a slight bulge of the lateral lobes and isthmus.

The techniques used to examine the thyroid gland include observation, palpation, and auscultation. Observation of thyroid function or possible dysfunction includes more than observation of the area where the thy-

roid gland is located. The effects of thyroid activity are widespread; therefore, observations of behavior, appearance, skin, eyes, hair, and cardiovascular status are important.

To inspect the thyroid gland, the examiner stands before the client and observes particularly the lower half of the neck first in normal position, next in slight extension, and then while the client swallows a sip of water (Fig. 11-9). The movements of the cartilages are easily observed. Any unusual bulging of thyroid tissue in the midline of the lobes or behind the sternocleidomastoid muscles should be noted; normally, none is seen. A good cross-light is helpful for observing subtle neck movements or ascending masses.

Following observation, the neck is palpated for the presence of an enlarged thyroid, for consistency of the gland, and for any nodules. The normal thyroid gland is not palpable. However, in a thin neck, the isthmus is occasionally palpable; in a short, stocky neck, even an enlarged gland may be difficult to palpate. Palpation may be done with the examiner standing either in front of or behind the client. Although there are several techniques used for palpation of the thyroid, the underlying principles for each technique include movement of the gland while the client swallows, adequate exposure of the gland by relaxation and manual displacement of surrounding structures, and comparison of one side of the gland with the other. The sternocleidomastoid muscles are strong and large, and the key is to relax them. The thyroid gland is fixed to the trachea and thus ascends during swallow-

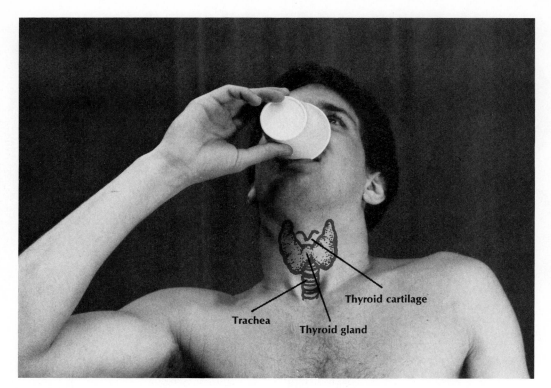

Figure 11-9

Observation for the thyroid gland with the neck in slight extension. The structures of the thyroid gland are more distinct during swallowing.

ing. This distinguishes thyroid structures from other neck masses. The examiner seeks to determine the gland's size, degree of enlargement, consistency, and surface characteristics, the presense of nodules, and the presence of a bruit.

Posterior approach. The client is seated on a chair or examining table while the examiner stands behind. The client is requested to lower the chin to relax the neck muscles. The examining fingers are curved anteriorly, so that the tips rest on the lower half of the neck over the trachea (Fig. 11-10). The client is asked to swallow a sip of water while the examiner feels for any enlargement of the thyroid isthmus. To facilitate examination of each lobe, the client is asked to turn the head slightly toward the side to be examined with the chin still lowered. For example, to examine the right thyroid lobe, the examiner has the client lower the chin and turn the head slightly to the right. With the fingers of the left hand, the examiner displaces the thyroid cartilage slightly to the right while the fingers of the right hand palpate the area lateral to the cartilage where the thyroid lobe lies to check for any enlargement (Fig. 11-11). The client is asked to swallow a sip of water during the procedure.

Anterior approach. The examiner stands in front of the client and, with the palmar surfaces of the

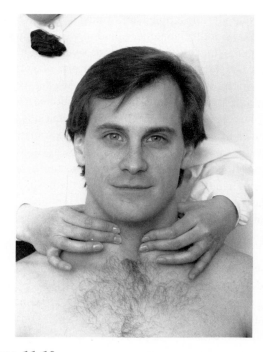

Figure 11-10

Posterior approach to thyroid examination. Standing behind the client, the examiner palpates for the thyroid isthmus by placing the palmar aspects of the fingertips over the lower portion of the trachea.

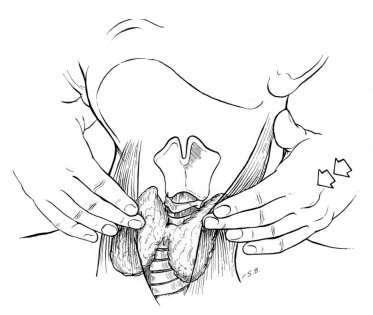

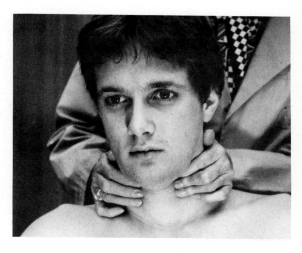

Figure 11-11

Posterior approach to thyroid examination. To examine the right lobe of the thyroid gland, the examiner displaces the trachea slightly to the right with the fingers of the left hand and palpates for the right thyroid lobe with the fingers of the right hand.

index and middle fingers, palpates below the cricoid cartilage for the thyroid isthmus as the client swallows a sip of water. In a procedure similar to the one used with the posterior approach, the client is asked to flex the head and turn it slightly to one side and then the other. The examiner palpates for the left lobe by displacing the thyroid cartilage slightly to the left with the left hand and examining for thyroid enlargement with the right hand (Fig. 11-12). Again, the examiner palpates the area and hooks thumb and fingers around the sternocleidomastoid muscle (Fig. 11-13). The procedure is repeated for the right side. The examiner may also palpate for thyroid enlargement on the right side by placing the thumb deep to and behind the sternocleidomastoid muscle while the index and middle fingers are placed deep to and in front of the muscle (Fig. 11-14).

If enlargement of the thyroid gland is detected or suspected, the area over the gland is auscultated for a bruit. In a hyperplastic thyroid gland, the blood flow through the thyroid arteries is accelerated and produces vibrations that may be heard with the bell of the stethoscope as a soft, rushing sound or bruit. (See Chapter 15 for further discussion of bruits.)

Thyroid tissue located in the retrosternal area may also become enlarged. This is not discernible by physical examination but should be considered if other physical findings suggest thyroid dysfunction.

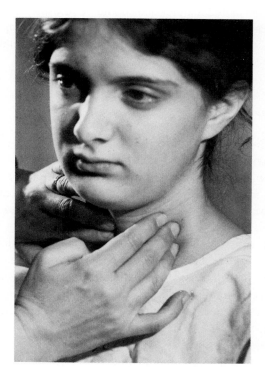

Figure 11-12

Anterior approach to thyroid examination. Standing in front of the client, the examiner uses the fingers of the left hand to displace the trachea slightly to the left while the fingers of the right hand palpate for the left thyroid lobe.

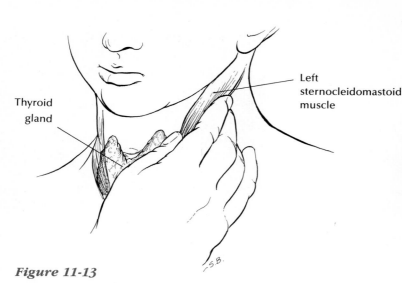

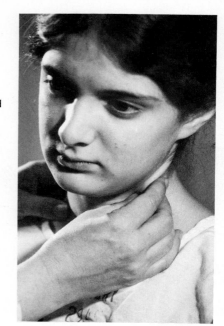

Figure 11-13

Anterior approach to thyroid examination. The examiner grasps around the left sternocleidomastoid muscle with the right hand to palplate for an enlarged left thyroid lobe.

The normal consistency of the thyroid may be described as "meaty" to firm or hard. The surface may be smooth or irregular. Palpable masses of 5 mm or larger are considered nodules and should be measured and their location described. The examiner should determine the size, shape, consistency, surface characteristics, and freedom of movement of the nodule.

Variations from Health

HEAD

Several conditions may result in abnormalities of the skull. For example, an abnormally large head in children may result from the accumulation of fluid in the ventricles of the brain (hydrocephalus). In adults a large head may result from osteitis deformans, wherein the bony thickness increases, or from excessive hormone secretion (acromegaly), wherein the skull becomes enlarged and thickened, the length of the mandible increases, the nose and forehead are more prominent, and the facial features appear coarsened. Local deformities of the skull may result from trauma or from the surgical removal of portions of the skull.

Sebaceous cysts may develop on the scalp. These result from the occlusion of sebaceous gland ducts and are palpable as smooth, rounded nodules attached to the scalp. The scalp should also be assessed for dandruff and for the presence of parasites.

The hair is subject to the influence of altered met-

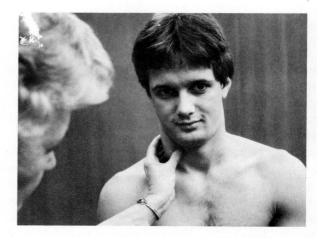

Figure 11-14

Anterior approach to thyroid examination. Examining for an enlarged right thyroid lobe, the examiner grasps and palpates around and deep to the right sternocleidomastoid muscle.

abolic conditions. The classic examples are the changes caused by thyroid disorders. In hypothyroidism, the hair is coarse, dry, and brittle; in hyperthyroidism, the hair becomes fine, silky, and soft. The thinning or loss of hair (alopecia) may be hereditary, especially in men, or be a side effect of drugs used to treat malignant tumors. This condition may also accompany prolonged illness or emotional stress.

In western societies, headache is a very common complaint. For the most part, headache, especially chronic headache, is only infrequently caused by organic disease. Yet it may also be the presenting symptom of severe illness such as cerebral hemorrhage, brain tumor, or meningitis. Whether the source is benign or malignant, a headache may be intense and quite debilitating. For clients in whom there is no demonstrable physical pathologic condition, the mechanism appears to be a disturbance of the function of the brain, of the blood supply to the brain, or of other structures of the head (Peatfield, 1986).

The various kinds of headaches may be divided into three main groups (Diamond and Dalessio, 1986):
• Vascular
• Muscle contraction
• Traction and inflammatory

Headache

Vascular headaches

This category includes migraine, cluster, hypertensive, and toxic vascular headaches. In all these types a process of vascular dilation provokes the headache. Vasoconstriction may also occur and be related to the sensory and motor phenomena that are sometimes experienced with migraine and cluster headaches.

Migraine headaches

Migraine headaches may begin in childhood, adolescence, or young adulthood (the 20s and 30s) and become chronic. They may occur at sporadic intervals during a lifetime, but with an identifiable pattern, as with the menstrual cycle. The location is often unilateral, but it may be generalized or may switch from one side to the other from one headache to the next. The pain may last for several hours to several days. The severity of the pain is often described as intense, pulsating, or throbbing. Prodromata, or warning signals, frequently precede the headache: they may be limited to visual symptoms such as flashing lights, scotomata (blind spots), hemianopsia (loss of vision on one side), or distorted perceptions of sizes and shapes of objects. Other prodromal events may include paresthesias or an aura. Symptoms that may occur simultaneously with the migraine headache include photophobia, nausea, and vomiting. Many factors have been implicated in the precipitation of migraine headaches, among which are fatigue, loss of sleep, prolonged hunger, menstruation, birth control pills, stress, bright sunlight, and foods or drugs containing vasoactive chemicals. Migraine headache is a familial illness. It occurs more frequently in females. A history of successful relief of pain with ergotamine tartrate indicates a migrainous condition. Reserpine may promote migraine headaches.

Cluster headaches

Cluster headaches tend to begin during the night several hours after the person falls asleep. They may be seasonal, occurring in the spring and fall and extending in repetitive clusters from several weeks to several months. The individual headache may last from several minutes to 2 to 4 hours. The pain is described as deep, burning, boring, knifelike and intense. Symptoms associated with cluster headaches include an ipsilateral modified Horner's syndrome, with ptosis and constriction of the pupil, lacrimation, flushing or blanching of the face, and nasal discharge. Cluster headaches are more frequent in males and generally occur during the third and fourth decades of life.

Hypertensive headaches

Hypertensive headaches are related to elevation in the systemic arterial blood pressure. They are typically present on awakening and generally remit as the day progresses. They may be generalized or occipital in location.

Toxic vascular headaches

Toxic vascular headaches may be produced by fever, ingestion of alcohol, poisons, or carbon dioxide retention.

Muscle contraction headaches

This type of headache, also referred to as "tension headache," is the most common type of head pain. It may result from psychogenic problems, such as depression and anxiety, or from organic problems, such as cervical arthritis. It is characterized by a dull, bandlike, constricting, and persistent pain that may last from hours to days or months. It tends to occur during early and middle adulthood in both males and females. It is typically bilateral and may be generalized to the frontal, parietal, temporal, or occipital area.

Traction and inflammatory headaches

Traction and inflammatory headaches include those caused by organic diseases of some structure of the head or neck, including the brain, meninges, arteries, veins, eyes, ears, teeth, nose and paranasal sinuses, jaw, and joints of the neck. They may be a result of infection, intracranial or extracranial lesions, occlusive vascular disorders, brain edema, abscesses, cerebral puncture, or inflammatory processes such as arteritis, encephalitis, or meningitis. The location of the headache depends on the nature of the underlying disorder.

Other Head and Neck Pains

Traumatic headaches

The postconcussion headache consists of a dull generalized pain and may be associated with other symptoms such as dizziness or lack of concentration. It may persist over weeks or months and may be made worse by straining or coughing.

Temporomandibular joint disease

Pain in the area of the temporomandibular joint (TMJ) (see Fig. 11-1) as a result of dislocation of the condyle, osteoarthritis, rheumatoid arthritis, or a myofacial pain symdrome is often localized to the neck and ear in the area adjacent to the joint. There is also limitation of motion of the jaw, muscle tenderness, and, in some cases, joint crepitus.

Polymyalgia rheumatica

The polymyalgia rheumatica syndrome is characterized by an aching pain and stiffness in the neck and shoulders, which may also extend to the upper arms, forearms, hips, and thighs. Aching is increased with motion, and the muscles may be tender.

Trigeminal neuralgia (tic douloureux)

Trigeminal neuralgia, or tic douloureux, is a neurologic abnormality caused by degeneration of or pressure on one or all of the three divisions of the trigeminal nerve, CN V (see Fig. 11-2). Dysfunction of the first divison, the ophthalmic, results in pain around the eyes and over the forehead; that of the second division, the maxillary, results in pain in the nose, cheek, and upper lip; and that of the third division, the mandibular, results in pain in the lower lip and side of the tongue. The pain is described as aching, burning, flashing, or stablike. These lancinating attacks of pain will often cause the person to wince with facial contractions. They may occur spontaneously or be evoked by pressure on the trigger zone on the face. They may also be initiated by cold air or a light touch on the cheek or by biting, chewing, laughing, swallowing, talking, yawning, or sneezing. An attack of pain is characterized by high-intensity pain for about 30 seconds followed by a period of abatement: this cycle may continue for hours. Trigeminal neuralgia affects persons in middle to late adulthood.

FACE

Changes in color, shape, symmetry, hair distribution pattern, or movement of the face may occur. In situations in which there is an increased amount of unsaturated hemoglobin in the body tissues, as may occur with cardiac or pulmonary disease, or in which there is a local stasis of circulation, various facial and head structures, including the lips, nose, cheeks, ears, and oral mucosa, may become bluish, or cyanotic. Facial pallor results from a decrease in local vascular supply, as in shock. The yellow color of jaundice results from an abnormal increase in bilirubin. Before jaundice is generally evident in the skin, it may be observed in the sclera and in the mucous membranes of the mouth under the tongue and on the palate. Localized color changes result from acne, moles, and scar tissue. More rare conditions associated with color alterations include lupus erythematosus, wherein an erythematous discoloration bridges the cheeks and nose, and conditions that alter the deposition of melanin, resulting in light or dark patchy areas.

Numerous situations may cause a change in facial shape. Edema, often initially evident in the eyelids, may result from cardiovascular or kidney disease. Thyroid disorders also affect the face: excessive function, hyperthyroidism, may be associated with an apparent protrusion of the eyeballs (exophthalmos) and with elevation of the upper lids, resulting in a staring or startled expression; diminished function, hypothyroidism, may lead to "myxedema facies," wherein the face is dull and puffy with dry skin and coarse features. As a result of increased adrenal hormone production (Cushing's syndrome) or secondary to the intake of synthetic adrenal hormones, "moon facies" may be observed, wherein the face is round and the cheeks quite red. Prolonged illness, dehydration, or starvation may produce a cachectic face, wherein the eyes, cheeks, and temples appear sunken, the nose appears sharp, and the skin is dry and rough.

Asymmetry or abnormal movements, or both, may result from facial nerve lesions. In Bell's palsy, a paralysis of the seventh cranial nerve, the eye on the affected side cannot close completely, the lower eyelid droops, the nasolabial fold is lost, and the corner of the mouth droops. Slight weakness may be present but is not evident when the face is at rest, so the examiner should carefully check facial muscle function.

In the women of some ethnic groups, increased facial hair is a normal finding. Elevated production of adrenal hormones may lead to excessive hair growth in the moustache and sideburn areas and on the chin. Hyperthyroidism causes thinning of the scalp hair and eyebrows.

NECK

Common abnormalities of the neck muscles include stiffness and pain. In tense individuals, some degree of muscle spasm may occur, and tenderness on palpation may

Table 11-2

Affects of hyperthyroidism and hypothyroidism on body structures and systems

Body system or structure	Hyperthyroidism	Hypothyroidism
General		
Weight	Loss	Gain
Temperature intolerance	Heat	Cold
Skin	Warm, moist, increased sweating, smooth texture, diffuse pigmentation, erythema	Cool, pale, dry, coarse, rough, scaly, itchy, doughy consistency
Hair	Fine texture, loss, inability to hold a permanent	Poor growth, loss, dry
Cardiovascular/pulmonary	Increased cardiac output, increased blood pressure, wide pulse pressure, tachycardia, atrial arrhythmias, systolic murmur, palpitations, angina, dyspnea, edema, increase in rate or depth of respirations; bruit may be heard over thyroid	Congestive heart failure, angina, slow pulse, pericardial or pulmonary effusion
Gastrointestinal	Indigestion, anorexia, polyphagia, diarrhea	Decreased appetite, constipation
Renal	Polydipsia, polyuria, urgency	Decreased output
Nervous	Restlessness, irritability, anxiety, memory loss, easy distractibility, decreased ability to concentrate	Decreased relaxation phase of deep tendon reflexes, depression
Muscular	Weakness, tremulousness	Stiffness, aching
Eyes	Lid lag and lid retraction giving startled or frightened look, tearing, conjunctival irritation	Periorbital puffiness
Reproductive		
Women	Hypomenorrhea, ammenorrhea	Menorrhagia
Men	Loss of libido, decreased potency	Decreased libido, decreased potency
Voice		Deep, hoarse
Hearing		Acuity may diminish

be elicited over the affected muscles. Stiffness of the neck may also result from vertebral disease or meningitis. Cervical arthritis produces limitation of motion, and central nervous system (CNS) disease involving irritation of the meninges is associated with pain on neck motion. NOTE: If there is any suspicion of traumatic neck injury, passive range of motion should never be done.

Thyroid gland: hyperthyroidism and hypothyroidism

The excessive amounts of thyroid hormone found in hyperthyroidism and the inadequate amounts of thyroid hormone found in hypothyroidism cause a wide variety of clinical findings in nearly every body system and in many structures. These findings are outlined in Table 11-2. With hyperthyroidism in younger individuals, in general the nervous symptoms dominate; with older individuals,

the cardiac and myopathic symptoms predominate. With hypothyroidism in the adult the early signs and symptoms of hypothyroidism are nonspecific and insidious. They may include lethargy, constipation, cold intolerance, and menorrhagia.

The presentation of hyperthyroidism in the elderly may differ from that in the younger person, and many of the symptoms of the dysfunction, such as anorexia, weight loss, weakness, and tremor, may be viewed as the result of other aging changes.

The thyroid gland may incur diffuse or local enlargement. Diffuse enlargement may occur to varying degrees. Symmetric thyroid enlargement may occur in areas where there is a deficiency of dietary iodine. Localized or nodular enlargement may consist of one or more nodules and may occur in either the lobes or the isthmus. Solitary nodules suggest carcinoma, particularly in younger people.

Health History
Head, Face and Neck

NOTE: A yes response to any question *must* be further investigated. Use the following indicators throughout the assessment: (1) onset (specific date, sudden or gradual), (2) duration, (3) frequency, (4) precipitating factors, (5) aggravating or alleviating factors, (6) treatment, and (7) outcome

Present status

1. Do you have headaches?
   a. Location
   b. Pain character: sharp, throbbing, piercing, intense
   c. Accompanying symptoms: photophobia, visual distortion, tearing, nausea/vomiting, diarrhea
2. Do you have facial pain?
   a. Location: specific area
   b. Pain character: aching, burning, flashing, stablike, constant
3. Do you have neck stiffness?
   a. Location
   b. Relation to injury or infection
   c. Limitation in movement

Past history

1. Have you ever had a head injury?
   a. Trauma type
   b. Loss of consciousness
   c. Accompanying symptoms: visual changes, lightheadedness, fainting, vertigo, behavior change
2. Have you ever had head, neck, or facial surgery?
   a. Type
   b. When
   c. Residual effects

4. Have you had a neck injury?
   a. Location
   b. Accident related
   c. Accompanying symptoms: tenderness, swelling, limitation in motion

Associated conditions

1. Do you have thyroid dysfunction?
   a. Associated symptoms: fatigue, lethargy, insomnia, irritability, nervousness, emotional changes, change in sleep patterns
2. Have you ever had a seizure?
   a. Type: grand mal, petite mal
   b. Medication prescribed
   c. Aura(s): sound, sight, smell
   d. Activity restrictions/employment affected

Family history

1. Is there a family history of seizure activity?
   a. Type
2. Do you have a family history of debilitating headaches?

Sample assessment record

Client states headache began gradually yesterday morning while painting in basement and is not relieved by aspirin. Complains of constant throbbing pain in center of forehead and around eyes. Denies neck stiffness, head or neck injury, neck/head surgery, and seizure activity. Denies symptoms of thyroid dysfunction and has negative family history of seizure activity or headaches.

BIBLIOGRAPHY

Dalessio DJ, editor: Wolff's headache and other head pain, ed 4, New York, 1980, Oxford University Press.

DeGroot LJ and others: The thyroid and its diseases, New York, 1984, John Wiley & Sons.

Diamond S and Dalessio DJ, editors: The practicing physician's approach to headache, ed 4, Baltimore, 1986, William & Wilkins.

Diamond S and Medina JL: In Appenzellar O, editor: The headache history—key to diagnosis in pathogenesis and treatment of headache, New York, 1976, Spectrum Publications.

Lance JW: Mechanism and management of headache, ed 4, London, 1982, Butterworth Scientific.

Peatfield R: Headache, Berlin, 1986, Springer-Verlag.

Solomon DH: In Van Middlesworth L, editor: Clinical examination of the thyroid in the thyroid gland, a practical clinical treatise, Chicago, 1986, Year Book Medical Publishers.

Thompson JM and others, editors: Clinical nursing, St Louis, 1986, The CV Mosby Co.

12

Assessment of the lymphatic system

OBJECTIVES

Upon successful review of this chapter, learners will be able to:

- Describe anatomy and physiology of the lymphatic system

- Outline history relevant to assessment of the lymphatic system

- State related rationale and demonstrate assessment of regional lymph nodes, including inspection and palpation techniques

- List characteristics pertinent to examination of lymph nodes or masses

- Recognize possible pathological conditions associated with location and characteristics of abnormal lymph nodes

- Identify possible pathological conditions related to lymphatic vessels

ANATOMY AND PHYSIOLOGY

The lymphatic system provides a defensive network against the invasion of microorganisms by capturing and destroying them. It also carries malignant cells from sites of neoplasm. Examination of the lymphatic system for superficial enlarged lymph nodes thus can provide an early indication of infection or malignancy. The lymphatic system consists of a network of collecting ducts, lymph fluid, and various tissues including the lymph nodes, spleen, thymus, tonsils, adenoids, and Peyer's patches in the intestines. Small aggregates of lymphoid tissue are also found in the lungs, the bone marrow, and the mucosa of the stomach and appendix.

The lymphatic vessels originate as microscopic, open-ended tubules or capillaries that merge to form large collecting ducts. Those then drain to specific lymph nodes; ducts from these lymph nodes eventually empty into the venous system at the subclavian veins (Fig. 12-1). The right subclavian vein receives the lymphatic trunk, which drains from the right side of the head and neck, right arm, and right side of the chest wall. The left subclavian vein receives lymph from the thoracic duct, the major vessel of the lymphatic system, which drains lymph from the remaining portion of the body. The entire lymph system is about 2% to 3% of total body weight.

The lymphatic and cardiovascular systems are closely related. The fluid and proteins that compose the lymphatic fluid, lymph, move originally from the vascular system to the interstitial spaces, where they are collected by the microscopic lymphatic tubules, which in turn return the various fluids and proteins to the cardiovascular system. The lymphatic capillary system is very extensive. All tissues supplied with blood vessels also possess lymphatic vessels, except the placenta and

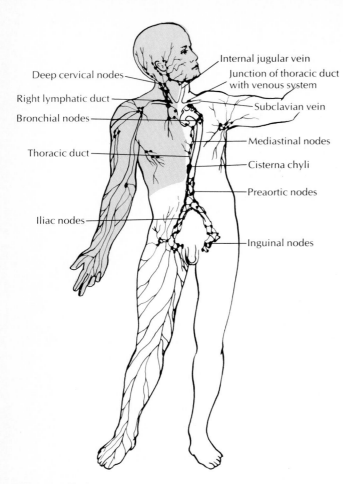

Figure 12-1

Lymphatic drainage pathways. Shaded area of the body is drained through the right lymphatic duct, which is formed by the union of three vessels: the right jugular trunk, the right subclavian trunk, and the right bronchomediastinal trunk. Lymph from the remainder of the body enters the venous system by way of the thoracic duct.

the brain. Also, many of the lymphatic vessels are located very near the vessels of the cardiovascular system.

The lymphatic system has no pumping device of its own, and its movement is much slower than that of the blood circulatory system. Factors affecting the movement of lymph include:

1. Compression of the lymphatic vessels by surrounding structures, especially contracting muscles
2. Respiratory movements, which move lymph forward in the thoracic duct
3. Propulsive action of the smooth muscles in the walls of the lymphatic vessels, lymph nodes, and collecting ducts
4. Arterial pulsations: most of the lymphatic vessels lie close to blood vessels; the deep lymphatic vessels accompany the veins and arteries, the pulsations of which can be transmitted to the lymphatic vessels

5. Negative pressure in the great vessels at the root of the neck
6. Peristaltic contractions of the intestines
7. Capillary blood pressure

The formation and flow of lymph can be increased by the following processes:

1. An increase in capillary pressure resulting from increased venous pressure due to venous stasis or obstruction
2. An increase in permeability of the capillary walls resulting from an increase in temperature, a decrease in oxygen supply, or the administration of histamine
3. Increases in metabolic activity, the muscular pumping effect, or glandular activity (little lymph is formed when an individual is given anesthesia or is on absolute bed rest)
4. Passive movements and massage, which facilitate the flow of lymph through the lymphatic vessels
5. Administration of hypertonic solutions, such as glucose and sodium chloride solutions

A slowing or stopping of lymph movement may be caused by any mechanical obstruction, which will dilate the system. Because the system is permeable, if it is obstructed, lymph may diffuse back into the vascular system, or collateral connecting channels may be established.

Lymph nodes typically occur in groups or centers. The superficial nodes lie in the subcutaneous connective tissues; the deeper nodes are beneath the muscular fascia or in various body cavities. Some nodes may have a diameter of 0.5 cm, but most are smaller. Their normal shape is round or oval. Normally, lymph nodes cannot be felt or seen. When the superficial lymph nodes are enlarged, they are accessible to physical examination by observation or palpation.

Lymph is a clear, sometimes opalescent to yellow-tinged fluid containing a variety of white blood cells, mostly lymphocytes, and occasional red blood cells. Sites of production of lymphocytes include the lymph nodes, tonsils, adenoids, bone marrow, and spleen. Some lymphocytes remain unchanged in the nodes; others differentiate into a variety of cells that remain in the lymphoid tissue or enter the lymph or the blood. Two types of lymph cells that enter the bloodstream are the B lymphocytes and the T lymphocytes. B lymphocytes have a life span of 3 to 4 days and are relatively small in number. T lymphocytes have a life span of 100 to 200 days and are more numerous. The number of lymphocytes increases in response to most viral infections and some bacterial infections.

Other tissues in the lymphatic system are the spleen, tonsils and adenoids, thymus, and Peyer's

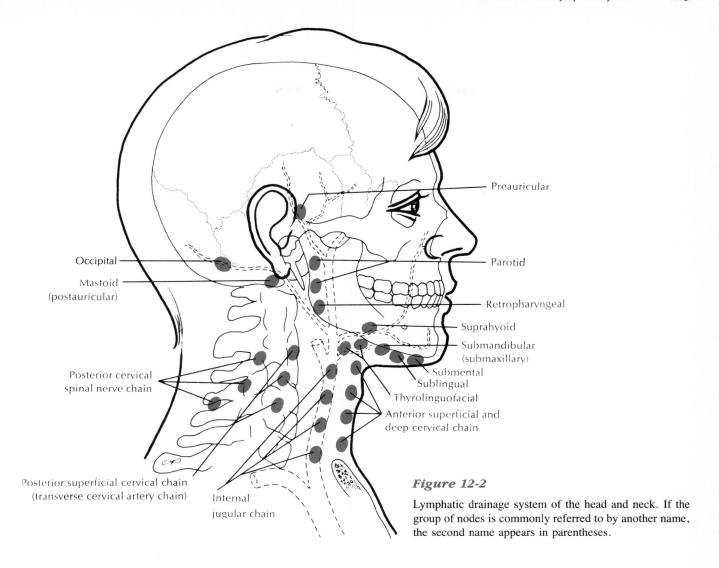

Figure 12-2

Lymphatic drainage system of the head and neck. If the group of nodes is commonly referred to by another name, the second name appears in parentheses.

patches. The spleen is located in the upper left quadrant of the abdomen between the stomach and the diaphragm. Early in life it is a blood-forming organ; later it serves as a storage site for red corpuscles and, with its blood filtering systems, as part of the body's defense system. The spleen may manufacture blood when the bone marrow is severely compromised. (See Chapter 16, Assessment of the Abdomen, for further information on the spleen.) The tonsils are located between the palatine arches on either side of the pharynx, just beyond the base of the tongue. They are composed mostly of lymphoid tissue and covered with mucous membrane. The adenoids lie at the nasopharyngeal border. Frequent viral or bacterial infection or allergic reactions enlarge the adenoids and obstruct breathing through the nasopharyngeal passageway. (See Chapter 9, Assessment of the Ears, Nose, and Throat, for further discussion of the tonsils and adenoids.)

The functions of the lymphatic system include (1) the movement and transport of lymph, (2) production of lymphocytes, (3) production of antibodies, (4) phagocytosis by the reticuloendothelial cells lining the sinuses of the lymph nodes, spleen, and liver, and (5) absorption of fat and fat-soluble substances from the intestines.

SUPERFICIAL LYMPH NODES BY REGION

Head and Neck

Head

Lymphatic drainage from the skin of the head, ears, nose, cheeks, and lips is delivered by the collecting ducts to the lymph centers of the head (Fig. 12-2).

The *occipital center* nodes receive the collecting ducts from the occipital region of the scalp and from the deep structures of the back of the neck.

The *postauricular, or mastoid, center* nodes are located over the outer surface of the mastoid process.

They drain the parietal region of the head and part of the ear.

The *preauricular center* nodes are situated in front of the tragus of the ear. The afferent ducts are from the forehead and upper face.

The nodes of the *parotid center* may be found on the surface of the parotid gland, within the tissue of the gland, or under the parotid fascia. The nodes of both the preauricular and parotid centers receive collecting ducts from the side of the head and the parotid gland as well as from the forehead, cheek, eyelids, ear, nose, upper lip, and eustachian tubes.

The *submandibular center* lies on the medial border of the mandible, following the mandibular branch of the facial nerve. This center receives collecting ducts from the chin, upper lip, cheek, nose, teeth, eyelids, part of the tongue, and floor of the mouth.

The nodes of the *retropharyngeal center* are found at the junction of the posterior and lateral walls of the pharynx near the location of the atlas. Lymph from the nasal cavity and from the accessory sinuses of the nose, palate, epipharynx, and nasopharynx is delivered to these nodes.

The *submental center* receives collecting ducts from the tongue. They are located in the submental triangle between the platysma and mylohyoid muscles. These nodes receive ducts from the gums, the floor of the mouth, and the anterior third of the tongue.

The *sublingual nodes* lie below the tongue and collect from the tongue.

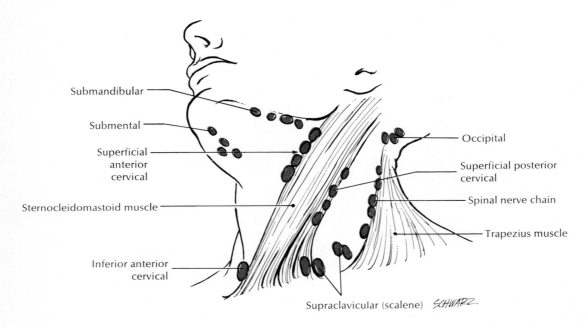

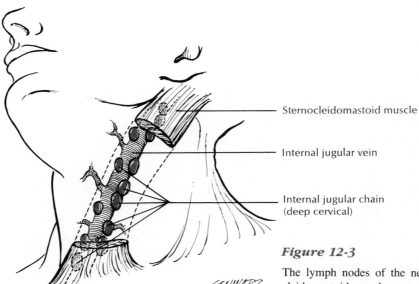

Figure 12-3

The lymph nodes of the neck. Note relationship to the sternocleidomastoid muscle.

Neck

The lymph nodes of the neck receive the lymph from the head and from the structures of the neck itself. These nodes are grouped serially and are referred to as chains (see Fig. 12-2; Fig. 12-3).

The *anterior superficial cervical chain* is located over and anterior to the sternocleidomastoid muscle and near but deeper than the external jugular vein. The nodes are beneath the platysma muscle and superficial cervical fascia and receive lymph from the skin and neck.

The nodes of the *thyrolinguofacial chain* are found between the lower margins of the posterior head of the digastric muscle and the thyrolinguofacial venous trunk. Lymph draining to this group is from the parotid, submaxillary, retrolaryngeal, prelaryngeal, pretracheal, and recurrent areas and from the tongue, palate, tonsils, thyroid and submaxillary glands, nose, pharynx, and outer and middle ear.

The *deep cervical chain* is made up of four chains of lymph nodes: the prelaryngeal chain, located anterior to the larynx; the prethyroid chain, situated anterior to the thyroid gland; the pretracheal and laterotracheal chain, located anterior and lateral to the trachea; and the recurrent chains found along the course of the recurrent laryngeal nerve. These nodes receive lymph from the larynx, thyroid gland, trachea, and upper part of the esophagus.

The *internal jugular chain* is made up of many lymph nodes that lie close to and along the jugular vein. The last of these nodes lie close to the thoracic duct.

The *spinal nerve chain* follows the external branch of the spinal nerve (cranial nerve [CN] IX). Collecting ducts from the posterior and lateral regions of the neck reach these nodes, as do those of the occipital and mastoid regions of the head.

The *posterior superficial cervical chain* follows the transverse cervical artery and vein. This chain terminates in the great lymphatic trunk on the right side and in the thoracic duct on the left side. Lymph from the subclavian, laterocervical, anterothoracic, and internal mammary regions reaches these nodes.

The *supraclavicular,* or scalene, nodes lie above the clavicle.

Lymph nodes that are involved with the drainage of the tongue and the ear are illustrated in Figs. 12-4 and 5.

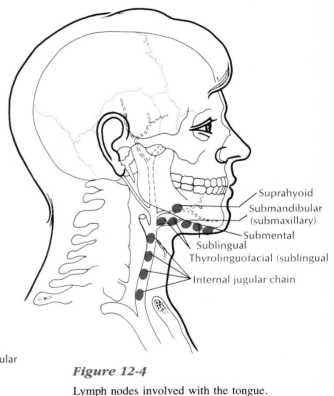

Figure 12-4

Lymph nodes involved with the tongue.

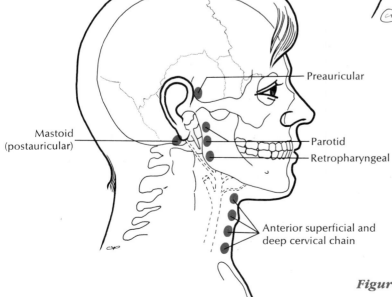

Figure 12-5

Lymph nodes involved with the ear.

Upper Extremity

A system of superficial and deep collecting ducts carries the lymph from the upper extremity to the infraclavicular (subclavian) lymphatic nodes (Fig. 12-6). The only peripheral center is the *epitrochlear center,* which receives some of the collecting ducts from the pathway along the ulnar artery and nerve. Lymphatics of the ulnar surface of the forearm, the fourth and fifth fingers, and the medial surface of the middle finger drain into the epitrochlear node. It is located at the elbow in a depression above and posterior to the medial condyle of the humerus.

Axilla

Five groups of lymph nodes are located in the axillary fossa (Fig. 12-7). All drain in an upward and medial direction toward the main lymph collecting channels.

The *axillary* (brachial) nodes receive collecting ducts from the upper extremity, deltoid region, and anterior wall of the chest, including part of the breast.

The *posterior* (scapular) nodes lie in the posterior aspect of the axilla and drain the posterior wall of the chest and the posteroinferior neck.

The *apical* (intermediate) nodes lie high in the axilla and receive ducts from the axillary and posterior lymph centers and from the chest wall, breast, and arm.

The *anterior axillary* (pectoral) group lies in the anterior aspect of the axilla and includes a superior group of two or three nodes found in the region of the third rib and the second and third intercostal spaces and an inferior group located over the fourth to sixth ribs. The ducts entering these nodes are from the breast and anterolateral chest wall and from the integument and muscles of the abdominal wall superior to the umbilicus.

The *infraclavicular* (subclavian) nodes are situated below the clavicle. Infections or malignancy of the upper extremity, breast, and chest wall may result in enlargement of these nodes.

Breast

Lymphatic drainage of the breast moves in several directions (Fig. 12-8). Cutaneous lymphatic drainage from the skin of the breast, excluding the areolar and nipple areas, flows into the axillary nodes. Lymph from the medial aspect of the skin of the breast may flow to the opposite breast. Lymph from the inferior portion of the breast can reach the deep lymphatic centers of the epigastric region and subsequently the liver and other abdominal regions and organs. Drainage from the areolar and nipple areas of the breast flows into the anterior axillary group of nodes. Lymphatic drainage from the deep mammary tissues flows into the anterior axillary nodes. Some of this lymph also flows into the infraclavic-

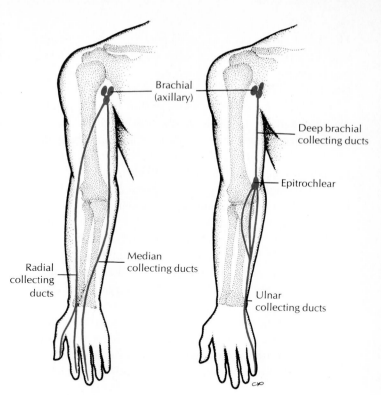

Figure 12-6

System of deep and superficial collecting ducts, carrying the lymph from the upper extremity to the subclavian lymphatic trunk. The only peripheral lymph center is the epitrochlear, which receives some of the collecting ducts from the pathways near the ulnar and radial nerves.

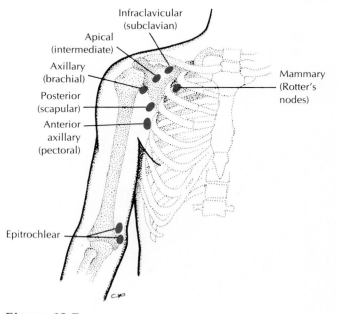

Figure 12-7

Five groups of lymph nodes may be distinguished in the axillary fossa.

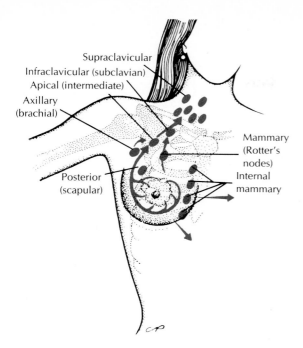

Figure 12-8

Lymphatic drainage of the breast.

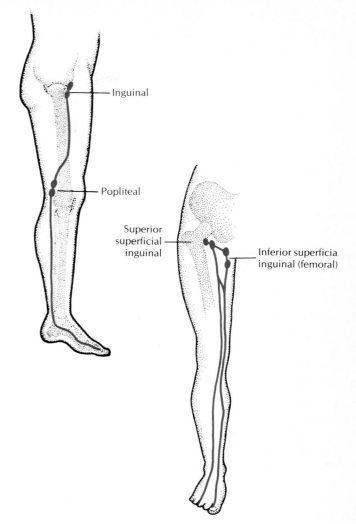

Figure 12-9

Lymphatic drainage of the lower extremity.

ular and supraclavicular nodes. Lymph from the retroareolar areas, medial glandular breast tissue, and lower glandular breast tissue drains into the substernal internal mammary nodes, which drain into the thorax and abdomen.

Lower Extremity

A system of superficial and deep collecting ducts drains the lymph from the leg (Fig. 12-9). The *popliteal lymph center* is located in the back of the knee. The afferent ducts to these nodes are from the heel and outer aspect of the foot. The majority of lymph drainage from the lower extremity is delivered to the *inguinal nodes*. There are two groups of superficial inguinal nodes: inferior and superior.

The inferior group is a group of large lymph nodes that receives lymph from the superficial regions of the leg and foot. These inguinal nodes lie below the junction of the saphenous and femoral veins. The superficial nodes lie along the course of the saphenous vein. The deep sublinguinal nodes lie medial to the femoral vein and follow the vessel into the abdomen.

The superior group lies along the inguinal ligament. The afferent ducts are from the abdominal wall inferior to the umbilicus, from the buttocks, and from the efferent vessels of the inferior center. Lymph from around the internal female genitalia drain into the pelvic and para-aortic nodes, which are deep and not accessible

to physical examination. The vulva and lower third of the vagina drain to the inguinal nodes. In the male, lymphatic drainage from the testes is also deep into the abdomen, inaccessible to physical examination. Lymph from the penile and scrotal surfaces drains to the inguinal nodes.

RELEVANT HISTORY

Relevant history would include fever, infections, fatigue, weakness, unexplained weight loss or gain, intravenous use of street drugs, tuberculosis and other skin testing, blood transfusions, use of blood products, chronic illness (cardiac, renal, malignancy, acquired immunodeficiency syndrome [AIDS]), and surgery with trauma to regional lymph nodes.

Present problems would include:
1. Enlarged nodes (client may refer to them as bumps, kernels, or swollen glands):
   a. Characteristics: location, onset, duration, quantity, tenderness
   b. Associated symptoms: pain, fever, redness
   c. Predisposing factors: infection, malignancy, trauma
2. Bleeding:
   a. Site: nose, mouth, rectal, skin
   b. Characteristics: onset, duration, frequency, amount, color
3. Swelling:
   a. Characteristics: location, onset, duration, intermittent or constant
   b. Predisposing factors: cardiac, hepatic, or renal disorder, venous insufficiency, infection, trauma, surgery
   c. Other symptoms: redness or discoloration, warmth, ulceration

EXAMINATION

The techniques of observation and palpation are used to examine the lymphatic system. The equipment used includes a centimeter ruler and tape measure. Examination of the lymphatic system is incorporated into the complete physical examination in each region of the body where superficial nodes might be palpated (Fig. 12-10).

The first step is inspection for enlarged lymph nodes, skin lesions, edema, erythema, and red streaks on the skin. The next step is to palpate gently the lymph node areas using the pads of the second, third, and fourth fingers in a gentle circular motion. Press lightly at first, increasing the pressure gradually. Heavy pressure can push the nodes into the deeper soft tissues so that their presence may be missed. Move the skin lightly over the underlying tissues rather than moving the examining fingers over the skin.

Any nodes detected should be described according to location, size, regularity, consistency, tenderness, mobility or fixation to surrounding tissues, and discreteness or matting (see boxed material). Palpable lymph nodes are generally not present in healthy individuals, but some people have a few discrete, mobile, small (less than 1 cm in diameter) nodes that are not clinically significant. Large, fixed, matted, inflamed, or tender lymph nodes indicate a problem. Nodes are described as matted if they are enlarged and close enough together so that they feel like a mass rather than like separate and discrete nodes. Enlarged nodes resulting from infection may be tender and matted, particularly if the infection persists. Enlarged nodes due to malignancy are generally not tender; they vary considerably in size, tend to be hard, and often show

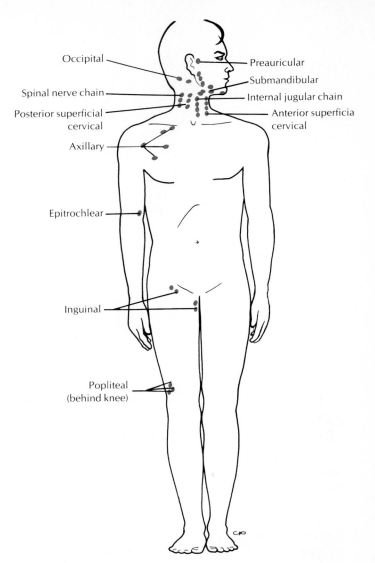

Figure 12-10

Areas to be examined for lymph nodes during the physical examination.

asymmetric involvement. When enlarged lymph nodes are found, the examiner must explore the areas drained by those nodes for signs of infection or malignancy.

Examination of Lymph Nodes by Region
Head and neck

The practitioner must establish a sequence such as the following one for examining the numerous nodal centers of the head and neck:
1. Preauricular—in front of the ear (Fig. 12-11)
2. Mastoid or posterior auricular—behind the ear over the mastoid process
3. Occipital—at the base of the skull posteriorly
4. Parotid—near the angle of the jaw
5. Submandibular—midway between the angle of the jaw and the tip of the mandible

---

Characteristics Assessed in Examination of Lymph Nodes

Location

Describe site specifically. Use imaginary body lines or axes and bony prominences to describe the location. Draw pictures where appropriate.

Size

Describe size in three dimensions (length, width, and thickness).

Shape

Describe as round or oval, regular or irregular.

Surface characteristics

Describe as smooth, nodular, irregular.

Consistency

Describe as hard, firm, soft, spongy, cystic.

Symmetry

Describe whether symmetric or asymmetric.

Fixation, mobility

Describe whether mass is mobile or fixed to surrounding structures.

Tenderness

Describe whether mass is present without palpation or elicited by palpation.

Erythema

Describe extent of color change if present.

Pulsatile nature

Describe pulsations if they are usually not palpable at this site. Auscultate all masses for bruits.

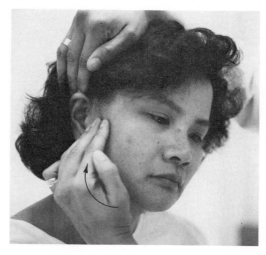

Figure 12-11

Palpation of the preauricular lymph nodes.

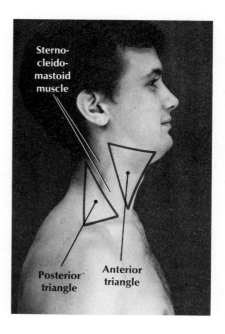

Figure 12-12

The conception of the triangles of the neck is useful in defining the location of palpable lymph nodes. The sternocleidomastoid muscle is the division line between the anterior and posterior triangles. The trapezius muscle marks the posterior border of the posterior triangle.

6. Submental—in the midline posterior to the tip of the mandible

   The neck can be divided into anterior and posterior triangles divided by the sternocleidomastoid muscle (Fig. 12-12). The practitioner then moves to the neck to examine the following:

1. Anterior superficial cervical chain—over and anterior to the sternocleidomastoid muscle, in the anterior triangle of the neck (Figs. 12-12 and 12-13).
2. Posterior cervical chain—along the anterior edge of the trapezius, in the posterior triangle of the neck (see Fig. 12-12; Fig 12-14).
3. Deep cervical nodes—deep to the sternocleidomastoid (These are difficult to examine, particularly if pressed too heavily. The examiner should probe gently with thumb and fingers around the muscle or hook the thumb and fingers around the muscle.)

4. Supraclavicular or scalene nodes—in the angle formed by the clavical and the sternocleidomastoid muscle (Fig. 12-15)

   It is useful to have the client bend the head forward or toward the side of the neck being examined to reduce muscle tension and enhance accurate palpation (Figs. 12-16 and 12-17).

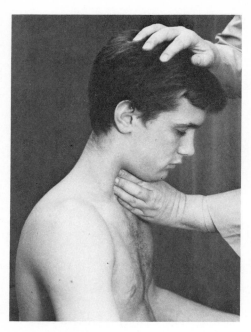

Figure 12-13

Palpation of the anterior triangle.

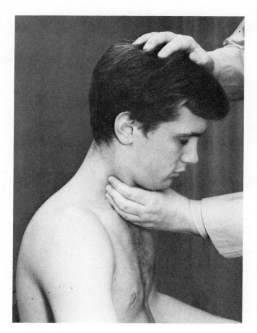

Figure 12-14

Palpation of the posterior triangle.

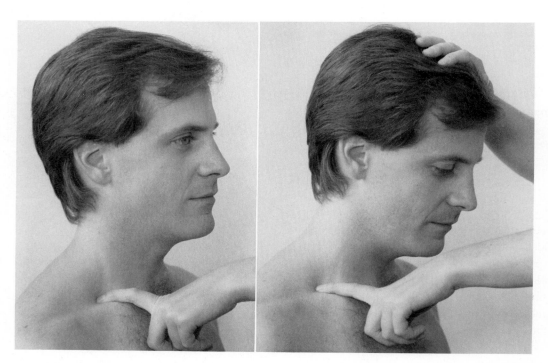

Figure 12-15

Palpation of the scalene triangle for the supraclavicular lymph nodes. The client is encouraged to relax the musculature of the upper extremities, so that the clavicles are dropped. The examiner's free hand is used to flex the client's head forward to obtain relaxation of the soft tissues of the anterior neck. The left index finger is hooked over the clavicle lateral to the sternocleidomastoid muscle.

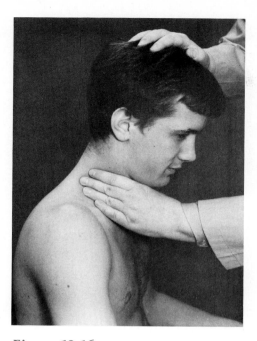

Figure 12-16

Flexing the neck to relax muscles.

Upper extremity

The epitrochlear node is palpated above and posterior to the medial condyle of the humerus (Fig. 12-18). The examiner should flex the client's arm to reduce muscle tension.

Axilla

Examination of the axillary lymph nodes is approached by palpating the apical, lateral, anterior, and posterior regions of the axilla. At the top are the apical (intermediate) nodes; medially are the axillary nodes; anteriorly are the anterior axillary (pectoral) nodes; and posteriorly are the posterior (scapular) nodes. To palpate the axillary lymph nodes, the examiner uses the arm to support the client's contralateral forearm or has the client's forearm rest on the examiner's forearm (Fig. 12-19). A deliberate, firm, and yet gentle touch will feel less ticklish to the client. The examiner palpates along the upper chest wall and deep into the axilla by gently rolling the soft tissue against the chest wall and muscles.

Breast

Examination of the lymph nodes of the breast and adjacent structures is described in Chapter 13, Assessment of the Breasts.

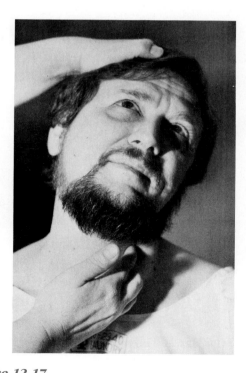

Figure 12-17

Bending the head toward the side being examined to relax muscles and soft tissue allows more accurate palpation for lymph nodes.

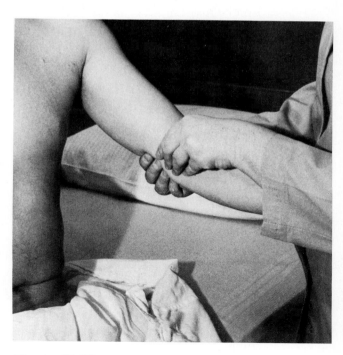

Figure 12-18

Palpation for the epitrochlear lymph nodes.

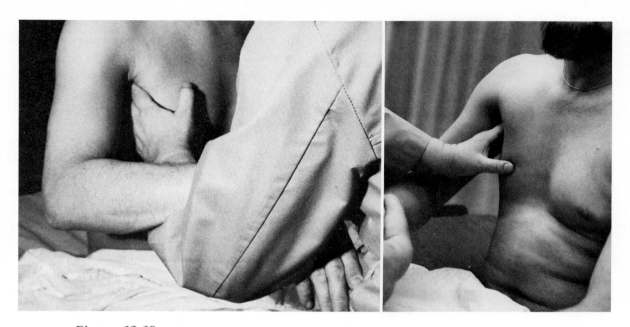

Figure 12-19

The soft tissues of the axilla are gently rolled against the chest wall and the muscles surrounding the axilla. Note two methods of supporting the client's arm.

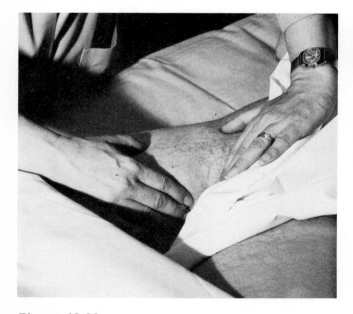

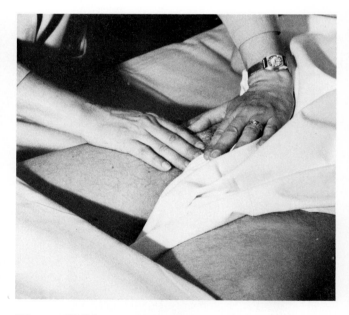

Figure 12-20

Palpation of the inferior superficial inguinal (femoral) lymph nodes.

Figure 12-21

Palpation of the superior superficial inguinal lymph nodes.

Lower extremity

The examiner palpates the inferior and superior superficial inguinal nodes while the client is lying down with the knee slightly flexed (Figs. 12-20 and 12-21). Also, the knee should be flexed when the popliteal nodes behind the knee are being examined.

COMMON ABNORMALITIES

Pathologic findings in the lymphatic system result from:
1. Localized or systemic infection
2. Metastatic cancer
3. Malignant lymphomas
4. Hypersensitivity reactions

Health History
Lymphatic System

NOTE: A yes response to any question *must* be further investigated. Use the following indicators throughout the assessment: (1) onset (specific date, sudden or gradual), (2) duration, (3) frequency, (4) precipitating factors, (5) aggravating or alleviating factors, (6) treatment received, and (7) outcome.

Present status

1. Do you have lumps under your arms, in your neck or groin?
   a. Description: hard, soft, constant, intermittent, moveable, fixed
2. Do you experience tenderness or pain under your arms, in your neck or groin?
   a. Description: constant, only when touched, dull, aching, interferes with movement
3. Do your legs swell?
   a. Description: pitting, nonpitting, affected by time of day, constant, intermittent, interferes with walking
4. Are you unusually fatigued or weak?
   a. Relation to activity
5. Do you use illicit street drugs?
   a. Type and route—describe
6. Does your skin itch?
   a. Location
   b. Accompanying rash present
7. Do you have night sweats?

Past history

1. Have you had Hodgkin's disease?
   a. Stage classification
2. Have you had a low grade fever?
   a. Degree of elevation
   b. At specific time of day

Associated conditions

1. Have you had an infection?
   a. Location
   b. Fever present
2. Have you had cancer?
   a. Location
   b. Residual effects
3. Have you had frequent sore throats?
4. Have you had a blood transfusion?
   a. When
   b. Reason
5. Have you had surgery on your spleen, underarms, groin, tonsils, adenoids, breast(s)?
   a. When
   b. Type
   c. Residual effects
6. Have you been diagnosed as having AIDS or AIDS-related complex?
7. Have you had heart disease?
   a. Type

Family history

1. Does any family member have a history of cancer, lymphomas, anemias, Hodgkin's disease?
2. Has anyone in your family had infectious mononucleosis?

Sample assessment record

Client states onset of fatigue was 3 months ago. States she is unable to work some days because of the fatigue. Has had night sweats and generalized itching over entire body for last 4 to 5 weeks. Denies having infection, sore throat, or fever but noted a slight swelling in the neck under the jaw in the last week. Denies any accompanying neck pain. Denies swelling in armpits, groin, or legs. Denies use of illicit drugs, receiving a blood transfusion, and any previous surgery. Negative family history for cancer, heart disease, or mononucleosis.

The location and characteristics of abnormal lymph nodes help to determine the site, origin, and cause of the disease. The clinical significance of a node depends, in part, on its location and on the client's age. Children are more likely than adults to develop generalized lymphadenopathy and more frequently have enlarged nodes with mild infections of the respiratory tract and skin. Children with no other physical findings frequently have enlarged neck nodes that may not be clinically signficant. Lymphadenopathy in the adult usually indicates more serious disease. The most frequent causes of node enlargement are acute and chronic infections and neoplastic disease. Enlarged nodes resulting from acute infection are firm and tender and may be discrete or matted. The overlying skin may be red and edematous. In chronic infection the nodes are nontender. The nodes associated with lymphoma are rubbery, firm, large, mobile and may not be tender. The nodes of metastatic cancer are hard, bound to surrounding tissue and thus immobile and nontender.

Variations from Health
Infection

Among the common infections associated with enlarged nodes in the neck are bacterial infections such as streptococcal pharyngitis and viral infections such as viral pharyngitis and infectious mononucleosis.

Generalized lymphadenopathy is frequently seen in individuals with AIDS and AIDS-related complex (ARC). This is often found early in the disease.

Neoplasms

Malignant lymphomas, including Hodgkin's disease, cause nodes to be large, discrete, nontender, and firm and rubbery. Such nodes may be localized to any area but are occasionally generalized. Chronic lymphocytic leukemia causes lymphadenopathy with the same characteristics as lymphoma, but the findings are usually generalized.

Lymph nodes of metastatic cancer are nontender, have firm to hard consistency, may be discrete or matted, and tend to be localized initially.

Lymphedema

Acquired lymphedema results from trauma to the ducts of regional lymph nodes, typically the axillary and inguinal nodes. Infection; surgical trauma as with radical mastectomy or groin dissection, especially when followed by radiation therapy; or the presence of a tumor leading to blockage can all cause lymphedema.

Congenital lymphedema is an uncommon disorder caused by hypoplasia and maldevelopment of the lymphatic system. This results in swelling and distortion of the extremities, which varies with the severity and distribution of the disease.

Painless swelling of the involved extremity is the earliest and most common indication of lymphedema.

Initially the swelling may subside at night, but as the process progresses and the subcutaneous tissue and skin become fibrotic, the swelling becomes permanent. Lymphedema is nonpitting, and the overlying skin will eventually thicken.

Acute lymphangitis

Acute lymphangitis is the inflammation of one or more lymphatic vessels characterized by pain, malaise, and possibly fever. One or more red streaks may follow the course of the lymphatic collecting duct(s) progressing up the extremity. The examiner should look for skin lesions or other portals of entry distal to the inflammation.

Any swelling of an extremity due to lymphedema or lymphangitis should be measured regularly at a fixed distance from some anatomic landmark, such as a bony prominence or a joint.

BIBLIOGRAPHY

Brady LW and others: Differentiating neck masses in children, Patient Care 18:12, 1984.

Brady LW and others: Causes of neck masses in young adults, Patient Care 18:30, 1984.

Brady LW and others: When an older adult develops a neck mass, Patient Care 18:56, 1984.

Haagensen CD and others: The lymphatics in cancer, Philadelphia, 1972, WB Saunders Co.

Mayerson HS: Lymph and lymphatic system, Springfield, Ill, 1968, Charles C Thomas, Publisher.

Zitelli BJ: Neck masses in children: adenopathy and malignant disease, Pediatr Clin North Am 28:813, 1981.

Zuelzer WW and Kaplan J: The child with lymphadenopathy, Semin Hematol 12:323, 1975.

13

Assessment of the breasts

OBJECTIVES

Upon successful review of this chapter, learners will be able to:

- Describe anatomy and physiology of the breasts through the life span

- State related rationale and demonstrate assessment of the breasts, including inspection and palpation techniques

- Outline history relevant to a breast examination

- Recognize abnormalities and common deviations of the breasts in men and women

- Describe procedures used to evaluate breast masses

- Identify breast cancer risk factors

ANATOMY AND PHYSIOLOGY

The breast is a modified sebaceous gland that is paired and located on the anterior chest wall between the second and third ribs superiorly, the sixth and seventh costal cartilages inferiorly, the anterior axillary line laterally, and the sternal border medially.

The functional components of the female breast consist of the acini or milk-producing glands, a ductal system, and a nipple (Fig. 13-1, *A*). The glandular tissue units are called lobes and are situated in circular, spoke-like fashion around the nipple. There are 15 to 25 lobes per breast. Each lobe is composed of 20 to 40 lobules, each containing 10 to 100 acini.

Much of the bulk of the breast is composed of subcutaneous and retromammary fat. The breast is fairly mobile but is supported by a layer of subcutaneous connective tissue and by Cooper's ligaments (Fig. 13-1, *B*). The latter are multiple fibrous bands that begin at the breast's subcutaneous connective tissue layer and run through the breast, attaching to muscle fascia.

Knowledge of the lymphatic drainage of the breast is critical because of the frequent dissemination of breast cancer through this system. There are three types of lymphatic drainage of the breast (Fig. 13-2).

Cutaneous lymphatic drainage is of lymph from the skin of the breast, excluding the areolar and nipple areas; this lymph flows into the ipsilateral axillary nodes (the mammary, scapular, brachial, and intermediate nodes). Lymph from the medial cutaneous breast area may flow to the opposite breast. Lymph from the inferior portion of the breast can reach the lymphatic plexus of the epigastric region and subsequently the liver and other abdominal regions and organs.

Areolar lymphatic drainage is of lymph formed in the areolar and nipple areas of the breast; this lymph

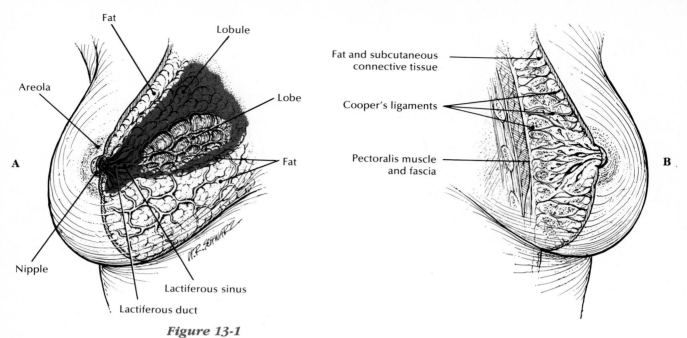

Figure 13-1

Female breasts. **A,** Internal structures. **B,** Supportive tissue structures.

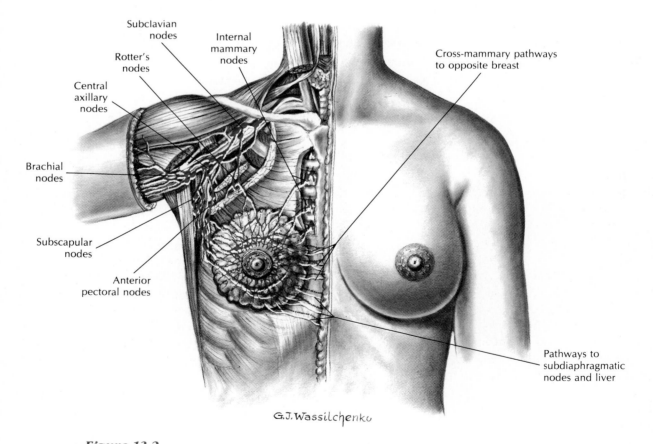

Figure 13-2

Lymphatic drainage of the breast.
(From Jensen MD and Bobak IM: Maternity and gynecologic care: the nurse and family, ed 3, St Louis, 1985, The CV Mosby Co.)

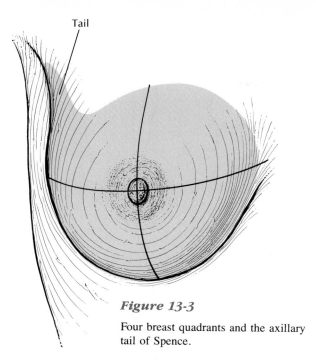

Tail

Figure 13-3

Four breast quadrants and the axillary tail of Spence.

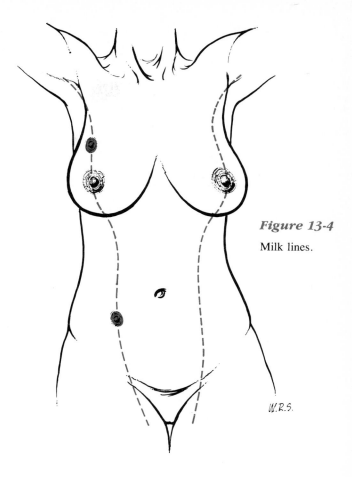

Figure 13-4

Milk lines.

flows into the anterior axillary group of nodes (the mammary nodes).

Deep lymphatic drainage is of lymph from the deep mammary tissues; this lymph flows into the anterior axillary nodes. Some of this lymph also flows into the apical, subclavian, infraclavicular, and supraclavicular nodes. Also, lymph from the retroareolar areas, medial glandular breast tissue areas, and lower glandular breast tissue areas communicates with lymphatic systems draining into the thorax and abdomen.

The largest portion of glandular breast tissue occurs in the upper lateral quadrant of each breast. From this quadrant there is an anatomic projection of breast tissue into the axilla. This projection is termed the axillary tail of Spence (Fig. 13-3). The majority of breast tumors are located in the upper lateral breast quadrant and in the tail of Spence.

On general appearance the normal breasts are reasonably symmetric in size and shape, although they are not usually absolutely equal. This symmetry remains constant at rest and with movement. The skin of the breast is the same as that of the abdomen or back. There may be a small number of scattered hair follicles around the areola. In light-complected persons a horizontal or vertical vascular pattern may be observed. This pattern, when normally present, is symmetric.

The areolae are pigmented areas surrounding the nipples. Their color varies from pink to brown, and their size varies greatly. Several or many sebaceous glands (termed Montgomery's tubercles or follicles) may be present on the areolar surface.

The nipples are round, hairless, pigmented, protuberant structures whose size and shape vary among women and in an individual woman depending on the state of contraction. Usually nipples are directed or "point" slightly upward and laterally.

Inversion of the nipple is an invagination or depression of its central portion. Inversion can occur congenitally or as a response to an invasive process.

During early embryonic development longitudinal ridges exist, extending from the axilla to the groin. Called "milk lines" (Fig. 13-4), these ridges usually atrophy, except at the level of the pectoral muscles, where a breast will eventually develop. In some women the ridges do not entirely disappear, and portions of the milk lines persist. This existence is manifested in the presence of a nipple, a nipple and a breast, or glandular breast tissue only. This congenital anomaly is termed a supernumerary breast or nipple.

The gross appearance and size of the normal female breast vary both among individuals and for an individual at various phases of development. The following describes breast development through a woman's life span (Fig. 13-5):

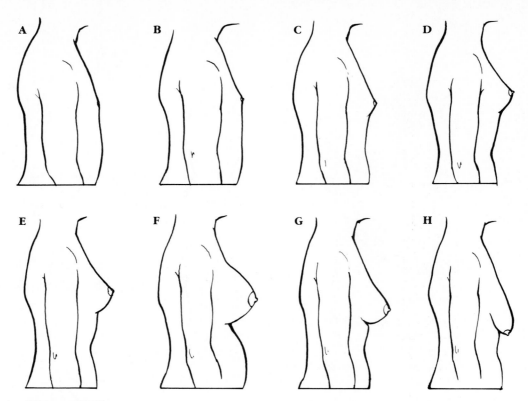

Figure 13-5

Appearance of the female breast in various life periods. **A,** Appearance before age 10. **B** to **D,** Appearance between ages 10 through 14. **E,** Appearance of the nulliparous, adult breast. **F,** Appearance of the breast during pregnancy. **G,** Appearance of the breast in a woman who has had a pregnancy. **H,** Appearance of the breast after menopause.

1. *Appearance before age 10:* There is little difference in gross appearance between male and female breasts. The nipples are small and slightly elevated. There is no palpable glandular tissue or areolar pigmentation.

2. *Appearance between the ages of 10 and 14:* The mammary tissues adjacent to and beneath the areola grow, resulting in an increased diameter of the areola and the formation of a "mammary bud." The nipple and breast protrude as a single mound. Breast development may normally begin or progress unilaterally. Next the general mammary growth and increases in diameter and pigmentation of the areola continue, resulting in further elevation of the breasts. The nipple begins to separate from the areola. Growth continues in the mammary tissues. The nipple and areola form a mound distinct from the globular shape of the rest of the breast.

3. *Appearance after age 14:* The shape of the adult female breast is gradually formed. The areola recedes into the general contour of the breast, and only the nipple protrudes. The size of the adult female breast is influenced by heredity, individual sensitivity to hormones, and nutrition.

4. *Appearance during the female reproductive years:* In response to hormonal changes during the menstrual cycle, there is a cyclic pattern of breast size change, along with nodularity and tenderness, that is maximal just before menses. The breast is smallest in days 4 through 7 of the menstrual cycle. During days 3 to 4 before the onset of menses, mammary tenseness, fullness, heaviness, tenderness, and pain are experienced by many women, and total breast volume is significantly increased.

5. *Changes in pregnancy:* The breast increases in size, sometimes to as large as two or three times the usual size. The areolae and nipples become more prominent and more deeply pigmented. The veins engorge, the Montgomery's glands become more apparent, and striae are often observed.

6. *Menopausal changes:* After menopause, the breast's glandular tissue gradually involutes, and fat is deposited in the breasts. Breast form becomes flabby and flattened.

   The male breast contains a nipple and an areola. Beneath the nipple is a small amount of breast tissue, which usually cannot be clinically differentiated from the other subcutaneous tissues.

EXAMINATION

Approach to the Examination

Some girls and women are embarrassed during the breast examination. The examiner should take care to ensure privacy for the examination and to avoid unnecessary exposure of the breasts. Explanation of the components of the examination can also assist to relieve discomfort.

During the health history preceding the physical examination, the examiner should assess the woman's level of knowledge and practice regarding breast self-examination. The examination provides an excellent opportunity for teaching self-examination and for reviewing the client's technique.

HELPFUL HINT: A small pillow or a folded towel will be needed for all examinations. A ruler and a glass slide and cytology fixative may be needed if there are abnormal clinical findings.

If the client has noticed a lump or change in one of the breasts, ask her to point out the area and to demonstrate the technique used to note the lump or change. The examiner can take special note of that area during the examination.

Many adolescent or adult male clients may not have had a breast examination previously and may be concerned that the examiner may have noticed a problem. Explanation to male clients that breast lesions are possible in men and that the breast examination is a routine component of a complete health assessment can decrease the possibility of worry and embarrassment. Often male clients have perspiration in the axilla and are embarrassed when a female examiner palpates the dampened area. A tissue may be offered to the male client to dry the area.

Inspection

Inspection and palpation are the techniques to examine the breast. For initial inspection, the client is seated on the side of the examination table and is uncovered to the waist. The breasts are observed for symmetry of shape and size, surface characteristics, and abnormal amount or distribution of hair.

Symmetry of shape and size

Normal female breasts are bilaterally similar in shape and size. However, frequently one breast is somewhat smaller than the other (Fig. 13-6). In males, breasts are normally even with the chest wall, except for obese men, whose breasts assume a bilaterally convex shape similar to female breasts.

Surface characteristics

Surface characteristics include hyperpigmentation, moles and nevi, edema, retraction or dimpling, focal vascular-

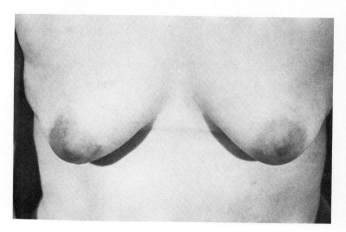

Figure 13-6

Observation of the breasts. These breasts have several characteristics that are deviations within normal limits: (1) the left breast is slightly larger than the right; (2) the direction of the nipples is slightly different; and (3) there are two indentations in the outer right breast.

ity, and lesions. The skin of the breasts appears smooth, and the surface contour should appear even and uninterrupted. Only the areola and nipple are normally hyperpigmented. Other portions of the breast are normally a color uniform with the individual's skin. Focal hyperpigmentation is an abnormal finding.

Moles and nevi are common. The client should be questioned about changes or problems with any common skin lesion noted.

Edema of the breast produces exaggeration of the skin pores, creating an orange-peel appearance of the breast called peau d'orange (Fig. 13-7, *B*).

Retraction, or dimpling, appears as a depression or pucker on the skin (Fig. 13-7, *A*). It usually is caused by the fibrotic shortening and immobilization or Cooper's ligament by an invasive process.

Vascular patterns should be diffuse and symmetric. Hypervascular patterns may be noted in pregnant, obese, and very fair-skinned individuals. Focal or unilateral patterns are abnormal and may be produced by dilated superficial veins from increased blood flow to a malignancy (Fig. 13-7, *A*).

The elastic fibers of the dermis may be damaged whenever the skin of the breasts is stretched rapidly, and observable striae, or stretch marks, are produced. Newly created striae are reddish; they become whitish with age.

Areolar area and nipple characteristics

After puberty, women may normally have a scattering of coarse, curly hair on the breasts, mostly near the areola. After puberty, males often have a dense mass of chest

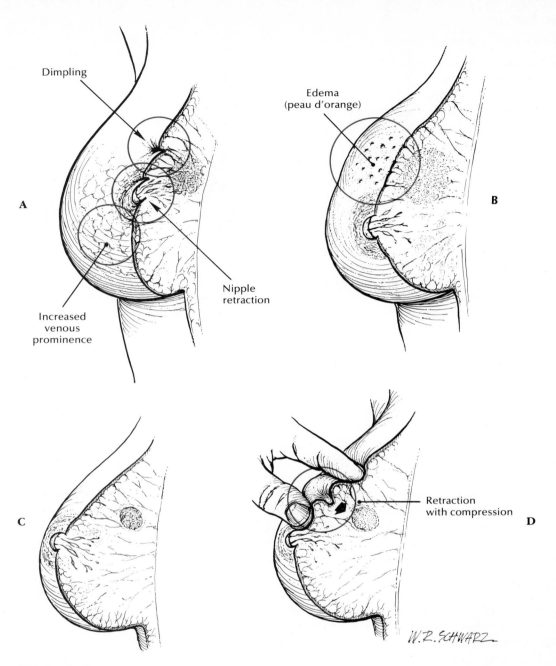

Figure 13-7

Abnormalities of the breast. **A,** Breast with dimpling, nipple retraction, and increased venous prominence. **B,** Breast with edema (peau d'orange or pigskin appearance). **C,** Breast with tumor; no retraction is apparent. **D,** Breast with tumor; retraction is apparent with compression.

hair around the areola. Male hair patterns in female clients are abnormal.

The areolar area is normally round or oval and bilaterally similar. Irregular placement of Montgomery's tubercles is common and normal. The areolar area can range from light pink to dark brown depending on the client's genetic skin color and hormonal influences. In pregnancy, the areolae enlarge and darken.

The areolar area is inspected for size, shape, sym-

metry, color, surface characteristics, bulging, and lesions. As mentioned previously, size, shape, and color can normally vary greatly in symmetric patterns. Any asymmetry, mass, or lesion should be considered abnormal.

If the breasts are symmetric, both nipples should be pointing laterally in the same way. The nipple is observed for size, shape, ability to erect, color, discharge, and lesions. The nipples should be round, equal in size,

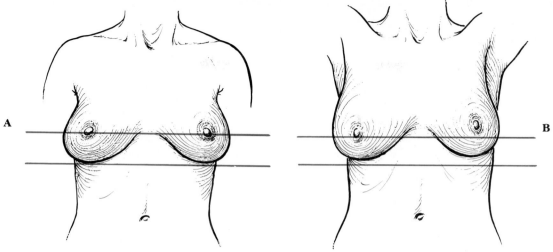

Figure 13-8

A, Breasts appear symmetric at rest. **B,** Breasts do not move symmetrically with arm elevation. The right breast is immobilized.

homogeneous in color, and have convoluted surfaces, which give them a wrinkled appearance. They should appear soft and smooth and have no crusting, cracks, or discharge.

Inversion of one or both nipples, if present from puberty, is normal; however, this condition may interfere with breast-feeding. Recent inversion of the nipple is probably retraction (see Fig. 13-7, *A*) and should be investigated.

Supernumerary nipples and areolar may appear along the milk lines (see Fig. 13-4). These lesions can vary in size, are the color of the individual's actual areolae, and are often mistaken for moles. Occasionally glandular tissue may accompany these lesions.

Paget's disease appears as a red glandular erosion of the nipple or as a nipple that is dry, scaly, or friable. The areola may also be affected. Paget's disease is a malignant condition requiring prompt therapy.

Breast secretions are normal in pregnancy or lactation. Other causes of discharge are mechanical nipple stimulation, drug influence, hypothalamic and pituitary disorders, and malignant and benign breast lesions. The discharge can be milky, watery, purulent, serous, or bloody. The method for determining the site of discharge production is discussed in the section on palpation.

Sitting positions for breast inspection

There are four major sitting positions of the client used for breast inspection. Every client should be examined in each position:

1. The client seated with arms at sides. The breasts are observed at rest and without movement to establish a baseline for comparison. Men are observed in this position only if they have unusually large breasts, in which case the other inspection positions will be used also.
2. The client is seated with arms abducted over the head. This maneuver creates tension on the suspensory ligaments and may accentuate asymmetry, retraction, and fixation.
3. The client is seated and pushes the hands into the hips (or pushes the palms together), simultaneously eliciting contraction of the pectoral muscles. This maneuver contracts the pectoral muscles and can reveal deviations in symmetry.
4. The client is seated and leans over while the examiner assists in supporting and balancing the client. During this maneuver, the breasts should hand evenly and symmetrically. It is especially useful in examining the movement and contour of large breasts.

While the client is performing these maneuvers, the breasts are carefully observed for symmetry, bulging, retraction, and fixation. An abnormality may not be apparent in the breasts at rest (Fig. 13-8, *A*), but a mass may cause the breasts, through invasion of suspensory ligaments, to fix, preventing them from upward or forward movement in positions 2 (Fig. 13-8, *B*) and 4. Position 3 specifically assists in eliciting dimpling if a mass has infiltrated and shortened suspensory ligaments.

The breasts are also observed with the client lying down, before the examiner palpates.

Palpation

The range of normal breast consistency is wide. The normal breast feels granular. This granularity is generalized and becomes more prominent with age.

The breasts normally feel somewhat "lumpy." This results from the configuration of the breast lobes, the fat and connective tissue between and supporting the lobes and other structures, and the irregular density of lobules. Thus, the consistency of breasts is not uniform. However, this variation of consistency should be noted uniformly through the breasts of an individual client.

The breasts feel relatively homogeneous in the young adolescent. The presence of progesterone in pregnancy and premenstrually causes the breasts to feel gen-erally nodular. Hormonally induced nodularity is bilateral and diffuse.

The primary purpose for the palpation of breasts is to discover masses. If a mass is discovered, it is assessed according to the characteristics shown in the box below.

The palpation portion of the examination of the breast begins with palpation for axillary, subclavicular, and supraclavicular lymph nodes. This is most effectively performed with the client in a sitting position. The lo-

---

Assessment of Breast Masses

1. *Location:* Masses are designated according to the quadrant in which they lie: upper outer, lower outer, upper inner, or lower inner (Fig. 13-9, *A*). When describing the mass in the client's record, one may find it helpful to draw the mass within a diagram of the breast (Fig. 13-9, *B*). Another method of describing location is to visualize the breast as the face of a clock; the nipple is center. A mass can be designated, for example, as being "5 cm from the nipple in the 8 o'clock position."
2. *Size:* The size should be approximated in centimeters in all its planes. For example, a mass may be ovoid, 3 cm wide, 2 cm long, and 1 cm thick.
3. *Shape:* The shape may be round, ovoid, irregular, or matted. Matting occurs in the presence of multiple lesions.
4. *Consistency:* The palpable consistency of a breast lesion may be soft, hard, solid, or cystic. One way to evaluate the consistency of a breast lesion is to palpate over the lesion with the pads of the index and middle fingers of the palpating hand (Fig. 13-10, *A*).

5. *Discreteness:* The borders of a mass are assessed to determine if they are sharp and well defined or irregular. To assess discreteness, the examiner attempts to palpate all the borders of the mass with the thumb and index finger of the palpating hand (Fig. 13-10, *B*).
6. *Mobility:* The movability of the mass within the breast is assessed as freely movable, or fixed. To assess mobility, the examiner uses the thumb and index finger of the examining hand to "hold" the mass, and then the mass is moved in all directions possible (Fig. 13-10, *C*). A fixed mass will not permit any movement.
7. *Tenderness:* The client is questioned regarding any discomfort with palpation.
8. *Erythema:* The area of skin overlying the mass is inspected for erythema.
9. *Dimpling over the mass:* The tissue over the mass is compressed to determine if this maneuver produces dimpling (Fig. 13-7, *D*).

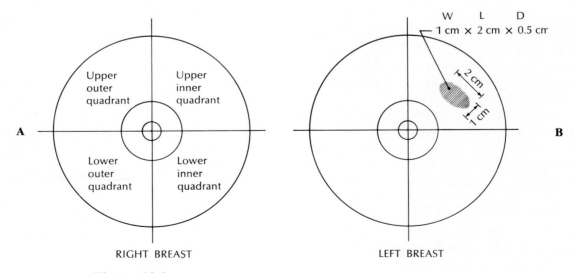

Figure 13-9

A, The four quadrants of the breast. **B,** Diagram of a mass within a breast.

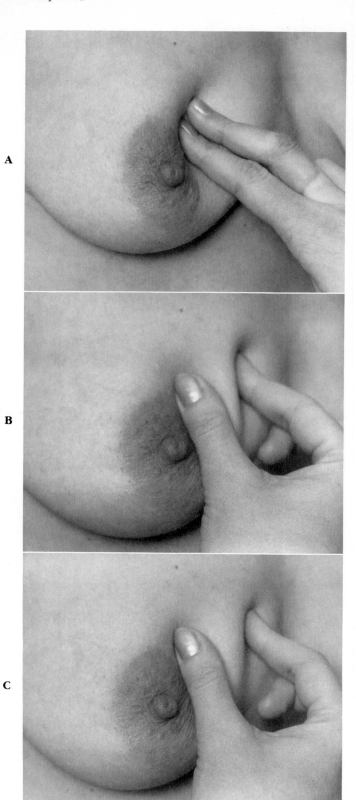

cation and palpation of the axillary, subclavicular, and supraclavicular nodes are described in Chapter 12 on assessment of the lymphatic system. To emphasize the importance of an adequate axillary area examination with each breast examination, this procedure is reviewed here.

In examining the axilla, the tissues can be best appreciated if the area muscles are relaxed. Contracted muscles may obscure slightly enlarged nodes. To achieve this relaxation while at the same time abducting the arm, the examiner supports the ipsilateral arm (Fig. 13-11).

The examiner should visualize the axilla as a four-sided pyramid and thoroughly palpate the following areas: (1) the edge of the pectoralis major muscle for the mammary group of nodes, (2) the thoracic wall for the intermediate group of nodes, (3) the upper part of the humerus for the brachial axillary group of nodes, and (4) the anterior edge of the latissimus dorsi muscle for the subscapular group of nodes.

The breasts are most effectively palpated with the client in a supine position. Because of time constraints on most physical examinations, it is not advised that all breasts be also palpated with the client in a sitting position. However, several groups of clients should also be examined in the sitting position: women with present or past complaints of breast masses, women at high risk of breast cancer, and women with pendulous breasts.

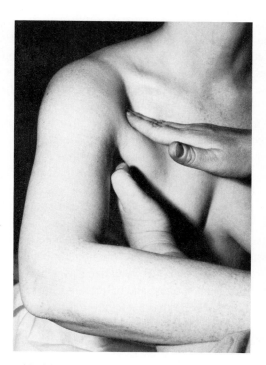

Figure 13-10

A, Palpating for consistency of breast lesion. **B,** Palpating for delineation of borders of breast mass. **C,** Palpating for mobility of breast mass.

Figure 13-11

Palpation of the axillary lymph nodes. (Note that the client's arm is supported on the examiner's arm.)

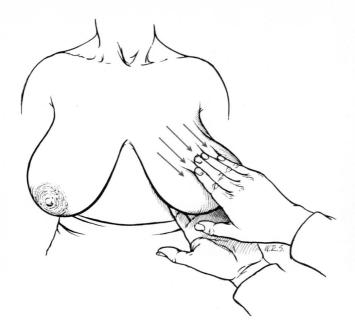

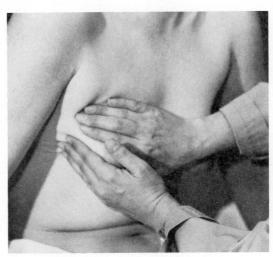

Figure 13-12

Bimanual palpation of the breasts.

With the client in a sitting position, small breasts can be examined by using one hand to support the breast while the other hand palpates the tissue against the chest wall. Pendulous breasts are palpated using a bimanual technique (Fig. 13-12). The inferior portion of the breast is supported in one hand while the other palpates breast tissue against the supporting hand.

The client is then asked to lie down. The breasts are palpated while they are flattened against the rib cage. If the breasts are large, several mechanisms can be employed to enhance this flattening. A small pillow or a rolled towel can be placed under the ipsilateral shoulder, or the client can abduct the ipsilateral arm and place her hand under her neck. Both maneuvers shift the breast medially. The humerus should be at least slightly abducted to allow for thorough palpation of the tail of Spence.

The breasts are then thoroughly palpated (Fig. 13-13). The examiner should develop a system of breast examination and habitually start and end at a fixed point on the breasts. The starting point is arbitrary. The breasts are palpated with the palmar surfaces of the fingers held together. The movements are smooth and back and forth or circular. The breast is visualized as a bicycle wheel with six or eight spokes, and palpation occurs along each spoke until the breast has been thoroughly surveyed (Fig. 13-14, A). Special attention is focused on the upper outer quadrant area and on the tail of Spence because about half of all breast cancers develop there (Fig. 13-15).

An alternate method of breast palpation is to consider the breast as a group of concentric circles with the nipple as the center. Palpation occurs along the circumferences of the circle, starting at the outermost circle, until the total breast area is adequately surveyed (Fig. 13-14, B).

The areolar areas are carefully palpated to determine the presence of underlying masses. Each nipple is gently compressed to assess for the presence of masses or discharge (Fig. 13-13, C). If discharge is noted, the breast is milked along its radii to identify the lobe from which the discharge is originating. Compression of the discharge-producing lobe will cause discharge to exude from the nipple.

If a client reports a breast nodule, the "normal" breast is examined first so that the baseline consistency of that breast will serve as a control when the reportedly abnormal one is palpated.

Mammary folds, crescent-shaped ridges of breast tissue found at the inferior portions of very large or pendulous breasts, may be confused with breast masses but are nonpathologic.

The sequence of the breast examination is illustrated in Fig. 13-16.

Despite improved mammographic techniques and their availability, a large portion of malignant breast lesions are found by women themselves. Therefore, the health-oriented examiner should assess each client's level of knowledge and practice related to breast self-examination. During the practitioner's examination of the breasts, the practitioner can describe the steps of the examination and the rationale for each step. A return demonstration by the client on her own breasts reinforces learning and memory of the procedure.

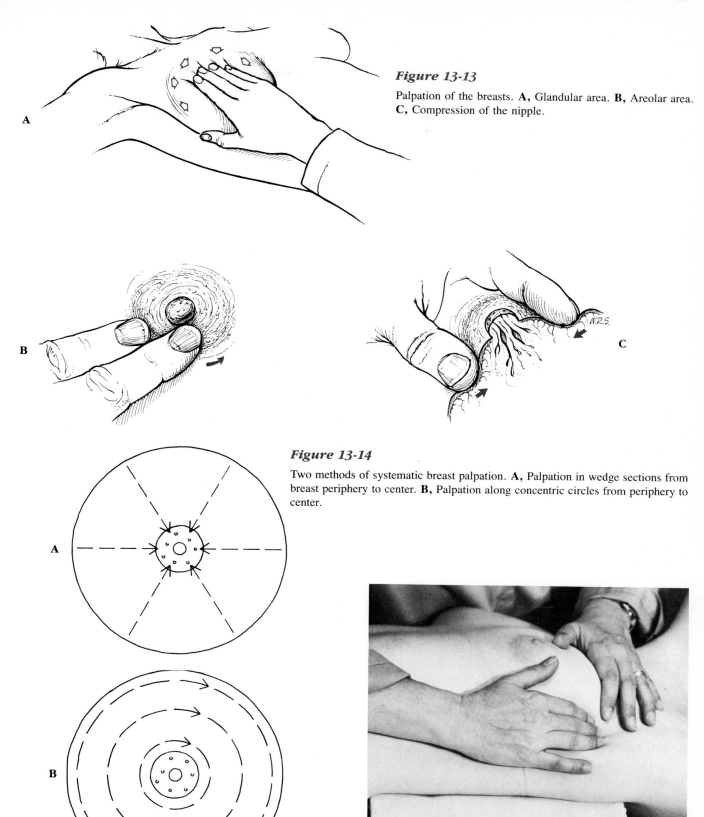

Figure 13-13

Palpation of the breasts. **A,** Glandular area. **B,** Areolar area.
C, Compression of the nipple.

Figure 13-14

Two methods of systematic breast palpation. **A,** Palpation in wedge sections from
breast periphery to center. **B,** Palpation along concentric circles from periphery to
center.

Figure 13-15

Palpation of the axillary tail of Spence.

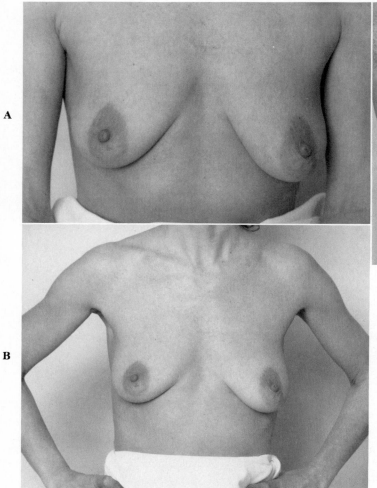

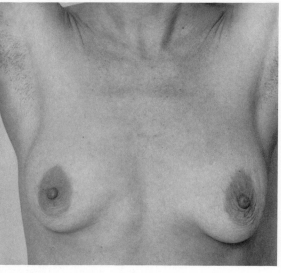

Figure 13-16

Sequence of the breast examination. **A,** Observation of the breasts at rest. **B,** Observation with client's arms overhead. **C,** Observation with client contracting pectoral muscles.

The following points should be emphasized in the teaching of breast self-examination:
1. The majority of breast lumps are not cancer.
2. The majority of cancerous breast lesions are curable.
3. Breasts should be examined each month between the fourth through the seventh day of the menstrual cycle, when the breasts are least congested.
4. Visual inspection and palpation should be done.
5. Visual inspection should be done in four arm positions and while the woman is stripped to her waist and looking at herself in a mirror. The four arm positions are: arms at rest, hands on hips and pressed into the hips contracting chest muscles, hands over the head, and torso leaning forward.
6. Many women prefer to do palpation in the shower when the soap and water assist the hands to glide easily over the skin. However, the examination of large breasts and the axilla is better done in a supine than a standing position. Therefore, supine examination is recommended, as well as the examination in the bath and shower.

7. The entire breast should be examined in a systematic way.
8. Specific examination of the nipple, through compression for discharge, and the areola, through palpation, should not be forgotten.
9. Any change should be reported to a health care provider as quickly as possible.

Special Examination Procedures

Further evaluation of breast masses is accomplished through the use of several recently developed techniques. These techniques are as follows:
1. *Mammography* is the technique of breast examination with low-energy radiography.
2. *Xerography* is mammography using a xerographic plate instead of film. The advantages of this technique are that radiation doses are smaller than with conventional mammography and the images produced are more distinct.
3. *Thermography* is a technique that measures temper-

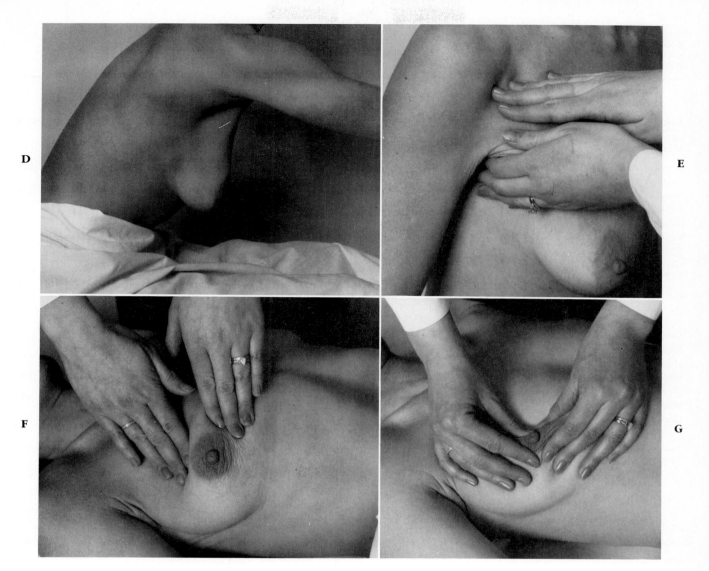

Figure 13-16, cont'd

D, Observation with client leaning forward. **E,** Palpation of axillary nodes (note: although not shown, the client's arm should be supported on the examiner's arm; palpation of the supraclavicular and subclavicular areas is not illustrated). **F,** Palpation of the glandular area. **G,** Palpation of the nipple and areolar areas.

ature distribution of the breast. Malignant lesions appear as "hot spots" in the breast.

Mammographic techniques have been improved tremendously in terms of safety and effectiveness during the past 10 years. Mammography is the major method of detecting nonpalpable breast lesions. Nonpalpable lesions are generally early, small, and local. Therefore, survival rates are increased with early detection.

The taking and interpretation of mammograms require specialized skill. Often mammography is offered through a community-based screening program. A baseline mammogram is recommended for all women between the ages of 35 and 40, followed by mammograms every 1 to 2 years for asymptomatic women aged 40 to 49. Yearly mammograms are recommended for women over age 50 (Porrath, 1986).

VARIATIONS FROM HEALTH

Breast Cancer

Although certain breast lesions have characteristic findings on inspection and palpation, diagnosis is not made by clinical examination but by surgical procedures and laboratory examinations. The practitioner is encouraged to learn distinguishing characteristics of breast lesions but not to rely on them for diagnosis.

Table 13-1

Risk factors for breast cancer in women

Factor	Differentiation of risk		Strength of factor
	High risk	**Low risk**	
Demographic factors			
Age	Old	Young	Strong
Marital status	Never married	Never married	Weak
Race	White	Black	Weak
Residence—country	North America, northern Europe	Asia, Africa	Strong
Residence—U.S. location	Northern United States	Southern United States	Weak
Residence—type	Urban	Rural	Weak
Socioeconomic status	Upper	Lower	Moderate
Personal history			
Age—menarche	Early	Late	Weak
Age—menopause	Late	Early	Weak
Age—first term pregnancy	>30 yr	<30 yr	Moderate
Family history—bilateral breast cancer	Present	Absent	Strong
Family history—breast cancer	Present	Absent	Moderate
History—Cancer in one breast	Present	Absent	Strong
History—Fibrocystic disease	Present	Absent	Moderate
History—Cancer in ovary or endometrium	Present	Absent	Moderate
History—Chest radiation	Large doses	Low exposure	Moderate
Oophorectomy	None	Present	Moderate
Premenopausal body build	Obese	Thin	Moderate

Adapted from Marchant DJ: Breast disease, New York, 1986, Churchill Livingstone.

The lesions of breast cancer are often solitary, unilateral, solid, hard, irregular, poorly delineated, nonmobile, painless, nontender, and located in the upper outer quadrants.

Breast cancer is a leading cause of death in women in the United States and also a leading cause of cancer morbidity. On the average one of every 13 women will develop breast cancer. Knowledge of factors indicating that a woman is at a higher than usual risk of cancer can assist in making decisions about screening programs and the frequency of general physical examinations.

A summary of risk factors for breast cancer in women is presented in Table 13-1. Women at increased risk should be taught to perform self-examination and should receive a professional physical examination at least once a year.

The American Cancer Society (Mammography Guidelines 1983) recommends the following breast cancer screening test schedule for asymptomatic women:

1. All women over age 20 should perform breast self-examination monthly.
2. Women between the ages of 20 and 40 should have a breast examination by a qualified health care pro-vider every 3 years, and women over age 40 should have an examination yearly.
3. All women should have a baseline mammogram between the ages of 35 and 39.
4. Asymptomatic women aged 40 to 49 should have a mammogram every 1 to 2 years.
5. All women over 50 should have a mammogram every year.

The Male Breast

Occurring most frequently in the areolar area, male breast cancer accounts for approximately 1% of all breast cancers. Every male client should be given a thorough breast examination with an adaptation of the technique used for female clients.

The male breast is observed with the man sitting. The various sitting positions used with the woman are unnecessary. Palpation of the breasts, nipple, and areolae can occur with the client supine. The palpation of the axillary nodes is an essential component of the examination of the male client.

Gynecomastia, enlargement of the male breast, is a frequently occurring multicausal condition. Causes in-

---

Health History
Breasts

NOTE: A yes response to any question *must* be further investigated. Use the following indicators throughout the assessment: (1) onset (specific date, sudden or gradual), (2) duration, (3) frequency, (4) precipitating factors, (5) aggravating or alleviating factors, (6) treatment received, and (7) outcome.

Present status

1. Do you do breast self-examination regularly?
   a. Monthly
   b. During menstrual cycle

Past history

1. Have you had pain or tenderness in your breast(s)?
   a. With menses
   b. Character of pain
   c. Lumps noted
   d. Nipple discharge
2. Have you had a mammography?
   a. At what age
   b. Date of last one
3. Have you ever had a lump in your breast(s)?
   a. Any lump changes
   b. Any lumps in armpits
   c. Pain associated with lumps

4. Have you had discharge from your nipples?
   a. Type: bloody, serous, purulent, causes nipple crusting, cracking, dryness, scaling

Associated conditions

1. Do you have high blood pressure or diabetes?
2. What age did your menses begin and end?
3. Have you ever been pregnant?

Family history

1. Is there a family history of breast cancer?
2. Is there a female family history of recurring breast cysts?

Sample assessment record

Admitted for biopsy of lump in right breast. Lump first noted yesterday during breast self-examination. No pain, swelling, redness, or nipple discharge. No other lumps ever noted. Has not ever had mammogram but had routine pap smear and breast exam by physician 4 months ago. Had two pregnancies. Started menses at age 13 and menopause at age 47. No familial history of breast cancer or cysts.

---

clude pubertal changes, hormonal administration, cirrhosis, leukemia, thyrotoxicosis, and drugs.

Benign Lesions of the Female Breast

Benign lesions account for approximately 70% to 80% of breast operations. The most commonly seen benign breast lesions are fibrocystic disease and fibroadenomas.

Fibrocystic disease is an exaggeration of the normal changes in the breasts during the menstrual cycle and is eventualy characterized by the formation of single or multiple cysts in the breasts. Fibrocystic disease develops in three stages:

1. The first stage is called *mazoplasia* and occurs in the late teens and early 20s. It is characterized by painful, tender, premenstrual breast swelling (chiefly in the axillary tails) that subsides after menses.
2. The second stage occurs in the late 20s and early 30s. The breasts exhibit multinodular changes, and sometimes a dominant mass can occur, which is usually described as a thickness rather than a lump.
3. Subsequently, cysts develop. The onset of cyst formation is often preceded by sudden dull pain, a full feeling, or a burning sensation in the breast.

The lesions of cystic disease are commonly bilateral, multiple, painful, tender, well delineated, and slightly mobile. The discomfort from and size of lesions increase premenstrually.

Fibroadenomas are benign lesions that contain both fibrous and glandular tissues. They are usually solitary and unilateral. They are generally palpated as mobile, solid, firm, rubbery, regular, well-delineated, nontender, painless lumps. Fibroadenomas are usually found in women between the ages of 15 and 35 and produce no premenstrual changes.

BIBLIOGRAPHY

Annonier C: Female breast examination, Berlin, 1983, Springer-Verlag.

Dunphy JE and Botsford TW: Physical examination of the surgical patient, ed 4, Philadelphia, 1975, WB Saunders Co.

Eggertsen SC, Berg AO, and Moe RE: An evaluation of individual components of breast self-examination, J Fam Pract 17:921, 1983.

Fogel CI and Woods NF: Health care of women: a nursing perspective, St Louis, 1981, The CV Mosby Co.

Gallagher S and others: The breast, St Louis, 1978, The CV Mosby Co.

Haagemen CD: Diseases of the breast, ed 3, Philadelphia, 1986, JB Lippincott Co.

Harris JR, Hellman S, Henderson IC, and Kinne DW: Breast diseases, Philadelphia, 1987, JB Lippincott Co.

Kishner R: Breast cancer: a personal history and an investigative report, New York, 1975, Harcourt Brace Jovanovich.

Mahoney LJ, Bird BL, and Cooke GM: Annual clinical examination: the best available screening test for breast cancer, N Engl J Med 301:315, 1979.

Mammography Guidelines 1983: Background statement and update of cancer-related check-up guidelines for breast cancer detection in asymptomatic women age 40 to 49, CA 33:255, 1983.

Marchant DJ: Breast diseases, New York, 1986, Churchill Livingstone.

Marty PJ, McDermott RJ, and Gold RS: An assessment of three alternate formats for promoting breast self-examination, Cancer Nurs 6:207, 1983.

National Cancer Institute: Breast cancer digest, Bethesda, Md, 1984, The Institute.

Oberst MJ: Testing approaches to teaching breast self-examination, Cancer Nurs 4:246, 1981.

Paulus DD: Imaging in breast cancer, CA 37:133-150, 1987.

Porrath S: The multimodality approach to breast imaging, Rockville, Md, 1986, Aspen Publishers.

Seidman H, Gelb SK, Silverberg E, et al: Survival experience in the breast cancer detection project, CA 37:258-290, 1987.

Venet L: Self-examination and clinical examination of the breast, Cancer 46:930, 1980.

14

Assessment of the respiratory system

OBJECTIVES

Upon successful review of this chapter, learners will be able to:

- Describe anatomy and physiology of the respiratory system
- State related rationale and demonstrate assessment of the respiratory system, including inspection, palpation, percussion, and auscultation techniques
- Outline history relevant to assessment of the respiratory system
- Recognize characteristics associated with

  Normal and abnormal fremitus

  Percussion tones

  Breath sounds
- Describe the origin and characteristics of adventitious sounds
- Describe findings frequently associated with common lung conditions

ANATOMY AND PHYSIOLOGY

The major purpose of the respiratory system is to supply the body with oxygen and eliminate carbon dioxide. This is accomplished through complex cooperation of many body systems that, in wellness, act in harmony. The actual transfer of oxygen and carbon dioxide between environmental gas and body liquid occurs in the alveoli, which are obviously not accessible to clinical examination. However, assessment of respiratory efficiency is accomplished by direct and indirect appraisal of structures supporting alveolar function.

The thoracic cage consists of a skeleton of 12 thoracic vertebrae, 12 pairs of ribs, the sternum, the diaphragm, and the intercostal muscles and is semirigid (Fig. 14-1). The skeletal parts of the thoracic cage consist of the ribs, the sternum, and the vertebrae. The ribs are paired. Anteriorly, the costal cartilages of the first seven ribs articulate with the body of the sternum, and the costal cartilages of the eighth to the tenth ribs are attached to the costal cartilages just above the ribs. The 11th and 12th ribs are termed "floating ribs" and are unattached anteriorly. The tip of the 11th rib is located in the lateral thorax, and the tip of the 12th rib is located in the posterior thorax. Posteriorly, all ribs articulate with the thoracic vertebrae.

The adult sternum is approximately 17 cm long and consists of three parts: the manubrium, the body, and the xiphoid process. The manubrium of the sternum articulates with and supports the clavicle. The manubrium and the body of the sternum articulate with the first seven ribs. None of the ribs articulates with the xiphoid. An anatomic landmark, the angle of Louis, is the junction of the manubrium and the body of the sternum. The second rib attaches to the sternum at the angle of Louis.

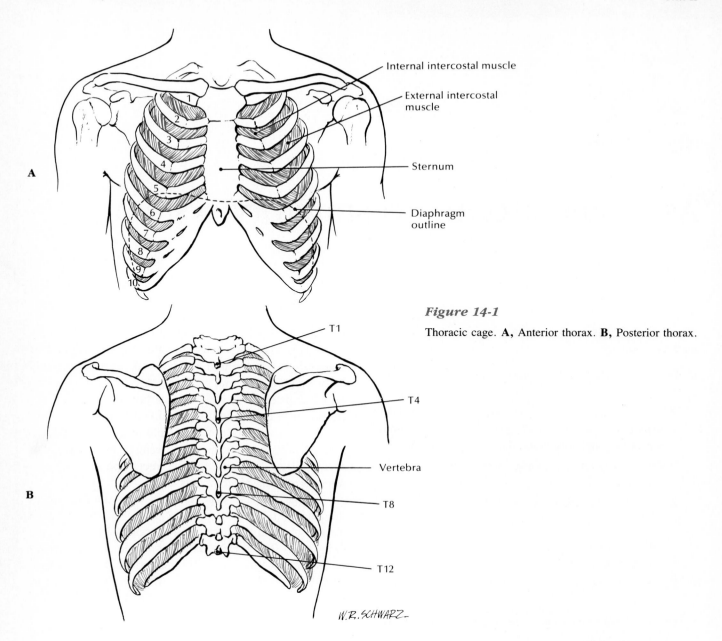

W.R.SCHWARZ

Figure 14-1

Thoracic cage. **A,** Anterior thorax. **B,** Posterior thorax.

The spaces between the ribs are termed *intercostal spaces* (ICS). They are named according to the rib immediately superior; for example, the space between the second and third rib would be the second ICS.

The thoracic cavity is divided into two distinct right and left pleural cavities, separated by the mediastinum, containing the heart and the other structures that connect the head with the abdomen. The pleural cavities are lined by serous membranes, the parietal and visceral pleurae. The parietal pleura lines the chest wall and the diaphragm; the visceral pleura lines the outside of the lung. The space between the pleurae contains a lubricating fluid.

The lungs are paired, asymmetric, conical organs that conform to the thoracic cavity. The right lung con-tains three lobes, and the left lung contains two.

Air reaches the lungs through a system of flexible tubes. Air enters through the mouth or nose, traverses the respiratory portion of the larynx, and enters the trachea. The trachea, approximately 10 to 11 cm long in the adult, begins at the lower border of the cricoid cartilage and divides into a left and right bronchus, usually at the level of T4 or T5 posteriorly and slightly below the manubriosternal joint anteriorly.

The right bronchus is shorter, wider, and more vertical than the left bronchus. The bronchial structures further subdivide into increasingly smaller bronchi and bronchioles. Each bronchiole opens into an alveolar duct from which multiple alveoli radiate (Fig. 14-2). Lungs in the adult contain approximately 300 million alveoli.

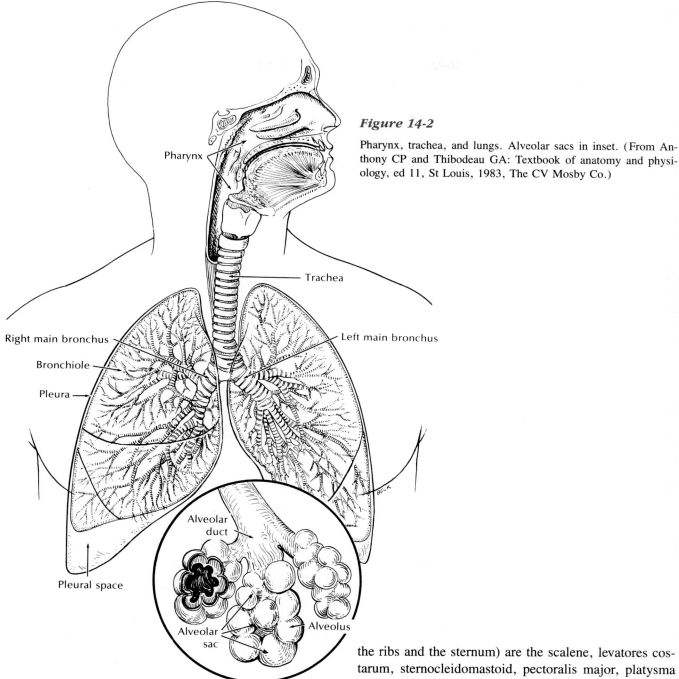

Figure 14-2

Pharynx, trachea, and lungs. Alveolar sacs in inset. (From Anthony CP and Thibodeau GA: Textbook of anatomy and physiology, ed 11, St Louis, 1983, The CV Mosby Co.)

The bronchi have both transport and protective purposes. Their cavities contain mucus, which entraps foreign particles and is continuously swept by ciliary action into the throat, where it can be eliminated.

The muscles used in inspiration can be divided into two types: primary and accessory (Fig. 14-3). The diaphragm and the external intercostal muscles are the primary muscles of respiration. Accessory muscles of respiration can be used voluntarily to facilitate or increase inspiration or expiration in both health and disease. The muscles used in forced inspiration (i.e., to assist in raising the ribs and the sternum) are the scalene, levatores costarum, sternocleidomastoid, pectoralis major, platysma myoides, and serratus posterior superior muscles. The muscles used in forced expiration or to assist in depressing the ribs are the rectus abdominis, external and internal oblique, the transverse abdominis, internal intercostals, serratus posterior inferior, and quadratus lumborum.

The thoracic cage is perpetually moving in the inspiratory and expiratory phases of respiration (Fig. 14-4). During inspiration, the diaphragm descends and flattens and the intercostal muscles contract. These maneuvers produce differences in pressure among the areas of the mouth, the alveoli, and the pleural areas; and air moves into the lungs. The intrathoracic pressure is de-

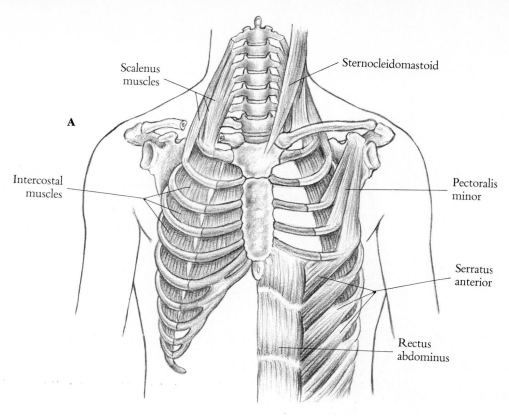

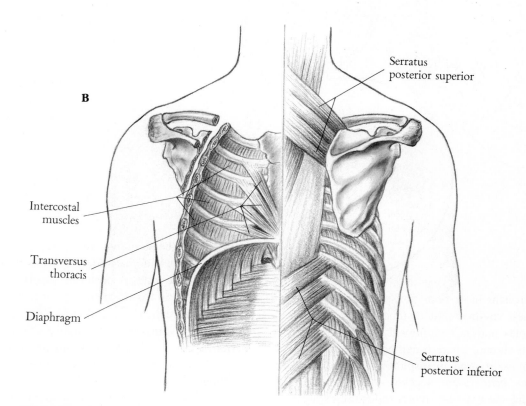

Figure 14-3

Muscles of ventilation. **A,** Anterior view. **B,** Posterior view. (From Seidel HM and others: Mosby's guide to physical examination, St Louis, 1987, The CV Mosby Co.)

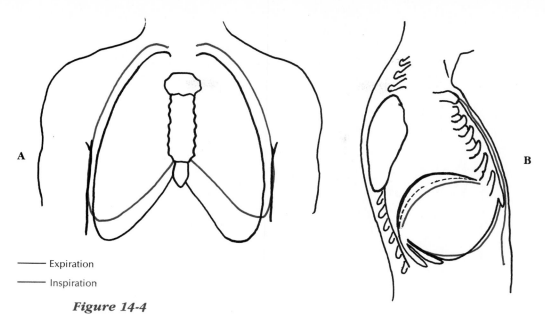

Figure 14-4

Movement of the thorax during respiration. **A,** Anterior thorax. **B,** Lateral thorax.

creased, the lungs are expanded, and the ribs flare, increasing the diameter of the thorax. The second to the sixth ribs move around two axes in a motion commonly termed the "pump handle" movement. The lower ribs move in a "bucket handle" motion. Because of the length and positioning of the lower ribs and because the lower interspaces are wider, the amplitude of movement is greater in the lower thorax.

Inspiration is opposed by the elastic properties of the respiratory system. Expiration is a relatively passive phenomenon. At the completion of inspiration, the diaphragm relaxes and the elastic recoil properties of the lungs expel air and pull the diaphragm to its resting position.

Topographic Anatomy

Topographic (surface) landmarks of the thorax assist the examiner in identifying the location of the internal, underlying structures and in describing the exact location of abnormalities (Fig. 14-5).

Manubriosternal junction (angle of Louis). The manubriosternal junction is the articulation between the manubrium and the body of the sternum and is an extremely useful aid in rib identification. This junction is named the angle of Louis. The angle of Louis is a visible and palpable angulation of the sternum.

The superior border of the second rib articulates with the sternum at the manubriosternal junction. The examiner can begin to palpate and count distal ribs and rib interspaces from this point. It should be reiterated that an ICS is numbered corresponding to the number of

the rib immediately superior to the space. In palpation for rib identification, the examiner should palpate along the midclavicular line rather than at the sternal border because the rib cartilages are very close at the sternum and the cartilages of only the first seven ribs attach directly to the sternum.

Suprasternal notch. The suprasternal notch is the depression above the manubrium.

Costal angle. The costal angle is the angle formed by the intersection of the coastal margins.

Midsternal line. The midsternal line is an imaginary line drawn through the middle of the sternum.

Midclavicular lines. The midclavicular lines are left and right imaginary lines drawn through the midpoints of the clavicles and parallel to the midsternal line.

Anterior axillary lines. The anterior axillary lines are left and right imaginary lines drawn vertically from the anterior axillary folds, along the anterolateral chest, and parallel to the midsternal line.

Vertebra prominens (seventh cervical vertebra). When the client flexes the neck anteriorly and the posterior thorax is observed, a prominent spinous process can be observed and palpated. This is the spinous process of the seventh cervical vertebra. If two spinous processes are observed and palpated, the superior one is C7 and the inferior one is the spinous process of T1. The counting of ribs is more difficult on the posterior than on the anterior thorax. The spinous processes of the vertebrae can be counted relatively easily from C7 to T4. From T4 the spinous processes project obliquely, causing the spinous process of the vertebra not to lie over its

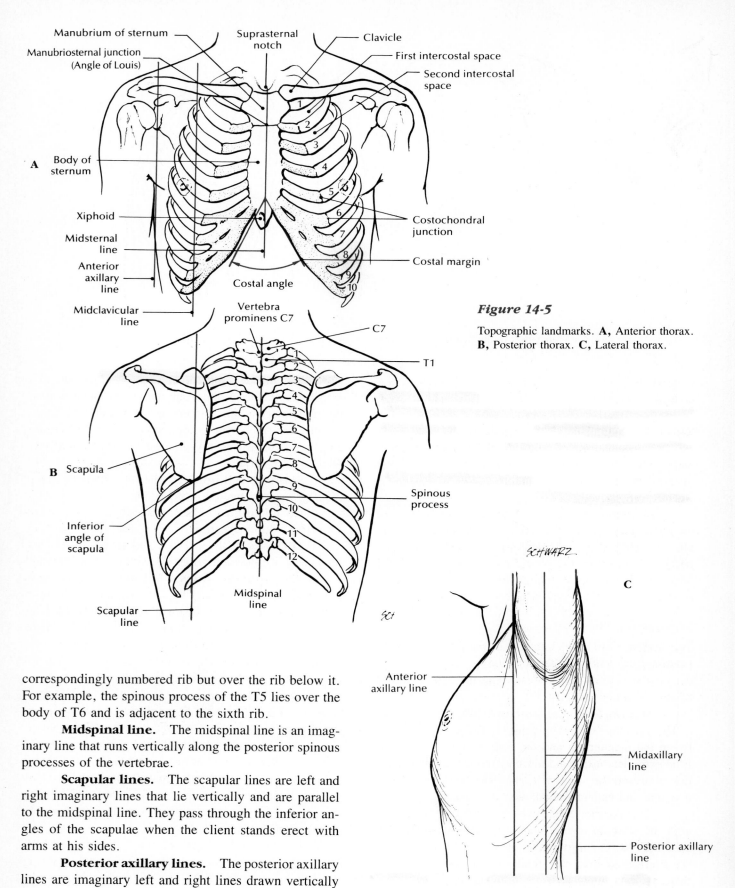

Figure 14-5

Topographic landmarks. **A,** Anterior thorax. **B,** Posterior thorax. **C,** Lateral thorax.

correspondingly numbered rib but over the rib below it. For example, the spinous process of the T5 lies over the body of T6 and is adjacent to the sixth rib.

Midspinal line.   The midspinal line is an imaginary line that runs vertically along the posterior spinous processes of the vertebrae.

Scapular lines.   The scapular lines are left and right imaginary lines that lie vertically and are parallel to the midspinal line. They pass through the inferior angles of the scapulae when the client stands erect with arms at his sides.

Posterior axillary lines.   The posterior axillary lines are imaginary left and right lines drawn vertically

A

Right upper lobe

Right middle lobe

Right lower lobe

Sixth rib

Trachea

Left bronchus

Left upper lobe

Cardiac outline

Left lower lobe

SCHWARZ

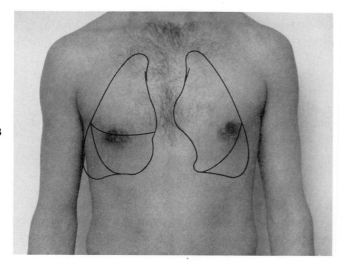

B

Figure 14-6

Anterior thorax. **A,** Internal organs and structures. **B,** Lung borders.

and organ parts of the respiratory system and other systems sharing the thoracic area (Figs. 14-6 to 14-9).

Lung borders. In the anterior thorax, the apices of the lungs extend for approximately 2 to 4 cm above the clavicles. The inferior borders of the lungs cross the sixth rib at the midclavicular line. In the posterior thorax, the apices extend to T1. The lower borders vary with respiration and usually extend from the spinous process of T10 on expiration to the spinous process of T12 on deep inspiration. In the lateral thorax, the lung extends from the apex of the axilla to the eighth rib of the midaxillary line.

Lung fissures. The right oblique (diagonal) fissure extends from the area of the spinous process of the third thoracic vertebra laterally and downward until it crosses the fifth rib at the right midaxillary line. It then continues anteriorly and medially to end at the sixth rib at the right and left midclavicular lines. The right horizontal fissure extends from the fifth rib slightly posterior to the right midaxillary line and runs horizontally to the area of the fourth rib at the right sternal border. The left oblique (diagonal) fissure extends from the spinous process of the third thoracic vertebra laterally and downward to the left midaxillary line at the fifth rib and continues anteriorly and medially until it terminates at the sixth rib in the left midclavicular line.

Border of the diaphragm. Anteriorly, on expiration, the right dome of the diaphragm is located at the level of the fifth rib at the midclavicular line and the

from the posterior axillary folds along the posterolateral wall of the thorax when the lateral arm is abducted directly from the lateral chest wall.

Midaxillary lines. The midaxillary lines are imaginary left and right lines drawn vertically from the apices of the axillae. They are approximately midway between the anterior and the posterior axillary lines and parallel to them.

• • •

The various landmarks and imaginery lines assist in determining the location of underlying structures and in describing the location of abnormal findings.

Underlying Thoracic Structures

When examining the respiratory system, the practitioner must maintain a mental image of the placement of organs

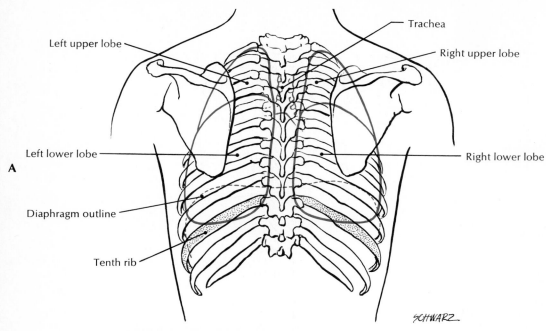

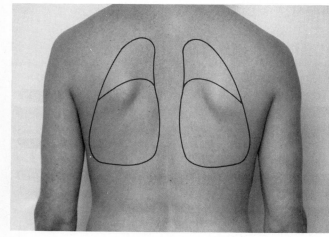

SCHWARZ

Figure 14-7

Posterior thorax. **A,** Internal organs and structures.
B, Lung borders.

left dome is at the level of the sixth rib. Posteriorly, on expiration, the diaphragm is at the level of the spinous process of T10; laterally, it is at the eight rib at the midaxillary line. On inspiration the diaphragm moves approximately 1.5 cm downward with the right side being slightly higher than the left side.

Trachea.   The bifurcation of the trachea occurs approximately just below the manubriosternal junction anteriorly and at the spinous process of T4 posteriorly.

EXAMINATION

Preparation and Equipment

Equipment needed for the respiratory system examination are (1) a stethoscope with a bell and diaphragm, (2) a marking pencil, and (3) a centimeter ruler. The exami-

nation should be performed in a warm, quiet, well-illuminated area that allows for privacy.

Inspection

Inspection is performed to (1) measure and assess pattern of respirations, (2) assess the skin and the overall symmetry and integrity of the thorax, and (3) assess thoracic configuration.

For adequate inspection of the thorax, the client should be sitting upright without support and uncovered to the waist. It is essential that the room lighting be adequate and that a mechanism for supplementary lighting be available for close inspection of small areas. The client must be warm and not observed by persons extraneous to the examination. Females may wish to have a gown or towel to cover their breasts while the posterior thorax is being examined.

The examiner first observes the general shape of the thorax and its symmetry. Although no individual is absolutely symmetric in both body hemispheres, most individuals are reasonably similar side to side. Using the client as a control whenever paired parts are examined is an excellent habit and will often yield significant findings.

The approach to the physical examination is regional and integrated. The examination of systems is combined in body regions when appropriate. Since the client is uncovered to the waist during the examination, a large portion of skin and tissue is accessible to inspec-

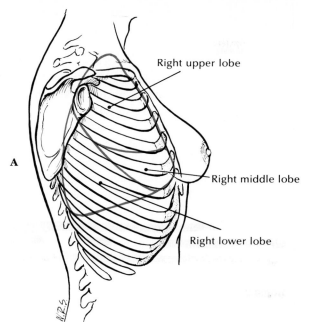

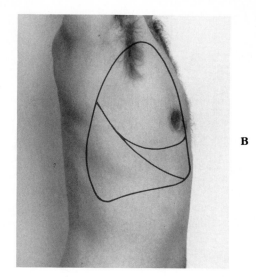

Figure 14-8

Right lateral thorax. **A,** Internal organs and chest structures. (Note the relationship of the breast to chest organs and structures.) **B,** Lung borders.

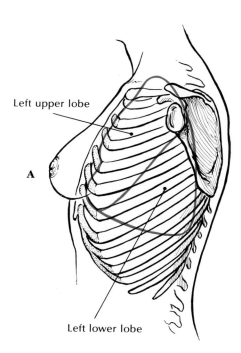

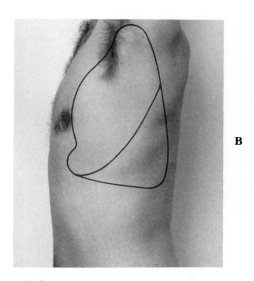

Figure 14-9

Left lateral thorax. **A,** Internal organs and chest structures. **B,** Lung borders.

tion. The observation of skin and underlying tissue provides the examiner with knowledge of the general nutrition of the patient. Common thoracic skin findings are the spider nevi associated with cirrhosis and seborrheic dermatitis (see Chapter 8 on skin assessment).

Thoracic configuration.   The anteroposterior diameter of the thorax in the normal adult is less than the transverse diameter at approximately a ratio of 1:2 to 5:7 (Fig. 14-10). In the normal infant, in some adults

with pulmonary disease, and in aged adults the thorax is approximately round. This condition is called barrel chest. The barrel chest is characterized by horizontal ribs, slight kyphosis of the thoracic spine, and prominent sternal angle. The chest appears as though it were in continuous inspiratory position. Other observed abnormalities of thoracic shape might include the following:

1. Retraction of the thorax. The retraction is unilateral, or of one side. *pneumothorax – collapsed*

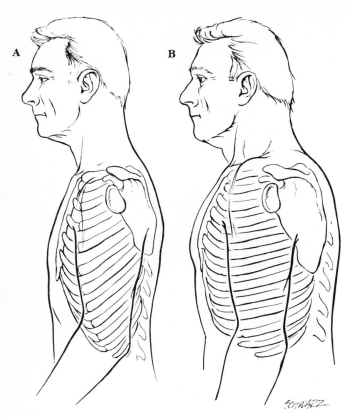

Figure 14-10

A, Client with normal thoracic configuration. **B,** Client with increased anteroposterior diameter. Note contrast in the angle of the slope of the ribs and the development of the accessory muscles of respiration in the neck.

2. Pigeon or chicken chest (pectus carinatum)—sternal protrusion anteriorly. The anteroposterior diameter of the chest is increased, and the resultant configuration resembles the thorax of a fowl.
3. Funnel chest (pectus excavatum)—depression of part or all of the sternum. If the depression is deep, it may interfere with both respiratory and cardiac function.
4. Spinal deformities. While the client is uncovered and the examiner is behind him or her the spine should be examined for deformities. (See Chapter 18 on musculoskeletal assessment for the specific techniques of spinal examination.)

    Ribs and interspaces. The reaction of interspaces on inspiration may indicate some obstruction of free air inflow. Bulging of interspaces on expiration occurs when there is obstruction to air outflow or may be the result of tumor, aneurysm, or cardiac enlargement. Normally, the costal angle is less than 90 degrees, and the ribs are inserted into the spine at about a 45-degree angle (see Fig. 14-1). In clients with obstructive lung diseases these angles are widened.

Pattern of respiration. Normally, men and children breathe diaphragmatically, and women breathe thoracically or costally. A change in this pattern might be significant. If the client appears to have labored respiration, the examiner observes for the use of the accessory muscles of respiration in the neck—the sternocleidomastoid, scalenus, and trapezius muscles—and for supraclavicular retraction. Impedance to air inflow is often accompanied by retraction of the intercostal spaces during inspiration. An excessively long expiratory phase of respiration accompanies outflow impedance and may be accompanied by the use of abdominal muscles to aid in expiration.

    The normal adult resting respiratory rate is 12 to 20 breaths per minute and is regular. The ratio of respiratory rate to pulse rate normally is 1:4. Tachypnea is an adult respiratory rate of over 20 breaths per minute; bradypnea is an adult respiratory rate of less than 10 breaths per minute.

    There are many abnormal patterns of respiration. Some of the commonly seen patterns are listed in Fig. 14-11. Dyspnea is a subjective phenomenon of inadequate or distressful respiration.

    Lips and nails. Inspection of the respiratory system examination includes observation of lips and nail beds for color and observation of the nails for clubbing. These phenomena are discussed in Chapter 7 on general assessment and in Chapter 15 on cardiovascular assessment.

Palpation

Palpation is performed to (1) further assess abnormalities suggested by the history or observation, such as tenderness, pulsations, masses, or skin lesions; (2) assess the skin and subcutaneous structures; (3) assess the thoracic expansion; (4) assess vocal (tactile) fremitus; and (5) assess the tracheal position.

    General palpation. The examiner should specifically palpate any areas of abnormality. The temperature and turgor of the skin should be generally assessed. The examiner then palpates the muscle mass and the thoracic skeleton. If the client has no complaints in relation to the respiratory system, a rapid, general survey of anterior, lateral, and posterior thoracic areas is sufficient. If the client does have complaints, all chest areas should be meticulously palpated for tenderness, bulges, or abnormal movements.

    Assessment of thoracic expansion. The degree of thoracic expansion can be assessed from the anterior or posterior chest (Fig. 14-12). Anteriorly, the examiner's hands are placed over the anterolateral chest with the thumbs extended along the costal margin, point-

TYPE OF RESPIRATION	DIAGRAM	DISCUSSION
Normal	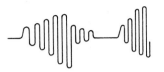	2-20/min in adults; regular in rhythm; ratio of respiratory rate to pulse rate is 1:4
Hyperventilation or Kussmaul's respiration		Increase in both rate and depth; hyperpnea is an increase in depth only
Periodic respiration	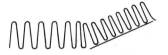	Alternating hyperpnea, shallow respiration and apnea; sometimes called Cheyne-Stokes respiration; frequently occurs in the severely ill
Sighing respiration		Deep and audible; audible portion sounds like a sigh
Air trapping		Present in obstructive pulmonary diseases; air is trapped in the lungs; respiratory level rises, and breathing becomes shallow
Biot's breathing	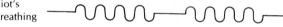	Shallow breathing interrupted by apnea; seen in some CNS disorders and in healthy persons

Figure 14-11

Characteristics of commonly observed respiratory patterns.

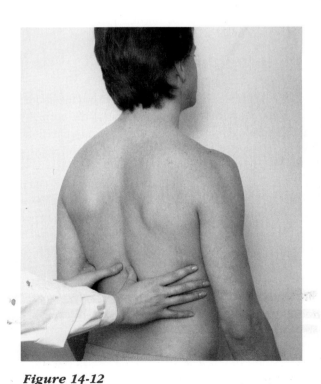

Figure 14-12

Palpation of thoracic excursion.

ing to the xiphoid process. Posteriorly, the thumbs are placed at the level of the tenth rib and the palms are placed on the posterolateral chest. The examiner feels the amount of the thoracic expansion during quiet and deep respiration and observes for divergence of the thumbs on expiration. Symmetry of respiration between the left and right hemithoraces should be felt as the thumbs are separated approximately 3 to 5 cm during deep inspiration.

Assessment of fremitus. Fremitus is vibration perceptible on palpation. Vocal or tactile fremitus is palpable vibration of the thoracic wall, produced by phonation.

The client is asked to repeat "one, two, three" or "ninety-nine" while the examiner systematically palpates the thorax (Fig. 14-13). The examiner can use the palmar bases of the fingers, the ulnar aspect of the hand, or the ulnar aspect of the closed fist. If one hand is used, it should be moved from one side of the chest to the corresponding area on the other side. If two hands are used for examination, they should be simultaneously placed on the corresponding areas of each thoracic side. See Table 14-1 for types of fremitus.

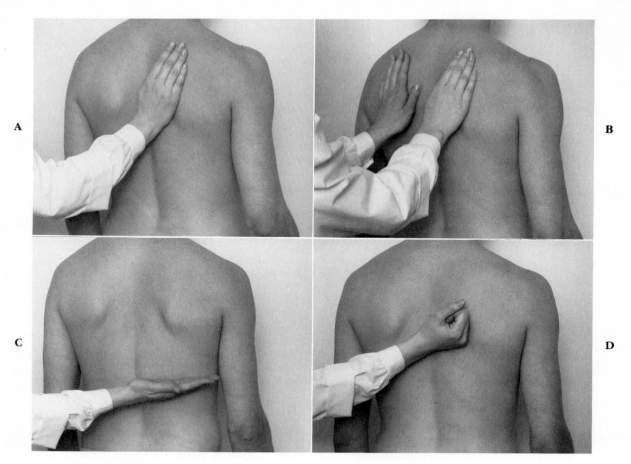

Figure 14-13

Palpation for assessment of vocal fremitus. **A,** Use of palmar surface of fingertips. **B,** Simultaneous application of the fingertips of both hands. **C,** Use of ulnar aspect of the hand. **D,** Use of ulnar aspect of the closed fist.

When examining the thorax, the practitioner must be mindful of the four parts for examination: the posterior chest, the anterior chest, the right and left lateral thoracic areas, and the apices. The examiner should move from the area of one hemisphere to the corresponding area on the other (right to left, left to right) until all four major parts are surveyed. During palpation for assessing fremitus and all subsequent procedures for examination of the respiratory system, all areas must be meticulously and systematically examined. Usually, the apices, posterior chest, and lateral areas can be examined with the practitioner standing behind the client.

Assessment of tracheal deviation. The trachea should be assessed by palpation for lateral deviation. The examiner places a finger on the trachea in the suprasternal notch, then moves the finger laterally left and right in the spaces bordered by the upper edge of the clavicle, the inner aspect of the sternocleidomastoid muscle, and the trachea. These spaces should be equal on both sides. In diseases such as atelectasis and pulmonary fibrosis, the trachea may be deviated toward the abnormal side. The trachea may be deviated toward the normal side in conditions such as neck tumors, thyroid enlargement, enlarged lymph nodes, pleural effusion, unilateral emphysema, and tension pneumothorax.

An alternate method of examining for tracheal deviation is as follows: the examiner stands in front of the seated client and places both hands around the client's neck with the thumbs in the spaces lateral to the trachea. Normally, both thumbs should palpate the straight borders of the trachea and equal spaces bilaterally.

Crepitations. In subcutaneous emphysema, the subcutaneous tissue contains fine beads of air. As this tissue is palpated, audible crackling sounds are heard. These sounds are termed *crepitations*.

Percussion

Percussion is the tapping of an object to set underlying structures in motion and consequently to produce a sound called a percussion note and a palpable vibration. Per-

Table 14-1

Characteristics of normal and abnormal tactile fremitus

Type of fremitus	Discussion of characteristics
Normal (moderate) fremitus	Varies greatly from person to person and depends on the intensity and pitch of the voice, the position and distance of the bronchi in relation to the chest wall, and the thickness of the chest wall. Fremitus is most intense in the second intercostal spaces at the sternal border near the area of bronchial bifurcation.
Increased vocal fremitus	May occur in pneumonia, compressed lung, lung tumor, or pulmonary fibrosis. (A solid medium of uniform structure conducts vibrations with greater intensity than a porous medium.)
Decreased or absent vocal fremitus	Occurs when there is a diminished production of sounds, a diminished transmission of sounds, or the addition of a medium through which sounds must pass before reaching the thoracic wall as, for example, in pleural effusion, pleural thickening, pneumothorax, bronchial obstruction, or emphysema.
Pleural friction rub	Vibration produced by inflamed pleural surfaces rubbing together. It is felt as a grating, is synchronous with respiratory movements, and is more commonly felt on inspiration.
Rhonchal fremitus	Coarse vibrations produced by the passage of air through thick exudates in the large air passages. These can be cleared or altered by coughing.

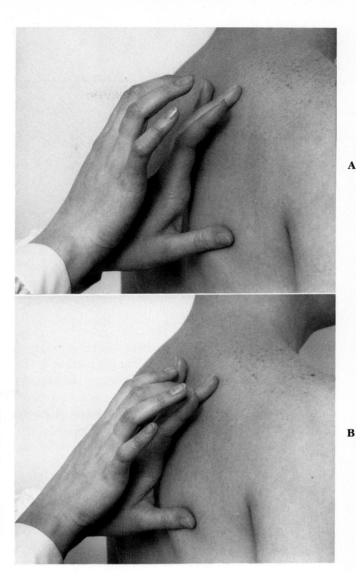

A

B

Figure 14-14

Indirect percussion. **A,** Positioning of the hands. **B,** Hand movement.

cussion penetrates to a depth of approximately 5 to 7 cm into the chest. Percussion is used in the thoracic examination to determine the relative amounts of air, liquid, or solid material in the underlying lung and to determine the positions and boundaries of organs. The techniques of percussion are discussed in Chapter 6, and the student is referred to that chapter for review.

Two techniques of percussion are immediate, or direct, percussion and mediate, or indirect, percussion. In *immediate,* or *direct, percussion* the examiner strikes the area to be percussed directly with the palmar aspect of two, three, or four fingers held together or with the palmar aspect of the tip of the middle finger. The strikes are rapid and downward; movement of the hand from the wrist is in rapid strokes. This type of percussion is not normally used in thoracic examination. It is useful in the examination of the thorax in the infant and the sinuses in the adult. *Mediate,* or *indirect, percussion* is the strik-

ing of an object held against the area to be examined (Fig. 14-14). The middle finger of the examiner's left hand (if the examiner is right-handed) is the pleximeter. The distal phalanx and joint and the middle phalanx are placed firmly on the surface to be percussed. Although most practitioners usually find that the area of the interphalangeal joint is the most effecitve pleximeter point for percussion, the quality of the percussion sound and the comfort of the examiner should serve as criteria for the selection of a pleximeter point. The examiner may find that a point between the proximal and the distal interphalangeal joints is more effective and comfortable. This alteration of technique is acceptable. In all cases, the point struck by the plexor should be pressed as tightly as possible against the patient, with all other areas of that

Table 14-2

Description of percussion tones

Tone	Intensity	Pitch	Duration	Quality	Normal location
Hyperresonance	Very loud	Very low	Long	Booming	Child's lung
Resonance	Loud	Low	Long	Hollow	Peripheral lung
Tympany	Loud	High	Medium	Drumlike	Stomach
Dullness	Medium	High	Medium	Thudlike	Liver
Flatness	Soft	High	Short	Extreme dullness	Muscle

hand held off the client's skin. The plexor is the index finger of the examiner's right hand or the index and middle fingers held together. For position see Fig. 14-14.

With the forearm and shoulder stationary and all movement at the wrist, the pleximeter is struck sharply with the plexor. The blow is aimed at the portion of the pleximeter that is exerting maximum pressure on the thoracic surface, usually the base of the terminal phalanx, the distal interphalangeal joint, or the middle phalanx. The blow is executed rapidly, and the plexor is immediately withdrawn. The plexor strikes with the tip of the finger at right angles to the pleximeter. One or two rapid blows are struck in each area. Bony areas are avoided; interspaces are used for percussion. The examiner compares one side of the thorax with the other.

With experience and study the practitioner will be able to differentiate among the five percussion tones commonly elicited on the human body. In the study of tones, the determination of four characteristics will assist in assessment and labeling:

1. *Intensity (amplitude):* the loudness or softness of the tone.
2. *Pitch (frequency):* relates to the number of vibrations per second. Rapid vibrations produce high-pitched tones; slow vibrations produce low-pitched tones. The greater the density of an object, the higher the frequency.
3. *Duration:* the amount of time a note is sustained.
4. *Quality:* a subjective phenomena relating to the innate characteristics of the object being percussed.

Table 14-2 lists and describes the commonly used descriptive terms for percussion tones elicited by percussion over the thorax and the normal location of such sounds in the thoracic region. Hyperresonance is an abnormal percussion tone in adults. Table 14-5 describes clinical assessment findings in several, common, respiratory system problems and provides examples of abnormal occurrence of the various percussion tones.

Fig. 14-15 is a percussion map for the normal chest. The procedure for thoracic percussion is as follows:

1. Percuss the apices to determine if the normal 5 cm area of resonance is present between the neck and shoulder muscles (Fig. 14-15).
2. Position the client with the head bent and the arm folded over the chest (Fig. 14-16). With this maneuver, the scapulae move laterally and more lung area is accessible to examination.
3. On the posterior chest percuss systematically at about 5-cm intervals from the upper to lower chest, moving left to right, right to left, and avoiding scapular and other bony areas; percuss the lateral chest with the client's arm positioned over the head (Fig. 14-17).
4. Measure the diaphragmatic excursion. Instruct the client to inhale deeply and hold the breath in. Percuss along the scapular line on one side until the lower edge of the lung is identified. Sound will change from resonance to dullness. Mark the point of change on each side at the scapular line. Then instruct the client to take a few normal respirations. Next, instruct the client to exhale completely and hold expiration. Proceed to percuss up from the marked point at the midscapular line to determine the diaphragmatic excursion in deep expiration. Repeat the procedure on the opposite side. Measure and record the distance between the upper and lower points in centimeters on each side. The diaphragm is usually slightly higher on the right side, and excursion is normally 3 to 5 cm bilaterally. Diaphragmatic excursion is usually measured only on the posterior chest (Fig. 14-18).
5. On the anterior chest, percuss systematically as done for the posterior chest.

In the actual examination, the practitioner would complete the examination of the apices and the posterior and lateral chest and would then percuss the anterior chest. A recommended sequence for the examination of the posterior, lateral, and anterior thoracic areas is illustrated in Fig. 14-19.

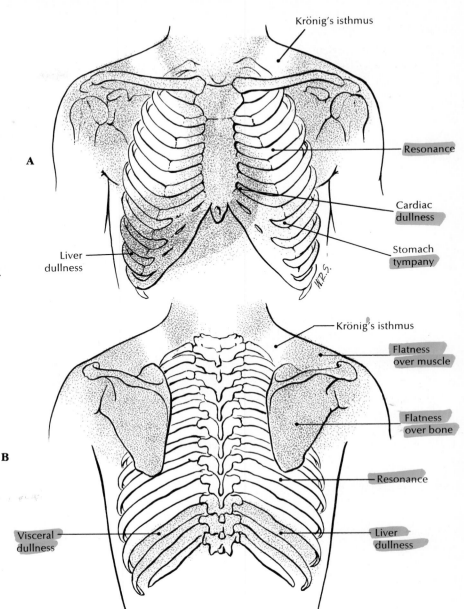

Figure 14-15

Percussion areas. **A,** Normal anterior chest. **B,** Normal posterior chest.

Auscultation

Through auscultation, the practitioner obtains information about the functioning of the respiratory system and about the presence of any obstruction in the passages. Auscultation of the lungs is accomplished with a stethoscope. The diaphragm of the stethoscope is usually used for the thoracic examination because it covers a larger surface than the bell and because the diaphragm is more appropriate for the high pitch of breath sounds.

The stethoscope is placed firmly, but not tightly, on the skin. Client or stethoscope movement is avoided because movements of muscle under the skin or movements of the stethoscope over hair will produce confusing extrinsic sounds.

Before beginning auscultation, the examiner should instruct the client to breathe through the mouth and more deeply and slowly than in usual respiration. The examiner systematically auscultates the apices and the posterior, lateral, and anterior chest (Fig. 14-19). At each application of the stethoscope, the examiner listens to at least one complete respiration. The examiner should observe the client for signs of hyperventilation and stop the procedure if the client becomes light-headed or faint. The process of auscultation includes (1) the analysis of breath sounds, (2) the detection of any abnormal sounds, and (3) the examination of the sounds produced by the spoken voice. As with percussion, the examiner should use a zigzag procedure, comparing the finding at each

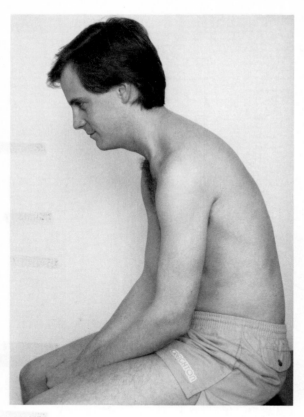

Figure 14-16

Position of the client for examination of the posterior thorax.

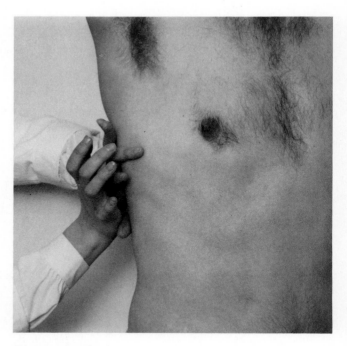

Figure 14-17

Position of the client for percussion of the lateral thorax.

Figure 14-18

Assessment of diaphragmatic excursion.

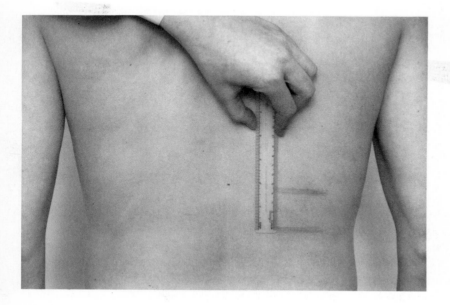

point with the corresponding point on the opposite hemi-thorax.

Breath sounds. Breath sounds are the sounds produced by the movement of air through the tracheo-bronchoalveolar system. These sounds are analyzed according to pitch, intensity, quality, and relative duration of inspiratory and expiratory phases. Table 14-3 outlines the types of sounds heard over the normal and the abnormal lung.

The sounds that are heard over normal lung parenchyma are called vesicular breath sounds. The inspiratory phase of the vesicular breath sounds is heard better

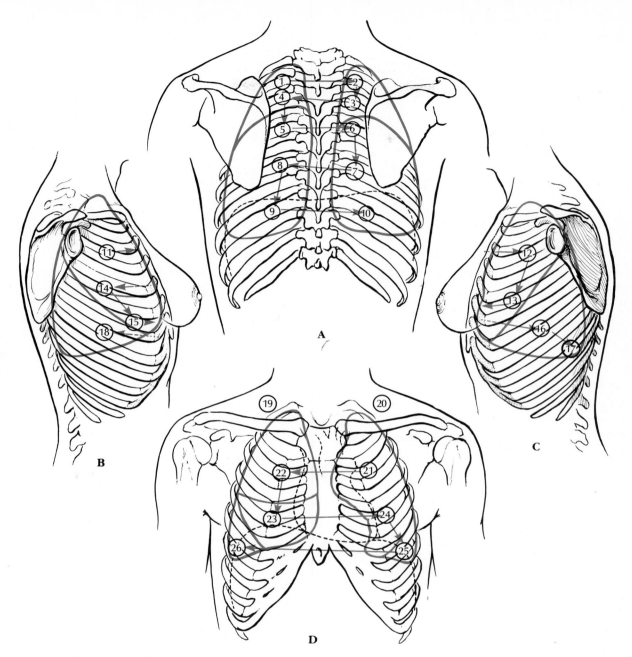

Figure 14-19

Routine for systematic percussion of the thorax. Numbers indicate a recommended sequence for percussion and auscultation during a routine screening examination. **A,** Posterior thorax. **B,** Right lateral thorax. **C,** Left lateral thorax. **D,** Anterior thorax.

than the expiratory phase and is about 2.5 times longer. These sounds have a low pitch and soft intensity.

Bronchovesicular breath sounds are normally heard in the areas of the major bronchi, especially in the apex of the right lung and at the sternal borders anteriorly and posteriorly at tip level between the scapula. Bronchovesicular breath sounds are characterized by inspiratory and expiratory phases of equal duration, moderate pitch, and moderate intensity. When bronchovesicular breath sounds are heard over the peripheral lung, an underlying pathologic condition is likely.

Bronchial breath sounds are normally heard over the trachea and indicate a pathologic condition if heard over lung tissue. They are high-pitched, loud sounds with shortened inspiratory and lengthened expiratory phases. The inspiratory and expiratory phases are audibly separated by a gap of silence.

Fig. 14-20 shows the various areas for assessing

Table 14-3

Characteristics of breath sounds

Sound	Duration of inspiration and expiration	Diagram of sound	Pitch	Intensity	Normal location	Abnormal location
Vesicular	Inspiration > expiration 5:2		Low	Soft	Peripheral lung	Not applicable
Bronchovesicular	Inspiration = expiration 1:1		Medium	Medium	First and second intercostal spaces at the sternal border anteriorly; posteriorly at T4 medial to scapulae	Peripheral lung
Bronchial (tubular)	Inspiration < expiration 1:2		High	Loud	Over trachea	Lung area

Table 14-4

Origin and characteristics of adventitious sounds

Sound	Diagram of sound	Origin	Characteristics
Crackles*—fine to medium		Air passing through moisture in small air passages and alveoli	Discrete, discontinuous; inspiratory; have a dry or wet crackling quality; not cleared by coughing; sound is simulated by rolling a lock of hair near the ear
Crackles*—medium to coarse		Air passing through moisture in the bronchioles, bronchi, and trachea	As above; louder than fine rales
Wheezes		Air passing through air passages narrowed by secretions, swelling, tumors, and so on	Continuous sounds; originate in the small air passages; may be inspiratory and expiratory but usually predominate in expiration; high-pitched, wheezing sounds
Rhonchi—sonorous		Same as wheezes	Continuous sounds; originate in large air passages; may be inspiratory and expiratory but usually predominate in expiration; low-pitched, moaning or snoring quality; coughing may alter sounds
Friction rubs		Rubbing together of inflamed and roughened pleural surfaces	Creaking or grating quality; superficial sounding; inspiratory and expiratory; heard most often in the lower antero-lateral chest (area of greatest thoracic expansion); coughing has no effect

*Crackles are also called rales or crepitations.

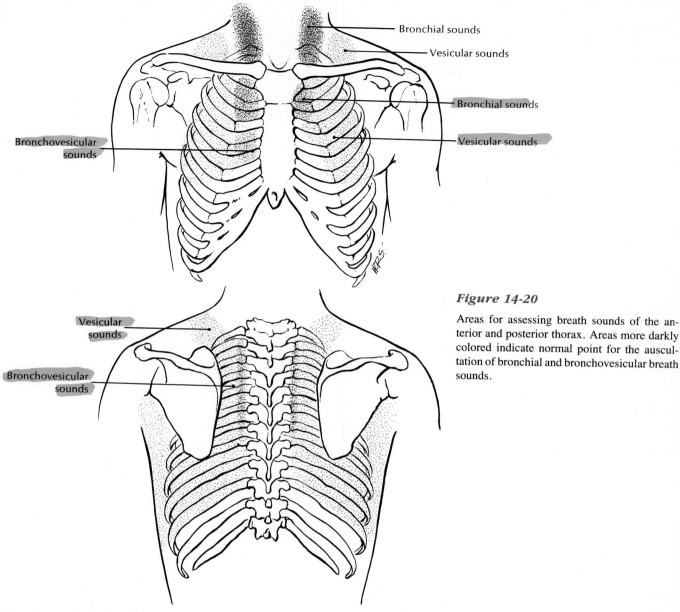

Figure 14-20

Areas for assessing breath sounds of the anterior and posterior thorax. Areas more darkly colored indicate normal point for the auscultation of bronchial and bronchovesicular breath sounds.

breath sounds of the anterior and posterior thorax.

Absent or decreased breath sounds can occur in (1) any condition that causes the deposition of foreign matter in the pleural space, (2) bronchial obstruction, (3) emphysema, or (4) shallow breathing.

Increased breath sounds, as from vesicular to bronchovesicular or bronchial, can occur in any condition that causes a consolidation of lung tissue.

Abnormal or adventitious sounds. Adventitious sounds are not alterations in breath sounds but abnormal sounds superimposed on breath sounds. Classification of these sounds varies among authorities; consequently, nomenclatures are arbitrary. Commonly used terms for adventitious sounds are described in Table 14-4.

A rale is a short, discrete, interrupted, crackling or bubbling sound that is most commonly heard during inspiration. Rales are thought to be produced by air passing through moisture in the bronchi, bronchioles, and alveoli or by air rushing through passages and aveoli that were closed during expiration and abruptly opened during inspiration. The pitch and location in the inspiratory phase of the rales are thought to indicate their site of production. Low-pitched, coarse rales occurring early in inspiration are thought to originate in the bronchi, as in bronchitis. Medium-pitched rales in midinspiration occur in diseases of small bronchi, as in bronchiectasis. High-pitched, fine rales are found in diseases affecting the bronchioles and alveoli and occur late in inspiration. The sound of rales is similar to the sound produced by hairs

Table 14-5

Assessment findings frequently associated with common lung conditions

Condition*	Breath sound	Description
Normal lung		The tracheobronchial tree and alveoli are clear; the pleurae are thin and close together; the chest wall is mobile
Asthma		Asthma is characterized by intermittent episodes of airway obstruction caused by bronchospasm, excessive bronchial secretion, or edema of bronchial mucosa
Atelectasis		Atelectasis is a collapse of alveolar lung tissue, and findings reflect the presence of a small, airless lung; this condition is caused by complete obstruction of a draining bronchus by a tumor, thick secretions, or an aspirated foreign body

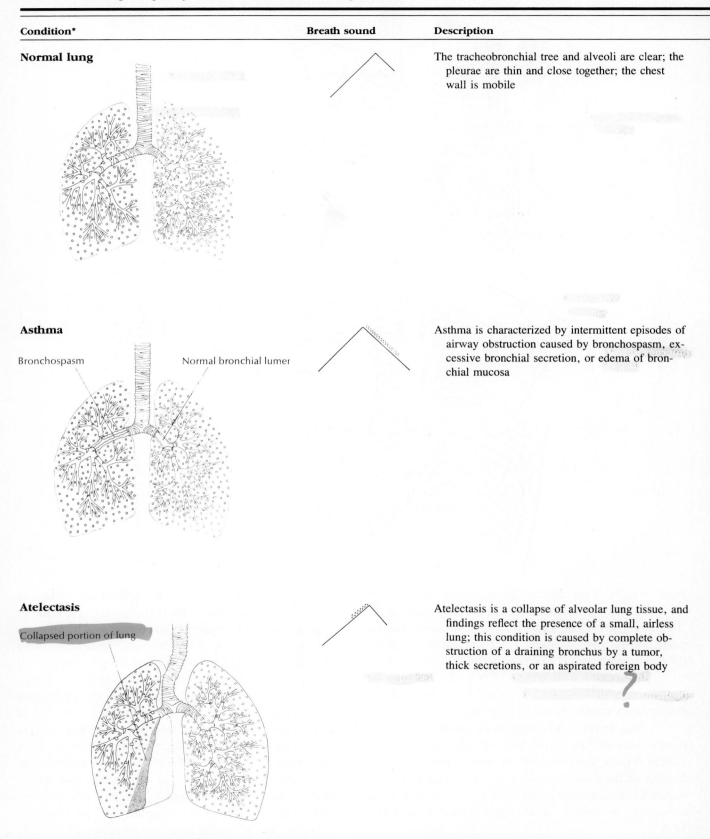

Asthma: Bronchospasm — Normal bronchial lumer

Atelectasis: Collapsed portion of lung

*Although some disease conditions are bilateral, one diseased lung and one normal lung are illustrated for each condition to provide contrast. When an abnormality is illustrated, the pathologic condition is illustrated on the left side and the normal lung is on the right side of the illustration.

Inspection	Palpation	Percussion	Auscultation
Good, symmetric rib and diaphragmatic movement	Trachea—midline Expansion—adequate Tactile fremitus—moderate Diaphragmatic excursion— 3 to 5 cm	Resonant	Breath sounds—vesicular Vocal fremitus—muffled Adventitious sounds—none, except for a few transient crackles at the bases
Cyanosis Air trapping with audible wheezing Use of accessory muscles of respiration	Tactile fremitus—decreased	Hyperresonant	Breath sounds—distant Vocal fremitus—decreased Adventitious sounds—wheezes
Less chest motion on affected side Affected side retracted, with ribs appearing close together Cough Rapid, shallow breathing	Trachea—shifted to affected side Expansion—decreased on affected side Tactile fremitus—decreased or absent	Dull to flat over collapsed lung Hyperresonant over the remainder of the affected hemithorax	Breath sounds—decreased or absent Vocal fremitus—varies in intensity, usually reduced or absent on affected side Adventitious sounds—fine, high-pitched crackles may be heard over the terminal portion of inspiration

Continued

Table 14-5

Assessment findings frequently associated with common lung conditions—*cont'd*

Condition	Breath sound	Description
Bronchiectasis Dilated bronchi		Bronchiectasis is abnormal dilation of the bronchi or bronchioles or both
Bronchitis—acute Bronchial inflammation with abnormal secretion		Acute bronchitis is an inflammation of the bronchial tree characterized by partial bronchial obstruction and secretions or constrictions; it results in abnormally deflated portions of the lung
Emphysema Abnormally distended alveoli		Emphysema is a permanent hyperinflation of the lung beyond the terminal bronchioles, with destruction of alveolar walls

Inspection	Palpation	Percussion	Auscultation
If mild, respirations are normal If severe, tachypnea Less expansion on affected side Cough with purulent sputum	Trachea—midline or deviated toward affected side Expansion—decreased on affected side Tactile fremitus—strong	Resonant or dull	Breath sounds—usually vesicular Vocal fremitus—usually muffled Adventitious sounds—crackles
If severe, tachypnea and cyanosis Rasping cough with mucoid sputum	Tactile fremitus—moderate or strong	Resonant	Breath sounds—vesicular Vocal fremitus—moderate Adventitious sounds—localized crackles, sibilant ronchi
Dyspnea with exertion Barrel chest Tachypnea Use of accessory muscles of respiration	Expansion—limited Tactile fremitus—weak	Resonant to hyper-resonant Diaphragmatic excursion—decreased	Breath sounds—decreased intensity; often prolonged expiration Vocal fremitus—muffled or decreased Adventitious sounds—occasional ronchi or wheezes; often fine crackles in late inspiration

Continued

Table 14-5

Assessment findings frequently associated with common lung conditions—*cont'd*

Condition	Breath sound	Description
Pleural effusion and thickening		Pleural effusion is a collection of fluid in the pleural space; if pleural effusion is prolonged, fibrous tissue may also accumulate in the pleural space; the clinical picture depends on the amount of fluid or fibrosis present and the rapidity of development; fluid tends to gravitate to the most dependent areas of the thorax, and the adjacent lung is compressed
Pneumonia with consolidation		Pneumonia with consolidation occurs when alveolar air is replaced by fluid or tissue; physical findings depend on the amount of parenchymal tissue involved
Pneumothorax		Pneumothorax implies air in the pleural space. There are three types of pneumothorax: (1) closed—air in the pleural space does not communicate with the air in the lung; (2) open—air in the pleural space freely communicates with the air in the lung; air in the pleural space is atmospheric; and (3) tension—air in the pleural space communicates with air in the lungs only on inspiration; air pressure in the pleural space is greater than atmospheric. Physical signs depend on the degree of lung collapse and the presence or absence of pleural effusion

Fluid in the pleural space

Consolidation

Air in the pleural space

Inspection	Palpation	Percussion	Auscultation
Tachypnea Decrease in the definition of the intercostal spaces on the affected side	Trachea—deviation toward normal side Expansion—decreased on affected side Tactile fremitus—weak or absent	Dull to flat	Breath sounds—decreased or absent Vocal fremitus—muffled or absent; if the fluid compresses the lung, sounds may be bronchial over the compression, and bronchophony, egophony, and whisper pectoriloquy may be present Adventitious sounds—pleural friction rub sometimes present
Tachypnea Guarding and less motion on affected side	Expansion—limited on the affected side Tactile fremitus—usually strong, but may be weak if a bronchus leading to the affected area is plugged	Dull to flat	Breath sounds—increased in intensity; bronchovesicular or bronchial breath sounds over affected area Vocal fremitus—increased bronchophony, egophony, whisper pectoriloquy present Adventitious sounds—inspiratory crackles terminal third of inspiration
Restricted lung expansion If large, tachypnea Bulging in the intercostal spaces on the affected side Cyanosis	Trachea—deviated toward normal side Expansion—decreased on affected side Tactile fremitus—absent	Hyperresonant	Breath sounds—usually decreased or absent; if open pneumothorax, have an amorphic quality Vocal fremitus—decreased or absent Adventitious sounds—none

Continued

Table 14-5

Assessment findings frequently associated with common lung conditions—*cont'd*

Condition	Breath sound	Description
Pulmonary fibrosis—diffuse		Pulmonary fibrosis is the presence of an excessive amount of connective tissue in the lungs; consequently, the lungs are smaller than normal and less compliant; the lower lobes are usually the most affected

Fibrotic portion of lung

being rolled between the fingers while close to the ear.

Rhonchi are continuous sounds produced by the movement of air through narrowed passages in the tracheobronchial tree. Rhonchi predominate in expiration because bronchi are shortened and narrowed during this respiratory phase. However, rhonchi can occur in the inspiratory as well as the expiratory phase of respiration, suggesting that lumen have been narrowed during both respiratory phases. As with rales, the pitch and location of rhonchi in the expiratory phase are thought to indicate their origins. Low-pitched rhonchi, sometimes called sonorous rhonchi and usually heard in early expiration, originate in the larger bronchi; high-pitched, sibilant rhonchi, sometimes called wheezes, originate in small bronchioles and often occur in late expiration.

A pleural friction rub is a loud, dry, creaking or grating sound indicative of pleural irritation. It is produced by the rubbing together of inflamed and roughened pleural surfaces during respiration and therefore is heard best during the latter part of inspiration and the beginning of expiration. Because thoracic expansion is greatest in the lower anterolateral thorax, pleural friction rubs are most often heard there.

If the client has rales, the examiner listens for several respirations in the areas in which the rales are heard to determine the effects of deep breathing. Also, the client is asked to cough, with the changes in adventitious sounds noted after coughing.

If the client has complained of respiratory difficulty and no adventitious sounds are heard, he or she is asked to cough; often, adventitious sounds are noted in posttussive breathing.

Voice sounds.   Vocal resonance is produced by the same mechanism that produces vocal fremitus. Resonance is transmitted voice sounds as heard by the stethoscope on the chest wall. Normal vocal resonance is heard as muffled, nondistinct sounds; it is loudest medially and is less intense at the periphery of the lung. Vocal resonance is assessed if there has been any respiratory abnormality detected on observation, palpation, percussion, or auscultation. The routine is the same systematic one previously used in the respiratory examination. The client says "one, two, three" or "ninety-nine" while the examiner surveys the thorax (see boxed material on p. 323).

The increase in loudness and clarity of vocal resonance is termed *bronchophony*. Special vocal resonance techniques are used when resonance is increased. These include tests for whispered pectoriloquy and egophony.

Whispered pectoriloquy is exaggerated bronchophony. The client is instructed to whisper a series of words. The words as heard through the stethoscope on the chest wall are distinct and understandable.

In *egophony*, the intensity of the spoken voice, as heard through the stethoscope applied to the chest wall, is increased and the voice has a nasal or bleating quality.

Inspection	Palpation	Percussion	Auscultation
Dyspnea on exertion Tachypnea Thoracic expansion diminished Cyanosis	Trachea—deviated to most affected side	Resonant to dull	Breath sounds—reduced or absent, bronchovesicular or bronchial Vocal fremitus—increased, whisper pectoriloquy may be present Adventitious sounds—crackles on inspiration and expiration

Voice Sound Assessment Techniques		
Client vocalization	**Normal auscultory finding**	**Abnormal auscultory finding**
"Ninety-nine" spoken "e- e- e" spoken "Ninety-nine" whispered	Muffled, nondistinct sound Muffled, nondistinct sound Barely audible, nondistinct sound	"Ninety-nine": bronchophony "a- a- a": egophony "Ninety-nine": whispered pectoriloquy

If the client says "e- e- e," the transmitted sound will be "a- a- a."

Decreased vocal resonance occurs in the same clinical situations as when vocal fremitus is decreased and breath sounds are absent. Vocal resonance is increased and whispered pectoriloquy and egophony may be present in any condition that causes a consolidation of lung tissue.

Variations from Health

Despite the heavy reliance on laboratory and x-ray findings in the diagnosis of respiratory problems, the examiner can derive reasonably sound diagnostic probabilities by compiling and analyzing the physical assessment data. Table 14-5 outlines the usual assessment findings in a variety of common problems.

Health History
Respiratory System

NOTE: A yes response to any question *must* be further investigated. Use the following indicators throughout the assessment: (1) onset (specific date, sudden or gradual), (2) duration, (3) frequency, (4) precipitating factors, (5) aggravating or alleviating factors, (6) treatment received, and (7) outcome.

Present status

1. Do you have a cough?
   a. Description: dry, hacking, hoarse, barking, whooping, moist, bubbling
2. Do you produce sputum when you cough?
   a. Description: color, amount, frequency, odor, bloody
3. Do you have shortness of breath?
   a. Associated symptoms: chest pain, choking
   b. Temperature
4. Do you or have you smoked tobacco?
   a. Amount and duration
5. Do you have allergies?
   a. Allergen: pollens, foods, medications, metals, animals hair/dander

Past history

1. Have you worked around lung irritants?
   a. Source: asbestos, coal dust, textiles, pollutants, grain, stone dust, dust
2. Have you had lung disease?
   a. Type: TB, cancer, pneumonia, emphysema, asthma

Associated conditions

1. Do you have heart disease?
2. Do you have renal disease?
3. Have you had a heart attack?

Family history

1. Does anyone in your family smoke?
2. Is there a family history of TB, asthma, lung cancer?

Sample assessment record

Client states lung emphysema was diagnosed 3 years ago. Is always short of breath but has been worse last 2 days. Is unable to climb stairs without resting and has difficulty walking on flat ground for one block. Uses oxygen at home at 2 liters per minute after meals, at night, and during any physical activity. Has moist cough several times daily that produces white or yellow sputum. When sputum is yellow, he takes prescribed Ampicillin as directed. Color of sputum has always cleared after taking medication. States sputum is now white. Smoked for 50 years but stopped 3 years ago when emphysema was diagnosed. Denies allergies and working with lung irritants. Denies TB, cancer, and familial lung disease. Denies heart and renal disease.

BIBLIOGRAPHY

Capel LH: Lung sounds: a new approach, Practitioner 219:633, 1979.

Carroll JL, Clayton JE, and Lemen RJ: The physiology and clinical usefulness of common pulmonary findings, Ariz Med 40:408, 1983.

Cherniak RM and Cherniak L: Respiration in health and disease, Philadelphia, 1983, WB Saunders Co.

Cotes JE: Lung function: assessment and application in medicine, ed 4, Oxford, 1979, Blackwell Scientific Publications.

Longe RL, Taylor AT, and Calvert JC: Physical assessment series: the thorax and the lungs, Drug Intell Clin Pharm 15:166, 1981.

Loudon RG: The lung exam, Clin Chest Med 8:265-272, 1987.

Mitchell RS and Petty TL, editors: Synopsis of clinical pulmonary disease, ed 3, St Louis, 1982, The CV Mosby Co.

Naylor CD, McCormack DG, and Sullivan SN: The midclavicular line: a wandering landmark, Can Med Assoc J 136:48-50, 1987.

Poe RH and Israel RH: Problems in pulmonary medicine for the primary physician, Philadelphia, 1982, Lea & Febiger.

Pulmonary terms and symbols: A report of the ACCP-ATS Joint Committee on Pulmonary Nomenclature, Chest 67:583, 1975.

Schreiber JR and others: Frequency analysis of breath sounds by phonopneumography, Med Instrum 15:331, 1981.

Slonim NB and Hamilton LH: Respiratory physiology, ed 4, St Louis, 1981, The CV Mosby Co.

Tattersfield AE and McNeil MW: Respiratory disease, London, 1987, Springer-Verlag.

Wilkins RL, Hodgkin JE, and Lopez B: Lung sounds: practical guide, St Louis, 1988, The CV Mosby Co.

Wilkins RL, Sheldon RL, and Krider SJ: Clinical assessment in respiratory care, St Louis, 1985, The CV Mosby Co.

Witkowski AS: Pulmonary assessment: a clinical guide, Philadelphia, 1985, JB Lippincott Co.

chapter

15

Assessment of the cardiovascular system

OBJECTIVES

Upon successful review of this chapter, learners will be able to:

- Describe anatomy and physiology of the heart and neck vessels

- Recognize variations of the first, second, third, and fourth heart sounds

- Recognize characteristics associated with heart murmurs

- Outline history relevant to assessment of the cardiac system

- State related rationale and demonstrate assessment of the cardiovascular system, including inspection, palpation, and auscultation

- Recognize abnormalities of jugular venous pressure and waves

- Recognize variations of the carotid arterial pulse

- Recognize characteristics and problems associated with
  Cardiac dysrhythmias
  Heart failure
  Ischemic heart disease
  Myocardial infarction
  Hypertension
  Cor pulmonale
  Infection and inflammation

This chapter covers those portions of the cardiovascular examination dealing with examination of the heart and the major neck vessels—the jugular veins and the carotid arteries. Assessment of the peripheral pulses and blood pressure measurement, which are also integral components of the cardiovascular examination, are described in Chapter 7, "General assessment, including vital signs."

The Heart

ANATOMY AND PHYSIOLOGY

In the examination of the heart and the subsequent description of findings, several anterior chest wall landmarks are important. These include the midsternal line; the midclavicular line; the anterior, middle, and posterior axillary lines; the suprasternal notch; and the ribs and intercostal spaces. The area of the chest overlying the heart and pericardium is known as the precordium. These landmarks are illustrated in Fig. 15-1.

The heart lies in the thoracic cavity within the mediastinum. The upper portion, consisting of both atria, lies at the top behind the upper portion of the body of the sternum; the lower portion, composed of both ventricles, is directed downward and toward the left. The upper portion is referred to as the base of the heart, and the lower left portion is referred to as the apex. The aorta, pulmonary arteries, and great veins are located around the upper portion, or base, of the heart.

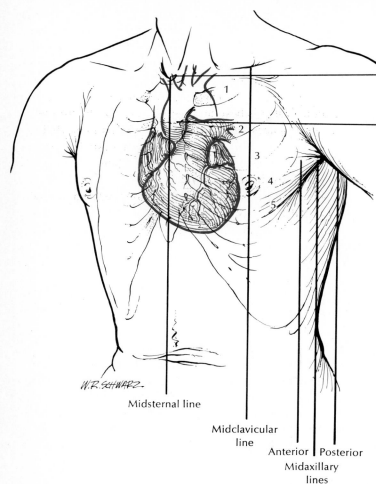

Suprasternal
notch

Angle of Louis

Midsternal line

Midclavicular
line

Anterior   Posterior
Midaxillary
lines

W.R.SCHWARZ

Figure 15-1

Chest wall landmarks.

Heart Chambers

Most of the anterior cardiac surface consists of the right ventricle, which lies behind the sternum and extends to the left of it. The left ventricle lies posterior to the right ventricle and extends further to the left, thus forming the left border of the heart and making up a small portion of the anterior cardiac surface. The right atrium lies slightly above and to the right of the right ventricle, and the left atrium occupies a posterior portion of the heart (Fig. 15-2). It is the contraction and thrust of the left ventricle that produces the normal apical impulse, sometimes referred to as the point of maximum impulse, that is located at or just medial to the midclavicular line in the fifth left intercostal space.

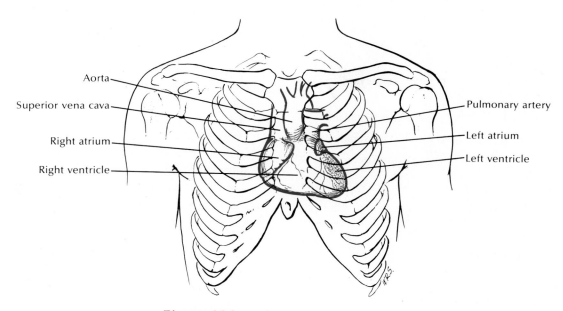

Aorta

Superior vena cava

Right atrium

Right ventricle

Pulmonary artery

Left atrium

Left ventricle

Figure 15-2

Position of the heart chambers and great vessels.

Heart Valves

The atrioventricular (AV) valves lie between the atria and ventricles; the right AV valve is the tricuspid valve, and the left is the mitral valve. The semilunar valves separate the ventricles from the great vessels, the aorta, and the pulmonary artery. On the right the pulmonic valve separates the right ventricle from the pulmonary artery, and on the left the aortic valve separates the left ventricle from the aorta. It is basically the closure of the heart valves that produces the normal heart sounds. (There is much discussion about the actual mechanism of heart sound production; it is thought that tensing of the muscular structures and flow of blood may be involved, as well as valve closure.)

Although the four valves are actually located rather close to each other in a small area behind the sternum (Fig. 15-3, *A*), the areas on the chest wall where their closure is best heard are not located directly over the valves but rather more in the direction of the flow of blood (Fig. 15-3, *B*). The sound produced by closure of the mitral valve is best heard at the apex, at the fifth left intercostal space (LICS) in the midclavicular line (MCL); the sound produced by closure of the tricuspid valve is best heard along the lower left sternal border (LSB) at the fourth left intercostal space; the sound produced by the aortic valve is heard best at the second right intercostal space (RICS) at the sternal border (SB); and the sound produced by the pulmonic valve is best heard at the sec-

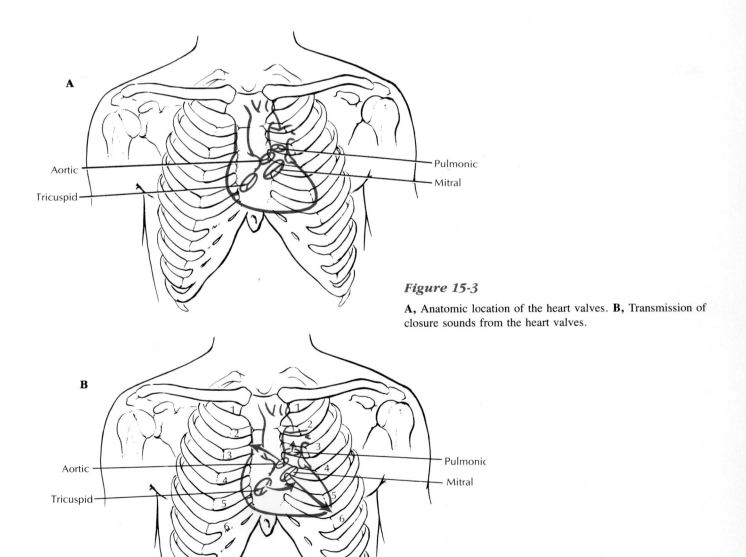

Figure 15-3

A, Anatomic location of the heart valves. **B,** Transmission of closure sounds from the heart valves.

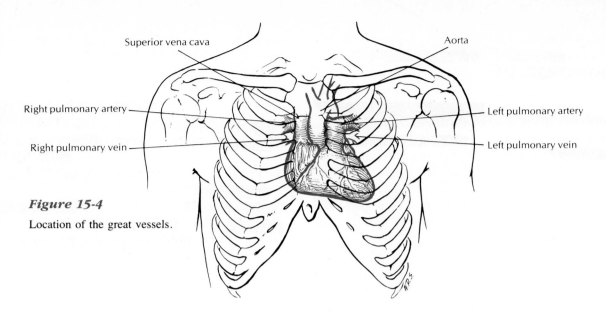

Figure 15-4

Location of the great vessels.

ond left intercostal space at the sternal border. The auscultatory valve areas can be summarized as follows:

Mitral valve: Fifth LICS at MCL
Tricuspid valve: Fourth LICS at SB
Aortic valve: Second RICS at SB
Pulmonic valve: Second LICS at SB

The Great Vessels

The great vessels lie at the top, or base, of the heart. The pulmonary artery extending from the right ventricle bifurcates quickly into its left and right branches. The aorta, extending from the left ventricle, curves upward over the heart, then backward and down. The superior and inferior venae cavae empty into the right atrium, and the pulmonary veins return blood to the left atrium. The relationship of these vessels to the heart chambers is shown in Fig. 15-4.

Pericardium

The pericardium is a tough, double-walled, fibrous sac encasing and protecting the heart. Several cubic centimeters of fluid are present between the inner and outer layers of the pericardium, providing for easy, low-friction movement. The outer layer of the pericardium is firmly attached to the diaphragm, sternum, pleura, esophagus, and aorta.

Variable Position of the Heart

The position of the heart in the thorax has a large range of normal and varies considerably with different body builds, chest configurations, and diaphragm levels. In an average-size person, the heart lies obliquely; one third of it lies to the right of the midsternal line, and two thirds of it lies to the left of it. In short, stocky persons the heart may tend to lie more horizontally; in tall, slender persons it may hang more vertically. In the rare condition of dextrocardia, the position of the heart is reversed and lies on the right side of the chest.

Cycle of Cardiac Events

The flow of blood, movements of the chambers and valves, pressure relationships, and electrical stimulation are discussed here briefly.

The cardiac cycle may be said to begin with the return of blood from the systemic circulation through the superior and inferior venae cavae to the right atrium and with the return of oxygenated blood from the lungs through the pulmonary veins to the left atrium (Fig. 15-5). Following ventricular systole, during which blood has been ejected from the ventricles, the AV valves open, allowing blood that has been collected in the atria to flow into the ventricles. Toward the end of this passive filling phase, or ventricular diastole, the atria contract, ejecting the remaining blood into the ventricles. Then ventricular contraction begins. As intraventricular pressure increases, the AV valves are forced closed, preventing regurgitation of blood to the atria and producing the first heart sound (S_1). During the early part of contraction, the volume of blood in the ventricle remains the same; this is called the period of isovolumic contraction. As the pressure continues to rise during ventricular contraction, a point is reached when the pressure in the left ventricle exceeds the pressure in the aorta; the semilunar valves are forced open, and blood is ejected into the aorta

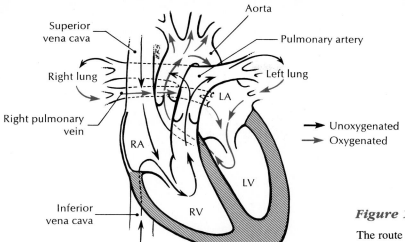

Figure 15-5

The route of blood flow through the chambers of the heart and the great vessels.

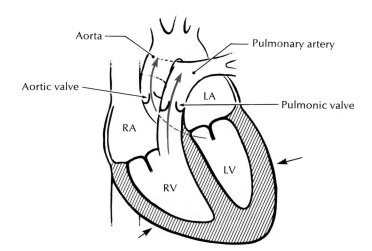

Figure 15-6

Ventricular systole. The ventricles contract, forcing the aortic and pulmonic valves to open; blood flows into the aorta and pulmonary artery.

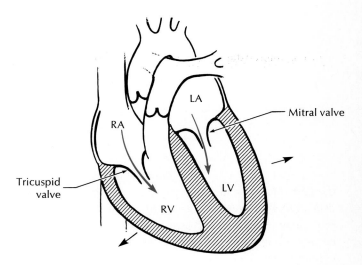

Figure 15-7

Ventricular diastole. The ventricles relax and the mitral and tricuspid valves open, allowing blood to flow from the atria to the ventricles.

(Fig. 15-6). (Events on the left side of the heart are used for describing the cycle. Right-sided events are similar but occur at much lower pressures.)

At the end of ejection, the ventricle relaxes, the pressure in the ventricle drops below the pressure in the aorta, and the semilunar valves snap shut, producing the second heart sound (S_2). Meanwhile, during ventricular systole the atria have been filling; as the ventricular pressure drops, the AV valves open, permitting the flow of blood into the ventricles once again (Fig. 15-7). Because of the manner in which myocardial depolarization occurs, events on the left side of the heart normally occur slightly before events on the right side. Therefore, in the production of S_1, mitral valve closure briefly precedes tricuspid valve closure. Similarly, in the production of S_2,

aortic valve closure precedes pulmonic valve closure. The pressure relationships and points of valve closure are illustrated in Fig. 15-8.

Normally, ventricular systole, the contraction phase, is slightly shorter than ventricular diastole, the relaxation or filling phase. At heart rates of about 120 beats per minute, the phases become nearly equal in length.

The electrical events stimulating and coordinating the mechanical events just described begin with an electrical discharge originating at the sinoatrial (SA) node, located in the right atrium. This electrical discharge then flows through the atria, producing atrial contraction. The impulse then travels to the AV node, located in the low atrial septum, and on through the bundle of His and its

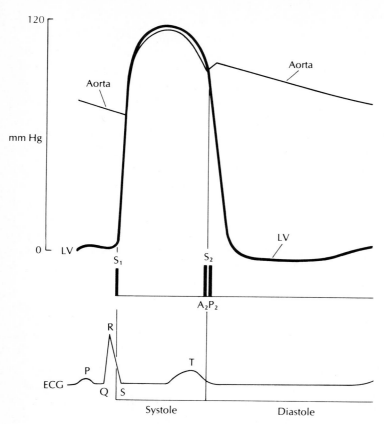

Figure 15-8

· Pressure curves of the left ventricle and aorta, S_1 and S_2, and the ECG.

branches in the myocardium, stimulating ventricular contraction. The SA node is the cardiac pacemaker, normally discharging between 60 and 100 impulses per minute. The passage of the electrical impulses is shown in the electrocardiogram (ECG) tracing below the pressure diagram in Fig. 15-8. The P wave represents spread of the impulse through the atria; the PR interval extends from the beginning of the P wave to the beginning of the QRS complex; it represents the time taken for the original impulse to pass from the SA node, through the atria and the AV node, to the ventricles. The QRS complex represents spread of the impulse through the ventricles; the T wave represents repolarization of the ventricles. Electrical stimulation briefly precedes the mechanical response.

Characteristics of Cardiovascular Sounds

All sounds, including those of cardiovascular origin, can be characterized by their frequency (pitch), intensity (loudness), duration, and timing in the cardiac cycle. All cardiovascular sounds are of relatively low frequency and require special concentration for perception by the human ear. Examples of heart sounds in the lower frequencies include the diastolic murmur of mitral stenosis and a third heart sound (S_3); the normal S_2 is of a slightly higher frequency, and the diastolic murmur of aortic or pulmonic valve insufficiency is of yet a higher frequency.

The intensity of cardiovascular sounds is widely variable. The range extends from sounds that can be heard only with great concentration and by careful "tuning in" to those that can be heard with the edge of the stethoscope barely touching the chest wall.

The duration of most cardiovascular sounds is very brief, usually much less than 1 second. In cardiac auscultation, both the duration of sounds and the periods of silence are important. Normally, S_1 and S_2 are very brief, lasting only fractions of a second; the intervals of silence, that is, systole and diastole, are longer. Diastole is longer than systole at a heart rate below 120 beats per minute; at faster rates the duration of diastole is diminished, and systole and diastole become about equal in duration.

The timing of any additional cardiac sounds is designated as occurring during either systole or diastole. Systole begins with S_1 and extends to S_2; diastole begins with S_2 and extends to the next S_1. A helpful method for determining S_1 and S_2 and thus differentiating systole and diastole is to palpate the carotid pulse while auscultating the heart. The carotid pulsation and S_1 are very nearly synchronous; S_1 only briefly precedes the carotid impulse.

Heart sounds are illustrated by vertical bars. The height of the bar indicates the relative loudness of the sound, and the width of the bar indicates the duration. For example, S_1 and S_2 as heard at the base and apex of the heart are illustrated as shown in Fig. 15-9.

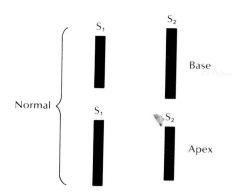

Figure 15-9

Relative loudness of S_1 and S_2 as heard over the base and apex of the heart.

The audibility of cardiac sounds is modified by the amount of interposed tissue between the sound at its point of origin and the outer chest wall. Large amounts of fat, muscle, or air, as in the obese, muscular, or emphysematous client, tend to dampen or diminish the heart sounds and cause them to sound more distant.

Heart sounds

First heart sound. The AV valves are forced closed as ventricular pressure rises, producing S_1. This sequence of events is similar on both sides of the heart, but pressures and pressure gradients are much greater on the left side, and the sounds produced by left-sided events are usually louder. Events on the left side usually slightly precede those on the right side because the left ventricular myocardium begins depolarization slightly earlier. S_1 can be heard over the entire precordium but is heard best at the apex and is usually louder than S_2 there (Fig. 15-9). At the base of the heart S_1 is usually louder on the left than on the right and on both sides is quieter than S_2. Usually both components of S_1, mitral and tricuspid valve closure, are heard as one sound. As a result of slight asynchrony in valve closure, however, a split S_1 may be audible and may be heard in the area where tricuspid valve closure is best transmitted, that is, at the fourth left intercostal space at the sternal border. Tricuspid valve closure may become louder as a result of pulmonary hypertension because of the increased right-sided pressures. Splitting of S_1 is neither as commonly nor as easily heard as splitting of S_2.

The frequency of S_1 is slightly lower than that of S_2, and its duration is slightly longer. Its occurrence can be timed with the apical impulse or with the carotid pulsation; it should not be timed with the radial pulse, because the time lapse is too great and leads to confusion.

Factors altering or influencing the loudness of S_1 may be extracardiac or cardiac. Extracardiac factors usually affect both S_1 and S_2. An increase in the amount of tissue interposed between the heart and the stethoscope, as found in obesity, emphysema, or the accumulation of pericardial fluid, will diminish the intensity of both S_1 and S_2. Cardiac factors influencing the intensity of S_1 consist of the position of the AV valves at the time of ventricular contraction, the structure of the valves, and the force and abruptness of ventricular contraction. If ventricular systole begins when the AV valves are still wide open, before they have time to "drift" or "float" close together, a loud S_1 results. This situation occurs when the PR interval is short, as accompanies hyperkinetic states such as exercise, anemia, fever, and hyperthyroidism. Conversely, a prolonged PR interval, during which the AV valves may begin to close and ventricular contraction is delayed, may result in a faint S_1. Even with a normal PR interval, S_1 may be diminished. With forceful atrial contraction into a noncompliant ventricle, a situation that may exist with hypertension, the pressure rise in the ventricle may cause the valve to close sooner; the valve may already be partially closed at the onset of ventricular contraction.

Changes in valve leaflet structure may alter the intensity of S_1. As a result of rheumatic fever, the mitral valve may become so fibrosed and calcified that only limited motion is possible and S_1 is diminished. However, if the valve leaflets retain some mobility, as they may with mitral stenosis, S_1 may be accentuated. Significant mitral stenosis may also increase S_1 because of the greater ventricular pressure needed to overcome the increase in atrial pressure. This produces an increased closing pressure and more abrupt closure. Abrupt ventricular contractions producing a more intense S_1 may also result from the hyperkinetic states mentioned earlier.

In the presence of a complete heart block, where the length of the PR interval is frequently changing, variation in the intensity of S_1 will occur.

Second heart sound. As ventricular systole is completed, pressure in the aorta and pulmonary artery exceeds ventricular pressure and the semilunar valves close. Vibrations produced by closure of the aortic and pulmonic valves are primarily responsible for S_2. Closure of the aortic valve is the loudest component of S_2 at both the right and left second intercostal spaces and is referred to as A_2; the sound produced by the pulmonic valve, referred to as P_2, is normally heard only in a small area centering around the second left interspace and can be identified as separate from the component of S_2 caused by aortic valve closure only when splitting of S_2 occurs. In children and adolescents P_2 may normally be accentuated, causing an increase in S_2 heard in the pulmonic area. A_2 and P_2 refer to the two components of S_2; they do *not* refer to any anatomic location on the chest wall.

S$_2$ is audible over the entire precordium but is best heard at the base of the heart and is louder there than S$_1$; at the apex it is quieter than S$_1$ (see Fig. 15-9). S$_2$ marks the beginning of diastole, normally the longer interval. It is slightly higher in frequency and shorter in duration than S$_1$.

Right ventricular systolic ejection time is very slightly longer than left ventricular systolic ejection time. Therefore, pulmonic valve closure, which marks the end of right ventricular ejection, occurs slightly later than aortic valve closure and is known as normal physiologic splitting of the second heart sound. This normal asynchrony of valve closure is increased during inspiration because of the decrease in intrathoracic pressure, which facilitates increased venous return to the right side of the heart and a further delay in pulmonic valve closure. During expiration, the disparity between left and right ejection times is decreased and splitting becomes less pronounced or nonexistent as the valves close nearly synchronously, producing a single sound (Fig. 15-10). Inspiratory splitting is commonly most marked at the peak of the inspiratory phase of respiration and is best determined during ordinary respiration. If the breath is held in inspiration, rather than sustaining the splitting, the ejection times again equalize and the split sound becomes single. Splitting will be evident only where pulmonic and aortic closure can be heard, that is, at the second left interspace.

The degree of splitting varies from one individual to another. In some individuals two distinct sounds are quite clear although very close in sequence (the splitting seems more like two parts of a single sound), whereas in others no splitting can be recognized. In some individuals clear splitting may be audible during inspiration, and a very slight degree of splitting is audible during expiration.

Variations in S$_2$ include changes in loudness and variations in splitting. In general, louder closure sounds result from higher closing pressure. In systemic hypertension, for example, louder aortic closure sounds occur; S$_2$ may become ringing or tambourlike and may become louder than S$_1$ at the apex. Exercise and excitement may also increase the pressure in the aorta and thus increase the aortic S$_2$. Conditions associated with pulmonary hypertension, including mitral stenosis and congestive heart failure, may produce an increased pulmonic S$_2$. A fall in systemic blood pressure, as occurs with shock, will produce a diminished aortic S$_2$. As was the case with S$_1$, pathologic changes in the valves will also affect the intensity of S$_2$. Semilunar valves that are injured but still flexible may increase S$_2$, whereas injured valves that

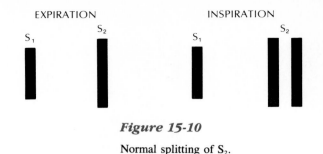

EXPIRATION   INSPIRATION

Figure 15-10

Normal splitting of S$_2$.

have become markedly thickened and calcified may diminish it.

Variations in splitting of S$_2$ include wide splitting, fixed splitting, and paradoxical splitting (Fig. 15-11). Conditions causing delayed electrical activation, on contraction or emptying, or both, of the right ventricle (e.g., right bundle branch block) also cause a delay in pulmonic valve closure. Wide splitting of S$_2$ exists with expiration; on inspiration, the splitting is even wider. Fixed splitting is associated with large atrial septal defects. Here, pulmonic closure is delayed because with each beat, the right ventricle is ejecting a larger volume than is the left ventricle. Presumably, right-sided filling cannot be further increased by inspiration, so the split sound remains relatively fixed. In contrast to delayed closure of the pulmonic valve with its resultant wide splitting, delayed closure of the aortic valve in a left bundle branch block may result in narrowed splitting or splitting where the normal sequence of sounds is reversed, so that pulmonic closure precedes aortic closure. This produces a paradoxical situation, wherein inspiration results in the two sounds' coming closer together and even fusing to a single sound and expiration results in more widely separated sounds. On expiration, pulmonic closure occurs first, followed by aortic closure; then on inspiration, when pulmonary valve closure is normally delayed, the pulmonic sound merges with the aortic sound.

Third heart sound.   During diastole there are two phases of rapid ventricular filling. The first is in early diastole and is a passive, rapid filling phase. When the AV valves open, after S$_2$, the blood stored in the atria flows rapidly into the ventricles. This rapid distention of the ventricles causes vibrations of the ventricular walls to occur. Known as the third heart sound (S$_3$) (Fig. 15-12), these vibrations are low in frequency and intensity and are best heard at the apex with the bell of the stethoscope. The sound may be accentuated by having the client assume the left lateral decubitus position. This sound is commonly heard in healthy children and young adults and in such instances is known as a physiologic S$_3$. However, in other circumstances, an S$_3$ is abnormal. For example, in an older person with heart disease an S$_3$

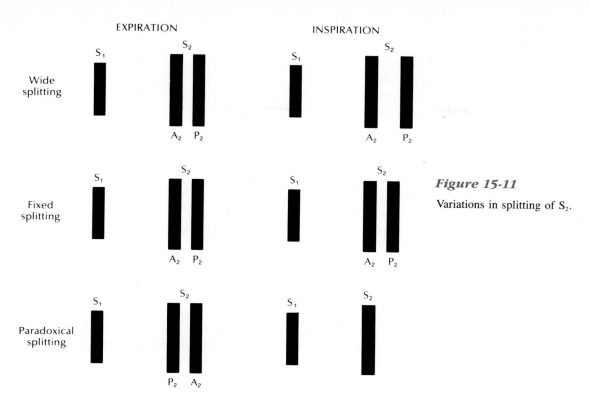

EXPIRATION

INSPIRATION

Wide splitting

Fixed splitting

Paradoxical splitting

Figure 15-11

Variations in splitting of S_2.

often signifies myocardial failure. In such a case S_3 contributes to the production of a ventricular or protodiastolic gallop.

Fourth heart sound. The second phase of rapid ventricular filling occurs after the first phase of passive filling. In late diastole, with atrial systolic ejection of blood into the ventricle, the second, active rapid filling phase occurs, just before S_1. The inflow of this phase, too, may cause vibrations of the valves, supporting structure, or ventricular walls, resulting in a late diastolic filling, or fourth, heart sound (S_4) (Fig. 15-13). It may be heard physiologically, especially in a young person with a thin chest wall, but is more rare in a normal client than is a physiologic S_3. An abnormal S_4 results from an increased resistance to filling secondary to either a change in compliance of the ventricle or to an increase in volume. Therefore, it may be associated with hypertensive cardiovascular disease, coronary artery disease, or aortic stenosis, wherein there may be decreased left ventricular compliance. It may be associated with severe anemia or hyperthyroidism, wherein there is an increased stroke volume.

S_4 is also a low-frequency, low-intensity sound, heard best with the bell at the apex shortly before S_1. It may also be well heard at the base. Care must be taken not to confuse an S_4 with a split S_1. The presence of an S_4 produces a sequence of sounds known as a presystolic gallop because of its timing in the cardiac cycle.

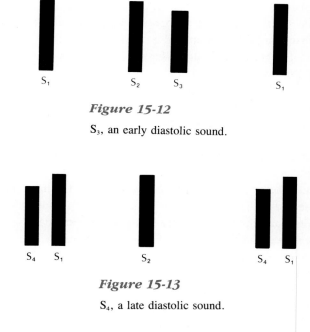

Figure 15-12

S_3, an early diastolic sound.

Figure 15-13

S_4, a late diastolic sound.

Summation gallop. When both phases of rapid ventricular filling become audible events as an S_3 and S_4, a quadruple rhythm results. As the heart rate increases and diastole becomes shorter, the two sounds come closer together and may be heard as one sound in diastole. Then there are three cardiac sounds: S_1 and S_2 and the summation sound of S_3 and S_4. This is known as a summation gallop.

Abnormal extra heart sounds. There are two extra heart sounds that always indicate an abnormality. Both sounds are produced by the opening of diseased valves. They are the opening snap of the mitral valve and the ejection click, or opening snap, of a semilunar valve. Pericardial friction rub also produces an extra cardiac sound.

Opening snap of the mitral valve. Opening of the mitral valve, normally a silent event, may become audible if it becomes thickened or otherwise altered, as by rheumatic heart disease. This sound occurs early in diastole, is high pitched and brief, and has a snapping or clicking quality (Fig. 15-14). It is usually best heard medial to the apex and toward the lower left sternal border and may radiate toward the base. It is always associated with a good, and often accentuated, S_1. It can be differentiated from an S_3 because it occurs earlier (temporally, mitral valve opening is before ventricular filling), is sharper and higher pitched, and radiates more widely. In the pulmonic area, the opening snap must be differentiated from a split S_2. A split S_2 is best heard in the second left intercostal space, and an opening snap is best heard between the apex and the lower left sternal border. Whereas respiration affects the splitting of S_2, an opening snap is not affected by respiration and will remain at a fixed interval after the aortic component of S_2.

The loudness of the opening snap is affected by the pressure in the left atrium and by the flexibility of the mitral valve. Higher left atrial pressures increase the loudness of the opening snap. Marked fibrosis and calcification of the valve decrease the mobility, and consequently, the sound produced.

Ejection click. Semilunar valve changes may also be associated with an opening sound. This sound occurs early in systole at the end of isovolumic contraction when semilunar valves open (Fig. 15-14). The aortic ejection click, the more common of the two, is heard both at the base and at the apex and does not change with respiration. Pulmonary ejection clicks are heard best at the second left interspace, radiate poorly, and change in intensity with respiration, increasing with expiration and decreasing with inspiration.

Pericardial friction rub. Inflammation of the pericardial sac causes the parietal and visceral surfaces of the roughened pericardium to rub against each other. This produces an extra cardiac sound of to-and-fro character with both systolic and diastolic components. One, two, or three components of a pericardial friction rub may be audible. A three-component rub indicates the presence of pericarditis and serves to distinguish a pericardial rub from a pleural friction rub, which ordinarily has two components. It resembles the sound of squeaky leather and is often described as grating, scratching, or rasping. The sound seems very

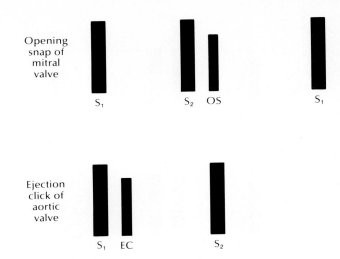

Figure 15-14

Opening snap of the mitral valve following S_2 and ejection click of the aortic valve following S_1.

close to the ear and may seem louder than or may even mask the other heart sounds. Friction rubs are usually best heard between the apex and sternum but may be widespread.

HEALTH HISTORY

Abnormalities of the heart and major blood vessels may be difficult to pinpoint as cardiovascular disease because they may produce symptoms affecting other body systems, such as the lungs, or may present in a location other than at or around the heart itself, such as anginal pain occurring in the jaw or teeth with minimal pain in the chest. Also, serious cardiac disorders may be present without causing symptoms, and some symptoms such as palpitations, difficulty breathing, and chest pain may be present in a client who does not have a cardiac disorder.

The client who complains of chest pain should be asked to indicate where the pain is located; pain of cardiac origin will often be indicated by placement of the hand over the sternal area, whereas pain from another source may be pointed to with one finger over a specific spot. If the client complains of difficulty breathing brought on by exertion, the practitioner should inquire exactly how much and what kind of exertion is required to bring on the symptom.

The healthy history for the system would include questions on the topics listed in the box on p. 335.

EXAMINATION

The division of the cardiac examination into the techniques of inspection, palpation, and auscultation is useful. Because the findings of inspection and palpation are

Weight changes: either gain or loss can be a cardiac symptom. Sudden weight gain can be a sign of fluid retention, whereas progressive loss in a client taking digitalis can be a sign of drug toxicity.

Fatigue: this may be a sign of heart failure or of excessive diuretic or other antihypertensive therapy. Diuretics may cause lowered serum sodium or potassium.

Insomnia: this may be a sign of heart failure in the elderly client.

Chest pain or chest pressure: either pain or pressure is a common cardiac symptom, although both may also be caused by noncardiac conditions. The practitioner should inquire about site, type, spread to other areas, duration, and precipitating factors. The pain of angina pectoris may be described as dull, pressing, squeezing, or burning. It is typically located substernally and may radiate down the inner side of the left arm or to the neck, jaw, teeth, or throat. It may be precipitated by cold, exercise or other exertion, stress, or eating. The symptoms of an acute myocardial infarction are similar to those of angina pectoris but may last longer and are not relieved by nitroglycerin. The client may also experience a cold sweat, may develop a cyanotic or ashen color, and may have nausea or vomiting.

Palpitations: the client may experience an awareness of the heart beating, which may also be described as skipping of heartbeats, a sensation of heart flutter, or a jumping sensation in the chest. Palpitations are usually caused by premature atrial or ventricular beats or by paroxysmal tachycardia in persons with AV block when the ventricular rate is irregular. Individuals with normal cardiac rhythm may also experience palpitations when the cardiac rate exceeds 90 beats per minute.

Dyspnea: breathlessness or the awareness of difficult breathing may be caused by a cardiac or a pulmonary disorder. Most clients with cardiac dyspnea complain of dyspnea brought on by exertion. Paroxysmal nocturnal dyspnea, where the client falls asleep normally but awakens in several hours with shortness of breath, is almost always a symptom of acute left-sided congestive heart failure.

Orthopnea: this is difficulty in breathing that decreases in the upright position.

Cough: this symptom is caused by congestion of the pulmonary system, commonly occurring with left-sided heart failure.

Hemoptysis: coughing up blood may also be caused by a cardiac or pulmonary disorder. Cardiac causes include mitral stenosis, acute pulmonary embolism and infarction, and pulmonary hypertension. There may be only slight streaks of blood in the sputum, or, if pulmonary edema is present, the sputum may be pink and frothy.

Gastrointestinal symptoms: anorexia, nausea, and bloating may be symptoms of right-sided heart failure or side effects of drugs, including digitalis, diuretics, and potassium salts. Vomiting may occur with acute right-sided heart failure, which causes stretching of the liver capsule, and may also occur with an acute myocardial infarction.

Nocturia: this is a common experience of clients with heart failure.

Headache: clients with systemic hypertension may experience dull, nagging headaches.

Tinnitus: clients with systemic hypertension may experience an intermittent or continuous buzzing in the ears.

Personal habits:
- Caffeine intake in coffee, tea, cola drinks, chocolate, and cocoa.
- Use of tobacco.
- Use of salt, including cooking and table salt and canned, processed, and packaged foods.
- Use of drugs, including digitalis, diuretics, nitrates, antiarrhythmics, anticoagulants, estrogen, contraceptive pills, phenothiazines, and tricyclic antidepressants (these can cause arrhythmias).
- Life-style patterns or coping with stress and distress.
- Family history of cardiac diseases, stroke, hypertension, or diabetes.

---

closely related and complementary to one another, these techniques are discussed together. Auscultation provides much valuable information about cardiac dynamics, but the practitioner must be cautious not to apply the stethoscope to the chest wall before performing the visual and palpatory examinations.

Several environmental considerations are basic to the cardiac examination. A quiet room is essential, because cardiac sounds are for the most part subtle and low pitched and are thus easily missed if outside noises prevail. The room should also provide privacy for the client and be warmed or cooled to a comfortable temperature. Equipment required for this portion of the physical examination includes a stethoscope equipped with both a bell and diaphragm, a centimeter ruler, a marking pencil,

and a good light source that can be directed tangentially across the chest wall.

Examination of the precordium is most effectively performed with the examiner standing on the client's right side. The complete assessment requires that the client be examined in the sitting, supine, and left lateral recumbent positions. Whereas inspection and palpation are performed primarily with the client in the supine position, thorough auscultation should be performed with the client in all three positions. Both sitting forward and lying in the left lateral position bring various parts of the heart closer to the chest wall, thus enhancing certain auditory findings.

It is important to remember that examination of the peripheral pulses, including the radial, brachial, femoral, popliteal, dorsalis pedis, and posterior tibial, is an essential component in the assessment of the cardiovascular system. Also included are the assessment of the abdominal aorta and assessment of the blood pressure in the upper and lower extremities in the sitting, standing, and lying positions. These components may be assessed during this portion of the examination or integrated with other portions of the physical examination.

Inspection and Palpation

Inspection and palpation of the precordium should be performed before the stethoscope is applied to the chest wall. It is sometimes tempting to use the stethoscope as the only means of assessing findings over the precordium, but much valuable information can be gained by using visual and tactile assessment procedures. These findings will enhance and may augment the auditory findings.

The purpose of both inspection and palpation is to determine the presence and extent of normal and abnormal pulsations over the precordium. These pulsations may be manifested as the apex beat (or apical impulse) or as heaves or lifts of the chest; they provide some reflection of myocardial and hemodynamic activity. Inspection and palpation together provide a useful method of assessing left, right, and combined ventricular hypertrophy. The visibility and palpability of those movements are affected by the thickness of the chest wall and by the type and amount of tissue through which the vibrations must travel.

Inspection

The chest wall and epigastrium are inspected while the client is in the supine position. A tangential light is helpful for observing subtle movements of the chest. The examiner stands to the client's right side and observes the chest for size and symmetry and then for any pulsations, retractions, heaves, or lifts. The location and timing of all impulses should be noted.

Apical impulse. The thrust of the contracting left ventricle may produce a visible pulsation in the area of the midclavicular line in the fifth left intercostal space. This is the normal apical impulse, and it is visibly evident in about half the normal adult population. It occurs nearly synchronously with the carotid impulse, and simultaneous palpation of a carotid artery is helpful in identifying it.

When visible, the apical impulse helps to identify an area very near the cardiac apex, thus giving some indication of cardiac size. With left ventricular hypertrophy or dilatation, or both, as may occur with systemic hypertension, the apical impulse may be located more

laterally or inferiorly, or both; for example, it may be located at the left anterior axillary line in the sixth left intercostal space.

Retractions. A slight retraction of the chest wall just medial to the midclavicular line in the fifth interspace is a normal finding. Marked or actual retraction of the rib is abnormal and may result from pericardial disease. Left ventricular hypertrophy is often accompanied by a systolic thrust, producing a "rocking" movement.

Heaves or lifts. When the work and forcefulness of the right ventricle is greatly increased, a diffuse lifting impulse is often produced along the left sternal border with each beat. This is referred to as a *lift* or *heave;* these terms are generally used interchangeably.

Palpation

The technique of palpation builds on and expands the findings gleaned from inspection. The entire precordium is palpated methodically, beginning at the apex, moving to the left sternal border, and then to the base of the heart (Fig. 15-15). Other areas may also be included if indicated, including the left axillary area, the epigastrium, and the right sternal border. During palpation the examiner is searching for the apical impulse at or near the apex and for any abnormal heaves, thrills, or retractions elsewhere on the precordium, indicating cardiac hypertrophy, dilatation, or murmurs. The abnormal flow of blood resulting in an audible murmur may also result in the palpatory sensation known as a thrill. It is rather like a rushing sensation beneath the fingers and has been likened to the feeling transmitted to the fingers placed over the larynx of a purring cat. As with inspection, the shape and thickness of the chest wall are important variables.

The client is in the supine position for this portion of the cardiac examination. The examiner should take adequate time to "tune in" or "warm up" to movements over the precordium, because many are faint and subtle and are perceived only after a "warming up" period. It is important to describe pulsations in relation to their timing in the cardiac cycle. This is facilitated by simultaneously palpating the carotid pulsation with the left hand while palpating the precordium with the right. All pulsations should be described in terms of their location in an interspace and their distance from the midsternal, midclavicular, or axillary lines.

Apical impulse. Although the thrust noted over the apex of the heart is sometimes referred to as the point of maximum impulse (PMI), this term is not recommended because the actual point or area of maximum

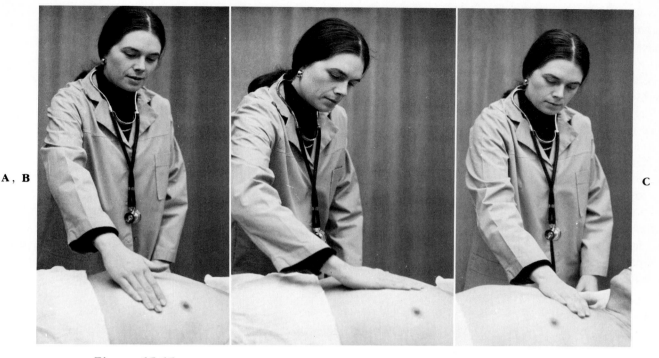

A , B   **C**

Figure 15-15

Palpation of the precordium. The examiner palpates three areas of the precordium. **A,** Over the apex. **B,** Over the left sternal border. **C,** Over the base of the heart.

impulse may not be located over the apical area. The term *apical impulse* is preferred. The presence, location, size, and character of the apical impulse should be assessed. The apical impulse is palpable in about half the normal adult population.

Standing to the right of the client and using the fingertips and palmar aspect of the right hand, the examiner palpates first over the apex, particularly in the area of the fifth interspace in the midclavicular line. Normally, the apical impulse is palpable in or just medial to the midclavicular line and is felt as a faint, short-duration, localized tap less than 2 cm in diameter. On occasion the apical impulse may be normally located lateral to the midclavicular line, for example, in association with a high diaphragm, as occurs with pregnancy. The outward movement of the normal impulse is not excessively forceful and is palpable only during the first part of systole. The amplitude of the apical impulse may seem to be increased in normal individuals with thin chest walls. Turning the client to the left lateral position may cause a normal impulse to seem abnormal in both amplitude and duration, since the apex is brought closer to the chest wall, thus accentuating its activities. In obese persons or those with an increased anteroposterior chest diameter, the apical impulse is not likely to be palpable. Conditions such as anxiety, anemia, fever, and hyperthyroidism may

produce an apical impulse increased in force and duration. Normally, systolic ejection may be associated with a slight retraction of the lower left parasternal area.

Apex area: left ventricular hypertrophy. Hypertrophy of the left ventricle typically produces an abnormally forceful and sustained outward movement during ventricular systole. In addition, the apex impulse may be displaced laterally and downward and may be increased in size. For example, the apical impulse may be found 4 cm lateral to the midclavicular line in the sixth intercostal space and may be 4 cm in diameter.

Generally, the degree of displacement of the impulse correlates with the extent of cardiac enlargement. In addition to an alteration in location and size, the impulse may become more diffuse and palpable in more than one interspace; also, the amplitude or forcefulness may be increased. Displacement tends to be maximal when there is both dilatation and hypertrophy. Conditions associated with a volume overload, such as mitral and aortic regurgitation and left-to-right shunts, tend to produce such dilatation and hypertrophy. Hypertrophy of the left ventricle without dilatation, as may occur with aortic stenosis and systemic hypertension, results in an apical impulse that is increased in force and duration but not necessarily displaced laterally; it may still be located in the midclavicular line. In some persons with left ventricular hypertrophy, the increased force and prolonged duration of the apical impulse produces a lifting sensation under the examiner's fingers.

Left sternal border: right ventricular hypertrophy. Right ventricular hypertrophy is less common than left ventricular hypertrophy. It may be detected on palpation as a diffuse, lifting systolic impulse along the lower left sternal border. This finding may be associated with a systolic retraction at the apex, resulting from displacement and rotation of the left ventricle posteriorly by the enlarged right ventricle. A diffuse lift, or heave, along the lower left sternum is associated, for example, with pulmonary valve disease, pulmonary hypertension, and chronic lung disease. A thrill may also be palpated in this area and is associated with ventricular septal defects. The palmar aspect of the examiner's right hand is placed over the left sternal border.

Base of the heart. The examiner's right hand rests over the base of the heart at the second left and right intercostal spaces at the sternal borders and feels for pulsations, thrills, or the vibrations of semilunar valve closure. Normally, the base is fairly "quiet" to palpation.

Aortic stenosis may be associated with a thrill palpable in the first and third right interspaces, as well as in the second right interspace. In persons with systemic hypertension, it may be possible to palpate the accentuated vibration of aortic valve closure at the time of S_2.

Pulmonic valve stenosis may be associated with a thrill in the second and third left interspaces near the sternum. In persons with pulmonary hypertension, pulsations may be palpated in the same area. The most common causes of abnormal pulsations in the pulmonary artery area are increases in pressure or flow in the pulmonary artery, such as in pulmonary hypertension or atrial septal defect. In some normal people with thin chest walls, it is possible to palpate a brief, slight pulsation in this area. Conditions such as anemia, fever, exertion, and pregnancy would accentuate this pulsation.

Percussion

The technique of percussion is of limited value in cardiac assessment. In the past, percussion was used to determine the borders of cardiac dullness, but the actual size of the heart is much more accurately determined by a chest roentgenogram, and ventricular hypertrophy is better determined by combined inspection and palpation. Variations in chest wall configuration and the type and amount of interposed tissue, such as air or fat tissue, alter and limit the accuracy of this procedure. The value of percussion is further limited in the assessment of right ventricular enlargement, since this condition causes substernal and anteroposterior enlargement, which is not accessible to the percussion note.

Auscultation

The stethoscope is a device that gathers and slightly amplifies sound before it is transmitted to the ears. A comfortable and properly fitting stethoscope is essential for adequate auscultation. Although the selection of proper earpieces for comfort and the best sound transmission is a matter of individual preference, several general guidelines are useful for making that selection. The earpieces should be large enouogh to provide a snug fit in the external canal and to block out extraneous room noises. Enough tension should be present to hold the earpieces tightly in place. The rigid metal tubing leading to the earpieces should be bent to angle in the same direction as the ear canal, that is, forward. The flexible tubing may be made of rubber or plastic, and it should be thick enough to keep out extraneous sounds; it should also be reasonably short, about 1 ft, because added length dampens the sound and decreases the efficiency of the stethoscope in transmitting higher frequencies.

The stethoscope chestpiece should be equipped with both a bell and a diaphragm, each of which selectively transmits different frequencies of sound. The valve facilitating a change between the two should be tight fitting, permitting a change without the admission of outside sound. The diaphragm accentuates the higher frequency sounds. It should be made of a fairly rigid substance and should be pressed firmly against the skin during auscultation, further enhancing faint, high-frequency sounds. In contrast to the diaphragm, the bell brings out the low-frequency sounds and filters out the high-frequency ones. It should be placed very lightly on the chest wall with just enough pressure applied to seal the edge. If greater pressure is applied to the bell against the chest wall, the skin becomes a relatively tight diaphragm, filtering out the lower-pitched sounds. Alternating the application of light and heavy pressure to the bell may be a helpful maneuver when listening to low-pitched murmurs or filling sounds. Most low-pitched sounds are diastolic filling sounds or murmurs and are often best heard with the client lying down, since orthostatic pooling on standing may cause such sounds to diminish in intensity. Although heart sounds are referred to as being of "high" or "low" frequency, these terms are relative. All heart sounds are generally low pitched (low frequency) and are in a range ordinarily difficult for the human ear to hear. Thus, any technique that improves audibility should be carefully implemented.

Satisfactory auscultation requires a quiet room; mechanical and conversational noises must be minimized. The room should be comfortably warm for the client so that shivering and subsequent muscular noises are avoided. The anterior chest should be exposed to the waist. The examining table should be adequately large

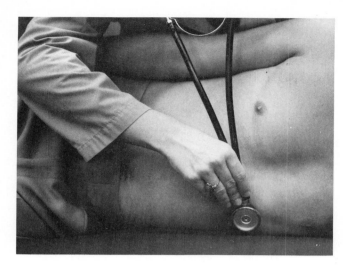

Figure 15-16

With the client lying in the left lateral position, the examiner listens for low-pitched diastolic sounds using the bell of the stethoscope.

for the client to change positions from sitting to supine to left lateral recumbent with ease. Auscultation in only one position is not adequate.

A systematic method of auscultation is essential; all precordial areas and each sound and pause must be attended to. One recommended system is to begin at the apex and "inch" the stethoscope toward the left sternal border and up the sternal border to the second left and then to the second right intercostal space. Another method consists of beginning the examination at the base of the heart at the second right intercostal space, where S_2 is always the loudest of the two heart sounds. This is particularly helpful if the heart sounds are heard as nearly equal in intensity at the apex. Auscultation should be performed using both the bell and the diaphragm and should cover the entire precordium and areas of radiation, such as the axillary area or carotid arteries, when indicated.

In each area examined, the examiner listens selectively to each component of the cardiac cycle; as with palpation, this usually requires a period of "warming up" or "tuning in" to the various cardiac events. First, the examiner notes the rate and rhythm of the heartbeat. Then, at each auscultatory area, the examiner concentrates initially on S_1, noting its intensity and variations therein, possible duplication, and the effects of respiration. The examiner then selects out S_2 and focuses on the same characteristics. Next, he or she concentrates on systole, then on diastole, listening first for any extra sounds and then for murmurs. The examiner must listen selectively for each component; it is impossible to listen for everything at once.

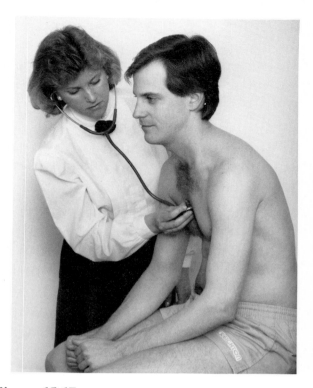

Figure 15-17

Using the diaphragm of the stethoscope while the client leans forward and holds the breath in full expiration, the examiner listens for high-pitched murmurs at the base of the heart.

If the initial part of the examination is performed with the client supine, the client is asked to roll to the left side; the examiner applies the bell lightly at the apex and listens for the presence or absence of low-frequency diastolic sounds, such as a filling sound or a mitral valve murmur (Fig. 15-16). The client is then asked to sit up and lean slightly forward. Pressing the diaphragm firmly against the chest, the examiner listens at both the second left and the second right intercostal spaces at the sternal border to detect the presence or absence of high-pitched diastolic murmurs of aortic or pulmonic valve insufficiency (Fig. 15-17). Listening is done during normal respiration and then with the client's breath held in deep expiration.

Neck Vessels

The vascular structures of the neck accessible for and included in the cardiovascular examination are the jugular veins and the carotid arteries. Examination of these vessels provides information on local states and also reflects the activity of the heart. The jugular veins are observed for pulse waves and pressure level; the carotid arteries are examined by inspection, palpation, and auscultation to assess the characteristics of their pulsations.

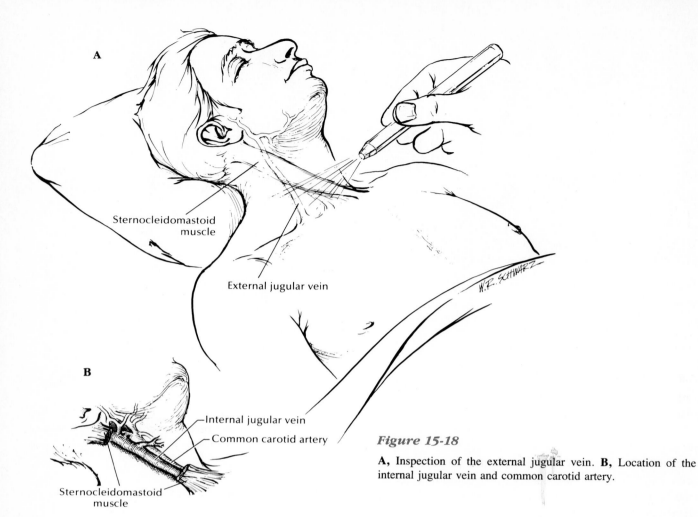

Sternocleidomastoid
muscle

External jugular vein

W.R. SCHWARZ

Internal jugular vein

Common carotid artery

Sternocleidomastoid
muscle

Figure 15-18

A, Inspection of the external jugular vein. **B,** Location of the internal jugular vein and common carotid artery.

JUGULAR VEINS

Venous pulse waves and venous pressure are assessed at the external and internal jugular veins. The external jugular veins lie superficially and are visible above the clavicle close to the insertion of the sternocleidomastoid muscles. The internal jugular veins are larger and lie deep to the sternocleidomastoid muscles near the carotid arteries; reflection of their activity may be visible on the skin overlying these vessels. Blood from the jugular veins flows directly into the superior vena cava. Fig. 15-18 illustrates the location of the external and internal jugular veins.

Venous return and the filling volume are important determinants of cardiac performance. These cannot be directly assessed on physical examination, but a general estimate can be made from observation of the jugular veins. The veins leading to the right side of the heart may be thought of as a system of distensible tubes with partially competent valves. Therefore, some judgment of the filling pressure of the heart may be made by observing the pressure level and the waveforms transmitted from

the heart. Observation of the two components of pressure level and pulse waves in the veins gives an indication of the dynamics of the right side of the heart.

When the normal person is in the sitting position, no jugular venous pulsations are visible; with the trunk elevated 45 degrees from horizontal, the jugular venous pulse does not rise more than 1 to 2 cm above the level of the manubrium. When the normal person is in the reclining position, the venous pulse becomes evident because gravity no longer prevents backflow from the heart and the veins become filled.

In the examination of the jugular veins the client is in the supine position. If this position is uncomfortable, the client's trunk may be elevated to a 45-degree angle. If the veins are very distended, it is best to examine them with the client in a sitting position. The veins or venous pulsations are more readily visible if the client's neck is slightly turned away from the side being examined, and the veins are observed with tangential lighting so that small shadows are cast. Clothing should be removed from the neck and upper thorax so that there is no constriction.

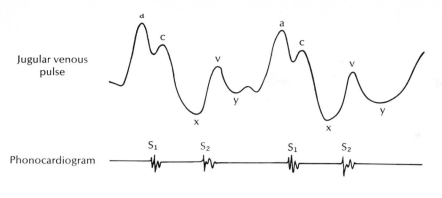

Jugular venous pulse

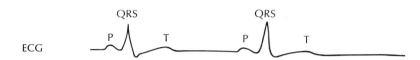

Phonocardiogram

ECG

Fig. 15-19

Jugular venous pulse waves in relation to S_1 and S_2 and the ECG.

The head and neck may rest comfortably on a pillow, but the neck should not be sharply flexed.

Jugular Venous Pulse

The normal venous pulse consists of three positive components—the a, c, and v waves—and two negative slopes—the x and y descents (Fig. 15-19). The a wave is frequently the highest part of the total pulse wave and is produced by atrial contraction. As the right atrium contracts, ejecting blood into the right ventricle, there is also a brief backflow of blood into the vena cava. This retrograde pulse wave is reflected in the jugular veins as the a wave. This wave occurs just before S_1; if an S_4 is present, it occurs at the peak of the a wave.

Two simultaneous events contribute to the production of the c wave: the impact of the adjacent carotid artery pulsation and the retrograde transmission of a pulse wave, caused by right ventricular systole and bulging of the closed tricuspid valve. The c wave occurs at the end of S_1.

The tricuspid valve remains closed during ventricular systole while blood from the systemic circulation continues to fill the vena cava and the right atrium. The increased volume in these structures leads to a pressure increase reflected in the jugular veins as the v, or passive filling, wave. This wave reaches a peak during late ventricular systole. Following this, the pressure in the right atrium begins to fall as the bulging of the tricuspid valve decreases, first during relaxation of the right ventricle and then as the tricuspid valve opens.

The x descent following the c wave is produced by downward displacement of the base of the ventricles (including the tricuspid valve) during ventricular systole and by atrial diastole. The y descent following the v wave is produced by the opening of the tricuspid valve and the subsequent rapid flow of blood from the right atrium to the right ventricle.

It is usually possible to discern the three positive and two negative waves of the jugular venous pulse when the heart rate is below 90 beats per minute and the PQ interval is normal. At more rapid heart rates, there is often a fusion or overlapping of some of the waves, and analysis of the waveform is difficult.

Abnormalities of waves

The a wave. The a wave, which may be the highest or most pronounced of the three positive waves, is increased when it becomes more difficult for the contracting right atrium to empty into the right ventricle. For example, in tricuspid valve stenosis the a wave is more prominent. When there is right ventricular enlargement resulting from severe pulmonary stenosis or pulmonary hypertension and the right atrium must contract more forcefully to fill it, an enlarged a wave also results.

Irregularly enlarged a waves result from complete AV block. When the atrium contracts against a closed tricuspid valve, giant (cannon) a waves are produced. In ventricular tachycardia, the cannon waves may occur irregularly, since the cause of their production—simultaneous atrial and ventricular systole and a closed tricuspid valve—does not accompany each beat.

The x descent and c and v waves. When the tricuspid valve is insufficient, backflow of blood from the right ventricle to the right atrium occurs during ventricular systole. This causes the x slope to become obliterated or replaced by the positive waves, the c and v waves, which then form the c-v wave. Thus, with the obliteration of a negative slope and the accentuation of the two positive waves, a large jugular venous pulse wave is produced. The c-v wave may become so enlarged as to resemble exaggerated arterial pulsations. Tricuspid insufficiency may be organic, resulting from rheumatic heart disease; or it may be produced in clients with generalized cardiac failure, wherein the right ventricle becomes so dilated that the tricuspid ring is stretched and regurgitation ensues.

The y descent. The tricuspid valve opens shortly after S_2, and the rapid filling phase of ventricular diastole begins. The characteristics of the y descent depend on several factors, including pressure and volume circumstances in the great vessels, the right atrium, and the right ventricle, and resistance to flow across the tricuspid valve. Tricuspid stenosis, therefore, would produce a slow y descent because it presents obstruction to right atrial emptying. In clients with severe heart failure in which the venous pressure is extremely high, a sharp, exaggerated y wave is produced.

Differentiation from carotid arterial pulsations

Because the internal jugular veins lies deep to the sternocleidomastoid muscle and close to the carotid artery, its pulsations may be confused with those produced by the common carotid artery. There are several means of differentiating these pulsations.

Quality and character of the pulse. In normal sinus rhythm, the jugular venous pulse has three positive waves and the carotid pulse has one positive wave. Usually, the venous pulse waves are more undulating than the brisk arterial waves. The examiner may be assisted in differentiating the two by palpating the carotid pulse on one side of the neck and observing the jugular venous pulse on the other.

Effect of respiration. With normal inspiration, intrathoracic pressure decreases, blood flow into the right atrium increases, and the level of the pulse wave in the neck veins descends. The opposite occurs during expiration. Respiration does not have this effect on the carotid pulsations.

Effect of changing position. Pulsations in the neck veins become more prominent when the client assumes the recumbent position and less prominent when the client is in the sitting position. Carotid pulsations are not affected by posture.

Effect of venous compression. The pulsations of the jugular veins are rather easily eliminated by applying gentle pressure over the vein at the base of the neck above the clavicle. This blocks the retrograde transmission of the venous pulse wave, leaving only the arterial pulsations.

Effect of abdominal pressure. Pressure applied by the examiner's hand over the client's abdomen may cause an increased prominence of the venous pulsations. The examiner presses, using the palm of the hand and applying moderately firm pressure over the upper right quadrant of the abdomen for 30 to 60 seconds. In normal persons there is slight, if any, increase in the venous pulsations. However, if there is right-sided heart failure, the jugular venous pulsations and distention may markedly increase as venous return to the heart is increased. Normally this maneuver produces no change in the carotid pulsations.

Jugular Venous Pressure

The level of the column of blood in the jugular veins reflects the volume and pressure circumstances on the right side of the heart. Both the external and internal jugular veins can be assessed. Although other mechanical techniques are available to evaluate venous pressure, inspection on physical examination remains a useful and reliable maneuver.

In a normal client examined in the supine position, full neck veins are normally visible. When the normal person is examined with the thorax elevated to a 45-degree angle from horizontal, the venous pulses should ascend no more than a few centimeters above the clavicle. With markedly elevated venous pressure, the neck veins may be distended as high as the angle of the jaw, even when the person is in the upright sitting position. The height of venous pressure may be estimated by measuring the distance that the veins are distended above the manubrium sterni.

The examiner should inspect the veins on both sides of the neck. When the venous pressure is generally increased, distention is noted on both sides; unilateral distention may occur as a result of kinking in the left innominate vein in some older clients. It may be necessary to change the position of the client to view the jugular venous pulse and pressure most clearly. The sternal angle, or angle of Louis, is used as a reference point. The vertical distance between the sternal angle and the highest level of the jugular pulsations is measured and recorded in centimeters (Fig. 15-20). The lower the client's head must be placed before the pulsations are visible, the lower the pressure; the higher the client's head must be placed before the upper level of the pulsations can be identified, the higher the venous pressure. Venous pressures greater than 3 to 4 cm above the sternal angle are abnormal. The level to which distention is observed and the position of the client should be noted.

Elevation of venous pressure may indicate congestive heart failure, constrictive pericarditis, or obstruction

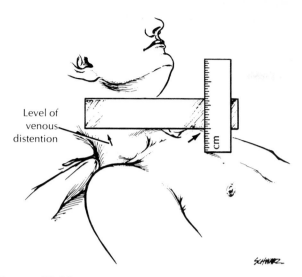

Figure 15-20

Measurement of jugular venous pressure. The arrows indicate the height of the jugular venous pressure in centimeters.

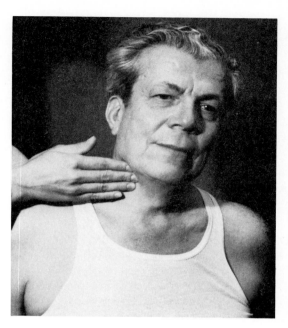

Figure 15-21

The examiner palpates the carotid pulse below and just medial to the angle of the jaw.

of the superior vena cava. The most common cause of elevated venous pressure is failure of the right ventricle resulting from left ventricular failure. As described earlier, the effect of applying increased abdominal pressure may increase the amount of venous distention in the presence of right-sided heart failure.

CAROTID ARTERIES

The techniques of inspection, palpation, and auscultation are used in examining the carotid arteries. The neck is observed for unusually large or bounding carotid pulses. The carotid arterial pulses are then palpated bilaterally, as are all the pulses, for rate, rhythm, equality, amplitude, and contour. The examiner palpates with the forefinger below and just medial to the angle of the jaw (Fig. 15-21). Only one side is examined at a time to avoid excessive carotid sinus massage, thus preventing unnecessary slowing of the pulse, and to avoid further embarassment of borderline circulation in older clients. The head should be rotated slightly toward the side being examined to relax the sternocleidomastoid muscle. The heart sounds may be used as reference points, and simultaneous auscultation of the heart is then helpful. S_1 and the carotid impulse are very nearly simultaneous events. The carotid arteries are auscultated with the bell of the stethoscope for bruits indicating local obstruction or for the sound of transmitted cardiac murmurs.

Carotid Arterial Pulse

The carotid arteries are the best arteries in which to assess several characteristics of the arterial pulse, for example,

whether the force is strong or weak, the rise and collapse rapid or slow, and the impulse double or single.

The normal carotid pulse consists of a single positive wave followed by a dicrotic notch (Fig. 15-22). The upstroke is smooth and rapid, the summit is dome shaped, and the downstroke is less steep than the upstroke. The dicrotic notch on the downstroke may not be palpable or may be only slightly palpable. It is often definitely felt in the otherwise healthy client during exercise, excitement, or fever.

The size or amplitude of the arterial pulse is determined by a variety of factors, including left ventricular stroke volume and ejection rate, peripheral resistance or distensibility, and pulse pressure. Clinically, abnormalities of the pulse size may be divided into two groups: exaggerated, or hyperkinetic, pulses and weak, or hypokinetic, pulses. During palpation, the examiner may gain an impression of the height of the pulse and the rate of change on the upstroke and downstroke.

Situations associated with a widened arterial pulse pressure—an increased stroke volume and decreased peripheral resistance—produce a hyperkinetic carotid pulse. The pulse may be large and strong with a normal contour (bounding pulse), or it may be characterized by a markedly high and rapid upstroke (water-hammer pulse) or by an extremely rapid downstroke (collapsing pulse). In the latter two cases, the peak of the pulse is short and rapid. The hyperkinetic pulse may be produced as the

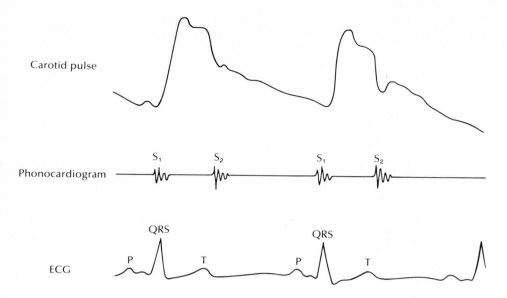

Carotid pulse

Phonocardiogram   S₁   S₂   S₁   S₂

ECG   QRS   P   T   P   QRS   T

Figure 15-22

The carotid pulse wave in relation to S₁ and S₂ and the ECG.

result of hyperdynamic or high-output states, such as occur with anxiety, exercise, fever, or pregnancy; as the result of hyperthyroidism or anemia; or as the result of abnormally rapid runoff of blood from the arterial system, such as occurs with abnormal shunting of blood (patent ductus arteriosus or septal defects) or with aortic insufficiency. Aortic insufficiency is a common organic cause of the hyperkinetic pulse in adults. With severe regurgitation, the pulse is described as water hammer and collapsing; a large volume of blood is rapidly ejected from and then returns to the left ventricle across the incompetent valve. Another cause of the hyperkinetic pulse in adults is a complete heart block with bradycardia and increased stroke volume.

The hypokinetic carotid pulse is associated with conditions wherein there is a diminished stroke volume of the left ventricle, increased peripheral vascular resistance, a narrowed pulse pressure, or resistance to flow across the cardiac valves. Examples of causes of a hypokinetic pulse include left ventricular failure resulting from myocardial infarction, constrictive pericarditis, and moderate or severe valvular aortic stenosis. In aortic stenosis, the pulse may demonstrate a slow upstroke, a delayed peak, and a small volume.

Pulses with double, rather than single, pulsations may be produced by combined aortic stenosis and insufficiency (pulsus bisferiens) or by lowered peripheral resistance and lowered diastolic pressure (dicrotic pulse).

A pulse that occurs at regular intervals but varies in amplitude (pulsus alternans) is produced by alterations in left ventricular contractile force, as may occur with left ventricular failure. Premature ventricular contractions coupled with previous normal beats produce a bigeminal pulse; that is, every alternate beat is premature.

Auscultation

Several conditions may produce a palpable carotid thrill associated with an audible bruit. These conditions include local obstruction of a carotid artery, a jugular vein—carotid artery fistula, and high-output state, such as occurs with severe anemia and thyrotoxicosis. Aortic valvular stenosis may cause a thrill to be referred to the carotid arteries. The bruits are heard by placing the bell of the stethoscope on the skin overlying the carotid artery and listening while the client holds his or her breath (Fig. 15-23). The bell of the stethoscope is used because the bruits are low-pitched sounds.

Cardiovascular Findings Associated with Hypertension

To assist the student clinician in organizing the examination around a prevalent cardiovascular problem, the various components of the history and physical examination of a client with elevated blood pressure, or hypertension, are presented here. Although approximately 90% of persons with hypertension have primary or essential hypertension, it is important to rule out potentially curable secondary causes; findings indicative of those causes are also included here.

Many persons with elevated blood pressure have no observable symptoms related to that abnormality, and it may be identified during a routine examination. Others, however, do describe one or several symptoms, most commonly a headache, which may be present on awakening and subside after the individual has been up for some time. Other early symptoms include light-headedness, dizziness, tinnitus, fatigue, weakness, nervousness, flushing sensations, and epistaxis. Later symptoms

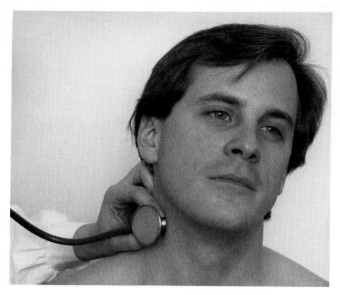

Figure 15-23

The examiner listens with the bell of the stethoscope for bruits over the carotid artery.

of hypertension are attributable to the effects of sustained high blood pressure on the heart, eyes, cerebral circulation, and kidneys. These symptoms may include, for example, dyspnea, orthopnea, paroxysmal nocturnal dyspnea, palpitations, chest pain, edema, eye fatigue, blurred vision, headache, weakness, numbness, tingling of the hands and feet, polyuria, nocturia, and flank pain.

The examiner should inquire about the presence of any of these symptoms. The client should also be asked about any family history of hypertension, the use of steroids, and, with women, the use of oral contraceptives or any previous hypertension associated with pregnancy.

Secondary causes of hypertension include coarctation of the aorta, primary hyperaldosteronism, Cushing's syndrome, pheochromocytoma, and renal vascular disease. Symptoms related to these causes include history of leg fatigue with coarctation of the aorta; episodes of muscular weakness, polyuria, nocturia, polydipsia, and intermittent paresthesias with primary aldosteronism; alteration of sexual function (amenorrhea, impotence), emotional lability, weakness, and backache with Cushing's syndrome; weight loss, palpitations, headache, nervousness, sweating, blanching, coldness of skin, nausea, vomiting, and abdominal pain with pheochromocytoma; and flank pain and urinary tract infections and symptoms with renal and renal vascular disease. A careful history for any of these symptoms of secondary hypertension should be obtained.

VARIATIONS FROM HEALTH

A vast array of disease processes can affect the heart and major blood vessels. Only a few of the more commonly encountered abnormal variations in the adult population will be covered here, including heart murmurs, dysrhythmias, heart failure, ischemic heart disease, and hypertension.

Heart Murmurs

A variety of conditions may result in the production of the more prolonged sound during systole or diastole known as a murmur. These are abnormal sounds produced by vibrations within the heart or in the walls of the large vessels. They tend to originate in the vicinity of the heart valve and are often best heard around the area of the valve responsible for their production.

Mechanisms of production

Three main factors related to murmur production are (1) increased flow rate of blood across normal valves, (2) forward flow through an irregular or constricted valve or into a dilated vessel or chamber, and (3) backflow, or regurgitant flow, through an incompetent or insufficient valve, a septal defect, or a patent ductus arteriosus (Fig. 15-24). In addition, a combination of these factors may prevail.

Murmurs are illustrated in a manner similar to the way in which they appear in a phonocardiogram, that is, with a series of vertical lines in systole between S_1 and S_2 or in diastole between S_2 and S_1. The lines are drawn to indicate the level of, and increase or decrease in, intensity of the sound. For example, a midsystolic ejection murmur that is crescendo-decrescendo is shown in Fig. 15-25, *A;* a holosystolic regurgitant murmur is shown in Fig. 15-25, *B.*

Valve alterations. The adequacy of opening and closure of the valves and of the orifice size determines many of the characteristics of murmurs. Heart valves that are functioning normally and competently permit the forward flow of blood and prevent backflow, or regurgitation. It is essential to understand the stations of the valves and flow patterns during systole and diastole. During ventricular systole, the mitral and tricuspid valves are closed, preventing backflow, and the aortic and pulmonic valves are open, permitting forward flow. During ventricular diastole, the mitral and tricuspid valves are open, permitting forward flow, and the aortic and pulmonic valves are closed, preventing backflow.

Stenotic valves prevent adequate forward flow; thus, a stenosed mitral or tricuspid valve interferes with normal flow during diastole, when the atrium empties blood into the ventricle. Mitral or tricuspid stenosis pro-

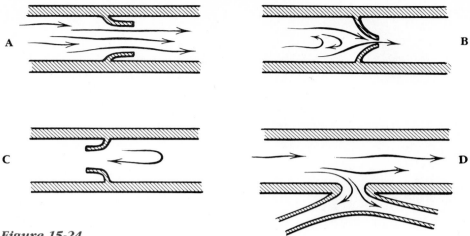

Figure 15-24

Mechanisms of murmur production. **A,** Increased flow across a normal valve. **B,** Forward flow through a stenotic valve. **C,** Backflow through an incompetent valve. **D,** Flow through a septal defect or arteriovenous fistula.

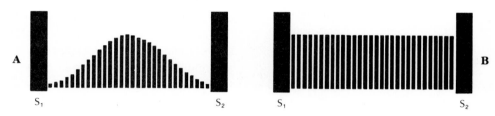

Figure 15-25

Systolic murmurs. **A,** Crescendo-decrescendo systolic ejection murmur. **B,** Holosystolic regurgitant murmur.

duces a diastolic murmur (Fig. 15-26, *A*). A stenosed aortic or pulmonic valve prevents adequate forward flow of blood during ventricular systole, when the blood is being forced from the ventricle into the aorta or pulmonary artery; thus aortic (or pulmonic) stenosis produces a systolic murmur (Fig. 15-26, *B*). Blood flowing through such a narrowed orifice meets resistance and produces vibrations.

Incompetent or insufficient valves fail to close completely during that phase of the cardiac cycle when their leaflets should be firmly approximated; they leave an aperture through which blood flows inappropriately back from the ventricles to the atria or from the aorta or pulmonary artery back to the ventricles. This regurgitation, or backflow, of blood produces vibrations of the valve and of parts of the myocardium, producing a murmur. An incompetent mitral or tricuspid valve permits the inappropriate backflow of blood from the ventricle to the atrium during ventricular systole, producing a systolic murmur (Fig. 15-27, *A*). An insufficient aortic or pulmonic valve permits the backflow of blood from the aorta or pulmonary artery to the ventricle during ventricular diastole, producing a diastolic murmur (Fig. 15-27, *B*).

Characteristics

Murmurs are classified and described according to several characteristics, including timing (systolic or diastolic), frequency, location, radiation, intensity, quality, and effects of respiration.

Timing. The timing of murmurs is according to their occurrence during either diastole or systole. At times, murmurs may occur during both phases of the cycle. The timing of the murmur may be further characterized as occurring during the entire phase of a cycle or, for instance, during early, mid-, or late systole. Murmurs that endure throughout systole are known as holosystolic or pansystolic murmurs; the same is true for diastolic murmurs. Early diastolic murmurs are known as protodiastolic, and late diastolic murmurs are called presystolic.

In general, systolic murmurs are caused by stenosed aortic or pulmonic valves or by incompetent mitral or tricuspid valves, and diastolic murmurs are produced by stenosed mitral or tricuspid valves or by incompetent aortic or pulmonic valves. It is important to remember, however, that not all murmurs result from valve defects; they may also be produced by alteration in the velocity

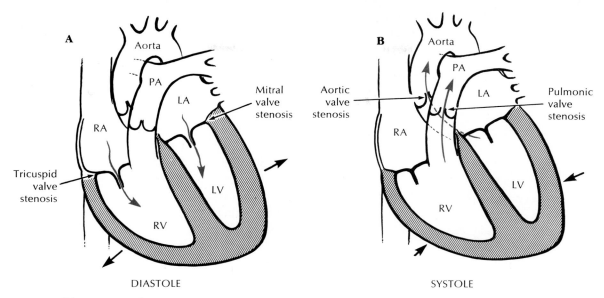

Figure 15-26

A, Mitral or tricuspid valve stenosis produces a diastolic murmur. **B,** Aortic or pulmonic valve stenosis produces a systolic murmur.

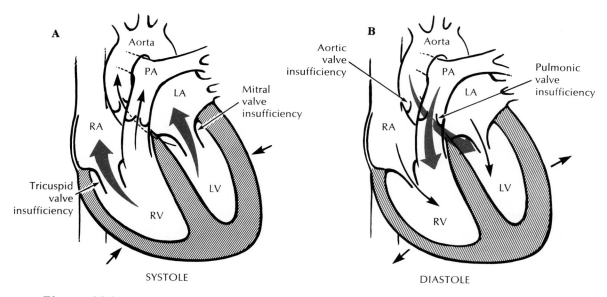

Figure 15-27

A, Mitral or tricuspid valve insufficiency produces a systolic murmur. **B,** Aortic or pulmonic valve insufficiency produces a diastolic murmur.

of flow, by changes in the vessels, and by defects in the myocardium.

Frequency. The frequency, or pitch, of murmurs varies from high to low. The main determining factor is the velocity of blood flow. Generally, when the rate of flow is rapid, a high pitch results; when the velocity is slow, the pitch is low. The pitch of a murmur is described as high, medium, or low.

Location. A murmur is described by means of anatomic landmarks according to where it is best heard.

Some are localized to small areas, whereas others are heard over large portions of the precordium. The location of a murmur is significant in terms of its site of production. The murmurs originating from valvular alterations are usually best heard in the area to which sounds from that valve are transmitted.

Radiation. Some murmurs radiate in the direction of the bloodstream by which they are produced. For example, the diastolic murmur of aortic insufficiency may be heard along the left sternal border. In this case, the blood leaks back from the aorta into the left ventricle. Other factors, such as the variation in sound transmission through various tissues, also influence radiation.

Intensity. The loudness of a murmur is described on a scale of one to six; one is the softest, and six is the loudest. The description of each level of loudness is as follows:

Grade I: Barely audible, very faint; can be heard only with special effort
Grade II: Clearly audible but quiet
Grade III: Moderately loud
Grade IV: Loud
Grade V: Very loud; may be heard with stethoscope partly off the chest
Grade VI: Loudest possible; audible with the stethoscope just removed from contact with the chest wall

It is important to note that although the grading of the loudness of a murmur is helpful, it is also a rather subjective description, dependent on the listener's auditory acuity.

The terms *crescendo* and *decrescendo* are used to describe the pattern of intensity reflecting changes in the flow rate. A crescendo-decrescendo murmur, for example, increases from quiet to louder and then decreases again. In the case of aortic stenosis, for example, the flow rate increases, reaches a peak, and then decreases, producing a crescendo-decrescendo systolic murmur with a rather harsh quality. The diastolic murmur of aortic insufficiency is a decrescendo, high-pitched, blowing murmur. The flow rate of blood leaking back into the ventricle from the aorta is approximately proportional to the decreasing pressure gradient between the aorta and the ventricle. Although the patterns of the various murmurs may not be that easily determined with the stethoscope, the murmurs do appear that way on the phonocardiogram.

Quality. Several descriptive terms are often used to characterize a murmur; these include *musical, blowing, harsh,* or *rumbling.* For example, the murmur of aortic stenosis may be described as harsh; the murmur of mitral insufficiency may be described as a long, blowing sound; and the murmur of mitral stenosis tends to be of a low, rumbling quality.

Effects of respiration. As mentioned earlier in this chapter, certain events on the right side of the heart are affected by respiration as a result of intrathoracic pressure changes and right-sided filling changes. Murmurs that originate on the right side of the heart are also subject to influence by these factors. The murmur of tricuspid insufficiency, for example, may increase with inspiration.

Systolic murmurs

Murmurs occurring during ventricular systole are a result of increased flow rate across normal valves or abnormal blood flow patterns across (1) the inflow tract (the AV valves), (2) the outflow tract (the semilunar valves), or (3) ventricle to ventricle (ventricular septal defect). Incompetent or insufficient AV valves do not prevent backflow of blood from the ventricles to the atria during ventricular systole and thus produce systolic regurgitant murmurs. These murmurs may last during all or part of systole. Insufficient AV valves may be the result of rheumatic valvular disease or papillary muscle dysfunction. Stenotic aortic or pulmonic valves make it difficult for the blood to flow from the ventricles to the aorta and pulmonary arteries during ventricular systole and thus produce systolic ejection murmurs. Because there is a short time interval between the closing of the AV valves (S_1) and the opening of the semilunar valves, systolic ejection murmurs will begin after the first heart sound, reflect the ejection of blood during systolic contraction, and end before the second heart sound. They are often called *midsystolic ejection murmurs.* Some systolic ejection murmurs are innocent, whereas others are pathologic. The abnormalities that cause a turbulent flow across these semilunar valves may be the result of dilatation or narrowing of the pulmonary artery or aorta, aortic or pulmonic valvular or subvalvular stenosis, or high output states such as anemia, thyrotoxicosis, or pregnancy.

Innocent systolic ejection murmurs are commonly heard in children and adolescents. They occur within a normal cardiovascular system and are not the result of any recognizable heart abnormality. They reflect the contractile force of the heart that results in greater blood flow velocity during early or mid-systole. Smaller chest measurements in the young also increase the audibility of these murmurs. Innocent systolic ejection murmurs may also occur with other high output states including pregnancy, anxiety, anemia, fever, and thyrotoxicosis.

Innocent systolic ejection murmurs are heard best with the bell held lightly against the chest in the pulmonic area (second left intercostal space) or around the lower left sternal border toward but not including the apex. They tend to be short, rarely extending through the entire systole, but begin shortly after the first heart sound and end well before the second heart sound (Fig. 15-28). They are softer than grade III, are of medium pitch, and have a blowing quality. They increase in held expiration, may change with position, and may be heard best when the client is in the recumbent position. The heart sounds remain unchanged.

These murmurs must be differentiated from pathologic systolic ejection murmurs that may result from mild

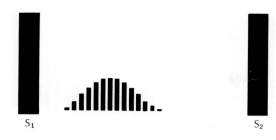

S_1 S_2

Figure 15-28

Innocent systolic murmur.

aortic or pulmonic stenosis or atrial or ventricular septal defects. A pansystolic or late systolic murmur indicates an organic problem.

Stenosis or obstruction of the aortic or pulmonic valves or deformity of the valves or adjacent vessels (the aorta and the pulmonary arteries) may cause *mid-systolic ejection murmurs*. The murmur of aortic valve stenosis or deformity begins after the first heart sound when the pressure in the ventricle is high enough to open the aortic and pulmonic valves, ends before the aortic and pulmonic valves close (S_2), and thus has a crescendo-decrescendo pattern (see Fig. 15-25, *A*). With less aortic deformity present, the murmur reaches a peak earlier in systole. The murmur is medium pitched and harsh, may be faint to loud, and is best heard with the diaphragm at the first or second right intercostal spaces with the client sitting up and leaning forward with the breath held in expiration. If the murmur is loud, it may be heard over the entire thorax and is often accompanied by a thrill. (A thrill is a palpable vibration often associated with a very loud murmur; it usually signifies a pathologic cardiac condition.) The existence of emphysema may cause the murmur to seem faint. Arrhythmias, shock, or heart failure causes the murmur to become softer.

The systolic murmur of aortic stenosis may be associated with a diminished second heart sound, an early ejection click, the sustained thrusting apical impulse of left ventricular hypertrophy, a slowly rising carotid pulse wave, and narrow pulse pressure. Rheumatic fever is the most common cause of aortic stenosis and valve deformity. Congenital deformities are another cause.

A basal systolic murmur associated with hypertension and arteriosclerotic roughening of the aorta and aortic valve are commonly heard in older people. This murmur is best heard at the second right intercostal space, is of medium pitch, has a rough quality, is usually not very loud, and is often transmitted to the apex. It is best heard with the client sitting up and leaning forward. Either the diaphragm or the bell may be used. The second heart sound is of normal or increased loudness.

Murmurs that occupy all of systole are called *ho-*

losystolic or *pansystolic*. They are associated with turbulent blood flow from a high-pressure to a low-pressure area, such as occurs with regurgitation from a ventricular chamber to an atrial chamber across an incompetent AV valve, or with leakage from the left to the right ventricle through a ventricular septal defect. The murmur will continue as long as there is a sufficient pressure gradient across the incompetent orifice beginning with the first heart sound and lasting up to the second heart sound (see Fig. 15-25, *B*).

Mitral regurgitation may result from malfunction of a number of structures including the valve ring or leaflets, the chordae tendineae, the papillary muscles, and the wall of the ventricle. This murmur is usually loudest at the apex; as the loudness increases, the sound may be transmitted to the axilla. It has a high pitch and a blowing quality and is best heard with the diaphragm of the stethoscope. If the murmur is faint, it may be heard better after exercise in the left lateral position or sitting up and leaning forward to the left. This murmur does not increase with inspiration. The first heart sound may be normal, increased, or decreased, depending on the condition of the mitral valve. The second sound may be normal or increased. A third heart sound may be present.

The murmur resulting from a ventricular septal defect is best heard at the fourth, fifth, and sixth interspaces at the left sternal border. It may radiate over the precordium but not to the axilla. It is high pitched and harsh and may be accompanied by a thrill. The size of the septal defect and the resistance in the pulmonary vessels determine the direction and velocity of flow during systole. With a small defect there may be greater resistance to pressure than with a larger defect, thus producing a louder holosystolic murmur.

Diastolic murmurs

Diastole is normally free of murmurs; therefore a murmur heard during this portion of the cardiac cycle almost always indicates heart disease. Causes of diastolic murmurs include insufficiency of the aortic or pulmonic valves, permitting abnormal backflow from the aorta and pulmonary arteries, or stenosis of the mitral or tricuspid valves, preventing an adequate forward flow of blood.

Diastolic murmurs may occur in early, middle, or late diastole. Early diastolic murmurs are usually produced by aortic or pulmonic valvular insufficiency or dilatation of the valvular ring. Mid- and late diastolic murmurs are usually caused by narrowed, stenosed mitral or tricuspid valves that obstruct the inflow or by an increased flow rate across the valves.

Aortic valve insufficiency is associated with a diastolic regurgitant murmur that begins with the aortic

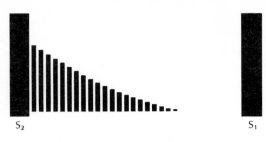

Figure 15-29

The diastolic murmur of aortic valve insufficiency.

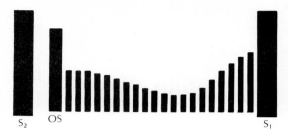

Figure 15-30

The diastolic murmur of mitral stenosis with opening snap of mitral valve.

component of the second heart sound at the time the aortic pressure exceeds the ventricular pressure. As the pressure in the aorta falls and the ventricles fill, the murmur decreases in intensity. This murmur begins loud in early diastole and then fades (Fig. 15-29), giving it a descrescendo character. It is high pitched and blowing and is best heard with the diaphragm with the client leaning forward in deep expiration. If the aorta is dilated, it may be loudest in the second right intercostal space. It may be accompanied by an aortic systolic murmur caused by increased flow, a third heart sound, a sustained thrusting apical impulse, and wide pulse pressure. The second heart sound may be increased or diminished depending on the condition of the aortic valve. This murmur is most commonly caused by rheumatic heart disease, but it may be caused by congenital valve disease.

Mitral stenosis is associated with a diastolic murmur that is produced by the flow of blood from the left atrium into the left ventricle and is most intense when that flow is greatest, that is, after the opening snap of the mitral valve. This is a mid-diastolic murmur. As the degree of stenosis increases, contraction of the auricle may force more blood across the valve and produce a presystolic accentuation of this diastolic murmur (Fig. 15-30). When faint or moderately loud, the murmur is low pitched and rumbling; as it becomes louder, it becomes more harsh. This murmur is generally heard only over a small area just medial to and above the apex or at the point of maximum impulse. It may be best heard when the client turns from the supine to the left lateral position. Exercise will increase the intensity of the murmur. The bell of the stethoscope should be held very lightly on the skin; heavy pressure on the bell may obliterate the sound of a faint mid-diastolic murmur.

Mitral stenosis is frequently associated with an increased first heart sound; there may also be an opening snap of the mitral valve. However, the first sound may be decreased and the opening snap absent if the valve and chordae tendineae are fibrosed or the mitral valve area is narrow in tight mitral stenosis.

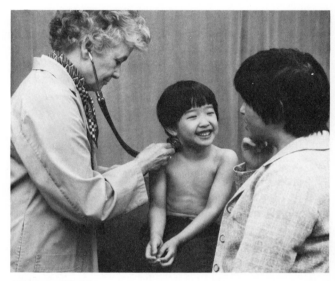

Figure 15-31

Venous hum. The venous hum is a continuous, low-pitched hum heard over the neck in many children; it is often best heard over the right supraclavicular space.

The *venous hum* is a continuous low-pitched hum heard over the neck in many children and some adults. It is produced by turbulent blood flow in the internal jugular veins. The venous hum is best heard over the supraclavicular spaces, more commonly on the right. It is heard better with the client sitting up and is accentuated on the right by having the client turn the head to the left and slightly upward (Fig. 15-31). The hum is loudest in diastole. Because it is produced by blood flow in the jugular veins, it can be stopped by applying gentle pressure over the internal jugular vein in the neck between the trachea and the sternocleidomastoid muscle at about the level of the thyroid cartilage.

Cardiac Dysrhythmias

Cardiac dysrhythmias, also known as arrhythmias, are disorders of heart rate and rhythm caused by a disturb-

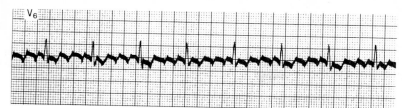

Figure 15-32

Regular atrial contractions occur at a rate so rapid that the conduction system cannot respond; thus the ventricular rate is slower.
(From Guzzetta CE and Dossey BM: Cardiovascular nursing: body-mind tapestry, St Louis, 1984, The CV Mosby Co.)

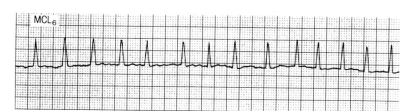

Figure 15-33

Dysrhythmic, irregular atrial contractions lead to irregular ventricular contractions. The heart sounds can be described as chaotic.
(From Guzzetta CE and Dossey BM: Cardiovascular nursing: body-mind tapestry, St Louis, 1984, The CV Mosby Co.)

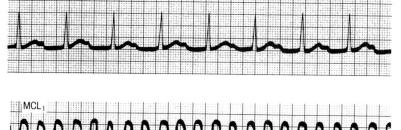

Figure 15-34

Conduction from the atria to the ventricles is partially or completely disrupted. The heart rate is slow.
(From Guzzeta CE and Dossey BM: Cardiovascular nursing: body-mind tapestry, St Louis, 1984, The CV Mosby Co.)

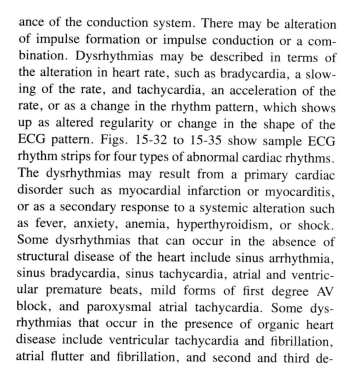

Figure 15-35

The source of the electrical impulse is an unusual focus somewhere in the ventricles. The heartbeat is rapid and relatively regular.
(From Guzzetta CE and Dossey BM: Cardiovascular nursing: body-mind tapestry, St Louis, 1984, The CV Mosby Co.)

ance of the conduction system. There may be alteration of impulse formation or impulse conduction or a combination. Dysrhythmias may be described in terms of the alteration in heart rate, such as bradycardia, a slowing of the rate, and tachycardia, an acceleration of the rate, or as a change in the rhythm pattern, which shows up as altered regularity or change in the shape of the ECG pattern. Figs. 15-32 to 15-35 show sample ECG rhythm strips for four types of abnormal cardiac rhythms. The dysrhythmias may result from a primary cardiac disorder such as myocardial infarction or myocarditis, or as a secondary response to a systemic alteration such as fever, anxiety, anemia, hyperthyroidism, or shock. Some dysrhythmias that can occur in the absence of structural disease of the heart include sinus arrhythmia, sinus bradycardia, sinus tachycardia, atrial and ventricular premature beats, mild forms of first degree AV block, and paroxysmal atrial tachycardia. Some dysrhythmias that occur in the presence of organic heart disease include ventricular tachycardia and fibrillation, atrial flutter and fibrillation, and second and third de-

gree AV block. Certain alterations of cardiac rhythm are frequently associated with certain underlying processes, such as atrial fibrillation in clients with thyrotoxicosis, mitral valve disease, and left atrial enlargement; and ventricular tachycardia in clients with ischemic heart disease. Other disturbances should alert the practitioner to the possibility of drug-related findings, such as excess digitalis, antiarrhythmics, diuretics, and catecholamines. The following electrolyte disturbances can also cause dysrhythmias:

Hyperkalemia ($\uparrow$ K): leads to AV block, impairment of intraatrial and intraventricular conduction with prolonged P waves and QRS complexes.

Hypokalemia ($\downarrow$ K): may lead to atrial and ventricular extrasystoles, coupled beats, tachycardia, mild atrioventricular and intraventricular conduction defects: severely lowered potassium may produce multifocal premature ventricular contractions deteriorating into ventricular fibrillation.

Hypercalcemia ($\uparrow$ Ca): decreases conduction velocity and shortens the refractory period leading to the development of coupled ventricular beats, ventricular tachycardia and ventricular fibrillation.

Heart Failure

Heart failure exists when an abnormality of myocardial function is responsible for the ventricles' inability to deliver adequate quantities of blood to the metabolizing tissues at rest or during normal activity. It may result from anatomic lesions of the heart valves or of the pericardium that produce interference in cardiac filling or emptying or from severe or prolonged disorders of cardiac rate or rhythm.

The term *congestive heart failure* has frequently been used because so many of the clinical manifestations of heart failure result from excessive accumulation of fluid. However, although diuretic therapy can often eliminate or markedly reduce the congestive manifestations, the underlying disorder of cardiac function may not be altered. Therefore, the term *heart failure* is preferred.

Heart failure may be caused by numerous conditions, including pulmonary embolism, infection, anemia, thyrotoxicosis, pregnancy, dysrhythmias, myocarditis, bacterial endocarditis, systemic hypertension, and physical, dietary, and emotional excesses.

Clinical manifestations of heart failure may include dyspnea, orthopnea, paroxsymal nocturnal dyspnea, fatigue, weakness, Cheyne-Stokes (periodic or cyclic) respirations, and cerebral symptoms including confusion, difficulty in concentration, and impaired memory.

With mild to moderate heart failure, the practitioner may find that the client may appear to be in no distress unless asked to lie flat for more than a few minutes. With more advanced heart failure, the pulse pressure may be diminished, reflecting a reduced stroke volume, and occasionally the diastolic arterial pressure may rise due to generalized vasoconstriction. The lips and nail beds may be cyanotic. The neck veins may be distended, and there may be basal pulmonary rales, dependent edema, ascites, congestive hepatomegaly, and jaundice.

Ischemic Heart Disease

Ischemic heart disease, also known as coronary artery disease, is the result of inadequate perfusion of a portion of the myocardium, most commonly caused by atherosclerosis of the coronary arteries. Atherosclerosis is a disorder of lipid metabolism characterized by deposits of fat-containing substances along the intima of blood vessels and by smooth muscle cell proliferation. Advanced atherosclerosis of the coronary arteries always leads to ischemic heart disease, but lesser amounts of atherosclerotic changes in the coronary arterial walls may exist without producing disease of the myocardium. The location and degree of atherosclerotic lesions are important in determining whether clinically evident ischemia will result. The extent of collateral circulation to the myocardium is another factor in the development of ischemic heart disease.

An inadequate blood supply to the myocardium results in mechanical and electrical alterations. Contractility of the myocardium is impaired; if it is limited to the ischemic portion, there is an asymmetric, inefficient pattern of contraction, with the affected portion bulging out while the rest of the ventricle contracts. Ventricular wall compliance may also be affected, thus impairing filling of the ventricle. Early electrical changes are in the repolarization process, which show up as inverted T waves and later by displacement of the ST segment. An additional significant consequence of an ischemic myocardium is ventricular irritability, which can result in premature ventricular systole, ventricular tachycardia, and ventricular fibrillation. Most sudden deaths from ischemic heart disease are from ventricular dysrhythmias.

Factors affecting the incidence and progression of ischemic heart disease include hypertension, elevated levels of low density lipoproteins (LDLs), elevated serum cholesterol, obesity, smoking, a sedentary life-style, diabetes, use of oral contraceptives, and personality characteristics such as aggressiveness, competitiveness, and an urgent sense of the passage of time. Symptomatic ischemic heart disease occurs predominantly in people over age 40, although it may also occur in young adults. Men are at greater risk than women for developing ischemic heart disease; however, this difference in susceptibility decreases with increasing age. Changes in lifestyle for women, which include taking on greater responsibilities in the workplace in addition to home and child-rearing responsibilities, and the trend to begin smoking at an earlier age, may increase the incidence of the disease among women.

Angina pectoris

Angina pectoris is a clinical syndrome characterized by chest pain, which is most commonly a manifestation of ischemic heart disease. The majority of individuals affected by angina pectoris are men in their 50s and 60s. A complete and detailed history of the anginal attacks is essential in assessing the client, since the physical examination of people with angina pectoris typically reveals little about the condition. The attacks will commonly be described as following a meal, exertion, or strong emotions.

The discomfort in the chest may be described as pain, but it is more typically described as aching, tightness, pressure, heaviness, burning, or a choking or squeezing sensation. It may be described as feeling like gas, indigestion, or heartburn. Anginal pain is not described as knifelike or sharp. Most individuals describe the location as retrosternal or slightly to the left of the sternum. It may radiate to the left shoulder and upper arm and may travel to the inner aspect of the left arm, elbow, wrist, fourth and fifth fingers, right shoulder, neck, jaw, or epigastric area. Occasionally, the pain may be experienced only in the area or areas of radiation and not in the typical substernal area. Anginal attacks usually last approximately 3 minutes but may last for 15 to 20 minutes if precipitated by extreme anger or an unusually heavy meal. The relationship of angina to exertion and emotion is significant, since these produce the discomfort and rest relieves it. Nitroglycerine also relieves the pain. Other symptoms that may accompany anginal pain include digestive disturbances, dizziness, dyspnea, faintness, pallor, palpitations, and sweating. Between episodes of angina, physical findings are usually normal; however, during an attack certain signs may be present, including a fourth heart sound, which indicates the increased amplitude of the presystolic expansion of the left ventricle, and a systolic murmur of mitral regurgitation, which indicates a dysfunction of the papillary muscles.

Myocardial infarction

Myocardial infarction most typically is characterized by severe pain, described by the individual as the worst pain ever experienced. It is more severe and lasts longer than the pain of angina pectoris. It usually involves the central portion of the chest and may radiate to the arms, abdomen, back, jaw, and neck. Associated symptoms may include sweating, weakness, nausea, vomiting, lightheadedness, restlessness, coolness of the extremities, and anxiety. Pain is not always present, however; some myocardial infarcts are painless.

The pulse is usually rapid, although some individuals develop bradycardia with heart rates of 40 to 50 beats per minute. The precordium is usually quiet, and the apical impulse may be difficult or impossible to palpate. Heart sounds are usually diminished, although they may be normal. An S_4 is the most common extra sound; an S_3 is less common. The apical systolic murmur of mitral regurgitation resulting from papillary muscle dysfunction may be present, as well as a pericardial friction rub.

Hypertension

Systemic hypertension is a sustained or intermittent elevation of the systolic or diastolic blood pressure to 160/95 mm Hg or over. Persons with a blood pressure reading of lower than 140/90 are considered normotensive, and those with a blood pressure reading between 140/90 and 160/95 are considered borderline hypertensive. Blood pressure level does vary with activity, both physical and emotional, and a single elevated reading does not indicate a diagnosis of hypertension; it does indicate that further assessment is needed.

Systemic hypertension affects about 15% of all Americans and remains one of the leading causes of death and disability among adults. It constitutes a major risk factor in the development of coronary, cerebral, and renal vascular disease. Early detection and intervention provide the possibility for controlling the hypertension and reducing the risks of organ involvement. Many individuals who have an elevated blood pressure are unaware of that fact; thus hypertension is often referred to as a "silent killer." Furthermore, many persons who are aware of their diagnosis do not receive adequate treatment or comply with a treatment regimen.

Classification

Hypertension may be classified according to type, that is, systolic or diastolic, and to cause, that is, primary (essential) and secondary.

Systolic hypertension (systolic pressure greater than 150 mm Hg) associated with increased output and increased pulse pressure can result from a loss of elastic tissue and arteriosclerotic changes that occur in the aorta and other large blood vessels with advancing age. It can also occur with a number of other conditions such as anxiety, fever, hyperthyroidism, anemia, aortic regurgitation, AV fistula, and complete AV block.

Systolic pressure represents the greatest pressure exerted by the blood against the arterial walls following ventricular contraction. Diastolic hypertension (diastolic pressure greater than 90 mm Hg) is a disease phenomenon reflecting the increased amount of pressure exerted on the arterial walls of the small arteries following aortic valve closure, the phase of ventricular relaxation. Increased diastolic pressure results from decreased arteriolar caliber, as with atherosclerosis and vasoconstriction, and with increased blood viscosity. Both conditions lead to increased vascular resistance.

Primary (essential) hypertension. Primary, or essential, hypertension is the most common form of hypertension, accounting for about 90% of persons with this health problem. Its cause remains unknown; however, two mechanisms probably involved in its development are overactive sympathetic nervous system stimulation, which accelerates cardiovascular function, and sodium and water retention by the kidneys. In this form of hypertension both systole and diastole are elevated. Blood pressure is determined by cardiac output and peripheral vascular resistance: an elevated blood pressure can result from an increase in either one or both factors. In the early stages of hypertension, there may be an increase in cardiac output, but over time the cardiac output may be normal or low with an elevation in peripheral vascular resistance. Other forms of hypertension of uncertain etiology include accelerated malignant hypertension and hypertension associated with toxemia of pregnancy.

Secondary hypertension.   Secondary hypertension results from numerous conditions, such as:
1. Renal parenchymal disorders
    a. Acute and chronic glomerulonephritis
    b. Chronic pyelonephritis
    c. Polycystic kidneys
2. Renovascular disorders
    a. Unilateral renal disease
    b. Arteriolar nephrosclerosis
    c. Diabetic nephropathy
3. Endocrine disorders
    a. Pheochromocytoma
    b. Adrenocortical hyperfunction
    c. Myxedema
4. Central nervous system disorders
    a. Cerebrovascular accidents
    b. Increased intracranial pressure
    c. Brain tumor
5. Coarctation of the aorta
6. Drug-induced hypertension
    a. Oral contraceptives, estrogens
    b. Thyroid hormones
    c. Amphetamines

Pathologic changes

Early hypertension is not associated with pathologic changes. Later, the arterioles and arteries develop sclerotic changes. The small vessel damage incurred over time causes structural damage to the heart, kidneys, and brain, resulting in a decreased blood supply to these organs and progressive functional impairment. The left ventricle develops hypertrophy and dilation due to the increase in peripheral resistance. This may lead to coronary insufficiency and myocardial infarction if the enlarged heart muscle exceeds its blood supply.

Symptoms

Patients with hypertension frequently exhibit no symptoms; however, occipital headaches, dizziness, and tinnitus are not uncommon. Epistaxis may occur if the blood pressure level rises suddenly. Vague precordial pains, palpitations, restlessness, and feelings of nervous tension may also be present.

Physical examination

During the early stages of hypertension, the physical examination may show minimal abnormalities, other than the elevation in the blood pressure. As the disease progresses, however, several organs may be affected. On palpation of the chest wall for cardiac findings, the apical impulse may be forceful and displaced beyond the left midclavicular line and downward, occupying a larger area than normal. On auscultation, an accentuated second sound at the base of the heart is commonly heard. An apical systolic murmur may appear because of the dilatation of the subvalvular structures of the mitral valve, producing functional mitral regurgitation. An aortic systolic murmur may also appear due either to dilatation of the aortic valve ring or to rapid flow of blood through a dilated aorta. Occasionally an aortic diastolic murmur may appear because of functional dilatation of the aorta with aortic valve regurgitation. Assessment of the effects of hypertension on other target organs includes:
1. Retinal examination for retinal arteriolar narrowing, hemorrhages, exudates, and papilledema
2. Examination of the neck for distended veins and carotid bruits
3. Examination of the abdomen for bruits, aortic dilation, and enlarged kidneys
4. Examination of extremities for diminished or absent peripheral pulses, edema, and bilateral inequality of pulses
5. Assessment for neurologic signs of cerebral thrombosis or hemorrhage

Findings associated with secondary causes of hypertension include:
1. *Pheochromocytoma:* weight loss, headache, palpitations, nervousness, excessive perspiration, blanching, coldness of skin, nausea, vomiting, and abdominal pain
2. *Coarctation of the aorta:* leg fatigue and diminished or absent lower extremity pulses, difference in blood pressure between the upper and lower extremities
3. *Cushing's syndrome:* truncal obesity, pigmented striae, alteration of sexual function (amenorrhea, impotence), emotional lability, weakness, and backache
4. *Hyperaldosteronism:* polyuria, nocturia, polydipsia, fatigue, intermittent paresthesias, and muscle cramps
5. *Renal and renal vascular disease:* flank pain and urinary tract infections

---

Health History
Cardiovascular

NOTE: A yes response to any question *must* be further investigated. Use the following indicators throughout the assessment: (1) onset (specific date, sudden or gradual), (2) duration, (3) frequency, (4) precipitating factors, (5) aggravating or alleviating factors, (6) outcome, and (7) treatment.

Present status

1. Do you have chest pain?
   a. Description: pressure, sharp, dull ache, tightness, burning, radiates to jaw, teeth, arms
   b. Associated symptoms: dizziness, dyspnea, faintness, pallor, palpitations, diaphoresis, cyanosis of lips, ears, nailbeds
2. Do you have shortness of breath?
   a. Associated symptoms: faintness or syncope
3. Do your feet or legs swell?
   a. Weight gain: amount, time span, affected by time of day
4. Does fatigue limit your activity?
   a. Description
   b. Associated symptoms: chest pain, shortness of breath
5. Do you have a sputum-producing cough?
   a. Description of sputum: frothy, white, bloody, yellow
6. Do you ever feel irregular heart beats?
   a. Type: skipping, rapid
   b. Associated symptoms: fainting, pain
7. Do you have high blood pressure?
   a. Associated symptoms: lightheadness/dizziness, ringing in ears, fatigue/weakness, nervousness, flushing, nosebleeds

Past history

1. Have you had chest pain?
   a. Type: dull, pressing, squeezing, tightness, heaviness, burning, indigestion, gas
2. Do you use tobacco, salt, or caffeine products?
   a. Amount
   b. Symptoms with use: swelling, shortness of breath
3. Have you had rheumatic heart disease?
   a. Current residual effects

Associated conditions

1. Have you had any illness that causes secondary hypertension?
   a. Type: renal disease, endocrine disease, CNS disorders, drug induced

Family history

1. Do you have family history or heart disease, stroke, diabetes, hypertension?
   a. Identification of relationship

Sample assessment record

Client states while clipping hedges a sudden heavy pressure occurred in mid-sternal region and radiated to teeth and jaws. Also had shortness of breath and diaphoresis. Denies swelling of extremities. Has shortness of breath with strenuous activity. Denies cough and irregular heart beat. Has been treated for hypertension for last 5 years. Does not smoke, adheres to a 2 gram salt diet and restricts caffeine intake to 1 cup of coffee daily. Denies rheumatic heart disease and other hypertensive sequela. States mother had hypertension and diabetes. She died at age 57 after a heart attack.

BIBLIOGRAPHY

American Heart Association: Examination of the heart (series of four), New York, 1967, The Association.

Andreoli KG and others: Comprehensive cardiac care, ed 6, St Louis, 1987, The CV Mosby Co.

Ayres SM, Gregory JJ and Buehler ME, editors: Cardiology: a clinicophysiologic approach, New York, 1971, Appleton-Century-Crofts.

Braunwald E, editor: Heart disease: a textbook of cardiovascular medicine, Philadelphia, 1984, WB Saunders Co.

Burch GE: A primer of cardiology, Philadelphia, 1971, Lea & Febiger.

Conner WE and Bristow JD, editors: Coronary heart disease: prevention, complications, and treatment, Philadelphia, 1985, JB Lippincott Co.

Goldberger E: Textbook of clinical cardiology, St Louis, 1982, The CV Mosby Co.

Guzzetta CE and Dosey BM: Cardiovascular nursing: body-mind tapestry, St Louis, 1984, The CV Mosby Co.

Harris R: Clinical geriatric cardiology, ed 2, Philadelphia, 1986, JB Lippincott Co.

Hurst JW, editor: The heart, ed 3, New York, 1974, McGraw-Hill Book Co.

McGurn WC: People with cardiac problems: nursing concepts, Philadelphia, 1981, JB Lippincott Co.

Pollock ML and Schmidt DH, editors: Heart disease and rehabilitation, ed 2, New York, 1986, John Wiley & Sons.

Ravin A: Auscultation of the heart, Chicago, 1977, Yearbook Medical Publishers.

Selzer A: Principles of clinical cardiology, Philadelphia, 1975, WB Saunders Co.

Underhill SL and others: Cardiac nursing, Philadelphia, 1982, JB Lippincott Co.

Wenger NK, Hurst JW and McIntyre MC: Cardiology for nurses, New York, 1980, McGraw-Hill Book Co.

chapter 16

Assessment of the abdomen

OBJECTIVES

Upon successful review of this chapter, learners will be able to:

- Describe anatomy and physiology of the abdomen and major abdominal organs

- State related rationale and demonstrate assessment of the abdomen, including anatomical mapping, inspection, auscultation, percussion, palpation, and ballottement

- Outline history relevant to an abdominal assessment

- Recognize possible pathological conditions associated with regional or quadrant pain and related symptoms

- State related rationale and demonstrate examination of the following abdominal structures
    Liver
    Gallbladder
    Spleen and pancreas
    Kidneys and bladder
    Umbilicus
    Musculature
    Vasculature

- Recognize signs and symptoms from other systems that influence abdominal assessment

ANATOMY AND PHYSIOLOGY

The abdomen, the largest body cavity, spans superiorly from the diaphragm to the lesser pelvis inferiorly. Its perimeter is bound anteriorly by the abdominal muscles, intercostal angle, and iliac and posteriorly by the vertebral column and lumbar muscles.

Because major body organs are contained in this large cavity, there is a greater susceptibility for organ dysfunction. Methodical and systematic evaluation is vital to distinguish variations from the norm.

Stomach

The stomach is located in the left quadrant of the abdomen, directly below the diaphragm. It is separated into three areas: the fundus, located above and to the left of the cardiac sphincter; the body, found directly below the fundus; and the pyloric antrum, positioned proximal to the pyloric sphincter.

Two sphincters regulate the flow of substances into and out of the stomach. The cardiac sphincter controls the inflow of food from the esophagus into the stomach. The pyloric sphincter regulates the outflow of chyme to the duodenum.

The primary functions of the stomach are to store food, to mix digestive enzymes and hydrochloric acid, and to liquify food into chyme. Protein breakdown is initiated with the conversion of protein to peptones.

Intestines

The small intestines fill a major section of the abdominal cavity and extend from the pyloric sphincter to the ileocecal valve. It consists of three segments: the duodenum, the top portion; the jejunum, the middle portion; and the ileum, the lower portion. At the duodenum, bile and pancreatic secretions are received from the common bile duct for digestion. Absorption then takes place through the walls of the small intestine.

The large intestines extend from the ileocecal valve to the anus. It is composed of three segments: the cecum with the vermiform appendix, the colon, and the rectum.

The cecum is located in the lower right quadrant of the abdomen. The vermiform appendix is a process extending off the lower part of the cecum. It is subject to infection and inflammation that can cause a rupture, expelling bacteria-laden substances into the abdominal cavity.

The colon frames the abdominal cavity. The ascending colon advances upward on the right side to the hepatic flexure. From there the transverse colon passes along the top of the abdominal ventral to the liver and stomach. The colon drops downward at the splenic flexure. Here the descending colon progresses to the brim of the pelvis where it unites with the sigmoid colon.

Liver

The liver lies primarily within the right hypochondrium and epigastrium with a small portion lying in the left hypochondrium regions of the abdomen. It is situated beneath the diaphragm. The rib cage covers a substantial part of the liver, leaving only the lower margin exposed. The liver spans the upper quadrant of the abdomen from the fifth intercostal space to slightly below the costal margin.

The liver performs many complex functions:
1. It produces and secretes bile.
2. It has a major role in regulating blood glucose levels.
3. It maintains an important part in protein, carbohydrate, and lipid metabolism.
4. It stores vitamins A, B_{12} and other B-complex vitamins, and D and various minerals such as iron and copper.
5. It synthesizes most plasma proteins such as serum albumin, serum globulin, fibrinogen, and blood-clotting factors.
6. It is instrumental in the detoxification of many substances, including drugs.

Gallbladder

The gallbladder is located on the inferior surface of the liver. A pear-shaped sac, it acts as a reservoir for bile from the liver. The gallbladder concentrates the bile by absorbing excess water through its walls.

The gallbladder is drained by the cystic duct. The cystic duct unites with the hepatic duct from the liver to form the common bile duct. From there, the common bile duct passes downward into the duodenum.

Pancreas

Just below the liver lies the pancreas. It is situated posterior to the greater curvature of the stomach in front of the first and second lumbar vertebrae.

The pancreas has both an exocrine and an endocrine function. The endocrine secretions from the islets of Langerhans produce insulin, glucagon, and gastrin. The exocrine secretions from the acinar cells produce bicarbonate and pancreatic enzymes necessary for digestion and absorption in the small intestine.

Spleen

Located to the left of the stomach and directly above the kidney in the left upper quadrant of the abdomen is the spleen. The spleen has numerous functions, but its four primary functions are as follows:
1. It acts as a blood reservoir for 1% to 2% of the red blood cell mass.
2. It removes old or agglutinated red blood cells and platelets.
3. It is partially responsible for iron metabolism.
4. It helps produce erythrocytes outside the bone marrow in the fetus and during bone marrow depression.

Kidneys, Ureters, and Bladder

Covered by peritoneum and embedded in fat, the kidneys are located in the dorsal part of the abdomen between the 12th thoracic and third lumbar vertebrae. The right kidney is slightly lower than the left. The kidneys measure approximately 11 cm long, 5 to 7.5 cm wide, and 2.5 cm thick.

The nephron is the working unit of the kidney. The nephron's structure consists of the glomerulus and the tubular system. Filtration occurs at the glomerular membrane whereas reabsorption and secretion of essential materials happens in the tubular system.

The kidneys are drained by the ureters and empty into the bladder. These tubes pass anteriorly along the psoas major muscles toward the pelvis. They enter the bladder at the posterolateral aspect. Peristaltic action propels the urine downward to the bladder.

Located behind the symphysis pubis in the anterior half of the pelvis is the bladder, which has a maximum storage capacity of 1000 to 1800 ml. Moderate distention is felt at approximately 250 ml of urine, with discomfort encountered at 400 ml. When distended, the bladder will rise above the level of the pubic bone.

Peritoneum

The peritoneum, a serous membrane, covers and protects the abdominal cavity. The peritoneum is divided into two layers, the parietal and visceral peritoneum. The parietal peritoneum lines the abdominal wall, and the visceral peritoneum covers the organs in the abdomen. The mesentery and omentum are two folds of the peritoneum. The mesentery encircles the jejunum and ileum, then attaches them to the posterior abdominal wall. In addition, it supports blood vessels, lymphatic vessels, lymph nodes, and nerves. The greater omentum is connected to the upper border of the duodenum, to the lower edge of the stomach, and to the transverse colon. It protects and insulates. The lesser omentum is attached between the liver and the stomach. Peritonitis is an inflammation of the peritoneum, often seen in rupture of an intra-abdominal viscus, such as the appendix.

EXAMINATION

Preparation for the Examination

Although physical assessment of the abdomen includes all the four methods of examination (inspection, auscultation, percussion, and palpation), palpation is the technique most useful in detecting abdominal pathologic conditions. Inspection is done first, followed by auscultation, since the movement or stimulation by pressure on the bowel occasioned by palpation and percussion is known to alter the motility of the bowel and generally to heighten the sounds.

Equipment

The only special equipment necessary for examination of the abdomen is a stethoscope; a metal, cloth, or plastic ruler or tape measure that will not stretch; a skin-marking pencil; examining table and light; small pillows; and drapes to cover the client.

Position

The position that the client assumes voluntarily is important to note. The individual with abdominal pain frequently draws up the knees to reduce tension on the abdominal muscles and to reduce intra-abdominal pressure. The client with generalized *peritonitis* lies almost motionless with the knees flexed.

Marked restlessness has been associated with biliary and intestinal colic and intraperitoneal hemorrhage.

Before positioning the client for the abdominal examination, the practitioner should be certain that the client has recently voided (the bladder is empty).

The optimum position of the client for the abdominal examination is *supine* with the abdominal muscles as relaxed as possible. Tension in the abdominal wall muscles is best avoided by placing the client's arms com-

fortably at his or her sides as opposed to extending them upward, as occurs in placing them behind the head. Contraction of the abdominal muscles may be further avoided by placing a small pillow beneath the knees to aid in maintaining the legs in slight flexion. Also, a small pillow placed beneath the head may add to the client's comfort.

The room should be sufficiently warm that the draped client does not shiver, thereby tensing the abdominal wall. A further advantage may be obtained by instructing the client to relax and to breathe quietly and slowly through the mouth. Explanation of the entire examination before beginning and support during the examination may help to ease tension.

The entire abdomen must be free of clothing. An examination gown may be folded up over the chest, or a small towel may be used to cover the breasts of women. A sheet may be folded downward to the level of the mons.

Health History

The health history provides information regarding the chief complaint, the medical history, the family history, the social history, and the environmental-occupational history. Any problems related to the organs, peritoneum, and vascular system in the abdominal cavity should be explored. See the sample health history on p. 386.

Inspection

A single source of light is used in inspection of the abdomen. The light may be directed at a right angle to the long axis of the client or may be focused lengthwise over the client, shining from the foot to the head. The examiner assumes a sitting position, *generally at the right side of the client;* the examiner's head is only slightly higher than the client's abdomen. The resultant shadow will be high, so that even small changes in contour will be highlighted, thereby increasing the likelihood of detection of a pathologic condition. The examiner should be familiar with the normal topography of the abdomen to avoid identifying normal contours as masses (see Fig. 16-7). The examiner should carefully focus attention on the abdomen to describe accurately the presence or absence of symmetry, distention, masses, visible peristaltic waves, and respiratory movements. If the presence of peristalsis is in question, the examiner should carefully study the abdomen for several minutes.

The client is instructed to take a deep breath, forcing the diaphragm downward and decreasing the size of the abdominal cavity. In this manner, masses such as

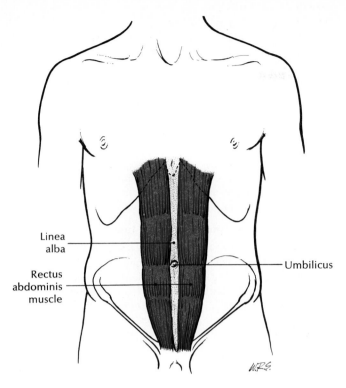

Figure 16-1

Rectus abdominis muscles. Separation of these muscles is called diastasis recti and may be detected by observation or palpation.

enlarged liver or spleen are made more obvious. The rectus muscles (Fig. 16-1) are prominent landmarks of the abdominal wall. *Diastasis recti abdominis* is a separation of rectus abdominis muscles. The separation may be palpated and may be observed as a ridge between the muscles when the intra-abdominal pressure is increased by raising the head and shoulders. The defect does not pose a threat to the functions of the abdominal structures. Diastasis recti abdominis generally occurs as a result of pregnancy or marked obesity.

The examiner should then inspect the abdomen from a standing position at the foot of the bed or examining table. Asymmetry of the abdominal contour may be more readily detected form this position.

Anatomic mapping

Definitive description of signs and symptoms of the abdomen is facilitated through two commonly used methods of subdivision (Figs. 16-2 and 16-3 and the boxes on p. 360). The most frequently used method divides the abdomen into four quadrants. An imaginary perpendicular line is dropped from the sternum to the pubic bone through the umbilicus, and a second line is dropped at a right angle to the first through the umbilicus.

For the most part, abdominal structures will be located in these quadrants as shown on p. 360.

Loops of the small bowel are found in all four quadrants. The bladder and the uterus are located at the lower midline.

The second method of establishing zones of the abdomen results in nine sections (see Fig. 16-3). This is accomplished by dropping two imaginary vertical lines from the midclavicles to the middle of Poupart's (inguinal) ligament, analogous to the lateral borders of the rectus abdominis muscles. At right angles to these lines, two imaginary parallel lines cross the border of the costal margin and the anterosuperior spine of the iliac bones. Essentially, the abdominal structures correlate with the zones shown on p. 360.

Certain anatomic structures have been used as landmarks to facilitate the description of abdominal signs and symptoms (Fig. 16-4). The following landmarks have been useful for this purpose: the ensiform (xiphoid) process of the sternum, the costal margin, the midline—drawn from the tip of the sternum through the umbilicus to the pubic bone, the umbilicus, the anterosuperior iliac spine, Poupart's (inguinal) ligament, and the superior margin of the os pubis (compare with the boxes on p. 360).

Abdominal structures protected by the rib cage that are examined in health assessment are the liver, stomach, and spleen (Fig. 16-5). These structures are evaluated by palpation and percussion.

Skin

The abdomen is an especially valuable area for observation of the skin, since it encompasses a relatively large expanse of skin. Inspection of the abdominal skin for pigmentation (particularly jaundice), lesions, striae, scars, dehydration, general nutritional status, venous patterns, and the condition of the umbilicus may yield valuable information about the client's general state of health.

Pigmentation. Because the skin of the abdomen is frequently protected from the sun by clothing, it may serve as a baseline for comparison with the pigmentation of the more tanned areas. Jaundice is more readily observed in this less-exposed skin. Irregular patches of faint tan pigmentation may be a result of von Recklinghausen's disease.

Lesions. The observation of skin lesions is of

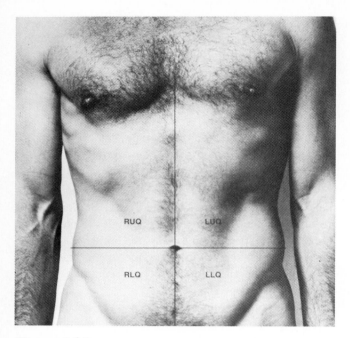

Figure 16-2

The four quadrants of the abdomen.
(From G.I. series: physical examination of the abdomen, Chapter 1, Inspection, Richmond, VA, 1981, AH Robins Co.)

Anatomic Correlates of the Four Quadrants of the Abdomen

Right upper quadrant	Left upper quadrant
Liver and gallbladder	Left lobe of liver
Pylorus	Spleen
Duodenum	Stomach
Head of pancreas	Body of pancreas
Right adrenal gland	Left adrenal gland
Portion of right kidney	Portion of left kidney
Hepatic flexure of colon	Splenic flexure of colon
Portions of ascending and transverse colon	Portions of transverse and descending colon

Right lower quadrant	Left lower quadrant
Lower pole of right kidney	Lower pole of left kidney
Cecum and appendix	Sigmoid colon
Portion of ascending colon	Portion of descending colon
Bladder (if distended)	Bladder (if distended)
Ovary and salpinx	Ovary and salpinx
Uterus (if enlarged)	Uterus (if enlarged)
Right spermatic cord	Left spermatic cord
Right ureter	Left ureter

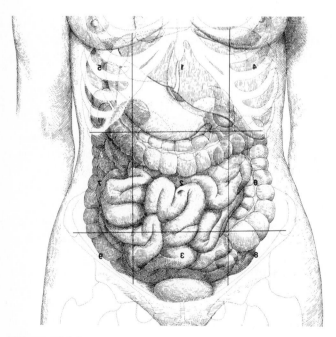

Figure 16-3

The nine regions of the abdomen. *1*, Epigastric; *2*, umbilical; *3*, hypogastric (pubic); *4* and *5*, right and left hypochondriac; *6* and *7*, right and left lumbar; *8* and *9*, right and left inguinal.
(From G.I. series: physical examination of the abdomen, Chapter 1, Inspection, Richmond, Va, 1981, AH Robins Co.)

Anatomic Correlates of the Nine Regions of the Abdomen

Right hypocondriac	Epigastric	Left hypochondriac
Right lobe of liver	Pyloric end of stomach	Stomach
Gallbladder		Spleen
Portion of duodenum	Duodenum	Tail of pancreas
Hepatic flexure of colon	Pancreas	Splenic flexure of colon
Portion of right kidney	Portion of liver	Upper pole of left kidney
Suprarenal gland		Suprarenal gland

Right lumbar	Umbilical	Left lumbar
Ascending colon	Omentum	Descending colon
Lower half of right kidney	Mesentery	Lower half of right kidney
Portion of duodenum and jejunum	Lower duodenum	Portions of jejunum and ileum
	Jejunum and ileum	

Right inguinal	Hypogastric	Left inguinal
Cecum	Ileum	Sigmoid colon
Appendix	Bladder	Left ureter
Ileum (lower end)	Uterus (in pregnancy)	Left spermatic cord
Right ureter		Left ovary
Right spermatic cord		
Right ovary		

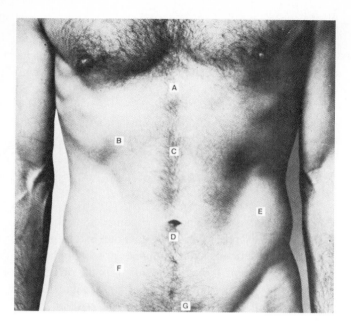

Figure 16-4

Landmarks of the abdomen. *A,* Ensiform (xiphoid) process of the sternum; *B,* costal margin; *C,* midline; *D,* umbilicus; *E,* antero-superior iliac spine; *F,* Poupart's ligament; *G,* superior margin of the os pubis.
(From G.I. series: physical examination of the abdomen, Chapter 1, Inspection, Richmond, Va, 1981, AH Robins Co.)

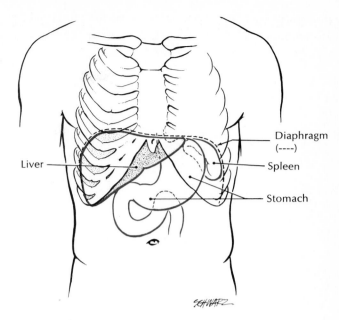

Figure 16-5

Abdominal structures protected by the rib cage. The liver, stomach, and spleen are examined by palpation and percussion.

particular significance, since gastrointestinal alterations are frequently associated with skin changes.

Generally, the skin lesions result from gastrointestinal disease. However, skin lesions and gastrointestinal disease may arise from the same cause. They may also occur without interrelationship.

Although the presence of small hard, painless nodules over a wide area of the abdomen may be a result of metastasis of malignancy, the nodules are generally not the result of carcinoma of the abdominal viscera.

Tense and glistening skin is often correlated with ascites or edema of the abdominal wall.

Striae. *Lineae albicantes,* or *striae,* are atrophic lines or streaks that may be seen in the skin of the abdomen following rapid or prolonged stretching of the skin that disrupts elastic fibers of the reticular layer of the cutis. Striae of recent origin are pink or blue but progress to silvery white. Striae occurring as a result of Cushing's disease, however, remain pink-purple. The stretching of abdominal skin may occur as a result of pregnancy (Fig. 16-6), an abdominal tumor, ascites, or obesity.

Scars. Inspection of the abdomen for scars may yield valuable data concerning previous surgery or trauma. The size and shape of scars are best described

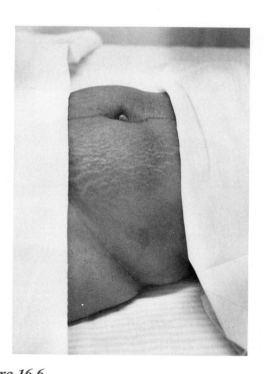

Figure 16-6

Striae of the abdominal wall resulting from stretching of the skin from pregnancy.

through the use of a drawing of the abdomen on which the landmarks or quadrants are shown and the dimensions noted in centimeters as in the following:

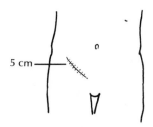

If the cause of the scar was not elicited in the history, the information is sought during inspection. The fact that the client has experienced a previous surgery should alert the examiner to the possibility that adhesions may be present.

Deep, irregular scars may indicate burns. Some individuals produce a dense overgrowth of fibrous tissue in the healing process. This overgrowth is called a *keloid* and consists of large, essentially parallel bands of dense collagenous material, separated by bands of cellular fibrous tissue. Keloid formation most frequently occurs following a traumatic injury or burn. Increased preva-lence of keloid formation has been noted in black individuals and those of Asian extraction.

Veins.   A fine venous network may be seen in the abdominal wall. Dilated veins are observed in vena cava obstruction.

Umbilicus.   The umbilicus is observed for signs of vena cava obstruction (dilated veins), umbilical hernia, metastatic carcinoma, and dampness or the smell of urine (patent urachus).

Contour

Contralateral areas of the normal abdomen are symmetric in contour and appearance. The contour of the normal abdomen is described as flat, rounded, or scaphoid. Contour is a description of the profile line from the rib margin to the pubic bone, viewed from a right angle to the umbilicus with the client in a recumbent position (Fig. 16-7).

A flat contour is one wherein the abdominal wall is viewed as an essentially horizontal plane from the rib margins to the pubic bone. The flat contour is seen in the muscularly competent and well-nourished individual.

A rounded contour is the description given the

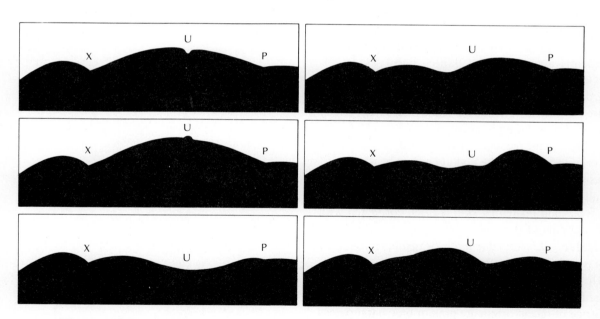

Figure 16-7

Abdominal profiles. **Left. Top,** Generalized distention, with umbilicus inverted: obesity or recent distention from gas. **Middle,** Generalized distention with umbilicus everted: chronic ascites, tumor, or umbilical hernia. **Bottom,** Scaphoid abdomen from malnourishment. **Right. Top,** Distention of lower half: ovarian tumor, pregnancy, or bladder. **Middle,** Distention of lower third: ovarian tumor, uterine fibroids, pregnancy, or bladder. **Bottom,** Distention of upper half: carcinomatosis, pancreatic cyst, or gastric dilatation. *X,* Xiphoid; *U,* umbilicus; *P,* pubis.
(From G.I. series: physical examination of the abdomen, Chapter 1, Inspection, Richmond Va, 1981, AH Robins Co.)

convex profile made by the abdominal wall to the horizontal plane. With the individual in the recumbent position, the maximum height of the convexity is at the umbilicus. However, when the individual stands, the convexity has its greatest height between the umbilicus and the symphysis pubis because of the pull of gravity. The rounded abdomen is normal in the infant or toddler, but in the adult it is generally caused by poor muscle tone or excessive subcutaneous fat deposits, or both. The rounded abdomen is often called the "spare tire" or "bay window" of middle age.

A scaphoid contour depicts a concave profile to the horizontal plane and may be seen in thin clients of all ages. The scaphoid contour reflects a decrease in fat deposits in the abdominal wall, as well as a relaxed or flaccid abdominal musculature.

If an umbilical or incisional hernia or diastasis recti abdominis is suspected, the client is instructed to raise his head from the pillow, increasing the intraabdominal pressure, which may cause the hernia to protrude. The rectus muscles will contract, and a separation will be revealed.

Distention is the term used for unusual stretching of the abdominal wall. Abdominal distention has frequently been described as resulting from fat (obesity), feces or flatus (constipation or intestinal obstruction), fetus (pregnancy), fibroid tumor (or other abdominal mass), or fluid (ascites). The presence of distention generally implies disease and therefore warrants further investigation. *Asymmetric distention* of the abdominal wall may be caused by hernia, tumor, cysts, or bowel obstruction. A mnemonic device for classifying the six common causes of distention are fluid, *flatulence,* fat, feces, fibroid tumor, and fetus—the six Fs.

Generalized, or *symmetric, distention* of the abdomen with the umbilicus in its normal inverted position is generally a result of obesity or recent pressure of fluid or gas within the hollow viscera. If the umbilicus is observed to be everted (umbilical hernia), ascites or underlying tumor may be the cause. Ovarian tumor, distended bladder, or pregnancy may be suspected if the distention is confined to the area between the umbilicus and the symphysis pubis; distention of the lower third of the abdomen suggests ovarian tumor, uterine fibroid tumor, pregnancy, or bladder enlargement (see Fig. 16-7). Possible causes of distention of the upper half of the abdominal wall include pancreatic cyst or tumor and gastric dilatation.

Movement

Respiratory movement. Observation of respiratory movement has more significance in the male client, since the female client manages gaseous exchange mainly with costal movement. On the other hand, the male client evidences essentially abdominal respiratory movement at rest. Peritonitis or other abdominal infection and disease may limit this abdominal respiratory action in the male client.

Whereas abdominal breathing is the mode in the child who is less than 6 or 7 years of age, the presence of abdominal respiratory movements in an older child may indicate respiratory problems. The absence of abdominal respiratory movements in the child who is younger than 6 suggests peritoneal irritation. Retraction of the abdominal wall on inspiration is called Czerny's sign and is associated with some central nervous system (CNS) diseases, such as chorea.

Visible peristalsis. Motility of the stomach and intestines may be reflected in movement of the abdominal wall in lean individuals, even in the absence of disease. However, when strong contractions are visible through an abdominal wall of average thickness, the possibility of bowel obstruction should be investigated. The abdomen is observed for several minutes from just above the level of the abdominal profile while the examiner sits at the client's side, gazing across the abdomen. Weak peristalsis may be augmented by percussing the abdomen. Peristaltic waves of the stomach and small intestine may be seen as elevated oblique bands in the upper left quadrant that move downward to the right. Several of these peristaltic waves occurring in rapid succession may produce a series of parallel bands or a "ladder effect."

Reverse peristalsis, observed in the upper abdomen in an infant, is seen as an undulation moving from left to right. This observation indicates the presence of pyloric stenosis or, more rarely, duodenal stenosis or malrotation of the bowel.

Before touching the abdomen, the examiner asks the client whether any of the abdominal areas are painful or tender. If the answer is positive, the indicated areas are treated with gentleness.

Pulsation. Pulsation of the abdominal aorta is visible through most of its length in vibration of the abdominal wall in thin persons. Pulsation of the aorta is visible in most persons in the epigastrium.

Auscultation

Auscultation of the abdomen precedes percussion because bowel motility, and thus bowel sounds, may be increased by palpation and percussion. The stethoscope and hands should be warmed; if they are cold, they may initiate a contraction of the abdominal muscles.

Auscultatory findings of diagnostic significance are those sounds originating from the viscera, the arterial system, the venous system, muscular activity, or parietal friction rubs. Light pressure on the stethoscope is sufficient to detect bowel sounds and bruits (Fig. 16-8). Because the abdominal intestinal sounds are relatively high pitched, the diaphragm of the stethoscope, which accentuates the higher-pitched sounds, should be used. However, the bell may be used in exploring arterial murmurs and venous hums.

Peristaltic sounds

The use of the diaphragm of the stethoscope to hear the sounds of air and fluid as they move through the gastrointestinal tract can provide valuable diagnostic clues relevant to the motility of the bowel. Normal bowel sounds are high-pitched, gurgling noises that occur approximately every 5 to 15 seconds. Some authorities suggest that the number is as high as 15 to 20 per minute, or roughly one bowel sound for each breath sound. However, peristaltic sounds may be quite irregular. Thus, it is recommended that the examiner listen for at least 5 minutes before concluding that no bowel sounds are present. The duration of a single sound may be less than a second or may extend over several seconds. The frequency of sounds is related to the presence of food in the gastrointestinal tract or to the state of digestion. Since bowel sounds are caused by the passage of fluids and gasses through the intestine, uninterrupted bowel sounds may be heard over the ileocecal valve 4 to 7 hours following a meal. A silent abdomen, that is, the absence of bowel sounds, indicates the arrest of intestinal motility. Stimulation of peristalsis may be achieved by flicking the abdominal wall with a finger (direct percussion). The examiner is advised to listen intently in each quadrant for several seconds before assuming the absence of bowel sounds.

Stomach sounds may be heard in a well child by rocking the child back and forth. The presence of fluid within the stomach may produce a splash.

The two significant alterations in bowel sounds are (1) the absence of any sound or extremely soft and widely separated sounds; and (2) increased sounds with a characteristically high-pitched, loud, rushing sound (borborygmi).

Decreased bowel sounds. Inhibition of motility of the bowel is accompanied by diminished or absent bowel sounds. Decreased motility occurs with inflammation, gangrene, or paralytic ileus. Peritonitis, electrolyte disturbances, the aftermath of surgical manipulation of the bowel, and late bowel obstruction are frequently accompanied by decreased peristalsis. In addition, diminished bowel sounds are often correlated with pneumonia.

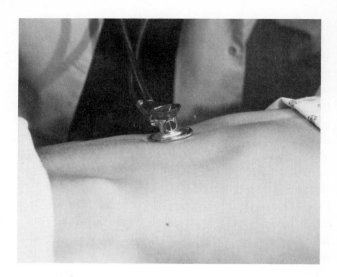

Figure 16-8

Auscultation for bowel sounds. Intestinal sounds are relatively high pitched; the diaphragm of the stethoscope is used.

Increased bowel sounds. Loud, gurgling *borborygmi* accompany increased motility of the bowel such as that which occurs with diarrhea. Sounds of loud volume also are heard over areas of a stenotic bowel. Sounds resulting from an early bowel obstruction are high pitched. These may be splashing sounds, similar to the emptying of a bottle into a hollow vessel. Fine, metallic, tinkling sounds are emitted as tiny gas bubbles break through the surface of intestinal juices. Increased motility may be the result of a laxative or gastroenteritis. Common pathologic conditions associated with increased bowel sounds are gastroenteritis and subsiding ileus.

Vascular sounds

Arterial sounds. *Bruits* are heard when an artery is partially obstructed, causing turbulent flow. A bruit that is heard while the client is in a variety of positions and with the bell of the stethoscope held lightly against the abdomen may indicate a dilated, tortuous, or constricted vessel (Fig. 16-9). Loud bruits detected over the aorta may indicate the presence of an aneurysm. The aorta is auscultated superior to the umbilicus. The locations of the aorta, renal arteries, and iliac arteries are illustrated in Fig. 16-10. Soft, medium- to low-pitched murmurs resulting from renal arterial stenosis may be heard over the upper midline or toward the flank.

For the hypersensitive client, particular care is devoted to listening over the center epigastrium and posterior flank for a bruit in the arterial tree. An epigastric bruit radiating laterally suggests renal artery stenosis.

Venous hums. A normal hum originating from the inferior vena cava and its large tributaries is continuously audible through the stethoscope. Its tone is me-

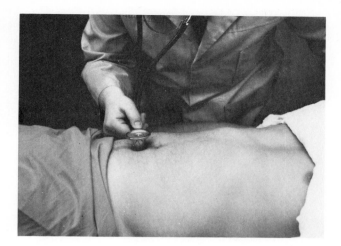

Figure 16-9

Auscultation for bruits is performed with the bell of the stethoscope held lightly against the abdomen.

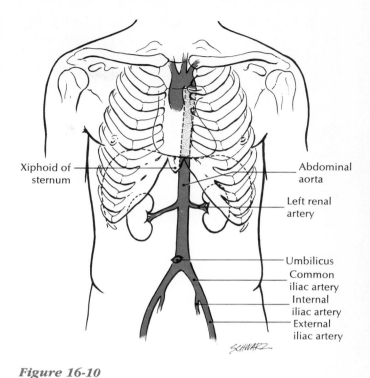

Figure 16-10

The abdominal aorta. Note location of renal and iliac arteries. These arteries and the aorta are auscultated for bruits.

dium pitched and is similar to a muscular fibrillary hum. In the presence of obstructed portal circulation, as from a cirrhotic liver, an abnormal venous hum may be detected in the periumbilical region. Pressure on the bell may obscure the hum. The hum may be accompanied by a palpable thrill.

Another pathologic hum accompanies the dilated periumbilical circulation of Cruveilhier-Baumgarten disease. The hum may be detected near the midline between the umbilicus and the xiphoid process. Hepatic angiomas may produce hums that can be auscultated over the liver.

Scratch test

The scratch test makes use of the difference in sound over solid as opposed to hollow organs. Actually a percussion technique, it is occasionally used to assess the size of the liver. The stethoscope is placed over the liver while the opposite hand scratches lightly over the abdominal surface with short, transverse strokes (Fig. 16-11). When the scratch occurs over the liver, the sound is magnified. Although the test is of questionable accuracy, it is thought to be of some value in assessing the individual with abdominal distention or spastic abdominal muscles.

Peritoneal friction rub

Peritoneal friction rub provides a rough, grating sound that resembles two pieces of leather being rubbed together. Because the liver and spleen have large surface areas in contact with the peritoneum, these two structures are most often the originating sites of the peritoneal friction rubs.

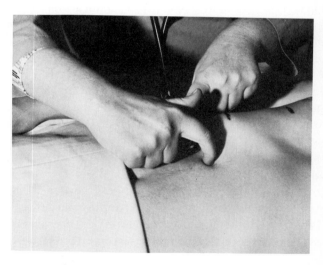

Figure 16-11

Scratch test in assessment of liver size. The stethoscope is placed over the liver while the other hand scratches lightly over the abdominal surface with short, transverse strokes; when the scratch is done over the liver, the sound is magnified.

Common causes of friction rubs include splenic infection, abscess, or tumor; these are heard best over the lower rib cage in the anterior axillary line. Deep respiration may emphasize the sound. Metastatic disease of the liver and abscess are the usual causes of peritoneal friction rubs located over the lower right rib cage.

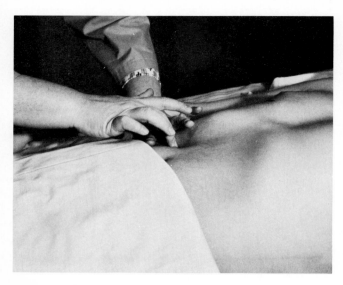

Figure 16-12

Percussion of the abdomen for evaluation of fluid, gaseous distention, and masses within the abdominal cavity.

Muscular activity sounds

A fibrillating muscle produces a hum that can be heard with a stethoscope. Both voluntary and involuntary contractions (as in muscle guarding of a painful area) produce this sound. The hum is often accentuated by palpation of the tender area.

Percussion

Percussion of the abdomen is aimed at detecting fluid, gaseous distention, and masses and in assessing solid structures within the abdomen (Fig. 16-12). The major contribution of this technique, in the absence of disease, is delineation of the position and size of the liver and spleen.

The entire abdomen should be percussed lightly for a general picture of the areas of tympany and dullness. Tympany will predominate because of the presence of gas in the large and small bowel, whereas resonance will be heard in some areas. Solid masses will percuss as dull, as will the distended bladder.

To lessen the chance of omitting any portion of the examination, the practitioner should establish a definite pattern or route to use habitually in percussing abdominal structures.

Assessment of the liver span

Percussion to determine the size of the liver is begun in the right midclavicular line at a level below the umbilicus (Fig. 16-13). The percussion is done over a region of gas-filled bowel (tympanitic) and progressed upward to-

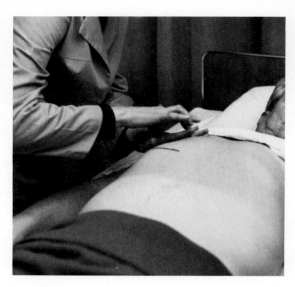

Figure 16-13

Percussion method of estimating the size of the liver in the midclavicular line. Lower border percussion is begun over a region of air- or gas-filled bowel and carried upward to the dull percussion note of the liver. The spot is marked. Upper border percussion is performed over the midclavicular line from an area of lung resonance to the first dull percussion note (generally the fifth to seventh interspace). The spot is marked.

ward the liver. The lower border of the liver is indicated by the first dull percussion note, and the site is marked on the abdomen. The upper border of liver dullness is ascertained by starting the percussion in the midclavicular line and examining caudally from an area of the lung resonance to the first dull percussion note (generally the fifth to seventh interspace). This spot is duly marked, and the distance between the two marks is measured in centimeters (Fig. 16-14). Other sites for measurement are the anterior axillary line and the midsternal line.

Suggested ranges of values for normal are 6 to 12 cm in the midclavicular line and 4 to 8 cm in the midsternal line (Fig. 16-15).

It is important to note that there is a direct correlation between body size (lean body mass) and liver span. It also must be remembered that men have larger livers than women. The mean midclavicular liver span in men is 10.5 cm, whereas it is 7.0 cm in women. A midclavicular liver span of 11 cm may indicate hepatomegaly in a 5-ft, 100 lb woman but may be within normal limits for a man.

Percussion of liver dullness is important in detecting atrophy of the liver, such as might occur in acute fulminating hepatitis.

A less accurate sign of an enlarged liver is the percussion or palpation of the liver edge 2 or 3 cm below

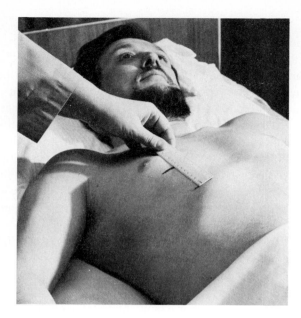

Figure 16-14

The distance between the two marks measured in estimating the liver span in the midclavicular line is normally 6 to 12 cm.

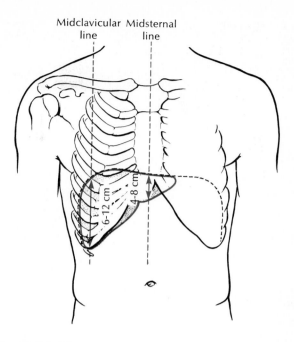

Figure 16-15

The range of liver span in the midclavicular and midsternal lines. The size of the liver shows a direct correlation to lean body mass. Thus, the mean clavicular liver span in men is 10.5 cm and in women 7.0 cm.

the costal margin in the midclavicular line because the upper border must be considered as well. The liver span is seen to be greater in men than in women and in the tall as opposed to the short individual. Error in estimating the liver span can occur when pleural effusion or lung consolidation obscures the upper liver border or when gas in the colon obscures the lower border.

On inspiration the diaphragm moves downward; thus, the span of liver dullness will normally be shifted inferiorly 2 to 3 cm. Pulmonary edema may also displace the liver caudally, whereas ascites, massive tumors, or pregnancy may push the liver upward. The liver assumes a more square configuration in cirrhosis of the liver, and the midclavicular and midsternal measurements may approach equality.

Percussion for tympany and dullness

Spleen. Splenic dullness can be percussed from the level of the sixth or ninth to the 11th rib just posterior to or at the midaxillary line on the left side.

Stomach. A lower-pitched tympany that that of the intestine is typical of the percussion note of the gastric air bubble. Percussion is performed in the area of the left lower anterior rib cage and in the left epigastric region to define the region occupied by the bubble. The percussion sounds of the stomach vary with the time the last meal was eaten.

Percussion for ascites (free fluid)

A technique for differentiating *ascites* from cysts or edema fluid in the abdominal wall is the percussion test for shifting dullness (Fig. 16-16).

Supine position. The client is placed in the supine position, and fluid dullness is percussed laterally in the flank while the abdomen medial to the dullness is tympanitic as a result of the presence of gas within the bowel. The line of demarcation between the dull and tympanitic sounds is marked, and the client is instructed to lie on his side. The ascites fluid will flow with gravity to shift the line of dullness closer to the umbilicus on the same side as the client is lying. A new line is marked, and the change is measured in centimeters. Subsequently, the client is turned to the opposite side and the change recorded. The test enables the examiner to detect free fluid and make a rough estimate of the volume.

Knee-chest position. Percussion of the periumbilical region of a client in the knee-chest position enables the examiner to detect smaller amounts of fluid than is possible with the individual supine.

Puddle sign. After maintaining the client in the knee-elbow position for several minutes so that ascitic fluid puddles over the umbilicus by gravity, the examiner percusses the umbilical area for the dull notes of fluid (Fig. 16-17).

Fist percussion

Another use of percussion in the abdominal examination is the use of fist percussion to vibrate the tissue rather than to produce sound (Fig. 16-18). The palm of the left hand is placed over the region of liver dullness and is struck a light blow by the fisted right hand. Tenderness elicited by this method is usually associated with hepatitis or cholecystitis. Fist percussion at the costovertebral junction is also useful in assessing renal tenderness. Fig. 16-19 demonstrates the relationship of the kidney to the costovertebral junction. The technique of direct fist costovertebral percussion is demonstrated in Fig. 16-20, and the indirect method is shown in Fig. 16-21.

Some disadvantage is recognized in the use of fist percussion to elicit renal tenderness. Even after warning the client, the blow sometimes is startling. Furthermore, the vibration may cause considerable pain and result in apprehension of further examination procedures. In addition, the examiner in standing behind the individual being examined is deprived of the opportunity to observe the client's response. Levinson (1982) has suggested the procedure of "flank lift" as a substitute for costovertebral fist percussion. With the client supine the examiner places both hands beneath the flanks and applies gentle and quick lifting. The person with renal inflammation will localize the pain. The stoical individual may only wince, but the presence of tenderness is confirmed. The lift can be graded in intensity, and there is less danger of hurting the client than with fist percussion.

Palpation

Following careful visual scrutiny, auscultation, and percussion, palpation is used to substantiate findings and to further explore the abdomen. Palpation is used to evaluate the major organs of the abdomen; these organs are examined with respect to shape, position and mobility, size, consistency, and tension. Thorough and systematic screening is performed to detect areas of tenderness, muscular spasm, masses, or fluid.

The client's position is checked to make sure that maximum relaxation has been achieved. The examiner's hands should be warm, and the examiner should use techniques for enhancing bodily and psychological relaxation. Observation that the client does not relax the abdominal muscles despite these maneuvers may justify the use of the technique in which the examiner exerts downward pressure on the lower sternum with the left hand while palpating with the other. The deeper inspiration that results inhibits abdominal muscle contraction. A suggestion for achieving relaxation in children is putting them into a tub of warm water, but this is not practical

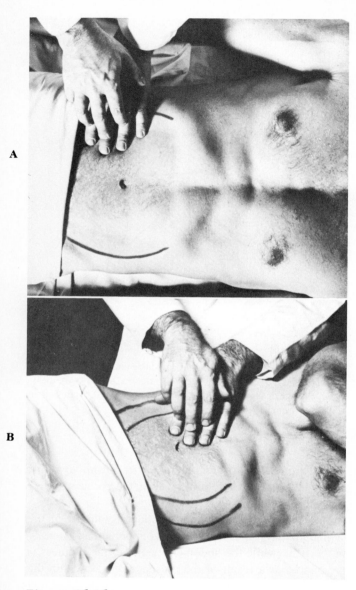

Figure 16-16

Test for shifting dullness. **A,** With the client on his back, the line of dullness is marked in both flanks. **B,** The client is rotated on one side and then the other, and the new levels of dullness are marked each time.

(From G.I. series: physical examination of the abdomen, Chapter 3, Percussion, Richmond, VA, 1981, AH Robins Co.)

A volume of free fluid in the peritoneal cavity greater than 2 liters can be detected by methods of shifting dullness. Ascites is caused by (1) diseases of the liver, such as cirrhosis and hepatitis; (2) diseases of the heart, such as congestive failure and constrictive pericarditis; (3) pancreatitis; (4) cancer, such as peritoneal metastases and ovarian tumors; (5) tuberculous peritonitis; and (6) hypoalbuminemia.

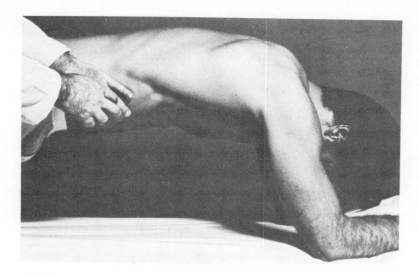

Figure 16-17

Elicitation of the puddle sign.
(From G.I. series: physical examination of the abdomen, Chapter 3, Percussion, Richmond, Va, 1981, AH Robins Co.)

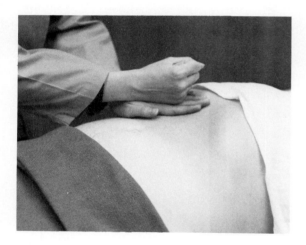

Figure 16-18

Fist percussion of the liver. The palm of the hand is placed over the region of liver dullness and is struck a light blow with the fisted right hand. Tenderness elicited by this method is usually a result of hepatitis or cholecystitis. Fist percussion may be used over the costovertebral junction to elicit renal tenderness. (See text for alternate methods.)

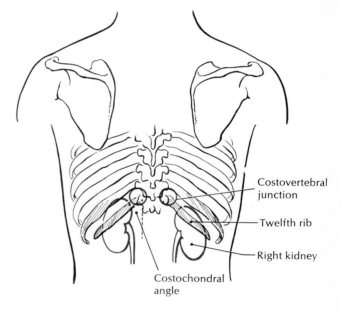

Figure 16-19

Relationship of the kidney to the 12th rib. Note the costovertebral junction.

for a screening examination. The examiner is at the right side of the client, and the fingers of the examining hand are approximated. Measurements are more accurately recorded in centimeters. The older method of describing distance in finger breadths invites error, since examiners' fingers are of varying diameters. The abdomen is explored in all four quadrants with both light and deep palpation. Light palpation is always done first.

Light palpation

Light palpation is gentle exploration performed while the client is in the supine position, with the examiner's hand parallel to the floor, the palm lying lightly on the abdomen, and the fingers approximated (Fig. 16-22). The fingers depress the abdominal wall approximately 1 cm without digging. This method of palpation is best for eliciting slight tenderness, large masses, and muscle

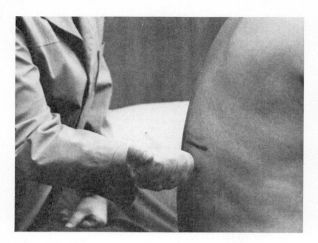

Figure 16-20

Direct percussion of the costovertebral junction to elicit tenderness related to the kidney.

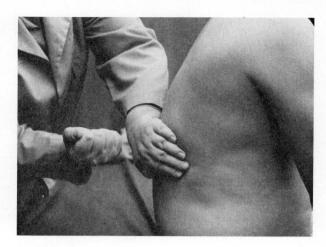

Figure 16-21

Indirect percussion of the costovertebral junction to elicit tenderness related to the kidney.

guarding. Frequently, an enlarged or distended structure may be appreciated with this light touch as a sense of resistance.

Areas of tenderness or guarding, or both, defined by light palpation will alert the examiner to proceed with caution in the application of more vigorous manipulation of these structures during the remainder of the examination.

Tensing of the abdominal musculature may occur because (1) the examiner's hands are too cold or are pressed too vigorously or deeply into the abdomen, (2) the client is ticklish or guards involuntarily, or (3) there is a subjacent pathologic condition, generally inflammatory. Rigidity is a borderlike hardness of the abdominal wall overlying peritoneal irritation. In generalized peritonitis, rigidity may be constant and hard.

• • •

Palpation should begin at a site distant from areas described as painful or that the examiner expects may be tender. Elicitation of pain may result in the client's refusing further examination. The palms are rested gently on the abdomen, and the fingers are flexed, repetitively moving systematically from one quadrant to another.

Assessment of hypersensitivity

Zones of hypersensitivity of sensory nerve fibers of the skin have been described and are thought to reflect specific zones of peritoneal irritation. These are called Head's zones of cutaneous hypersensitivity (Fig. 16-23). Although research has not provided proof for all the zones, clinical reliance has been demonstrated for the

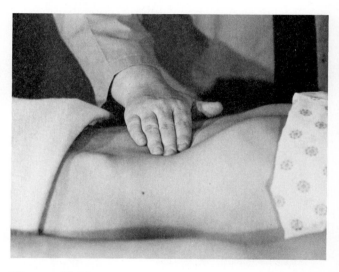

Figure 16-22

Light palpation is performed with the hand parallel to the floor and the fingers approximated. The fingers depress the abdominal wall about 1 cm. This method of palpation is recommended for eliciting slight tenderness, large masses, and muscle guarding.

zone shown for the appendix in cases of appendicitis and for the midepigastrium in the individual with peptic ulcer.

Evaluation of this hypersensitivity may be achieved in two ways. One method is to stimulate gently with the sharp end of an open safety pin, a wisp of cotton, or the fingernail (Fig. 16-24). The second method is to gently lift a fold of skin away from the underlying musculature (Fig. 16-25). The alert client may be able to verbalize the reaction to this stimulation, or changes in facial expression (grimacing) may indicate the increased sensation the individual is experiencing.

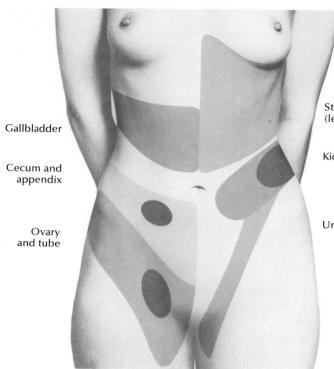

Gallbladder

Cecum and
appendix

Ovary
and tube

Stomach
(left half only)

Kidney

Ureter

Figure 16-23

Head's zones of cutaneous hypersensitivity.
(From G.I. series: physical examination of the abdomen, Chapter
2, Palpation, Richmond, Va, 1981, AH Robins Co.)

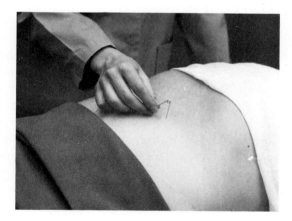

Figure 16-24

Assessment of superficial pain sensation of the abdomen.

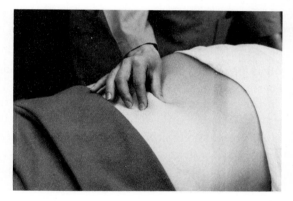

Figure 16-25

Assessment of hypersensitivity by lifting a fold of skin away from
the underlying musculature.

Assessment of muscle spasticity

Involuntary muscle contraction or spasticity may indicate
peritoneal irritation. Further palpation is done to determine whether the spasticity is unilateral or on both sides
of the abdomen. Generalized and boardlike contraction
is thought to be typical of peritonitis. Further definition
is achieved by asking the client to raise the trunk from
a horizontal position without arm support. The experience
of unilateral pain in response to this maneuver may further pinpoint the areas of spasticity. This mechanism may
also help to differentiate muscle contraction from ab-

dominal mass; as the head is raised, the hand would be
moved away from an abdominal mass. Rigidity and tenderness over McBurney's point and in some cases over
the entire right side strongly suggest appendicitis. Acute
cholecystitis is frequently accompanied by rigidity of the
right hypochondrium.

Moderate palpation

The side of the hand rather than the fingertips is used in
moderate palpation (Fig. 16-26). This method obviates
the tendency to dig into the abdomen with the fingertips,

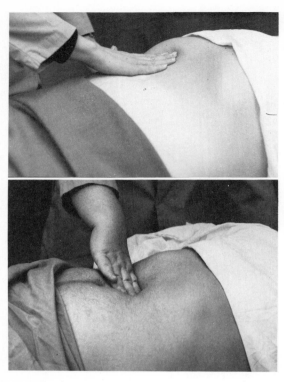

Figure 16-26

Moderate palpation is performed with the side of the hand. This method of palpation is particularly useful in assessing organs that move with respiration, such as the liver and spleen.

as well as the resultant discomfort and involuntary guarding that may accompany such focal probing.

The sensation produced by palpating with the side of the hand is particularly useful in assessing organs that move with respiration, such as the liver and the spleen. The organ is felt during normal breathing cycles and then as the client takes a deep breath. On inspiration the organ will be pushed downward against the examining hand.

Tenderness not elicited by gentle palpation may be perceived by the client on deeper pressure.

Deep palpation

Deep palpation is indentation of the abdomen performed by pressing the distal half of the palmar surfaces of the fingers into the abdominal wall (Fig. 16-27). The abdominal wall may slide back and forth while the fingers are moving back and forth over the organ being examined. Deeper structures, such as retroperitoneal organs (the kidneys), or masses may be felt with this method. Tenderness of organs not elicited by light or moderate palpation may be uncovered with this method. In the absence of disease, the pressure produced by deep palpation may produce tenderness over the cecum, the sigmoid colon, and the aorta.

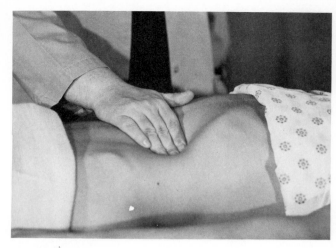

Figure 16-27

Deep palpation is performed by pressing the distal half of the palmar surfaces of the fingers into the abdominal wall. Deep structures such as the retroperitoneal organs are assessed by deep palpation.

The technique of deep palpation may help to give more specific information concerning a lesion or mass detected by lighter palpation.

Bimanual palpation

Superimposition of one hand. Bimanual palpation with superimposition of one hand may be used when additional pressure is necessary to overcome resistance or to examine a deep abdominal structure. In this method one hand is superimposed over the other, so that pressure is exerted by the upper hand while the lower hand remains relaxed and sensitive to the tactile sensation produced by the structure being examined. Generally, for the right-handed examiner the left hand is the lower, or examining, hand while the right hand applies pressure exerted by the tips of the left fingers on the terminal interphalangeal points of the examining fingers (Fig. 16-28). The technique is recommended because the palpating hand is less sensitive if it must be used to exert pressure at the same time.

Trapping technique. Both hands may be used to establish the size of a mass. The mass is trapped between the examining hands for measurement.

Detection of a pulsatile mass. Pulsation may be sensed in the fingertips of both hands as they are pushed apart as a pulsatile flow expands a structure such as the aorta; pulsation may also be felt in a mass held between the examining hands. This palpatory finding indicates that the structure being felt is pulsating rather than transmitting pulsation. The normal aorta is approximately 2.5 to 4 cm wide, whereas an aneurysm is a good deal broader. As noted previously, a bruit is generally heard

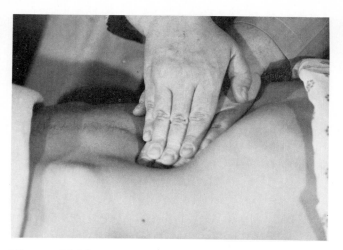

Figure 16-28

Bimanual palpation with superimposition of one hand. Pressure is exerted by the upper hand while the lower hand remains relaxed and sensitive to tactile stimulation.

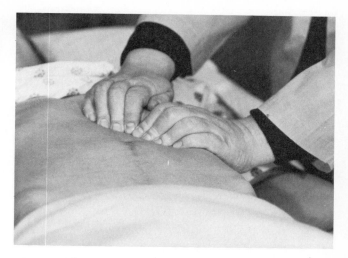

Figure 16-29

Bimanual palpation with the hands side by side. Descent of the liver or spleen (as above) is often measured by hooking the fingers over the costal margin from above. This technique is called the Middleton technique and is used to examine the spleen.

over an aneurysm. The most common physical finding in clients with an abdominal aneurysm is the presence of an expansile, pulsating mass, more than 95% of which are located inferior to the renal arteries but generally at or above the umbilicus. Femoral pulses are usually present but are markedly damped in amplitude. More than half of clients with abdominal aneurysms are asymptomatic; thus the mass might be discovered during a screening physical examination. Although more than 80% of abdominal aneurysms can be palpated, small aneurysms in the markedly obese client may not be felt.

Hands approximated (side by side). Minimum descent of the liver or spleen below the costal margin is occasionally detected by hooking the fingers over the costal margin from above while standing beside the thorax, facing the client's feet (Fig. 16-29). This procedure is called the Middleton technique and is used to examine the spleen.

The outline of a tubular structure such as the sigmoid colon or cecum can frequently be more specifically outlined with the hands side by side, rolling the fingers over the structure.

Palpation to elicit rebound tenderness

Rebound tenderness is a symptom of peritoneal irritation. To provoke rebound tenderness, the approximated fingers are pushed gently but deeply in a region remote from that suspected of tenderness and then rapidly removed. The maneuver as illustrated in Fig. 16-30 is being performed over *McBurney's point* and might elicit rebound tenderness related to appendicitis. The rebound of the structures indented by palpation causes a sharp stabbing sensation of pain on the side of the inflammation. This sensation

of pain following the withdrawal of pressure is a sign of peritoneal irritation. The test may be repeated over to the side of the suspected disease. The test is best performed near the conclusion of the examination, since the production of severe pain or muscle spasm may interfere with subsequent examination. Voluntary coughing by the client may produce the same results.

Many examiners consider the elicitation of rebound tenderness by palpation as a crude and painful technique. The resultant severe pain and muscle spasm not only interfere with subsequent examination but may interfere with trust in the client-clinician relationship. Light percussion can be used to produce vibration, which produces a mildly uncomfortable response in the presence of peritoneal inflammation. The technique is reputed to be able to localize very small areas of peritoneal inflammation, in some cases as small as a quarter.

Ballottement

Ballottement (Fig. 16-31) is a palpation technique used to assess a floating object. Fluid-filled tissue is pushed toward the examining hand so that the object will float against the examining fingers. This is the technique used to determine by abdominal palpation whether the head or the breech of the fetus is in the fundus of the uterus.

Single-handed ballottement. Single-handed ballottement is performed with the fingers extended in a straight line with the forearm and at a right angle to the abdomen. The fingers are moved quickly toward the mass or organ to be examined and held there. As fluid or other

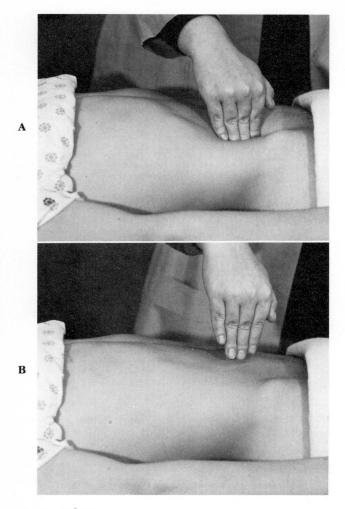

Figure 16-30

Palpation to elicit rebound tenderness. **A,** Deep pressure is applied to the abdominal wall. **B,** On release of pressure, a sensation of pain would indicate peritoneal irritation. This is a test for appendicitis. In this case, the test for rebound tenderness is being performed over McBurney's point and may elicit tenderness related to appendicitis.

structures are displaced, the mass will move upward and be felt at the fingertips. Some examiners prefer this technique for examination of the spleen.

Bimanual ballottement. Bimanual ballottement is accomplished by using one hand to push on the anterior abdominal wall to displace contents to the flank while the other receives the mass or structure pushed against it and feels the dimensions.

Demonstration of ascites by palpation

The presence of large amounts of fluid within the peritoneal cavity allows the elicitation of a fluid wave (Fig. 16-32). To test for the presence of a fluid wave, the client is placed in a supine position. The examiner places the

Table 16-1

Characteristics of abdominal masses related to common pathologic conditions

Description of mass	Possible pathologic condition
Descends on inspiration	Liver, spleen, or kidney mass
Pulsatile mass	Abdominal aneurysm, tortuous aorta
Movable from side to side, not head to foot	Mesenteric or small bowel mass
Complete fixation	Tumor of pancreatic or retroperitoneal origin

palmar surface of one hand firmly against the lateral abdominal wall and taps the contralateral wall with the other hand. An assistant places the edge of one hand and lower arm firmly in the vertical midline of the client's abdomen to damp vibrations that might otherwise be transmitted through the tissues of the anterior abdominal wall.

Palpation for abdominal masses

All the quadrants of the abdomen are examined systematically by palpation. For the most part, bimanual examination with the hands superimposed is the technique most useful. Initially, light palpation is used; the examiner then proceeds to deep palpation.

The characteristics of an abdominal mass are carefully described. Of particular importance are consistency, regularity of contour movement with respiration, and mobility (Table 16-1). A sketch of the anterior abdominal wall with all its bony landmarks and the umbilicus may be the most efficient way to convey location, shape, and size.

Difficulties in determining that a palpable mass is in the anterior abdominal wall rather than in an intraabdominal position may be resolved by asking the client to flex the abdominal muscles. Masses in the subcutaneous tissue will continue to be palpable, whereas those in the peritoneal cavity will be more difficult to feel or will be pushed out of reach altogether.

Normal abdominal structures occasionally mistaken for masses are:
1. Lateral borders of the rectus abdominis muscles
2. Uterus
3. Feces-filled ascending colon
4. Feces-filled descending colon and sigmoid colon
5. Aorta
6. Common iliac artery
7. Sacral promontory

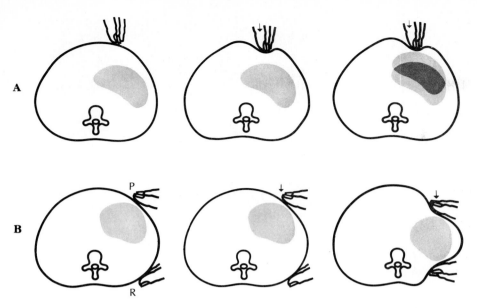

Figure 16-31

Ballottement. **A,** Single-handed ballottement: **B,** Bimanual ballottement: *P,* Pushing hand; *R,* receiving hand.
(From G.I. series: physical examination of the abdomen, Chapter 2, Palpation, Richmond, Va, 1981, AH Robins Co.)

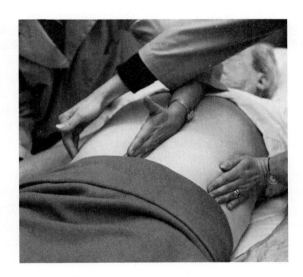

Figure 16-32

Test for presence of a fluid wave.

Palpable bowel segments. The presence of feces within the bowel frequently contributes to the examiner's ability to palpate the cecum, the ascending colon, the descending colon, and the sigmoid colon. The feces-filled cecum and ascending colon produce a sensation suggestive of a soft, boggy, rounded mass. The client may complain of cramps resulting from stimulation of the bowel by the movements of palpation.

Examination of the Specific Abdominal Structures

Palpation is a useful technique for identification and assessment of the specific abdominal structures. A systematic approach, always beginning at the same area, is suggested so that the examiner not skip any part of the abdomen. Since most examiners approach the client from the right, the liver may prove to be the most convenient structure to palpate first.

Liver

Two types of bimanual palpation are recommended for palpation of the liver. The first of these is superimposition of the right hand over the left hand. The client is asked to breathe normally for two or three breaths and then to breathe deeply. The diaphragm is exerted downward in inspiration and will push the liver toward the examining hand. The liver usually cannot be palpated in the normal adult. However, in extremely thin but otherwise well individuals, it may be felt at the costal margin. When the normal liver margin is palpated, it feels regular in contour and somewhat sharp. Descriptions of the abnormal liver are listed in Table 16-2.

In the second technique, the left hand is placed beneath the client at the level of the 11th and 12th ribs and upward pressure is applied to throw the liver forward toward the examining right hand. The palmar surface of the examiner's right hand is placed parallel to the right costal margin. As the client inspires, the liver may be felt to slip beneath the examining fingers.

Tenderness over the liver may be demonstrated by placing the palm of one hand over the lateral costal margin and delivering a blow to that hand with the ulnar surface of the other hand, which has been curled into a fist (see Fig. 16-18).

Whichever technique is chosen, the initial attempt to palpate the liver should be done slowly, carefully, and gently so that the liver margin is not missed.

Table 16-2

Characteristics of hepatomegaly related to common pathologic conditions

Description of liver	Possible pathologic condition
Smooth, nontender	Portal cirrhosis
	Lymphoma
	Passive congestion of the liver
	Portal obstruction
	Obstruction of the vena cava
	Lymphocytic leukemia
	Rickets
	Amyloidosis
	Schistosomiasis
Smooth, tender	Acute hepatitis
	Amebic hepatitis or abscess
	Early congestive cardiac failure
Nodular	Late portal cirrhosis
	Tertiary syphilis
	Metastatic carcinoma
Hard	Carcinomatosis

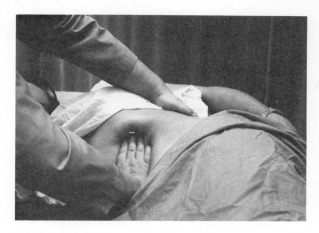

Figure 16-33

Assessment of the spleen.

Gallbladder

Whereas the normal gallbladder cannot be felt, a distended gallbladder may be palpated below the liver margin at the lateral border of the rectus muscle. The cystic nature of the mass helps in the identification of the gallbladder. There is, however, a good deal of variation in the location of the left border; it may be found either more medially or more laterally.

An enlarged, tender gallbladder indicates cholecystitis, whereas a large but nontender gallbladder suggests obstruction of the common bile duct.

Murphy's sign is helpful in determining the presence of cholecystitis through bimanual examination. While performing deep palpation, the examiner asks the client to take a deep breath. As the descending liver brings the gallbladder in contact with the examining hand, the client with cholecystitis will experience pain and stop the inspiratory movement. Pain may also occur in the client with hepatitis.

Spleen

The spleen is generally not palpable in the normal adult. Since the spleen is normally soft and is located retroperitoneally, it is frequently difficult to palpate. Turning the client on the right side (to gain gravitational advantage) brings the spleen downward and forward and thus closer to the abdominal wall and is often employed in the examination.

With the client in the supine position, three techniques of palpation are useful. In the first technique, the right hand is placed flat on the client's abdomen in the upper left quadrant with the fingers delving beneath the costal margin and toward the anterior axillary line (Fig. 16-33). The left hand is stretched over the client's abdomen and brought posterior to the client in the flank below the costal margin. This hand is used to exert an upward pressure that will displace the spleen anteriorly.

The Middleton technique for examination of the spleen is performed with the examiner standing on the client's left side, facing the client's feet. The fingers are hooked over the costal margin, pressing upward and inward at the anterior axillary line (see Fig. 16-29). On inspiration the spleen may be felt at the fingertips. The client may assist by placing the left fist under the left 11th rib.

Either of these techniques may be used while the client lies on the right side to throw the spleen forward and flexes the knees to relax the abdomen. Some authorities recommend that the client lie on the left side during splenic palpation; they propose that lying on the left side more effectively relaxes the abdominal musculature.

The technique of one hand superimposed over the other may also be used to palpate the spleen. Again, the examiner stands at the client's left side, facing the client's feet. The fingers are hooked over the costal margin, and the uppermost hand is used to apply pressure while the lower hand is used as a sensing device. Again, the client is asked to breathe in and out while the examiner focuses on the inspiratory phase in an attempt to feel the contour of the spleen.

Splenic enlargement is described by the number of centimeters the spleen extends below the costal margin:

(1) slight is 1 to 4 cm below the costal margin, (2) moderate is 4 to 8 cm below the costal margin, and (3) great is more than 8 cm below the costal margin.

The spleen may also be percussed. Normally, splenic dullness may be percussed from the 6th or the 9th to the 11th rib in the midaxillary line or posterior to the line. The span of normal splenic dullness does not exceed 7 cm.

A practical technique is to begin percussion at the 10th rib just posterior to the midaxillary line and to percuss in several directions from dull to resonance or tympany to outline the edges of the spleen.

When the spleen has normal dimensions, resonance may be percussed over the lowest left intercostal space between the anterior and midaxillary lines both during inspiration and expiration. However, a finding of resonance on expiration and dullness on inspiration probably denotes splenic hypertrophy. It is important to note that a full stomach or a colon packed with feces may percuss dull and therefore mimic splenic enlargement.

Enlargement of the spleen may best be described by a drawing of the anterior abdomen indicating the relative site and shape of the spleen in relation to the costal border and the umbilicus (Fig. 16-34).

Pancreas

The pancreas cannot be palpated in the normal client because of its small size and retroperitoneal position. However, a mass of the pancreas may occasionally be felt as a vague sensation of fullness in the epigastrium.

Kidney

Palpation of the kidney is best accomplished with the client in the supine position and with the examiner standing on the client's right side. For the left kidney, the examiner reaches across the client with the left arm, placing the hand behind the client's left flank (Fig. 16-35). The left flank is elevated with the examiner's fingers, displacing the kidney anteriorly. With the kidney optimally positioned, the right palmar surface of the examiner's other hand is used in deep palpation through the abdominal wall.

The kidneys are not palpable in the normal adult, and only the lower pole of the right kidney can be felt in very thin persons. In the elderly, as muscles lose tone and elastic fibers are lost, the kidneys may be more readily palpated. The left kidney is generally not palpable.

The examiner remains on the client's right side to examine the right kidney. The right flank is similarly elevated with the left hand, and the right hand is used to

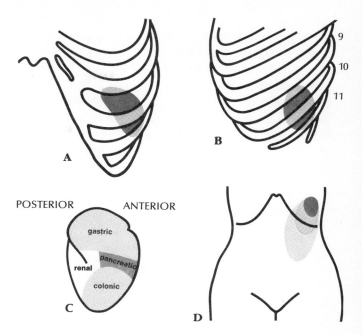

Figure 16-34

Normal (**A, B, C**) and enlarged (**D**) spleen. **A,** Anterior view. **B,** Left lateral view. **C,** Regions of spleen (anterior view) that touch other viscera. **D,** Directions of splenic enlargement. (From G.I. series: physical examination of the abdomen, Chapter 2, Palpation, Richmond, Va, 1981, AH Robins Co.)

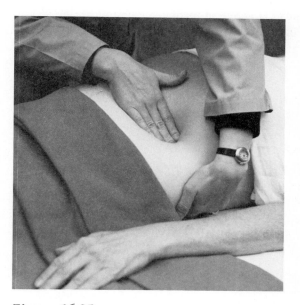

Figure 16-35

Assessment of the left kidney.

palpate deeply for the right kidney. The lower pole of the right kidney may be felt as a smooth, rounded mass that descends on inspiration.

Differentiation between splenic and kidney enlargement may be accomplished by percussion. The percussion note over the spleen is dull, since the bowel is displaced downward, whereas resonance is heard over the kidney because of the intervening bowel (Fig. 16-36). In addition, the free edge of the spleen is sharper in contour and tends to enlarge caudally and to the right.

Urinary bladder

The urinary bladder is not palpable in the normal client unless it is distended with urine. When the bladder is distended with urine, it may be felt as a smooth, round, and rather tense mass. Percussion may be used to define the outline of the distended bladder, which may extend up as far as the umbilicus.

Umbilicus

The umbilicus is observed for relationship to skin surface, hernia, inflammation, or signs of bleeding. The normal umbilicus is recessed below the skin surface.

Umbilical hernia. Whereas umbilical hernia noted in children is seen directly at the umbilical opening centrally located in the linea alba, the adult defect is often apparent above an incomplete umbilical ring and may be called paraumbilical.

The examination for hernia is done by pressing the index finger into the navel. The fascial opening may feel like a sharp ring, and there is a soft center. The umbilicus may be everted by marked intra-abdominal pressure from masses, pregnancy, or large amounts of ascitic fluid.

Sr. Mary Joseph's nodule. Carcinoma originating in the abdomen and particularly in the stomach may metastasize to the navel. The metastatic lesion is called Sr. Mary Joseph's nodule.

Patent urachus. On occasion the urinary tract of the fetus, which extends from the apex of the bladder to the umbilicus, does not fibrose. The result is an umbilicourinary fistula called a patent urachus. The client may report dampness or the smell of urine at the umbilicus.

Cullen's sign. Free blood in the peritoneal cavity may produce a blue hue at the umbilical opening, which is known as *Cullen's sign.*

Abdominal reflexes

The reflex is elicited by using a key, the base end of an applicator, or a fingernail and gently stroking the abdominal skin over the lateral borders of the rectus abdominis muscles toward the midline (Fig. 16-37). This maneuver is repeated in each quadrant. With each stroke, contraction of the rectus abdominis muscles is observed, coupled with pulling of the umbilicus to the stimulated side.

The reflex may be weak or absent in the individual

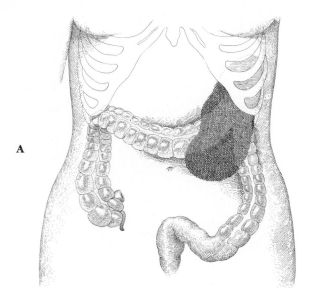
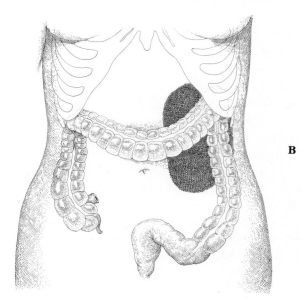

Figure 16-36

Differentiation of enlarged spleen (**A**) from enlarged left kidney (**B**).
(From G.I. series: physical examination of the abdomen, Chapter 3, Percussion, Richmond, Va, 1981, AH Robins Co.)

who has sustained a good deal of stretching of the abdominal musculature. Thus, the practitioner may be unable to obtain the abdominal reflex in the multiparous or obese client. The reflex may also be absent in the normal, aging client. Absence of the reflex may indicate a pyramidal tract lesion.

Changes in vascular patterns: venous engorgement

In health, the veins of the abdominal wall are not prominent, but in the malnourished individual the veins are more easily visible because of decreased adipose tissue. The venous return to the heart is cephalad in the veins above the umbilicus and caudal below the navel. Direction of flow may be demonstrated by placing the index fingers side by side over a vein, pressing laterally, and separating the fingers (Fig. 16-38). A section of the vein may be emptied. One finger is removed, and the time for filling is measured. The blood is milked from a short section of the vein, the other index finger is removed, and the time for filling from this side is measured. The flow of venous blood is in the direction of the faster filling.

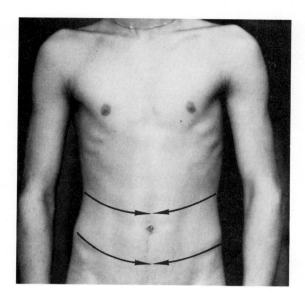

Figure 16-37

Stimulus sites for abdominal reflexes. All four quadrants must be tested.

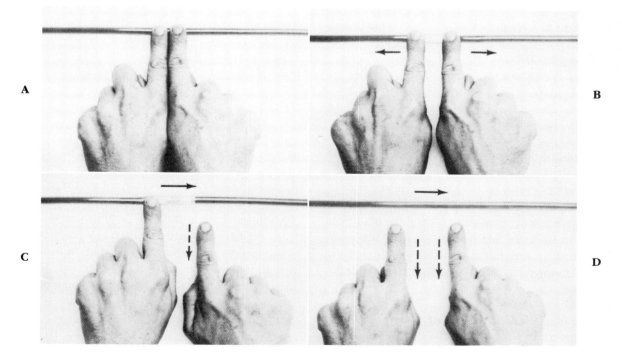

Figure 16-38

Procedure for detecting the direction of venous flow. **A,** Press the blood from the vein with two index fingers in apposition. **B,** Slide the two index fingers apart, milking the blood from the intervening segment of vein. **C,** Release the pressure form one end of the segment to observe the time for refilling from that direction. **D,** Repeat the procedure, but release the other end to observe the time of filling. The flow of venous blood is in the direction of the faster filling.

(From G.I. series: physical examination of the abdomen, Chapter 2, Palpation, Richmond, Va, 1981, AH Robins Co.)

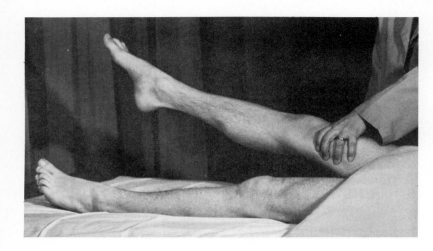

Figure 16-39

Iliopsoas muscle test.

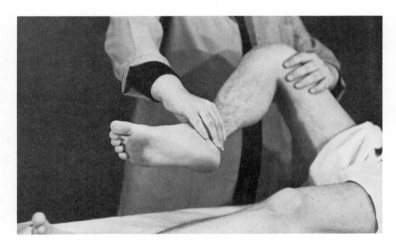

Figure 16-40

Obturator muscle test.

Reversal of flow or an upward venous flow in the veins below the umbilicus accompanies obstruction of the inferior vena cava, whereas superior vena cava obstruction promotes downward flow in the veins above the navel. A pattern of engorged veins around the umbilicus is called caput medusae and is occasionally seen as an accompaniment to emaciation or to obstruction of the superior or inferior vena cava, the superficial vein, or the portal vein.

Tests for irritation resulting from appendicitis

Iliopsoas muscle test.   An inflamed or perforated extrapelvic appendix may cause contact irritation of the lateral iliopsoas muscle. To elicit an indication of involvement, the client is placed in a supine position and asked to flex the lower extremity at the hip. The examiner simultaneously exerts a moderate downward pressure over the lower thigh (Fig. 16-39). With psoas muscle

inflammation, the client will describe pain in the lower quadrant. A more sensitive test of psoas muscle irritation is performed with the client lying on the left side. Pain is elicited through all positions of full extension of the right lower limb at the hip.

Obturator muscle test.   A perforated intrapelvic appendix or pelvic abscess adjacent to it may cause irritation of the obturator internus muscle. This pain is demonstrated with the client in the supine position. The client is asked to flex the right extremity at the hip and at the knee to 90 degrees. The examiner grasps the ankle and rotates internally and externally (Fig. 16-40). A complaint of hypogastric pain indicates obturator muscle involvement.

Back

The final step in the abdominal examination is inspection of the back with the client in the sitting position (Fig. 16-41). The flanks in the normal individual are sym-

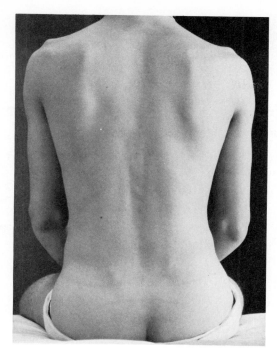

Figure 16-41

Inspection of the back with the client in the sitting position is the final step in the abdominal examination.

metric. Fullness or asymmetry may be a result of renal disorders. Ecchymoses of the flanks *(Grey Turner's sign)* are associated with retroperitoneal bleeding and may be associated with hemorrhagic pancreatitis. Unilateral flank pain or tenderness suggests renal or ureteral disease such as stone, tumor, infection, or infarct.

The costovertebral margin is percussed for tenderness (see the section on fist percussion).

VARIATIONS FROM HEALTH

Tables 16-3 to 16-6 list the history, signs, and symptoms of conditions associated with the abdomen.

Signs and symptoms of intestinal obstruction and of peritoneal irritation are shown in the boxes above.

Abdominal pain

Tables 16-7 and 16-8 list possible pathologic conditions based on descriptions of abdominal pain and its onset.

Referred pain or somatic pain from intra-abdominal structures

Pain related to abdominal structures may be sensed in remote body surface regions (compare with Table 16-9). The explanation for this phenomenon is that as pain is

---

Signs and Symptoms of Intestinal Obstruction

Distention
Hyperactive bowel sounds of high-pitched, tinkling character
Minimum rebound tenderness
Pain

Signs of proximal obstruction

Acute onset
Vomiting (marked)
Frequent bouts of pain
Distention (minimal)

Signs of distal obstruction

Onset may be more gradual
Less marked vomiting
Less frequent bouts of pain
Distention (marked)

Signs and Symptoms of Peritoneal Irritation

Boardlike, increased rigidity of abdominal wall
Silent bowel sounds
Tenderness and guarding
Severe focal pain
Palpable abdominal rigidity
Positive obturator test
Positive iliopsoas test
Nausea, vomiting
Shock-diaphoresis (requires emergency attention)
Hypotension

---

intensified, increased afferent impulses lower the client's pain threshold and excite secondary sensory neurons in the spinal cord. Thus, contact may be established between afferent visceral fibers and somatic nerves of the same embryologic dermatome. An example of this is pain sensed in the top of the shoulder caused by abdominal lesions or peritonitis. The diaphragm, which is irritated in this case, originates in the region of the fourth cervical nerve and derives its nerve supply from the third, fourth, and fifth cervical nerves. The shoulder is innervated by the fourth cervical nerve. Thus, shoulder pain may be a valuable clue in diagnosing perforated ulcer, hepatic abscess, pancreatitis, cholecystitis, ruptured spleen, pelvic inflammation, and hemorrhage into the peritoneum. Other examples of referred pain are noted in Fig. 16-42.

Table 16-3

Conditions associated with the right lower quadrant of the abdomen

Condition	History	Symptoms	Signs
Appendicitis	Children (except infants) and young adults	Anorexia Nausea Pain: early vague epigastric, periumbilical, or generalized pain after 12-24 hours; RLQ at McBurney's point	Signs may be absent early Vomiting Localized RLQ guarding and tenderness after 12-24 hours Rovsing's sign: pain in RLQ with pressure RLQ, iliopsoas sign Obturator sign White blood cell count 10,000 mm^3 or shift to left Low-grade fever Cutaneous hyperesthesia in RLQ Signs are highly variable
Mesenteric adenitis	Young person with history of respiratory infection	Lower abdominal pain May have normal appetite	Tenderness in RLQ Peritoneal irritation signs rare
Perforated duodenal ulcer	Prior history	Abrupt onset pain in epigastric area or RLQ	Tenderness in epigastric area or RLQ Signs of peritoneal irritation Heme-positive stool Increased white blood cell count
Cecal volvulus	Seen most frequently in the elderly	Abrupt severe abdominal pain	Distention Localized tenderness Tympany
Strangulated hernia	Any age Women: femoral Men: inguinal	Severe localized pain If bowel obstructed, generalized pain	If bowel obstructed, distention

Ectopic pregnancy (1% of all pregnancies)	Woman of child-bearing age
	Previous tubal pregnancy or pelvic inflammatory disease
	Missed menstrual period
	Spotting
		Symptoms of pregnancy, i.e., breast changes
		Lower abdominal pain
		Referred pain to shoulder
		Nausea
			Unruptured
			  Tenderness: cervical
			  Mass: adnexal or cul-de-sac
			Ruptured
			  Shock
			  Distention
			  Rigidity
			Mass: cul-de-sac
			Fever

Pelvic inflammatory disease	Woman
	
	Exposure to infection
		Lower abdominal pain
		
		Dyspareunia
			Tenderness: adnexal and cervical (chandelier sign)
			Cervical discharge
			Endocervical smear
			  Gonococcus in one third to one half of cases
			  Chlamydial and anaerobic bacteria cause remainder

Tubal abscess	Woman Exposure to infection Dyspareunia	Lower abdominal pain Mass: adnexal	Fever

Table 16-4

Conditions associated with the right upper quadrant of the abdomen

Condition	History	Symptoms	Signs
Liver hepatitis	Any age, often young blood product user	Fatigue Malaise Anorexia	Hepatic tenderness Hepatomegaly Bilirubin elevated Jaundice
	Drug addict	Pain in RUQ Low-grade fever May have severe fulminating disease with liver failure	Lymphocytosis in one third of cases Liver enzymes elevated Hepatitis A or B or antibodies to the viruses may be found
Acute hepatic congestion	Usually elderly with congestive heart failure Pericardial disease Pulmonary embolism	Symptoms of congestive heart failure	Hepatomegaly Congestive heart failure
Biliary stones, colic	"Fair, fat, forty" (90%) but can be 30 to 80 years of age	Anorexia Nausea Pain severe in RUQ or epigastric area Episodes last 15 minutes to hours	Tenderness in RUQ Jaundice
Acute cholecystitis	"Fair, fat, forty" (90%) but may be 30 to 80 years of age	Severe RUQ or epigastric pain Episodes prolonged up to 6 hours	Vomiting Tenderness in RUQ Peritoneal irritation signs Increased white blood cell count
Perforated peptic ulcer	Any age	Abrupt RUQ pain	Tenderness in epigastrium and/or right quadrant Peritoneal irritation signs Free air in abdomen

Table 16-5

Conditions associated with the left upper quadrant of the abdomen

Condition	History	Symptoms	Signs
Splenic trauma	Blunt trauma to LUQ of abdomen	Pain: LUQ pain of the abdomen often referred to the left shoulder (Kehr's sign)	Hypotension Syncope Increased dyspnea X-ray studies show enlarged spleen
Pancreatitis	Alcohol abuse Pancreatic duct Obstruction Infection Cholecystitis	Pain in LUQ or epigastric region radiating to the back or chest	Fever Rigidity Rebound tenderness Nausea Vomiting Jaundice Cullen's sign Turner's sign Abdominal distention Diminished bowel sounds
Pyloric obstruction	Duodenal ulcer	Weight loss Gastric upset Vomiting	Increasing dullness in LUQ Visible peristaltic waves in epigastric region

Table 16-6

Conditions associated with the left lower quadrant of the abdomen

Condition	History	Symptoms	Signs
Ulcerative colitis	Family history Jewish ancestry	Chronic, watery diarrhea with blood mucus Anorexia Weight loss Fatigue	Fever Cachexia Anemia Leukocytosis
Colonic diverticulitis	Over age 39 Low-residue diet	Pain that recurs in LUQ	Fever Vomiting Chills Diarrhea Tenderness over descending colon

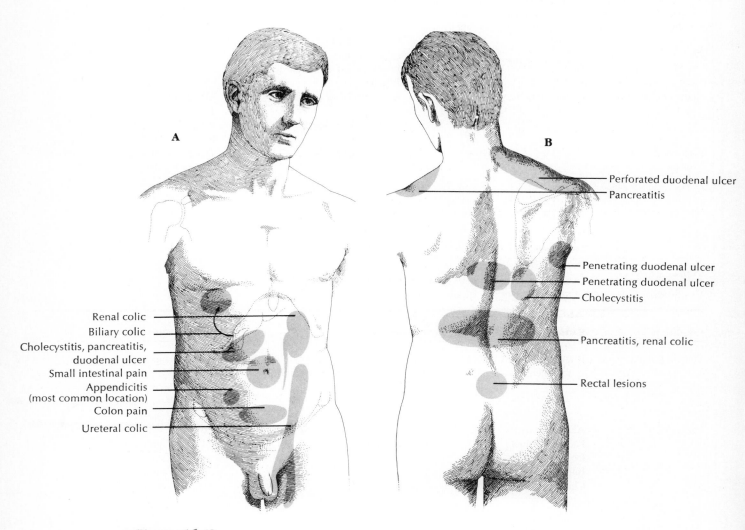

Figure 16-42

A, Common areas where abdominal pain is referred or perceived—anterior view. **B,** Common areas where abdominal pain is referred or perceived—posterior view.

(From G.I. series: physical examination of the abdomen, Chapter 2, Palpation, Richmond, Va, 1981, AH Robins Co.)

Table 16-7

Nature of abdominal pain

Description of pain	Possible pathologic condition
Burning	Ulceration (peptic)
Cramping	Biliary colic
Severe cramping (colic)	Appendicitis with fecalith
Aching	Appendiceal inflammation
Knifelike	Pancreatitis
Radiation of pain	See Fig. 16-42

Table 16-8

Onset of abdominal pain

Description of onset	Possible pathologic condition
Gradual onset	Infection
Acute onset	
Awakening client from sleep	Duodenal ulcer
Loss of consciousness	Acute pancreatitis
	Perforated ulcer
	Ruptured ectopic pregnancy
	Intestinal obstruction (strangulated)

Table 16-9

Symptoms or signs elicited in other systems that may focus the abdominal examination

Symptom or sign	Possible pathologic condition	Symptom or sign	Possible pathologic condition
Shock	Acute pancreatitis, ruptured tubal pregnancy	Flank tenderness	Renal inflammation, pyelonephritis
	Obstruction		Renal stone
Mental status deficit	Hemorrhage—duodenal ulcer		Renal infarct
	Abdominal epilepsy		Renal vein thrombosis
Hypertension	Aortic dissection	Leg edema	Iliac obstruction, pelvic mass
	Abdominal aortic aneurysm		Renal disease
	Renal infarction		Renal vein thrombosis
	Glomerulonephritis	Lymphadenopathy	Hepatitis
	Vasculitis		Lymphoma
Orthostatic hypotension	Hypovolemia—blood loss, fluid loss		Mononucleosis
Pulse deficit	Aortic dissection	Jaundice	Liver-biliary disease
	Aortic aneurysm or thrombosis		Excessive hemolysis
Bruits	Aortic dissection	Dark yellow to brown urine	Liver-biliary disease
	Aortic aneurysm		Blood as a result of kidney stone, infarct, glomerulonephritis, or pyelonephritis
	Dissection or aneurysm of arteries— splenic, renal, or iliac	Fever (103° F) and chills	Peritonitis
Low output cardiac symptoms			Pelvic infection
Atrial fibrillation	Ischemia of the mesentery		Cholangitis
Valvular disease, congestive heart failure	Embolus		Pyelonephritis
Pleural effusion	Esophageal rupture	White blood cell count >10,000 mm³ or shift to left (more than 80% polymorphonuclear cells) >20,000 mm³	Appendicitis (95%)
	Pancreatitis		Acute cholecystitis (90%)
	Ovarian tumor		Localized peritonitis
			Bowel strangulation
			Bowel infarction

Health History
Abdomen

NOTE: A yes response to any question *must* be further investigated. Use the following indicators throughout the assessment: (1) onset (specific date, sudden or gradual), (2) duration, (3) frequency, (4) precipitating factors, (5) aggravating or alleviating factors, (6) treatment received, and (7) outcome.

Present status

1. Do you have abdominal pain?
   a. Location
   b. Severity
   c. Type: burning, knifelike, sharp, cramping, aching, radiating
   d. Associated symptoms: fever, diarrhea, anorexia
2. Do you have nausea and vomiting?
   a. Emesis characteristics
   b. Nausea precedes vomiting or vice versa
   c. Projectile vomiting

Past history

1. Have you had a change in eating habits?
   a. Description: appetite change, weight loss or gain, difficulty swallowing, indigestion, specific food sensitivities or intolerances
2. Have you had any change in bowel habits?
   a. Stool description: color, odor, amounts, consistency, pain
3. Do you routinely use cathartics or enemas?
   a. Type
   b. Reason for use
4. Have you had any change in urination?
   a. Description: burning, color, odor, frequency

5. Have you had any bleeding?
   a. Tarry or black stools
   b. Blood in emesis or urine
6. Has your abdomen ever been distended?
   a. Description
7. Have you had abdominal surgery?
   a. Type
   b. When performed
   c. Residual effects

Associated conditions

1. Have you been exposed to any infectious diseases?
   a. Hepatitis
   b. Sexually transmitted diseases
   c. Foreign travel

Family history

1. Is there a family history of liver or kidney disease, colorectal cancer, malabsorption syndrome, peptic ulcer?

Sample assessment record

Client states sharp pain began yesterday in lower right quadrant and has been constant since. No precipitating, aggravating, or alleviating factors can be identified. Complains of constant nausea since onset but denies vomiting. Has no appetite and had a 10 pound weight loss in the last month. Indigestion is constant and unrelieved by antacid. Denies bowel habit change and routine use of cathartics or enemas. Denies any urination changes, tarry stools, and abdominal distention. Had uncomplicated appendectomy in 1980. Denies exposure to infectious diseases and has no family history of liver or kidney disease.

BIBLIOGRAPHY

Bowers AC and Thompson JM: Clinical manual of health assessment, ed 3, St Louis, 1988, The CV Mosby Co.

Given BA and Simmons SJ: Gastroenterology in clinical nursing, ed 4, St Louis, 1984, The CV Mosby Co.

Johnson LR: Gastrointestinal physiology, ed 3, St Louis, 1985, The CV Mosby Co.

Seidel HM and others: Mosby's guide to physical examination, St Louis, 1987, The CV Mosby Co.

Thompson JM and others: Mosby's manual of clinical nursing, ed 2, St Louis, 1989, The CV Mosby Co.

17

Assessment of the anus and rectosigmoid region

OBJECTIVES

Upon successful review of this chapter, learners will be able to:

- Describe anatomy and physiology of the rectosigmoid region

- Outline history relevant to rectosigmoid examination

- State related rationale and demonstrate assessment of the anus and rectum, including inspection and palpation techniques

- Describe the assessment of stool characteristics and related pathological conditions

- Describe procedures used to detect rectosigmoid pathology

- Identify possible pathological conditions of the rectosigmoid region

ANATOMY AND PHYSIOLOGY

The terminal gastrointestinal tract is termed the *rectosigmoid region* and includes the anus, the rectum, and the caudal portion of the sigmoid colon.

The anal canal is the final segment of the colon; it is 2.5 to 4 cm long and opens into the perineum (Fig. 17-1). The tract is surrounded by the external and internal sphincters, which keep it closed except when flatus and feces are passed. These sphincters are laid down in concentric layers. The striated external muscular ring is under voluntary control, whereas the internal, smooth muscle sphincter is under autonomic control. The internal sphincter is innervated from the pelvic plexus; sympathetic stimulation contracts the sphincter; parasympathetic stimulation relaxes it. The distal portion of the external sphincter extends past the internal sphincter and may be palpated by the examining finger.

The stratified squamous epithelial lining of the anus is visible to inspection, since it extends beyond the sphincters, where it merges with the skin. The junction is characterized by pigmentation and the presence of hair. From an internal view of the anal canal, columns of mucosal tissue, which extend from the rectum and terminate in papillae, may be identified; these anal columns, or columns of Morgagni, fuse to form the pectinate, or dentate, line. Spaces between these columns are called crypts. The anal columns are invested with cross channels of anastomosing veins, which form mucosal folds known as anal valves. These anastomosing veins form a ring known as the zona hemorrhoidalis. When dilated, these veins are called internal hemorrhoids. The lower section of the anal canal contains a venous plexus, which has only minor connection with the zona hemorrhoidalis and drains downward into the inferior rectal veins. Varicosed veins of this plexus are known as external hemorrhoids.

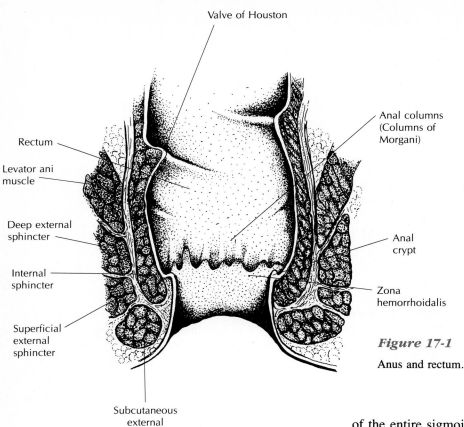

Valve of Houston

Rectum

Levator ani
muscle

Deep external
sphincter

Internal
sphincter

Superficial
external
sphincter

Subcutaneous
external
sphincter

Anal columns
(Columns of
Morgani)

Anal
crypt

Zona
hemorrhoidalis

Figure 17-1

Anus and rectum.

of the entire sigmoid colon and of the other portions of the colon.

Thus, internal hemorrhoids are encountered superior to the pectinate line and are characterized by the moist, red epithelium of the rectum, whereas external hemorrhoids are located inferior to the pectinate line and have the squamous epithelium of the anal canal or skin as their surface tissue.

The rectum is encountered as the portion of the gastrointestinal tract superior to the anal canal. It is approxiately 12 cm long and is lined with columnar epithelium. Superiorly, the rectum has its origin at the third sacral vertebra and is continuous with the sigmoid colon. Its distal end dilates to form the rectal ampulla, which contains flatus and feces. Four semilunar transverse folds (valves of Houston) extend across half the circumference of the rectal lumen. The purpose of the valves is not clear. It has been suggested that the valves serve to support feces while allowing flatus to pass. The rectum ends where the muscle coats are replaced by the sphincters of the anal canal.

The sigmoid colon has its origin at the iliac flexure of the descending colon and terminates in the rectum. Approximately 40 cm long, it is accessible to examination with the sigmoidoscope. Flexible fiber-optic instruments have made possible inspection of the mucosal surfaces

EXAMINATION

The purposes of the rectal examination include assessment of anorectal status and assessment of the accessible pelvic viscera as well as assessment of the male prostate gland and seminal vesicles or additional assessment of the female genitalia. The methods of the rectal examination include inspection and palpitation.

The rectal examination is an important component of every comprehensive physical examination. Additionally, a rectal examination is indicated whenever the client complains of symptoms that may indicate a problem or dysfunction with the region (see the box on p. 389).

In addition to historical information, the client may give some indication of a problem by particular movements; for example, shifting from one buttock to the other, which alleviates the discomfort of a thrombosed hemorrhoid.

Preparation

Most clients experience a significant amount of embarrassment and apprehension about the rectal examination—they may be concerned about the cleanliness of the area, the exploration of troubling symptoms, or pain. These fears can cause spasms of the anal sphincters and buttocks, making the examination unnecessarily uncomfortable. The following interventions may alleviate some client anxieties and facilitate client cooperation to enable as thorough and comfortable an examination as possible:

1. Teach the client relaxation techniques—remind the client to continue slow, deep breaths during the examination.
2. Advise the client about the potential of unusual sensations, especially feelings that defecation or passing gas is imminent, but reassure the client that such an accident is very unlikely.
3. Proceed with the examination in a sympathetic but confident manner.
4. Maintain gentleness in approach, avoiding undue force while allowing time for relaxation, but not withdrawing the examining hand until the examination is complete.
5. Drape the client to avoid unnecessary exposure of genitalia.

The client may be examined in one of the following positions:

1. *Left lateral or Sims' position* (Fig. 17-2): The client lies on the left side with the superior thigh and knee flexed, bringing the knee close to the chest. The client's left hip should rest on a small firm pillow or sandbag placed immediately adjacent to the side of the examination table, allowing the buttocks to be elevated and to project slightly over the edge of the table. The client's trunk should lie obliquely across the table top so that the head rests on a pillow near the opposite edge. The hips should be flexed to an angle slightly less than 90 degrees, placing the lower leg close to the opposite side of the table and parallel to its edge. The right side of the body should be displaced slightly forward. In this position the rectal ampulla is pushed down and posteriorly and thus is advantageously aligned for the detection of rectal masses. However, the upper rectum and pelvis structure tend to fall away in this position.

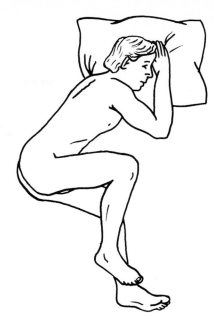

Figure 17-2

Position for rectal exam. *Note: Illustration for position only.* During actual examination, all clients should be appropriately draped. Additionally, a sandbag or pillow placed under the left hip would facilitate positioning.

2. *Knee-chest position:* The client is kneeling on the examining table with the shoulders and head in contact with the examining table. The knees are positioned more widely apart than the hips. The angle at the hip is 75 to 80 degrees. The size of the prostate gland is best assessed with the client in this position. This is an uncomfortable position and embarrassing for female clients especially.
3. *Standing position:* The client stands over the examining table with hips flexed and the trunk resting on the table. Prostate evaluation is facilitated in this position. This is the most commonly used position for examination of the prostate gland.
4. *Lithotomy position:* The position is used with female clients for a screening rectal examination following a pelvic examination. The client is supine with knees flexed and feet elevated and supported in stirrups.
5. *Squatting position:* The client squats on a firm flat surface with the examiner behind the client. Rectal prolapse may frequently be brought out in this position, and some lesions of the rectosigmoid region and pelvis may be felt in this position only.

For all rectal examinations, the examiner should wear two gloves throughout the examination.

The following supplies and equipment should be available for every rectal examination:

- Water-soluble lubricant
- Disposable gloves
- A good source of light
- A penlight
- Material for testing stool for occult blood

A review of related history is shown in the box opposite.

Inspection

The buttocks are carefully spread with both hands to examine the anus and the tissue immediately around the anus. This skin is more pigmented and coarse than the surrounding perianal skin and is also moist and hairless. The examiner visually assesses the perianal region for skin tags, lesions, scars or inflammation, perirectal abscesses, fissures, sentinel piles from rectal fissures, external hemorrhoids or fistula openings, condyloma acuminatum (viral warts), tumors, and rectal prolapse.

The client is asked to strain downward as though defecating, so that with slight pressure on the skin, rectal fissures, rectal prolapse, polyps, or internal hemorrhoids might be identified. Abnormal findings are described by locating them in terms of a clock, with the 12 o'clock position toward the symphysis pubis.

The sacrococcygeal area is inspected for pilonidal cyst or sinus. The pilonidal area is inspected for dimples (at the tip of the coccyx), sinus openings, or the presence of inflammation. The pilonidal area is felt for tenderness, induration, or swelling.

The skin of the pilonidal sinus may have abundant hair growth. The accumulation of secretions often leads to infection, which is generally accompanied by a foul-smelling discharge and local tenderness. The sinus may be simply blocked up by secretions, so that a tumescence is observed, which is tender to palpation.

Palpation

The examiner's nondominant hand is used to spread the buttocks apart. If the sphincter tightens, the client should be instructed and reassured; when the sphincter relaxes, the examination is continued. Painful lesions or bleeding may prevent completion of the examination.

While the client strains downward, the pad of the lubricated, gloved index finger is gently placed against the anal verge; firm pressure is exerted until the sphincter begins to yield, and the finger is then slowly inserted in the direction of the umbilicus as the rectal sphincter relaxes (Fig. 17-3). The client is asked to tighten the sphincter around the examining finger to provide a measurement of muscle strength of the anal sphincter. Hypertonicity of the external sphincter may occur with anx-

---

Review of Related History

General historical data

1. Medications
2. Diet
3. Activity-sleep patterns
4. Bowel habits and changes in habits
5. Past history of problems in the region, including trauma, hemorrhoids, and lesions
6. Family history of cancer in the region or in the gastrointestinal tract
7. Current signs or symptoms of problems in the region or in the gastrointestinal tract

If bowel function changes

1. Stools—number per day, consistency, color, presence of mucus, blood, fat, or unusual odor.
2. Timing of onset—association with diet, illness, changes in daily patterns, stress, or other patterns
3. Accompanying symptoms—flatus, nausea, vomiting, distention, cramping,

If regional anal discomfort (e.g., pain, itching, burning)

1. Association with body position, e.g. sitting, standing, walking, lying down
2. Association with defecation or straining with stool
3. Presence of blood, mucus, or other unusual substance

If rectal bleeding

1. Color—bright red, dark red-burgundy-black
2. Amount—on tissue, spotting in toilet, or active bleeding
3. Relationship to defecation and changes in stool and bowel habits
4. Associated gastrointestinal and regional symptoms

---

ious, voluntary or involuntary contraction or as a result of an anal fissure or other local pathologic condition. A relaxed or hypotonic sphincter is seen occasionally after rectal surgery or may be due to a neurologic deficiency. The subcutaneous portion of the external sphincter is palpated on the inner aspect of the anal verge. The palpating finger is rotated to examine the entire muscular ring. The intersphincteric line is marked by a palpable indentation. Palpation of the deep external sphincter is performed through the lower part of the internal sphincter, which it surrounds. Assessment of the levator ani muscle is accomplished by palpating laterally and posteriorly where the muscle is attached to the rectal wall on one side and then the other (Fig. 17-4).

The anal canal is short. The distance from the anal verge to the anorectal junction is less than 3 cm, a distance roughly equivalent to the distance from the fingertip to

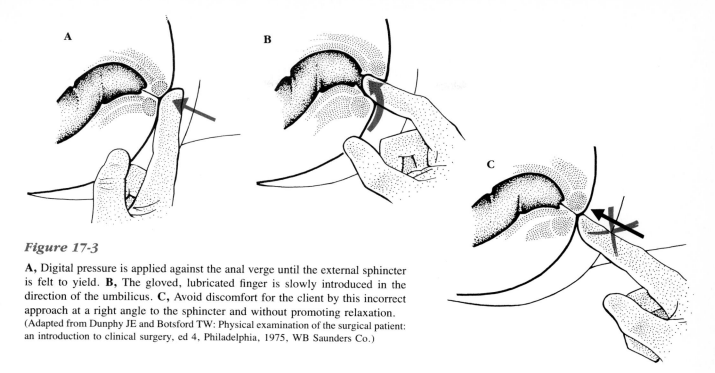

Figure 17-3

A, Digital pressure is applied against the anal verge until the external sphincter is felt to yield. **B,** The gloved, lubricated finger is slowly introduced in the direction of the umbilicus. **C,** Avoid discomfort for the client by this incorrect approach at a right angle to the sphincter and without promoting relaxation.
(Adapted from Dunphy JE and Botsford TW: Physical examination of the surgical patient: an introduction to clinical surgery, ed 4, Philadelphia, 1975, WB Saunders Co.)

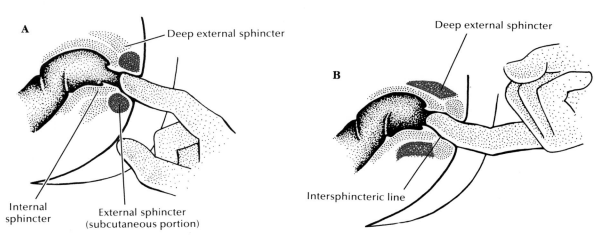

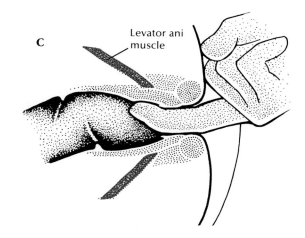

Figure 17-4

The subcutaneous portion of the external sphincter is palpated, **A,** followed by digital exploration of the deep external sphincter, **B, C,** Palpation of the levator ani muscle.
(Adapted from Dunphy JE and Botsford TW: Physical examination of the surgical patient: an introduction to clinical surgery, ed 4, Philadelphia, 1975, WB Saunders Co.)

Table 17-1

Assessment of stool characteristics

Description of the stool	Possible explanation
Yellow or green	Severe diarrhea, sterilization of bowel by antibiotics, diet high in chlorophyll-rich vegetables, and use of the drug calomel
Light tan, gray	Absence of bile pigments as may be found in blockage of the common bile duct, pancreatic insufficiency, obstructive jaundice, and diets high in milk or fat and low in meat
Black, tarry	Bleeding into the upper gastrointestinal tract, ingestion of iron compounds or bismuth preparations, and high proportions of meat in the diet
Red	Bleeding from the lower gastrointestinal tract, some foods such as beets
Translucent mucus on stool	Spastic constipation, nucleus colitis, emotional disturbance, and excessive straining
Bloody mucus	Neoplasm or inflammation of the rectal canal
Mucus with pus and blood	Ulcerative colitis, bacillary dysentery, ulcerating cancer of the colon, and acute diverticulitis
Fat in stool	Malabsorption syndromes, enteritis and pancreatic diseases, surgical removal of a section of the intestine, steatorrhea, and chronic pancreatic disease

the interphalangeal joint. The posterior wall of the rectum follows the curve of the coccyx and sacrum and feels smooth to the palpating finger. The mucosa of the anal canal is palpated for tumor or polyps. The coccyx is palpated to determine mobility and sensitivity.

The examining finger is able to palpate a distance of 6 to 10 cm of the rectal canal. A bidigital palpation of the sphincter area may yield more information than would be obtained by probing with the index finger alone. This is accomplished by pressing the thumb of the examining hand against the perianal tissue and moving the examining index finger toward it. This is a useful technique for detecting a perianal abscess and for palpating the bulbourethral (Cowper's) glands.

Rectal valves may be misinterpreted as protruding intrarectal masses, especially when they are well developed.

The lateral walls of the rectum may be palpated by rotating the index finger along the sides of the rectum. The ischial spines and sacrotuberous ligaments may be identified through palpation.

The prostate gland is situated anterior to the rectum; therefore, palpation through the mucosa of the anterior wall of the rectum allows the examiner to assess the size, shape, and consistency of the prostate gland. The client is asked to bear down so that a mass not otherwise reached might be pushed downward into the range of the examining finger.

The prostate gland, a bilobed structure, has a normal diameter of approximately 4 cm. The palpating finger identifies the smooth lateral lobes separated by a central groove. The prostate is approximately 2.5 cm long, and the presence of nodules is noted. The prostate should feel firm and smooth. The client should be asked to report tenderness to touch. (See Chapter 21 for assessment of male genitalia.)

The normal cervix can be felt as a small round mass through the anterior wall of the rectum. (See Chapter 22 for assessment of the female genitalia.)

Examination of the Stool

On withdrawal of the examining finger, the nature of any feces clinging to the glove should be examined (Table 17-1). The presence of pus or blood is noted. Bright red blood in small or large amounts may be from the large intestine, the sigmoid colon, the rectum, or the anus. However, the stool may be burgundy if the bleeding occurred in the ascending colon. Colonic bleeding may be suspected when blood is mixed with the feces, whereas rectal bleeding is probably occurring when the blood is observed on the surface of the stool. The presence of a good deal of blood in the stool may be associated with marked malodor.

A black, tarry stool (melena) results from bleeding in the stomach or small intestine; the blood is partially digested during its passage to the rectum. On the other hand, the black color may result from ingested iron compounds and bismuth preparations.

A small quantity of the feces is subjected to a chemical test for the presence of occult blood. Minimum abrasions of the gastrointestinal tract are thought to be responsible for blood loss of 1 to 3 ml daily in the feces. The loss of more than 50 ml from the upper gastrointestinal tract will produce melena. To detect quantities less than 50 ml or to determine whether black stools actually do contain blood, several reagents may be used.

Other Investigative Techniques

Anoscopy

Use of an anoscope for a more complete examination of the anal canal and internal hemorrhoidal zone.

Proctoscopy

Use of a proctoscope to visualize the anus and lower rectum. Approximately 9 to 15 cm of the lower intestinal tract can be visualized. The warmed and lubricated instrument is passed with the obturator for its full length. The obturator is removed, and the proctoscope is removed slowly while the examiner observes for ulcers, inflammation, strictures, or the cause of a palpable mass. Biopsy may be performed through the tube.

Sigmoidoscopy

Visual examination of the upper portion of the rectum that cannot be felt with the examining finger is possible with a sigmoidoscope, which allows direct visualization of the lower 24 cm of the gastrointestinal tract. This examination is partic-

ularly important, since half of all carcinomas occur in the rectum and colon. The early detection of polyps and malignant lesions may result in early and successful treatment of an otherwise fatal disease.

Manometry

This technique measures intraluminal pressure by a balloon probe attached to a catheter connected to a pressure transducer and a polygraph.

Sphincter electromyography

Needle or surface electrodes are used to detect the contractile activity of striated muscle and to obtain separate recordings from the external sphincter and from the puborectalis muscle.

Defecography and balloon proctography

Radiology investigations designed to image the rectum and the pelvic floor at rest and during contraction and defecation.

Tests for detecting blood in the feces rely on substances that detect peroxidase as an indication of hemoglobin content through color change in the stool specimen tested. Various reagent substances have been used to detect occult blood. Their sensitivity varies as follows:

1. Orthotoluidine (Hematest, Occultest)—10 times more sensitive than benzidine.
2. Benzidine—10 or more times sensitive than guaiac.
3. Guaiac (Hemoccult)—the least sensitive.

A single positive result does not necessarily confirm gastrointestinal bleeding. A positive result is an indication to repeat the test at least three times while the client follows a meatless, high-residue diet.

The various commercially prepared screening tests for occult blood are packaged with complete instructions for use. The steps of the Hematest are presented here as an example of the various tests, most of which are similar:

1. After the digital examination, a bit of the feces on the glove of the examining finger is wiped on a square of filter paper supplied with the kit.
2. The filter paper with the stool smear is placed on a glass slide.
3. A reagent tablet is placed in the center of the smear on the filter paper.
4. One drop of water is placed on the tablet, and the water is allowed to soak into the tablet for 5 to 10 seconds. Then a second drop of water is added, which should run from the tablet onto the specimen and the filter paper.

5. After two minutes, the filter paper will turn blue if the test is positive. The color on the tablet itself or color appearing after 2 minutes is irrelevant.

If the screening test is positive, the client is retested after 48 to 72 hours. The client is instructed to refrain from eating meat, poultry, fish, turnips, and horseradish during the next testing period. Additionally, the client may need to temporarily discontinue the use of the following: iron preparations, bromides, iodides, rauwolfia derivatives, indomethacin, colchicine, salicylates, phenylbutazone, oxyphenylbutazone, bismuth compounds, steroids, and ascorbic acid.

Additional Procedures

The presence of a pathological condition detected by the digital examination may be further explored by one of the procedures shown in the box above.

VARIATIONS FROM HEALTH

Pilonidal Cyst or Sinus

Pilonidal sinus is generally first diagnosed between the ages of 15 and 30, even though it is thought to be a congenital lesion. It is located superficial to the coccyx or lower sacrum. The sinus opening may look like a dimple, with another very small opening in the midline. In other cases a cyst is observed and may be palpated; in more advanced conditions a sinus tract may be palpated. The area may become erythematous, and a tuft of hair may be observed. The ingrowth of the hairs is probably the cause of infection, cyst, and fistula formation.

Pruritus Ani

Excoriated, thickened, and pigmented skin may result from chronic inflammation of pruritus ani. The itching and burning of the rectal area are most often traceable to pinworms in children and to fungal infections in adults. Diabetic clients are particularly vulnerable to fungal infections. A dull, grayish pink color of the perianal skin is a characteristic of fungal infections. The radiating folds of skin may appear enlarged, and the skin may be cracked or fissured. Pruritus ani characterized by dry and brittle skin is thought to be related to psychosomatic disease.

Rectal Tenesmus

Rectal tenesmus is the painful straining at stool associated with spasm of anal and rectal muscles; the client complains of a distressing feeling of urgency. The client is questioned concerning the nature of the stool. A hard, dry stool indicates constipation. A bloody, diarrheal stool might indicate ulcerative colitis. Rectal fissure may be the cause of tenesmus with normally constituted stools. Tenesmus may also be a symptom experienced by the client with a perirectal inflammation, such as prostatitis.

The client who complains of constant rectal pain is examined carefully for thrombosed rectal hemorrhoids.

Fecal Impaction

Fecal impaction is the accumulation and dehydration of fecal material in the rectum. When motility of the rectum is inhibited, the normal progression of feces does not occur and more water is reabsorbed through the bowel wall. The feces become hard and difficult to pass and may lead to complete obstruction. Fecal impaction is observed in individuals with chronic constipation and in individuals who have retained barium following gastrointestinal x-ray examination. The client complains of a sense of rectal fullness or urgency. Frequent small, liquid-to-loose stools may occur in incomplete obstruction. The dehydrated fecal mass is easily felt on palpation.

Anal Fissure

A thin tear of the superficial anal mucosa, generally weeping, may be identified by asking the client to perform Valsalva's maneuver. The fissure is most commonly (more than 90%) found in the posterior midline of the anal mucosa and less frequently in the anterior midline (Fig. 17-5).

Anal fissure is generally the result of the trauma such as that associated with the passage of a large, hard stool. The client may complain of local pain, itching, or

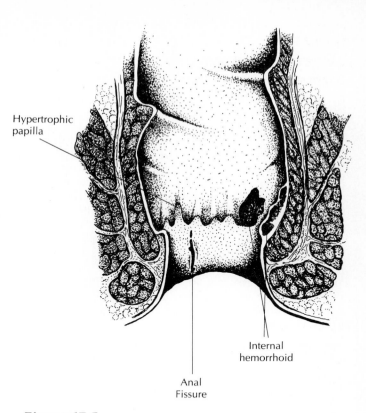

Figure 17-5

Common problems of the anus and rectum.

bleeding. Pain generally accompanies the passage of stool, and blood may be observed on the stool or on the toilet tissue. The inspection finding may include a sentinel skin tag or ulcer through which the muscles of the internal sphincter may be visible at the base. Because the examination is painful to the client, making it difficult to relax the anal muscle, local anesthesia may be necessary.

Fistula in Ano

A tract from an anal fissure or infection that terminates in the perianal skin or other tissue is termed an anorectal fistula; it usually has its origin from local crypt abscesses. The fistula is a chronically inflamed tube made up of fibrous tissue surrounding granulation tissue and may frequently be palpated. The external opening is generally visible as a red elevation of granulation tissue. Local compression may result in the expression of serosanguinous or purulent drainage. Palpation (bidigital) is best accomplished with a finger in the anorectal cavity compressing the tissue against the thumb on the skin surface. The fistulous tract feels like an indurated cord.

The site from which drainage from an anal infection occurs can be identified by relating the location of the external opening of the fissure to the anus (Table 17-2 and Fig. 17-6).

Table 17-2

Location of fistula site related to the external opening

	External opening	Location in the anus
Goodsell's rule	Posterior to a line between the ischial tuberosities	Posterior
	Radial from the drainage site	Anterior
Salmon's law	Posterior to the anus or more than 2.5 anterior or lateral	Posterior
	Anterior or less than 2.5 cm lateral	Anterior

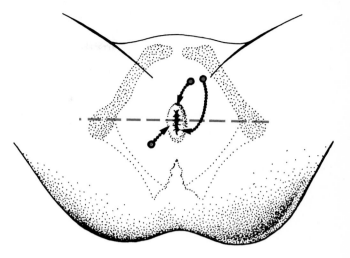

Figure 17-6

Salmon's law. Fissure location related to the aperture of the fistula. (Adapted from Dunphy JE and Botsford TW: Physical examination of the surgical patient: an introduction to clinical surgery, ed 4, Philadelphia, 1975, WB Saunders Co.)

Hemorrhoids

Hemorrhoids are dilated congested veins of the hemorrhoidal group. The swelling is associated with increased hydrostatic pressure in the portal venous system. The pressure associated with hemorrhoids correlates highly with pregnancy, straining at stool, chronic liver disease, and sudden increases in intra-abdominal pressure. Bowel habits also play a role in that hemorrhoids frequently occur with diarrhea or incomplete bowel emptying. Local factors such as abscess or tumor may also contribute to venous stasis.

Hemorrhoidal skin tags are ragged, flaccid, skin sacs located around the anus. These skin tags cover connective tissue sacs and are the locus of resolved external hemorrhoids. Clients describe these tags as painless. Internal hemorrhoids occur proximal to the pectinate line (see Fig. 17-5), whereas external hemorrhoids are those that are seen distal to this boundary. External hemorrhoids are covered by skin or anal squamous tissue.

External hemorrhoids are often accompanied by pain, particularly if the skin is stretched by a sudden increase in mass; since the mass is located near the sphincter muscles, spasm is not uncommon. External hemorrhoids often cause itching and bleeding on defecation. These dilated veins may not be apparent at rest but may appear as bluish, swollen areas at the anal verge when thrombosed. A thrombosed hemorrhoid is one in which blood has clotted, both within and outside the vein.

Internal hemorrhoids generally do not cause pain unless they are complicated by thrombosis, infection, or erosion of overlying mucosal surfaces. Discomfort is increased if the hemorrhoids prolapse through the anal opening. Bleeding may occur from the internal hemorrhoids with or without defecation. Proctoscopy is generally necessary for their identification.

Rectal Polyps

Rectal polyps, which feel like soft nodules, are encountered frequently. They may be pedunculated (on a stalk) or sessile (irregularly moundlike, growing from a relatively broad base, and closely adherent to the mucosal wall). Because of their soft consistency, they may be difficult or impossible to identify by palpation. Proctoscopy is usually necessary for identification, and a biopsy is performed to identify malignant lesions. A pedunculated rectal polyp occasionally prolapses through the anal ring.

Rectal Prolapse

Internal hemorrhoids are the type most commonly identified because of mucosal tissue prolapsing through the anal ring. The pink-colored mucosa is described as appearing like a doughnut or rosette. In the older client, however, protruding mucosa may herald eversion or prolapse of the rectum. Incomplete prolapse involves only mucosa, whereas complete rectal prolapse involves the sphincters.

The prolapse of tissue through the anal ring is described by the client as occurring on exercise or while straining at stool. Frequently, the client describes being able to push the mass back in with digital pressure. Inspection reveals a red, bulging, mucosal mass protruding through the anal ring.

Anal Incontinence

The loss of the voluntary ability to control defecation is called incontinence. The loss may range from the invol-

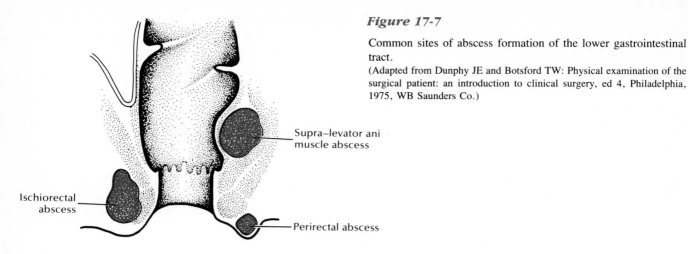

Figure 17-7

Common sites of abscess formation of the lower gastrointestinal tract.
(Adapted from Dunphy JE and Botsford TW: Physical examination of the surgical patient: an introduction to clinical surgery, ed 4, Philadelphia, 1975, WB Saunders Co.)

Supra–levator ani muscle abscess

Ischiorectal abscess

Perirectal abscess

Health History

Anus and Rectum

NOTE: A yes response to any question *must* be further investigated. Use the following indicators throughout the assessment: (1) onset (specific date, sudden or gradual), (2) duration, (3) frequency, (4) precipitating factors, (5) aggravating or alleviating factors, (6) treatment received, and (7) outcome.

Present status

1. Do you have rectal discomfort?
   a. Description: pain; burning; itching; swelling; associated with sitting, standing, walking, lying down; occurs with defecation
2. Do you have unusual stools?
   a. Description of consistency and color: hard, soft, semiformed, liquid, foamy, mucoid, fatty, bloody, tarry, black, yellow, grey
3. Do you have abdominal pain?
   a. Location
   b. Description: sharp, dull, cramping
   c. Associated symptoms: nausea, vomiting, flatus, abdominal distention
4. Do you have voluntary control of defecation?
   a. Limitations

Past history

1. Have you had changes in sleep or activity patterns?
   a. Description of change
2. Have you had alterations in bowel habits?
   a. Description: constipation, diarrhea, burning, straining, number of stools per day
3. Have you had a rectal infection?
   a. Type
   b. Associated symptoms: drainage
4. Have you had rectal bleeding?
   a. Color: black, tarry, bright red

5. Have you had rectal trauma?
   a. Description
6. Have you had rectal surgery?
   a. Description
   b. Residual effects

Associated conditions

1. Have you had gallbladder problems?
   a. Description
2. Are you on a special diet?
   a. Type: vegetarian, low or high meat, high or no milk, high or low fat
3. Are you on medication?
   a. Specific type

Family history

1. Do you have a family history of colorectal cancer or hemorrhoids?
2. Do you have a family history of malabsorption syndromes, ulcerative colitis, Chron's disease, or other forms of colitis?

Sample assessment record

Client states hemorrhoids were diagnosed several months ago. Continues to have rectal discomfort, itching, and small amounts of bright red blood in stools at times. States stools tend to be hard and sometimes grey. Denies abdominal pain and changes in sleep or activity patterns. No defecation control problems. Has frequent constipation and strains at stool. Has two to three stools per day. Denies rectal infection or trauma. Has no history of gallbladder problems. Is on a high fiber diet supplemented with prescribed stool softeners and drinks six to eight glasses of fluid per day. Negative family history for cancer, hemorrhoids, and colon disease or disorders.

untary passage of flatus to complete loss of sphincter tone. The loss of fecal gases or liquids may also occur in the presence of a normal sphincter in hyperdynamic bowel states.

Abscesses or Masses

Abscesses of the lower gastrointestinal tract that may be identified by physical examination (Fig. 17-7) include:

1. *Perirectal abscess:* This abscess may be palpated as a tender mass adjacent to the anal canal. The increased temperature of the mass may be helpful in identifying the inflammatory process.
2. *Ischiorectal abscess:* This abscess may be palpated as a tender mass protruding into the lateral wall of the anal canal.
3. *Supra–levator ani muscle abscess:* This abscess may be felt by the examining finger as a tender mass in the lateral rectal wall.

The presence of a mass in the rectum deserves special attention, since nearly half those discovered are malignant. The client frequently denies pain or other symptoms. Early lesions are felt as small elevations or nodules with a firm base. Ulceration of the center of the lesion results in a crater that may be palpated. An ulcerated carcinoma may be identified through palpation by its firm, nodular, rolled edge. The lesion of carcinoma is described by including annular or tubular shape, degree of fixation, and distance from the anus. The consistency of the malignant mass is often stony and hard, and the contour is irregular. Extension of metastatic carcinoma from the peritoneum to the pelvic floor is described as a rectal shelf. It is palpated as a hard, nodular ridge.

BIBLIOGRAPHY

Beahrs OH, Higgins GA, and Weinstein JJ, editors: Colorectal tumors, Philadelphia, 1986, JB Lippincott Co.

Corman ML: Colon and rectal surgery, ed 2, Philadelphia, 1984, JB Lippincott Co.

Cherry DA and Rothenberger DA: Pelvic floor physiology, Surg Clin North Am 68:1217-1230, 1988.

Fischbach FT: A manual of laboratory diagnostic tests, ed 10, Philadelphia, 1984, JB Lippincott Co.

Goldberg SM, Gordon PH, and Nivatvongs S: Essentials of anorectal surgery, Philadelphia, 1980, JB Lippincott Co.

Ger R: Surgical anatomy of the pelvis, Surg Clin North Am 68:1202-1216, 1988.

Goliger J: Surgery of the anus, rectum, and colon, London, 1984, Bailliere Tindall.

Gordon PH: The anorectum: anatomic and physiologic considerations in health and disease, Gastroenterol Clin North Am 16:1-15, 1987.

Kirsner JB and Shorter RG, editors: Diseases of the colon, rectum, and anal canal, Baltimore, 1988, Williams & Wilkins.

Kodner IJ, Fry RD, and Roe JP, editors: Colon, rectal, and anal surgery: current techniques and controversies, St Louis, 1985, The CV Mosby Co.

Localio SA, Eng K, and Coppa GF: Anorectal, presacral, and sacral tumors: anatomy, physiology, pathogenesis, and management, Philadelphia, 1987, WB Saunders Co.

Payne JE: Symptoms and the diagnosis of bowel cancer: a critical view, Med J Aust 148:505-507, 1988.

Raufman JP and Straus EW: Endoscopic procedures in the AIDS patient: Risks, precautions, indications, and obligations, Gastroenterol Clin North Am 17:495-506, 1988.

Spratt JS, editor: Neoplasms of the colon, rectum, and anus: mucosal and epithelial, Philadelphia, 1984, WB Saunders Co.

Schrock TR: Diseases of the anorectum. In Sleisenger MH and Fordtran JS, editors: Gastrointestinal disease, ed 4, Philadelphia, 1986, WB Saunders Co.

Stearns MW, editor: Neoplasms of the colon, rectum, and anus, New York, 1980, John Wiley & Sons.

18

Assessment of musculoskeletal system

OBJECTIVES

Upon successful review of this chapter, learners will be able to:

- Describe anatomy and physiology of the musculoskeletal system

- Outline history relevant to examination of the musculoskeletal system

- State related rationale and demonstrate assessment of the musculoskeletal system, including measurement, positioning, inspection, palpation, and tests of function

- Recognize usual findings and variations of
  Joint motion and angles
  Spinal contour and body alignment
  Muscle strength and tone
  Range of motion
  Gait

- Correlate body movements with associated muscles and motor nerves

- Describe procedures used to detect musculoskeletal abnormalities

- Recognize possible pathological conditions related to the musculoskeletal system

The skeletal system is made up of 206 bones and the joints by which they articulate. Bone, cartilage, and connective and hematopoietic (myeloid) tissues make up this system. These structures (1) provide support for the body, (2) allow movement as those muscles attached to the bones shorten in contraction (thereby pulling the bones), and (3) provide for the formation of red blood cells.

The musculoskeletal system is composed of more than 600 voluntary or striated muscles and constitutes the principal organ of movement as well as a repository for metabolites. The muscle mass accounts for as much as 40% of the weight of the adult man.

It is the partial contracture of skeletal muscle that makes all the characteristic postures of human beings possible, including the upright position that distinguishes the anthropoid.

The joint, with its synovial membrane, capsule, ligaments, and the muscles that cross it, is considered the functional unit of the musculoskeletal system. This discussion of musculoskeletal assessment assumes that the practitioner has an understanding of the anatomy and physiology of the joints involved.

The examination of neuromuscular coordination begins as the practitioner first meets and observes the client, and it continues as the client advances into the room, sits, rises from a sitting position, climbs onto the examining table, lies down, and rolls over. The practitioner should note the speed, coordination, and strength of motion and particularly note clumsy, awkward, or involuntary movements as well as tremor or fasciculation. An estimate of muscle strength may be gained from the

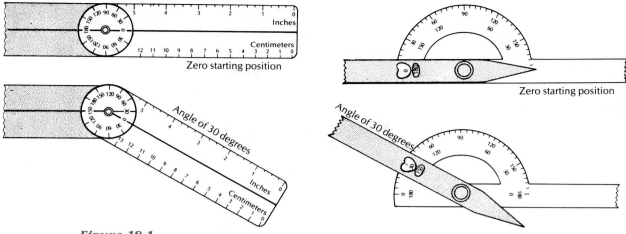

Figure 18-1

Goniometers used to measure joint motion. The extended anatomic position is accepted as zero degrees.
(From American Academy of Orthopaedic Surgeons Joint motion: method of measuring and recording, Chicago, 1965. The Academy.)

client's handshake. During the interview the flamboyance or paucity of gesture may provide valuable clues to the client's personality and general mobility.

The client's chief complaint may indicate the direction for emphasis of the physical assessment. The individual with a chief problem of bodily deformity, paralysis, weakness, or pain associated with movement causes the examiner to focus attention on the bones, joints, and muscles as the possible sites of disorder.

EQUIPMENT FOR MUSCULOSKELETAL ASSESSMENT

A cloth or metal tape measure that will not stretch and a *goniometer*—a protractor with movable arms that is used to measure the range of joint motion—are necessary for this examination (Fig. 18-1).

ASSESSMENT

The structure and function of the body's equipment for movement are explored essentially through the techniques of inspection and palpation of the joints and muscles, assessment of active and passive ranges of motion, and tests for muscle strength.

As in previously described assessments, the cephalocaudal (head to toe) organization for examination is used in examination of the bones, joints, and muscles. This organization provides order and aids in avoiding omissions. Side-to-side comparison is used as the basic criterion for assessment.

Thorough assessment of the musculoskeletal system can only be accomplished through the appropriate

---

Equipment

Nonstretchable tape measure
Goniometer
Examining table

Promote the Client's Comfort

Provide a warm room
Provide adequate lighting
Assist client to disrobe as needed
Protect the client's modesty
Explain each procedure before beginning
Provide short, clear instructions
Arrange for extra examination time for older or handicapped clients
Stabilize the joints during the examination by having the client sit or lie down
Properly sequence the examination to minimize position changes from sitting to lying

---

exposure of the client. The ambulatory individual can best be examined in shorts or swimming trunks. In this manner the extremities and spine are available for examination. Modesty may be protected for the female client by allowing her to wear a brassiere or some other abbreviated form of chest cover. An effort is made to protect the client's modesty, but a fully clothed client cannot be examined accurately.

Figure 18-2

The body is inspected, both anterior (**A**) and posterior (**B**) surfaces, for symmetry of contour and size, gross deformities, swelling, ecchymosis, or other discoloration.

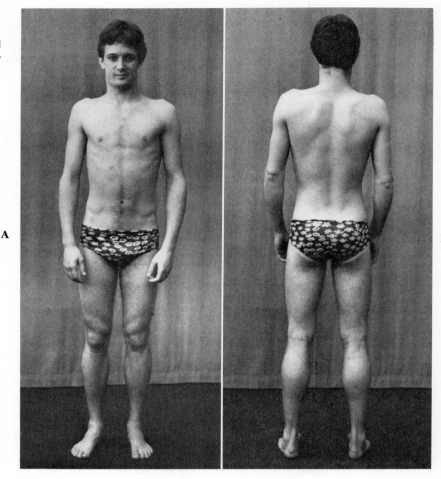

A   B

For each examination the client should be in the position that provides the greatest stability of joints.

General Inspection

General inspection of the musculoskeletal system includes a visual scanning for symmetry, contour, size, involuntary movement of the two sides of the body, gross deformities, areas of swelling or edema, and ecchymoses or other discoloration (Fig. 18-2).

The posture, or stance, and body alignment are viewed from both in front of and behind the client. The structural relationships of the feet to the legs and the hips to the pelvis are noted, as are those of the upper extremities, shoulder girdle, and upper trunk.

A deformity is an abnormality in appearance. *Varus* and *valgus* are terms used to describe an angular deviation from the normal structure of an extremity. The reference point is the midline of the body. Genu varum (bowlegs) is the lateral deviation of the leg from the midline (Fig. 18-3). Genu valgum (knock-knees) is deviation of the leg toward the midline (Fig. 18-4).

The shape of the spine is assessed, and its structural apposition to the shoulder girdle, thorax, and pelvis are ascertained. The normal spinal curvatures are concave at the cervical area, convex at the thoracic area, and concave at the lumbar area.

Scoliosis is a deformity of the spine seen as a lateral deviation (Fig. 18-5). This angling of the spine produces a downward slant of the thoracic cage on the affected side and an upward tilt of the pelvis on the contralateral side. A rotary deformity of the rib cage occurs as well. The ribs protrude posteriorly on the convex side of the spine. A hump or "razorback" may be observed. The protrusion may be made more obvious by asking the client to bend over to touch the toes. It is best observed from behind the client (Fig. 18-6).

Structural scoliosis, which is due to vertebral rotation, tends to become more prominent as the client bends forward. Functional scoliosis, which compensates for structural abnormalities other than those associated with the vertebral column, disappears when the client bends forward.

Kyphosis is a flexion deformity (Fig. 18-7, *B*). When the angle of the defect is sharp, the apex is called a gibbus.

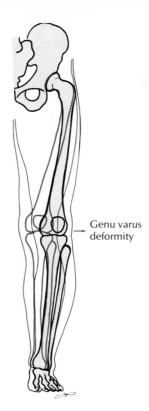

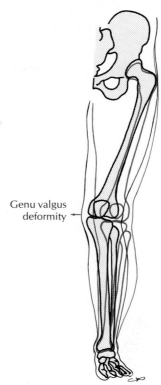

Genu varus
deformity

Genu valgus
deformity

Figure 18-3

Varus deformity of the leg: lateral deviation from the midline (bowleg). This condition was called valgus deformity in earlier times. Red outline figure shows normal position; black, the deformity.

Figure 18-4

Valgus deformity of the leg: deviation of the leg toward the midline (knock-knee). This condition was called varus deformity in earlier times. Red outline figure shows normal position; black, the deformity.

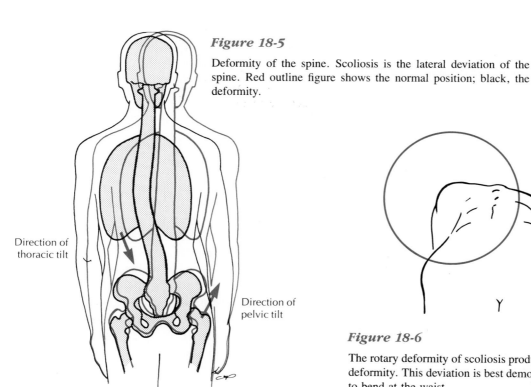

Figure 18-5

Deformity of the spine. Scoliosis is the lateral deviation of the spine. Red outline figure shows the normal position; black, the deformity.

Direction of
thoracic tilt

Direction of
pelvic tilt

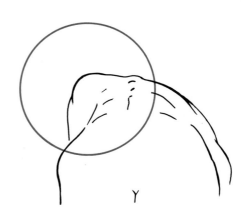

Figure 18-6

The rotary deformity of scoliosis produces a hump or "razor back" deformity. This deviation is best demonstrated by asking the client to bend at the waist.

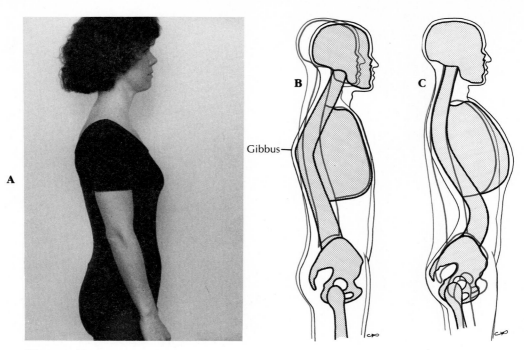

Figure 18-7

A, Normal curvature of the spine. **B,** Deformity of the spine. Kyphosis is flexion of the spine. When the angle of the defect is sharp, the apex is called a gibbus. **C,** Deformity of the spine. Lordosis (swayback) is extension of the spine. It is most commonly found in the lumbar area. Red outline figure shows the normal position; black, the deformity.

Lordosis (swayback) is an extension deviation of the spine commonly in the lumbar area (Fig. 18-7, *C*).

Measurement of the extremities

The musculoskeletal examination frequently includes the measurement of the extremities for length and circumference. Measurements of length are made to verify the symmetry of two limbs or to determine whether limbs are in normal range. The measurements are made with the client lying relaxed on a hard surface (examining table) with the pelvis level and the hips and knees fully extended and with both hips equally adducted. Frequently, apparent discrepancies in limb size are a result of position.

The length of the upper extremity is the distance from the tip of the acromion process to the tip of the middle finger; the shoulder is adducted and the other joints are at neutral zero (anatomic position—limb in extension). The length of the lower extremity is the distance from the lower edge of the anterosuperior iliac spine to the tibial malleolus (Table 18-1).

Measurement of muscle mass

The muscles are examined for gross hypertrophy or atrophy. Only in the markedly obese client are changes in

Table 18-1

Anatomic guideposts for measuring extremities

Area	From	To
Entire upper extremity	Tip of acromion process	Tip of middle finger
Upper arm	Tip of acromion process	Tip of olecranon process
Forearm	Tip of olecranon process	Styloid process of ulna
Entire lower extremity	Lower edge of antero-superior iliac spine	Tibial malleolus
Thigh	Lower edge of antero-superior iliac spine	Medial aspect of knee joint
Lower leg	Medial aspect of knee	Tibial malleolus

muscle mass difficult to assess. The difference in the firm, hypertrophic muscle of the athlete and the limp, atrophic muscle of the paralytic is obvious both on inspection and on palpation with the finger. Although muscle size is largely a function of the use or disuse of the muscle fibers, changes in the size of muscles may indicate disease. Malnutrition and lipodystrophy tend to reduce muscle size and markedly weaken the strength of contraction. Lack of neutral input resulting from lesions of the spinal cord or peripheral motor neuron may reduce muscle size by as much as 75% of the normal volume; this may occur over as short a time as 3 months. Measurements taken of limbs at their maximum circumference may provide a baseline for comparison when swelling or atrophy are suspected on in subsequent routine examination.

The limbs should be in the same position and the muscles in the same state of tension each time measurements are performed. Several corresponding points may be measured above and below the patella and olecranon process. Some clinics routinely measure at 10 cm below and at points 10 and 20 cm above the midpatella to provide uniformity. At any rate, a small diagram showing the points measured (Fig. 18-8) will obviate ambiguity. Differences in symmetry or of limb size at different times of less than 1 cm are not significant (Fig. 18-9).

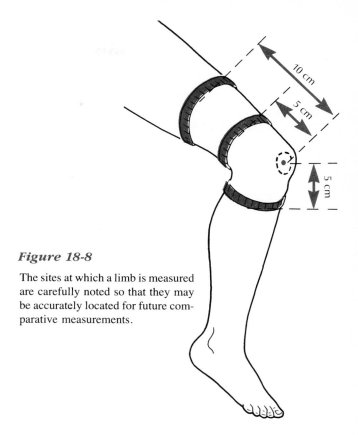

Figure 18-8

The sites at which a limb is measured are carefully noted so that they may be accurately located for future comparative measurements.

Assessment of Gait

Gait is evaluated in both phases—the stance and the swing—for rhythm and smoothness. *Stance* is considered to consist of three processes: (1) heel strike—the heel contacts the floor or ground; (2) midstance—body weight is transferred from the heel to the ball of the foot; and (3) push-off—the heel leaves the ground (see Chapter 7, General Assessment).

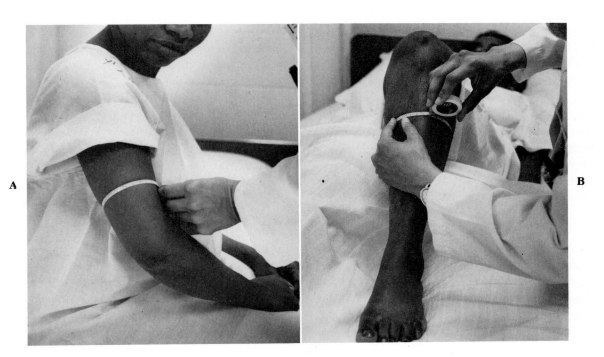

A

B

Figure 18-9

A, Measurement of upper mid-arm circumference. **B,** Measurement of mid-gastrocnemius circumference.

The *swing* phase also consists of three processes: (1) acceleration; (2) swing through—the lifted foot travels ahead of the weight-bearing foot; and (3) deceleration—the foot slows in preparation for the heel strike.

The description of the observation of the client's gait should include: *phase* (conformity); *cadence* (symmetry, regular rhythm); *stride length* (symmetry, length of swing); *trunk posture* (related to phases); *pelvic posture* (related to phases); and *arm swing* (symmetry, length of swing).

If pain is present, it should be described in relationship to the phases of gait.

Examination of Bones and Joints

Bones

Bones are examined for deformity or tumors. Bones are also examined for integrity by testing resistance to a deforming force. Palpation of the bone is performed to assess the presence of pain or tenderness. Tenderness of a bone may indicate tumor, inflammation, or the aftermath of a trauma. Frequently, traumatic injuries are associated with damage to both bone and nerve. Paralysis of the ulnar and median nerves in the hand is frequently the result of a hand injury and may result in a clawlike posture of the hand.

Joints

Signs and symptoms of disorders. Pain, swelling, partial or complete loss of mobility, stiffness, weakness, and fatigue are the signs and symptoms most frequently associated with disorders of the joints. Joint disease may be indicated by skin that feels warm, is red, has lesions, or is ulcerated. In the condition of psoriatic arthritis the lesions and the nails have been shown to be involved in about 50% of cases. Pitting is the most commonly recognized change. There may be isolated pitting of a single nail or the pitting may be *uniformly* distributed across the nails.

Pain. *Pain* is the symptom that most frequently causes the client to seek help, and understanding the character of the pain may be helpful in determining its cause in the physical assessment of the involved joints. The client should be encouraged to try to recall those events occurring before the onset of pain because most individuals tend to forget minor injuries or unusual physical activity in the weeks before the pain began. The client is unlikely to correlate symptoms and signs of infection in the months before with his current joint pain. The nature of the onset of pain is also important because rheumatoid symptoms are known to begin gradually, whereas gouty attacks are characterized by sudden onset that frequently wakes the client from sleep.

The client frequently has difficulty in localizing the pain associated with joint disease. His description may involve large areas of the body, that is, "my neck" (while moving the hand from the head to the thoracic vertebra), "my back," or "all down my arm." This difficulty in localizing the pain may be related to whether the pain is deep or superficial and whether a nerve is involved.

The locations or distribution of the pain may also provide valuable information. Rheumatoid involvement is known to be migratory, that is, involving first one joint, which improves, then another. On the other hand, most infectious arthritis is confined to one joint. The joint involvement in rheumatoid arthritis tends to be symmetric, whereas that of gout, psoriatic arthritis, and Reiter's syndrome tends to occur initially in one or two joints but becomes polyarticular in later stages. Spondylitis is first detected in the spine and then spreads to peripheral joints (centrifugal spread), whereas rheumatoid arthritis starts peripherally in the hands and feet and then involves the large joints of the hips, shoulders, and spine in the later stages of the disease (centripetal spread).

The time that pain occurs may also be diagnostic. The individual with osteoarthritis generally reports that the pain is made worse by increased use of the affected joint and, thus, frequently has pain later in the day or when tired. The individual with rheumatoid arthritis generally reports stiffness and pain that occurs early in the morning and some improvement when the part is exercised.

Questions directed to a description of referred pain may provide helpful. Spinal nerve root involvement is frequently felt in peripheral tissues. For instance, lumbosacral nerve root irritation (sciatica) may be experienced as pain in the thigh or the knee on the involved side. The area of referred pain corresponds with the segmental innervation of the structures. The description of this type of pain may include words associated with paresthesias, that is "prickling," "like an electric shock," "pins and needles," and "numbing." Pain of muscle origin may be described by such words as "pulled" or "charley horse." Joint pain descriptions may be noted along a spectrum from dull, aching, or stiff to excruciating and intolerable.

A knowledge of those measures known to alleviate the pain may also be valuable diagnostically. Some of these have already been discussed, for example, exercise for rheumatoid arthritis and rest for osteoarthritis.

Limitation of range of motion. The client may voluntarily limit the motion of a joint in response to pain. Spasm of the muscles involved in the movement of a joint may limit its motion. Mechanical obstruction to movement may accompany bony overgrowth and scar tissue. Limitation of motion in a joint is accompanied by weakness and atrophy of the muscles that are involved.

Decreased range of motion is observed in joints in which there is inflammation of surrounding tissues, arthritis, fibrosis, or bony fixation (ankylosis).

Deformity. Deformities of the joint include absorption of tissues, flexion contracture, and bony overgrowth. Absorption may produce a flail joint such that the bones making the joint move erratically. Deformities result from scarring phenomena following inflammation and infection.

Swelling. The amount of swelling of the joint may range from difficult to detect to visually evident fluid within the joint, that is, visible or palpable as a bulging of the joint capsule. Pressure on the sac at one point causes the fluid within to shift and may lead to bulging at another site. The sac may feel from soft to tense, and the involvement may be symmetric or unilateral. Frequently, the swelling is fusiform. Redness, warmth, swelling, and pain in a joint are the classic descriptors of an inflammatory process. The inflammation may be within the joint itself or in the soft tissue surrounding it. Swelling may also result from intra-articular effusion, synovial thickening, or bony overgrowth. The swelling may also result from the deposition of fat in the region adjacent to the joint.

The synovial membrane is not palpable in normal joints. The palpation of a "boggy" or "doughy" consistency generally indicates a thickened or otherwise abnormal synovial membrane.

Heberden's or Bouchard's nodes of the fingers or bony spurs, particularly in the knees, are typical of osteoarthritis.

Tenderness. Inflammatory processes cause joints to be tender. Arthritis, tendonitis, bursitis, and osteomyelitis are associated with tenderness in and around a joint. An attempt should be made to determine the anatomic structure that is tender.

Increased temperature. Heat over a joint indicates inflammation and suggests rheumatoid arthritis. Symmetric comparison of joints for temperature is indicated when one joint is hot. The backs of the fingers are used when comparing temperature.

Redness. Vasodilation or inflammation is noted in the skin overlying a tender joint affected by septic arthritis and gouty arthritis.

Crepitation. Crepitation (crackling or grating sounds) produced by motion of the joint is caused by irregularities of the articulating surfaces. The coarseness of surface may involve the cartilage or the bony capsule.

Inspection and palpation

A systematic assessment of individual joints may be made during the performance of the head to toe physical examination, or all the joints may be examined at a pre-

---

Inspection

Inspect the joints before proceeding with palpation to note areas that should be treated with caution. Record:
- Swelling
- Redness
- Deformity
- Subcutaneous nodules
- Tumors

Palpation

Ask the patient whether the joint is painful or tender before palpating. Palpate painful and tender joints lightly. Record:
- Pain
- Tenderness
- Swelling
- Increased temperature
- Crepitation

---

selected time during the examination. As with all bilateral structures, the paired joints should be compared.

The sequence for performing the examination of the joints is inspection, palpation, range of active motion, range of passive motion, and muscle strength testing. The examiner may use this sequence in a coordinated examination of each joint.

The assessment begins with inspection of the joint for swelling, redness, deformity, subcutaneous nodules, or tumors. Presence of any observed abnormalities guides the examiner in palpation. Joints are palpated for the presence of pain, tenderness, swelling, increased temperature, and crepitation. Painful and tender joints are palpated lightly.

The joints that are given special consideration are the temporomandibular, sternoclavicular, manubriosternal, shoulder, elbow, wrist, hip, knee, and ankle.

Temporomandibular joint. The temporomandibular joint is the articulation between the mandible and the temporal bone (Fig. 18-10). The joint is divided into two cavities as a fibrocartilaginous disk. Swelling is observed as a tumescence over the joint but must be considerable to be visible. Palpation is accomplished by placing the fingertips anterior to the external meatus of the ear. In the normal joint, there is a depression over the joint. Swelling may make this indentation difficult to feel. The jaw is palpated while it is moved through its range of motion: opening and closure of the mouth, protrusion (jutting of the jaw), retrusion (tucking in of chin), and side-to-side sliding of the mandible. The normal range of distance between the upper and lower incisors is 3 to 6 cm. Lateral motion of the jaw may be measured by asking the client to protrude the jaw and move it from side to side. The distance is measured by the distance that the midline of the lower lip deviates in each direction. The normal range of motion is 1 to 2 cm (Fig. 18-11). "Clicks" may be heard on movement and may be regarded as normal.

Sternoclavicular joint. The sternoclavicular joint is located at the juncture of the clavicle and the manubrium of the sternum. The joint is divided into two synovial cavities by a disk of cartilage and fibrous material. The joint is reinforced by a fibrous capsule and

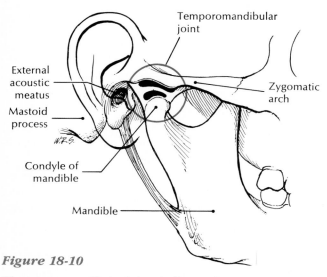

Figure 18-10

The temporomandibular joint. A fibrocartilaginous disk divides the articulation point into two synovial cavities. Note the proximity to external acoustic meatus.

ligaments (Fig. 18-12). The obtuse angle formed by the junction of the manubrium and body of the sternum is called the angle of Louis and has been used as a landmark for counting the ribs. Observation of this joint is readily accomplished because there is little tissue overlying it. Swelling, redness, bony overgrowth, and dislocation are not difficult to see. Swelling of the joint appears as a smooth, round bulge. Although this joint is often overlooked, it is often involved following surgery of the neck. Palpation is done with the fingertips. Movements of the shoulder depend on the normal function of this joint. Inflammation of the sternoclavicular joint may result in pain on movement of the shoulder girdle.

Manubriosternal joint. The hyaline cartilage–lined joint covers the articular surface of the second rib and those of the manubrium and body of the sternum (see Fig. 18-12). Little tissue overlies this joint. Observation is the only technique of examination because movement of the joint is minimal.

Shoulder joint (glenohumoral). The shoulder joint is a ball-and-socket joint that is the articulation of the humerus and the glenoid fossa of the scapula (Fig. 18-13). Protection of the joint is afforded by muscles and ligaments. A fibrous capsule surrounds the joint completely. Overlying these structures is the subacromial bursa. The portion of the bursa that lies beneath the deltoid is called the subdeltoid bursa. The clavicle and the acromion process of the scapula are articulated by the acromioclavicular joint. Inspection may reveal anterior dislocation of the shoulder as flattening of the lateral

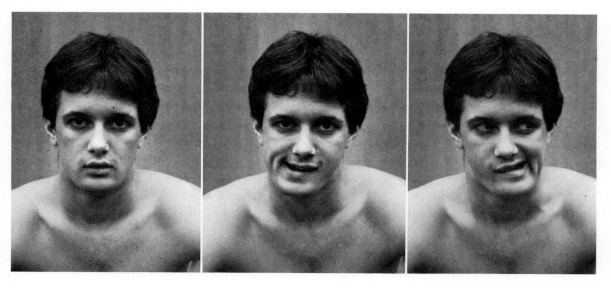

Figure 18-11

Lateral motion is determined by asking the client to move the lower jaw from side to side. The distance measured is the distance the midline of the lower lip deviates in each direction. The midline of the stationary upper lip may be used as the baseline.

aspect of the shoulder. Swelling of the joint as a result of fluid collection may be observed only when the amount of fluid is moderate to large. Visible swelling is generally observed over the anterior aspect of the shoulder. Palpation should include the joint and bursal sites. In the event that neoplasia or infection is suspected, the axilla

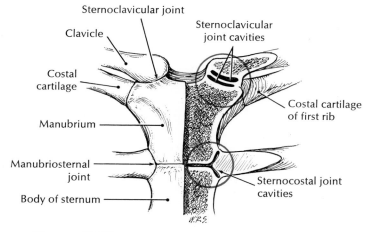

Figure 18-12

The sternoclavicular joint is divided into two synovial cavities. Movement of the shoulder girdle may cause pain when these joints are diseased. The manubriosternal joint examination is largely by inspection and palpation, since these joints move minimally.

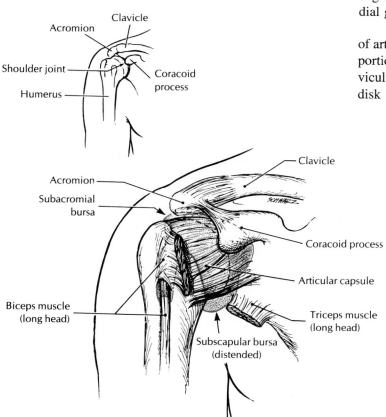

is palpated for lymph nodes. Special attention is also given to the tendons of the teres minor and infraspinatus muscles (called the rotator cuff). These tendons are palpated for swelling, nodes, tears, and pain. The client is instructed to adduct the arm by bringing it over the chest. The examiner, standing in front of the client, puts the thumb on the anterior surface of the joint and the tips of the fingers on the posterior aspect. The client is asked to move the humerus backward about 20 degrees. Moving behind the client and with the fingertips over the head of the humerus, the examiner asks the client to move the arm behind the body (internal rotation) with the hand between the scapulae.

Elbow joint. The elbow is the articulation of the humerus, radius, and ulna (Fig. 18-14). The three articulating surfaces are enclosed in a single synovial cavity. The synovial membrane is generally only palpable on the posterior aspect of the joint. Radial and ulnar ligaments provide protection to the joint. The olecranon bursa is the largest bursa of the elbow, although several smaller bursae are present. Swelling and redness are easily observed over the posterior aspect of the elbow. Palpation is accomplished with the tips of the fingers while applying pressure on the opposite side of the joint with the thumb of the dominant hand and while supporting the arm with the other. The client's arm is flexed 70 degrees. Joint swelling is most often palpable in the medial groove (Fig. 18-15).

Wrist joint. The wrist joint contains the points of articularion between the distal radius and the proximal portions of the following carpal bones: scaphoid or navicular, lunate, and triangular (Fig. 18-16). An articular disk divides the radius from the ulnar bone and also

Figure 18-13

The shoulder joint.

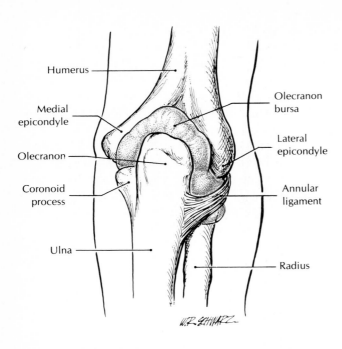

Figure 18-14

The elbow joint, posterior view.

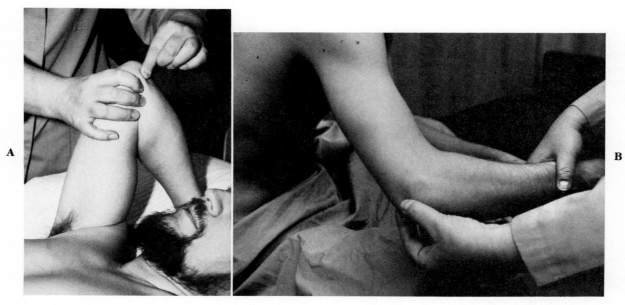

Figure 18-15

A, Examination of the extensor surface of the elbow joint in the supine position. **B,** Examination of the extensor surface of the elbow joint in the sitting position.

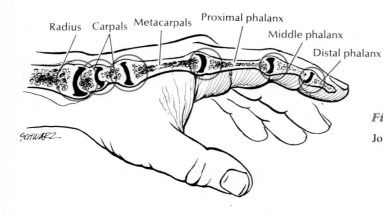

Figure 18-16

Joints articulating the bones of the wrist and hand.

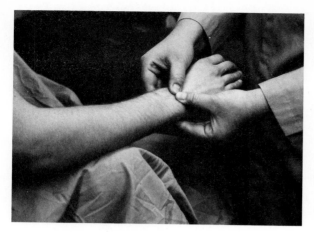

Figure 18-17

Examination of the wrist.

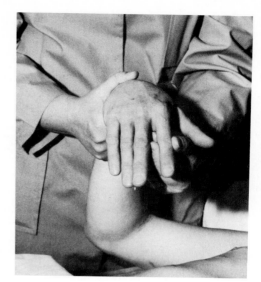

Figure 18-18

Palpation of the joints of the finger.

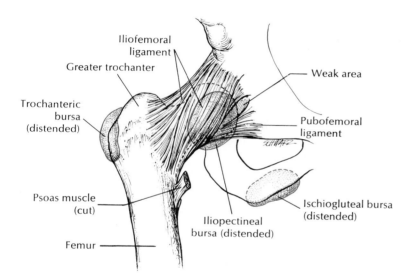

Iliofemoral ligament

Greater trochanter

Weak area

Trochanteric bursa (distended)

Pubofemoral ligament

Psoas muscle (cut)

Ischiogluteal bursa (distended)

Iliopectineal bursa (distended)

Femur

Figure 18-19

The hip joint.

separates the radius from the wrist joint. The wrist joint is protected by a fibrous capsule and ligaments. The joint is lined by synovial membrane. Swelling of the wrist joint is most frequently observed on the dorsal surface distal to the ulnar tip. Two hands for palpation are used such that the thumb and index fingers are opposed on either side of the wrist. Enough pressure is applied to outline bony and soft tissue structures (Fig. 18-17).

Carpal, metacarpal, and phalangeal joints. The joints between the carpal, metacarpal, and phalangeal bones are also examined by observation and palpation. Swelling is easily observed over the dorsal surface of the hand because there is little tissue over the joints. The thumb and index fingers are used to palpate the entire perimeter of each of these joints (Fig. 18-18).

Thickening of the flexor tendon sheath (seen in carpal tunnel syndrome) of the median nerve may lead to feelings of numbness and paresthesia. The thickness

of the sheath may be observed on the palmar surface of the wrist. In addition, tests may elicit these altered sensory phenomena. In the first of these tests, the client is asked to maintain palmar flexion for 1 minute. The experience of numbness and paresthesia over the palmar surface of the hand and the first three fingers and part of the fourth is called Phalen's sign. The symptoms resolve quickly after the hand is returned to the resting position. The second test consists of tapping over the median nerve (palmar aspect of wrist). The client's sensation of tingling or prickling is known as Tinel's sign.

Hip joint. The hip joint is the articulation of the acetabulum and the femur (Fig. 18-19). It is a ball-and-socket joint, protected by a fibrous capsule and ligaments. Three bursae reduce friction in the hip: (1) the trochanteric, between the posterolateral greater trochanter and the gluteus maximus; (2) the ileopectineal, between the anterior surface of the joint and the iliopsoas muscle;

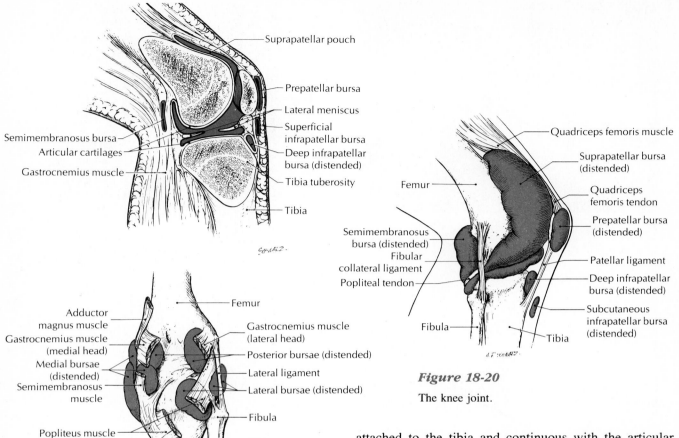

Figure 18-20

The knee joint.

and (3) the ischiogluteal, situated over the ischial tuberosity. Inspection of the hip joint includes an assessment of gait. Antalgic limp is characteristic of disease that produces pain in a hip joint. Antalgic limp is seen as a body tilt toward the involved diseased hip such that the weight of the body is directly over the hip. This decreases the need for abductor muscle movement and thus may decrease muscle spasm. If the abductor muscles are weak, that is, unable to support the pelvis, the unaffected hip may move downward such that the weight is borne on that side. This is called Trendelenburg's limp.

The synovial cavity of the hip is generally not palpated, even with it is distended. The bursae are not palpable unless they are swollen. Swelling and tenderness are the diagnostic findings of pathologic conditions of these structures.

Knee joint. The knee joint is the articulation of the femur, tibia, and patella (Fig. 18-20). The lining of the joint is a fibrous membrane. Synovial membrane covers the articular surface of the femur and tibia with folds to the patella. The medial and lateral menisci are fibrocartilaginous disks whose outside edges (horns) are

attached to the tibia and continuous with the articular capsule. The medial convexity of the femur rotates with the inner portion of the meniscus attached to it. A spiral distortion of the menisci occurs on rotation, making them susceptible to rupture. The surfaces of the menisci have no synovial membrane. They are thought to aid the spread of synovial fluid, and this may account for their existence. An anterior pouch in the knee joint that separates the patella and quadriceps tendon and muscle from the femur is called the suprapatellar pouch.

The bursae of the knee are numerous. On the anterior knee the prepatellar bursa lies immediately in front of the patella. The superficial infrapatellar bursa lies anterior to the patellar ligament, while the deep infrapatellar bursa is behind the ligament. Those of the posterior knee include the two gastrocnemius bursae, one of which separates the lateral head of the gastrocneminus muscle from the articular capsule and the other of which separates the medial head of the gastrocnemius muscle from the articular capsule. In addition, there is a large bursa separating the medial head of the gastrocnemius muscle from the semimembranosus muscle.

Inspection of the knee should be made with the client walking (to observe gait), sitting, and supine with knees extended. The examiner should be familiar with the normal contour of the knee, because loss of the con-

Figure 18-21

A, Knee effusion. **B,** Examination of the suprapatellar pouch.

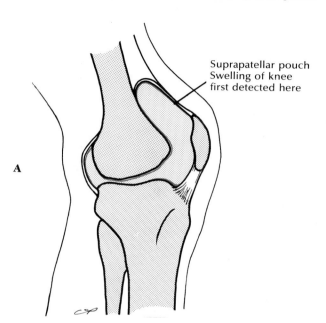

Suprapatellar pouch
Swelling of knee
first detected here

A

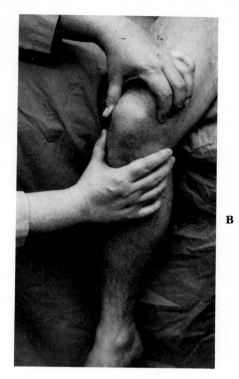

B

tour may occur with swelling. The client may voluntarily maintain the knee at 15 to 20 degrees of flexion because the knee joint is at maximum capacity at this angle, and thus pain is reduced. Swelling as a result of synovitis is most apparent at the suprapatellar pouch. Swelling as a result of meniscal cysts is observed at the lateral or the medial joint surface. Popliteal swelling is more obvious when the knee is extended. Swelling of the knee observed on the anterior aspect of the knee is called "housemaid's knee."

Palpation of the knee may be performed with the client in the sitting or supine position, whichever affords more comfort for the client. Palpation of the suprapatellar pouch (Fig. 18-21) is accomplished with the thumb and fingers of one hand while the other hand is used to push the contents of the articular cavity upward. To do this the thumb is placed on the lateral surface of the joint to the patella with fingers on the other lateral surface such that the arch formed by the thumb and fingers is below the patella. An inward and upward pressure thus applied moves fluid upward into the suprapatellar bursa. The examining hand is placed about 10 cm above the patella and moves gradually to the patella.

A second procedure for the palpation of the knee (Fig. 18-22) involves applying downward pressure over the suprapatellar pouch to localize the synovial fluid in the lower portion of the articular cavity. The other hand is used to palpate the lateral and medial joint surfaces with the fingers while steadying with the thumb. In in-

stances when considerable fluid is in the suprapatellar pouch, ballottement of the patella may be possible (Fig. 18-23). Ballottement is accomplished by applying downward pressure with one hand while the patella is pushed backward against the femur with a finger of the opposite hand. The popliteal region may be examined with the client in the prone position or standing. Swelling of the joint in the popliteal region is called Baker's cyst and is generally an extension of the articular cavity.

Sprains or tears of the ligaments are the most common injuries of the knee. Two sets of ligaments play a role in movement of the knee. They are the anterior and posterior cruciate ligaments and medial and lateral collateral ligaments. The anterior cruciate ligament limits extension and rotation, while the posterior stabilizes the femur against forward dislocation. The collateral ligaments prevent lateral dislocation of the knee. Abnormal movements of the knee may indicate dislocation. The tears may be palpated in the assessment of the knee.

Indications of pathologic conditions of menisci include (1) pain or tenderness on the lateral surfaces of the knee joint; (2) popping, snapping, or grating sounds with movement; and (3) inability to fully extend the knee. The medial meniscus is more often injured than the lateral.

Tests for a foreign body in the knee. An attempt is made to elicit *Apley's sign* (Fig. 18-24) in the client who is suspected of having a loose object in the knee joint or who has given a history of knee joint locking. The

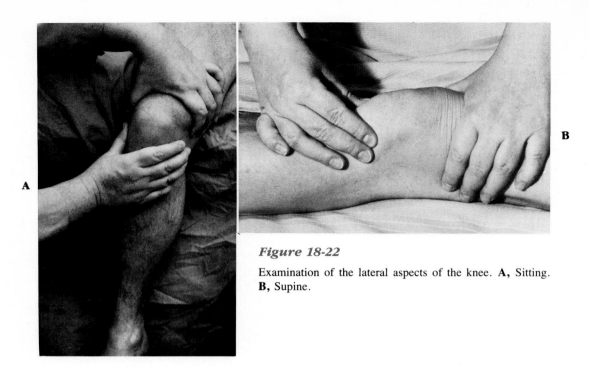

Figure 18-22

Examination of the lateral aspects of the knee. **A,** Sitting. **B,** Supine.

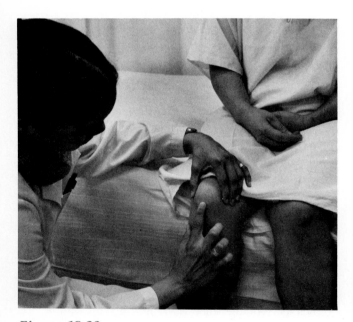

Figure 18-23

Ballottement of the patella.

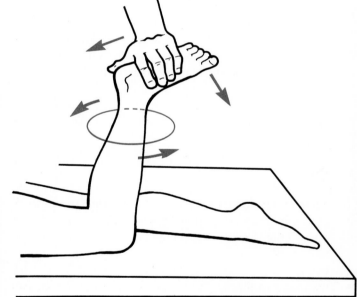

Figure 18-24

Elicitation of Apley's sign.

client assumes the prone positon with the suspected knee flexed to 90 degrees. The tibia is firmly opposed to the femur by exerting downward pressure on the foot. The leg is rotated externally and internally. Locking of the knee (positive sign) or the sound of clicks may indicate that a loose body, such as torn cartilage, is trapped in the articulation. Clicks or popping sounds are generated as the object escapes.

An attempt is made to elicit *McMurray's sign* (Fig. 18-25) in the individual who says he "feels something in the knee joint" or complains that "sometimes it just won't bend." The test may be performed with the client in the sitting position and while obtaining as much flexion of the suspected knee as possible. The leg is internally rotated while it is slowly being extended with one hand. The other hand is used to provide resistance at the medial aspect of

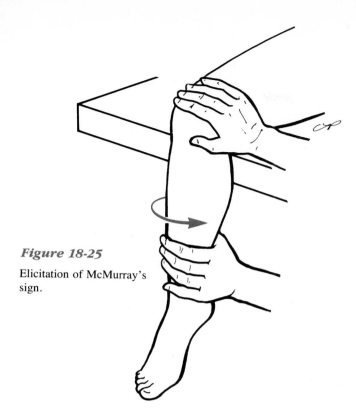

Figure 18-25

Elicitation of McMurray's
sign.

the knee. Extension of the knee may not be possible (positive
sign) if a loose body impedes its movement. The procedure
may be repeated employing external rotation and resistance
applied to the lateral aspect of the knee.

Ankle and foot joints.   The ankle joint is the
articulation between the tibia, fibula, and the talus (Fig.
18-26). The capsule is lined with synovia. The ankle
joint is protected by ligaments on the medial and lateral
surfaces but not on the anterior or posterior surfaces.

Talocalcaneal joint.   The joint between the
talus and calcaneus bones is called the talocalcaneal or sub-
talar joint. The forward extension of the joint cavity is the
articulation of the talus and the navicular bones. Articular
capsules lined with synovial membrane separate the remainder of the tarsal, metatarsal, and phalangeal bones of
the foot.

Inspection of the ankle and foot is made with the
client standing, walking, and sitting (not bearing weight).
Swelling is best observed over the dorsal aspect of the foot
because there is less tissue over the bone. Hallux valgus is
lateral deformity of the great toe such that it may lie above
or below the second toe. The metatarsophalangeal joint is
distorted in such a way that the first metatarsal bone is angled
medially. A callus or bursal distention generally occurs at
the joint. Hammer toe is a result of hyperextension of the
metatarsophalangeal joint and flexion of the proximal phalangeal joint (fig. 18-27).

Palpation of the ankle and foot is best accomplished with the fingertips of one hand while holding the

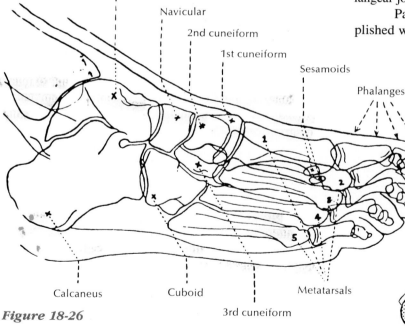

Figure 18-26

Bones of the ankle and foot.
(From Mann RA: DuVries' surgery of the foot, ed 5, St Louis, 1984,
The CV Mosby Co.)

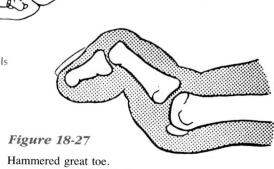

Figure 18-27

Hammered great toe.
(From Mann RA: DuVries's surgery of the foot, ed 5, St Louis, 1984,
The CV Mosby Co.)

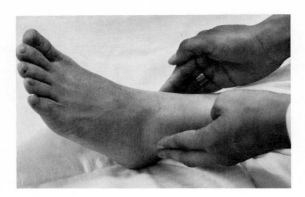

Figure 18-28

Examination of the ankle joint.

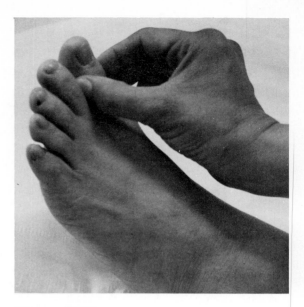

Figure 18-29

Examination of the joint of the toe.

foot behind the ankle with the other (Fig. 18-28). The metatarsal and phalangeal joints are palpated with the fingers on the anterior surface and the thumb on the sole surface (Fig. 18-29).

Results of examination of these joints may be conveniently summarized on a diagram by circling the joint involved (Fig. 18-30) and briefly noting any pathologic condition.

Straight leg–raising test. The straight leg–raising test (Fig. 18-31) is useful in defining herniated lumbar disk as the cause of sciatic nerve pain. The test is indicated for those individuals who complain of low back pain or of pain that radiates down the leg. The test is performed with the client lying on his back on a firm surface. The leg and thigh should be as relaxed as possible. The extended leg is raised behind the heel maintaining the heel and the foot in dorsiflexion until the client complains of pain. The foot is then dorsiflexed. Pain induced in this manner is caused by pressure on the dorsal roots of the lumbosacral nerves and is characteristic of herniated disk. The other leg is treated similarly, and results are compared. In the normal person, the leg may be flexed to 90 degrees without pain. Nerve root irritation is suggested by pain in lumbar, hip, or posterior leg or by muscle spasm.

In flexion of the hip in the normal individual the lumbar spine flattens in the lumbar region. For the individual with an immobile hip, continued flexion of the lumbar spine is seen when the leg is raised. Extending the leg stretches the ligaments and extensor muscles of the hip. Pain may indicate a pathologic condition in these structures.

Measurement of the range of joint motion

A standardized method for measuring and recording joint motion has been published by the American Academy of

Orthopaedic Surgeons (1965) (Table 18-2). The range of motion is described in degrees of deviation from a defined neutral zero point for each joint. The position of neutral zero is that of the extended extremity or anatomic position.

Seven types of joint motion have been defined: flexion, extension, abduction, adduction, internal rotation, external rotation, and circumduction (Figs. 18-32 to 18-35).

Flexion is the bending of the joint to approximate the bones it connects, thereby decreasing the joint angle. *Extension* is the straightening of a limb so that the joint angle is increased, the placement of the distal segment of a limb in such a position that its axis is continuous with that of the proximal segment, or the pulling or dragging force exerted on a limb in a direction away from the body.

Abduction is the movement of a limb away from the midline of the body or one of its parts. *Adduction* is the movement of a limb toward the central axis of the body or beyond it.

Internal rotation is the turning of the body part inward toward the central axis of the body. *External rotation* is the turning of the body part away from the midline.

Circumduction is the movement of a body part in a circular pattern. This is not a singular motion but a combination of the other motions.

Muscles are categorized according to the type of joint movement produced by their contraction. Muscles,

Text continued on p. 424.

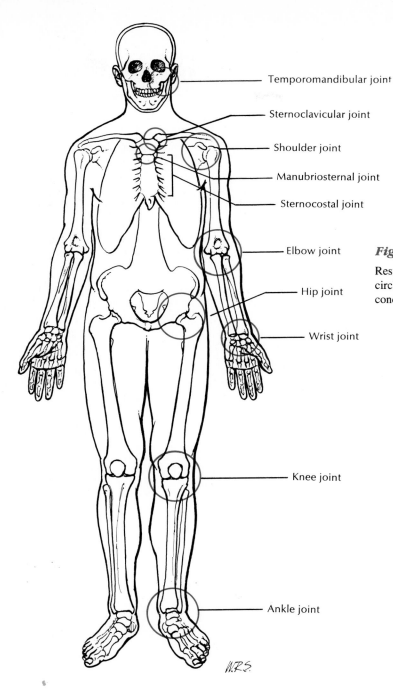

Temporomandibular joint

Sternoclavicular joint

Shoulder joint

Manubriosternal joint

Sternocostal joint

Elbow joint

Hip joint

Wrist joint

Knee joint

Ankle joint

Figure 18-30

Results of the examination of joints may be summarized by circling the joint involved and briefly noting the pathologic condition.

Figure 18-31

Straight leg-raising test.

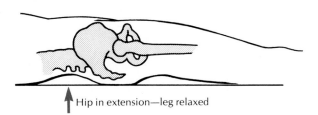

Hip in extension—leg relaxed

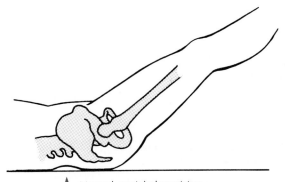

Normal, straight leg raising flattens the lumbar spine

Table 18-2

Testing for range of joint motion

Neck

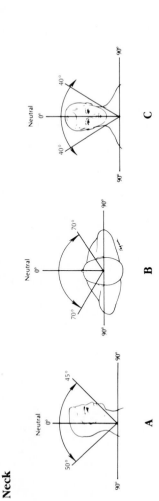

A B C

Figure 1

Range of motion of the cervical spine. **A**, Flexion and extension. These motions are usually designated by degrees, but the examiner may indicate the distance the chin lacks from touching the chest. **B**, Rotation. This is estimated in degrees from the neutral position or in percentages of motion, as compared to individuals of similar age and physical build. **C**, Lateral bend. This motion is also measured in degrees but can be indicated by the number of inches the ear lacks from reaching the shoulder.

From American Academy of Orthopaedic Surgeons: Joint motion: method of measuring and recording, Chicago, 1965, The Academy.

Trunk

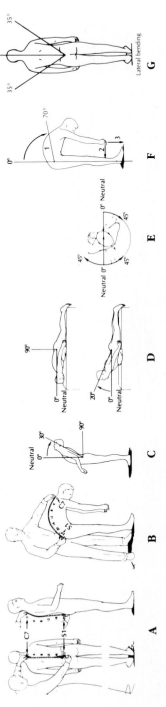

A B C D E F G

Figure 2

Range of motion of the spine. **A** and **B**, Steel tape measure method. This is perhaps the most accurate clinical method of measuring true motion of the spine in flexion. The flexible steel or plastic tape adjusts very accurately to the thoracic and lumbar contours of the spine. **A**, With the client standing, the 1-in marker of the tape is held over the spinous process C7 and the distal tape over the spinous process S1. **B**, As the client bends forward, if the lumbar curve reverses and the spinous processes spread, this will be indicated by lengthening of the measured distance from C7 to S1. In the normal healthy adult there is an average increase of 4 in in forward flexion. If the client bends forward with the back straight (as in rheumatoid spondylitis), the tape will not record motion. The examiner can record motion of the thoracic spine per se by measuring from the spinous process C7 to the spinous process T12. Likewise, motion of the lumbar spine can be measured from T12 to S1. Usually, if the total spine lengthening in flexion is 4 in, the examiner will find that 1 in occurs in the dorsal spine and 3 in occur in the lumbar spine. **C**, Client standing (extension). **D**, Client lying prone (extension). **E**, Rotation of spine. **F**, Client bending forward (flexion). *1*, Degrees of inclination of trunk (note reversal of lumbar curve) **G**, Client standing (lateral bending).

From American Academy of Orthopaedic Surgeons: Joint motion: method of measuring and recording, Chicago, 1965, The Academy.

Shoulder

Figure 3

Range of motion of the arm at the shoulder. **A,** Forward flexion (or forward elevation) and backward extension. *Forward flexion* is the forward upward motion of the arm in the anterior sagittal plane of the body from zero to 180 degrees. The opposite motion to the zero position may be termed "depression" of the arm. *Backward extension* is the upward motion of the arm in the posterior sagittal plane of the body from zero to approximately 60 degrees. **B,** Horizontal flexion and horizontal extension. *Horizontal flexion* is the motion of the arm in the horizontal plane anterior to the coronal plane across the body. This motion is measured from zero to approximately 130 or 135 degrees. *Horizontal extension* is the horizontal motion posterior to the coronal plane of the body. **C,** Abduction and adduction. *Abduction* is the upward motion of the arm away from the side of the body in the corneal plane from zero to 180 degrees. *Adduction* is the opposite motion of the arm toward the midline of the body or beyond it in an upward plane from zero to 50 degrees.
From American Academy of Orthopaedic Surgeons: Joint motion: method of measuring and recording, Chicago, 1965, The Academy.

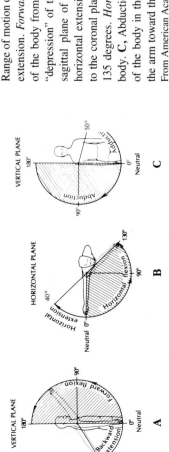

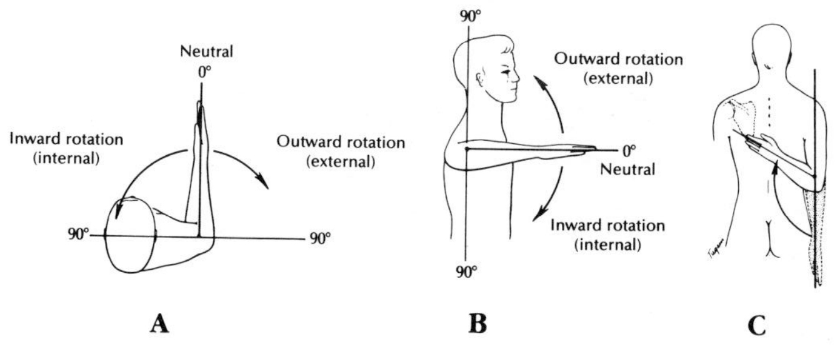

Figure 4

Rotation of the shoulder. **A,** Rotation with arm at side of body. Inward and outward rotation is recorded in degrees of motion from the neutral starting point. **B,** Rotation in abduction. Rotation in this position is less than with the arm at the side of the body. It is recorded in degrees of motion from the zero starting point. **C,** Internal rotation posteriorly. A clinical method of estimating function is the distance the fingertips reach in relation to the scapula or the base of the neck.
From American Academy of Orthopaedic Surgeons: Joint motion: method of measuring and recording, Chicago, 1965, The Academy.

Figure 5

Range of motion of the shoulder girdle. **A,** Flexion and extension. Forward flexion and backward extension of the shoulder girdle are measured in degrees from the neutral starting position. This is primary motion of the scapula and the clavicle. **B,** Elevation and depression. Upward motion of the shoulder girdle in elevation is measured in degrees. The opposite downward motion may be described as "depression" of the shoulder. Rotatory motion in the shoulder girdle is possible but cannot be accurately measured. It can be estimated in percentage of motion compared with individuals of similar age and physique.
From American Academy of Orthopaedic Surgeons: Joint motion: method of measuring and recording, Chicago, 1965, The Academy.

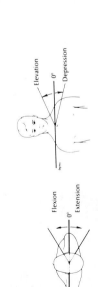

Continued.

Table 18-2

Testing for range of joint motion—cont'd

Elbow

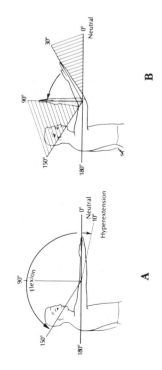

A

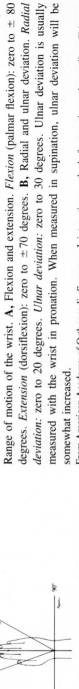

B

Figure 6

Range of motion of the elbow. **A**, Flexion and hyperextension. *Flexion:* zero to 150 degrees. *Extension:* 150 degrees to zero (from the angle of greatest flexion to the zero position). *Hyper-extension:* measured in degrees beyond the zero starting point. This motion is not present in all individuals. When it is present, it may vary from 5 to 15 degrees. **B**, Measurement of limited motion. (The unshaded area indicates the range of limited motion.) Limited motion may be expressed in the following ways: (1) the elbow flexes from 30 to 90 degrees (30° → 90°); (2) the elbow has a flexion deformity of 30 degrees with further flexion to 90 degrees.

From American Academy of Orthopaedic Surgeons: Joint motion: method of measuring and recording, Chicago, 1965, The Academy.

Forearm

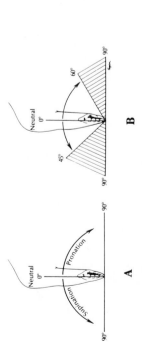

A

B

Figure 7

Range of motion of the forearm (elbow and wrist). **A**, Pronation and supination. *Pronation:* zero to 80 or 90 degrees. *Supination:* zero to 80 or 90 degrees. *Total forearm motion:* 160 to 180 degrees. Individuals may vary in the range of supination and pronation. Some individuals may reach the 90-degree arc, whereas others may have only 70 degrees plus. **B**, Limited motion. *Supination:* 45 degrees (0 → 45°). *Pronation:* 60 degrees (0 → 60°). *Total joint motion:* 105 degrees.

From American Academy of Orthopaedic Surgeons: Joint motion: method of measuring and recording, Chicago, 1965, The Academy.

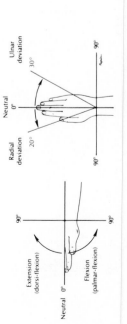

A

B

Figure 8

Range of motion of the wrist. **A**, Flexion and extension. *Flexion* (palmar flexion): zero to ± 80 degrees. *Extension* (dorsiflexion): zero to ± 70 degrees. **B**, Radial and ulnar deviation. *Radial deviation:* zero to 20 degrees. *Ulnar deviation:* zero to 30 degrees. Ulnar deviation is usually measured with the wrist in pronation. When measured in supination, ulnar deviation will be somewhat increased.

From American Academy of Orthopaedic Surgeons: Joint motion: method of measuring and recording, Chicago, 1965, The Academy.

Thumb

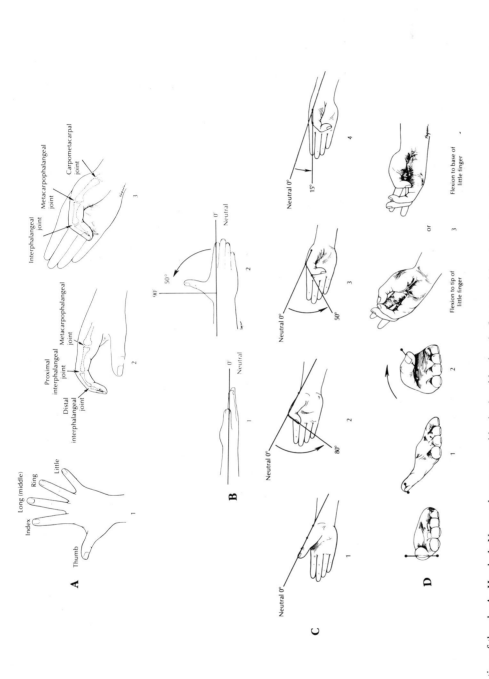

Continued.

Figure 9

Hand and range of motion of thumb. **A,** Hand. *1,* Nomenclature: to avoid mistaken identity, the fingers and thumb are referred to by name rather than by number. Anatomic nomenclature is used for joints of the fingers and thumbs. *2,* Joints of the fingers. *3,* Joints of the thumb. **B,** Abduction. *1,* Zero starting position: the extended thumb alongside the index finger, which is in line with the radius. *Abduction* is the angle created between the metacarpal bones of the thumb and index finger. This motion may take place in two planes. *2,* Abduction parallel to the plane of the palm (extension). **C,** Flexion. *1,* Zero starting position: the extended thumb. *2,* Flexion of the interphalangeal joint: zero to ±80 degrees. *3,* Flexion of the metacarpophalangeal joint: zero to ±50 degrees. *4,* Flexion of the carpometacarpal joint: zero to ±15 degrees. **D,** Opposition. Zero starting position *(far left)*: the extended thumb in line with the index fingers. *Opposition* is a composite motion consisting of three elements: *1,* abduction, *2,* rotation, and *3,* flexion. This motion is usually considered complete when the tip, or pulp, of the thumb touches the tip of the fifth finger. Some surgeons, however, consider the arc of opposition complete when the tip of the thumb touches the base of the fifth finger. Both methods are illustrated. From American Academy of Orthopaedic Surgeons: Joint motion: method of measuring and recording, Chicago, 1965, The Academy.

Table 18-2

Testing for range of joint motion—cont'd

Fingers

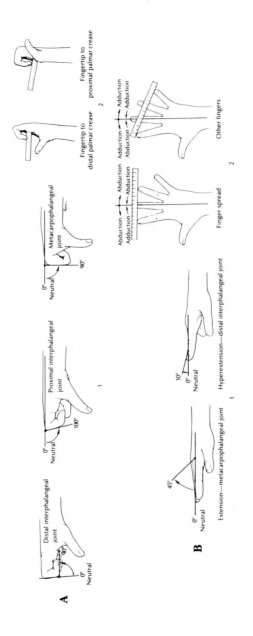

Figure 10

Range of motion of the fingers. **A,** Flexion. *1,* This motion can be estimated in degrees or in centimeters. Flexion is a natural motion in all joints of the fingers. *2,* Composite motion of flexion. This motion can be estimated by a ruler as the distance from the tip of the finger (indicate midpoint of pad and nail edge) to the distal palmar crease (*left*) (this measures flexion of the middle and distal joints) and the proximal palmar crease (*right*) (this measures the distal, middle, and proximal joints of the fingers). **B,** Extension, abduction, and adduction. *1,* Extension and hyperextension. Extension is a natural motion at the metacarpophalangeal joint, but it is an unnatural one in the proximal interphalangeal joint and in the distal interphalangeal joint. *2,* Abduction and adduction. These motions take place in the plane of the palm away from and to the long or middle finger of the hand. This can be indicated in centimeters or inches. The spread of fingers can be measured from the tip of the index finger to the tip of the little finger (*right*). Individual fingers spread from tip to tip of indicated fingers (*left*).

From American Academy of Orthopaedic Surgeons: Joint motion: method of measuring and recording, Chicago, 1965, The Academy.

Hip

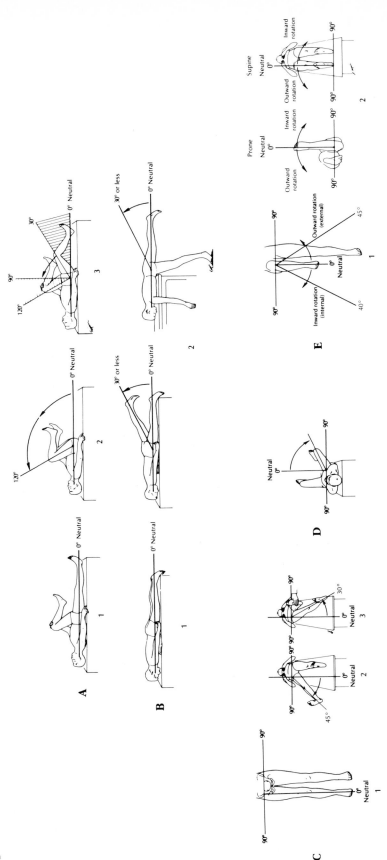

Figure 11

Range of motion of the hip. **A,** Flexion. *1,* Zero starting position of the right hip: client is supine on a firm, flat surface with the opposite hip held in full flexion. This flattens the lumbar spine and demonstrates a flexion deformity of the hip if present. *2,* Flexion. The motion is recorded from zero to 110 or 120 degrees. The examiner should place one hand on the iliac crest to note the point at which the pelvis begins to rotate. *3,* Limited motion in flexion. Limited motion is noted as in the elbow and knee: the hip flexes from 30 to 90 degrees (30° → 90°); the hip has a flexion deformity of 30 degrees with further flexion to 90 degrees. **B,** Extension. *1,* Zero starting position: client is prone on a firm, level surface. *2,* The upward motion of the hip is measured in degrees from the zero starting position. Two methods are commonly used. *Left,* With the client prone and a small pillow under the abdomen, the leg is extended with the knee straight or flexed. *Right,* With the opposite extremity flexed over the end of the examining table, the hip is extended. This method is a more accurate method of measuring extension. There is an anatomic question whether extension is present in the hip at all. Extension as seen from examination is that deviation of the extremity past the zero position and reflects some back motion. **C,** Abduction and adduction. *1,* Zero starting position: client is supine with the legs extended at right angles to a/transverse line across the anterosuperior spine of the pelvis. *2,* Abduction. The outward motion of the extremity is measured in degrees from the zero starting position to 45 degrees. *3,* Adduction. In measuring adduction the examiner should elevate the opposite extremity a few degrees to allow the leg to pass under it zero to 30 degrees **D,** Abduction in flexion. Abduction can be measured in degrees at any level of flexion. Usually, this is carried out in 90 degrees of flexion. **E,** Rotation. *1,* Rotation in flexion. Zero starting position: client is supine with the hip and knee flexed 90 degrees each and the thigh perpendicular to the transverse line across the anterosuperior spine of the pelvis. *Inward (internal) rotation* is measured by rotating the leg away from the midline of the trunk with the thigh as the axis of rotation, thus producing inward rotation of the hip 40 degrees. *Outward (external) rotation* is measured by rotating the leg toward the midline of the trunk with the thigh as the axis of rotation, thus producing outward rotation of the hip 45 degrees. *2,* Rotation in extension. Zero starting position: with client prone (*left*), the knee is flexed to 90 degrees and is perpendicular to the transverse line across the anterosuperior spine of the pelvis. *Inward rotation* is measured by rotating the leg outward. *Outward rotation* is measured by rotating the leg inward. Rotation in extension can also be measured with the client supine (*right*).

From American Academy of Orthopaedic Surgeons: Joint motion: method of measuring and recording, Chicago, 1965, The Academy.

Continued.

Table 18-2

Testing for range of joint motion—cont'd

Knee

KNEE

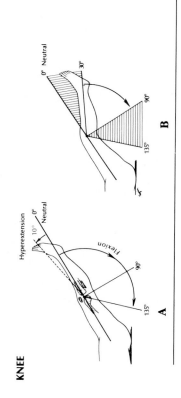

A

B

Figure 12

Range of motion of the knee. **A,** Flexion. Zero starting position: the extended straight knee with client either supine or prone. *Flexion* is measured in degrees from the zero starting point. *Hyperextension* is measured in degrees opposite to flexion at the zero starting point. **B,** Measurement of limited motion of the knee. The terminology for recording limited motion of the knee is similar to that of the elbow and hip: (1) the knee flexes from 30 to 90 degrees (30° → 90°); (2) the knee has a flexion deformity of 30 degrees with further flexion to 90 degrees.

From American Academy of Orthopaedic Surgeons: Joint motion: method of measuring and recording, Chicago, 1965, The Academy.

Ankle

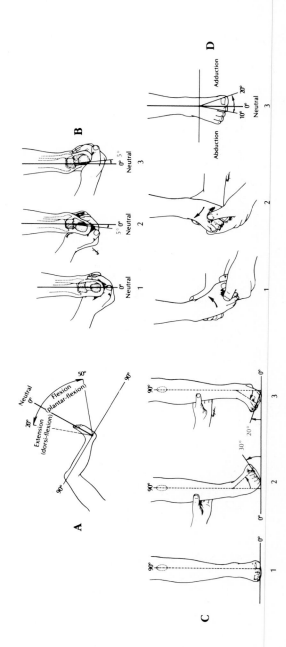

Figure 13

Range of motion of the ankle and foot. **A,** Extension (dorsiflexion) and flexion (plantar flexion). These motions are measured in degrees from the right-angle neutral position or in percentages of motion compared with the opposite ankle. *1,* Zero starting position: the heel is in line with the midline of the tibia. *2,* Inversion. The heel is grasped firmly in the cup of the examiner's hand. Passive motion is estimated in degrees or percentages of motion by turning the heel inward. *3,* Eversion. This motion is estimated by turning the heel outward. **C,** Motions of the forepart of the foot (active motion). *1,* Zero starting position: the foot is in line with the tibia in the long axis from the ankle to the knee. The axis of the foot is directed medially. This motion includes supination, adduction, and some degree of plantar flexion. The foot is compared with the opposite foot. *2,* Active inversion 30 degrees. The foot is the second toe. *2,* Active inversion 30 degrees. This motion can be estimated in degrees or expressed in percentages compared with the opposite foot. *3,* Active eversion 20 degrees. The sole of the foot is turned to face laterally. This motion includes pronation, abduction, and dorsiflexion. NOTE: Problems exist when the foot motions are divided into forefoot and hindfoot descriptions. Care must be made to record motions pertaining to that part of the foot described or to the whole foot, as the case may be. **D,** Motions of the forepart of the foot (passive motion). *1,* Inversion. The examiner carries the foot passively through the motions of active inversion. The heel must be held firmly by the examiner's hand, with the other hand turning the foot inward. *2,* Eversion. The examiner passively turns the foot outward in pronation, abduction, and slight dorsiflexion. *3,* Adduction and abduction. These passive motions are obtained by grasping the heel and moving the forepart of the foot inward or outward. This motion must take place in the plane of the sole of the foot.
From American Academy of Orthopaedic Surgeons: Joint motion: method of measuring and recording, Chicago, 1965, The Academy.

Great toe

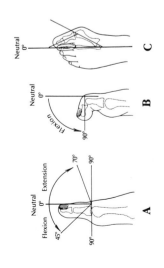

Figure 14

Range of motion of the great toe.* **A,** Flexion and extension of the great toe. Zero starting position: the extended great toe is in line with the first metatarsal bone. **B,** Flexion and extension are present at the metatarsophalangeal joint, and flexion only is present at the interphalangeal joint. **C,** The degree of deformity of the great toe in this instance, hallux valgus, may be measured in degrees of abduction of the metatarsal bone and in degrees of adduction of the proximal and distal phalanges.
From American Academy of Orthopaedic Surgeons: Joint motion: method of measuring and recording, Chicago, 1965, The Academy.

Lateral four toes

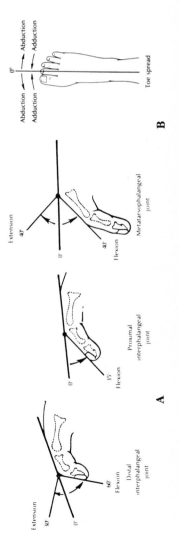

Figure 15

Range of motion of the lateral four toes. **A,** Second to fifth toes. Motion in flexion is present in the distal, middle, and proximal joints of the toes. Extension is present at the metatarsophalangeal joint. These motions can be simply expressed in degrees. **B,** Abduction and adduction (toe spread). This can be measured in relation to the second toe, which is the midline axis of the foot.
From American Academy of Orthopaedic Surgeons: Joint motion: method of measuring and recording, Chicago, 1965, The Academy.

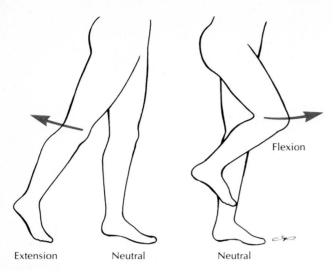

Figure 18-32

Joint motion. *Left,* Extension of the right knee and hip, increasing the joint angle. *Right,* Flexion of the right knee and hip, decreasing the joint angle.

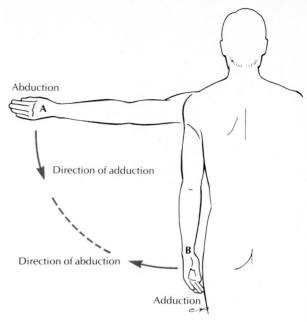

Figure 18-33

Joint motion. Abduction is the movement of a limb away from the midline of the body, as seen in position *A.* Position *B* illustrates an arm in adduction, the movement of a limb toward the central axis of the body.

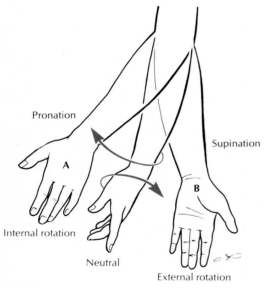

Figure 18-34

Joint motion. Internal rotation is the turning of a body part inward toward the midline, as seen in position *A.* Position *B* illustrates external rotation, the turning of a body part away from the midline.

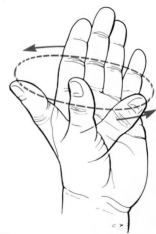

Figure 18-35

Joint motion. Circumduction is the movement of a body part in a circular pattern.

thus, are flexors, extensors, adductors, abductors, internal rotators, external rotators, or circumflexors. Muscles shorten on contraction and in so doing exert pull on the bones to which they are attached to move them closer together. Most muscles attach to two bones that articulate at an intervening joint. Generally, one bone moves while the other is held stable. This is caused by simultaneous shortening of other muscles. The body of the muscle that produces movement of an extremity generally lies proximal to the bone that is moved.

Goniometry and *arthrometry* are the terms used to describe the measurement of joint motion. The practitioner should learn to use the goniometer to measure the range of motion and to communicate the findings to other health team professionals.

The two arms of the *goniometer* are a protractor and a pointer that are joined at the zero point of the protractor (see Fig. 18-1). The hinge should provide sufficient friction that the instrument remains in position when picked up for reading after being set against the joint. The scale should be easily read from a distance of 18 in. Some goniometers have full-circle scales, whereas others have half-circle scales. The length of the arms is generally about 6 in so that it can be easily carried.

Range of motion is described as active when the client moves the joint and passive when the examiner provides the motion.

Active motion. Active joint motion that is smooth and painless through its complete range generally indicates the absence of any advanced lesion. Less muscle tension and joint compression are produced by the voluntary movement of the joints through their range of motion than when the joints are moved against resistance as in the strength tests. Therefore, the range of active motion should be assessed before muscle strength, since the more marked contraction may induce pain in the client, which may skew the test results.

Should the range of active motion of a given joint be less than the range of passive motion, further investigation should focus on true weakness, joint stability, pain, malingering, or hysterical weakness as possible causes.

Passive motion. The examiner moves the relaxed joint through the limits of its movement. When the range of motion is limited, the examiner explores further to determine whether there (1) is an excess of fluid within the joint; (2) are loose bodies in the joint; or (3) is joint surface irregularity or contracture of the muscle, ligaments, or capsule. Moving the joint through the range of its motion may also reveal hypermobility of the joint. In this case, further examination is directed toward differentiating among (1) a connective tissue disruption such as the relaxation of the ligaments that occurs in Marfan's syndrome, (2) a ligamentous tear, and (3) an intra-articular fracture. An example of how this information might aid in diagnosis would be seen in a joint that could be flexed to a smaller angle with passive movement than with active flexion. Such a finding would probably indicate a problem related to the musculature rather than a problem within the joint causing a block in the flexion.

Recording range of motion

The box on p. 426 summarizes joint movements and the maximum expected angles of movement. Limited joint motion may be recorded from the angle of the starting position to the maximal angle reached during movement (i.e., 20 degrees → 50 degrees, see Table 18-2).

Testing by functional group

The movement of the neck and the trunk may be examined in functional groups to determine muscle strength and the range of joint motion. The full range of motion may not be assessed as part of the screening examination unless the history or other parts of the physical examination indicate that muscular or neural dysfunction is a possible problem for the client.

Special tests of musculoskeletal function

Although the following tests are described separately, they may be incorporated into the systemic evaluation of the client, which progresses in a cephalocaudal direction.

Screening examination

In the screening examination, joints are actively carried through the ranges of motion and the results described as full range of motion. Joints that do not exhibit full range of motion are measured with the goniometer, and the results are recorded. Limitations in full range of motion may be an expected finding in older individuals.

Examination of the Muscles

Muscles are examined in symmetric pairs, that is, first one and then the other for equivalence in size, contour, tone, and strength. The contralateral, matching muscle pairs should be uniformly positioned while they are examined. They are examined both at rest and in a state of contraction.

The assessment sequence is inspection, palpation, and testing of muscle strength. The examination of functional muscle groups may be incorporated into examination of the joints.

Inspection and palpation

The muscles are inspected for symmetry of size and contour. Asymmetry, noted as hypertrophy or atrophy, is measured for verification (see previous discussion, pp. 402-403).

Palpation is used to detect swelling, localized temperature changes, and marked changes in shape. The consistency of the muscle on palpation is noted.

Muscle tone, or tonus, is the tension present in the resting muscle. It is also seen in the slight resistance

Principles of Muscle Examination	
Observe	Size, contour
	Bilateral symmetry
	Involuntary movement
Palpate	Tone
Test	Muscle strength against resistance

felt when the relaxed limb is passively moved.

While palpating the muscle, the examiner should be alert to fasciculations, which are involuntary contractions or twitchings of groups of muscle fibers.

The client should be requested to tell the examiner of any sensation while the muscles and tendons are being felt. The client's descriptions of pain or tenderness on palpation are recorded.

Tendon stretch reflexes, described in Chapter 20 on neurologic assessment, are generally altered in muscle disease, especially if the peripheral nerves are involved. For instance, the tendon reflexes are diminished in muscular dystrophy and polymyositis in proportion to the loss of muscle strength. A lengthened reflex cycle is characteristic of hyperthyroidism, whereas a shortened period indicates the hypermetabolic state.

Recording of data

The chart on pp. 427 and 428 provides a listing of clinically testable muscles. Although the methodical record-

---

Recording Range of Motion in Degrees

Cervical spine			**Fingers**	
Flexion	45		Flexion—distal interphalangeal joint	90
Extension	50		Flexion—proximal interphalangeal joint	100
Rotation (right)	70		Flexion—metacarpophalangeal joint	90
Rotation (left)	70		Extension—metacarpophalangeal joint	45
Lateral bending (right)	40		Hyperextension—distal interphalangeal joint	10
Lateral bending (left)	40		Abduction (measure from tips of fingers)	Varies
Spine			Adduction	Varies
Forward flexion (C7 to S1 = 4 in)	70		**Hip**	
Extension (standing)	30		Flexion (knees bent)	110-120
Extension (lying)	20		Extension	30
Rotation (right)	45		Abduction	45
Rotation (left)	45		Adduction	30
Lateral bending (right)	35		Internal rotation (hip and knee flexed)	40
Lateral bending (left)	35		External rotation (hip and knee flexed)	45
Shoulder			**Knee**	
Forward flexion	180		Flexion-extension	135
Backward extension	60		Hyperextension	10
Horizontal flexion	130-135		**Ankle**	
Horizontal extension	40		Dorsiflexion	20
Abduction	180		Plantarflexion	50
Adduction	50		Inversion hind foot (passive)	5
Internal rotation	90		Eversion hind foot (passive)	5
External rotation	90		Inversion	30
Elbow			Eversion	20
Flexion-extension	150		Abduction forefoot (passive)	10
Hyperextension	0-15		Adduction forefoot (passive)	20
Forearm (elbow and wrist)			**Great toe**	
Pronation	80-90		Flexion—metatarsophalangeal joint	45
Supination	80-90		Extension—metatarsophalangeal joint	70
Wrist			Flexion—interphalangeal joint (passive)	90
Extension	80		**Lateral four toes**	
Flexion	70		Flexion—distal interphalangeal joint	60
Radial deviation	20		Extension—distal interphalangeal joint	30
Ulnar deviation	30		Flexion—proximal interphalangeal joint	35
Thumb			Flexion—metatarsophalangeal joint	40
Abduction	50		Extension—metatarsophalangeal joint	40
Flexion—interphalangeal joint	80		Abduction	Varies
Flexion—metacarpophalangeal joint	50		Adduction	Varies
Flexion—carpometacarpal joint	15			
Opposition to tip or base of little finger				

ing of data for each muscle is painstaking, it serves as a baseline for subsequent changes and does indicate that the muscle was actually tested.

Screening test for muscle strength

Although muscle weakness in adults is generally mild and transitory, it may be the outcome of musculoskeletal, neurologic, metabolic, or infectious problems. Therefore, an evaluation is necessary. A simple screening test has been suggested that can be performed in less than 5 minutes and allows the examiner to find nearly any muscle or reflex abnormality.

Muscle strength may be assessed throughout the full range of motion for each muscle or goup of muscles. However, several screening examinations have been designed. One is described in Table 18-3. The usual method

Left							Right			
Range of motion	Tone	Fasciculation	Strength				Range of motion	Tone	Fasciculation	Strength
				Face:						
				Neck:	Flexor	Sternocleidomastoid				
					Extensor group					
				Trunk:	Flexor	Rectus abdominis				
					Rotators	Right oblique internal abductor Left oblique internal abductor Left oblique external abductor Right oblique external abductor				
					Extensors	Thoracic group Lumbar group				
					Pelvic elevator	Quadratus lumbar				
				Scapula:	Abductor	Serratus anterior				
					Elevator	Trapezius (superior)				
					Depressor	Trapezius (inferior)				
					Adductors	Trapezius (middle) Rhomboid major and minor				
				Shoulder:	Flexor	Deltoid (anterior)				
					Extensors	Latissimus dorsi Teres major				
					Abductor (to 90°)	Deltoid (middle)				
					Horizontal abductor	Deltoid (posterior)				
					Horizontal adductor	Pectoralis major				
					Rotators	Lateral rotator group Medial rotator group				
				Elbow:	Flexors	Biceps brachii Brachialis				
					Extensor	Triceps brachii				
				Forearm:	Extensors	Supinator group				
						Pronator group				
				Wrist:	Flexors	Flex. carpi radialis Flex. carpi ulnaris				
					Extensors	Ext. carpi rad. longus and brevis Ext. carpi ulnaris				

Adapted from Daniels L and Worthingham C: Muscle testing: techniques of manual examination, ed 4, Philadelphia, 1980, WB Saunders Co.

Continued

Left

Right

Range of motion	Tone	Fasciculation	Strength				Range of motion	Tone	Fasciculation	Strength
				Fingers:	MP flexors	Lumbricales				
					IP flexors (first)	Flex. digit. superficialis				
					IP flexors (second)	Flex. digit. profundus				
					MP extensors	Ext. digit. communis				
					Adductors	Interossei palmares Interossei dorsales				
					Abductors	Abductor digiti minimi Opponens digiti minimi				
				Thumb:	MP flexor	Flex. poll. brevis				
					IP flexor	Flex. poll. longus				
					MP extensor	Ext. poll. brevis				
					IP extensor	Ext. poll. longus				
					Abductors	Abd. poll. brevis Abd. poll. longus				
					Adductors	Adductor pollicis Opponens pollicis				
				Hip:	Flexor	Iliopsoas				
					Extensor	Gluteus maximus				
					Abductor	Gluteus medius				
					Adductor group					
					Rotators	Lateral rotator group Medial rotator group				
				Knee:	Flexors	Biceps femoris Inner hamstrings				
					Extensor	Quadriceps femoris				
				Ankle:	Plantar flexors	Gastrocnemius Soleus				
				Foot:	Invertors	Tibialis anterior Tibialis posterior				
					Evertors	Peroneus brevis Peroneus longus				
				Toes:	MP flexors	Lumbricales				
					IP flexors (first)	Flex. digit. brevis				
					IP flexors (second)	Flex. digit. longus				
					MP extensors	Ext. digit. longus Ext. digit brevis				
				Hallux:	MP flexor	Flex. hall. brevis				
					IP flexor	Flex. hall. longus				
					MP extensor	Ext. hall. brevis				
					IP extensor	Ext. hall. longus				

Gait:

Table 18-3

Screening test for muscle strength

Muscles tested	Client activity	Examiner activity	Muscles tested	Client activity	Examiner activity
Ocular muscu-lature			Biceps	Flex arm	Pull to extend arm
			Triceps	Extend arm	Push to flex arm
Lids	Close eyes tightly	Attempt to resist closure	Wrist muscula-ture	Extend hand	Push to flex
				Flex hand	Push to extend
Yoke muscles	Track object in six cardinal positions		Finger muscles	Extend fingers	Push dorsal surface of fingers
Facial muscula-ture	Blow out cheeks	Assess pressure in cheeks with fingertips		Flex fingers	Push ventral surface of fingers
	Place tongue in cheek	Assess pressure in cheek with fingertips		Spread fingers	Hold fingers together
			Hip muscula-ture	In supine position raise extended leg	Push down on leg above the knee
	Stick out tongue, move it to right and left	Observe strength and coordination of thrust and extension	Hamstring, gluteal, abductor, and adductor muscles of leg	Sit and perform alternate leg crossing	Push in opposite direction of the crossing limb
Neck muscles	Extend head backward	Push head forward	Quadriceps	Extend leg	Push to flex leg
	Flex head forward	Push head backward	Hamstring	Bend knees to flex leg	Push to extend leg
	Rotate head in full circle	Observe mobility, coordination	Ankle and foot muscle	Bend foot up (dorsiflexion)	Push to plantar flexion
	Touch shoulders with head	Observe range of motion		Bend foot down (plantar flexion)	Push to dorsiflexion
Deltoid	Hold arms upward	Push down on arms	Antigravity muscles	Walk on toes	
				Walk on heels	

of testing is manual and subjective. Resistance is applied to the muscles; the client is placed in the position that best allows movement through the full range. The muscle contractions are graded according to the examiner's judgment of the client's responses. The test allows for a systematic testing of muscle groups from head to toe. While walking into the examining room and undressing, the client is carefully observed for cues to neurologic and motion deficit and to ascertain that the chief complaint is verifiable by physical evidence. The following procedure may then be used:

1. The examiner assesses the ocular musculature by asking the client to close the eyes tightly as the examiner attempts to open the lids. The client is instructed to look up, down, right, and left as the examiner checks for lid lag and appropriate tracking of the eyes.

2. The examiner assesses the facial musculature by asking the client to blow out the cheeks while the examiner assesses the pressure against the fingers held

against the resultant cheek bulge. The client is then asked to put the tongue into the cheek, and the tension created in this bulge is tested. The client is then asked to stick out the tongue and to move it to the right and left.

3. The examiner assesses the neck musculature by asking the client to extend the head backward while standing erect as the examiner attempts to break the extension (Fig. 18-36). The client is then asked to bend the chin toward his chest forcefully as far as possible while the examiner attempts to bend the chin upward. The client is asked to touch each shoulder with the head and to rotate the head in a full circle.

4. The examiner tests the deltoid muscles by asking the client to hold the arms upward while the examiner tries to push them down. The client is asked to extend the arms while examiner attempts to press them down.

5. The examiner tests the biceps by asking the client to fully extend the arms and then to try to flex them

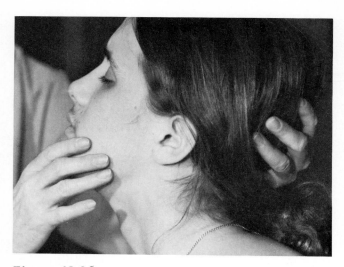

Figure 18-36

Assessment of the neck musculature. The client flexes his head backward while the examiner attempts to break the extension.

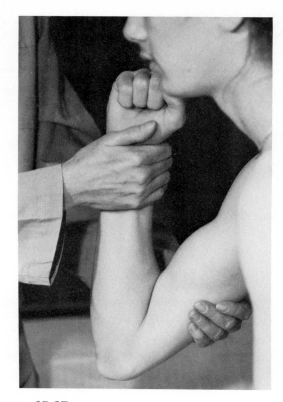

Figure 18-37

Assessment of biceps strength. The client flexes his arm while the examiner attempts to pull the arm into extension.

while the examiner attempts to pull them into extension (Fig. 18-37).

6. The examiner tests the triceps by asking the client to flex the arms and then to extend them while the examiner attempts to push them into a flexed position (Fig. 18-38).

7. The examiner assesses the wrist and finger musculature by asking the client to extend the hand and then to try to resist the examiner with the hand up, alternately with the fingers out or together, in an attempt to flex the wrist (Fig. 18-39). The handshake provides a measure of the strength of grasp (Fig. 18-40). Finger strength is assessed by pushing on the dorsal surface of the fingers while the client tries to extend them and on the ventral surface while he or she tries to flex the fingers further. Finger strength may be assessed by trying to move the fingers together as the client attempts to spread them (Fig. 18-41).

8. The examiner assesses hip strength by asking the client to assume the supine position and then to raise the extended leg while the examiner attempts to hold it down.

9. The examiner assesses the hamstring, gluteal, abductor, and adductor muscles of the leg by asking the client to sit and perform alternate leg crossing (Fig. 18-42).

10. The examiner tests quadriceps muscle strength by asking the client to extend a leg stiffly as the examiner tries to bend it (Fig. 18-43).

11. The examiner assesses the hamstring muscles by asking the client to bend the knees as the examiner tries to straighten them (Fig. 18-44).

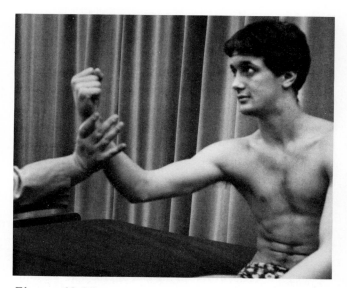

Figure 18-38

Assessment of triceps strength. The client attempts to extend his arm while the examiner attempts to push the arm into a flexed position.

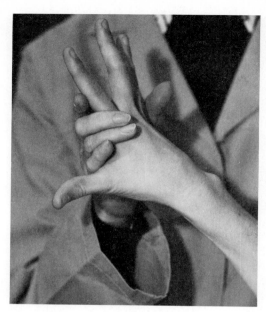

Figure 18-39

Assessment of wrist strength. The client pushes against the examiner's hand in an attempt to flex the wrist.

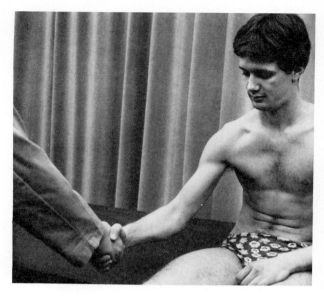

Figure 18-40

The handshake provides a measure of the strength of the hand grasp.

12. The examiner assesses the ankle and foot musculature by asking the client to exert upward foot pressure and then big toe pressure against the examiner's hands.

13. The client is asked to walk naturally for a short distance to observe gait (if the examiner has not already done so). Then the client is asked to take a few steps on the toes and a few steps on the heels.

The following criteria for recording the grading of muscle strength have been frequently used:

Functional level	Lovett scale	Grade	Percentage of normal
No evidence of contractility	Zero (0)	0	0
Evidence of slight contractility	Trace (T)	1	10
Complete range of motion with gravity eliminated	Poor (P)	2	25
Complete range of motion with gravity	Fair (F)	3	50
Complete range of motion against gravity with some resistance	Good (G)	4	75
Complete range of motion against gravity with full resistance	Normal (N)	5	100

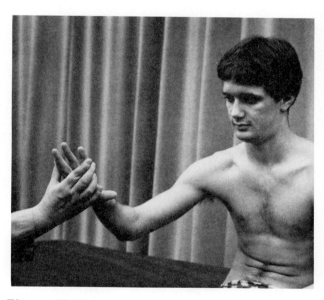

Figure 18-41

Finger strength is assessed as the examiner resists the client's attempts to spread them.

Some examiners prefer simple descriptive words such as *paralysis, severe weakness, moderate weakness, minimum weakness,* and *normal.* Disability is considered to exist if the muscle strength is less than grade 3; external support may be required to make the involved part functional, and activity of the part cannot be achieved in a gravity field.

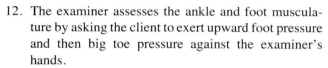

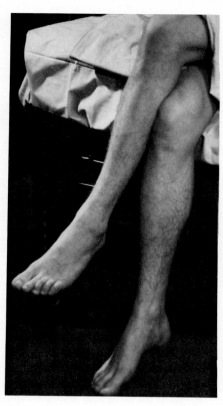

Figure 18-42

Alternate leg crossing for assessment of hamstring, gluteal, abductor, and adductor muscle strength.

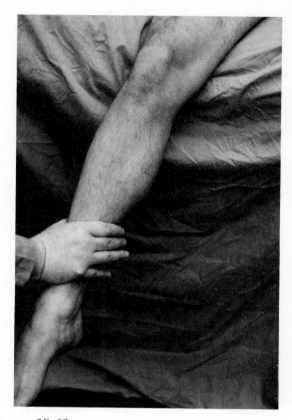

Figure 18-43

Assessment of quadriceps muscle strength. The client attempts to straighten the leg while the examiner attempts to flex it.

Figure 18-44

Assessment of hamstring muscle strength. The client flexes his knees while the examiner tries to straighten them.

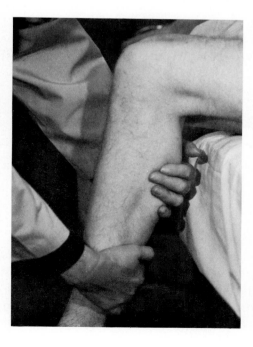

There is an expectation that muscle strength will be greater in the dominant arm and leg. Movements should be coordinated and painless.

The musculoskeletal screening test is the only one performed unless the examiner suspects a musculoskeletal problem. Another example of the screening examination has been developed by the house staff of Mayo Clinic as described in the boxed material on page 433. Full testing for muscle strength is described in Table 18-4.

Survey of Motor Function

	Right	Left
Arise from chair, arms folded		
Walk on toes	_____	_____
Walk on heels	_____	_____
Hop	_____	_____
Squat fully and rise		
Lift foot to step	_____	_____
Step up on step	_____	_____
Abduct arms to horizontal	_____	_____
Reach overhead (full extension)	_____	_____
Wing scapulae	_____	_____

Supine position

Lift head off table
Hands on occiput, rise to a
  sitting position
  Flex thigh, lifting extended   _____   _____
  leg

Prone position

Fully extend neck
Lift head and shoulders off table, hands on buttocks

The survey has been designed by the house staff of Mayo Clinic and may be used as a substitute for specific tests of muscle strength for very young children and for adults who are unable to cooperate with specific muscle testing. The survey is judged to be of greatest value in conditions defined by muscle weakness.

Distinction Between Upper and Lower Motor Neuron Involvement

A concept of clinical importance in the examination of the musculoskeletal system is the distinction between upper and lower motor neuron involvement. The cells of the upper motor neurons are in the cortex and terminate in the brainstem (corticobulbar tract) or cross over in the anterior gray horn of the medulla and end in the spinal cord (corticospinal tract). The corticobulbar fibers terminate in cranial nerve nuclei.

The corticospinal axons passing through the medullary pyramids are termed pyramidal tracts. Lower motor neurons include cranial nerve nuclei, their axons, anterior horn cells of the cord, and their axons.

Lesions of the upper motor neuron produce a spasticity or hypertonicity of the affected muscles, and muscle strength is not diminished. Tendon stretch reflexes are brisk, and Babinski's sign is present if the lesion is in the corticospinal tract. Atrophy occurs only with disuse of the muscles. By contrast, lesions of the lower motor neurons produce flaccidity or loss of muscle tone. The hypotonus leads to atrophy. Fasciculations are seen. Tendon reflexes are depressed or absent.

The distinctions between the two types of nerve involvement can often be made by palpation of the muscle and tests for muscle strength.

VARIATIONS FROM HEALTH

Muscle Weakness

The client who has difficulty in walking up steps or getting up from the sitting position, who is able to rise only by pushing off with the hands and arms or by pulling up by grasping some nearby furniture, may have a problem involving the shoulder or hip girdle musculature. Further tests would be needed to ascertain the presence of muscular dystrophy, myasthenia gravis, parkinsonism, or polymyositis. Myasthenia gravis may be more strongly suspected if the following are true: (1) The client is instructed to sit back and relax for a few minutes, after which he can rise easily; (2) the client is a woman in her 20s or a man in his 50s or 60s; (3) muscle atrophy is not present; and (4) the client has a ptosis or extraocular muscle weakness resulting in diplopia.

The presence of myasthenia gravis may be conclusively determined in the client with ptosis by the use of the Tensilon test, which is performed in the following manner. The examiner injects 2 mg of edrophonium chloride (Tensilon) while watching the client's eyelids. If there is no change after a minute, the examiner injects another 8 mg. In 90% of clients who have myasthenia gravis the ptosis is markedly improved, since muscle strength increases following the injection.

The client who has polymyositis may have pain, muscle atrophy, or a rash, particularly around the eyelids, as well as low-grade fever.

Parkinsonism may be the underlying cause when the aging client has difficulty rising from a chair. This impression may be substantiated if the client says stiffness is a problem. The examiner should be alert in this case for signs of flexion posture, slow and intermittent movement, frequent tremor, masked facies, or movement of several joint units at one time because these signs are also characteristic of Parkinson's disease.

Viral, upper respiratory tract infections may be suspected in the individual who has a mild elevation in temperature and whose chief complaint revealed that he had no symptoms only a day or so before but now feels weak, almost unable to move.

If the initial examination fails to demonstrate muscular or neural disease, the possibility of fatigue should be considered.

The client who complains of intermittent bouts of muscle weakness should be methodically and carefully investigated for ischemic attacks, disorders of glucose metabolism (diabetes), anemia, and serum electrolyte

Text continued on p. 461.

Table 18-4

Testing for muscle strength

Movement	Muscles	Motor nerves	Positions for testing	Instructions and tests for muscle strength
Neck				

Flexion	Prime mover: sternocleido-mastoid (Fig. 1*)
	Accessory muscles
	  Scalenus anterior
	  Scalenus medius
	  Scalenus posterior
	  Rectus capitis anterior
	  Longus capitis
	  Longus colli
	  Infrahyoid group
		Spinal accessory nerve (cranial XI)
		Cervical 2, 3
			Standing, sitting, supine	"Bend your head to touch your chin to your chest." Resistance is applied to the forehead. Pressure is exerted over the tip of the xiphoid process to obviate the tendency to contract the abdominal muscles to raise the chest (Fig. 2).

Extension	Prime movers (Fig. 3*)
	  Trapezius (superior fibers)
	  Semispinalis capitis
	  Semispinalis cervicis
	  Splenius capitis
	
	  Splenius cervicis
	
	  Spinalis capitis
	  Spinalis cervicis
	  Longissimus capitis
	  Longissimus cervicis
	  Accessory muscles
	  Levator scapulae
	  Multifidi
	  Obliquus capitis
	  Rectus capitis posterior
		Spinal accessory nerve (cranial XI)
		Cervical 3, 4
		Dorsal rami of spinal nerves
		Dorsal rami of spinal nerves
		Dorsal rami of middle and lower cervical nerves
		Dorsal rami of middle and lower cervical nerves
		Adjacent spinal nerves
		Adjacent spinal nerves
		Adjacent spinal nerves
		Adjacent spinal nerves
			Standing, sitting, prone	"Bend your head back as far as possible."
				"Lift your head up as far as you can." Resistance is applied to the occipital prominence (Fig. 4).

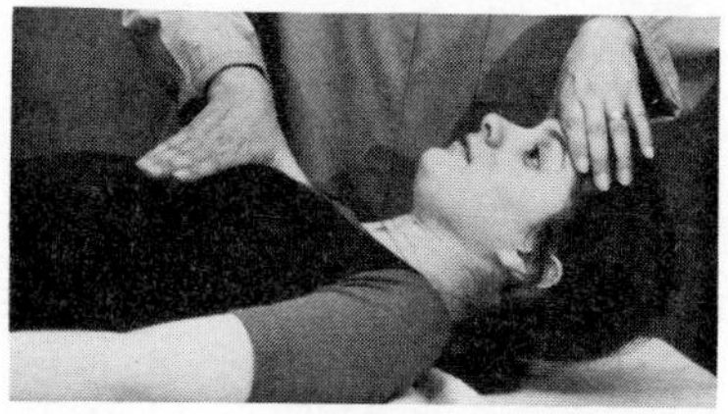

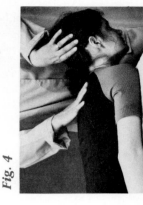

Fig. 2

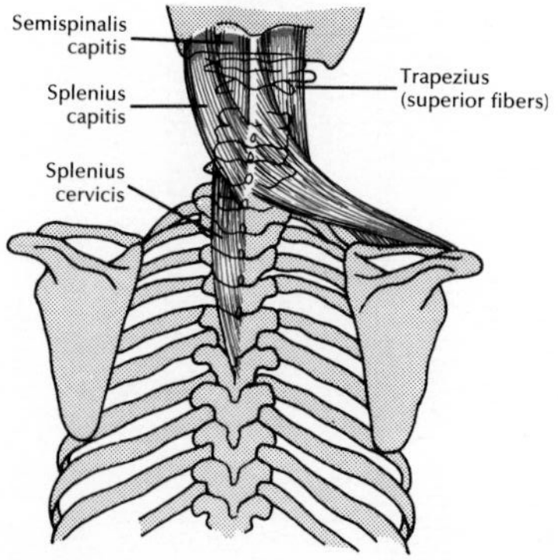

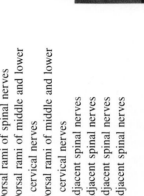

Fig. 4

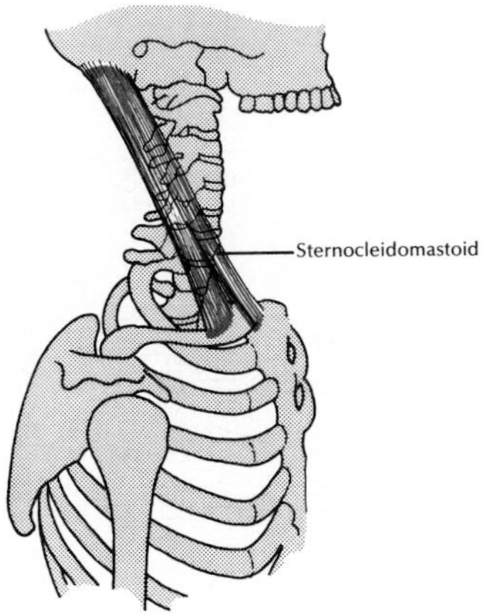

Sternocleidomastoid

Fig. 1

Semispinalis capitis Splenius capitis Splenius cervicis Trapezius (superior fibers)

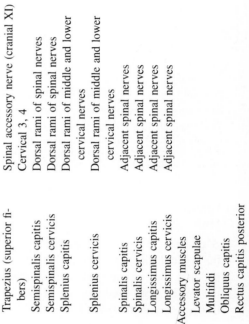

Fig. 3

Rotation

Motion	Muscles	Nerve	Position	Instructions
Anterolateral	Prime mover: sternocleidomastoid (see Fig. 1) Accessory muscles Scalenus anterior Scalenus medius Scalenus posterior Rectus capitis anterior Longus capitis Longus colli Infrahyoid group	Spinal accessory nerve (cranial XI) Cervical 2,3	Standing, sitting, supine	"Bend your head forward and turn your head as far as you can to the right (left)." "Bend your head so that your ear is close to your chest." Resistance is applied to the right (left) temple.
Posterolateral	Prime movers (see Fig. 3) Trapezius (superior fibers) Semispinalis capitis Semispinalis cervicis Splenius capitis Splenius cervicis Spinalis capitis Spinalis cervicis Longissimus capitis Longissimus cervicis Accessory muscles Levator scapulae Multifidi Obliquus capitis Rectus capitis posterior	Spinal accessory nerve (cranial XI) Cervical 3, 4 Dorsal rami of spinal nerves Dorsal rami of spinal nerves Dorsal rami of middle and lower cranial nerves Dorsal rami of middle and lower cranial nerves Adjacent spinal nerves Adjacent spinal nerves Adjacent spinal nerves Adjacent spinal nerves	Standing, sitting, prone	"Bend your head back and turn your head to the right (left)." Resistance is applied to the right (left) occiput.
Lateral bend	Prime mover: sternocleidomastoid (see Fig. 1) Accessory muscles Scalenus anterior Scalenus medius Scalenus posterior Rectus capitis anterior Longus capitis Longus colli Infrahyoid group	Spinal accessory nerve (cranial XI) Cervical 2, 3	Standing, sitting, supine	"Bend your head so that your right (left) ear touches your shoulder. Do not bring your shoulder up to meet your ear." Resistance is applied to the right (left) temporal bone.

Continued

*Adapted from Daniels L and Worthingham C: Muscle testing: techniques of manual examination, ed 4, Philadelphia, 1980, WB Saunders Co.

Table 18-4

Testing for muscle strength—*cont'd*

Movement	Muscles	Motor nerves	Positions for testing	Instructions and tests for muscle strength
Trunk				
Flexion	Prime mover: rectus abdominis (Fig. 5*) Accessory muscles Obliquus internus abdominis Obliquus externus abdominis	Intercostal nerves (thoracic 6-12, lumbar 1)	Standing Supine (knees not bent)	"Bend over; touch your toes" (Fig. 6). "Try to sit up without using your hands." Legs are stabilized (Fig. 7). Two important signs may be elicited in assessing abdominal muscle strength: 1. Beevor's sign, upward movement of the umbilicus on contraction of the abdominal muscles, is associated with comparative weakness of the lower abdominal muscles in relation to the upper abdominal muscles. 2. Hyperextension of the lumbar spine when the client tries to rise to a sitting position occurs when strong hip flexors are contracted in the presence of weak abdominal muscles.

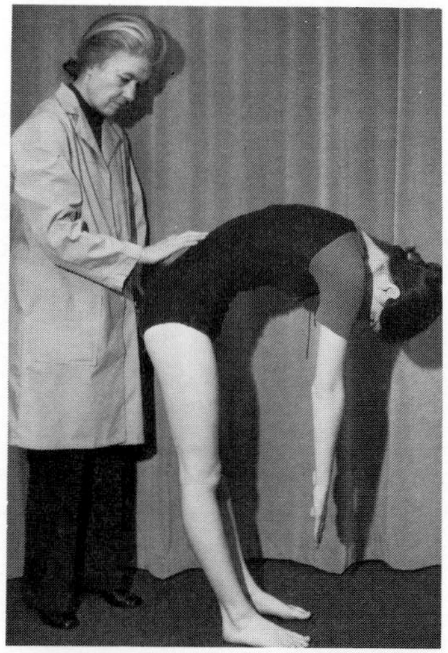

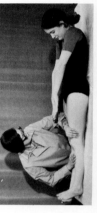

Fig. 6

Fig. 7

Rectus abdominis

Aponeurosis of internal oblique
Aponeurosis of external oblique
Conjoined tendon

Pyramidalis
Spermatic cord

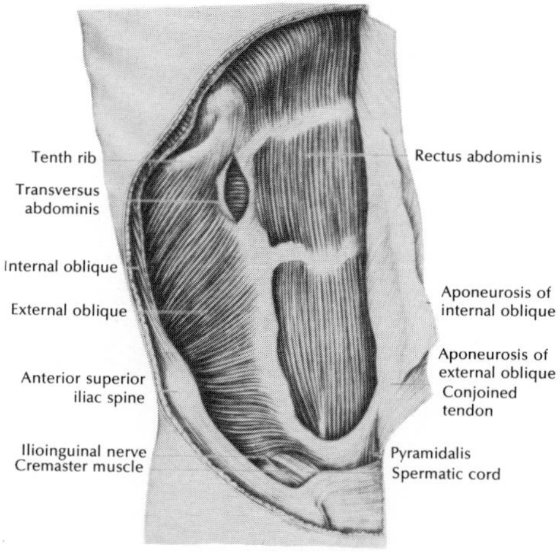

Tenth rib
Transversus abdominis
Internal oblique
External oblique
Anterior superior iliac spine
Ilioinguinal nerve
Cremaster muscle

Fig. 5

Continued

Extension	Standing	Prime movers (Fig. 8†)		"Bend your head and shoulders back as far as you can."
	Prone	Longissimus thoracis	Adjacent spinal nerves	"Lift your head and shoulders up from the table without using your hands."
		Iliocostalis thoracis	Adjacent spinal nerves	Pelvis is stabilized. Resistance is applied between the scapulae (Fig. 9).
		Spinalis thoracis	Adjacent spinal nerves	
		Iliocostalis lumborum	Adjacent spinal nerves	
		Quadratus lumborum	Thoracic 12, lumbar 1	
		Accessory muscles		
		Rotators		
		Multifidi		
		Simispinalis		

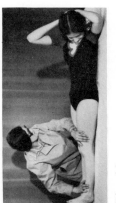

Fig. 9

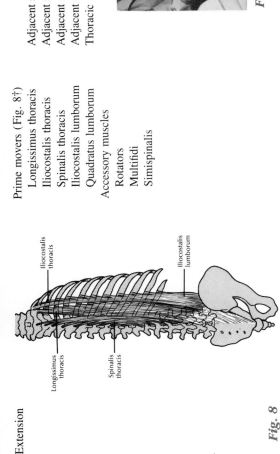

Iliocostalis thoracis
Longissimus thoracis
Spinalis thoracis
Iliocostalis lumborum

Fig. 8

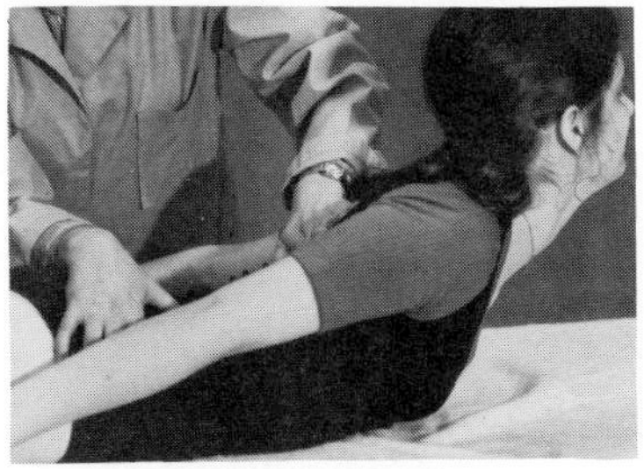

Rotation	Sitting (hips flexed)	Prime movers (Fig. 10†)		"Twist your right [left] shoulder to the opposite knee."
	Supine (hands behind head, legs stabilized)	Obliquus externus abdominis	Intercostal nerves (thoracic 8-12)	"Turn your right [left] shoulder to the opposite knee" (Fig. 11)
		Obliquus internus abdominus	Intercostal nerves (thoracic 8-12)	Resistance may be applied against the right (left) anterior shoulder.
		Accessory muscles		
		Rectus abdominis		
		Latissimus dorsi		
		Semispinalis		
		Multifidi		
		Rotators		

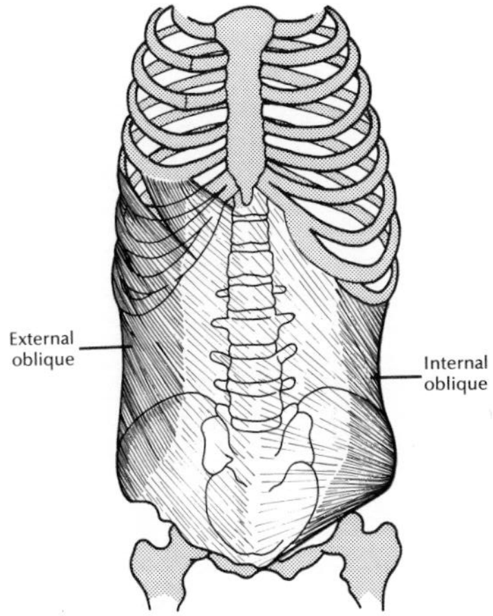

Fig. 11

Internal oblique
External oblique

Fig. 10

*From Francis CC and Farrell GL: Integrated anatomy and physiology, ed 3, St Louis, 1957, The CV Mosby Co.
†Adapted from Daniels L and Worthingham C: Muscle testing: techniques of manual examination, ed 4, Philadelphia, 1980, WB Saunders Co.

Table 18-4

Testing for muscle strength—*cont'd*

Movement	Muscles	Motor nerves	Positions for testing	Instructions and tests for muscle strength
Trunk—cont'd				
Elevation	Prime movers (Fig. 12*) Quadratus lumborum Iliocostalis lumborum Accessory muscles Obliquus internus abdominis Obliquus externus abdominis Latissimus dorsi Abductor muscles of hip	Thoracic 12; lumbar 1, 2 Adjacent spinal nerves	Supine (legs together) Standing	"Try to lift your right (left) hip toward your shoulder." Resistance is applied by the examiner holding the ankle (Fig. 13). "Thrust your right (left) hip forward and up."

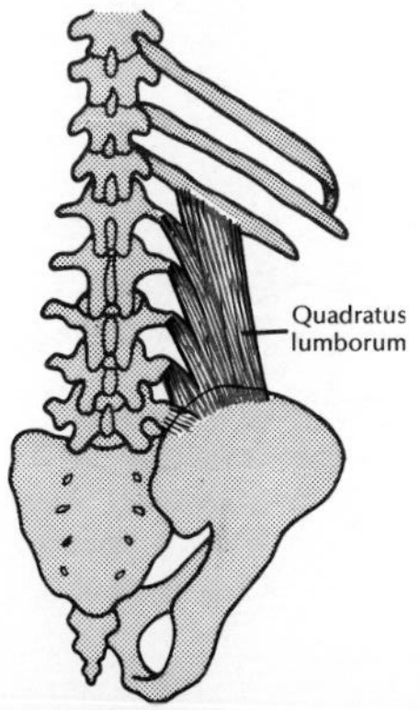

Fig. 13

Quadratus lumborum

Fig. 12

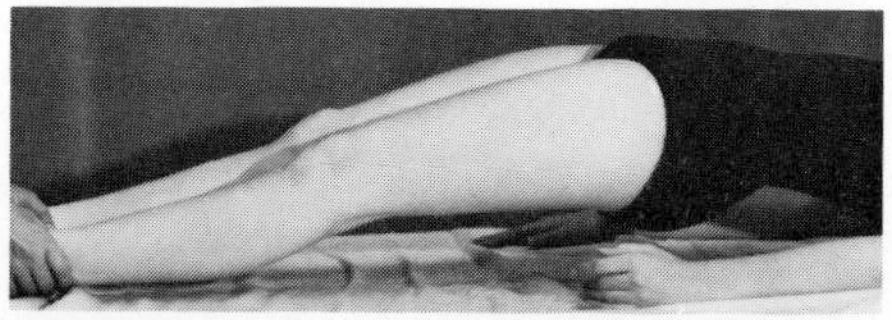

Shoulder: part 1

Forward flexion

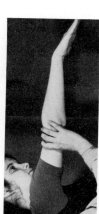

Deltoid (anterior fibers)
Coracobrachialis

Fig. 14

Prime movers (Fig. 14*)
Deltoid (anterior fibers)
Coracobrachialis
Accessory muscles
Deltoideus (middle fibers)
Pectoralis major (clavicular fibers)
Biceps brachii

Axillary nerve (cervical 5, 6)
Musculocutaneous nerve (cervical 6, 7)

Standing, sitting, supine

"Move your arms forward and up."
Resistance is applied at the level of the interior angle of the scapula on the upper side of the arm (Fig. 15).

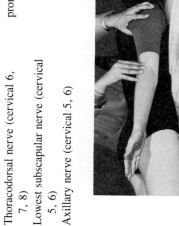

Fig. 15

Backward extension

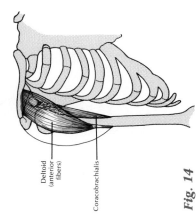

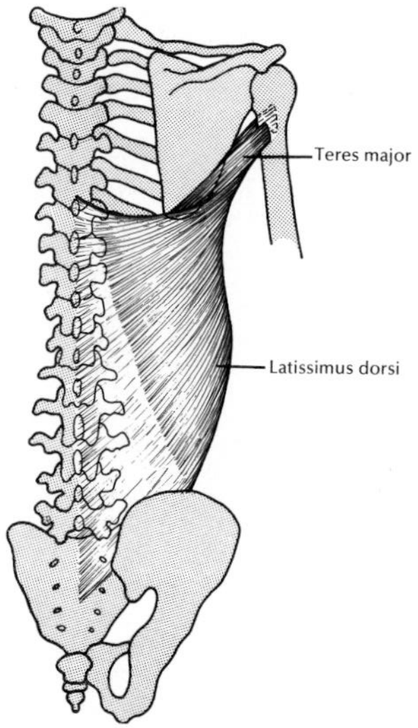

Teres major

Latissimus dorsi

Fig. 16

Prime movers (Fig. 16*)
Latissimus dorsi

Teres major

Deltoideus
Accessory muscles
Teres minor
Triceps brachii (long head)

Thoracodorsal nerve (cervical 6, 7, 8)
Lowest subscapular nerve (cervical 5, 6)
Axillary nerve (cervical 5, 6)

Standing, sitting, prone

"Move your arms downward and back."
"Clasp your arms behind your back."
Resistance is applied to the posterior aspect of the arm proximal to the elbow (Fig. 17).

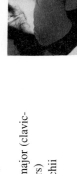

Fig. 17

Continued

*Adapted from Daniels L and Worthingham C: Muscle testing: techniques of manual examination, ed 4, Philadelphia, 1980, WB Saunders Co.

Table 18-4
Testing for muscle strength—*cont'd*

Movement	Muscles	Motor nerves	Positions for testing	Instructions and tests for muscle strength
Shoulder: part 1—cont'd				
Abduction	Prime movers (Fig. 18*) Deltoideus (middle fibers) Supraspinatus Accessory muscles Deltoideus (anterior and posterior fibers) Serratus anterior	Axillary nerve (cervical 5, 6) Suprascapular nerve (cervical 5)	Standing, sitting (scapula stabilized)	"Lift your arm straight out and to your side, away from your body." Resistance is applied to the superior aspect of the arm proximal to the elbow (Fig. 19).
Horizontal adduction	Prime mover: pectoralis major (Fig. 20*) Accessory muscle: deltoid (anterior fibers)	Medial and internal pectoral nerves (cervical 5, 6, 7, 8; thoracic 1)	Standing, sitting, supine (arm abducted)	"Bring your straight arm over your chest." Resistance is applied on the medial side of arm proximal to the elbow (Fig. 21).

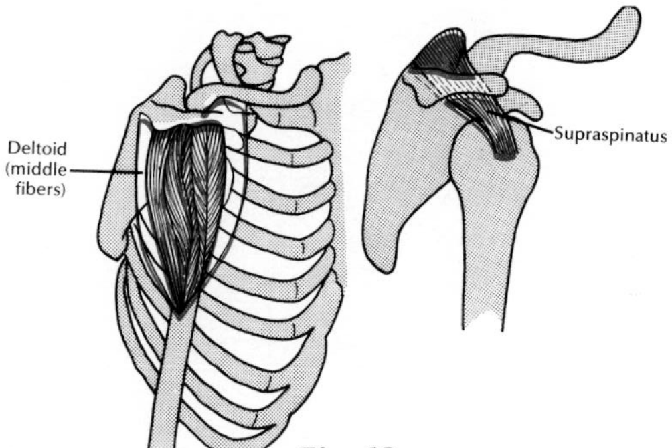

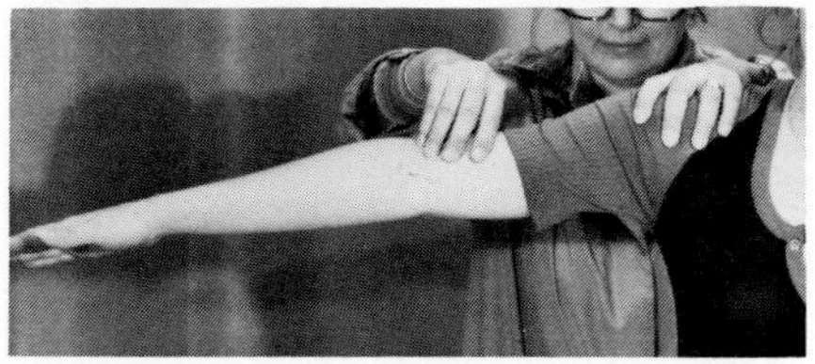

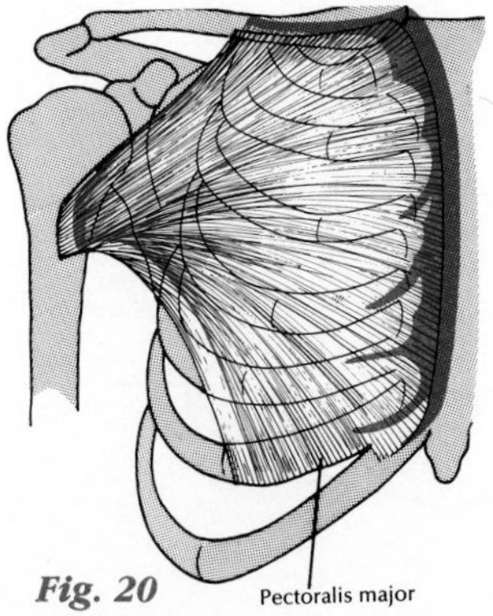

Supraspinatus

Deltoid (middle fibers)

Fig. 18

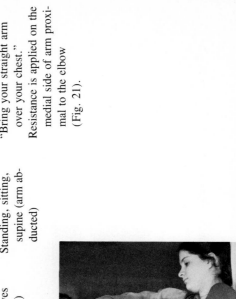

Fig. 19

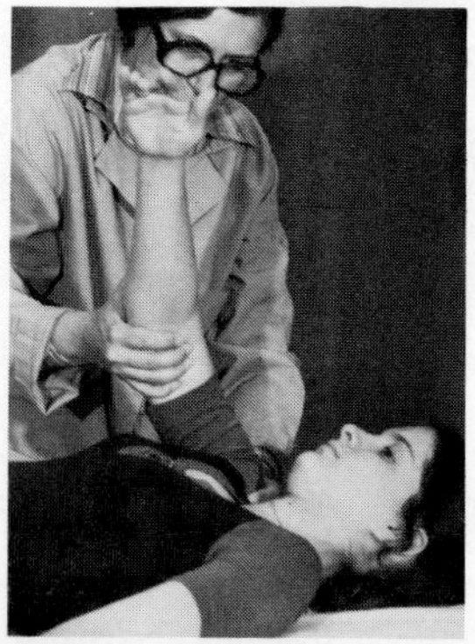

Fig. 21

Pectoralis major

Fig. 20

	Prime mover	Nerve	Position	Instructions
Horizontal abduction	Prime mover: deltoideus (posterior fibers) (Fig. 22*) Accessory muscles Teres minor Infraspinatus	Axillary nerve (cervical 5, 6)	Standing, sitting, prone (scapula stabilized, arm adducted)	"Keeping your arm at shoulder height, move it backward as far as you can." Resistance is applied on the posterior surface of the arm proximal to the elbow (Fig. 23).

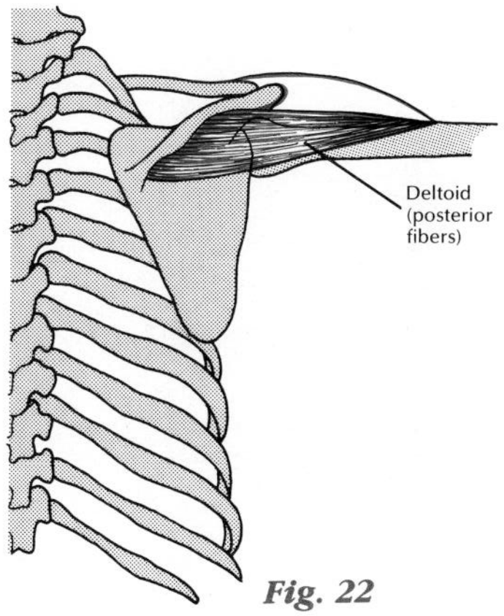

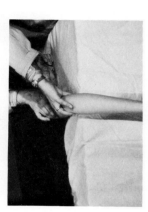

Deltoid (posterior fibers)

Fig. 22

Fig. 23

Shoulder: part 2

Rotation

	Prime movers	Nerve	Position	Instructions
Internal	Prime movers (Fig. 24*) Subscapularis Pectoralis major Latissimus dorsi Teres major Accessory muscle: deltoideus (anterior fibers)	Upper and lower subscapular nerves (cervical 5, 6) Medial and lateral pectoral nerves (cervical 5, 6, 7, 8; thoracic 1) Thoracodorsal nerve (cervical 6, 7, 8) Lowest subscapular nerve (cervical 5, 6)	Standing, sitting, prone (scapula stabilized)	"Rotate your shoulder inward, swing your arm backward with your palm upward, and point your fingers toward the ceiling." Resistance is applied to the volar surface of the wrist (Fig. 25).

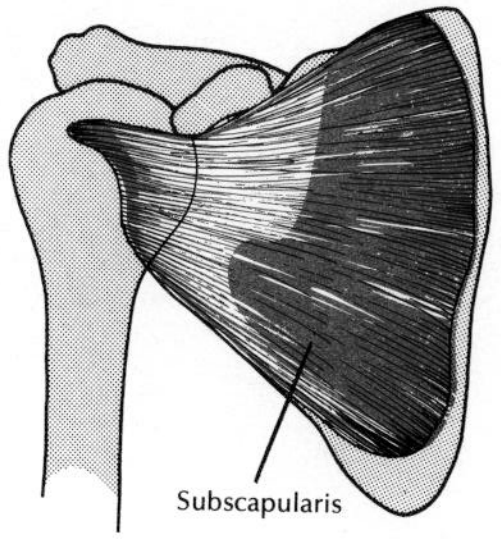

Subscapularis

Fig. 24

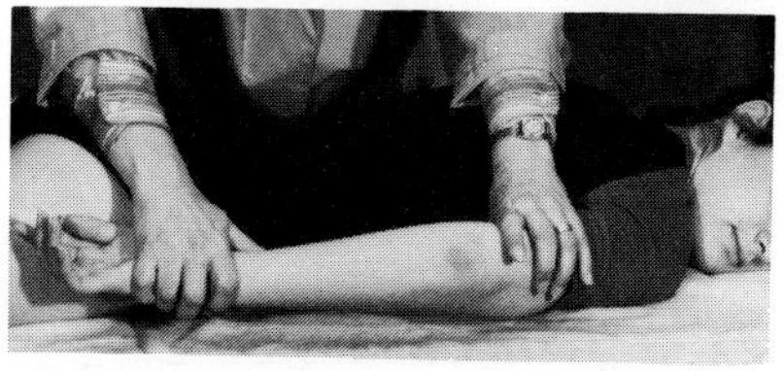

Fig. 25

Continued

*Adapted from Daniels L and Worthingham C: Muscle testing: techniques of manual examination, ed 4, Philadelphia, 1980, WB Saunders Co.

Table 18-4

Testing for muscle strength—*cont'd*

Movement	Muscles	Motor nerves	Positions for testing	Instructions and tests for muscle strength

Shoulder: part 2—cont'd

Movement	Muscles	Motor nerves	Positions for testing	Instructions and tests for muscle strength
External	Prime movers (Fig. 26*) Infraspinatus Teres minor Accessory muscle: deltoideus	Suprascapular nerve (cervical 5, 6) Axillary nerve (cervical 5)	Standing, sitting, prone (scapula stabilized)	"Rotate your shoulder outward with your palm facing you posteriorly; bring your arm upward as if throwing a ball behind you." Resistance is applied to the dorsum of the wrist (Fig. 27).
Scapular abduction and upward rotation	Prime mover: serratus anterior (Fig. 28*)	Long thoracic nerve (cervical 5, 6,7)	Standing, sitting	"Push your arm upward and forward as if pushing open a door." Resistance is applied with a hand at the wrist and elbow, making pressure toward the chest (Fig. 29).

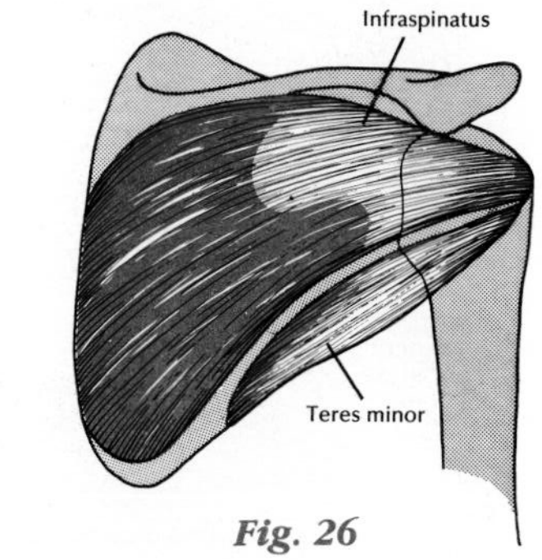

Fig. 26

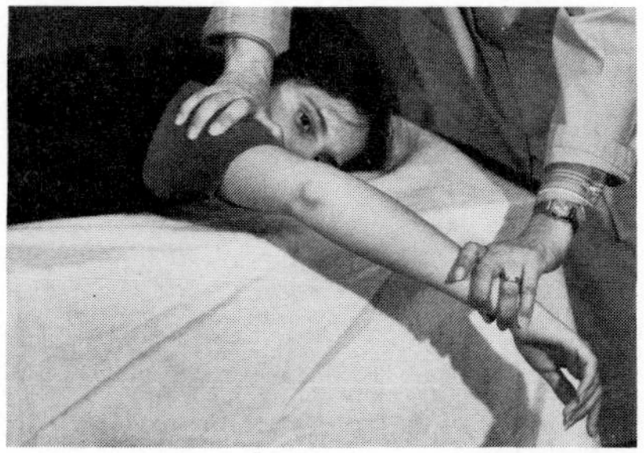

Infraspinatus

Teres minor

Fig. 27

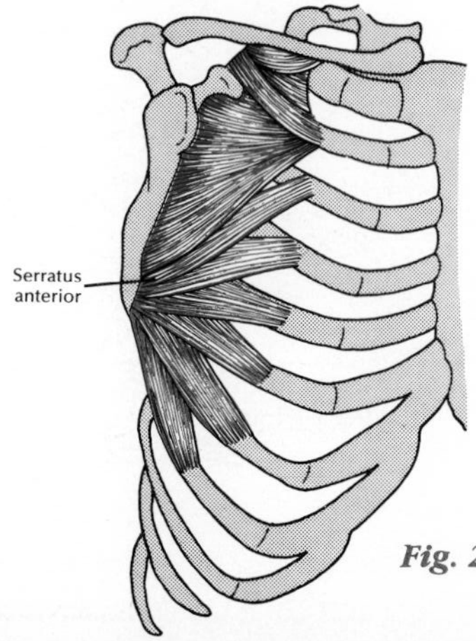

Fig. 28

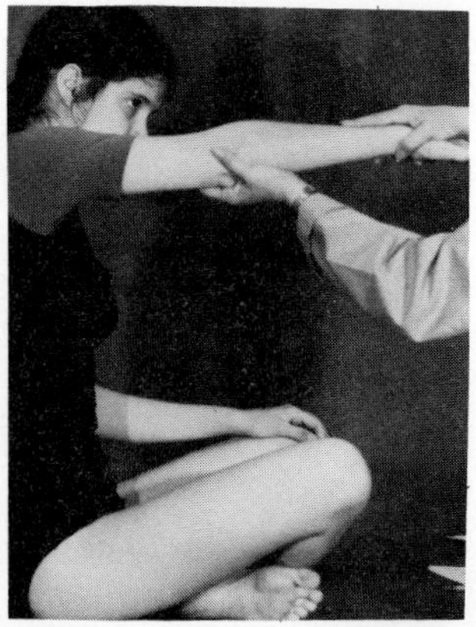

Serratus anterior

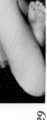

Fig. 29

Shoulder: part 3

Scapular adduction

Fig. 30

Prime movers (Fig. 30*)
Trapezius (middle fibers)

Rhomboideus major
Rhomboideus minor
Accessory muscle: trapezius (upper and lower fibers)

Spinal accessory nerve (cranial XI)
Cervical 3, 4
Dorsal scapular nerve (cervical 5)
Dorsal scapular nerve (cervical 5)

Standing, sitting, prone

"Try to bring your shoulder blades together in back." Resistance is applied over the posterior shoulder (Fig. 31).

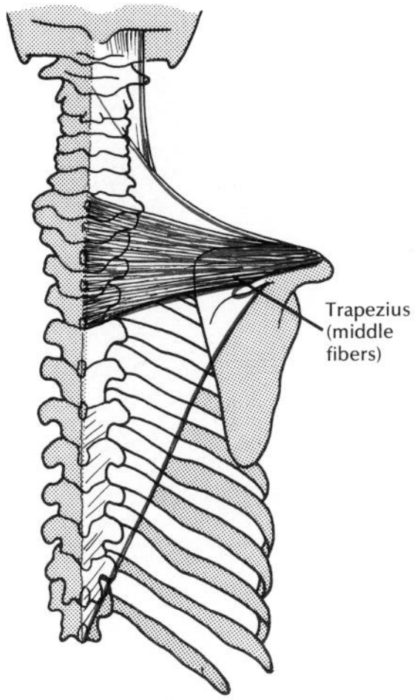

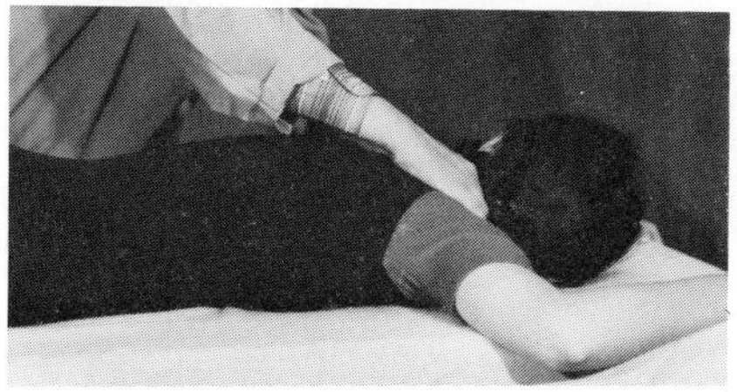

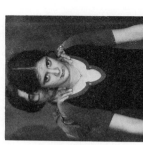

Fig. 31

Scapular elevation

Fig. 32

Prime movers (Fig. 32*)
Trapezius (superior fibers)
Levator scapulae
Accessory muscles
Rhomboideus major
Rhomboideus minor

Spinal accessory nerve (cranial XI)

Cervical 3, 4

Standing, sitting, lying

"Shrug your shoulders." "Hunch your shoulders against my hand." Resistance is applied to the superior aspect of the shoulder centered over the trapezius muscle (Fig. 33).

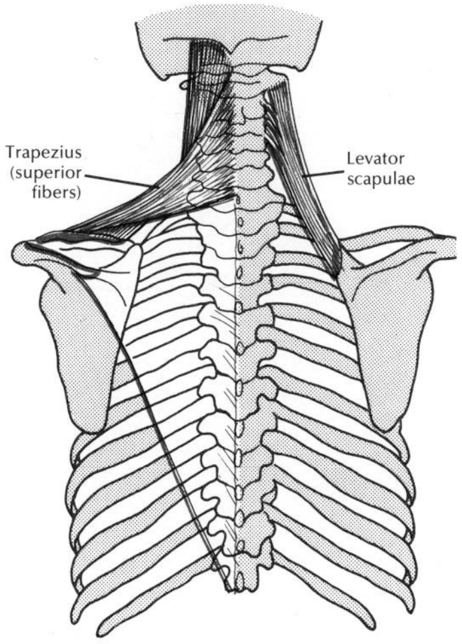

Fig. 33

Continued

*Adapted from Daniels L and Worthingham C: Muscle testing: techniques of manual examination, ed 4, Philadelphia, 1980, WB Saunders Co.

Table 18-4

Testing for muscle strength—*cont'd*

Movement	Muscles	Motor nerves	Positions for testing	Instructions and tests for muscle strength
Scapular depression and adduction	Prime mover: trapezius (inferior fibers) (Fig. 34*)	Spinal accessory nerve (cranial XI) Cervical 3, 4	Standing, sitting, prone	"Lift your arm and bring your shoulder blade down and close against your back chest wall. Bring the shoulder blade down against the chest." Upward pressure is applied against the deltoid muscle (Fig. 35).
Adduction and downward rotation	Prime movers (Fig. 36*) Rhomboideus major Rhomboideus minor	Dorsal scapular nerve (cervical 5) Dorsal scapular nerve (cervical 5)	Standing, sitting, prone (arm adducted over back in medial rotation)	"Lift up your arm. Concentrate on your elbow." Resistance is applied over the scapula (Fig. 37).

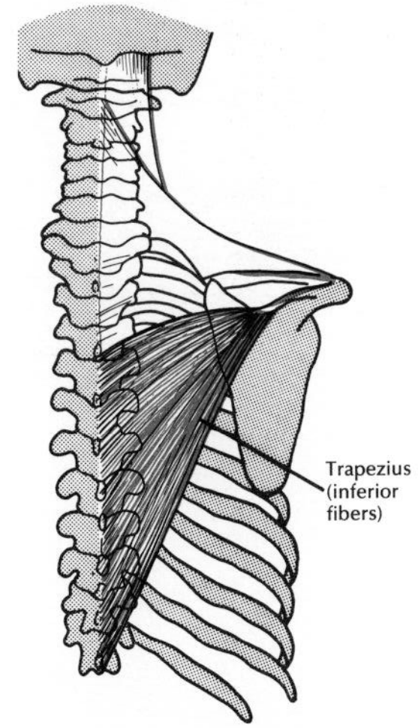

Fig. 34

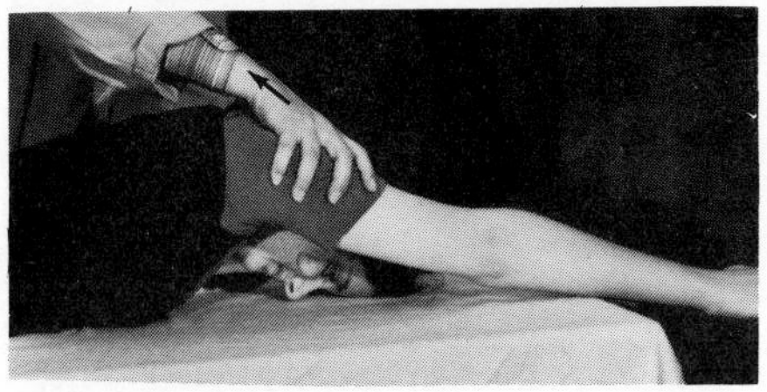

Fig. 35

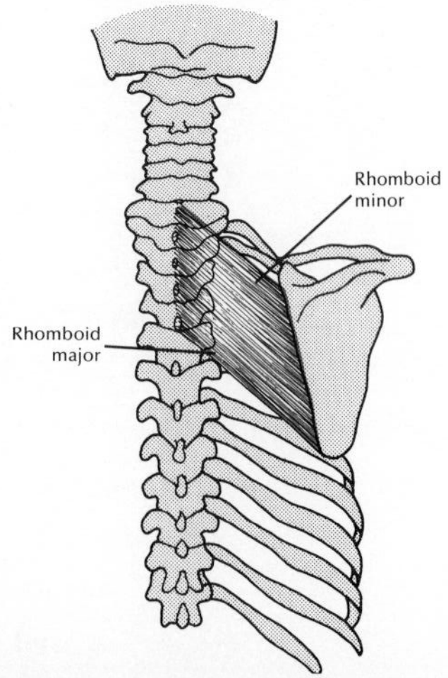

Fig. 36

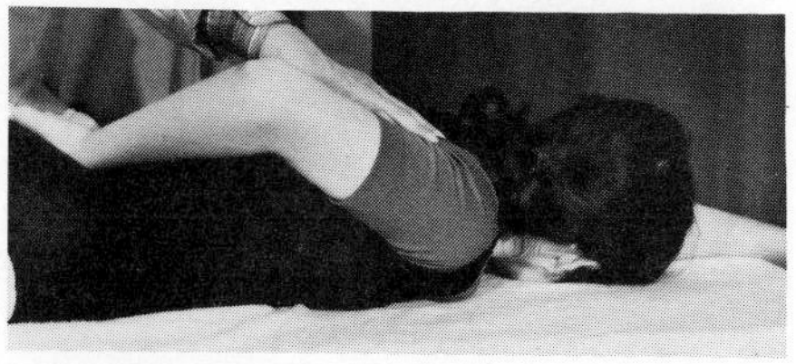

Fig. 37

Elbow

Flexion

Prime movers (Fig. 38*)
Biceps brachii

Brachialis

Brachioradialis
Accessory muscles: flexor muscles of forearm

Musculocutaneous nerve (cervical 5, 6)
Musculocutaneous nerve (cervical 5, 6)
Radial nerve (cervical 5, 6)

Standing, sitting, supine (arm extended)

"Move your right (left) hand to your right (left) shoulder."
"Make a fist; try to bring your fist to your shoulder."
Resistance is applied to the lower arm (Fig. 39).

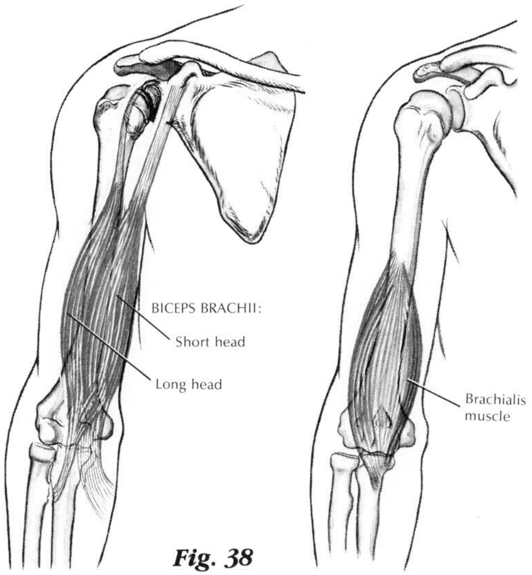

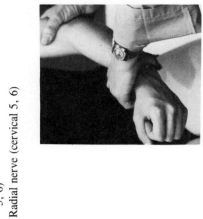

Brachialis muscle

BICEPS BRACHII:
Short head
Long head

Fig. 38

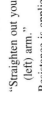
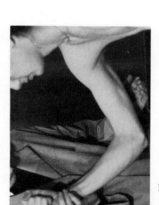

Fig. 39

Extension

Prime mover: triceps brachii (Fig. 40*)
Accessory muscles
Anconeus
Extensor muscles of forearm

Radial nerve (cervical 7, 8)

Standing, sitting, supine (arm flexed)

"Straighten out your right (left) arm."
Resistance is applied to the dorsal surface of the arm (Fig. 41).

TRICEPS BRACHII:
Long head
Lateral (short) head
Medial head

Fig. 40

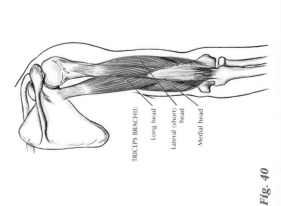

Fig. 41

Continued

*From Anthony CP and Thibodeau GA: Textbook of anatomy and physiology, ed 11, St Louis, 1983, The CV Mosby Co.

Table 18-4

Testing for muscle strength—*cont'd*

Movement	Muscles	Motor nerves	Positions for testing	Instructions and tests for muscle strength
Forearm				
Pronation	Prime movers (Fig. 42*) Pronator teres Pronator quadratus Accessory muscle: flexor carpi radialis	Median nerve (cervical 6, 7) Median nerve (cervical 8, thoracic 1)	Standing, sitting, supine (elbow flexed, hands extended, palms up)	"Rotate your right (left) hand inward so that your palm is downward." Resistance is applied at the base of the thumb on the volar surface (Fig. 43)
Supination	Prime movers (Fig. 44†) Biceps brachii Supinator Accessory muscle: brachioradialis	Musculocutaneous nerve (cervical 5, 6) Radial nerve (cervical 6)	Standing, sitting, supine	"Rotate your right (left) hand outward so that the palm is upward." Resistance is applied on the base of the thumb or over the surface of the hand on the dorsal surface (Fig. 45).

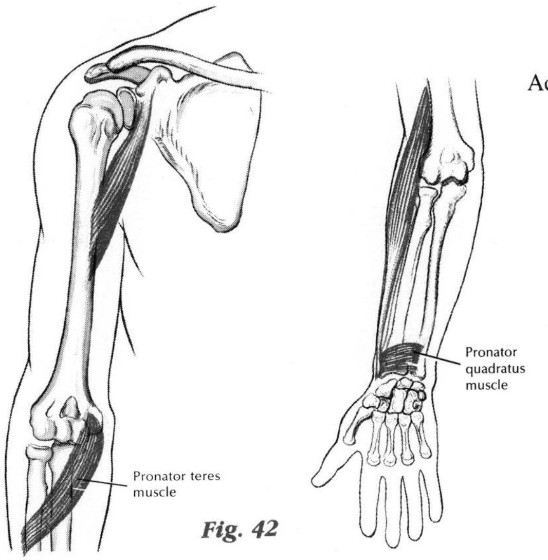

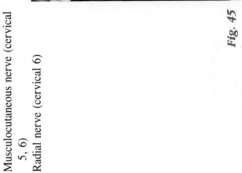

Fig. 43

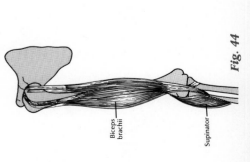

Fig. 45

Pronator quadratus muscle

Pronator teres muscle

Fig. 42

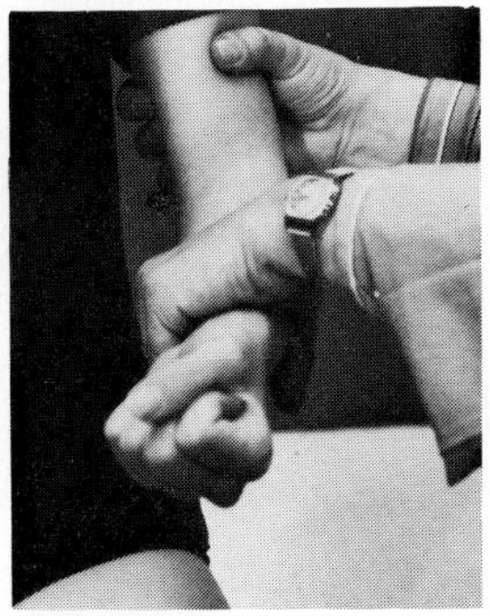

Biceps brachii

Supinator

Fig. 44

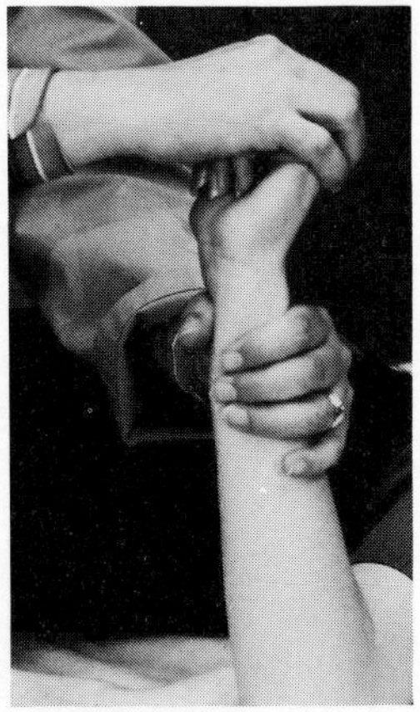

Wrist

Flexion

Prime movers (Fig. 46*)
Flexor carpi radialis
Flexor carpi ulnaris
Accessory muscle: palmaris longus

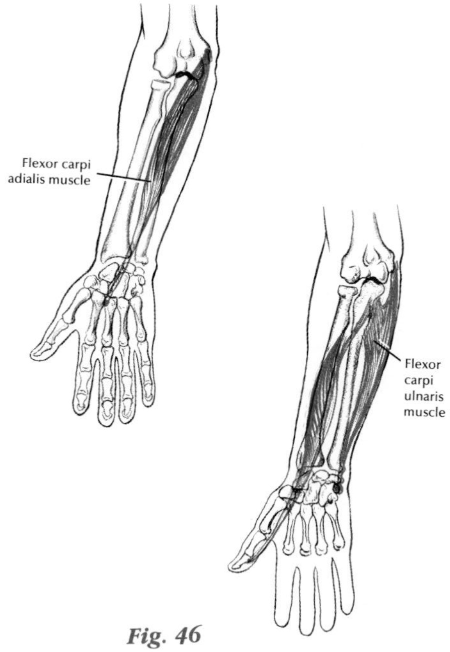

Medial nerve (cervical 6, 7)
Ulnar nerve (cervical 8, thoracic 1)

Standing, sitting, supine (unextended)

"Bend your right (left) hand down toward you." Resistance is applied to the volar surface of the hand (Fig. 47).

Fig. 46

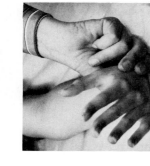

Fig. 47

Extension

Prime movers (Fig. 48†)
Extensor carpi radialis longus
Extensor carpi radialis brevis
Extensor carpi ulnaris

Radial nerve (cervical 6, 7)
Radial nerve (cervical 6, 7)
Radial nerve (cervical 6, 7, 8)

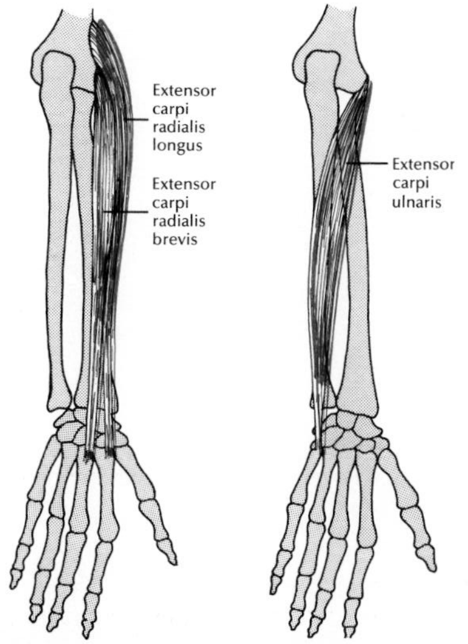

Standing, sitting, supine (wrist flexed)

"Bend your right (left) hand back on itself." Resistance is applied on the dorsal surface of the hand (Fig. 49).

Fig. 48

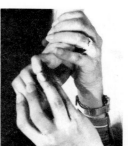

Fig. 49

Continued

*From Anthony CP and Thibodeau GA: Textbook of anatomy and physiology, ed 11, St Louis, 1983, The CV Mosby Co.
†Adapted from Daniels L and Worthingham C: Muscle testing: techniques of manual examination, ed 4, Philadelphia, 1980, WB Saunders Co.

Table 18-4

Testing for muscle strength—*cont'd*

Movement	Muscles	Motor nerves	Positions for testing	Instructions and tests for muscle strength
Thumb				
Flexion of joints Metacarpophalangeal Interphalangeal	Prime movers (Fig. 50*) Flexor pollicis brevis Flexor pollicis longus	Median nerve (cervical 6, 7) Ulnar nerve (cervical 8, thoracic 1)	Standing, sitting, supine (thumb extended)	"Bend your right (left) thumb to touch your palm." Resistance is applied to the thenar eminence—the dorsal surface of the distal phalanx (Fig. 51).
Extension of joints Metacarpophalangeal Interphalangeal	Prime movers (Fig. 52*) Extensor pollicis brevis Extensor pollicis longus	Radial nerve (cervical 6, 7) Radial nerve (cervical 6, 7, 8)	Standing, sitting, supine (thumb flexed)	"Straighten out your thumb as if thumbing a ride." "Thumb your nose." Resistance is applied to the dorsal surface of the distal phalanx (Fig. 53).

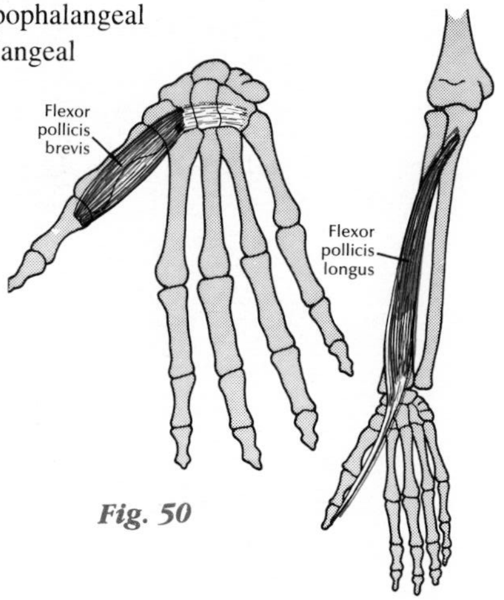

Fig. 51

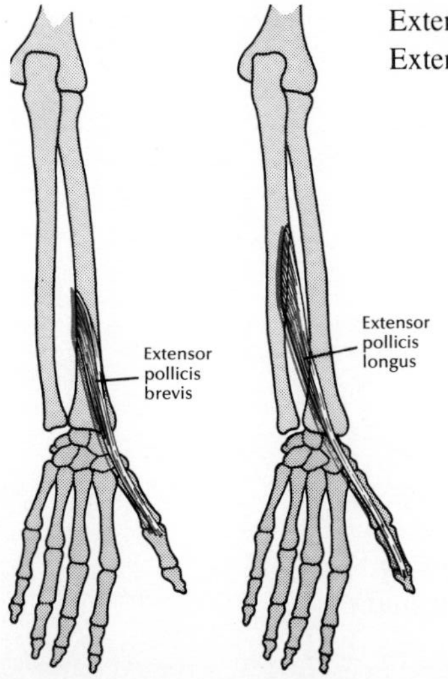

Fig. 53

Fig. 50

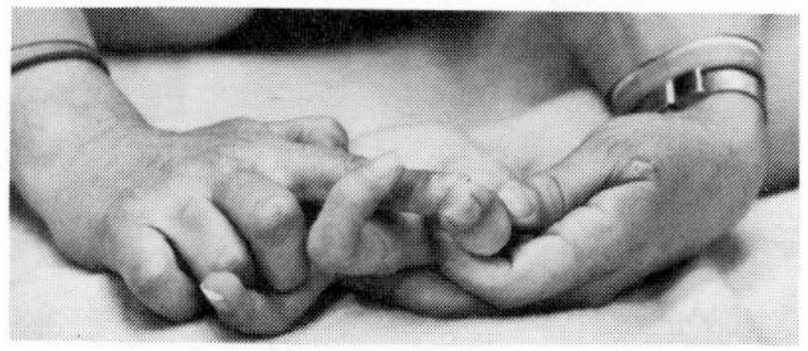

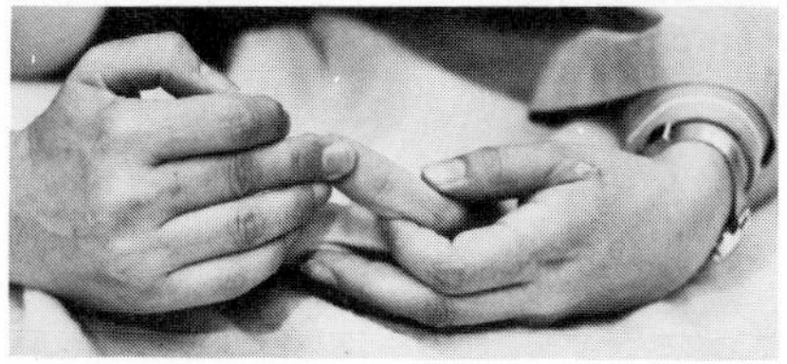

Fig. 52

	Prime movers	Nerve supply	Patient position	Instructions
Abduction 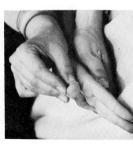 Abductor pollicis brevis / Abductor pollicis longus *Fig. 54*	Prime movers (Fig. 54*) Abductor pollicis longus Abductor pollicis brevis Accessory muscle: palmaris longus	Radial nerve (cervical 6, 7) Median nerve (cervical 6, 7)	Standing, sitting, supine (arms extended, may have hands in clapping position)	"Raise your right (left) thumb to the ceiling." Resistance is applied to the dorsal surface of the thumb (Fig. 55). 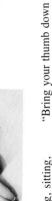 *Fig. 55*
Adduction 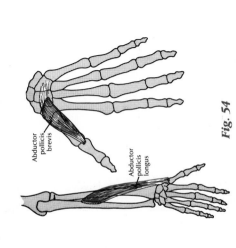 Adductor pollicis *Fig. 56*	Prime movers (Fig. 56*) Adductor pollicis oblique Adductor pollicis transverse	Ulnar nerve (cervical 8, thoracic 1) Ulnar nerve (cervical 8, thoracic 1)	Standing, sitting, supine	"Bring your thumb down against the index finger." Resistance in applied against the terminal phalanx.
Opposition 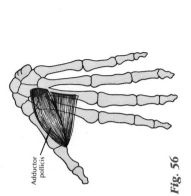 Opponens digiti minimi / Opponens pollicis *Fig. 57*	Prime movers (Fig. 57*) Opponens pollicis Opponens digiti minimi	Median nerve (cervical 6, 7) Ulnar nerve (cervical 8, thoracic 1)	Standing, sitting, supine	"Touch the top of the right (left) thumb to the tip and then to the base of the little, ring, middle, and index fingers." Resistance is applied to the palmar surfaces of the thumb and fingers (Fig. 58). 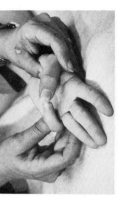 *Fig. 58*

Continued

*Adapted from Daniels L and Worthingham C: Muscle testing: techniques of manual examination, ed 4, Philadelphia, 1980, WB Saunders Co.

Table 18-4

Testing for muscle strength—*cont'd*

Movement	Muscles	Motor nerves	Positions for testing	Instructions and tests for muscle strength
Fingers				
Flexion of joints				
Metacarpophalangeal	Prime movers (Fig. 59*) Lumbricales Dorsal interossei Palmar interossei Accessory muscles Flexor digiti minimi brevis Flexor digitorum superficialis Flexor digitorum profundus	Ulnar nerve (cervical 8) Ulnar nerve (cervical 8) Ulnar nerve (cervical 8, thoracic 1)	Standing, sitting, supine	"Bend your fingers at the first [proximal] joint." Resistance is applied to the palmar surface of the proximal phalanges (Fig. 60).
Proximal interphalangeal	Prime mover: flexor digitorum superficialis	Median nerve (cervical 7, 8; thoracic 1)	Standing, sitting, supine	"Bend your fingers at the middle joint." "Crook your fingers." Resistance is applied to the palmar surface of the middle phalanges.
Distal interphalangeal	Prime mover: flexor digitorum profundus	Ulnar nerve (cervical 8, thoracic 1)	Standing, sitting, supine	"Bend your distal finger joint." "Crook your finger." Resistance is applied to the pad of the finger (Fig. 61).

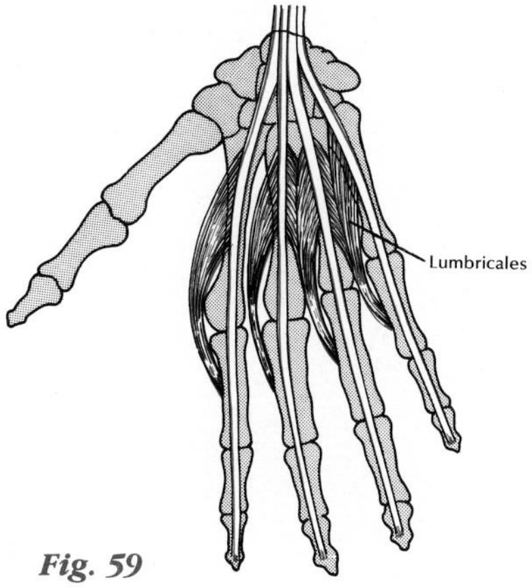

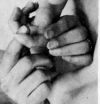

Fig. 60

Lumbricales

Fig. 59

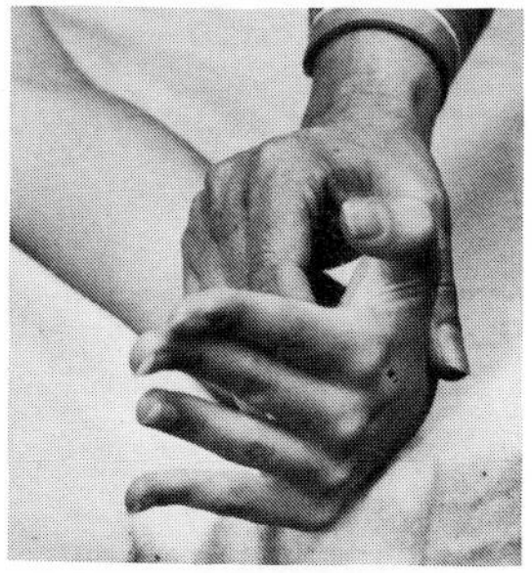

Fig. 61

Extension of metacarpophalangeal joints

Prime movers (Fig. 62*)		Standing, sitting, supine (fingers flexed)
Extensor digitorum communis	Radial nerve (cervical 6, 7, 8)	"Straighten out your fingers."
Extensor indicis proprius	Radial nerve (cervical 6, 7, 8)	Resistance is applied to the dorsal surface of the proximal and distal phalanges (Fig. 49).
Extensor digiti minimi	Radial nerve (cervical 7)	

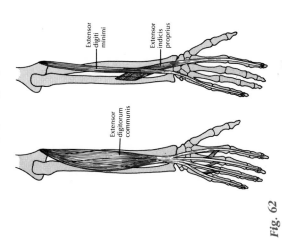

Fig. 62

Abduction

Prime movers (Fig. 63*)		Standing, sitting, supine (fingers together)
Interossei dorsales	Ulnar nerve (cervical 8, thoracic 1)	"Spread your fingers as far apart as possible."
Abductor digiti minimi	Ulnar nerve (cervical 8)	Pressure is exerted against the outside surfaces of the fingers being tested to resist spread of the fingers (Fig. 64).

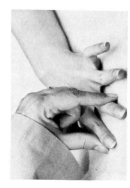

Fig. 64

Fig. 63

Adduction

Prime movers: interossei palmares (Fig. 65*)	Ulnar nerve (cervical 8, thoracic 1)	Standing, sitting, supine (fingers apart)
		"Put your fingers together. Press them hard against each other."
		An attempt is made to pull them apart (Fig. 66).

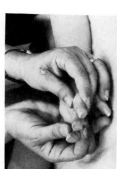

Fig. 66

Continued

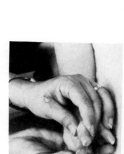

*Adapted from Daniels L and Worthingham C: Muscle testing: techniques of manual examination, ed 4, Philadelphia, 1980, WB Saunders Co.

Table 18-4

Testing for muscle strength—*cont'd*

Movement	Muscles	Motor nerves	Positions for testing	Instructions and tests for muscle strength
Hip				
Flexion	Prime movers (Fig. 67*)		Sitting, supine	"Draw your knees up to your chest."
	Psoas major	Femoral nerve (lumbar 2, 3)		"Bend your right (left) knee up to your chest."
	Iliacus	Femoral nerve (lumbar 2, 3)		Resistance is applied to the anterior surface of the leg proximal to the knee (Fig. 68).
	Accessory muscles			
	Sartorius			
	Rectus femoris			
	Tensor fasciae latae			
	Pectineus			
	Adductor brevis			
	Adductor longus			
	Adductor magnus (oblique fibers)			
Extension	Prime movers (Fig. 69†)		Prone	"Lift your right (left) leg toward the ceiling."
	Gluteus maximus	Inferior gluteal nerve (lumbar 5; sacral 1, 2)		Resistance is applied to the dorsal surface of the leg proximal to the knee (Fig. 70).
	Semitendinosus	Sciatic nerve (lumbar 4, 5; sacral 1, 2)		

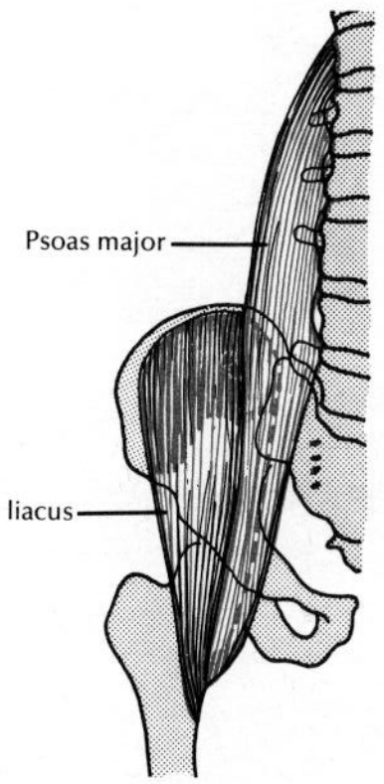

Fig. 67

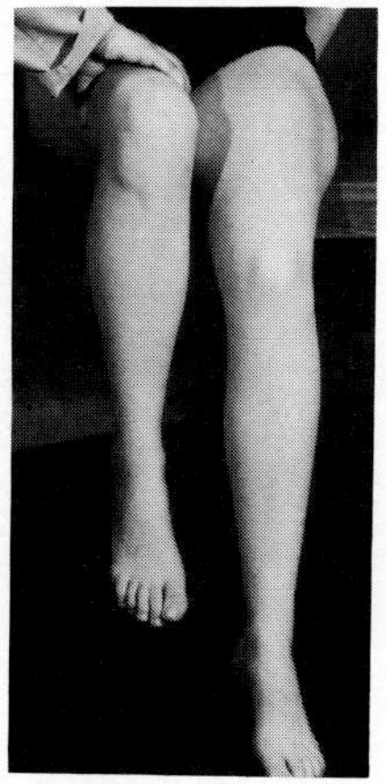

Psoas major

Iliacus

Fig. 68

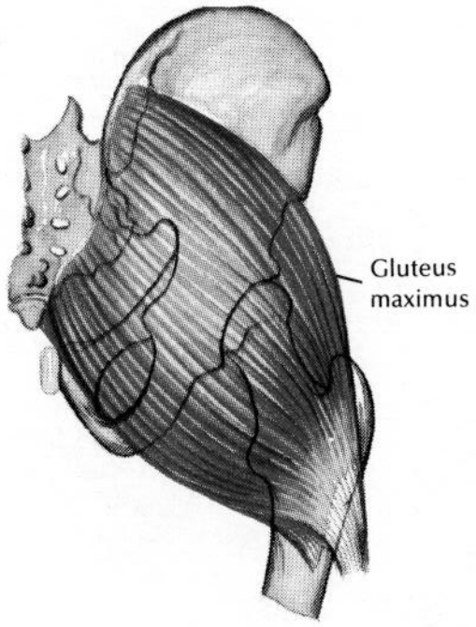

Gluteus maximus

Fig. 69

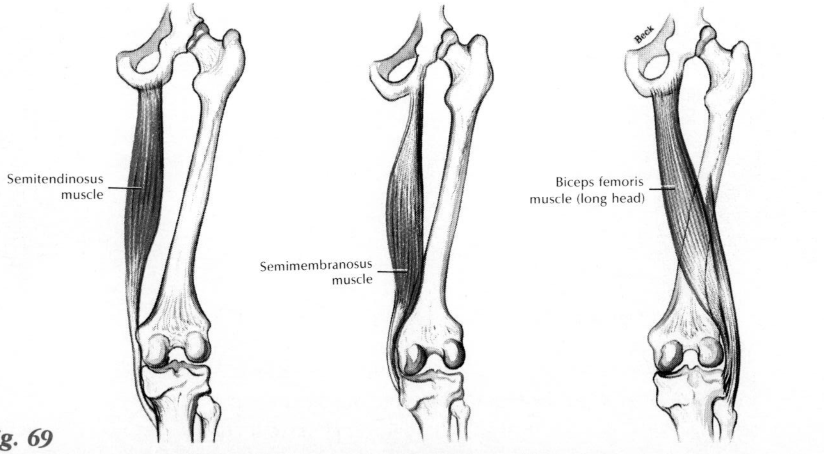

Semitendinosus muscle

Semimembranosus muscle

Biceps femoris muscle (long head)

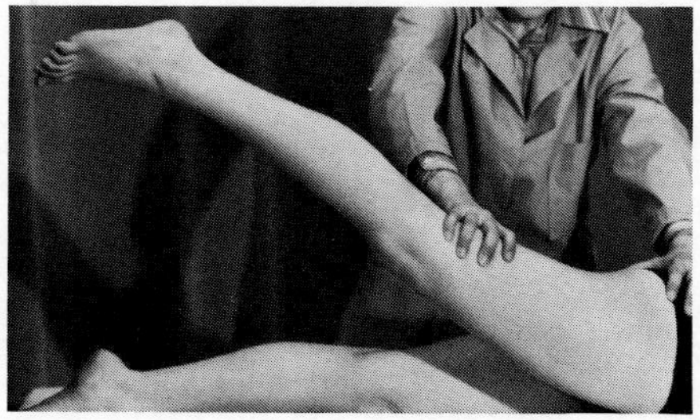

Fig. 70

Abduction

Semimembranosus — Sciatic nerve (lumbar 5; sacral 1, 2)

Biceps femoris (long head) — Sciatic nerve (sacral 1, 2, 3)

Prime mover: gluteus medius (Fig. 71†) — Superior gluteal nerve (lumbar 4, 5; sacral 1)

Accessory muscles
Gluteus minimus
Tensor fasciae latae
Gluteus maximus (upper fibers)

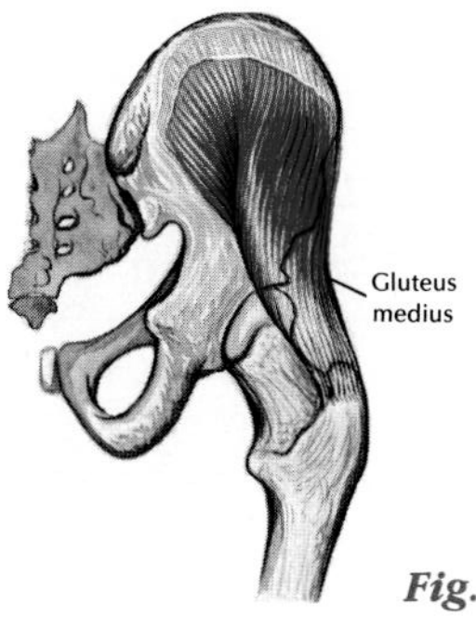

Gluteus medius

Fig. 71

Fig. 72

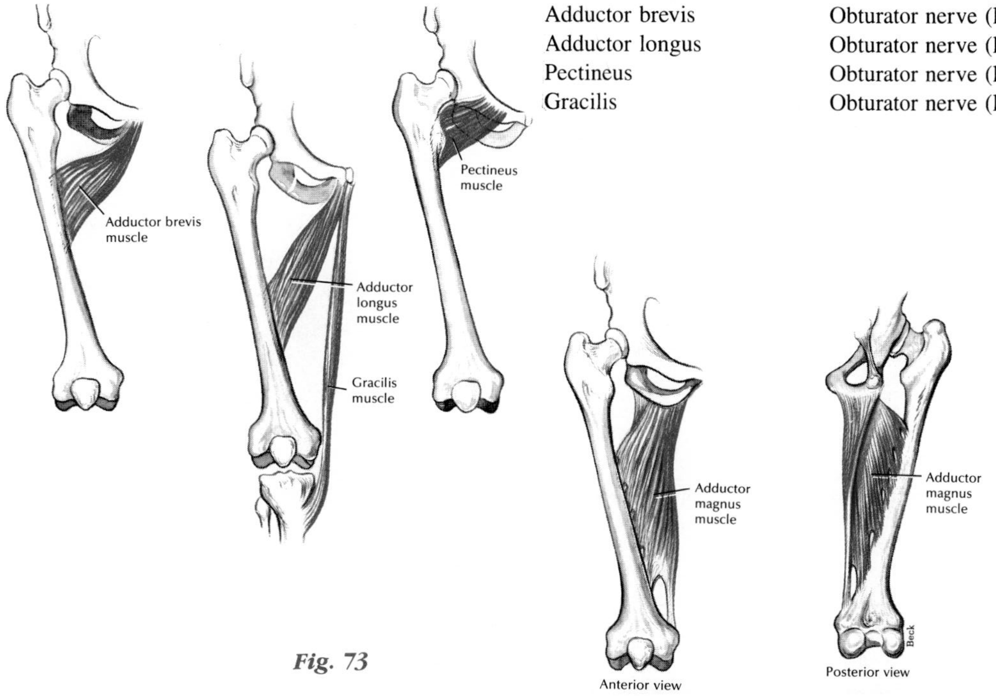

Lateral lie

"Move your upper leg toward the ceiling."
Resistance is applied to the lateral surface of the upper leg (Fig. 72).

Adduction

Prime movers (Fig. 73†)
Adductor magnus — Obturator nerve (lumbar 3, 4)
Adductor brevis — Obturator nerve (lumbar 3, 4)
Adductor longus — Obturator nerve (lumbar 3, 4)
Pectineus — Obturator nerve (lumbar 2, 3, 4)
Gracilis — Obturator nerve (lumbar 3, 4)

Pectineus muscle

Adductor longus muscle

Gracilis muscle

Adductor brevis muscle

Adductor magnus muscle

Adductor magnus muscle

Beck

Anterior view

Posterior view

Fig. 73

Fig. 74

Lateral lie, legs apart

"Try to bring your legs together."
Resistance is applied to the medial surface of the thighs proximal to the knees (Fig. 74).

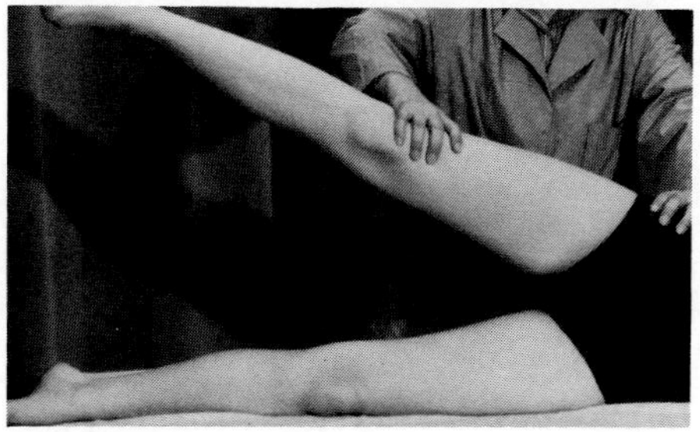

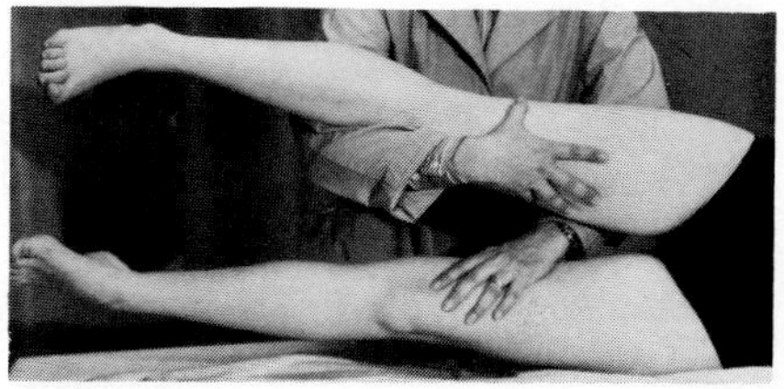

Continued

---

*Adapted from Daniels L and Worthingham C: Muscle testing: techniques of manual examination, ed 4, Philadelphia, 1980, WB Saunders Co.
†From Anthony CP and Thibodeau GA: Textbook of anatomy and physiology, ed 11, St Louis, 1983, The CV Mosby Co.

Table 18-4

Testing for muscle strength—*cont'd*

Movement	Muscles	Motor nerves	Positions for testing	Instructions and tests for muscle strength
Hip—cont'd				
Rotation (knees extended) Internal	Prime movers (Fig. 75*) Gluteus minimus	Superior gluteal nerve (lumbar 4, 5; sacral 1)	Sitting (legs about a foot apart at ankle)	"Pivot your right hip inward—your foot will move away from your body."
	Tensor fasciae latae	Superior gluteal nerve (lumbar 4, 5; sacral 1)		Resistance is applied toward the midline at the lateral surface of the ankle (Fig. 76).
	Accessory muscles Gluteus medius (anterior fibers) Semitendinosus Semimembranosus			
External	Prime movers (Fig. 77†) Obturator externus Obturator internus	Obturator nerve (lumbar 3, 4) Obturator nerve (lumbar 5; sacral 2, 3)	Sitting	"Rotate your hip outward; your foot will turn in." Resistance is applied to the medial aspect of the ankle (Fig. 78).
	Quadratus femoris	Obturator nerve (lumbar 5; sacral 1)		
	Piriformis	Obturator nerve (sacral 1, 2)		
	Gemellus superior	Obturator nerve (lumbar 5; sacral 1, 2, 3)		
	Gemellus inferior	Obturator nerve (lumbar 5; sacral 1)		
	Gluteus maximus	Obturator nerve (lumbar 5; sacral 1, 2)		
	Accessory muscles Sartorius Biceps femoris (long head)			

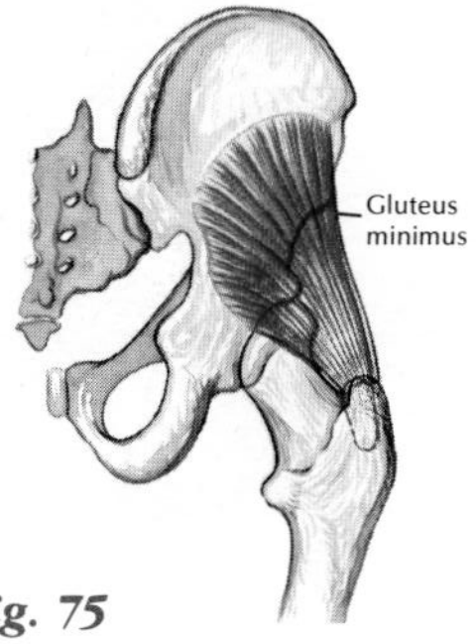

Fig. 76

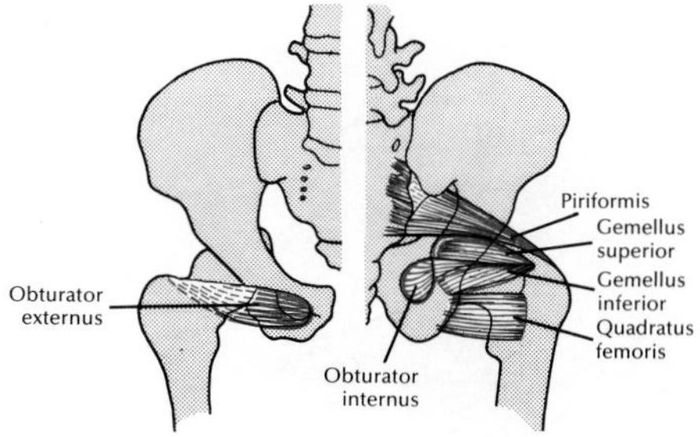

Fig. 78

Gluteus minimus

Fig. 75

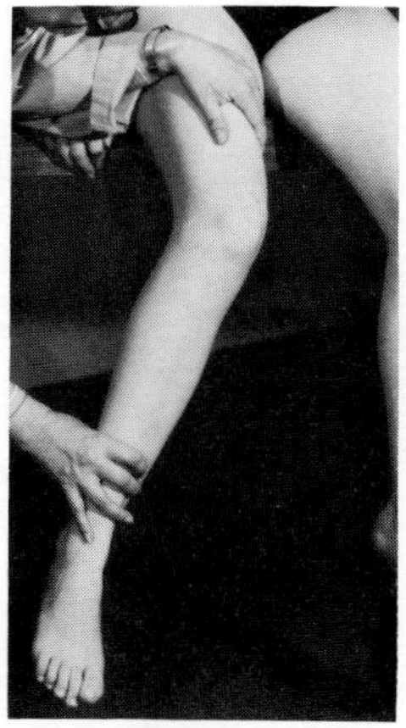

Piriformis
Gemellus superior
Gemellus inferior
Quadratus femoris
Obturator internus
Obturator externus

Fig. 77

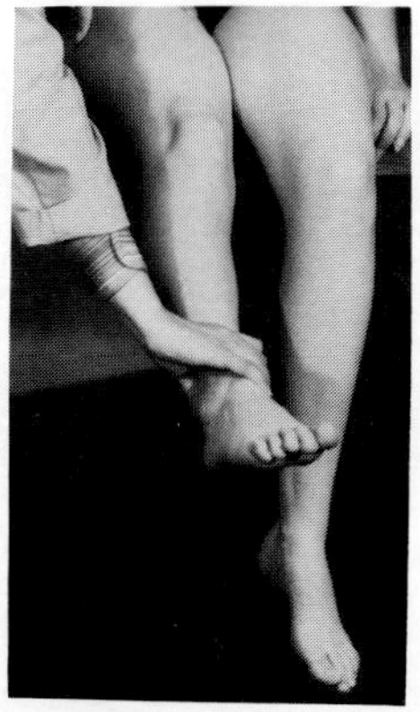

Movement	Patient position	Instructions	Nerve	Muscles
Rotation (knees flexed)	Supine (knees flexed)	"Rotate your knees outward. Bend them toward the table. Bring them as close as you can to the table." Resistance is applied to the lateral aspects of the knees.	Femoral nerve (lumbar 2, 3, 4)	Prime mover: sartorius Accessory muscles External rotators of hip Flexors of hip, knee
Abduction	Supine	"Bend your knees out." Resistance is applied to the upper outer aspect of each leg.	Superior gluteal nerve (lumbar 4, 5; sacral 1)	Prime mover: tensor fasciae latae Accessory muscles Gluteus medius Gluteus minimus
Knee Flexion	Prone	"Bend your right (left) leg. Try to touch your heel to the back of your leg." Resistance is applied to the dorsal aspect of the ankle (Fig. 80).	Sciatic nerve (sacral 1, 2, 3) Sciatic nerve (lumbar 4, 5; sacral 1, 2) Sciatic nerve (lumbar 4, 5; sacral 1, 2, 3) Sciatic nerve (lumbar 4, 5; sacral 1, 2, 3)	Prime movers (Fig. 79*) Biceps femoris (long head) Biceps femoris (short head) Semitendinosus Semimembranosus Accessory muscles Popliteus Sartorius Gracilis Gastrocnemius

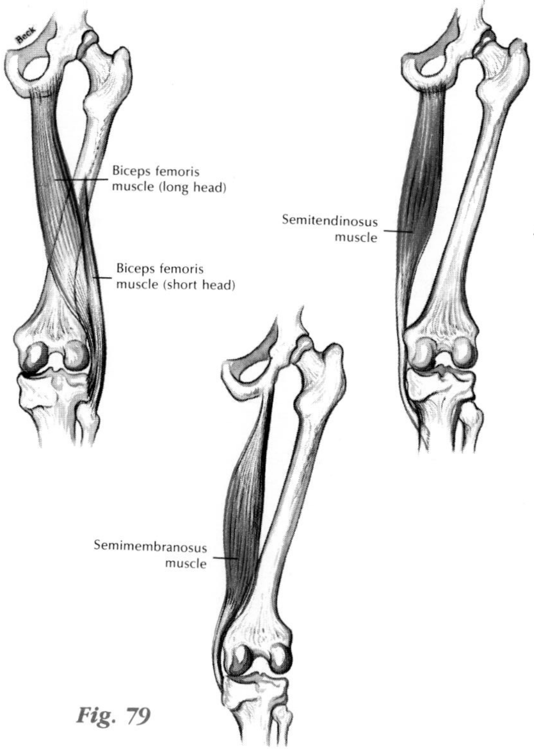

Fig. 80

Fig. 79

Biceps femoris muscle (long head)
Biceps femoris muscle (short head)
Semitendinosus muscle
Semimembranosus muscle

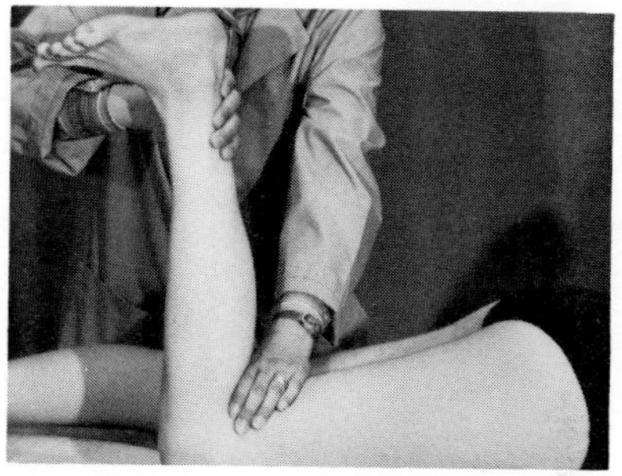

Continued

*From Anthony CP and Thibodeau GA: Textbook of anatomy and physiology, ed 11, St Louis, 1983, The CV Mosby Co.
†Adapted from Daniels L and Worthingham C: Muscle testing: techniques of manual examination, ed 4, Philadelphia, 1980, WB Saunders Co.

Table 18-4

Testing for muscle strength—*cont'd*

Movement	Muscles	Motor nerves	Positions for testing	Instructions and tests for muscle strength
Knee—cont'd				
Extension	Prime movers (Fig. 81*) Rectus femoris Vastus intermedius Vastus medialis Vastus lateralis	Femoral nerve (lumbar 2, 3, 4) Femoral nerve (lumbar 2, 3, 4) Femoral nerve (lumbar 2, 3, 4) Femoral nerve (lumbar 2, 3, 4)	Sitting	"Straighten out your right (left) leg." Resistance is applied against the anterior aspect of the ankle.

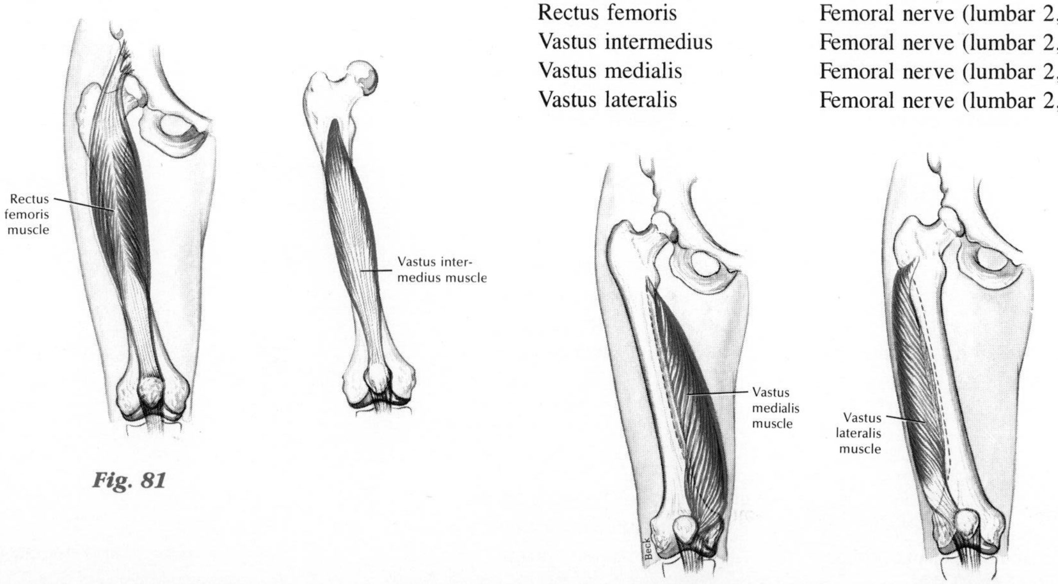

Fig. 81

Ankle

Dorsiflexion	Prime mover: tibialis anterior (Fig. 82†)	Deep peroneal nerve (lumbar 4, 5; sacral 1)	Sitting, supine	"Bend your toes toward your knees." Resistance is applied to the dorsal aspect of the foot.
	Prime mover: tibialis posterior (Fig. 82)	Deep peroneal nerve (lumbar 5; sacral 1)	Sitting, supine	"Rotate your right (left) foot toward the left (right) foot. Turn it as far as you can." Resistance is applied to the medial aspect of the foot at the first metatarsal joint.
Plantar flexion	Prime movers (Fig. 83†) Gastrocnemius Soleus Accessory muscles Tibialis posterior Peroneus longus Peroneus brevis Flexor hallucis longus Flexor digitorum longus Plantaris	Tibial nerve (sacral 1, 2) Tibial nerve (sacral 1, 2)	Sitting, supine	"Point your toes away from you (downward) as far as you can." Resistance is applied to the ball of the foot (Fig. 84).

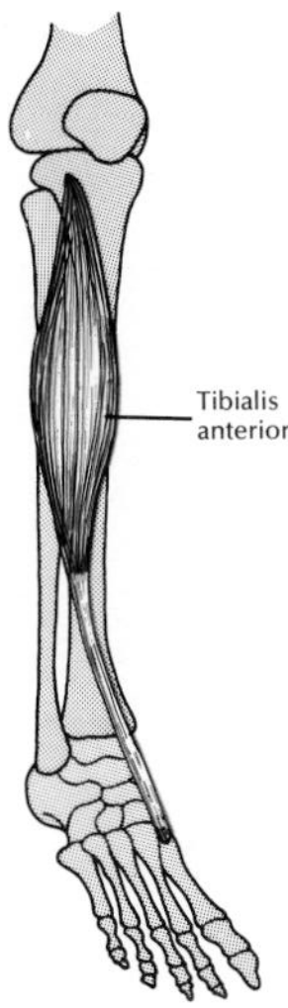

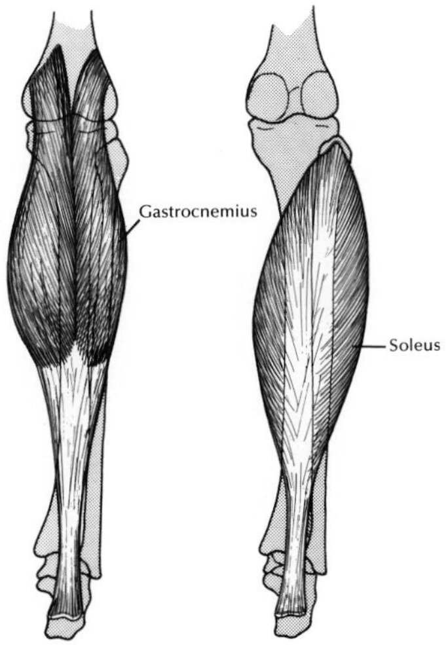

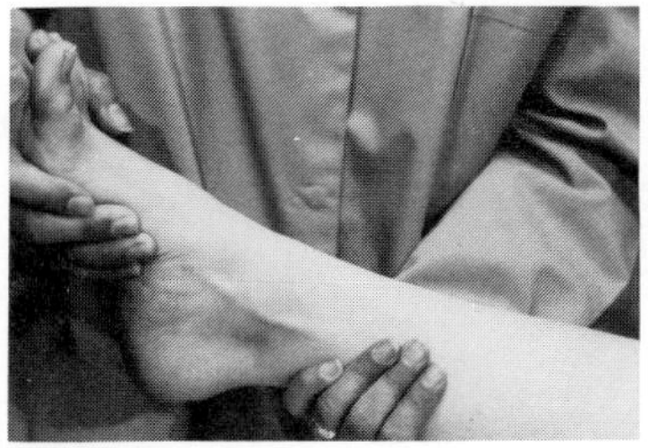

Fig. 84

Fig. 82

Fig. 83

Continued

*Adapted from Daniels L and Worthingham C: Muscle testing: techniques of manual examination, ed 4, Philadelphia, 1980, WB Saunders Co.
†From Mann RA: DuVries' surgery of the foot, ed 4, St Louis, 1978, The CV Mosby Co.

Table 18-4

Testing for muscle strength—*cont'd*

Movement	Muscles	Motor nerves	Positions for testing	Instructions and tests for muscle strength
Foot				
Inversion	Prime mover: tibialis posterior (Fig. 85*) Accessory muscles Flexor digitorum longus Flexor hallucis longus Gastrocnemius (medial head)	Tibial nerve (lumbar 5, sacral 1)	Sitting, supine	"Point your toes, then rotate them inward." Resistance is applied against the medial aspect of the first metatarsal bone (Fig. 86).
Eversion	Prime movers (Fig. 87*) Peroneus longus Peroneus brevis Accessory muscles Extensor digitorum longus Peroneus tertius	Superficial peroneal nerve (lumbar 4, 5; sacral 1) Superficial peroneal nerve (lumbar 4, 5; sacral 1)	Sitting, supine	"Point your toes and rotate them outward." Resistance is applied against the lateral aspect of the fifth metatarsal bone.

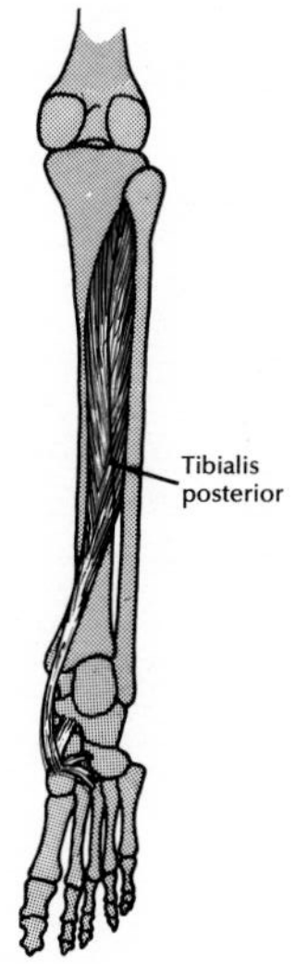

Tibialis posterior

Fig. 85

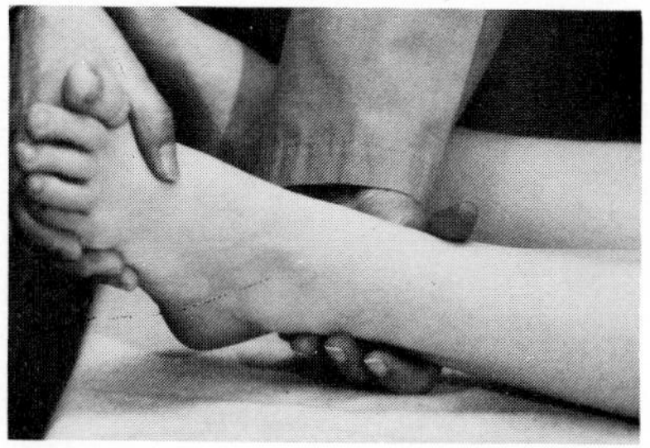

Fig. 86

Peroneus brevis

Peroneus longus

Fig. 87

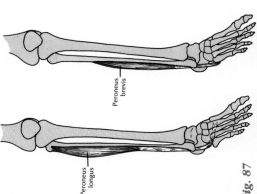

Great toe

Flexion of joints

Metatarsophalangeal

Prime mover: flexor hallucis brevis (Fig. 88*†)
Accessory muscle: flexor hallucis longus

Medial plantar nerve (lumbar 4, 5; sacral 1)

Sitting, supine

"Bend your right (left) big toe down."
"Curl your toe."
Resistance is applied to the plantar side of the toe (Fig. 89).

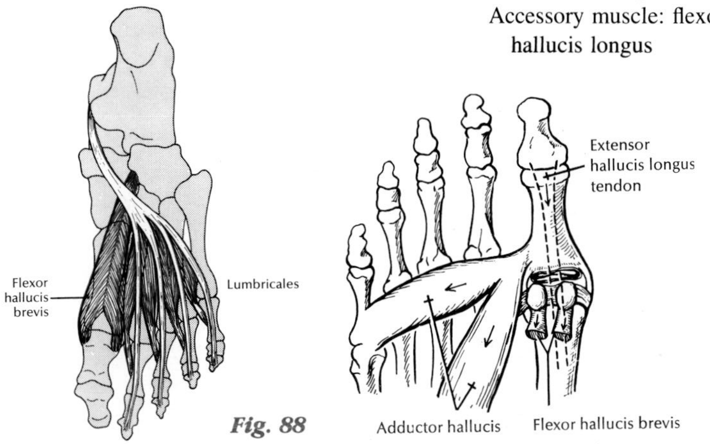

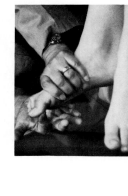

Fig. 89

Fig. 88

Labels (Fig. 88): Extensor hallucis longus tendon, Flexor hallucis brevis, Adductor hallucis, Lumbricales, Flexor hallucis brevis

Interphalangeal

Prime mover: flexor hallucis longus (Fig. 90*†)

Tibial nerve (lumbar 5; sacral 1, 2)

Sitting, supine

"Bend your right (left) big toe down."
"Curl your toe."
Resistance is applied to the plantar surface of the distal phalanges.

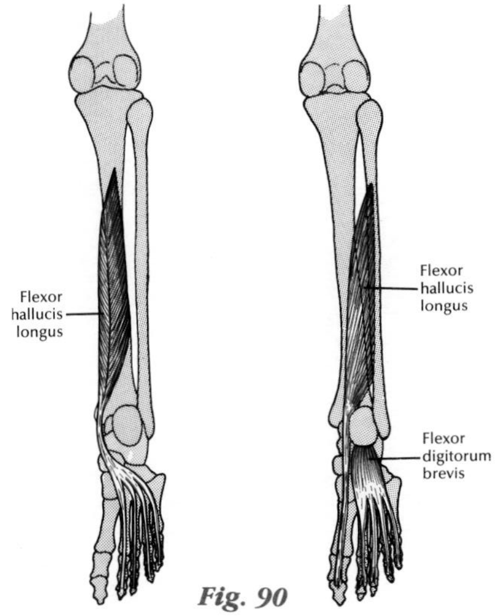

Fig. 90

Labels (Fig. 90): Flexor hallucis longus, Flexor digitorum brevis, Flexor hallucis longus

Continued

*Adapted from Daniels L and Worthington C: Muscle testing: techniques of manual examination, ed 4, Philadelphia, 1980, WB Saunders Co.
†From Mann RA: DuVries' surgery of the foot, ed 4, St Louis, 1978, The CV Mosby Co.

Table 18-4
Testing for muscle strength—*cont'd*

Movement	Muscles	Motor nerves	Positions for testing	Instructions and tests for muscle strength
Toe—cont'd.				
Extension of metatarsophalangeal joint	Prime movers (Fig. 91*) Extensor digitorum longus; Extensor digitorum brevis	Deep peroneal nerve (lumbar 4, 5; sacral 1); Deep peroneal nerve (lumbar 5; sacral 1)	Sitting, supine	"Bend your right (left) big toe upward." Resistance is applied to the dorsum of the toe (Fig. 92).
Lateral four toes Flexion of toe joints Metatarsophalangeal	Prime mover: lumbricales (Fig. 88) Accessory muscles Interossei dorsales and plantares; Flexor digiti quinti brevis; Flexor digitorum longus; Flexor digitorum brevis	Medial plantar nerve (lumbar 4, 5); Lateral plantar nerve (sacral 1, 2)	Sitting, supine	"Bend all your toes downward." Resistance is applied to the plantar surface of the proximal phalanges.
Proximal interphalangeal	Prime mover: flexor digitorum brevis (Fig. 90)	Medial plantar nerve (lumbar 4, 5)	Sitting, supine	"Bend your toes downward." Resistance is applied to the plantar surface of the medial phalanges.

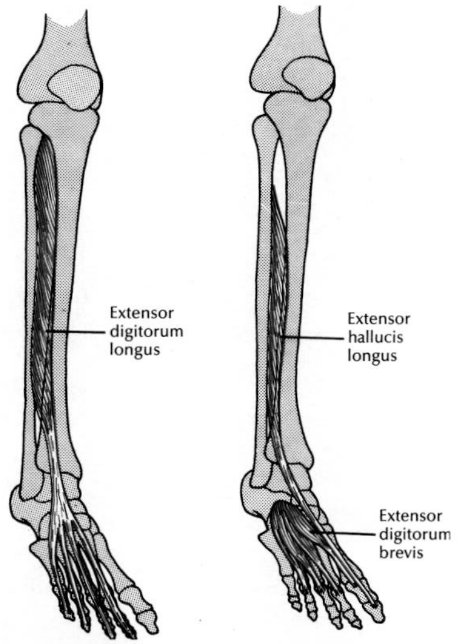

Fig. 92

Extensor digitorum longus

Extensor hallucis longus

Extensor digitorum brevis

Fig. 91

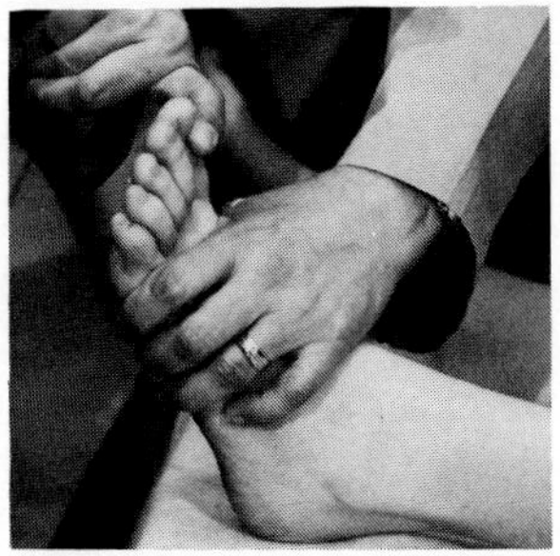

Distal interphalangeal	Prime mover: flexor digitorum longus (Fig. 90)	Tibial nerve (lumbar 5, sacral 1)	Sitting, supine	"Bend your toes downward." Pressure is applied to the plantar surface of the distal phalanges (Fig. 93).
Extension of metatarsophalangeal joint	Prime movers (Fig. 91) Extensor digitorum longus Extensor digitorum brevis	Deep peroneal nerve (lumbar 4, 5; sacral 1) Deep peroneal nerve (lumbar 5; sacral 1)	Sitting, supine	"Straighten out your toes. Point your toes upward." Resistance is applied to the dorsum of the proximal phalanges.

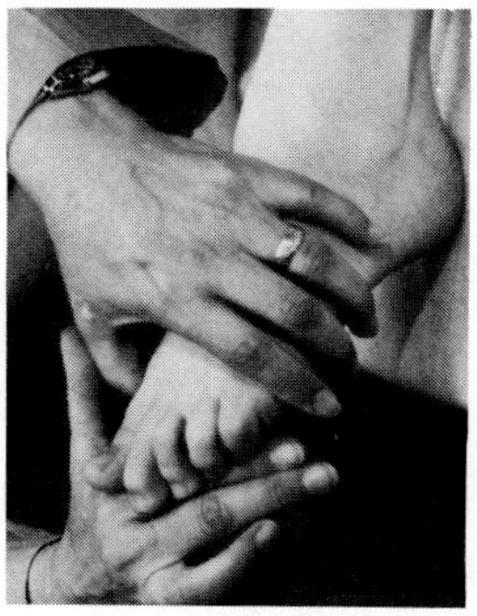

Fig. 93

*From Mann RA: DuVries' surgery of the foot, ed 4, St Louis, 1978, The CV Mosby Co.

(Continued from p. 433)

disturbances, particularly of potassium or calcium ion concentrations.

Transient ischemic attacks (TIAs) may cause a focal episode of motor dysfunction related to vascular disease, such as arteriosclerosis or essential hypertension. It is particularly important to listen for bruits over the neck vessels in the elderly client with muscle weakness, since these bruits might strengthen the impressions of vascular disease.

Clinical correlation of signs of muscle weakness and disease entities have shown that each neuromuscular disease has a general predilection for a particular group of muscles. A given pattern of weakness, then, suggests the possibility of a certain disease and excludes others. An example lies in the adage that peripheral muscle involvement in the extremities is of muscular origin, whereas distal disease is of neuropathic origin. Further explanation of the correlation of assessment data with underlying disease processes appears in Table 18-5.

Hypokalemia

Since the ratio of the concentrations of potassium ion of the intracellular milieu to the extracellular fluid determines the rate of cell firing, a deficit of this ion is accomplished by disorders of structure and function in muscular and neural tissues. Both skeletal and smooth muscles are affected by hypokalemia. The client complains of varying degrees of weakness and lassitude. Extreme hypokalemia may be accompanied by muscular paralysis. Some other signs that will help confirm hypokalemia as the cause of muscle weakness are abnormalities in motor and secretory activities of the gastrointestinal tract, changes in electrocardiograms, and dilute urine. Some of the conditions known to be correlated with a deficiency of this ion are diarrhea, excessive losses in the urine resulting from the use of chlorothiazide or mercurial diuretics or steroid hormones, Cushing's syndrome, and primary aldosteronism.

Age-related muscle weakness

Wasting of muscles and a decrease in muscle strength have been traditionally attributed to the aging process. Histologically, the muscle tissue shows increased amounts of collagen initially, followed by fibrosis of connective tissue.

Involuntary Contraction of Skeletal Muscles

Fasciculations

Fasciculations are the visible, spontaneous contraction of a number of muscle fibers supplied by a single motor nerve filament. Visible dimpling or twitching may be

Table 18-5

Topographic patterns of muscle palsy

Muscle weakness or paralysis	Signs	Possible cause
Ocular	Diplopia	Myasthenia gravis
	Ptosis	Thyroid disease
	Strabismus	Ocular dystrophy and botulism
Bifacial	Inability to smile	Myasthenia gravis
	Inability to expose teeth	Facioscapulohumeral dystrophy
	Inability to close eyes	Guillain-Barré syndrome
Bulbar	Dysphonia	Myasthenia gravis
	Dysarthria	Myotonic dystrophy
	Dysphagia	Botulism
	Hanging jaw facial weakness (may or may not be present)	Diphtheria
		Poliomyelitis
		Early polymyositis
Cervical	Inability to lift head from pillow (hanging head syndrome)	Polymyositis
		Dermatomyositis
	Weakness of posterior neck muscles	Progressive muscular dystrophy
Bibrachial	Weakness, atrophy, and fasciculations of hands, arms, and shoulders (hanging arm syndrome)	Amyotrophic lateral sclerosis
Bicrural	Lower leg weakness	Diabetic polyneuropathy
	Floppy feet	
	Inability to walk on heals and toes	
Limb-girdle	Inability to raise arms	Polymyositis
	Inability to rise from sitting position	Dermatomyositis
	Difficulty in climbing stairs without use of arms	Progressive muscular dystrophy
	Waddling gait	
Distal limb	Foot-drop with steppage gain	Familial polyneuropathy
	Weakness of all leg muscles	
	Wrist-drop—weakness of handgrips ("claw hand") (later sign)	
Generalized or universal	Limb and cranial muscle weakness (acute in onset and periodic)	Electrolyte imbalance
		Hypokalemia
		Hypocalcemia
		Hypomagnesemia
	Slow onset and progressive paralysis	Motor system disease
	Atrophy	
	Fasciculations of limb and trunk muscles	
	No sensory loss	
	Paralysis developing over several days	Guillain-Barré syndrome
	Mild degree of generalized weakness	Glycogen storage diseases
		Vitamin D deficiency
Single muscles or groups of muscles	Inability to contract affected muscles	Thyrotoxic myopathy (almost always neuropathic)

seen, although there is usually insufficient power generated to move the joint.

Fasciculations during muscular contraction (twitching) occur in conditions of irritability that result in poorly coordinated contraction of small and large motor units. Benign fasciculation occurs in the normal individual and is characterized by normal muscle strength and size. Rarely, myokymia, a rippling appearance of the muscle occasioned by numerous fasciculations, is noted in a normal individual.

Fascicular twitches that occur during rest in a client with exaggerated muscular weakness and atrophy are characteristic of a peripheral motor neuron disorder. Generalized fascicular twitching occurring in a progressive, wavelike patttern over an entire muscle and progressing to complete paralysis is characteristic of certain

Table 18-6

Tremor classification

Cause	Type and rate of movement	Description
Anxiety	Fine, rapid, 10 to 12 per second	Irregular, variable
		Increased by attempts to move part; decreased by relaxation of part
Parkinsonism	Fine, regular, or coarse, 2 to 5 per second	Occurs at rest
		May be inhibited by movement
		Involves flexion of finger and thumb "pill rolling"
		Accompanied by rigidity, "cogwheel" phenomena, bradykinesia
Cerebellar tremor	Variable rate	Evident only on movement (most prominent on finger-to-nose test)
		Dysmetria (seen when client is asked to pat rapidly—pats are of unequal force and do not all arrive at same point)
Essential or senile	Coarse, 3 to 7 per second	Involves the jaw, sometimes the tongue, and sometimes the entire head
Metabolic		Disappears on complete relaxation or in response to alcohol
		Variable
		Client is obviously ill; if illness is a result of hepatic failure, client will have other signs, such as palpable liver, spider nevi

types of poisoning (organic phosphate) and of poliomyelitis.

Cramps, spasm (Table 18-6)

Muscular spasm may occur at rest or with movement and may occur in the normal individual with metabolic and electrolyte alterations. Cramping is commonly noted following excessive sweating and with hyponatremia, hypocalcemia, hypomagnesemia, and hyperuricemia. Diseases that magnify these alterations are correlated with the presence of muscle spasm. A continuous spasm that is heightened by attempts to move the affected muscles is seen in tetanus and following the bite of the black widow spider.

Paravertebral muscle spasm is often responsible for low back pain.

Tetany. Hypocalcemia, as well as hypomagnesemia, may cause the involuntary spasms of skeletal muscle that resemble cramping. The calcium deficit causes depolarizaton of the distal segments of the motor nerve; furthermore, there is a change within the muscle fibers themselves, since nerve section or block does not prevent these tetanic contractions. Tetanic cramps can be elicited by percussing the motor nerve leading to a muscle group at frequencies of 15 to 20 per second. *Chvostek's sign* is the spasm of the facial muscles produced by tapping over the facial nerve near its foramen of exit. The instability of the neuromuscular unit is heightened by hyperventilation (alkalosis) and hypoxia (ischemia).

Trousseau's sign is the production of tetany of the carpal muscles following occlusion of the blood supply to the arms by a tourniquet. The client may also describe tingling and prickling paresthesia resulting from the stimulation of sensory nerve fibers. Electromyographical tracings show fast-frequency doublets and triplets of motor unit potentials. Tetany in its mildest form affects the distal musculature in the form of carpopedal spasm but may involve all the muscles of the body except those of the eye.

Muscle cramp. Muscle cramp frequently occurs after a day of vigorous exercise. As the feet cool, a sudden movement may trigger a strong contraction of the foot and leg. The musculature is visible, and the muscle feels hard on palpation. The spasm will cease in response to stretch of the fibers. In the case of the gastrocnemius muscle, the stretch can be achieved by dorsiflexion of the foot. Occasionally massage is helpful in relaxing the spasm. Fasciculations may frequently be observed before and after the cramp and are further evidence of the hyperexcitability of the neuromuscular unit. Electromyogram recordings show high-frequency action potentials during the cramp. These muscle spasms have greater frequency when the client is dehydrated or sweating and in the pregnant client.

The cause of the pain associated with muscle cramp has not been determined but is thought by some to be caused by the increased metabolic needs of the hyperactive muscles and to the collection of the metabolic waste products such as lactic acid within the muscle.

Muscle Enzyme Levels

Destructive diseases of striated muscle fibers result in the loss of enzymes from the intracellular compartment of the muscle. The enzymes enter the blood and can be measured. The usual laboratory analysis of serum enzymes includes alkaline phosphatase, lactic dehydrogenase (LDH), serum glutamic oxaloacetic transaminase (SGOT), and creatine phosphokinase (CPK). Enzymes are found in all tissues. Since high concentrations of these enzymes are found in the heart and liver, elevated serum level values may result from myocardial infarction or hepatitis. However, CPK, although present in the heart and brain, is most concentrated in the striated muscle. The level may rise from a normal level of 0 to 65 international units (IU) to more than 1000 IU in clients with destructive lesions of the striated muscles.

Myalgia

"I hurt all over" is frequently the chief complaint for the diffuse muscle pain that accompanies many types of systemic infection, for example, influenza, measles, rheumatic fever, brucellosis, dengue fever, or salmonellosis. Soreness and aching are other descriptive terms for this type of involvement. Little is known of the cause. *Fibromyositis* (myogelosis) is the term used to describe the inflammation of the fibrous tissue in muscle, fascia, and nerves. The client may complain of pain and tenderness in a muscle after exposure to cold, dampness, or minor trauma.

Firm, tender zones occasionally several centimeters in diameter are found on palpation. Palpation, active contraction, or passive stretching increases the pain. Intense pain localized to a smaller group of muscles may be a result of epidemic myalgia, also called pleurodynia, "painful neck," or "devil's grip." Intense pain at the beginning of neurologic involvement has been seen in poliomyelitis and herpes zoster.

The pain of poliomyelitis is described as marked during the initial involvement of the nerve, whereas the later sensation of the paralyzed muscle is said to be one of aching. The segmental pattern of the intense pain of

---

Health History
Musculoskeletal

NOTE: A yes response to any question *must* be further investigated. Use the following indicators throughout the assessment: (1) onset (specific date, sudden or gradual), (2) duration, (3) frequency, (4) precipitating factors, (5) aggravating or alleviating factors, (6) treatment received, (7) outcome.

Present status

1. Do you have joint pain or stiffness?
   a. Location: area, migratory or confined to one joint, symmetrical
   b. Description: prickling, numbing, pulled, charley horse, dull, aching, affected by time of day
2. Do you have other joint symptoms?
   a. Description: popping, grating, heat, swelling, redness
3. Do you have pain in your muscles?
   a. Description: aching, sharp, dull
   b. Associated symptoms: swelling, changes in strength
4. Do you have any joint, bone, or muscle disability that requires assistance?
   a. Type: physical therapy, use of supportive devices, moderation of normal ADL or dependence on others for ADL needs

Past history

1. Have you had any change in your strength or coordination?
   a. Description: new clumsiness, awkwardness, or loss of dexterity; spasms, tremors, or involuntary movement; paralysis; weakness; cramps

2. Have you had any bone surgery?
   a. Type: restored or maintained function, prevented or corrected deformity, relieved pain

Associated conditions

1. Do you have any other illness that affects your muscles?
   a. Description: TIA, glucose disorders, anemias, electrolyte (calcium or potassium) disturbances

Family history

1. Do you have a family history of muscular dystrophy, osteoporosis, rheumatoid arthritis, or other types of arthritis?

Sample assessment record

Client complains of dull lower back pain that often radiates down right leg. Sharp lower back pain began two weeks ago after falling off a curb. Pain subsided but then radiated down right leg when standing. Is more prevalent while walking up stairs. Requires assistance with bathing and household chores. Has had severe muscle spasms and increased weakness in right leg muscles. Today developed burning sensation in right foot. Admits slight improvement when lying supine with head slightly elevated and knees flexed. Denies past history of spinal injuries or other systemic illnesses. Has no family history of osteoporosis or arthritis.

herpes zoster is caused by the inflammation of spinal nerves and dorsal root ganglia that occurs 3 to 4 days before the skin eruption.

The initial symptoms of rheumatoid arthritis may be diffuse muscular soreness and aching, which may antedate the joint involvement by weeks or months. The muscles are tender, and the client describes the pain as occurring not at the time of activity but hours later. An increased sedimentation rate or a positive latex fixation test may support the conclusion of rheumatoid involvement.

Electromyography

The electromyogram is the graph generated from the electrical potential of individual muscles. The test is accomplished by inserting needles directly into the muscle being studied and recording the potential with the muscle at rest, with slight voluntary contractions, and at maximum flexion. Whereas the heart can be sampled from a number of surface electrode positions, the skeletal muscles are variable in size, widely separated, and numerous. Therefore, no small number of leads can give an adequate picture of their activity. Furthermore, surface electrodes yield only a summation of the underlying activity. To ascertain the bursts of individual muscle units, sterile needle electrodes must be used to register the activity.

Thus, the electromyogram must be done for one muscle at a time. Information obtained from the tracing is useful in determining neural adequacy of the muscle and the presence of intrinsic muscle disease.

Muscle Biopsy

Muscle biopsy was first used by Cachenne in 1868. Currently the use of muscle biopsy is believed to be indicated for five clinical problems: (1) atrophy of the muscle that is progressive (when doubt exists whether the disease is myogenic or neurogenic); (2) localized inflammatory disease of the muscle wherein biopsy may contribute to isolating the causative agent, thus allowing institution of the appropriate therapeutic regimen; (3) certain metabolic diseases wherein the histologic or biologic data, or both, thus provided may help to identify the disease; (4) fever associated with many visceral and cutaneous lesions wherein biopsy of the muscle may reveal further connective tissue and vascular involvement to support the conclusions of a generalized involvement; and (5) trauma wherein the biopsy may further define the degree of nerve and muscle injury.

BIBLIOGRAPHY

Adams RD and Kakulas BA: Diseases of the muscle: pathological foundations of clinical myology, ed 4, Philadelphia, 1985, Harper & Row, Publishers.

American Academy of Orthopaedic Surgeons: Joint motion: method of measuring and recording, Chicago, 1965, The Academy.

Beetham W and others: Physical examination of the joints, Philadelphia, 1965, WB Saunders Co.

Daniels L and Worthingham C: Muscle testing: techniques of manual examination, ed 4, Philadelphia, 1980, WB Saunders Co.

Enneking WF and Sherrard MG: Physical diagnosis of the musculoskeletal system, Gainesville, Fla, 1969, Storter Printing Co.

Goodgold J and Eberstein A: Electrodiagnosis of neuromuscular diseases, Baltimore, 1978, Williams & Wilkins.

Hoppenfield S: Physical examination of the spine and extremities, New York, 1976, Appleton-Century-Crofts.

Knapp ME: Electromyography, Postgrad Med 47:213, 1970.

Layzer RB and Rowland LP: Cramps, N Engl J Med 285:31, 1971.

Mann RA, editor: DuVries surgery of the foot, ed 5, St Louis, 1984, The CV Mosby Co.

McCarty DJ, editor: Arthritis, ed 9, Philadelphia, 1979, Lea & Febiger.

Moosa A: Paediatric electrodiagnosis, Arch Dis Child 46:149, 1972.

Polley HF and Hunder GG: Physical examination of the joints, Philadelphia, 1978, WB Saunders Co.

Rosse C and Clawson D: Introduction to the musculoskeletal system, New York, 1970, Harper & Row, Publishers.

Walton J, editor: Disorders of voluntary muscle, ed 4, New York, 1981, Churchill Livingstone.

Yates DA: The electrodiagnosis of muscle disorders, Proc R Soc Med 65:617, 1972.

chapter

19

Assessment of mental status

OBJECTIVES

Upon successful review of this chapter, learners will be able to:

- Describe the structure and purpose of the mental status examination

- Delineate therapeutic interaction skills to help elicit data

- Describe the role of the nursing process in conducting a mental status examination

- Outline a mental health examination to assess mental status

- Recognize characteristics and possible pathology associated with agnosia, speech, and mental status disorders

- Describe tests and procedures used to detect variations in
  Level of consciousness
  Personality and emotional status
  Visual-motor and sensory function
  Cognitive abilities

- Differentiate DSM-III-R diagnostic terminology from NANDA-approved diagnoses

The *mental status examination* is an organized collection of observational data that reflect an individual's current psychological and physiologic functions at that moment. The body of the examination includes the description of the client's *appearance,* general *behavior, affect, mood, motor activity, speech, orientation, thought processes, judgment,* and *memory.* The examiner also observes the individual's *perception* of his or her condition, *attitudes* displayed during the examination, and responses evoked by the examiner. An initial physical assessment may be conducted, as well as evaluation of risk factors.

The major focus of the mental status examination is the identification of the individual's strengths and capabilities for interaction with the environment, such as the ability to initiate and sustain meaningful relationships and to attain happiness and satisfaction congruent with sociocultural life-style. Thus, a thorough background is obtained that includes the client's educational and physical development, occupational role, economic status, relationships, responsibilities felt toward family, work, or school, *stressors* (actual or perceived), goals (attainable and unrealistic), and support systems (individuals and affiliations). A preliminary treatment plan is designed and modified as more data are collected (Table 19-1).

THE INTERVIEW

The interview is the initial and most important tool used to obtain information about the individual's health assessment. It is a richer, more flexible method of collecting behavioral data than are questionnaires or computers. It allows the examiner more time to use all the senses to explore specific topics and concerns identified by the client through verbal and nonverbal responses.

Table 19-1

Assessment of mental status

Mental status

Appearance: _____
Affect: _____
Mood: _____
Speech: _____
Orientation: _____   Memory: _____
Concentration: _____
Thought Process: _____   Delusions: _____
Hallucinations: _____   Judgment: _____
Strengths: _____

Physical assessment (By patient report):   (By examination)

EYES, EARS, NOSE, THROAT: _____   _____

CARDIOVASCULAR: _____   _____

RESPIRATORY: _____   _____

GASTROINTESTINAL: _____   _____
GENITOURINARY: _____   _____
SKELETAL: _____   _____
INTEGUMENTARY: _____   _____
CENTRAL NERVOUS SYSTEM/MOTOR: _____   _____

Safety assessment (Indicate yes or no):

Suicide risk: _____   Homicidal threat: _____   Smoking risk: _____
Impulse control adequate: _____   Fall risk (confused, hypomaniac, disability or poor gait): _____
Medical risk (if yes, define): _____

Preliminary treatment plan (Mark as indicated):

Orient to reality: _____   Push participation: _____
Provide support: _____   Rapid tranquilization: _____
Provide structure: _____   Teach social skills: _____
Maintain safety on unit: _____   Medication education and compliance: _____
Allow regression/space: _____   Outpatient referral: _____
Behavioral contract: _____   Needs placement or living orientation: _____
Medical needs (List or put N/A): _____

_____   _____   _____
(R.N. signature)   (Date)   (Time)

Modified from RN orientation manual, Alvarado Parkway Institute, LaMesa, Calif.

Although it is critical to identify behaviors that form *themes* or *patterns* indicating disruptions in mental health processes, responses elicited during a single interview are only samples of the individual's thoughts and feelings. Such behaviors may represent early defining characteristics of a deeper problem requiring further exploration of the client's mental status, or they may simply be individual or cultural *idiosyncrasies*.

A client with a saddened facial expression, slumped shoulders, and lowered voice tone may be demonstrating some features of a *depressive* illness or may be reacting to some very real concerns. Fears regarding illness, family responsibilities, attitudes of others, and financial worries are some variables that can alter a client's feelings and behaviors.

In many cultures mental illness is perceived as a

character weakness or a personal failure. Such beliefs can invoke feelings of guilt, shame, and powerlessness and a loss of self-esteem, all of which are bound to produce negative behaviors. A client who demonstrates *hyperactive* behaviors, such as pacing back and forth, chain-smoking, or rapid speech or breathing patterns, although manifesting many symptoms of *anxiety* or *mania,* may also be reacting to similar fears and perceptions as the individual who appeared depressed.

Role of the Practitioner

Although methods of data collection, assessment, and evaluation of a client's mental status vary among facilities, conduction of the initial mental health interview is now widely accepted as a role for the professional nurse. Reports in the literature reveal that in recent years, many baccalaureate and associate degree nursing programs have made great strides toward integration of psychosocial, developmental, cultural, and sexuality concepts within their curricula. Also, nurses throughout history have communicated therapeutically with clients across the life span as an integral feature of their approach to care.

Method of Interviewing

The best method of interviewing a client to elicit facts and feelings for history is by asking both *closed-* and *open-ended questions* appropriately in a matter-of-fact manner while maintaining good *eye contact* and an *open posture.* Closed-ended queries are frequently used to obtain facts.

> How long have you been at your present job?
> Do you get along well with your co-workers?

Open-ended questions are often used to elicit perceptions, thoughts, and feelings.

> Tell me how you feel about your work.
> How does your illness affect your co-workers?

Responses obtained from closed-ended questions often prompt the examiner to use the open-ended approach to elicit more substantive information. This is well-illustrated in the above examples.

Active listening is a skill that has been successfully implemented by nurses of every culture in all situations throughout history. The examiner who allows the client sufficient time to respond to queries while appearing alert, interested, and unhurried may not be actively listening, although the above strategies are all correct.

For active listening to be successful, the examiner must *reflect* back the client's words and behaviors when-

ever appropriate, throughout the interview, to let the client know she or he is really attending to the client's feelings. Reflection can be used by *restating* or repeating the client's words and by offering observations of the client's behaviors. The client then has an opportunity to *clarify* his or her position by accepting or rejecting the examiner's impressions. The more an examiner can *validate* a client's responses, the greater the opportunities for accurate problem identification and high-quality care.

Acknowledgment of the client's responses can be elicited through the use of *general leads,* such as "uh-huh" or "go-on" or by simple nodding of the head at appropriate intervals. A more complete description of *facilitative communication* strategies can be found in Chapter 1.

The use of *therapeutic communication* skills in interviewing provides the examiner with more opportunities to observe the client's levels of awareness, *cognitive* function, and *affective* state. Questions are directed toward obtaining as much data as possible about the client's symptoms, such as dysfunctional thoughts and behaviors, the family, medical history, life situation, and support systems.

In assessing the client's mental status, the examiner focuses on the symptoms, on how the client views them, and on how disruptive they are to the client and others. The evolution of the symptoms is traced, and the examiner compares and contrasts them with observation of the client's current behaviors. Because the data reported by the client may change with each examination, or the client's words may signify different meanings to different examiners, it is imperative to document a client's behaviors and words accurately, succinctly, and in *measurable,* descriptive terms, using short, direct quotes only when it enhances the client's meaning or clarifies the situation.

(Correct) Client smoked 1/2 pack of cigarettes in 30 minutes. He paced across the room 4-5 times and stated "I'm really feeling nervous" twice.
(Incorrect) Client chain-smoked during interview. He appeared agitated and verbalized his anxiety.

The choice of words used to describe behavior during the interview should be carefully selected, since some words hold negative connotations for most people. For example, a client with rapid body movements may find it more acceptable to be termed overactive or *hyperactive* than to be called agitated or "hyper." A client who is quick to anger may balk at being labeled *hostile,* but probably would not object to being called overly sensitive or even hypersensitive.

It is also important to consider the effects of prescription medications and illicit drugs on the client's mental processes and behaviors. Communication barriers related to age or culture can often be bridged through the use of qualified interpreters, friends, or family members. It is crucial, however, that information derived from sources other than the client be evaluated in terms of these individuals' relationship with the client. Clients with speech or auditory problems related to such conditions as *aphasia,* deafness, or birth impairments may be helped to communicate through the use of sign language experts, alphabet boards, writing, drawing, or gesturing.

Appraisal of a client's mental status is an ongoing process that can be built into any interview. The method of interviewing can be enhanced by an examiner who uses keen behavioral observations to assess the client's individual needs and employs facilitative communication skills to meet those needs.

PHYSICAL APPEARANCE AND BEHAVIOR

The examiner carefully observes the client's physical appearance, manner of dress, facial expression, and body posture as a measure of mental function. Assessment of neurologic status is composed of the way the client looks, acts, and feels (see Chapter 7 on general assessment). Particular attention is given to posture.

Assessment of Motor Behavior—Movement
Posture, behavior, and reaction time

Posture is important in providing clues to the client's feelings. The client who walks slowly into the room, barely lifting the feet, and who slumps in the chair while avoiding the examiner's glance may be eloquently portraying a lack of affect or depression. Conversely, the person who bounds into the room, energetically shaking the examiner's hand while rapidly glancing around the room, may be demonstrating the significant overreaction of mania. The individual with tense muscles and furrowed brow, or the furtive, darting eyes and wet handshake, should alert the examiner to the probability of anxiety.

Jerky motor movements, *shuffling (parkinsonism) gait,* muscle rigidity *(dystonia), facial grimacing,* and motor restlessness *(akathisia)* may be *extrapyramidal side effects (EPSE),* resulting from *neuroleptic medications* that block *dopamine,* a *neurotransmitter* responsible for smooth muscle movement.

With each interchange, the speed and appropriateness of the client's motor movements and reactions are evaluated on an imaginary continuum of *poverty of movement* to hyperactivity. Symptomatology and patterns of behavior indicating specific disorders or pathologic

states are further explored to corroborate the examiner's initial impressions.

Coordination

General coordination of movement is assessed through observing the client's gait. To evaluate the complex acts of coordination, the examiner may give the client simple phrases to write and simple geometric figures to draw. The client is asked to draw more fundamental figures such as a circle, square, or triangle, followed by more complex figures such as a house or flower. Persons with *Alzheimer's disease* or brain damage from other sources are unable to make accurate copies of the figures.

The *Bender-Gestalt visual-motor test,* designed by Lauretta Bender, adapted from designs used by *Wertheimer* in his studies of *Gestalt psychology,* is useful for both children and adults. A child younger than 3 years is not expected to produce any of the test's designs meaningfully; a child aged 4 years, however, should be able to produce some of them, albeit poorly. This skill should progressively improve, with reasonable accuracy and organization demonstrated by ages 10 through 12. Studies show that test results may also illustrate pathologic conditions in adults such as organic brain disease, *mental retardation,* aphasias, *psychoses,* anxiety disorders, and malingering.

Test material consists of nine individual designs, each printed against a white background on a separate card. The client can use all the time needed to copy each design as he or she views it. *Memory* function is not tested during this phase. During the recall phase (after 45 to 60 seconds) the client is asked to reproduce as many of the designs as possible from memory. This phase tests the person's visual memory. It is often helpful to note the client's level of function by comparing the results of the two test phases.

The result of psychological tests for brain damage assessment produce greater reliability than behavioral observations, although both examine the same functions, such as the speed of response, level of *comprehension,* and use of language. Visual memory and *psychomotor skills,* not readily elicited in the general examination, are assessed in depth during *neuropsychological testing* and thus provide additional information about other aspects of intellect and personality (Table 19-2).

A more in-depth description of psychological tests can be found in Kaplan and Sadock, pp. 126-136.

Grooming and Apparel

Failure of the client to give reasonable attention to grooming and personal cleanliness is a clue to underlying emo-

Table 19-2

Tests for assessing brain damage

Category	Subcategories	Remarks
General scales	Wechsler scales (WAIS, WISC, WPSSI) Stanford-Binet Halstead-Reitan battery	Given the availability of adequate normative standards in relation to the patient's educational and cultural background, a performance significantly below expectations should raise the question of cerebral damage. This generalization applies to both adults and children.
Reasoning and problem solving	Shipley abstractions Raven progressive matrices Gorham proverbs Elithorn perceptual mazes Porteus mazes Goldstein-Scheerer sorting tests Wisconsin card-sorting test	Performance level is closely related to educational background and premorbid intellectual level. In general, the clinical application of these tests is more useful in the case of educated patients. If specific language and perceptual defects can be ruled out as determinants of defective performance, failure suggests frontal lobe involvement or diffuse cerebral disease.
Memory and orientation	Repetition and reversal of digits Visual memory for designs Auditory memory for words or stories Visual memory for words or pictures Temporal orientation	For complete assessment, a number of memory tasks (auditory versus visual, verbal versus nonverbal, immediate versus recent) should be given. Defects in temporal orientation suggestive of impairment in recent memory may be elicited.
Visuoperceptive and visuo-constructive	Identification of hidden figures Discrimination of complex patterns Facial recognition Inkblot interpretation Block design construction Stick arranging Copying designs Three-dimensional block construction Responsiveness to double visual stimulation	These tasks are useful indicators of the presence of cerebral disease. Analysis of qualitative features of performance and comparison of performance level with the status of language and reasoning abilities often provide indications with regard to locus of the lesion.
Somatoperceptual	Finger recognition Right-left orientation Responsiveness to double tactile stimulation	These are useful indicators of the presence and locus of cerebral disease.
Language	Token test Controlled word association Illinois test of psycholinguistic abilities Diagnostic reading tests	Test performance depends on educational background, and clinical interpretation must allow for this and other possibly significant factors. In adult patients, defective performance (particularly in relation to other abilities) suggests dysfunction of the cerebral hemisphere that is dominant for language. In children, defective performance does not have this localizing significance but does raise the question of the presence of cerebral damage. Performance on verbal reasoning tests, such as Shipley abstractions and Gorham proverbs, may also disclose specific impairment in language function.
Attention, concentration, and motor abilities	Simple and choice reaction time Visual vigilance Imitation of movements Motor impersistence	These are useful behavioral indicators of the presence and sometimes the locus of cerebral disease that deserve more extensive clinical application.

From Kaplan HI and Sadock BJ: Modern synopsis of comprehensive textbook of psychiatry/IV, ed 4, Baltimore, 1985, Williams & Wilkins, p 133.

tional problems. Thus an unclean body; dirty, unkempt hair or nails; and a disheveled, neglected appearance in a previously well-groomed individual are clues that further exploration is needed.

The individual (male or female) who presents with carelessly, brightly, or *bizarrely* applied makeup may be demonstrating symptoms of mania and warrants further exploration by the examiner. However, lack of cosmetics may have no clinical significance if the client has an allergy to makeup or if she never uses it. The person who suddenly fails to wear previously used cosmetics concomitantly with a deteriorating appearance is in need of further examination.

The client's clothing is observed to determine its appropriateness to time, place, age, and life-style. Bright yellows and reds have been associated with *euphoria,* whereas drab olive green and black have been linked with depression. However, such information must be evaluated along with other relevant symptomatology and not viewed in isolation.

Attention is also given to amount and type of jewelry and style of hair and dress. The female who wears overtly masculine clothing and has closely cropped hair may be giving a message of her sexual identity, exhibiting the unisex nature of dress so popular nowadays, or simply demonstrating her preferred, unique fashion style. *Symbolic* jewelry, such as the peace sign or religious figures, may be the client's way of making a statement about a value-belief system. Such adornments may be supportive during times of stress and *psychic* vulnerability.

Deterioration or drastic changes in an individual's grooming occur in anxiety, depression, mania, *schizophrenia,* and *organic mental disorders.* One-sided neglect has been observed in clients with lesions or tumors in the parietal area of the brain. Bowel and bladder functions should also be evaluated as part of this examination.

Interaction with the Examiner

The practitioner makes an overall assessment of whether the client is cooperative, recalcitrant, friendly, hostile, or ingratiating. The examiner is alert to her or his own feelings *(autodiagnosis),* whether or not the reasons for them are consciously understood. Discussion of feelings with qualified staff is helpful in validating them.

The client who invokes a sense of fear and foreboding in the examiner must be observed closely and assessed for potential for violence until further evaluation either corroborates or invalidates such feelings. It is useful to determine if this individual elicits similar feelings in others so that steps can be taken to improve the individual's relationships in the *milieu.*

Speech

The client's manner of speech may offer clues about his or her thought processes. Comprehension of and ability to use the spoken language may be evaluated during the assessment interview. The individual's responses to the examiner's questions and instructions give valuable information about the client's comprehension and willingness to cooperate.

Please change into this gown.
Sit on this chair facing me.

The nature of the client's responses is also important. The mentally healthy individual answers questions frankly. Failure to answer a question, *circumlocution,* and other evasive replies, and undo or unwarranted criticism of the examiner should be noted.

Rapid-fire conversation should be noted, as well as slow and halting delivery. These observations should be mentally positioned on a continuum of poverty of speech to hyperactive verbal behavior. The client who monopolizes the interview should also be assessed further. Slow, monotonous speech is characteristic of parkinsonism. The client, just as the professional, chooses the words he feels are best suited to his companion and the situation. Thus, the words chosen by the client usually reveal his general intelligence, educational level, social status, and level of functioning.

Articulation is assessed. This includes fluency, ease of expression, rhythm, hesitancies, stuttering, and repetitiousness. The omission or addition of letters, syllables, and words, or their transposition, and the misuse of words suggest aphasia. The client may attempt to express his thoughts nonverbally (pantomime) to avoid revealing that he has forgotten a word. Repetitious, abnormal thought patterns are recorded. These include *neologisms, verbigeration,* or *echolalia*—symptoms noted in schizophrenia.

Disorders of the structures responsible for speech may be evident during conversation with the client. These include the following:
1. *Dysphonia:* Difficulty or discomfort in making laryngeal speech sounds, such as hoarseness. *Dysphonia puberum* is difficulty in controlling laryngeal speech sounds that occur as the larynx enlarges in puberty.
2. *Dysarthria:* Difficulty in articulating single sounds or phonemes of speech; individual letters *(f, g, r);* labials—sounds produced with the lips *(b, m, w,* rounded vowels) (cranial nerve [CN] VII); gutterals—sounds produced in the throat (CN X); and linguals—sounds produced with the tongue *(l, t, n)* (CN XII). Dysarthria may be demonstrated by asking the client

Table 19-3

Classification of aphasias

Type of aphasia	Site of lesion	Speech or language disorder
Broca's aphasia (expressive speaking)	Left inferior third frontal convolution (Broca's area) (Fig. 19-1)	Nonfluent Agrammatical Difficulty in finding words to no oral expression skills—apraxia Writing generally impaired Comprehension retained
Wernicke's aphasia (auditory receptive)	Posterior portion superior temporal gyrus Part of second temporal gyrus	Normal to hyperfluent Emphasis on verbs Neologism Jargon Gibberish Impaired auditory comprehension Does not recognize his own speech errors Difficulty in repeating phrases after the examiner
Global	Diffuse large lesion May involve both Broca's and Wernicke's areas	Language skills inconsistent Recurrent repetition of phrases—fluent
Anomia	Area of angular gyrus	Fluent Grammatical Reduced rate resulting from difficulty in finding words Pauses Circumlocution Impaired comprehension of isolated nouns and verbs General auditory comprehension retained
Transcortical sensory	Lesion isolating angular gyrus from the remainder of brain	Echos interviewer's speech Does not initiate speech Increased ability to preserve and recite memorized material Markedly impaired reading and writing
Transcortical motor	Frontal lobe, anterior to Broca's area	Does not initiate speech No spontaneous speech—short answers to questions Repetition intact Comprehension preserved

to repeat a phrase such as "Methodist Episcopal" or by asking him to read a short paragraph containing all of these letters.

3. *Dysprosody:* Difficulty in speech such that inflection, pronunciation, pitch, and rhythm are impaired.

Aphasia

Aphasia is a general term for a dysfunction or loss of ability to express thoughts by speech, writing, symbols, or signs or to interpret *sensory* input (Table 19-3). These disorders are caused by lesions of the brain (Fig. 19-1). The term *aphasia* excludes those disturbances of expression related to abnormalities of neurons to the muscles of speech, disorders of the anatomical structures that participate in the production of speech and mental im-

pairment. Aphasia encompasses *agnosia,* the inability to recognize once-familiar objects, and *apraxia,* the inability to carry out purposeful activity related to language. The most common cerebral pathologic condition associated with aphasia is vascular disease. Although the cerebral hemispheres share equal responsibility in controlling the two sides of the body in general, language requires the simultaneous input of both and is controlled by one. The hemisphere in which language is controlled is called the dominant hemisphere. It has been demonstrated that 95% of these individuals who are right-handed and have a language deficit have lesions of the left cerebral hemisphere, whereas 70% of left-handed individuals with language impairment also have a lesion of the left cerebral hemisphere.

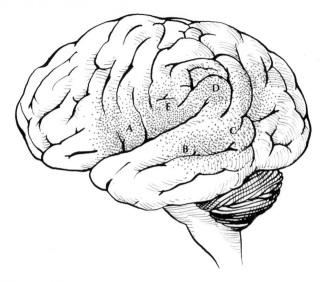

Figure 19-1

Aphasic zone of the left cerebral hemisphere. Neurologic deficits include *A,* middle and inferior frontal gyri and lower precentral gyrus: anarthria, alexia, contralateral facial weakness; *B,* supramarginal gyrus: generalized aphasia, hemianesthesia, hemianopia; *C,* angular gyrus: aphasia with reading disturbance, quadrantanopsia, hemiplegia, hemianesthesia; *D,* posterior, superior, and middle temporal gyri: sensory aphasia, paraphasia, jargon aphasia; and *E,* includes island of Reil: severe aphasia, anarthria, right hemiplegia.

Aphasia may be evaluated during the initial interview with the client. The ability of the client to comprehend auditory verbal stimuli may be tested against the client's ability to answer questions and carry out instructions. Visual verbal function is assessed from the client's ability to read and to explain the content he has read (see boxed material above). Further evaluation is made by asking the client to identify familiar objects or geometric figures.

The client may be able to express himself in some forms of speech when his free-flowing conversational speech is impaired. Some of these are included in Table 19-4.

Agnosia

Agnosia is a general term for the dysfunction or loss of ability to interpret sensory stimuli. These disorders have been termed *receptive aphasia.* Individuals with visual agnosia have the primary reception of the visual image but are unable to associate the previous experience that allows interpretation of what is being viewed. Specific cerebral cortical regions make it possible for the individual to recognize visual, auditory, and tactile stimuli. Testing for tactile interpretation is assessed during the neurologic examination (Table 19-5).

Clinical Indications of Aphasia Involving Speech

Hesitations
Omission or addition of letters, syllables, or words
Substitution of words with inappropriate implication
Circumlocution
Neologism
Using some words again and again—lack of variety in vocabulary
Use of nonverbal language to substitute for a word
Syntactical error (disturbance of balance or rhythm of words in sequence); can write better than speak
Semantic errors (inability to interpret metaphors, the connotation of words)
Severe aphasia:
   Inability to speak
   Repetition of single word or phrase

Table 19-4

Speech types that may be retained in aphasia

Speech type	Description of speech type
Emotional speech	Swearing, exclamations, oaths
Automatic speech	Nursery rhymes, poems, other series of words learned in early life, days of the week
Singing	Singing may be possible while speech is not

Apraxia

Comprehension is normal in apraxia. *Ideational apraxia* is the term for loss of ability to formulate the ideational concepts necessary to carry out a skilled motor act. The individual is unable to conceive the idea or retain it. This dysfunction accompanies diffuse cerebral disorders, such as arteriosclerosis.

Motor apraxia is decline of kinesthetic motor patterns necessary to a motor act. This impairment may be related to a lesion of the precentral gyrus.

Ideomotor apraxia is the term used to define the situation in which an individual has lost the skills for a given complex act but may retain conditioned habits. These old patterns may be performed repetitiously *(perseverance).* This may be associated with disease of the supramarginal gyrus of the parietal lobe on the dominant side of the brain. Apraxias not related to language are tested at the time of the neurologic assessment.

Writing

The client may be asked to write his or her name or address or may be allowed to write anything. As with verbal expression, aphasia may be indicated by the omission or addition of letters, syllables, or words. Mirror writing has been interpreted as a symptom of dysfunction related to cerebral dominance. A recently completed letter or other example of writing by the client may give valuable information regarding thought processes. *Agraphia* is the term used to describe a disturbance in writing. When agraphia is the only symptom present, it may be the result of a cerebral lesion of the second frontal convolution or the region of the angular gyrus and occipital lobe.

The writing observed in clients with *Parkinson's disease* is small and constricted, known as micrographia. Uncoordinated writing is seen in persons with cerebellar disease.

Cognitive Processes

The *sensorium* is assessed for *consciousness, orientation,* attention span, *recent* and *remote memory,* insight, and judgment.

State of consciousness, awareness

The first step in the evaluation of the client's sensorium is the determination of the state of consciousness, that is, the individual's awareness and responsiveness to his experiences.

Consciousness may be regarded as the individual's awareness of the stimuli from his environment and within himself. Clinical appraisal is more reliable for assessing the awareness of the client to external variables, since these can be checked against the examiner's impressions. However, the client may give a very informative discussion of his internal feelings.

The levels of conscious perception are thought to be a function of the conscious *ego.* The awareness of self and environment, which is called consciousness, may be affected by the nature and the amplitude of the stimuli received by the individual. Thus, the awareness of feelings and reactions have been described to be different for those excluded from external stimuli and reacting signals from the self only; that is, for those individuals with perceptual deprivation. Consciousness may also be impaired by internal stimuli (fear, rage) and by some pathophysiologic changes (fever, pain). The unconscious ego may also interfere with the client's level of consciousness. Clients with acute anxiety may dissociate or fail to perceive both internal and external stimuli.

More precise description of consciousness is obtained by differentiating between field of consciousness and clarity of consciousness. *Field of consciousness* is the range or area of stimuli perceived. *Clarity of consciousness* is the intensity or clarity of perception. An example of the differences in these two aspects is seen in the depressed individual. Although the depressed individual may not attend to all of the events in his milieu, he is clear in his perceptions of those he does describe;

Table 19-5

Tests for agnosia

Type	Description	Test	Site of lesion
Olfactory	Inability to recognize once-familiar smells	Identify volatile, easily recognized substances: Coffee Vanilla Oil of lemon	Prepiriform lobe
Visual	Inability to recognize once-familiar colors	Identify: color, geometric figures, pictures, sides of body, parts of body	Occipital and adjacent parietal lobe
Auditory	Inability to recognize once-familiar tones, music, sounds	Identify: musical melody, ringing of bell	Temporal lobe—lateral and superior and adjacent to parietal lobe (Wernicke's area)
Tactile	Inability to recognize once-familiar objects by feeling them (stereognosis)	Identify object held in hand such as: coins, key, comb	Superior parietal lobe
Body parts	Inability to recognize body part (somatagnosia) or to determine laterality (individual may ignore or not use the part)	Identify body parts by name as right or left	Posteroinferior parietal lobe

field of consciousness is narrowed, but clarity of consciousness remains intact.

A disturbance in consciousness results in lack of clarity or in confusion of the client's awareness of self or the environment. The examination of consciousness may focus on four areas of awareness: awareness of one's internal state, subject-object differentiation, clarity of ego boundaries, and body awareness.

If the normal client is able to describe how he is feeling—his *internal state*—in words that are clear and logical to the examiner, his awareness of inner life experience is considered intact.

The client who is confused concerning time and place may have poor *subject-object differentiation*, fre-

quently confusing one object for another or persons for inanimate objects.

Disruption of *ego boundaries* implies that the individual is hazy about his perception of the origin of stimuli—whether they are of an external, subconscious, or conscious origin. This is normal in the developing child. The infant views himself and the nuturing mother figure as one and the same. This lack of clarity of ego boundaries is also typical of some religious rituals practiced by adults. Blurred ego boundaries are common in clients with psychosis.

The mentally healthy person is alert to the *parameters of his body* and its performance. Although there is considerable variation from one individual to another, the

Table 19-6

Levels of consciousness (responsiveness)

	Behaviors
Conscious	Appropriate response (rate and quality) to external and internal stimuli
	Oriented to *time, place,* and *person*
Confusion	Inappropriate response to stimuli and decrease in attention span and memory
	Reactions to simple commands may be retained
Lethargy (hypersomnia)	Drowsiness or increased sleeping time
	Can be aroused; responds appropriately
	May fall immediately asleep again
Delirium	Confusion associated with disordered perception and decreased attention span, motor and sensory excitement
	Reactions to stimuli are inappropriate
	May have marked anxiety
Coma	Loss or lowering of consciousness
Stage I (stupor)	Arousable for short periods to verbal, visual, or painful stimuli
	Simple motor and verbal response to stimuli (shutting eyes, protruding tongue)
	Responses slow
	Corneal and pupillary reflexes sluggish
	Deep tendon reflexes and superficial reflexes unaffected
	Pathological reflexes may be obtained
Stage II (light coma)	Simple motor and verbal (moaning) response to painful stimuli
	Motor response generally flexion (avoidance) or mass movement
Stage III (deep coma)	Decerebrate posturing to painful stimuli (extension of body and limbs and pronation of arms)
Stage IV	Muscles flaccid
	Eyes do not react to light
	Apneic; on ventilator
	Superficial and some spinal reflexes (deep tendon reflexes) may be present
Brain death	Two EEG tracings 24 hours apart indicate absence of brain waves ⎫
	Cerebral function absent 24 hours ⎪
	Failure of cerebral perfusion ⎬ All must be present
	Expert opinion rules out hypothermia or drug toxicity ⎭
Syncope	Temporary loss of consciousness (partial or complete) associated with increased rate of respiration, tachycardia, pallor, perspiration, coolness of skin
Fugue state	Dysfunction of consciousness (hours or days) wherein the individual carries on purposeful activity that he does not remember (afterward)
Amnesia	Memory loss over time or for specific subjects
	Individual affected responds appropriately to external stimuli

well person can readily distinguish himself from the environment.

Levels of consciousness.   The following sections deal with alterations in levels of consciousness including assessment of the individual in *coma*. The reader may prefer to study this material after learning more about health assessment, particularly neurologic assessment.

The levels of consciousness (responsiveness) are generally described according to the behavior exhibited by the individual. Table 19-6 includes a useful categorization of the levels of consciousness.

Clinical states frequently mistaken for coma include the following:

"Locked-in state"—client's face and limbs are totally paralyzed but may be differentiated by other signs.

Hysteria

Catatonic state—increased limb tone to passive motion (waxy flexibility) is a sign that may help to differentiate this condition.

Negativism

Many systems of classification of coma have been devised. The *Glasgow Coma Scale* (1974) is an assessment tool that relies totally on behavioral evaluation. The advantage in the use of such a tool is that words having different meanings to various individuals are avoided, for example, "stupor," "semicomatose," or "obtunded." Thus, reliability in evaluation of coma is enhanced. A score is obtained by weighing behaviors (Table 19-7). A person with normal consciousness would obtain a score of 14.

Response to pain may be the only indication of sensory stimulation. Painful stimuli include pinching of skin, pricking with a pin, pressure over supraorbital notches (oculosensory reflex), pinching the skin of the neck (ciliospinal reflex), pressure over knuckles, pressure (squeezing muscle masses or tendons), particularly the gastrocnemius (calf muscle). The client may respond by extension of limbs, facial grimacing, or withdrawal. Flexion responses are considered withdrawal responses and therefore purposeful. Nonpurposeful responses are mass reactions or extension of limbs. This scale is particularly useful in the ongoing care of hospitalized clients in coma (Table 19-8 and boxed material below).

Causes of Coma	
Toxic and metabolic	**Disorders involving physical damage to the brain**
Exogenous toxins	Tumor
Alcohol	Edema
Drugs	Stroke
Metabolic	Intracerebral hemorrhage
Uremia	Contusion
Hepatic failure	
Hypoxia	
Hypercapnia	
Hypercalcemia	

Table 19-7

Glasgow coma scale—record of individual recovering from coma

	Score		Day 1	Day 2	Day 3	Day 4	Day 5
Eye opening response	Spontaneous opening	4					X
	To verbal stimuli	3				X	
	To pain	2	X	X	X		
	None	1					
Most appropriate verbal response	Oriented	5					X
	Confused	4					
	Inappropriate words	3				X	
	Incoherent	2		X	X		
	None	1	X				
Most integrated motor response (arm)	Obeys commands	5				X	X
	Localizes pain	4		X	X		
	Flexion to pain	3					
	Extension to pain	2	X				
	None	1					
TOTAL SCORE			5	8	8	11	14

Table 19-8

Assessment of the individual in coma

Assessment category	Examination	Possible findings	Possible underlying conditions
General inspection	Appearance	Chronic or acute illness	
		Emaciation	
		Dehydration	
	Odor	Fruity breath	Ketosis
		Alcohol	Alcoholic toxication
	Position	Opisthotonos	Meningitis
Skin	Color	Pallor	Hemorrhage; anemia
		Florid	Hypertension; polycythemia
		Flushing	Fever; acute alcoholic intoxication
		Cyanosis	Cardiorespiratory disease
		Cherry red	Carbon monoxide poisoning
		Sweating	Hypoglycemia; lysis of fever
		Uremic frost of nose and lips	Uremia
		Jaundice	Hepatic or biliary disease
		Petechiae	Blood dyscrasias
		Dependent edema on ankles	Cardiac, renal disease
		Signs of injury—especially head bruises, Battle's sign, hematoma, laceration	Injury
			Trauma—most frequent cause of coma
Vital signs	Blood pressure	Increase	Hypertension; renal disease
		Decrease	Shock
	Temperature	Increase	Infection
		Decrease	Increased intracranial pressure
	Pulse	Tachycardia	Fever; hyperthyroidism
		Bradycardia	Increased intracranial pressure
			Heart block
		Bounding	Hypertension
	Respiration	Cheyne-Stokes respiration	Neural lesion; central respiratory structures
		Kussmaul's ventilation	Diabetic acidosis
		Posthyperventilation apnea of 15 to 30 seconds	Brain damage
		Respiratory ataxia	Lesion of medulla
		Hyperventilation	Hypoxia; acidosis; lesion of brain, reticular area
Neurological	Sensory	Impairment of orientation, attention span, memory	
		May have illusions, delusions, hallucinations	
		Pain response—purposeful avoidance; withdrawal of limbs moving away from midline; arms triple flexed	
Cranial nerves	CN II, optic	Ophthalmoscopic examination of fundus	
		Papilledema	Increased intracranial pressure
		Hemorrhages and exudates	Uremia
	CN III, oculomotor PERRLA (pupils equal, round, reactive to light and accommodation)	Palpebral fissure decreased	CN III paralysis
		Pupils pinpoint in size	Toxic states, especially morphine; thrombosis or hemorrhage of basilar artery; lesion of the pons
		Miosis	Unilateral lesions of brainstem
		Unequal pupil size	Head trauma; alcohol toxicity; diabetic coma; uremia; carbon monoxide poisoning
		Diminshed light relfex	

Continued

Table 19-8

Assessment of the individual in coma—*cont'd*

Assessment category	Examination	Possible findings	Possible underlying conditions
		Anisocoria such that pupil dilated and not reactive to light on side of lesion resulting from increased intracranial pressure	Supratentorial lesion, that is, brain tumor, abscess, subdural hematoma, skull fracture with middle cerebral artery hemorrhage
		Mydriasis	
	CN V, sensory motor	Diminished response to painful stimuli	
		Diminished response of corneal reflex	
		Diminished response of jaw jerk reflex	
	CN VII, motor	Diminished response to corneal reflex	
		Chvostek's sign	Tetany
		Facial paresis, palpebral fissure increased in width in deep coma; eyes open; shallow nasolabial fold; droop of mouth; puffing of cheek on expiration and retraction on inspiration	
	CN VIII, auditory (auditory-palpebral reflex) vestibular	Diminished response to sound	
		Diminished blinking in response to loud noise	
		Nystagmus at rest	
		Diminished caloric nystagmus	
	CN IX, X	Diminished palatal and pharyngeal reflexes—causes stertorous respiration, swallowing difficulties	
		Impaired laryngeal function; tone of voice altered	
		Diminished cough reflex	
Motor status	Involuntary movement	Tremors, twitches, spasms, convulsions	Epilepsy, cerebral lesions
	Symmetry of motion		
	Paralysis	One side flaccid, becoming spastic with hyperactive stretch reflexes	Cerebral lesions
		Face—lower portion only	Cerebral lesion
	Position of limbs	Flaccid, decreased tone	Recently paralyzed
		Spasticity	Cerebral lesions
		1. Early flaccid paralysis, deep tendon reflexes and superficial reflex normal or diminished extensor plantar	
		2. Later—deep tendon responses hyperactive; superficial reflexes absent; extension of arms, legs, plantar	
Reflexes	Deep tendon reflexes (DTRs)	Diminished or abolished DTRs	Deep coma
		First, flaccid paralysis	
		Tonic neck reflex, decerebrate rigidity	Brainstem lesions
Meningeal involvement		Nuchal rigidity	Meningeal irritation
		Kernig's sign	Infection
		Brudzinski's sign	

Orientation

Orientation is assessed from the client's awareness of person, place, and time.

A typical kind of protocol used in obtaining this information is as follows:

Person
What is your name? Address? Telephone number?
Do you know who I am?
Do you know what my job is?
Place
Tell me where you are. What is the name of this place?
Do you know the name of the town you are in?
Who brought you here?
Time
Do you know what day this is? Month? Year?

The degree of *disorientation* is recorded. Descriptions should include enough data to allow the reader to know if the client has no awareness of a particular parameter, limited or dysfunctional awareness, or exact perception.

Time orientation is the one most frequently disordered in clients with mental disease. The feeling that time is passing slowly is characteristic of anxious or depressed clients who tend to underestimate the passage of time. On the other hand, *obsessive-compulsive* individuals are highly cognizant of the exact time. A disturbance in time orientation is an early finding in organic mental disorders, as well as toxic or metabolic effects of the central nervous system.

A disturbance of place orientation may accompany organic mental disorders or schizophrenia. An individual may not be oriented as to person in the aftermath of cerebral trauma or seizures or in *amnesic fuguelike* states.

Loss, disappointment, and emotional pain are experienced by most individuals following a stressful situation. They may demonstrate feelings of *depersonalization* or withdrawal and deny the reality of what is happening to them. These are temporary, functional defenses against anxiety. But the well-integrated person is generally able to accept the circumstances causing his pain when the stress abates. The client who is mentally vulnerable, however, may become progressively more withdrawn or depersonalized, or develop amnesia.

The individual with schizophrenia may demonstrate marked withdrawal, isolation, *symbolism,* or *grandiose gestures*. In addition, his body image may be distorted as to shape and movement, as well as feelings of weight.

Attention span

An appraisal of the individual's attention span includes the examiner's description of the client's abilities to maintain interest and to concentrate.

The attention span is one of the first functions of the sensorium to become affected. Allowing the client to talk over a short period of time will illustrate his stream of consciousness. The continuity of ideas is evaluated. The client's response to questions and directives will demonstrate his attentiveness to the environment. When a new idea is introduced in the interview, the well-integrated client processes this alteration and responds appropriately. The client may be given a series of numbers to repeat immediately or asked to memorize two or three sentences and repeat them back at a later time in the interview. Sometimes a fictitious name and address are used.

Attention span may be impaired in most individuals who are fatigued, anxious, or chemically impaired. In many pathologic states attention span is shortened. The client may be easily *distractible, confused,* or negativistic.

Memory

Memory is a function of general cerebral competence. Impairment of memory occurs in both neurologic and psychiatric disorders. Some general questions that may help the examiner elicit a disorder in memory are as follows:

Have you noticed any loss of memory?
How well do you remember what you are told? What has happened to you?
Do you remember those things that happened years ago best or those that happened today or yesterday?

Immediate memory (verbalized remembering immediately after presentation). Immediate memory is tested by digit recall. Two sample tests follow:

Please allow me to test your memory skills. I'd like you to repeat these numbers after me:
7, 4
9, 6, 5, 3
8, 9, 4, 1, 5
3, 8, 7, 4, 1, 6

I will say some numbers; you say them backward. For instance, I say *8, 2;* you say *2, 8:*
3, 8
7, 2, 0
5, 9, 2, 7

The average individual can generally repeat five to seven digits forward and four to six digits backward.

Recent memory may be impaired in temporal lobe trauma, senile dementia, Alzheimer's disease, and *Korsakoff's psychosis*.

Recent memory (verbalized remembrances after several minutes to an hour). Examples of questions and exercises for assessing recent memory are as follows:

How long have you been here?
Why did you come here?
What were you doing before you came here?
What time did you get up today?
How many meals have you eaten today?
What did you eat for breakfast today?

The client may be given some simple information and asked to reproduce it after a few minutes.

Remote memory (verbalized remembrances after hours, days, or years). The client may also be given three to five unrelated words to remember and repeat back. Examples of questions for assessing remote memory are as follows:

Where were you born?
Tell me the name of the high school you attended.
What was your mother's maiden name?

Remote memory is lost in widespread cortical damage such as the late stages of dementia. It may be dysfunctional in schizophrenic illnesses.

In testing for memory the examiner does not ask questions for which he does not have access to answers. Memory loss in organic dementia may involve disorders for immediate and recent events while clients may be able to recall events from childhood with accuracy. Memory disturbances are observed in febrile and toxic conditions, as well as in mania and anxiety. Frontal lobe lesions are often associated with memory loss.

Amnesic conditions are those in which memory is lost for a specific period of time or for certain life situations. In spite of memory loss the individual with amnesia remains aware of his environment. Amnesia is frequently associated with posttrauma periods and epileptic disorders.

Confabulation is an attempt by the client to "fill in the gaps" with fabricated or made-up answers when he is unable to remember.

Abstraction ability. To assess abstraction ability, the examiner may ask the client to give the meaning of familiar proverbs:

A bird in the hand is worth two in the bush.
People in glass houses should not throw stones.
When the cat's away, the mice will play.
Don't count your chickens before they hatch.
A rolling stone gathers no moss.
A stitch in time saves nine.

Similarities. The following exercises may be used to assess the client's ability to determine similarities:

Tell me how the following are like each other: bird and butterfly; dog and goldfish; fish and plankton; window and door; German person and Swiss person; pencil and typewriter.
Try to finish these comparisons for me: beer is to glass as coffee is to _____; engine is to airplane as pedal is to _____ .

The assessment of the ability to define the subtle but essential differences between objects or between events is the objective in testing the perception of dissimilarities. Some examples of items that may be used to assess this ability are as follows:

Tell me how these objects differ: a bush and a tree; a rock and a plant.

Lesions of the left hemisphere of the brain may impair the client's abilty to recognize similarities and to discriminate objects and events.

Ability to learn (comprehension). The ability to learn includes abilities in perception retention, association (interpretation), and recent memory. The processes are thought of as registration, storage, and retrieval. The client is given an address or a sentence that does not contain familiar associations. The material may be presented in writing or may be spoken. The client is asked to remember the content verbatim:

Listen to me carefully, I am going to give you an address that I want you to remember. Later on, I will ask you to repeat it for me: Apartment 13, Dover Hill Building.

Or the client might be given a sentence such as the Babcock sentence:

One thing a nation must have in order to become rich and great is a large and secure stock of wood.

Or the rest may consist of four unrelated words. An approximate 5- to 10-minute interval is allowed before the client is asked to repeat the material.

Computation. The following exercise may be used to assess the client's computational abilities.

Subtract 7 from 100. Continue on subtracting 7 from the resulting remainder.

The ability to calculate may be impaired in diffuse brain disease and lesions of the angular gyrus. The person with healthy cerebral function is able to complete the computation in 1½ minutes with less than four errors.

Organic mental disorders may be one reason for slowness in computation or increased numbers of errors. However, computation skills may be impaired in depression or anxiety.

Ability to read. A copy of a current newspaper or popular periodical may be used to determine the client's reading skills. The examiner should be certain that the client is wearing corrective lenses if they are needed for reading.

Impairment of the ability to read is called *dyslexia*.

General knowledge—general information

Health assessment may include an evaluative estimate of what the client has learned in school and an estimate of his awareness of current events. The examiner should *match* his *inquiries* to the *educational, sociocultural,* and *life experiences of the client.* The client might be asked questions about well-known national leaders such as the president, capitals of countries, or names of oceans. The questions of current events should include generally known phenomena. The examiner might base these questions on recent newspaper headlines that deal with important current issues.

Intellectual level

The examiner has obtained several criteria that are a part of human *intellectual* capacity: vocabulary, memory, calculation, reading, writing, and general knowledge. There is no need, in a screening assessment, to administer intelligence tests. However, the incorporation of selected items from the *Stanford-Binet test* may provide enough information to allow the examiner to further assess whether referral is necessary. It has been suggested that test items be selected from the 10-year-old level for initial presentation and then move to progressively more difficult tasks.

The intellectual level of the client may be deduced from his perceptive grasp of the comments and questions directed toward him, his level of general information and vocabulary, his exercise of logic, range and originality of thought, and cultural attainments.

Higher intellectual functions of *judgment,* analysis, synthesis, and abstraction are impaired in acute brain injury even when specific receptive, expressive, or memory functions are intact. On the other hand, cognitive abilities may remain operant when specific expressive and memory functions are impaired.

Expressive functions are speaking, drawing, writing, and other physical movement, including nonverbal behaviors. All mental activity must be inferred from the expressive functions. Disorders of the expressive functions are known as *apraxias* (see Table 19.2 for tests assessing brain damage).

Judgment

Judgment is a skill that encompasses all the cognitive processes necessary for evaluation, assessment, and decision making, particularly those in which two or more experiences are related to one another. The individual who is able to evaluate a situation and determine the appropriate reaction(s) is said to have good judgment or

reasoning ability. Assessment of judgment is accomplished through evaluation of the client's expressed attitudes to his social, physical, occupational, and domestic status and his plans for the future. Judgment may be considered intact if the client's business affairs are in order and he is meeting social and family obligations. The client might also be asked to explain how he would respond in certain social situations.

Simple tests of reasoning ability include an explanation of the meaning of abstractions. Judgment may be impaired in highly charged emotional states, mental retardation, organic mental disorder, schizophrenia, anxiety, and mania.

Two examples of questions that elicit judgment skills are:

What would you do if you were in a theater when fire broke out?

What would you do if you found four, stamped, addressed envelopes?

Thought processes

Thought processes are the individual's subjective ideations, comprehensions, and interpretations based on life experiences. The examiner must rely on the client's verbal and nonverbal expressions in drawing conclusions about his or her ability to think logically and coherently and in a goal-directed sequence. The client who jumps from one thought to another in an *illogical* sequence with no connection between the thoughts may be demonstrating *loose associations,* a symptom often seen in clients with *schizophrenia.* A client who rapidly skips from one complete idea to another without relationship to the preceding content may be manifesting *flight of ideas,* a symptom commonly observed in clients with *bipolar disorder, manic phase.*

The examiner must carefully observe the client's *affect* to see whether it is *congruent* with the client's verbal content. For example, a client who expresses little or no emotion while verbalizing the desire for self-harm or harm to others is demonstrating an incongruence between affect and verbal content. Such *mood-incongruence* has been noted in persons with schizophrenia. On the other hand, the individual with an obviously saddened affect who expresses *suicidal ideations* is demonstrating *mood-congruence,* a symptom more often noted in persons with *major depression.* In any case, both types of clients need immediate attention and further exploration of symptoms.

Disturbances in thought processes are noted in the form of thinking, the stream of thought, and the thought content. *Dereism* or dereistic thinking emphasizes a client's disconnection from reality and reflects an illogical form of thinking. The person's mental activity is incongruent with universally accepted laws of logic and experience. The individual with schizophrenia often expresses dereistic thoughts derived from internal stimuli, based on illogical premises.

My mother is blonde and an alcoholic; therefore all blonde women are alcoholics.

Autism or autistic thinking emphasizes a client's preoccupation with inner thoughts, *daydreams, fantasies, delusions,* and *hallucinations* that reflect unusual thought content and occur after disconnection from reality. Autistic traits such as daydreams or fantasies can be noted in persons considered more shy or introverted than usual, but the manner of speech used by the client with schizophrenia is conspicuously *stilted* by *bizarre* choices of words or phrases, inaudibility, or inappropriate shouting, all very specific clues to the diagnosis.

Variation from the usual rate or nature of association is considered a disturbance in the stream of thought. *Magical thinking,* extreme *intellectualization, circumstantiality, preservation, stereotypy, thought blocking,* or *thought insertion* are specific examples of disturbed thought stream.

Other disturbances in form, stream, or flow of thought are *tangential thinking, clang associations, pressure of speech, the aphasias, mutism,* and *contrete* versus *abstract thinking.* The rate of speech is also examined, since it is critical to contrast the associative stream of the manic individual with the *catatonic excitement* of the schizophrenic client. The client with schizophrenia draws on an inner repertoire of inaccessible thoughts, while the person with mania expresses words and ideas based on an outer, more accessible repertoire. Although schizophrenic clients tend to be more disorganized in their thinking, individuals with either disorder may demonstrate *psychotic* thought processes.

In depressed states, the flow of associations may slow down as an ongoing result of extreme sadness and *dysphoria.* Should the client's despair reach extreme proportions, the clinical picture could resemble the mutism of a catatonic schizophrenic.

The examiner also searches for signs of *phobias, obsessions,* or *compulsions,* all symptoms of disturbances in thought content that represent types of *anxiety disorders* or *personality disorders. Somatic* complaints may reflect either anxiety or depression and need further exploration of degree and type. *Levels of consciousness, orientation to person, place, and time,* and *recent versus remote memory* are also analyzed to rule out *organic mental disorders* or *neurologic disease.*

Common signs and symptoms illustrating alterations in mental health functioning are generally those that are uselessly repetitive, disabling, or uncomfortable for the client and others in the environment. Typical examples of thought disorders are delusions and hallucinations, often associated with schizophrenia, but also demonstrated in affective disorders such as major (unipolar) depression with psychotic features and bipolar disorder, manic phase. Delusions and hallucinations can also occur as a result of alcohol or chemical abuse, organic mental disorders, and brain disease. Refer to the Glossary at the end of this text for a more definitive list of symptoms commonly used to describe alterations in mental health function.

Emotional status, affect

Affect is defined as the external observable manifestation of emotion, whereas mood is the internally experienced emotion or feeling state. The examiner is generally able to develop an estimate of the client's prevailing mood and emotional status or affective state from verbal and nonverbal behaviors. Affects may be described as *labile,* repeated, rapid, and abruptly shifting. Affective responses, the feelings associated with ideas, are noted throughout the interview process. The examiner observes the *appropriateness* and degree of affect to a given idea as well as the range of affect to a variety of situations. A range of affect may be described as broad (mentally healthy), restricted (constricted), *blunted,* or *flat.*

The depressed individual may demonstrate a blunted affect. The depressed person who expresses suicidal feelings needs immediate attention. Flat or *bizarre affect* may be seen in clients with schizophrenia. *Apathy* may be observed in persons with organic mental disorder.

An interview protocol to assist the examiner in bringing out feelings of clients who resist offering spontaneous data is described (see the box on p. 484). It is important to note that the client's mood and affect may be altered in both organic and psychogenic disorders.

Insight

Insight is the client's ability to perceive himself realistically and to understand himself. The evaluation of insight involves the assessment of the client's understanding of and attitude toward the cause and nature of his illness. Simple questions such as "Why did you decide to come here (name of health care facility) at this time?" allow the client to explain in his own words his comprehension of his health status and his realization of physical and mental symptoms.

It is important to elicit the individual's attitude and willingness to accept professional advice and treatment. When an apparent lack of insight is found, the examiner should attempt to determine if a real loss has occurred or whether the client may be attempting to hide his problems. Insight may be lost in the euphoria of mania, or may be ascribed to external sources in paranoia.

The data elicited in the chief complaint and present illness may provide the examiner with information about the client's insight. Helpful questions used in concluding the analysis of the chief complaint are:

Have you noticed any change in yourself, or in your outlook on life?
Have you noticed any change in your feelings?

The appraisal of emotional status includes an investigation of the client's life situation and personality (general coping behavior). An example of an interview protocol to elicit this information follows:

Queries	Frequently recorded responses
Present (chief) complaint	
Tell me why you are here.	
Present illness	
When did you last feel well?	
What changes have you noted in yourself?	
When did you first notice the problem?	
How long did it last?	
What do you feel is causing the problem?	
Have you had any other troubling bodily or psychological feelings (symptoms)?	
How are you sleeping? Eating?	
Do you feel better in the morning or in the evening?	
Have you gained or lost any weight?	
Family history	
How old is your father? Is he employed?	
What does [did] he do for a living?	
How old is your mother? Is [was] she employed?	
Did either your father or your mother have any other marriages?	
How well did they get along?	
Tell me about their personality [temperament]?	Affectionate, warm easygoing, strict, cold, always worried, always in debt, drunk all the time
How did you feel about your parents?	
Was your home a comfortable place?	
Did any of your family have any emotional problems? Ever need to see a doctor because of a nervous problem?	

Queries	Frequently recorded responses
Childhood and premorbid personality	
What were you like as a child?	Friendly; happy; nervous; jumpy; shy; selfconscious; delicate; enuresis; nail biting; fears—of the dark, small rooms, open spaces, high places, crowds; depressed; loner; read all the time; hated sports; successful; unsure of self
How did your parents [brothers, sisters] describe you to others?	
What did your teachers think of you?	
Did you like to be with people?	
Tell me how you would describe yourself.	
Medical history	
Have you ever been diagnosed as having a disease? *If yes,* Explain this to me.	
Psychological history	
Have you ever been in counseling or treatment for an emotional problem?	
Recent stress	
Have you had any recent cause for grief?	
Have you been bereaved over the loss of a loved person?	
Are all your relatives and friends in good health?	
Are there any problems with your job?	
Is money a problem for you?	
Are there problems in your marriage? Love life?	
Education	
Where did you go to school?	
Wat was the highest grade you attended?	
How did you feel about school?	
How well did you do in school?	Overachievement, truancy, suspension
Employment	
What kind of work do you do?	
Where have you worked and how long at each job?	Long periods of unemployment, frequent job turnover
Have you ever served in a military service?	
Do you enjoy working?	
How do you get along with your boss? People who work for you?	
Delinquency	
Have you ever been in trouble with school? The police?	
Is your sexual relationship satisfactory to you? *If no;* How do you manage?	Masturbation, homosexuality, extramarital intercourse
Do you have any extramarital relationships?	

Queries

Frequently recorded responses

Social milieu
Tell me about your friends.

Support systems
Who would you turn to if you were in trouble?
Do you feel that you need someone to turn to?

Insight
Do you consider yourself different now than before your problem began?
What do you think about your problem?
Do you think you are sick? *If yes;* Do you think you will get over it?
Do you think you need help?
In what way would you change if you had a choice?
Do you think the same way now that you always have?
Do your thoughts come slower [faster] than they used to?

Drug history
Have you ever been given a prescription for medicine by a doctor? *If yes,* Tell me about it.
Have you ever used drugs available in the street? *If yes,* How much? How long? Are you taking drugs now?

Grass (marijuana), uppers, downers, cocaine, crack, crystal, hash, tic (phencyclidine [PCP]), horse (heroin)

Do you drink beer? Wine? Whiskey? How much? How long? *or* How much and what are you drinking these days?
Do you drink soda pop? How much?

Marital history
How old is your wife [husband]?
How long have you been married?
How do you feel about your marriage?

Hate to go home, often go out with the guys

How many children do you have?
Were there any other pregnancies?
How do you get along with your children?
What kinds of things do you do as a family?
How many times were you engaged?
Were you ever married before? *If yes,* Tell me about it.

Interview Protocol

General questions

How do you feel inside?
How have your spirits been?
Do you feel this way most of the time?
Are you in good spirits, happy (unhappy) most of the time?
Do you let others know how you feel? *If no;*
Are you afraid to let people know how you feel?
Can you control how you feel?
When do you feel the best, in the morning or in the evening?
How do you feel life has treated you?
Do you enjoy your life?
Is life worth living for you?
What does the future look like? *If no;*
Does everything look hopeless? Do you think you will see tomorrow?
What plans have you made for the future?
Have you ever considered hurting yourself *If yes;* Did you follow through and actually harm yourself? *If yes;* How did you do it?
Do you have any plans for self-harm now? *If yes;* What are your plans?
Do you think about dying? *If yes;* How often?
Refer to the Glossary for a list of terms commonly used to describe mood and affect.

Draw-a-person test

Self-drawings made by the client on blank pieces of paper may help the examiner in evaluation of body image. ("Draw yourself for me.") The drawing is inspected with special reference to size of image, the facial expression (affect), the activity of the figure, the amount and nature of detail, and the diminution or exaggeration of body parts. Another useful device is that of asking the client to fill in an outline of the human body. ("Draw your insides.") The heart, lungs, and intestines are the structures most frequently added. The placement and size of the organs drawn by the client may provide clues of their meaning to him (Fig. 19-2).

Once a symptom has been identified as a chief complaint (i.e., phobia, depression, compulsion, psychosomatic dysfunction), the history relevant to its development is explored. The individual's previous personality (characteristic behavior pattern) is explored in relation to behaviors that led to the exacerbation of the symptom in response to stress. In addition, the potential for resolution of the problem is identified; that is, the individual's personal, social, and environmental resources are determined.

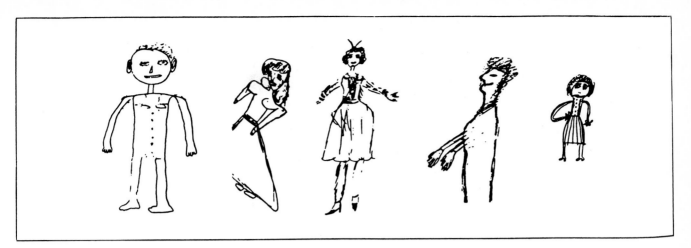

Figure 19-2

Examples of the Draw-a-Person test done by five women who had been hospitalized for two years.
From Spire RH: An experimental study of the use of photographic self-image confrontation as a nursing procedure in the care of
chronically ill schizophrenic female patients. (Project in partial fulfillment of MS degree, State University of New York at Buffalo)
1967, pp 243, 248, 249, 251, 256.

Coping behaviors or strategies

In an evaluation of the individual's resources for adjusting to life's experiences, it is valuable to know the coping behaviors he or she has found helpful in reducing stress, such as contact sports, jogging, meditation, and reading.

The examiner must be aware that unconscious defense mechanisms such as denial and protection are the ego's method of protecting the organism from overwhelming anxiety and may be adaptive. When used frequently and rigidly, dysfunctional behavior may result. (See Glossary.)

Organic brain syndromes

Organic brain syndrome describes symptomatology not differentiated in terms of etiology indicating medical or neurologic dysfunction causing an impairment of orientation, memory, or other mental functions (see boxed material opposite). Affective symptoms, delusions, hallucinations, and obsessions may also be present. An acute brain syndrome *(delirium)* is one of short duration that is usually reversible. A chronic brain syndrome *(dementia)* is long standing and often progressive in nature, with a less favorable prognosis. Organic mental disorder is a defined organic brain syndrome with a known etiology.

Affective (mood) disorders

The client with an affective disorder runs the gamut from depression to exaggerated *euphoria* or mania. The highs and lows show little correlation with the life situation (see boxed material on p. 486).

Organic Brain Syndrome:
Characteristic Symptoms and Signs

Acute delirium	**Dementia**
Impairment of consciousness	May be disoriented
Delusions possible	Attention span impaired
Hallucinations possible	Judgment impaired
May be disoriented	Recent memory impaired
Attention span impaired	Mood swings
Judgment impaired	Irritability—lability
Mood swings	Deterioration of personal habits
Recent memory impaired	Unclouded sensorium
Restlessness	Organic mental disorder
Anxiety	Alzheimer's disease
Fear	

During the down mood period, the client evidences such symptoms as *anorexia,* insomnia, sense of worthlessness, sense of being a burden, and thoughts of self-destruction. On the high mood cusp the client may describe flights of ideas or hyperactivity.

Primary affective disorders pertain to clients who have had no previous psychiatric disorders. *Secondary affective disorders* are ascribed to clients who have been previously diagnosed with a psychiatric illness.

A *bipolar disorder* is diagnosed when mania is present or indicated by history whether or not depression occurs. Depression occurring in the absence of mania is known as *major depression (unipolar).*

Affective (Mood) Disorders: Characteristic Symptoms and Signs

Mania

Euphoria
Irritability (sometimes)
Flight of ideas—generally comprehensible
Distractibility
Delusions possible (may be of grandeur)
Passivity—sensation that body is under external control
Depersonalization

Somatic

Hyperactivity
Rapid speech rate
Rhyming
Punning—sarcasm
Decreased sleep

Depression

Dejection
Discouragement
Despondency
Depression
Feeling of being down in the dumps, blue (dysphoria)
Irritability
Fearfulness
Loss of interest in daily activities
Social withdrawal
Guilt
Inability to focus thoughts
Indecisiveness
Recurring preoccupation with suicide, death
Thoughts of self-destruction
Hopelessness—powerlessness
Feeling of gloomy future, impending doom
Loss of interest in sexual activity
Delusions possible (frequently involving self-deprecation)

Somatic

Pain
Tachycardia
Dyspnea
Gastrointestinal dysfunction
Anorexia
Constipation
Sleep disorders
Insomnia
Hypersomnia
Lack of energy
Psychomotor retardation
Frequent crying
Impotence (in men)
Restlessness
Pacing, wringing of hands
Somatic symptoms involving physical distortions, e.g., a rotting gut or heart of stone

Schizophrenia: Characteristic Symptoms and Signs

Poor prognosis

Delusions
Hallucinations; symptoms develop slowly
Clear sensorium
Chronic disorder
Blunted, shallow (flat), or inappropriate affect
Catatonic motor behavior
Waxy flexibility; periods of immobility
Repeated grimacing, posturing
Disordered thought processes

Good prognosis

Delusions
Hallucinations
Clear sensorium
Symptoms transitory
Symptoms develop abruptly
More likely to show affective responses, usually depression
Recovery is usual
Good premorbid social/occupational functioning
Probable precipitating stressor
No family history

The client with an affective disorder often tells the examiner that "something is wrong with my mind."

Paranoid ideations have been reported in clients with affectve disorders. Such thoughts appear to be augmented ideas of reference related to the feeling of worthlessness and delusions depicting physical distortions (bizarre somatization).

The periods of illness may last from a few days to several years, and the client appears to function well in the interim.

Primary affective disorders are most frequently first diagnosed when the client is about 40, whereas the client with a bipolar affective disorder may be in his 30s.

Clients being treated with tricyclic antidepressant drugs may have complaints of side effects, such as blurred vision, dry mouth, or orthostatic hypotension. On the other hand, symptoms of severe headaches or hypertension in a patient taking monoamine oxidase inhibitors (MAOIs) should alert the examiner to obtain a thorough food and drug history, since the combination of MAOIs with certain foods or drugs may be associated with these potentially serious side effects. Lithium, a drug commonly used to control mania, can cause tremor, thirst, and GI upset among other symptoms. An accurate drug history and knowledge of toxic effects are critical. (Refer to current professional pharmacology text for more information on drugs used to treat mental disorders.)

Schizophrenic disorders

Hallucinations and delusions are the diagnostic signposts of schizophrenia. They are critical symptoms used in the diagnosis and classification of schizophrenic disorders (see the box above). Both delusions and hallucinations represent an internal modification of the environment to meet the desires or needs of the client. The presence of hallucinations may be suspected in the person who adopts listening attitudes or appears preoccupied.

Two classifications of these disorders are described in the literature related to prognosis. Schizophrenic disorders with a poor prognosis include *chronic schizophrenia*, and *process schizophrenia*. Schizophrenic disorders with a good prognosis include *schizophreniform* and *schizoaffective disorders* and *acute, reactive schizophrenia*.

The client's use of language is a valuable identifying characteristic of individuals with schizophrenia. They have been noted to use the same set of syntactic, semantic, and discourse patterns as mentally healthy individuals but not as proficiently. Furthermore, the person with schizophrenia appears to ignore the listener, whereas most people generally base the organization and content of their remarks on the last remark(s) of the person with whom they are talking. Schizophrenic individuals tend not to maintain this relationship, and to ignore their listener's lack of awareness to the subjects that they have newly introduced.

The development of schizophrenia may occur over a long period of time.

A schizoid personality is said to exist in the client who is markedly shy, withdraws from social relationships, and is unable to establish close personal relationships. This behavior is generally noted in adolescence, though delusions and hallucinations generally begin in the 20s.

The schizophreniform disorders are abrupt in onset and occur without a psychiatric history before the present illness.

Anxiety

The client demonstrating symptoms of severe or panic anxiety has recurrent periods of abrupt onset anxiety that terminate without intervention. The client complains of fright without a known object. The autonomic nervous system is activated.

Characteristic symptoms and signs include:

Palpitations	Headache
Breathlessness, smothering	Fatigue, weakness
Dyspnea	Paresthesias
Nervousness	Tremors, shakiness
Dizziness	Sighing
Faintness	Nausea and vomiting
Feeling of impending doom	Abdominal cramps
	Diarrhea
	Flatus

The age of onset extends from midadolescence through the early 30s.

Hysteria

Hysteria is a disorder characterized by multiple somatic symptoms. Examples of such complaints include gastro-intestinal disturbances, pains (dysmenorrhea, headaches, back pain), anxiety, sexual problems, and conversion symptoms. The symptoms often defy the boundaries of what is commonly known about pathophysiology. The descriptions are often vividly portrayed or markedly exaggerated, or both, so that these clients often spend a good deal of time in hospitals and undergo many surgical procedures. Because there are often many vague symptoms, the history may be difficult to report or record, so verbatim documentation may provide accuracy. Conversion symptoms are idiopathic symptoms that indicate neurologic disorders such as amnesia, unconsciousness, paralysis, anesthesias, or blindness.

Hysteria is most commonly first seen in the teens. The incidence is higher in women than in men.

Obsessive-compulsive disorder

Obsessions are long-lasting, unwilled, troubling thoughts or impulses that usually do not interest the individual and serve no purpose but cannot be ignored. *Compulsions* are the behaviors that result from the obsessions. The behaviors are repetitive, performed in a ritualistic stereotyped pattern. Thus, an obsessive-compulsive disorder is said to exist in the presence of obsessions and compulsions when no other disorder is evident. Other terms for this include *psychasthenia, phobic-ruminative state*, and *obsessional state*. Compulsions serve to decrease the anxiety which is caused by the obsessive thoughts and may be adaptive, although the individual can become dysfunctional if they persist.

Definitions

obsessional convictions Magical formulations ("If I have my purse here, nothing can happen to me.")

obsessional fears Repeated feelings of fright, particularly of disease, filth, sharp instruments

obsessional ideas Words, phrases, or rhymes that recur in the thought processes of the individual, frequently interrupting other thought sequences

obsessional images Recurrent imagined scenes, often dealing with sexual acts or excreta

obsessional impulses Irresistible thoughts related to self-injury, to injury of others, or to some other embarrassing behavior

obsessional rituals Recurrent, stylized actions; protocols for washing or combing hair, eating

obsessional rumination Prolonged reflection on a subject without reaching a decision

phobia A highly disturbing, recurring, and unrealistic fear; may relate to any situation or object

Antisocial personality

The antisocial personality describes an individual who has displayed a pattern of antisocial, delinquent, or criminal behavior. The stage is set for this type of personality disorder in childhood. Early symptoms include restlessness, a short attention span, and defiance of discipline. A history of poor school and work adjustment is the rule. Promiscuous sexual behavior and conversion symptoms are frequently observed.

The acute appearance of psychiatric symptoms in a person whose history reveals that affect and behavior had been normal before this occurrence is commonly seen in frontal and temporal lobe tumor, hydrocephalus, and cortical atrophy. The most common symptom found in these individuals is depression.

PSYCHOANALYSIS CONCEPTS AND MENTAL HEALTH

Psychoanalytic theory conceptualizes mental functioning as processes occurring within the id, ego, and superego. The id, ego, and superego are considered psychic forces for which no anatomic structure or physiologic function is directly comparable. The id integrates instinctual primitive impulses arising from the biologic organization of the person and manifested in the mind. The id provides psychic energy for biologic forces. Although the id has multiple drives, they are broadly categorized as sexual and aggressive drives. The id operates on the infantile pleasure principle.

The ego is the name given to those mental processes that function to (1) bring awareness of stimuli affecting the individual from the internal (ego and superego) and external environment, (2) integrate the stimuli, and (3) initiate the activities (defense mechanisms) that will maintain the internal and external adaptation. The ego operates on the reality principle. It serves as a moderator between the id and superego.

The superego is the moral judge of the other mental functions, operating on the basis of right, wrong, reward, punishment, good, or bad. The parts of the superego that operate at the conscious level correspond to the conscience.

Psychologic conflict is viewed as the presence of contradictory and incompatible psychologic drives and forces present in the human mind at one time. Intrapsychic conflict is caused by incompatible drives between psychic structures, whereas external conflict exists between the mind and the external environment. The psychic structures and external forces are constantly changing. Thus, the ego is changing, altering defense mechanisms, to maintain a steady state. The amplitude of internal drives varies with age.

The id drives related to sexual activity are moderately strong during the oedipal phase, decline in latency, increase significantly in puberty, and decrease somewhat throughout the remainder of life. The superego

is moderately intense in latency, declines in adolescence, and undergoes some alteration in the moral grids used to judge mental functions. The antisocial personality is believed to operate on an "underdeveloped" superego.

Healthy or "Normal" Mental Functioning

The ego develops more flexibility and is more efficient in maintaining adaptation with maturity. Hartman describes health as the degree of adaptation the individual has to internal and external environments. Saperstein also saw normality in terms of adaptation. He described flight, dependency, and self-sufficiency as the defenses used to adapt to the culture.

Freud described normality as the average presentation of the ego.

. . . only normal on the average. His ego approximates that of the psychotic in some part or another and to a greater or lesser extent; and the degree of its remoteness from one end of the series and its proximity to the other will furnish us with a provisional measure of what we have so indefinitely termed alteration of the ego.

Jones stated that a normal mind did not exist. However, he described a normal mind as having four characteristics: (1) a capacity for adaptation to reality; (2) object relationships or interactions with other people must include positive, friendly feelings (ambivalence and narcissism being resolved); (3) primitive drives are neutralized so that energy is used in productive pursuits; and (4) a capacity for enjoyment, self-containment, happiness, and freedom from anxiety. Jones did not believe these characteristics could be fully attained but could be used to determine degrees of normality.

Essler posited that a normal ego was one that would respond to therapy with a disillusion of symptoms. He believed that absolute normality could not exist. He further declared that psychoanalytical theory was the best method with which to gauge normality. A normal person would be able to free associate, would be aware of feelings and thoughts without resistance, and would respond to interpretation by relinquishing symptoms. Essler said that the ability to function was central to the concept of health.

Reider discussed social factors in the development of a neurotic drive for normalcy and defined normal behavior as a defense against anxiety. Gitleson described how normality could be used as a narcissistic defense through identification with the aggressor that the person perceives in society.

Klein saw normality as a well-integrated personality characterized by the following:
1. Emotional maturity—The individual can accept substitute gratification for infantile wishes and can enjoy pleasures without conflict.

2. Strength of character—Positive introjects and identifications dominate over negative identifications.
3. Capacity to deal with conflicting emotions—Love and hate can both be present, but the capacity for love predominates.
4. Balance between internal life and adaptation to reality—The individual shows insight and understanding of internal processes.
5. Composite of various parts of personality.

Klein stated that total integration never exists.

Saul viewed mental health as emotional maturity—the capacity to love and to be a good and responsible spouse, parent, and citizen—to have given up infantile helplessness and need for love.

Erikson described the development of the individual by behavioral definitions of the various stages of life. It was Erikson's opinion that the ego is faced with numerous conflicts and disruptions. Normal persons are those who adapt to the conflicts at each stage of life.

Glover described the normal person as one free of symptoms—able to love someone other than himself and work in a productive manner. He stated that the normal person had reconciled his internal drive to reality.

Menninger ascribes mental health to an individual who has adjusted to the world and other individuals with maximum effectiveness and happiness. Characteristics of the mentally healthy individual include an even temper, alert intelligence, pleasant disposition, and socially appropriate behavior.

Eric Fromm defined mental health as the ability to love and to create, to have a sense of one's self-identity, and to grasp reality.

Grotejohn emphasized the family interactions in the development of a normal ego identity.

Michaels stated that from a psychoanalytical point of view, a normal person does not exist. He agrees that basic theories of psychoanalysis propose that mental conflict is present in all persons and that normal people are relatively "neurotic."

Psychiatric Literature

Engel has objected to the idea of a dichotomy between health and illness. Engel focused on the interrelationships of mind and body in exploring the origin of psychosomatic illness.

Levine also discussed the relative nature of normality and stated that it could be defined by employing statistical averages for specific groups, intellectual and physical normality, absence of neurotic and psychotic symptoms, and emotional maturity.

Szasz and other psychiatrists have questioned whether mental illness exists. His particular concern was with calling maladaptive behavior mental illness.

The 1987 edition of the American Psychiatric Association's *Diagnostic and Statistical Manual of Mental Disorders III-R* says as a basic concept that

there is no satisfactory definition that specifies precise boundaries for the concept "mental disorders." Nevertheless it is useful to present concepts that have influenced the decision to include certain conditions as mental disorders . . . typically associated with a painful symptom (distress) or impairment in one or more important areas of functioning (disability).

Psychiatric Classification Systems

Psychiatric classification was initiated in 1896 by Kraepelin, who was the first to use the term *dementiapraecox*, now known as schizophrenia. Bleuler described schizophrenia, delineating the primary and secondary symptoms. Psychiatrists defined diagnostic categories. Clients were considered to be healthy if the signs and symptoms of a syndrome could not be found.

The absence of symptoms is equated with health. Many psychiatrists are now skeptical of a single cause of a mental illness and have studied alternative explanations including developmental history, early life experiences, stressors, and physiologic and biochemical alterations.

The first edition of the American Psychiatric Association's *Diagnostic and Statistical Manual of Mental Disorders,* known as DSM, was published in 1952. DSM-III appeared in 1980. DSM-III-R (revised edition) was published in 1987.

Features of the DSM-III-R include a multiaxial diagnostic system that requires that each client or case be assessed on five different axes, each one requiring a different class of information (American Psychiatric Association, 1987).

The purpose of the multiaxial system is to ensure attention to certain types of disorders, aspects of the environment, and areas of function that might be overlooked if the focus were on assessing a single presenting problem (see boxed material on p. 490).

Nursing Diagnosis is a statement that describes a client's health state or an actual or potential alteration in one's life processes (biologic, psychologic, sociocultural, developmental, and spiritual). The nurse uses the nursing process to identify and synthesize clinical data and to order nursing interventions to reduce, eliminate, or prevent health alterations (health promotion), actions in the legal and educational domain of nursing practice.

The North American Nursing Diagnosis Association (NANDA) is in the process of identifying, defining, and describing a classification system of nursing diag-

---

Axes

Axis I: Clinical syndromes; the entire classification of mental disorders.
(295.32) Schizophrenia, paranoid type, chronic.
V-Codes: Conditions not attributable to a mental disorder that are the focus of treatment.
(V-15.81) Noncompliance with medical treatment
Axis II: Developmental and personality disorders
(315.40) Developmental coordination disorder (child)
(308.81) Narcissistic personality disorder (adult)
Axis III: Physical disorders, conditions, or findings current or relevant to understanding or management of care.
(780.50) Insomnia related to a known organic factor.
Axis IV: Severity of psychosocial stressors occurring in the year preceding the current problem, evaluated on a scale of none (1) to catastrophic (6).
Axis V: Global assessment functioning (GAF)
Permits examiner to indicate overall judgment of the client's psychosocial and occupational functioning on a scale of highest level of function (90) to least level of function (1). Ratings are made for two time periods—current and highest level of function in past 3 months.

Adapted from American Psychiatric Association: Diagnostic and statistical manual of mental disorders, ed III-R, Washington DC, 1987, The Association.

Table 19-9

Medical and nursing diagnoses associated with disruptions in relatedness

Medical diagnostic class	Nursing diagnostic class
Schizophrenic disorders	Disruptions in relatedness
Personality disorders	

Associated medical diagnoses (DSM-III-R)	Associated nursing diagnoses (NANDA)
Schizophrenia	Anxiety
Paranoid	Impaired verbal communication
Catatonic	Ineffective coping
Disorganized	Family
Undifferentiated	Individual
Residual	Alteration in family process
Personality disorder	Impaired adjustment
Paranoid	Impaired social interaction
Schizoid	Self-care deficit
Schizotypal	Disturbance in self-concept
Antisocial	Sensory-perceptual alteration
Borderline	Altered thought processes
Dependent	

Adapted from Stuart G and Sundeen S: Principles and practice of psychiatric nursing, ed 3, St Louis, 1987, The CV Mosby Co.

---

noses. The eighth conference on the classification of nursing diagnoses was held in March 1988.

The Council on Psychiatric and Mental Health Nursing of the American Nurses' Association is developing a classification of phenomena of concern to psychiatric mental health nurses.

Nursing and medical diagnoses may complement each other but they remain separate entities. Nursing diagnoses can be formulated based on the client's maladaptive responses whether or not a medical diagnosis exists. In the medical model of psychiatry, the health problems are the mental disorders, from which many nursing diagnoses may emerge (Table 19-9).

Sample Protocol for Eliciting Psychiatric Symptoms

Questions leading to the elucidation of psychiatric symptoms might include the following:

Disturbing events

How did you feel at the time?

Hallucinations

Have you heard [sounds, voices, messages], seen [lights, figures], smelled [strange, bad, good odors], tasted [strange, bad, good tastes], or felt [touching, warm, cold sensation] anything that others who were present did not? If no one was present, would I have been able to have the same impressions from the experience?

What are the voices like? What do they say? (To determine if they instruct client to harm self or others)

Delusions

Do you feel that someone or something outside you is controlling you in some way? Are you able to control other people?

Do you feel that you are being watched? Followed?

Are people talking about you? *If yes,* Explain to me how you know.

Do you have anything to feel guilty about?

Do you feel you are a bad person?

Obsessions

Do you have some thoughts that keep coming back again and again? *If yes,* Tell me about them. How often? Are they pleasant [frightening] thoughts? Can you make them stop?

Compulsions

Are there some things you find yourself doing over and over? *If yes,* Tell me about them. How often? Can you stop doing these things?

Do you have someone or something outside you that is forcing you to do these things?

Do you find yourself checking and rechecking to make sure water is turned off? Gas? To make sure the doors are locked?

Somatic symptoms

Do you ever feel a lump in your throat?
Do you have difficulty swallowing? Speaking?
Have you ever been paralyzed?
How do your bowels function?
How is your appetite?
Do you have headaches?
Do you have enough energy to do all the things you would like to do?

Health History
Mental Status

NOTE: A yes response to any question *must* be further investigated. Use the following indicators throughout the assessment: (1) onset (specific date, sudden or gradual), (2) duration, (3) frequency, (4) precipitating factors, (5) aggravating or alleviating factors, (6) treatment received, and (7) outcome.

Present status

1. What are your concerns or symptoms?
   a. Description: fear, sadness, guilt, shame, anxiety, powerlessness, loss of self-esteem
2. Have you noticed recent changes in yourself?
   a. Description: anxiety, weight loss or gain, irritability, passivity, discouragement, guilt, indecision, rapid speech, pain, dyspnea, anorexia, insomnia, hypersomnia, restlessness, decreased sexual activity, faintness, headache, tremors, nausea, vomiting, diarrhea
3. Do you currently use or abuse illicit or prescription drugs or alcohol?
   a. Type
   b. Amount
   c. Why
4. Do you feel you are able to adequately care for yourself?
   a. Hygiene or ADL
   b. Financial transactions
   c. General communications
5. Are you employed?
   a. Type of work
   b. Number of absences in last year
   c. Reason for absences
6. Do you have difficulty fulfilling work expectations?
   a. Description of difficulties

Past history

1. Have you used or abused illicit or prescription drugs or alcohol in the past?
   a. Type
   b. Amount
   c. Why

2. Has your relationship with your family changed?
   a. Description: discord, withdrawal, physically abusive or abused, estrangement, separation or divorce
3. Have you ever considered harming yourself or others?
   a. Who, when, how, where
4. Have you had ECT treatments?
   a. When
   b. How many

Associated conditions

1. Have you had trauma to your head?
   a. Type
   b. When
   c. Causative factor
   d. Change in consciousness
   e. Residual effects
2. Have you had brain surgery?
   a. Type
   b. When
   c. Residual effects

Family history

1. Does anyone in your family have a diagnosed psychiatric disorder?

Sample assessment record

Client states wife died 3 months ago after a short illness and since then he has felt sad and lonely. Admits to insomnia since her death. He falls asleep easily but awakens after an hour or two then sleeps only intermittently and finally arises at dawn. He feels tired and listless all day. Has gained 10 pounds due to increased intake of junk and fast foods because he doesn't cook for himself. Also admits to drinking five to seven beers daily for the past 3 months but denies ever using or abusing drugs. Does not socialize with old friends because he feels he can't fit in anymore. Works on an assembly line and has had no absences in last 5 years. Is able to meet work requirements. Denies past episodes of mental illness and has no suicidal ideation. Denies having head trauma and brain surgery.

BIBLIOGRAPHY

American Psychiatric Association: Diagnostic and statistical manual of mental disorders, ed III-R, Washington DC, 1987, The Association.

Boettcher EG and Alderson SF: Psychotropic medications and the nursing process, J Psychosoc Nurs Ment Health Serv 20:11, 1982.

Carpenito LJ: Nursing diagnosis application to clinical practice, Philadelphia, 1989, JB Lippincott Co.

Cavenar JO Jr and Brodie HKH: Signs and symptoms in psychiatry, Philadelphia, 1983, JB Lippincott Co.

Chusid JG: Correlative neuroanatomy and functional neurology, ed 16, Los Altos, Calif, 1976, Lange Medical Publications.

Cihlar C: Mental status assessment for the E.T. nurse: psychologic impact of physical trauma, J Enterostomal Ther 13:49–53, 1986.

Daube JR and Sandok BA: Medical neurosciences, Boston, 1978, Little, Brown & Co.

Dawson DFL, Bartolucci G, and Blum HM: Language and schizophrenia: toward a synthesis, Comparative Psychiatry 21(1):81, 1980.

DeJong RN: The neurologic examination, ed 4, New York, 1979, Harper & Row.

Dreikurs R: Psychodynamics, psychotherapy and counseling, Chicago, 1967, Alfred Adler Institute.

Fieve RR and Dunner DL: Unipolar and bipolar affective states. In Flach FF and Draghi SC, editors: The nature and treatment of depression, New York, 1975, John Wiley & Sons.

Green C: The development of a conceptual framework for mental handicap nursing practice in the United Kingdom, Nurse Ed Today 8:9–17, 1988.

Hedlund JL and Vieweg BW: Automation in psychological testing, Psychiatr Ann 18: 1988.

Hume AJA, Barker PJ, Robertson W, and Swan J: Manic depressive psychosis: an alternative therapeutic model of nursing, J Adv Nurs 13:93-98, 1988.

Imboden JB and Chapman U: Psychiatric evaluation of the medical patient. Practical psychiatry in medicine, part 16, J Fam Pract 10:4, 1980.

Kaplan H and Sadock B: Comprehensive textbook of psychiatry/V (vol. 1 and 2), Baltimore, 1988, Williams & Wilkins.

Kolb LC: Modern clinical psychiatry, ed 9, Philadelphia, 1977, WB Saunders Co.

Lewis A: Mechanisms of neurological disease, Boston, 1976, Little, Brown & Co.

Lezak M: Neuropsychological assessment, New York, 1976, Oxford University Press.

Loomis ME and others: Development of a classification system for psychiatric mental-health nursing: individual response class, Arch Psychiatr Nurs 1:1, 1987.

Masserman JH and Schwab JJ: The psychiatric examination, New York, 1974, Intercontinental Medical Book Corp.

Mayo Clinic and Foundation: Clinical examinations in neurology, ed 4, Philadelphia, 1976, WB Saunders Co.

Morrison E, Fisher L, and Wilson H: NSGAE: Nursing adaptation, a proposed axis VI or DSM-III, J Psychosoc Nurs 23:8, 1985.

Nicholi AM Jr, editor: The Harvard guides to modern psychiatry, Cambridge, Mass, 1978, Belknap Press.

North American Nursing Diagnosis Association (NANDA): The eighth conference on the classification of nursing diagnosis, St. Louis, 1988, NANDA.

Schmidt RF: Fundamentals of sensory physiology, New York, 1978, Springer-Verlag New York.

Strahl MO and Lewis ND, editors: Differential diagnosis in clinical psychiatry, New York, 1972, Science House.

Strub RL and Black FW: The mental status examination in neurology, Philadelphia, 1979, FA Davis Co.

Stuart GW and Sundeen SJ: Principles and practice of psychiatric nursing, ed 3, St Louis, 1987, The CV Mosby Co.

Teasdale G and Jennett B: Assessment of coma and impaired consciousness: a practical scale, Lancet 2:81, 1974.

Wilson HS and Kneisl CR: Psychiatric nursing, ed 3, Menlo Park, Calif, 1988, Addison-Wesley Publishing Co.

Woodruff RA, Goodwin DW, and Guze SB: Psychiatric diagnosis, Oxford, 1984, Oxford University Press.

20

Assessment of the neurologic system

OBJECTIVES

Upon successful review of this chapter, learners will be able to:

- Describe anatomy and physiology of the neurologic system

- State related rationale and demonstrate examination of the neurologic system, including
  Cranial nerve function
  Proprioception and cerebellar function
  Reflexes
  Sensory function
  Review of musculoskeletal system

- Recognize possible pathological conditions related to the neurological system

- Correlate cranial nerves with their functions, assessment, makeup, and components

The neural system provides integration for all the functions of the body, but the system also derives its homeostatic balance from the appropriate functioning of the peripheral organs. The cells of the central nervous system (CNS), for example, depend on an adequate supply of glucose for their metabolic processes, and this supply can be maintained only when those tissues that play a role in intermediary metabolism function well. This balance makes neurologic assessment a part of all the components of the history and the physical examination.

The neurologic system controls cognitive and voluntary behavioral processes and the subconscious and involuntary bodily functions of the organism (see boxed material below). The major functions of the nervous system are reception (sensory), integration, and adaptation. That is, the normal nervous system receives stimuli from the environment, compares the adaptive processes necessary to adjustment to the environment with the functions the body is currently employing, and effects changes as necessary to ensure homeokinesis or survival.

Equipment needed for neurologic assessment includes vials of coffee and tobacco, for olfactory assessment and vials of glucose solution (sweet), salt solution, vinegar or lemon juice (sour), and quinine (bitter) for taste assessment. Test tubes of water are used to assess hot and cold temperature perception. Also necessary are an ophthalmoscope, a Snellen's chart for visual acuity, a Rosenbaum pocket-vision screener, a tuning fork, a reflex hammer, a tongue blade, an applicator, and a wisp of cotton.

The *mental status examination* is an integral part of the neurologic examination. In the context of the total assessment of health, however, this appraisal occurs much earlier in the examination. Most examiners make

---

Neurologic Physical Examination

The neurologic physical examination may be performed as five areas of investigation:
1. Assessment of cranial nerve function
2. Assessment of proprioception and cerebellar function
3. Musculoskeletal assessment (see Chapter 18)
4. Assessment of sensory function
5. Assessment of reflexes

---

assessments of mental status while obtaining the client's history and do special tests immediately afterward (see the boxed material above).

CRANIAL NERVE FUNCTION

CN I: Olfactory Nerve

The olfactory nerve is sensory in function and makes possible the sense of smell, or olfaction.

Processes

The peripheral neurons of the olfactory nerve are bipolar neurons. The ciliated, distal neurons penetrate the nasal mucosa in the roof of the nose, the upper septum, and the medial wall of the superior nasal concha. Unless the individual sniffs or inspires deeply, most of the inspired air does not contact the olfactory epithelium; during normal respiration, inspired air does not rise this high in the nares. Deep inspiration or sniffing causes a sudden rush of air into the upper nose and initiates swirling or turbulence of air around the olfactory mucosa. The central, unmyelinated axons are grouped in 15 to 20 bundles that pass through the cribriform plate of the ethmoid bone to synapse within the olfactory bulb. The second-order neurons course posteriorly from the bulb to the olfactory trigone, where they divide into medial and lateral striae. The medial striae terminate in the cortex of the medial subcallosal gyrus and the inferior portion of the cingulate gyrus. The lateral striae terminate in the uncus, the anterior portion of the hippocampal gyrus, and amygdaloid nucleus. Testing the sense of smell is an examination of the integrity of the entire system. When the same odor is smelled continuously, the olfactory cells are thought to be fatigued because a decreased awareness of odor is reported on long exposures.

Clinical examination

The client is asked to close the eyes (if the substance can be identified visually), occlude one nostril, and attempt to identify familiar substances with the open one, sniffing

or inhaling deeply. The substances should be mildly aromatic (volatile oils and liquids) and unambiguous, such as coffee, cigarettes, soap, peanut butter, toothpaste, oranges, vanilla, chocolate, and oils of wintergreen, lemon, lime, almond, and cloves. It has been shown that the most easily identified substances are coffee, oil of almond, chocolate, and oil of lime. Strongly aromatic compounds should be avoided in determining olfactory function because the vapors may prevent the perception of weaker substances. Substances that stimulate either gustatory receptors or trigeminal branches of the nasal mucosa should also be avoided, including chloroform, oil of peppermint, camphor, ammonia, alcohol, and formaldehyde.

The substances are housed in test tubes that are kept closed until the examiner is prepared to present them to the client.

The client is asked whether they smell anything and, if so, then attempts to identify the substance. The process is repeated for each nostril to determine symmetry (Fig. 20-1).

Cranial Nerves and Their Functions

I Olfactory	Sense of smell
II Optic	Visual acuity
III Oculomotor	Movement of eye muscles
	Upper lid opening
	Pupillary reflexes
IV Trochlear	Movement: superior oblique eye muscles
V Trigeminal	Sensory for face
	Motor to muscles of mastication
VI Abducens	Movement of lateral rectus eye muscle
VII Facial	Motor to muscles of facial expression
	Sensory: taste, anterior two thirds of tongue
VIII Acoustic	Auditory acuity
	Position in space: balance
IX Glossopharyngeal	Sensory position in space
	Motor to uvula
	Soft tissue of palate
	Sensory: taste in posterior one third of tongue
X Vagus	Motor to muscles of pharynx, larynx
XI Hypoglossal	Motor to tongue
XII Spinal accessory	Motor to sternocleidomastoid muscles and trapezius muscles

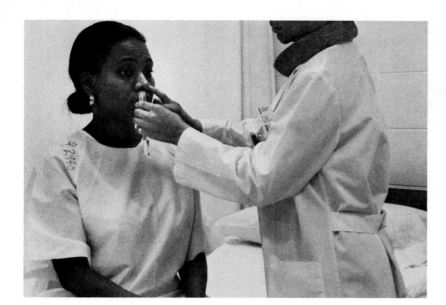

Figure 20-1

Testing for ability to smell. The client is asked to sniff as the test tube containing the test substance is placed beneath the nostril. The examiner holds the other nostril closed.

Both the number of substances used as stimuli and the number of correct responses should be recorded, along with differences in sensitivity from one nostril to the other.

If the client has difficulty identifying substances, ascertain whether they are able to smell anything at all. In addition, determine whether the client's nasal passages are patent.

Anosmia is the loss of the sense of smell or the inability to discriminate vapors. Diminution of the ability to smell is termed *hyposmia*. The client is not always aware of a deficit in olfaction. A pathophysiologic condition of the nasal mucosa or olfactory bulb or tract can interfere with the sensation of smell.

The individual with an impaired sense of smell also has difficulty in identifying flavors. Since the tongue has receptors for only sweet, salt, sour, and bitter, these must be regarded as the true tastes and will be retained in hyposmia and anosmia. However, flavor perception is a synthesis of odor, taste, and perceptions from stimulation of end organs in the mouth and pharynx. The individual with CN I involvement may complain only of loss of the sense of taste. The examiner should note that olfactory acuity is thought to be more acute before eating than after a meal.

The mucosal surfaces are examined when the client has difficulty in smelling, since an inflammation of the mucous membranes (viral, bacterial) decreases the sense of smell. Allergic rhinitis and excessive cigarette smoking commonly cause anosmia or hyposmia.

Lesions of the sinuses may result in distortion or hallucinations of smell but do not result in a loss of olfactory sensation. Unilateral loss of smell may be an early indication of a neoplasm involving the olfactory bulb or tract. Total anosmia may follow head trauma, especially fractures involving the cribriform plate. *Parosmia* is a perversion of the sense of smell that sometimes accompanies trauma or tumors of the uncus. Olfactory hallucinations that are offensive are known as *cacosmia*.

CN II: Optic Nerve

The optic nerve is described in Chapter 10 on eye assessment (note the sections on examination of visual acuity, visual fields, the pupils—tests of pupillary constriction, retinal fields, and the optic disc). Fig. 20-2 illustrates an examination for unilateral protrusion of an eye.

CN III: Oculomotor Nerve, CN IV: Trochlear Nerve, CN VI: Abducens Nerve

The oculomotor, trochlear, and abducens nerves are also described in Chapter 10 (note the sections on neuromuscular and extraocular muscle function—tests of eye movement).

Doll's head maneuver (vestibular oculogyric reflex)

Rapid turning of the head to one side results in ocular deviation to the contralateral side. In deep coma or other conditions resulting in paralysis of the oculomotor nerves or muscles, conjugate gaze to the contralateral side may be diminished or lost.

CN V: Trigeminal Nerve

The trigeminal nerve is motor to the muscles of mastication and sensory to the face and to the mucosa of the

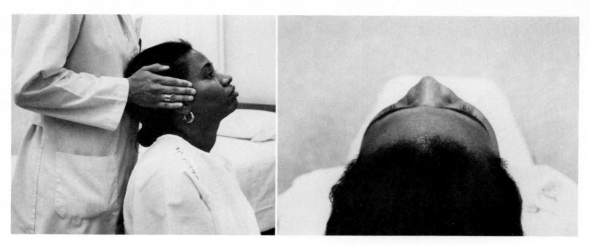

Figure 20-2

An examination for unilateral protrusion of an eye. The examiner stands behind the client and slowly extends the neck. The eyelashes should be sighted simultaneously for both eyes if they are similar in size and position.

nose and mouth in perceiving touch, temperature, and pain.

The nuclei of the trigeminal nerve are located in the midportion of the pons. The bulk of the cell bodies of the sensory portion of the trigeminal nerve lies in the gasserian ganglion, with the remainder in the mesencephalic nucleus. The sensory fibers to the gasserian ganglion are contained in one of the three proximal divisions of the nerve: ophthalmic, maxillary, or mandibular (Fig. 20-3). Peripheral nerve endings of the ophthalmic branch are sensory to the cornea, conjunctiva, upper lid, forehead, bridge of the nose, and scalp as far posteriorly as the vertex. The maxillary division of CN V conducts sensation from the skin of the lateral aspect of the nose, cheek, upper teeth, and jaw and from the mucosa of the lower nasal cavity, nasopharynx, hard palate, and uvula. The mandibular division contains the motor fibers that innervate the masseter, temporal, pterygoid, and digastric muscles. This division is also sensory to the skin of the lower jaw, pinna of the ear, anterior portion of the external auditory canal, side of the tongue, lower gums, lower teeth, floor of the mouth, and buccal surface of the cheek.

Afferent fibers from the gasserian ganglion enter the lateral portion of the pons and bifurcate into ascending and descending branches. The ascending branches pass to the main sensory nucleus responsible for the sensation of touch and to the mesencephalic nucleus that serves proprioception from the muscles of mastication and the periodontal membrane. The descending branch provides sensations of pain and temperature. The motor nucleus is located in the midcentral pons.

The muscles of mastication are evaluated by asking the client to bite down with as much force as possible.

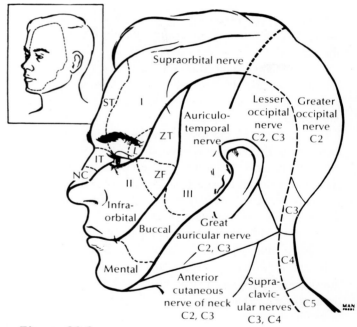

Figure 20-3

Cutaneous fields of the head and upper part of the neck. Inset shows the area of sensory loss in the face following resection of the trigeminal nerve. The cutaneous fields of the three branches of the trigeminal nerve are identified as *I*, ophthalmic; *II*, maxillary; and *III*, mandibular.
(From Haymaker W and Woodhall B: Peripheral nerve injuries, ed 2, Philadelphia, 1959, WB Saunders Co.)

The masseter muscles (Fig. 20-4) are evaluated by palpation, as are the temporal muscles (Fig. 20-5). Resistance is applied with downward pressure on the chin.

The pterygoid muscles may be examined by asking the client to press the jaw laterally against the examiner's hand with the mouth slightly open.

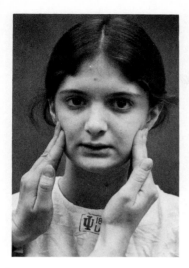

Figure 20-4

Palpation of the masseter muscles for size, strength, and symmetry to test CN V.

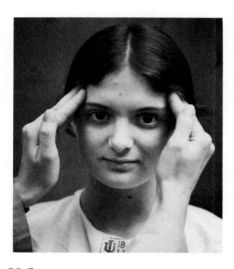

Figure 20-5

Palpation of the temporal muscles for size, shape, and symmetry to test CN V.

Atrophy of the muscle is recorded. Deviation of the jaw to one side indicates that the muscles of the side to which it is pulled are stronger than those of the opposite side. The individual is able to move the jaw to the unparalyzed side but not to the paralyzed side. The client may be asked to bite on a tongue blade; the position of the upper and lower incisors is compared to measure any deviation. An idea of the extent of weakness of the muscle might be gained by asking the client to move the jaw toward the weak side. Muscle tone and strength are also assessed, with the muscles observed for *fasciculations*.

The usual tests of sensation (see "Sensory function") are employed on both sides of the face, taking care that each division of the nerve is tested. Both skin and mucous membranes are examined. A wooden applicator may be used to touch various areas of the mucosa inside the mouth to test sensitivity to touch. The trigeminal nerve contains the afferent fiber for the corneal reflex (see Chapter 10 on eye assessment) and both the afferent and efferent fibers for the jaw closure reflex (described later in this chapter).

Motor pathophysiology

Myasthenia gravis. The weakness and ready fatigability of muscles that occur in myasthenia gravis may involve the muscles of mastication, making chewing difficult or impossible.

Amyotrophic lateral sclerosis. Degeneration of the motor nucleus of the trigeminal nerve may occur in amyotrophic lateral sclerosis, resulting in weakness and atrophy of the muscles of mastication. The client may be unable to chew or close the mouth.

Tetanus. Rigidly spastic muscles are frequently observed in tetanus infections. Spasm of the muscles of mastication is called lockjaw.

Sensory pathophysiology

Neuritis. Painful neuritis is caused by infection, vitamin deficiencies, and chemical irritants. When pain is severe, there is radiation over the three branches of the trigeminal nerve.

Trigeminal neuralgia (tic douloureux). Trigeminal neuralgia is characterized by excruciating pain of the lips, gums, or chin. The regions of pain may map out one of the divisions of the trigeminal nerve. These zones are supraorbital, infraorbital, and inferior to the labial fold midway to the angle of the jaw. Sharp pain may be elicited by applying pressure at the point where the trigeminal nerve emerges from the bone. Cold may also precipitate the pain. The condition generally occurs in elderly people. Clinical examination does not reveal impairment of sensory or motor function.

Herpes zoster (shingles). The gasserian ganglion, just as any ganglion of the body, may be affected by the herpesvirus. A characteristic papulovesicular rash generally involving the ophthalmic division may be observed. The vesicles are located over the forehead, eyelid, and cornea. These lesions may later ulcerate and keratinize. A neuralgia may remain after the rash has disappeared, and sensation may be lost from the involved area.

CN VII: Facial Nerve

The facial nerve is a motor to the facial muscles and sensory to taste sensation of the anterior two thirds of the tongue. It also conducts exteroceptive sensation from the eardrum area and proprioceptive information from the muscles it supplies. Visceral sensation from the salivary glands and mucosa of the mouth and pharynx is also conducted by CN VII. The facial nerve also carries parasympathetic fibers that stimulate secretion of the salivary glands, the lacrimal glands, and the mucosa of the nose, palate, and nasopharynx. The reticular formation of the pons is the location of the motor nucleus of the facial nerve.

Taste sensation is mediated by the taste buds of the tongue, and the sensation is conducted through the lingual nerve; the neurons of the lingual nerve have their cell bodies in the geniculate ganglion. Gustatory sensation is then conducted through the sensory portion of the intermediate nerve to the solitary tract of the pons.

The muscles controlled by the motor component of the facial nerve play a role in all the voluntary and involuntary movements of the face, except for movements of the jaw. The client's face is inspected for indications of facial muscle weakness, such as drooping of one side of the mouth, flattening of the nasolabial fold, and laxity of the lower eyelid.

The client is asked to perform the following facial movements: elevate the eyebrows, wrinkle the forehead by looking upward, frown (Fig. 20-6), smile or show the teeth (in this test, in addition to the facial muscles, the platysma muscle of the neck is noted) (Fig. 20-7), puff out the cheeks against the pressure of the examiner's fingers (Fig. 20-8), or whistle. The examiner evaluates the movements for muscle strength and symmetry. The client is told to close the eyes, first lightly and then tightly, while the examiner tries to open them. The platysma muscle is checked by asking the client to open the mouth slightly and to "jut out" the jaw.

In infants the facial muscles are evaluated during crying, while the practitioner evaluates tone and notes any atrophy and fasciculations.

Taste sensation for the anterior two thirds of the tongue is mediated through the sensory component of the facial nerve (CN VII) and is the only aspect of sensation that is tested. To test taste sensation, solutions of the following substances are applied with an applicator or pipette to the appropriate region of the lateral aspect of the tongue: sweet, salty, sour (vinegar, lemon juice), and bitter (quinine) (Figs. 20-9 and 20-10). A different applicator is used for each substance, and the client is allowed a sip of water in between testing to avoid mixing tastes. In addition, the tongue should remain protruded

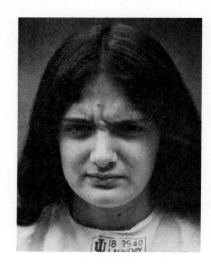

Figure 20-6

Test of CN VII. Client's ability to frown is inspected as a function of the facial muscles.

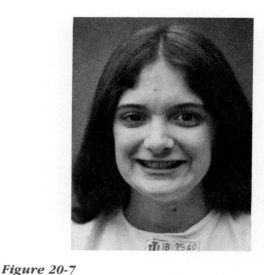

Figure 20-7

Test of CN VII. Client's ability to expose the teeth is inspected as a function of the facial muscles and platysma muscle of the neck.

throughout each test to avoid spreading the test substance over the tongue. The client is given a card with the words *salty, sweet, sour,* and *bitter* and asked to point to the one that best describes the solution on the tongue. Each substance is used twice. Both sides of the tongue must be assessed for each taste sensation. The number of tests and the number of correct responses are recorded.

The facial nerve also innervates the submandibular, submaxillary (sublingual), and lacrimal glands. However, the functions of salivation and lacrimation are generally not tested as a part of the routine physical examination.

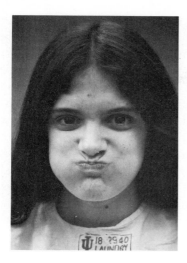

Figure 20-8

Test of CN VII. Client's ability to puff out the cheeks is inspected as a function of the facial muscles.

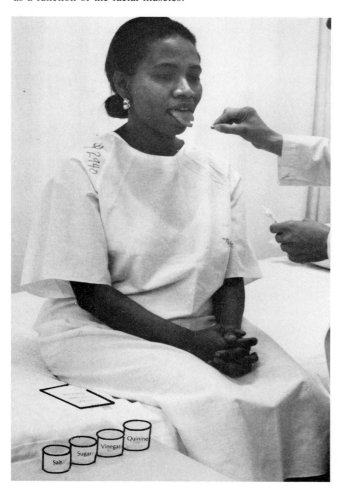

Figure 20-10

Solutions that will elicit the taste modalities are salty (saline solution), sweet (sugar), sour (vinegar or lemon juice), and bitter (quinine). The solutions are applied one at a time to the appropriate sensory area of the tongue.

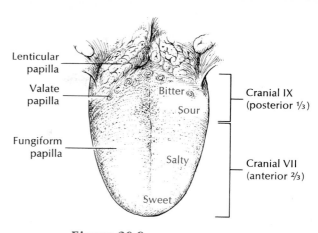

Figure 20-9

Localization of taste buds of tongue.

Motor pathophysiology

Motor weakness of CN VII is defined by the location of the particular lesion. Corticobulbar or upper motor neuron lesions are those that involve the motor cortex. The motor neurons supply the face or the axons of those neurons that form the corticobulbar tracts coursing through the internal capsule, cerebral peduncle, or pons. Corticobulbar paralysis is rarely complete and is contralateral to the lesion. The nuclear center of the brain that controls the upper part of the face receives both contralateral and ipsilateral fibers. The lower portion of the face, however, receives only contralateral fibers.

Chvostek's sign is produced by tapping the facial nerve. A positive response is a brisk contraction of the facial muscles that are innervated distal to the point of contact with the nerve. This may be elicited with a finger or a reflex hammer. The sign is seen in hypocalcemia and in hypoparathyroidism.

Peripheral nerve facial palsy of acute onset and unknown cause is called *Bell's palsy*. Evidence of this lower motor neuron disorder is seen when only one eye closes as the client attempts to close both eyes. Observation of a flat nasolabial fold may add to this suspicion. When the client attempts to raise the eyebrows, the eyebrow on the affected side will not raise and the forehead does not wrinkle. Other lower motor neuron weakness may result in partial or complete paralysis of an entire side of the face or a flat facial expression. The client may exhibit epiphora (overflow of tears), be unable to hold fluids orally because of a sagging mouth, or be unable to pronounce such labials as *b*, *m*, or *w*.

Upper motor neuron paralysis (hemiparesis) is rarely complete and is a possibility if the nasolabial folds appear flat when the client closes the eyes. In this case, both eyebrows raise and the forehead wrinkles. In upper motor neuron pathologic conditions, involuntary contractions of the facial muscle such as smiling may show normal strength, whereas voluntary contractions such as retracting the corner of the mouth may prove to be weak or absent. There may also be paralysis of eyelid closure (widening of palpebral fissure) or weakness of lid closure.

Sensory pathophysiology: ageusia

Ageusia is the loss of taste or the lack of ability to discriminate sweet, sour, salty, and bitter tastes. The nature of the loss of taste sensation may aid in making a diagnosis. For example:

1. Unilateral loss of taste may be caused by lesions of the solitary tract and its nucleus.
2. Bilateral ageusia may be caused by pathophysiologic phenomena occurring near the midline of the pons.
3. Hallucinations or perversions of taste may be caused by lesions of the uncus.

CN VIII: Acoustic Nerve

The acoustic nerve has two divisions: the vestibular and the cochlear.

Vestibular division

Neurons of the vestibular division of CN VIII are bipolar. The cell bodies are located in the vestibular ganglion. Peripheral fibers terminate in the neuroepithelium of the semicircular canals, utricle, and saccule, while the central portion terminates in the medulla in the vestibular nucleus. Axons from the cell bodies located in the vestibular nucleus terminate in the spinal cord (vestibulospinal tract) to produce reflex movements of the trunk and limbs, also contributing to the medial longitudinal fasciculus to produce conjugate eye movements in response to head movements. Fibers also terminate in the cerebellum, providing changes in muscle tone.

Tests for vestibular functions are *not routine* in the physical examination. The three types of stimuli used are caloric, rotational, and electrical. These stimuli produce changes in the flow of endolymph in the vestibular structures.

Bárány's test (caloric). The client is placed in a sitting position with the head tilted 60 degrees in extension (backward). The ear is irrigated with 5 to 10 ml of ice water (32° to 50° F) or 100 to 200 ml of cold water (68° F). The response of an individual with normal vestibular apparatus tested in the right ear is nausea, dizziness, and nystagmus. Horizontal nystagmus with the slow component to the right is normal. The slow phase is in the direction of endolymph flow. In addition, the client is tested for past pointing by asking the client to

touch the index finger to the examiner's. Past pointing and falling to the right occur in normal subjects. There will be no response in persons who have no vestibular function. The individual who has hyperirritability of the vestibular system may show vestibular responses to less strong stimuli, such as turning the head from side to side; the symptoms of vertigo and nausea will be stronger, and vomiting may occur.

Nylen-Bárány test. The Nylen-Bárány test is an examination for positional nystagmus. With the client's head hanging 45 degrees backward over the head of the examining table and 45 degrees to one side, the examiner observes for nystagmus. The client's head is then turned in the opposite direction, and the observation is repeated.

Bárány chair rotation test. The client is rotated ten times in 20 seconds and stopped suddenly. The examiner observes for nystagmus and postural deviation and checks for past pointing. Nystagmus, past pointing, and postural deviation are in the direction of the movement of the chair in the normal subject. Vertigo, the hallucination of continued movement, is in the opposite direction.

Electronystagmography. With this process, nystagmus may also be recorded from differences in electrical potential.

Vertigo is the most common symptom of vestibular disease. Any of the responses to the vestibular function tests, such as nausea, dizziness, or nystagmus, may be present in labyrinth disease. Nystagmus may be horizontal, vertical, or rotary. The causes of disease of the semicircular canals may include inflammation, hemorrhage, edema, and pressure alterations. Vertigo may also result from disorders of the cortex or other central nervous system structures.

Labyrinthitis and hemorrhage into the labyrinth have been termed *Meniere's disease,* even though this term is more correctly applied to the presence of excessive endolymph or edema.

Cochlear division

Tests for cochlear function (Fig. 20-11) are described in Chapter 9 on ears, nose, and throat assessment (note testing of auditory function—audiogram, Weber, and Rinne tests).

CN IX: Glossopharyngeal Nerve, CN X: Vagus Nerve

The glossopharyngeal and vagus nerves are closely related both anatomically and physiologically. These nerves are tested clinically as a unit.

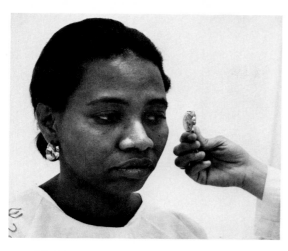

Figure 20-11

Gross test of hearing to assess cochlear function. The ticking watch is moved away from the ear until the client no longer hears it.

The glossopharyngeal nerve contains sensory and motor fibers. The sensory fibers arise from the posterior third of the tongue, middle ear, and eustachian tube and have their cell bodies in the petrosal ganglia and terminate in the solitary tract in the medulla. From the solitary tract, fibers connect with the cells of the superior salivary nucleus. Motor fibers arise from the upper portion of the ambiguous nucleus in the medulla to innervate the stylopharyngeus muscle.

The glossopharyngeal nerve is sensory for taste for the posterior third of the tongue and conveys general sensation from the tonsillar and pharyngeal mucosa. It also has afferent sensory fibers for the carotid sinus and body. Testing for taste sensation is conducted for the posterior tongue when the anterior tongue is examined (see CN VII; facial nerve).

The vagus nerve is sensory for the walls of the gastrointestinal viscera (to the transverse colon) and for the heart, lungs, and aortic bodies. The vagus is a motor nerve to the palate, pharynx, larynx, and the thoracic and abdominal visceral organs.

Testing of vagal function can be difficult. The clinical examination focuses on the musculature of the palate, pharynx, and larynx. The soft palate is inspected for symmetry. The uvula is identified, and any deviation from the midline is recorded (Fig. 20-12). Unilateral weakness is characterized by the dropping of the affected side and the absence of the arch on that side.

The client is asked to say, "Ah." The palate should rise symmetrically. The palatal reflex is elicited by stroking the mucous membrane of the soft palate with an applicator. The side touched retracts upward.

The gag reflex is obtained by touching the posterior wall of the pharynx with an applicator or a tongue

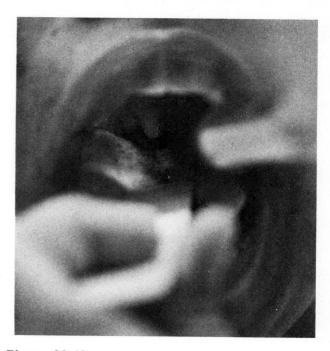

Figure 20-12

Test of glossopharyngeal and vagal nerve function. Uvula is observed in midline.

blade. The response includes elevation of the palate and contraction of the pharyngeal muscles.

Swallowing is evaluated by giving the client a small quantity of water to drink and observing while it is swallowed. Retrograde passage of water through the nose while drinking indicates a weakness of the soft palate wherein the nasopharynx is not closed off during the swallow.

In the presence of a lesion of the vagus nerve, the uvula and soft palate deviate to the unaffected side, since the muscles on the intact side are unopposed.

The client who is hoarse or who complains of a problem with vocalization is examined by indirect laryngoscopy. A laryngeal mirror and headlight allow visualization of the vocal cords.

CN XI: Spinal Accessory Nerve

Cell bodies of the spinal accessory nerve are located in the gray matter of the first five cervical cord segments and give off axons to the sternocleidomastoid and trapezius muscles, providing these muscles with motor innervation.

To test the spinal accessory nerve, the symmetry, size, and strength of these muscles are evaluated.

For assessment of the sternocleidomastoid muscle, the client is asked to turn the head to one side and push the chin in the same direction against the resistance of

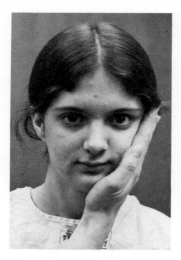

Figure 20-13

Assessment of the symmetry, size, and strength of the sternoclei-domastoid muscle in test of CN XI. The client is asked to turn the head to one side to push the chin against the resistance of the examiner's hand. The contralateral sternocleidomastoid muscle will stand out as it contracts. The muscle is palpated to assess tension.

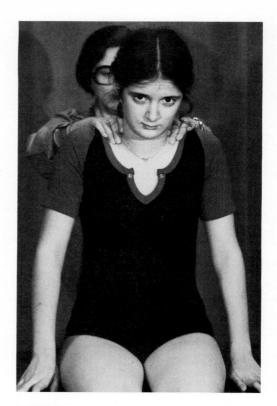

Figure 20-14

Assessment of the symmetry, size, and strength of the trapezius muscles in test of CN XI. The client shrugs the shoulders against the resistance of the examiner's hands.

the examiner's hand. The contralateral sternocleidomas-toid muscle will stand out and may be inspected and palpated (Fig. 20-13).

For assessment of the trapezius muscles, the client is asked to shrug the shoulders while the examiner exerts downward pressure against the muscles. As the muscles contract, they may be evaluated for strength and symmetry (Fig. 20-14).

The trapezius muscles may be further tested by asking the client to raise the arms to a vertical position. Weakness of the trapezius muscles makes this position difficult to achieve.

Neck trauma is the most frequent cause of dysfunction of the spinal accessory nerve. Radical neck dissection is often followed by symptoms of CN XI damage.

Torticollis is a condition of intermittent or constant contraction of the sternocleidomastoid muscle wherein the head is flexed forward and the chin is rotated away from the affected side.

CN XII: Hypoglossal Nerve

The nucleus of the hypoglossal nerve is in the medulla and provides motor fibers to both the extrinsic and the intrinsic muscles of the tongue, making possible articulation of lingual speech sounds and swallowing.

The tongue is inspected for size (atrophy), symmetry, and fasciculations. Deviation to the affected side is characteristic of unilateral peripheral nerve damage

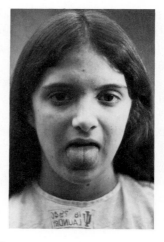

Figure 20-15

Assessment for symmetry, size, strength, and fasciculations of the muscles of the protruded tongue in test of CN XII.

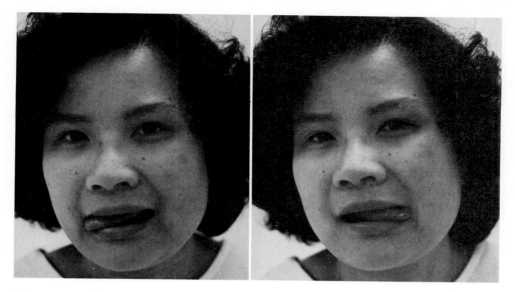

Figure 20-16

The client moves the tongue from side to side, progressively increasing the speed of motion.

because of the dominance of the genioglossus muscle on the unaffected side. The posterior fibers of this muscle push the tongue toward the opposite side.

The client is asked to stick out the tongue as far as possible. The examiner notes the client's ability to stick the tongue straight out, the strength of the movement, and how far out the client sticks the tongue (Fig. 20-15). The client also moves the tongue rapidly in and out and from side to side (Fig. 20-16). Upper motor neuron disease may result in slowness of alternate movements. In another test, the client curls the tongue upward as if to touch the nose and downward as if to lick the chin surface. The client may also be tested for muscle strength by asking him or her to push out the cheek with the tongue while the examiner pushes against it from the outside (Fig. 20-17).

The examiner tests lingual speech sound by giving the client a phrase for repetition that includes a number of words containing *l, t, d,* or *n.*

Table 20-1 is a summary of the cranial nerves, including their functions, assessment, makeup, and components.

PROPRIOCEPTION AND CEREBELLAR FUNCTION

The proprioceptive system of the nervous system maintains posture, balance, and other acts of coordination. The neural structures that are involved in proprioception are the posterior columns (gracilis and cuneatus) of the spinal cord, the cerebellum, and the vestibular apparatus. The posterior columns carry stimuli from the proprio-

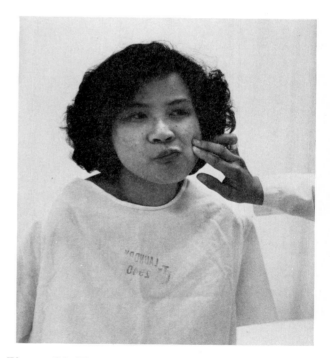

Figure 20-17

The strength of the tongue may be assessed by asking the client to push against the inner surface of the cheek with as much strength as possible. The examiner palpates the external surface of the cheek simultaneously.

Table 20-1
The cranial nerves

Nerve	Function	Clinical test	Cells of origin	Major components	Afferent	Efferent
I Olfactory	Smell	Odor applied to one nostril	Olfactory epithelium	Olfactory filaments	Visceral special Smell	
II Optic	Vision	Visual acuity: Snellen's chart; Visual fields: confrontation, tangent screen, perimeter	Retinal ganglion cells	Optic nerves Optic chiasm Optic tracts	Somatic special Vision	
III Oculomotor	Upward, downward, medial eye movement	Eye movement	Nucleus 3	Oculomotor nerve		Somatic Extraocular muscles Levator palpebrae Superior rectus Inferior rectus Inferior oblique
	Lid elevation	Lid movement				
	Pupil constriction	Pupillary response to light and accommodation	Edinger-Westphal nucleus	Oculomotor nerve Ciliary ganglion Ciliary nerves		Visceral general Intrinsic eye muscles, iris, ciliary muscle
IV Trochlear	Downward, medial eye movement	Eye movement	Nucleus 4	Trochlear nerve		Somatic Superior oblique muscle
V Trigeminal	Sensory Face Scalp Nasal mucosa Buccal mucosa	Corneal reflex Sensation Face Anterior scalp Nasal mucosa Buccal mucosa	Gasserian ganglion	Ophthalmic nerve Maxillary nerve Mandibular nerve	Somatic general Sensory Anterior half of scalp Face Buccal mucosa Dura, anterior, and middle fossa	
	Jaw muscles		Mesencephalic Nucleus 5	Motor root	Proprioception Muscles of mastication	
	Motor Masseter muscle Temporal muscle Digastric muscle	Muscle strength of masseter and temporal muscles; muscles palpated with jaw clenched	Motor nucleus 5	Motor root		Visceral special Muscles for mastication
VI Abducens	Lateral eye movement	Eye movement	Nucleus 6	Abducens nerve		Somatic lateral rectus

Nerve	Function	Assessment	Nucleus/Ganglion	Branch/Nerve	Type	Type
VII Facial						
Sensory						
External ear	Sensation	Geniculate ganglion	Intermediate nerve / Ramus of vagus nerve	Somatic general	
Taste: anterior two thirds of tongue	Taste: sweet, salty, sour	Geniculate ganglion	Intermediate nerve / Chorda tympani nerve	Visceral special	Visceral special
Deep facial	Sensation, deep facial		Lingual nerve / Intermediate nerve	Visceral general	
Motor						
Facial movement / Scalp muscle / Auricular muscle / Stylohyoid muscle / Digastric posterior belly	Corneal reflex / Facial movement: client frowns, wrinkles forehead, shows teeth	Motor nucleus 7	Temporofacial branch / Cervicofacial branch		
Salivation: submaxillary glands, sublingual glands		Superior salivary nucleus	Intermediate nerve / Chorda tympani nerve / Lingual nerve / Submaxillary ganglion	Visceral general	Visceral general
Lacrimation: lacrimal glands / Mucous membrane / Nasopharynx		Superior salivary nucleus	Intermediate nerve / Petrosal nerve / Sphenopalatine ganglion		Visceral general
VIII Acoustic						
Vestibular		Vestibular ganglion	Vestibular nerve	Somatic special	
Hearing	Audiometry	Spiral ganglion of cochlea	Cochlear nerve	Somatic special	
IX Glossopharyngeal						
Sensory						
External ear (part)		Superior ganglion	Ramus of vagus nerve	Somatic general	
Taste: posterior third of tongue	Taste: sweet, salty, sour	Petrosal ganglion		Visceral special	
Carotid: reflexes, baroreceptors and chemoreceptors, sinus, body			Carotid sinus nerve	Visceral special	
Motor						
Pharynx: gag reflex, swallowing, pharyngeal muscles	Gag test: give drink; watch swallow	Petrosal ganglion / Ambiguous nucleus	Pharyngeal branch / Lingual branch / Pharyngeal plexus	Visceral special	Visceral special
Parotid gland: salivation		Inferior salivatory nucleus	Tympanic nerve / Petrosal nerve	Visceral general	Visceral general

Continued

Table 20-1

The cranial nerves—*cont'd*

Nerve	Function	Clinical test	Cells of origin	Major components	Afferent	Efferent
X Vagus	Sensory					
	External ear (part)		Jugular ganglion		Somatic general	
	Pharynx		Nodose ganglion		Visceral general	
	Thoracic and abdominal viscera					
	Aortic arch			Carotid sinus nerve	Visceral special	
	Chemoreceptors					
	Baroreceptors					
	Motor					
	Swallowing, gag reflex		Ambiguous nucleus	Pharyngeal plexus		Visceral special
	Pronation	Observe speech		Laryngeal nerves		Visceral special
	Cardiac slowing		Dorsal motor nucleus 10			Visceral special
	Bronchoconstriction					Visceral general
	Gastric secretion					Visceral general
	Peristalsis					Visceral general
						Visceral special
XI Accessory	Motor					
	Swallowing: pharyngeal muscles	Give drink; watch swallow	Ambiguous nucleus	Cranial root		Visceral special
	Turning of head: sternocleidomastoid muscles	Client turns head against resistance	Ventral horn C2 Ventral root branch	Spinal root		
	Elevation of shoulders: trapezius muscles	Client shrugs shoulders against resistance	Ventral horn C3, 4 Ventral root branch			Visceral special
XII Hypoglossal	Motor					
	Muscles that move tongue: hypoglossus, genioglossus, styloglossus	Client sticks out tongue, moves tongue from side to side Observe speech	Nucleus 12	Hypoglossal nerve		Somatic

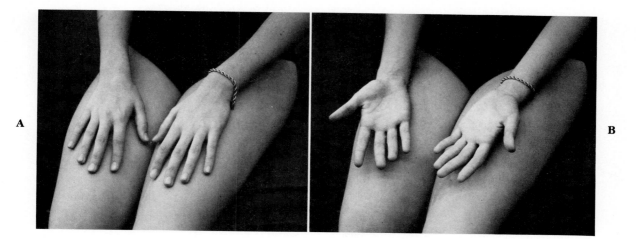

Figure 20-18

Test for dysdiadochokinesia (cerebellar function)—pronation (**A**) and supination (**B**) of the hands, with progressively more rapid movement.

ceptors in muscle tendons and joints. The posterior columns also carry fibers for touch sensation and two-point discrimination. Deficit of function of the posterior column impairs muscle and position sense. Clients with such an impairment are often observed to be watching their own arm and leg movements to know the position of the limbs from these visual clues.

The cerebellum functions primarily in the integration of muscle contractions for the maintenance of posture. Loss of cerebellar function results in *dyssynergia* (impairment of muscle coordination or of the ability to perform movements smoothly), intention tremor, or hypotonia.

Abnormalities of muscle tone, gait, speech, and nystagmus in lateral gaze may also indicate cerebellar dysfunction. Disburbances in the timing of movements may also be evident.

The vestibular system is concerned with righting movements. Vestibular disease is characterized by vertigo, nausea, and vomiting. A subjective phenomenon, vertigo is the illusion of movement of the individual or the environment. Nausea and vomiting frequently accompany vertigo. Nystagmus is also frequently associated with vertigo and may be vertical, horizontal, or rotary.

Ataxia is the impairment of position sense. Ataxia is more severe if visual images are excluded in posterior column disease but not in cerebellar dysfunction.

The client with a *cerebellar gait* walks with a wide base; the trunk and head are held rigidly; the legs bend at the hips; arm movements are not coordinated with the stride; the client lurches and reels, frequently falling.

The client with *cerebellar speech* has slow, hesitant, or dysarthric verbalization.

Jerking movements are noted in the client with a *cerebellar sitting posture* as the client attempts to maintain balance.

The client with proprioceptive or cerebellar dysfunction may experience difficulty with the following tests of posture or coordination.

The client is asked to pat the knees with the palms of the hands followed by the backs of the hands at an ever-increasing rate. The client with cerebellar disease has difficulty with rapid patting and supination-pronation alterations. The problem involves both smooth control of muscles and the starting and stopping of motion (Fig. 20-18). Clumsiness of movement and irregular timing are characteristic of affected individuals.

A test for *dysdiadochokinesia,* the ability to stop a movement and replace it by a movement in the opposite direction, is the pronation and supination test. The arms may be outstretched or flexed at the elbow. The movements are performed as rapidly as possible (see Fig. 20-18). Any movement may be tested that involves the alternated action of agonists and antagonists.

Accuracy of movement direction may be tested by asking the client to touch the nose with the index finger of first one hand and then the other with the eyes closed (Fig. 20-19). The client is then asked to repeat this activity several times while gradually increasing the speed of performance.

The client may be asked to touch the nose and then the examiner's finger at a distance of about 18 in (Figs. 20-20 and 20-21). This maneuver is also repeated with increasing speed. The finger-to-finger test involves asking the client to spread the arms broadly and then to bring them together in the midline. It is done slowly and then rapidly, with the eyes open and then closed. The

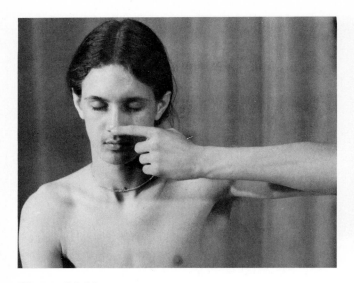

Figure 20-19

Test of cerebellar function. The client is asked to alternately touch the nose with the tip of the index finger of each hand, repeating the motion with increasing speed.

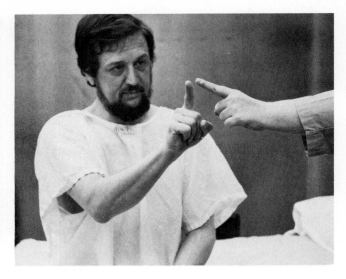

Figure 20-20

Test of cerebellar function. The client is asked to touch the examiner's finger, which is placed about 18 in from the client's eye.

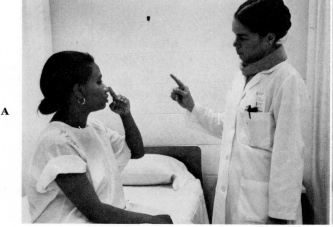

A

B

Figure 20-21

Test of cerebellar function. **A,** The client is asked to touch her nose with an index finger and then,
B, to touch the examiner's index finger at a distance of about 18 in, repeating the motion with increasing speed.

client is asked to pat and then use a polishing motion on the examiner's hand, progressively increasing the speed (Figs. 20-22 and 20-23).

In a test for rapid, skilled movement, the client touches each finger of one hand to the thumb of the same hand as rapidly as possible (Fig. 20-24).

The client is also asked to run the heel of each foot down the opposite shin (Fig. 20-25).

The client may be asked to draw a figure eight in the air while lying on the back.

While lying on the back, the client is asked to touch the ball of each foot to the examiner's hand. The

client is also asked to touch the examiner's finger with the large toe (Fig. 20-26).

In the Romberg test, the client is asked to stand with the feet together, first with eyes closed and then with them open, and is evaluated for swaying movement (Fig. 20-27). Slight swaying is normal. The examiner stands close enough to the client to prevent falling. The client who demonstrates Romberg's sign is asked to hop in place on one foot and then the other (Fig. 20-28).

Gait is assessed as the client walks with the eyes closed and then with them open.

The client is asked to stand on one foot and then

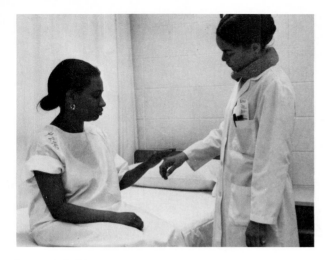

Figure 20-22

Test of cerebellar function. The client is asked to pat the examiner's hand, progressively increasing the speed of motion.

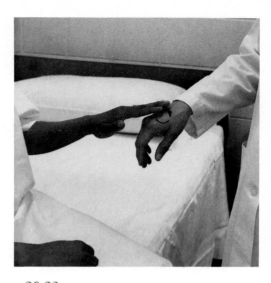

Figure 20-23

Test of cerebellar function. The client is asked to make a polishing (circular) motion on the volar surface of the examiner's hand, progressively increasing the speed of motion.

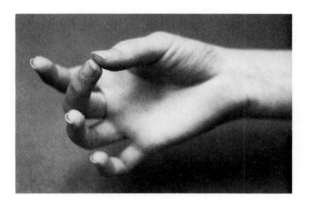

Figure 20-24

Test of cerebellar function. The client is asked to touch each finger of one hand to the thumb of the same hand as rapidly as possible.

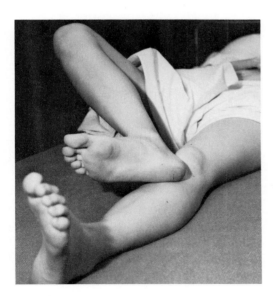

Figure 20-25

Test of cerebellar function. The client is asked to run the heel of each foot down the opposite shin.

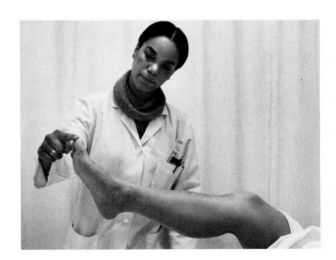

Figure 20-26

Test of cerebellar function. The client is asked to touch the examiner's finger with the large toe.

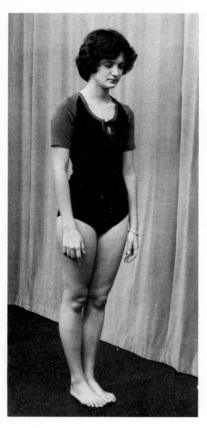

Figure 20-27

Test of the proprioceptive system. Romberg test—individual should be able to stand with eyes closed and feet together without swaying for approximately 5 seconds.

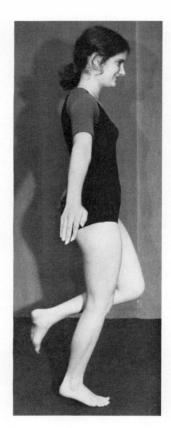

Figure 20-28

Test of the proprioceptive system. The client who has demonstrated Romberg's sign is asked to hop in place on one foot and then the other.

the other. The normal client is able to do this for about 5 seconds with the eyes closed (Fig. 20-29).

The client who is reasonably steady may be asked to do a knee bend from a standing position without support (Fig. 20-30).

The client is asked to walk a straight line, placing the heel of the leading foot against the toe of the other foot (Fig. 20-31).

The client is asked to pull against the resistance of the examiner's hands, and the client's hands are released without warning. The client with cerebellar disease may have difficulty in starting and stopping movement. Thus, there may be excessive after-movement or rebound, so that the client hits themselves.

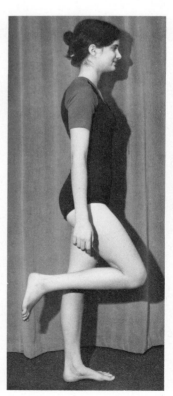

Figure 20-29

Test of the proprioceptive system. The client is asked to stand on one foot and then the other. The normal individual is able to do this for about 5 seconds with the eyes closed.

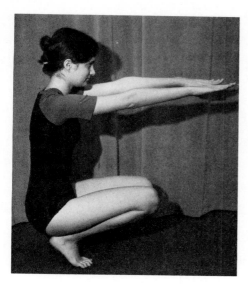

Figure 20-30

Test of the proprioceptive system. The client is asked to do a knee bend without support.

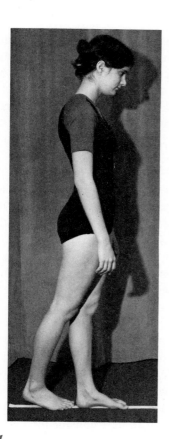

Figure 20-31

Test of the proprioceptive system. The client is asked to walk a straight line placing heel to toe.

Comparison of Disorders of the Cerebellum, Posterior Columns, and Vestibular Neurons

Cerebellar dysfunction

Ataxia not made worse in darkness or with eyes closed
Clumsiness
Poor coordination
Decomposition of movement
Dysmetria
Dysdiadochokinesia
Scanning speech
Hypotonia
Asthenia
Tremor
Nystagmus

Posterior column dysfunction

Ataxia made worse in darkness or with eyes closed
Positive Romberg's sign
Inability to recognize limb position
Astereognosis
Loss of two-point discrimination
Loss of vibratory sensation

Vestibular dysfunction

Nystagmus
Nausea
Vomiting
Ataxia

The terms *decomposition of movement, dysdiadochokinesia,* and *dysmetria* may be useful in recording observations of cerebellar or proprioceptive dysfunction (see the boxed material above).

SENSORY FUNCTION

The equipment needed for sensory testing includes a cotton wisp or soft brush, a safety pin, test tubes for cold and warm water, a tuning fork, and calipers or a compass with dull points.

Although it is not necessary to evaluate sensation over the entire skin surface, stimuli should be applied strategically so that the dermatomes and major peripheral nerves are tested. A minimum number of test sites would include areas on the forehead, cheek, hand, lower arm, abdomen, foot, and lower leg.

As a general rule, the more distal area of the limb is checked first. In the screening examination the nerve may be assumed to be intact if sensation is normal at its most peripheral extent. If evidence of dysfunction is found, the site of the dysfunction must be localized and mapped. This means determining the boundaries of the

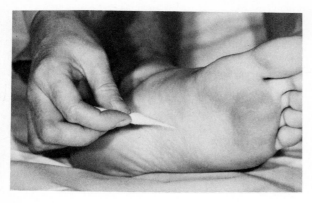

Figure 20-32

Test of sensation of light touch using a wisp of cotton applied firmly enough to stimulate the sensory nerve endings but not so much that the skin is indented.

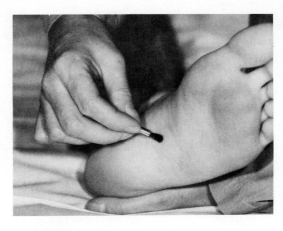

Figure 20-33

Test of light touch sensation using a soft brush.

loss of sensation. A lucid method of recording would include a sketch of the region involved and a description of the sensory change.

The intensity of the stimulus is kept to a minimum level on initial application. Gradual increases in magnitude may be made until the client is aware of the stimulus.

Variation in sensitivity of skin areas is seen in the normal client, so that a stronger stimulus is required over the back, the buttocks, and areas where the skin is heavily cornified. Symmetry of sensation is established by checking first one spot and then its mirror image area.

The client's eyes should be closed during evaluation of sensory modalities. The visual cuing that occurs when the client is able to see the examiner apply the stimulus may lead to false-positive responses in the client who is highly sensitive to suggestion.

HELPFUL HINT: Ensure that both the examiner and the client are rested, since if either is fatigued results may be erroneous. Inattention or low motivation may be interpreted as a sensory loss.

Vary testing sites and timing in stimulus application to avoid predictability.

Anesthesia, hyperesthesia, hypoesthesia, and *paresthesia* may be useful in describing and recording sensory dysfunction.

Light Touch Sensation

Light touch and deep touch are mediated by different nerve endings. Sensory fibers for simple touch enter the spinal cord and travel upward before crossing to enter the anterior spinothalamic tract to the thalamus. Light touch is the sensory system that is least often obtunded.

Both anterior spinothalamic tracts must suffer destruction before transmission of light touch is lost.

Light touch is tested by touching the skin with a wisp of cotton (Fig. 20-32) or a soft brush (Fig. 20-33). Pressure is applied in such a way that sensation is stimulated but not enough to perceptibly depress the skin. The client is instructed to say, "Yes," or "Now," when feeling the skin being touched. The hair of the skin should be avoided when testing for touch sensation in the skin. The follicles are innervated with sensory fibers that are stimulated by movement of the hair. Instances of distortion of sensation or *anesthesia* are recorded.

The client is asked to point to the spot where they were touched (tactile localization [point localization]).

Pain Sensation

Pain and temperature fibers both travel in the dorsolateral fasciculus for a short distance, after which they cross and continue to the thalamus in the lateral spinothalamic tract.

Superficial pain.   The evaluation of the sensory perception of superficial pain and pressure may be conducted through the use of the sharp and full points of a safety pin (Figs. 20-34 and 20-35); however, recent studies have indicated a risk of infection with safety pins and some examiners use the hub (dull) and point (sharp) of a hypodermic needle. The client is asked to say, "Sharp," "Dull," or "Can't tell," when he or she feels the pin touch the skin. At least 2 seconds should be allowed between successive tests to avoid summation effects (several successive stimuli perceived as one). Pain sensation may be lost in the presence of lesions of the tegmentum of the brainstem.

Deep pressure.   Deep pressure is tested over the eyeball, Achilles tendon, forearm, and calf muscles.

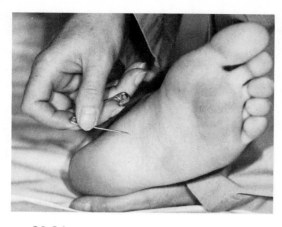

Figure 20-34

Evaluation for superficial pain using the sharp point of a safety pin.

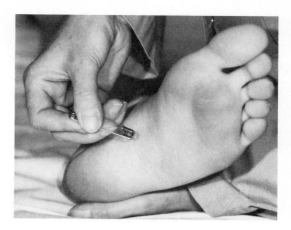

Figure 20-35

Alternate use of the dull end of the pin for evaluation of pain.

Temperature Sensation

In the screening examination, temperature assessment need not be done when pain sensation is found to be within normal limits. When it is performed, the stimuli are tubes filled with warm and cold water that are rolled against the skin sites to be tested. The examiner tests the stimuli on his or her own skin to avoid burning the client and to provide a comparison. The client is asked to say, "Hot," "Cold," or "Can't tell." The tubes are applied to a sufficient number of areas to ascertain that all dematomes are included.

Vibration Sensation

The normal client is able to distinguish vibration when the base of a vibrating tuning fork is applied to a bony prominence such as the sternum, elbow, or ankle. The client perceives the vibration as a buzzing or tingling sensation.

The greatest sensitivity to vibration is seen when the tuning fork is vibrating between 200 and 400 cycles per second (cps). A large tuning fork is suggested, since the decay of vibration occurs more slowly in the larger instrument.

After the client closes the eyes, the vibrating tuning fork may be applied to the clavicles, spinous processes, elbows, finger joints, knees, ankles, and toes (Fig. 20-36). The client is asked to say, "Yes," or "Now," (1) when first feeling the vibrations and (2) when the vibrations stop. The examiner must emphasize to the client the importance of signifying the cessation of the feeling of vibration. The examiner may damp the vibrations of the tuning fork to move along more rapidly.

Vibratory sensation is diminished in the older client (after 65 years of age), particularly in the extremities.

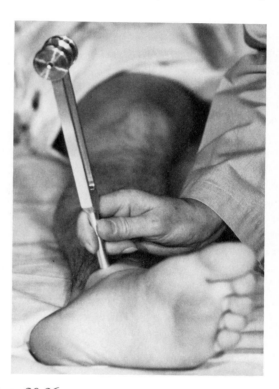

Figure 20-36

Test of sensitivity to vibration. The base of the vibrating tuning fork is applied to bony prominences such as the sternum, elbow, or ankle.

Tactile Discrimination

Tactile discrimination requires cortical integration. Three types of tactile discrimination that are tested clinically include (1) *stereognosis,* (2) *two-point discrimination,* and (3) *extinction.* Afferent fibers for vibration, proprioception, and stereognosis are found to take one of three courses after entering the spinal cord: they (1) synapse immediately with motor cells to form a reflex arc, (2)

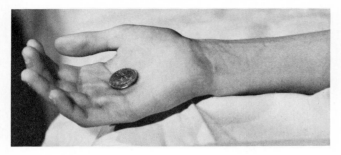

Figure 20-37

Test for stereognosis. The normal client can discriminate a familiar object (coin, key) by touching and manipulating it.

run superiorly in the dorsal column to the cerebellum, or (3) travel in dorsal columns to the medulla and cross-run to the thalamus.

Stereognosis. Stereognosis is the act of recognizing objects on the basis of touching and manipulating them. This is a function of the parietal lobes of the cerebral cortex. Objects used to test stereognosis should be universally familiar items, such as a key or coin (Fig. 20-37).

Two-point discrimination. Two-point discrimination is defined as the ability to sense whether one or two areas of the skin are being stimulated by pressure. This may be done with pins. One pin is held in each hand, and both are applied to the skin simultaneously. The client is asked if he or she feels one or two pinpricks. This determination may also be accomplished using calipers or a compass with dull points (Fig. 20-38).

In the adult client there is considerable variability of perceptual ability over the different parts of the body. The following are minimum distances between the two points of the calipers at which the normal adult can sense simultaneous stimulation:

Tongue: 1 mm
Fingertips: 2.8 mm
Toes: 3 to 8 mm
Palms of hands: 8 to 12 mm
Chest, forearms: 40 mm
Back: 40 to 70 mm
Upper arms, thighs: 75 mm

Extinction. The normal client, when touched in corresponding areas on both sides of the body, perceives touch in both areas. The failure to perceive touch on one side is called the extinction phenomenon. Impairment of the extinction phenomenon is frequently noted in lesions of the sensory cortex.

Kinesthetic Sensation (Position Awareness)

Kinesthetic sensation is that facilitated by proprioceptive receptors in the muscles, tendons, and joints. Perception

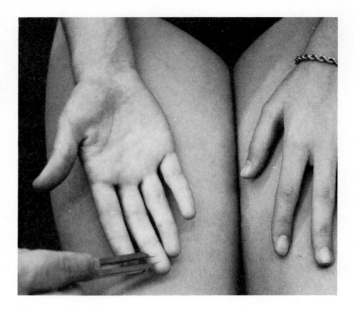

Figure 20-38

Test for two-point discrimination.

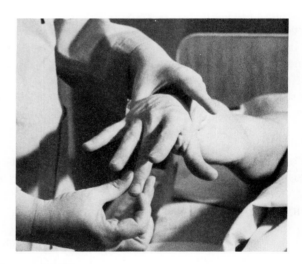

Figure 20-39

Test of kinesthetic sensation. The normal client can discriminate the position of body parts. With the client's eyes closed, the examiner changes the position of a finger. The client describes how the position was changed.

of the position, orientation, and motion of limbs and body parts is obtained from kinesthetic sensations.

With the client's eyes closed and the joint in a neutral position, the examiner changes the position of one finger of the client's hand. The joint must be held at the lateral aspect. The client is asked to describe how the position of the finger was changed. The finger is always moved to a neutral position before it is moved again (Fig. 20-39). This procedure may be done for any joint.

Table 20-2

Patterns of sensory loss

Pathologic involvement	Common cause	Characteristics
Peripheral nerve	Metabolic disorders, such as diabetes or nutritional deficiencies	Peripheral structures more frequently involved—"glove and stocking" involvement—may involve all sensory modalities
Specific peripheral nerve or root	Trauma Vascular occlusion	May map area of sensory loss specific to area innervated by the nerve and distal to the pathologic lesion
Dorsal root		Loss of sensation in the segmented distribution (dermatome)
Spinal cord—hemisection (Brown-Séquard's syndrome)	Trauma Medullary lesion Extramedullary lesion	Loss of pain and temperature perception on contralateral side, one or two segments below the lesion Loss of position sense, two-point discrimination, and vibratory sensation on ipsilateral side below the lesion
Brainstem	Trauma Neoplasm Vascular occlusion	Loss of pain and temperature sensation on contralateral side of body, ipsilateral side of face
Thalamus	Trauma Neoplasm Vascular occlusion	Loss of sensory modalities on contralateral side of body
Cortex—lesions of post-cortical cortex	Trauma Neoplasm Vascular occlusion	Loss of discriminatory sensation on contralateral side of body Loss of position sense, two-point discrimination, or stereognosis

Graphesthesia

The normal client can discern the identity of letters or numbers inscribed on the palm of the hand, back, or other areas with a blunt object.

Patterns of Sensory Loss

Loss of discriminatory sensation may indicate a lesion of the posterior columns or sensory cortex. Bilateral sensory loss in both lower extremities suggests a peripheral neuropathy, such as diabetic neuropathy. Often the pattern of sensory loss is useful in establishing a diagnosis. Some common patterns of sensory deficit are described in Table 20-2.

Sensory loss resulting from disease in a single peripheral nerve may be mapped over the skin surface distribution of that nerve. The nerves most commonly involved in disease include the medial, radial, ulnar, sciatic, femoral, and peroneal nerves. The examiner should be knowledgeable of the sensory, motor, and reflex distribution of these and other major nerves (Fig. 20-40). Body surface projections of the major nerves are seen in Fig. 20-41.

Figure 20-40

Areas of sensory loss from peripheral nerve lesions.
(From Prior A and Silberstein JS: Physical diagnosis: the history and examination of the patient, ed 4, St Louis, 1973, The CV Mosby Co.)

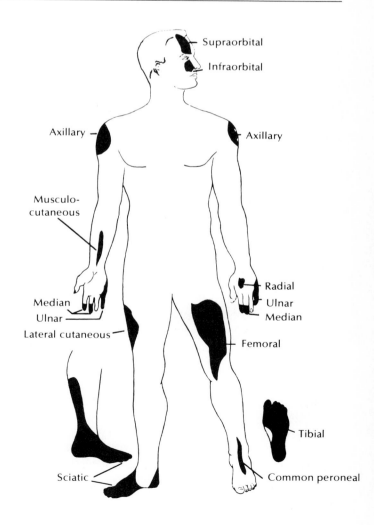

Supraorbital
Infraorbital
Axillary — — Axillary
Musculo-cutaneous
Median — Radial
Ulnar — Ulnar
Median
Lateral cutaneous — Femoral
Sciatic — Tibial
Common peroneal

Figure 20-41

Cutaneous fields of peripheral nerves from the anterior
(A) and posterior (B) aspects.
(From Haymaker W and Woodhall B: Peripheral nerve
injuries, ed 2, Philadelphia, 1959, WB Saunders Co.)

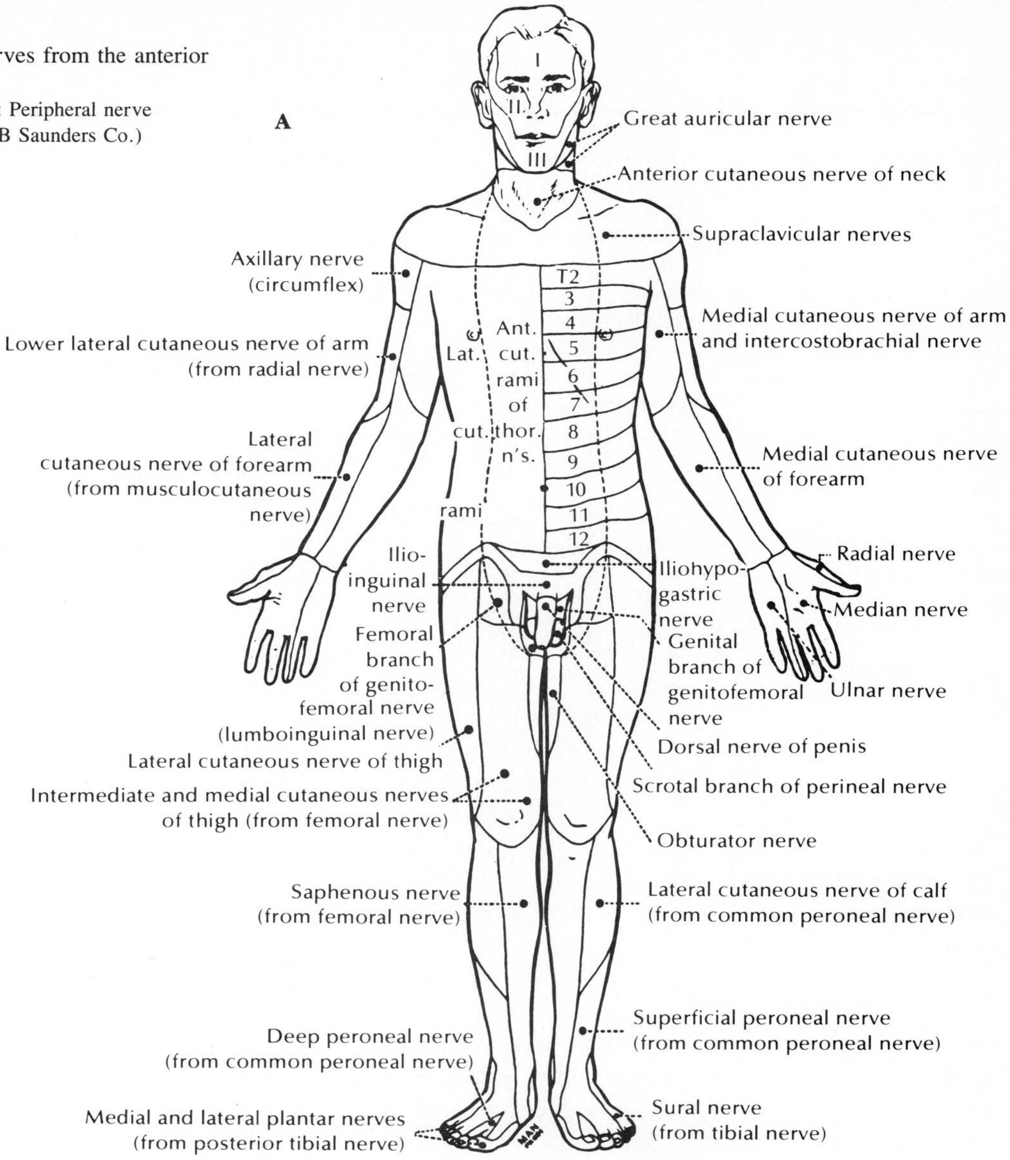

A

Great auricular nerve

Anterior cutaneous nerve of neck

Supraclavicular nerves

Axillary nerve
(circumflex)

Medial cutaneous nerve of arm
and intercostobrachial nerve

Lower lateral cutaneous nerve of arm
(from radial nerve)

Lateral
cutaneous nerve of forearm
(from musculocutaneous
nerve)

Medial cutaneous nerve
of forearm

Radial nerve

Median nerve

Ilio-
inguinal
nerve

Iliohypo-
gastric
nerve

Femoral
branch
of genito-
femoral nerve
(lumboinguinal nerve)

Genital
branch of
genitofemoral
nerve

Ulnar nerve

Lateral cutaneous nerve of thigh

Dorsal nerve of penis

Intermediate and medial cutaneous nerves
of thigh (from femoral nerve)

Scrotal branch of perineal nerve

Obturator nerve

Saphenous nerve
(from femoral nerve)

Lateral cutaneous nerve of calf
(from common peroneal nerve)

Superficial peroneal nerve
(from common peroneal nerve)

Deep peroneal nerve
(from common peroneal nerve)

Medial and lateral plantar nerves
(from posterior tibial nerve)

Sural nerve
(from tibial nerve)

Pathophysiologic conditions involving the dorsal root may result in sensory loss distributed over the dermatome for that root (Fig. 20-42). Clear description of sensory loss for a given segment may be difficult to obtain, since a good deal of sensory overlap occurs between the distribution of one root and another.

Both nerve and root sensory loss may result from disease involving a plexus. This phenomenon is frequently observed for the brachial plexus. Superior brachial plexus lesions involve C5 and C6, resulting in sensory loss in the shoulder and in the lateral arm and forearm. In addition, there may be weakness of the shoulder muscles. Inferior brachial plexus lesions involve C8 and T1, resulting in sensory loss of the medial surface of the arm and in weakness of the arm muscles.

Pathophysiologic conditions of the thalamocortical fibers on the cortex result in a loss of those cortical integrating functions (kinesthesia, two-point discrimination, stereognosis). Cortical mapping of the brain is seen in Fig. 20-43; the cortical integrating center for peripheral sensory phenomena is in the postcentral gyrus. Gross perceptions of vibration, pain, temperature, and crude touch may be retained.

The client's degree of awareness is often recorded in relation to the manner in which they react to external stimuli according to the following: alert, cooperative, orientation intact, responds to spoken words and commands, responds to tactile stimuli, responds to painful stimuli, does not respond to stimuli.

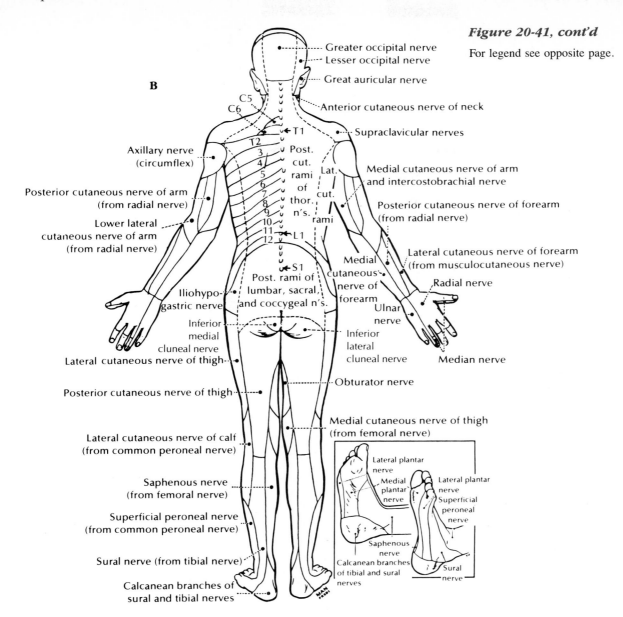

B

Greater occipital nerve
Lesser occipital nerve
Great auricular nerve
C5
C6
Anterior cutaneous nerve of neck
T1
T2
Supraclavicular nerves
Axillary nerve
(circumflex)
3
4
Post.
cut.
rami
of
thor.
n's.
Lat.
cut.
rami
Medial cutaneous nerve of arm
and intercostobrachial nerve
Posterior cutaneous nerve of arm
(from radial nerve)
5
6
7
8
9
Posterior cutaneous nerve of forearm
(from radial nerve)
Lower lateral
cutaneous nerve of arm
(from radial nerve)
10
11
12
L1
S1
Lateral cutaneous nerve of forearm
(from musculocutaneous nerve)
Medial
cutaneous
nerve of
forearm
Radial nerve
Post. rami of
lumbar, sacral,
and coccygeal n's.
Ulnar
nerve
Iliohypo-
gastric nerve
Inferior
medial
cluneal nerve
Inferior
lateral
cluneal nerve
Median nerve
Lateral cutaneous nerve of thigh
Posterior cutaneous nerve of thigh
Obturator nerve
Medial cutaneous nerve of thigh
(from femoral nerve)
Lateral cutaneous nerve of calf
(from common peroneal nerve)
Lateral plantar
nerve
Medial
plantar
nerve
Lateral plantar
nerve
Superficial
peroneal
nerve
Saphenous nerve
(from femoral nerve)
Superficial peroneal nerve
(from common peroneal nerve)
Sural nerve (from tibial nerve)
Saphenous
nerve
Calcanean branches
of tibial and sural
nerves
Sural
nerve
Calcanean branches of
sural and tibial nerves

Figure 20-41, cont'd

For legend see opposite page.

REFLEXES

Deep Tendon Reflex

The skeletal muscles contract when they are stretched by contraction of the antagonistic muscle, by the pull of gravity, or by external manipulation. The muscles will also contract when their tendons are stretched. These principles form the basis for an understanding of the deep tendon reflex (DTR). Afferent fibers for the reflex arise from both the muscle itself and the tendon.

Muscle spindles or fusiform capsules have been identified in abundance in skeletal muscles, particularly in antigravity muscles. The spindles are capsules surrounding two to ten specialized muscle cells known as intrafusal fibers; these spindles are parallel with surrounding muscles and are attached to them by connective tis-

sue. Both ends of the intrafusal fiber consist of striated contractile tissue, whereas the central portion, the nuclear bag, is expanded and nucleated. These bags are innervated, but primary afferent fibers are stimulated to carry impulses when the bag is stretched or otherwise deformed. On reaching the spinal cord, these action potentials activate the alpha motor neurons. The alpha motor neurons terminate at the end-plates of the skeletal muscle and stimulate their contraction (Fig. 20-44).

Afferent nerve fibers (gamma afferent fibers) encased in a fibrous capsule are called Golgi tendon organs or tendon end organs and are found in the tendons of skeletal muscles. Stretching of the muscle deforms and activates these afferent nerves, which end on and inhibit the alpha motor neurons. The threshold for activation of

ANTERIOR VIEW

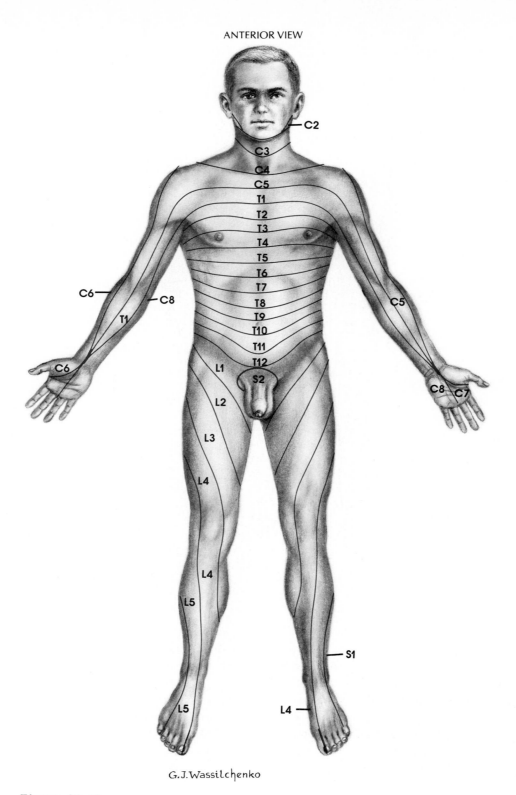

G.J.Wassilchenko

Figure 20-42

Dermatomes of the body. Each dorsal (sensory) spinal root innervates one dermatome. The first cervical nerve usually has no cutaneous distribution. The trigeminal nerve (CN V) supplies most of the general somatic sensory innervation to the anterior part of the head.
(From Rudy EB: Advanced neurological and neurosurgical nursing, St Louis, 1984, The CV Mosby Co.)

POSTERIOR VIEW

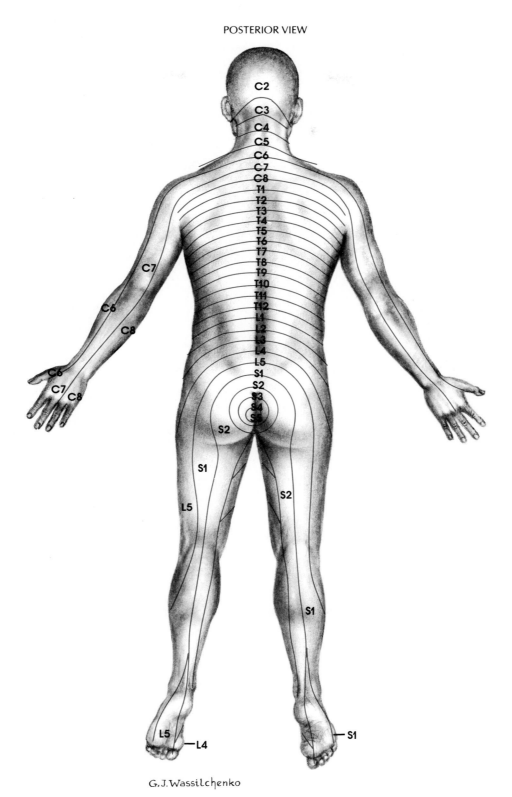

G.J.Wassilchenko

Figure 20-42, cont'd

For legend see opposite page.

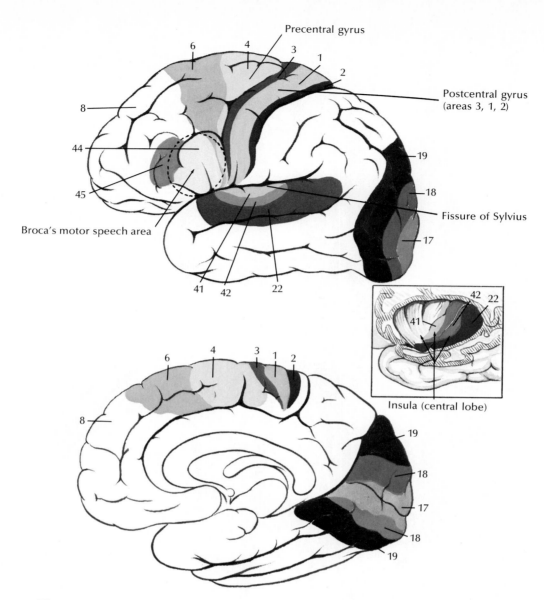

Figure 20-43

Maps of the human cortex. Identity of each numbered area is determined by structural differences in the neurons that compose it. Some areas whose functions are best understood are the following: areas *3, 1,* and *2,* somatic sensory areas; area *4,* primary motor area; area *6,* secondary motor area; area *17,* primary visual area; areas *18* and *19,* secondary visual areas; areas *41* and *42,* primary auditory areas; area *22,* secondary auditory area. Area *44* and the posterior part of area *45* constitute the approximate location of Broca's motor speech area.
(From Anthony CP and Kolthoff NJ: Textbook of anatomy and physiology, ed 9, St Louis, 1975, The CV Mosby Co. Modified from Brodmann K: Feinere Anatomie des Grosshirns, In Handbuch der Neurologie, Berlin, 1910, Springer-Verlag.)

the Golgi organs is significantly greater than that of the muscle spindles, and these organs are thought to modulate excessive stretching through inhibition of the muscle spindle (autoinhibition).

Another cell that may inhibit reflex contraction of a muscle is the Renshaw cell, an interneuron between axons of motor nerves. The full nature of this inhibition is not understood.

Golgi efferent nerves terminate in the muscle spindles and may regulate their sensitivity.

Fig. 20-45 illustrates the tendon reflex, using patellar tendon reflex as an example. The patellar tendon of the quadriceps muscle, an extensor muscle of the upper leg, is attached to the tibia. Deforming this tendon with a reflex hammer causes the muscle to be stretched, activating the muscle spindles, and thereby the primary

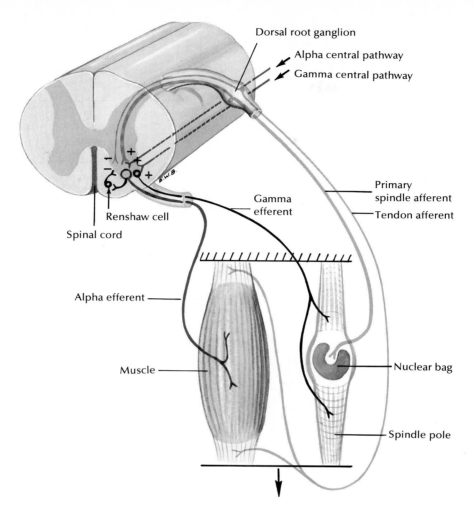

Figure 20-44

Neural basis for the stretch reflex. Afferent fibers from muscle spindle and tendon organs and efferent fibers to muscle and spindle (gamma fibers) are shown. Excitation is indicated by plus signs, inhibition by minus signs. The Renshaw cell is an interneuron that provides recurrent inhibition to the active motoneuron pool. Muscle is rigidly fixed at the upper end and subject to stretch in the direction of the arrow at the lower end.

(From Schottelius BA and Schottelius DD: Textbook of physiology, ed 18, St Louis, 1978, The CV Mosby Co.)

afferent nerve, in terminating on the alpha motor nerve in the cord segment (L3 and L4). The action potential thus stimulates the alpha efferent fibers, resulting in shortening of the quadriceps muscle, which pulls up the tibia to extend the leg. Dysfunction of the tendon reflex, then, could be attributed to lesions of the afferent or efferent arc of the nerve or to lesions of the muscle, tendon, or spinal segment involved.

Assessment of the DTRs allows the examiner to obtain information about the function of the reflex arcs and spinal cord segments without implicating other cord segments or higher neural structures.

Reflexes may be altered in pathophysiologic changes involving the sensory pathways from the tendons and muscles or the motor component, that is, the corticospinal or corticobulbar pathways (upper motor neuron), or the anterior horn cells or their axons (lower motor neuron).

The best muscle contraction is obtained in testing deep muscle tendons when the muscle is slightly stretched before the tendon is stretched (tapped with the reflex hammer).

Augmentation of the reflex may be obtained by isometrically tensing muscles not directly involved in the reflex arc being tested. For example, the client may be asked to clench the fists or to lock the fingers together and pull one hand against the other (Jendrassik's maneuver) (Fig. 20-46) as the examiner attempts to elicit reflexes in the lower extremity. To reinforce the reflex arcs of the upper extremities, the client may be asked to clench the jaws or to set the quadriceps.

Elicitation of Reflexes

Three categories of reflexes are described: (1) DTRs, elicited by deforming (tapping) a tendon (synonyms are muscle stretch reflexes, muscle jerks, and tendon jerks); (2) superficial or cutaneous reflexes, obtained by stimulating the skin; and (3) pathologic reflexes, which are usually present only in disease.

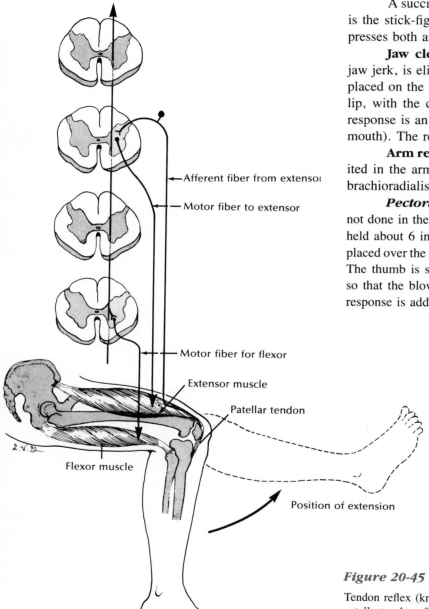

Reflexes may be graded for the record as follows:

4⁺ or + + + +	Brisk, hyperactive, clonus of tendon associated with disease
3⁺ or + + +	More brisk than normal, not necessarily indicative of disease
2⁺ or + +	Normal
1⁺ or +	Low normal, slightly diminished response
0	No response

The symmetry of the reflex from one side of the body to the other is also recorded. Differences in response on one side of the body may be helpful in locating the site of the lesions.

A succinct method of recording the reflex findings is the stick-figure representation (Fig. 20-47). This expresses both amplitude and symmetry well.

Jaw closure reflex.   The maxillary reflex, or jaw jerk, is elicited by tapping; the examiner's thumb is placed on the midline of the client's chin but below the lip, with the client's mouth slightly open. The normal response is an elevation of the mandible (closure of the mouth). The reflex may be difficult to demonstrate.

Arm reflexes.   Reflexes that are frequently elicited in the arms are the pectoralis, biceps, triceps, and brachioradialis reflexes and finger flexion.

Pectoralis reflex.   The pectoralis reflex test is not done in the screening examination. The client's arm is held about 6 in from the body. The examiner's thumb is placed over the tendon while the hand encircles the shoulder. The thumb is struck with the reflex hammer (Fig. 20-48) so that the blow is transmitted to the tendon. The normal response is adduction of the arm.

Figure 20-45

Tendon reflex (knee jerk or patellar tendon reflex). Note that the patellar tendon of the extensor muscle is attached to the tibia below the knee.
(From Schottelius BA and Schottelius DD: Textbook of physiology, ed 18, St Louis, 1978, The CV Mosby Co.)

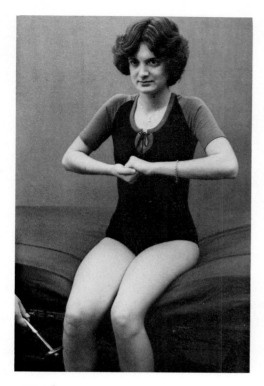

Figure 20-46

Augmentation maneuver for deep tendon reflexes.

Biceps reflex (Fig. 20-49). The client's arm is flexed at the elbow. The examiner's thumb is placed over the biceps tendon. The thumb is struck with the reflex hammer with a slight downward thrust to augment the tendon stretch. The normal response is flexion of the arm at the elbow.

Triceps reflex (Fig. 20-50). The client's arm is flexed at the elbow. The triceps tendon is tapped with the reflex hammer. The normal response is extension of the arm or straightening.

Brachioradialis reflex (Fig. 20-51). The client's arm is placed in a relaxed position. The styloid process (bony prominence on the thumb side of the wrist) or the radius is dealt a blow with the percussion hammer after palpation for the tendon (best elicited 3 to 5 cm above

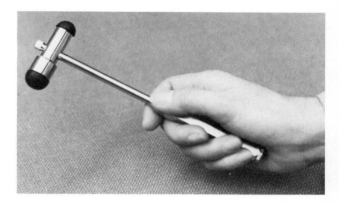

Figure 20-48

The percussion hammer is held between the thumb and index finger.

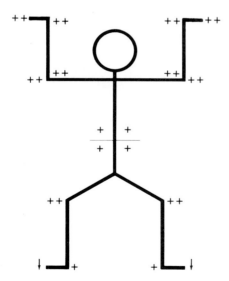

Figure 20-47

Stick figure drawing for recording reflexes. These are the reflexes usually tested in the screening examination; " + + " values shown here are normal.

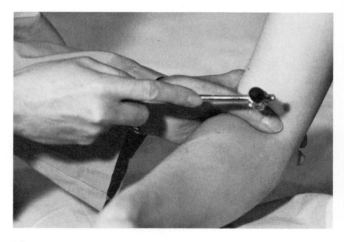

Figure 20-49

Elicitation of the biceps reflex. A downward blow is struck over the thumb, which is situated over the biceps tendon. The normal response is flexion of the arm at the elbow.

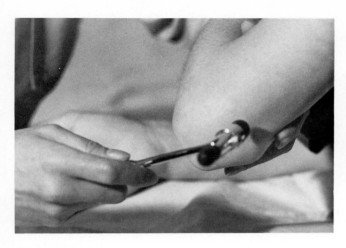

Figure 20-50

Elicitation of the triceps reflex. With the arm flexed at the elbow, the triceps tendon is tapped with the percussion hammer. The normal response is straightening or extension of the arm.

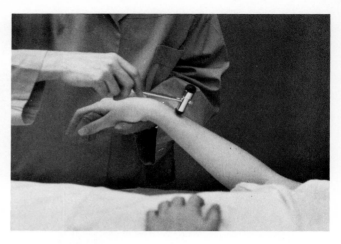

Figure 20-51

Elicitation of the brachioradialis reflex. The styloid process is dealt a blow with the percussion hammer. The normal response is flexion of the arm at the elbow and slight flexion of the fingers.

the wrist). The normal response is flexion of the arm at the elbow (pronation, supination) and at the forearm. The fingers of the hand may also flex (Fig. 20-52).

Finger flexor reflex (finger-thumb reflex). The client's arm is placed so that the wrist is relaxed and pronated. The fingers are slightly flexed at the metacarpophalangeal joint but relaxed. A tap is delivered to the fingertips. Flexion of the fingers is accompanied by flexion of the distal phalanx of the thumb.

Lower limb reflexes.   Reflexes commonly elicited in the lower limb are the patellar, Achilles tendon, and plantar reflexes.

Patellar reflex (Fig. 20-53).   The tendon is located directly inferior to the patella, or kneecap. With the legs of the client hanging freely over the side of the bed or chair or with the client in a supine position, the tendon is dealt a blow with the percussion hammer. The normal response is extension or kicking out of the leg as the quadriceps muscle contracts.

Achilles tendon reflex (Fig. 20-54).   The client's foot is held in the hand in a slightly dorsiflexed position. The Achilles tendon is delivered a blow with the percussion hammer. The normal response is plantar flexion of the foot.

Plantar reflex (Fig. 20-55).   Plantar reflexes are superficial reflexes. A key, pin, half a tongue blade, an applicator stick, or the handle portion of the reflex hammer may be used to elicit the reflex. The stimulus is applied to the lateral border of the client's sole, starting at the heel and continuing to the ball of the foot and then proceeding at a right angle over the ball of the foot toward the great

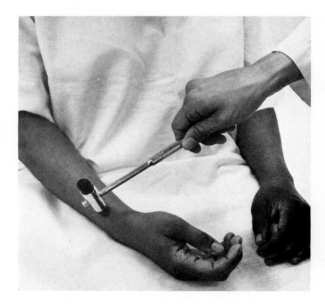

Figure 20-52

Elicitation of the brachioradialis reflex in the sitting position. The normal response is flexion of the arm at the elbow and slight flexion of the fingers.

toe. The normal response (negative Babinski's reflex) is flexion of all the toes (Fig. 20-56).

Before the child can walk, fanning and extension of the toes are the normal response.

Babinski's reflex is dorsiflexion of the great toe and fanning of the other toes (Fig. 20-57). Lesions of the pyramidal tract or motor nerves may be present in the client when Babinski's reflex is found.

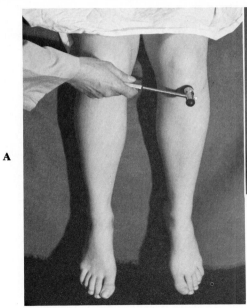

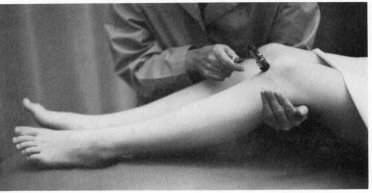

A

B

Figure 20-53

Elicitation of the patellar reflex. With the legs hanging freely over the side of the bed (**A**) or with the client in a supine position (**B**), a blow with the percussion hammer is dealt directly to the patellar tendon, inferior to the patella. The normal response is extension or kicking out of the leg.

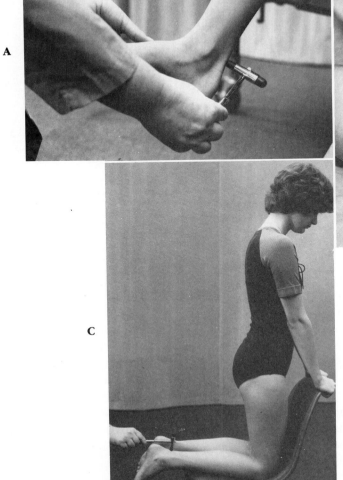

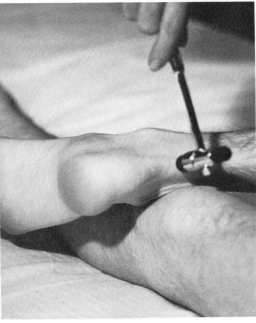

A

B

C

Figure 20-54

Elicitation of the Achilles tendon reflex. **A**, Sitting. **B**, Lying down. **C**, Kneeling on chair. The Achilles tendon is struck with the percussion hammer while the foot is slightly dorsiflexed. The normal response is plantar flexion of the foot. Both hip and knee are flexed, and the hip is rotated externally.

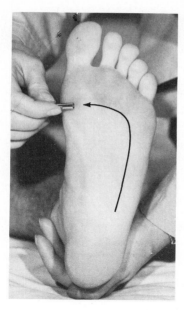

Figure 20-55

Elicitation of the plantar reflex. A hard object is applied to the lateral surface of the sole, starting at the heel and going over the ball of the foot, ending beneath the great toe. Extension or dorsiflexion of the great toe and fanning of the others is a positive Babinski's reflex.

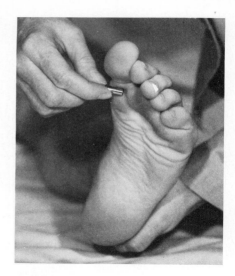

Figure 20-56

Normal response (negative Babinski's reflex) to plantar stimulation: flexion of all the toes.

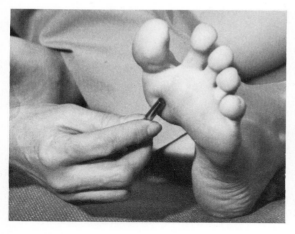

Figure 20-57

Elicitation of a positive Babinski's reflex: dorsiflexion of the great toe and fanning of the other toes.

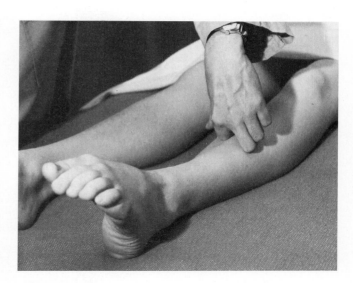

Figure 20-58

Elicitation of Oppenheim's reflex. Plantar flexion of the toes is obtained by running the index finger and thumb firmly down the tibial surface in a caudal direction.

If the examiner has difficulty in obtaining the plantar response, a similar reflex may be elicited by stimulating the lateral aspect of the dorsum of the foot. The *Chaddock sign* is the positive response (dorsiflexion of the great toe and fanning of the other toes) to this stimulus.

Other tests for eliciting the plantar response are the *Gordon reflex* (elicited by squeezing the calf muscles), *Oppenheim's reflex* (elicited by moving the thumb and index finger simultaneously and firmly over the tibial

surface in a caudal direction) (Fig. 20-58), and *Schäffer's reflex* (elicited by squeezing the Achilles tendon).

Abdominal reflexes.   See Chapters 16 and 17 on assessment of the abdomen and rectosigmoid region.

Cremasteric reflex.   The client's inner thigh is stimulated with a sharp object, such as a key or the stick end of an applicator, or with cold or hot water. The expected response is retraction (elevation) of the testis on the same side, as the cremaster muscle contracts.

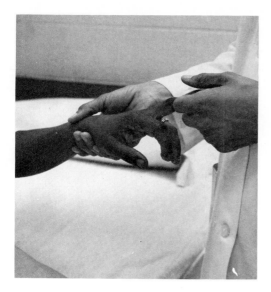

Figure 20-59

Preparation for elicitation of finger flexion reflex by Hoffman's method. The middle finger is extended to stretch the flexor tendons. The examiner then depresses the distal phalanx and allows it to flip up sharply. Flexion of the thumb or the other fingers may indicate pyramidal tract lesion.

Gluteal reflex. The client's buttocks are spread, and the perianal area is stimulated. The normal response is contraction of the anal sphincter.

Reflexes elicited in disease states

Wartenberg's reflex. The examiner grasps the flexed fingers of the client with the flexed examining fingers. Both individuals pull against the other; in doing so, the normal client will extend the thumbs. The individual with upper motor neuron disease will adduct and flex the thumb.

Finger flexor reflex. In *Trömner's method,* the metacarpophalangeal joint of the middle finger is extended (to stretch the flexor tendons). The palmar side of the distal phalanx is flicked by the examiner.

In *Hoffmann's method* (Fig. 20-59), the examiner depresses the distal phalanx and allows it to flip up sharply. A positive response is recorded if flexion of the thumb and other fingers is observed. This reflex is normally not elicited. Hoffmann's sign is the name given to the reflex when it is elicited. The presence of a pyramidal lesion may be suspected.

Grasp reflex (Fig. 20-60). The examiner places the index and middle finger in the client's palm, entering between the thumb and the index finger. The examiner's fingers are gently withdrawn, pulling the fingers across the skin of the client's palm. A positive response consists of the client's grasping the examiner's fingers. Present in in-

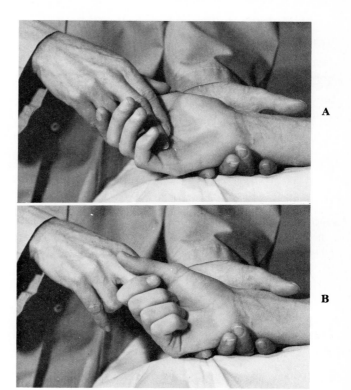

A

B

Figure 20-60

Elicitation of the grasp reflex. **A,** The examiner places the index and middle finger in the client's palm and gently withdraws them. **B,** A positive response consists of the client's grasping the examiner's fingers.

dividuals with widespread brain damage, the grasp reflex is normal in infants less than 4 months of age.

Loss of Reflexes

With loss of or diminution of reflexes on the same side, the examiner might suspect corticospinal lesions (Tables 20-3 and 20-4).

The reappearance of primitive reflexes such as Babinski's reflex also indicates a corticospinal pathologic condition.

Loss of sensation from a segment (dermatome) coupled with loss of reflexes suggests lesions in the sensory arc. Tabes dorsalis (neurosyphilis) produces this form of disorder.

VARIATIONS FROM HEALTH

Early Indications of Interruptions of the Corticospinal Tract

The examiner may elicit the *pronation sign* by asking the client to extend the arms at the level of the shoulders with the palms upward (Fig. 20-61). The arm on the

Table 20-3

Deep tendon reflex and muscle changes in upper and lower motor neuron lesions

Lesion	Common cause	Characteristics
Upper motor neuron lesion (cortico-spinal tract)	Cerebrovascular occlusion	Brisk reflexes
	Neoplasm—cerebral hemispheres	Contralateral arm and leg muscle spasticity—more marked in the flexors in arm and leg extensors
	Amyotrophic lateral sclerosis	Muscle weakness—disuse atrophy of those muscles that oppose the spastic muscles
	Deficiency diseases, pernicious anemia	Hyperreflexia
	Trauma	Babinski's sign present; clonus frequently seen
Lower motor neuron lesion (anterior horn cell, somatic motor part of cranial nerves)	Poliomyelitis	Hyporeflexia
	Amyotrophic lateral sclerosis	Diminution or absence of deep tendon reflexes
		Muscle atrophy
	Neoplasm	Muscle weakness, fasciculation, and fibrillation of muscle
	Trauma	Babinski's sign—diminished or absent

Table 20-4

Reflexes commonly tested in the physical examination

Reflexes	Segmental level	Reflexes	Segmental level
Deep tendon		**Superficial**	
Jaw	Pons	Corneal	Pons
Biceps	Cervical 5, 6	Palatal	Medulla
Triceps	Cervical 6, 7, 8	Pharyngeal	Medulla
Brachioradialis	Cervical 5, 6	Abdominal (upper)	Thoracic 7, 8, 9
Patellar	Lumbar 2, 3, 4	Abdominal (lower)	Thoracic 12; lumbar 1
Achilles	Sacral 1, 2	Cremasteric	Lumbar 1, 2, 3
		Gluteal	Lumbar 4, 5
		Plantar	Lumbar 4, 5; sacral 1, 2

affected side will drift downward and pronate.

The examiner may elicit *Barré's sign* by asking the client to flex the knees 90 degrees while in the prone position (Fig. 20-62). The affected leg will move downward.

Fine movements of the hands, such as picking up coins or pencils, are done slowly when there are lesions of the corticospinal tract. The ability to touch the thumb to the fingers is performed less rapidly.

Cortical Lesions

Disturbance in the ability to discriminate objects or symbols by means of the senses, assuming the individual previously had this skill, is termed *agnosia*. *Visual agnosia,* caused by lesions of the occipital cortex, is the inability to recognize objects. *Auditory agnosia,* caused by lesions below the sylvian fissure, is the inability to recognize familiar sounds. *Tactile agnosia,* caused by lesions of the parietal lobe, is the inability to recognize objects by feeling them.

A disturbance in the recognition of body parts is termed *autotopagnosia.*

An individual's lack of sight to his or her disease is termed *anosognosia.*

Lesions of the Cerebral Hemisphere Dominant for Language

Aphasia, the inability to comprehend or use language symbols, is caused by a disorder of the cortical areas necessary to speech or by neural connections in the ce-

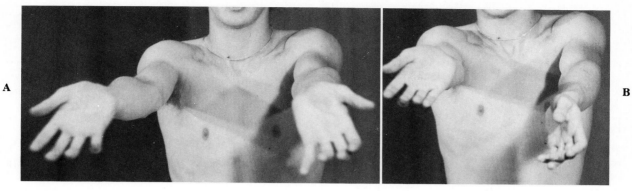

Figure 20-61

Elicitation of the pronation sign. **A,** The client is asked to extend the arms at shoulder height with the palms upward. **B,** Frequently in disease of the corticospinal tract, the affected arm will drift downward and pronate.

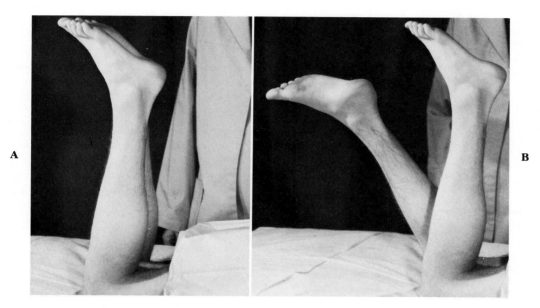

Figure 20-62

Elicitation of Barré's sign. **A,** The client is asked to lie on the abdomen, flexing the legs at a 90-degree angle. **B,** Frequently in disease of the corticospinal tract, the affected leg will drift downward.

rebral hemisphere dominant for speech: aphasia encompasses *dysarthria* and *dysphonia*. *Nonfluent aphasia* is the inability to produce words in either spoken or written form. The client with *fluent aphasia* can produce words but frequently chooses inappropriate words *(paraphasia)* or makes errors in content, occasionally creating words.

Lesions of the Cerebral Hemisphere Not Dominant for Language

A disturbance in the ability to perform a purposeful act when comprehension is intact is termed *apraxia*. For example, given a fork, the client may be unable to use it to eat; the client may be unable to dress or button a shirt. *Constructional apraxia* is the inability to draw or construct forms of two or three dimensions.

Signs of Meningeal Irritation

Meningeal irritation most commonly results from infection or intracranial hemorrhages. The following signs indicate the need for laboratory work to confirm the diagnosis.

Nuchal rigidity (stiff neck) is a common sign of meningitis and may be demonstrated through the use of cervical flexing.

Screening Physical Examination

When performing a neurologic screening examination, complete only those tests that will provide information on possible deficits. If abnormalities are identified, a more comprehensive examination is required.

Cerebral function

Observe appearance and behavior for appropriateness to the occasion and situation.

Assess mental status for orientation to person, place, and time; attention span; and calculation.

Elicit cognitive abilities of recent and remote memory as well as abstract reasoning.

Assess emotional stability through affect and mood, thought content, and idea expression.

Assess communication skills, expressive and receptive, for fluency, speech articulation, and clarity of thought conveyance.

Cranial nerves
Olfactory (1)

Test each nostril separately for the ability to identify a familiar odor.

Assess visual fields.

Optic (II)

Testing each eye individually, while the client looks straight ahead, have the individual indicate when the examiner's finger comes into peripheral vision range.

Assess visual acuity: use the Snellen or Rosenbaum chart.

Oculomotor nerve (III), trochlear nerve (IV), and abducens nerve (VI)

Examine eye for the six cardinal points of gaze, pupillary size and shape, direct and consensual pupillary response, accommodation, and opening of the eye lid.

Trigeminal nerve (V)

Sensory: Testing each side of the face, touch the forehead, cheeks, and jaw with a cotton swab, test tubes of warm and cold water, and a sharp pin.

Test the corneal reflex by touching the cornea with cotton or gauze.

Motor: Palpate the masseter and temporal muscles while the individual's teeth are clenched.

Facial nerve (VII)

Sensory: Place sugar, vinegar, salt, and quinine separately on the anterior two thirds of the tongue.

Motor: Assess facial muscles for strength and symmetry by asking the individual to raise the eyebrows, frown, smile, puff out the cheeks, close eyes tightly against resistance, and show the teeth.

Acoustic nerve (VIII)

Assess hearing acuity by covering one ear and move a ticking watch or whisper near other ear. (If acuity is suspect, perform Weber's and Rinne's tests next.)

Assess speech and swallowing.

Glossopharyngeal nerve (IX) and vagus nerve (X)

Examine the palatal arch for symmetric elevation while the individual opens mouth and says "Ah." Assess swallowing for smoothness and coordination and speech for articulation. Elicit the gag reflex.

Spinal accessory nerve (XI)

Inspect and palpate the trapezius and sternocleidomastoid muscles for symmetry and size. Have the individual raise the shoulders against resistance. Then have the individual turn the head against resistance.

Hypoglossal nerve (XII)

Inspect the tongue for atrophy, fasciculations, and alignment while it is sticking out. Have the individual press the tongue against the inside of the cheek while the examiner assesses its strength.

Cerebellar function and proprioception
Test for diadochokinesia (pronation and supination test)

With arms outstretched or flexed at the elbow, the individual rapidly pronates and supinates the hands; assess for smoothness of movement.

Test for movement direction accuracy

Finger-to-nose test: Have the individual rapidly touch the tip of the nose with the index finger of one hand, then the other. This should be performed with eyes open, then closed.

Heel-to-knee test: Have the individual run the heel of each foot down the leg, knee to foot, while in a supine position.

Romberg test: While standing with feet together and eyes closed, the individual stands for 5 seconds. Evaluate for gross swaying.

Motor function

Assess gait, posture, and smoothness of extremity movement while individual walks with eyes opened and closed.

Assess muscles bilaterally for tone, size, strength, and involuntary movement.

Sensory function

With the client's eyes closed, evaluate bilaterally for:

Touch sensation

The skin is touched lightly with a cotton swab.

Pain sensation

Use a pin to have individual identify sharp and dull pressure.

21

Assessment of the male genitalia

OBJECTIVES

Upon successful review of this chapter, learners will be able to:

- Describe anatomy and physiology of the male genitalia and inguinal region throughout the life span
- Outline history relevant to assessment of the male genitalia and inguinal region
- State related rationale and demonstrate assessment of the male genitalia and inguinal region, including inspection and palpation techniques
- Recognize abnormalities and common deviations of the male genital and inguinal region
- Describe diagnostic techniques used to assess scrotal abnormalities and related causative factors
- Compare characteristics of inguinal and femoral hernias

Male Genitalia

The examination of the genital organs of any client is usually preceived by both the client and the practitioner as being different from the examination of other body parts. Previously, most primary care providers for men were men. However, currently and increasingly in the future, many will be female. Therefore, the presentation in this chapter of the examination of the male genitalia emphasizes the approach by a female practitioner.

First, the female practitioner should feel emotionally comfortable with the examination. If she does not, she should routinely refer this part of the physical examination to a male practitioner. Next, if she is comfortable with the examination, she must accept that the male client may be reluctant to have his genitalia examined by a woman. Cajoling a client into an uncomfortable procedure may destroy futher rapport; his wishes in the situation should be respected. In most clinical settings, there is a male practitioner present who would be available for a few minutes to examine the male genitalia. Our experience has been that most male clients are agreeable to examination by a woman; if there is discomfort, it is usually on the examiner's part. It is therefore recommended that the beginning female examiner critically analyze her own feelings, fears, and beliefs; attempt male genital examination under supervision and with several cooperative clients; and then reexamine her feelings.

Rarely a male client will have an erection during examination of the genitalia regardless of the sex of the examiner. If this does occur, the most appropriate response is to reassure the client that an erection sometimes occurs and that the examiner is not offended and to proceed with the examination.

Characteristically the genital and rectal examinations are the last portions of the physical assessment. The examination should be preceded by a thorough history of the urinary system and a history of sexual functioning. As with the female client, questioning about sexual activity or performance while the genitalia are being handled may be perceived by the client as evaluative or provocative.

ANATOMY AND PHYSIOLOGY

The following is a review of the anatomy of the male genitalia (Fig. 21-1), which generally includes the penis, the scrotum, the testicles, the epididymides, the seminal vesicles, and the prostate.

The shaft of the penis is formed by three columns of erectile tissue bound together by heavy fibrous tissue to form a cylinder. The dorsolateral columns are called the corpora cavernosa; the ventromedial column is called the corpus spongiosum, and this column contains the urethra. Distally the penis terminates in a cone-shaped entity called the glans penis. The glans penis is formed by an extension and expansion of the corpus spongiosum penis, which fits over the blunt ends of the corpora cavernosa penis. The corona is the prominence formed where the glans joins the shaft. The urethra traverses the corpus spongiosum, and the external urethral orifice is a slitlike opening located slightly ventrally on the tip of the glans.

The skin of the penis is thin, hairless, darker than other skin, and only loosely connected to the internal parts of the organ. At the area of the corona, the skin forms a free fold, called the prepuce or foreskin. When allowed to remain, this flap covers the glans to a variable extent. Often the prepuce is surgically removed in circumcision (Fig. 21-2).

The scrotum is a deeply pigmented cutaneous pouch, containing the testes and parts of the spermatic cords (Fig. 21-3). The sac is formed by an outer layer of thin, rugous skin overlying a tight muscle layer. The left side of the scrotum is often lower than the right side because the left spermatic cord is usually longer. Internally the scrotum is divided into halves by a septum; each half contains a testis and its epididymis and part of the spermatic cord. The testes are ovoid and are suspended vertically, slightly forward; they lean slightly laterally in the scrotum. The mediolateral surfaces are flattened.

Figure 21-1

Male pelvic organs.
From Anthony CP and Thibodeau GA: Anatomy and physiology, ed 12, St Louis, 1987, The CV Mosby Co.)

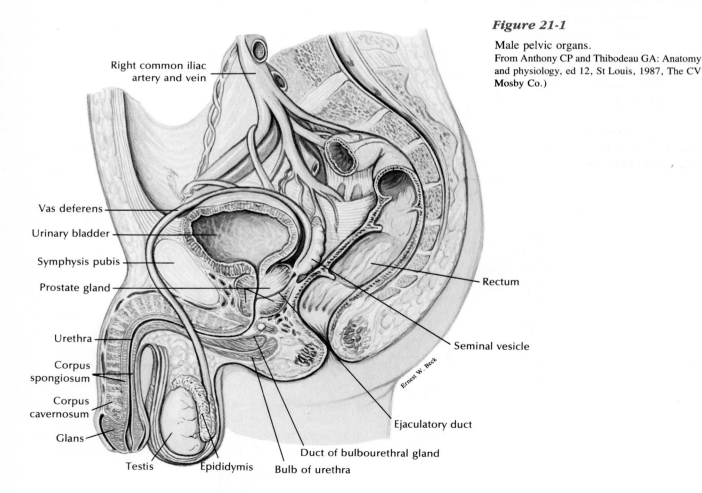

Right common iliac artery and vein

Vas deferens

Urinary bladder

Symphysis pubis

Prostate gland

Urethra

Corpus spongiosum

Corpus cavernosum

Glans

Testis   Epididymis   Bulb of urethra

Duct of bulbourethral gland

Ejaculatory duct

Seminal vesicle

Rectum

Each is approximately 4 to 5 cm long, 3 cm wide, and 2 cm thick.

The epididymis is a comma-shaped structure that is curved over the posterolateral surface and upper end of the testis; it creates a visual bulge on the posterolateral surface of the testis. The ductus deferens (or vas deferens) begins at the tail of the epididymis, ascends the spermatic cord, travels through the inguinal canal, and eventually descends on the fundus of the bladder (see Fig. 22-1).

The prostate, a slightly conical gland, lies under the bladder, surrounds the urethra, and measures approximately 4 cm at its base or uppermost part, 3 cm vertically, and 2 cm in its anteroposterior diameter. The prostate gland has been compared with the chestnut in size and shape. It has three lobes, left and right lateral lobes and a median lobe. These lobes are not well demarcated from each other. The median lobe is the part of the prostate that projects inward from the upper, posterior area toward the urethra. It is the enlargement of this lobe that causes urinary obstruction in benign prostatic hypertrophy.

The posterior surface of the prostate is in close contact with the rectal wall and is the only portion of the gland accessible to examination. Its posterior surface is slightly convex; a shallow median furrow divides all except the upper portions of the posterior surface into right and left lateral lobes.

The seminal vesicles are a pair of convoluted pouches, 5 to 10 cm long, which lie along the lower posterior surface of the bladder, anterior to the rectum (Fig. 21-4).

The testes produce both spermatozoa and testosterone. The epididymides serve as receptacles for storage, maturation, and transit of sperm. The vas deferens serves as a mechanism of transit from each epididymis to the seminal vesicles. The prostate produces the bulk of ejaculatory fluid. The temperature of the testes is controlled by the muscular layer of the scrotum, which controls the distance of the testes from the body. Spermatogenesis requires temperatures below 37° C. Therefore, the scrotum appears low in hot weather and high in cold weather.

The penis serves as the terminal excretory organ for urine and, with erection, as the means of ejaculating sperm. The physiologic process of erection occurs when the two corpora cavernosa become engorged with approximately 20 to 50 ml of blood through decreased venous outflow and increased arterial dilatation. Orgasm is a major, pleasurable sensation accompanying emission of secretions from the epididymes, the vas deferens, the seminal vesicles, the prostate, and the penis.

EXAMINATION

Preparation for the Examination

Usually the genital examinations are the last portions of a physical assessment. In preparation, the examiner should advise the client of the purpose of and procedures used in the examination and should assemble the needed equipment. In the case of a male genital examination, the equipment needed includes gloves and a penlight for transillumination of any potential mass. The client may be lying (with the examiner standing) or standing (with the examiner sitting or standing for various portions of the examination) and should have trousers and shorts removed.

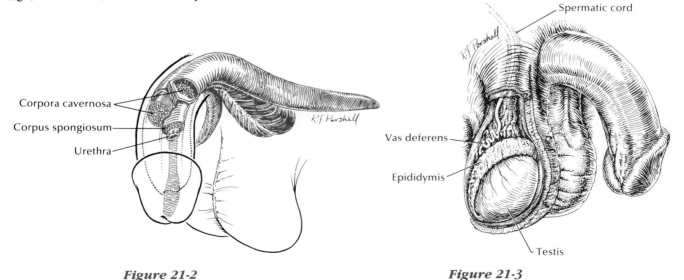

Figure 21-2
Circumcised penis.

Figure 21-3
Scrotum and scrotal contents.

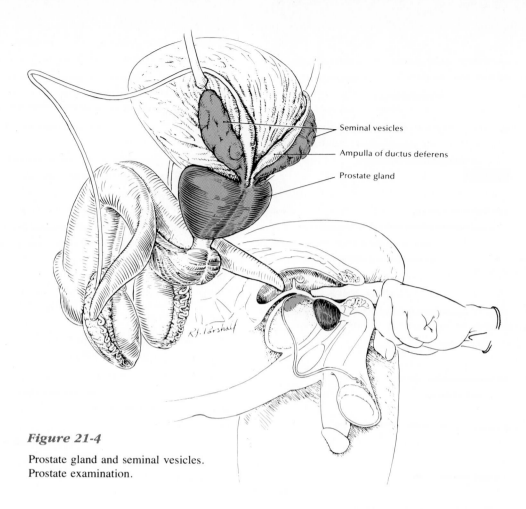

Figure 21-4

Prostate gland and seminal vesicles.
Prostate examination.

Seminal vesicles

Ampulla of ductus deferens

Prostate gland

Preparation for Male Genital Examination

Explanation of purposes and procedures
Client: stripped below the waist
Equipment: gloves, penlight for transillumination

The techniques of inspection and palpation are used to examine the male genitalia. Inspection and palpation occur consecutively for each portion of the genitalia.

After the inguinal and genital areas are exposed, the skin, hair, and gross appearance of the penis and scrotum are inspected. Examination of the skin, nodes, and hair distribution are discussed elsewhere in this text. The size of the penis and the secondary sex characteristics are assessed in relationship to the client's age and general development. If inflammation or lesions are observed or suspected, gloves are used for the examination.

The onset of the appearance of adult sexual characteristics is extremely variable. Pubic hair appears and the testes enlarge between the ages of 12 and 16 years. Penile enlargement and the onset of seminal emission normally occurs between the ages of 13 and 17 years. Table 21-1 contains a summary of developmental changes in the male genital system.

An ambulatory, cooperative client can assist in the examination by handling the penis and scrotum during inspection. The examiner must do all the handling for the debilitated client. The examiner is reminded to examine all the surfaces, including the posterior surfaces, of the male genitalia.

Penis

The color of the penis ranges from pink to light brown in whites and from light brown to dark brown in blacks. The penis is observed for lesions, nodules, swelling, inflammation, and discharge. If the client is uncircumcised, he is requested to retract the prepuce from the glans, and the glans and foreskin are examined carefully. If the uncircumcised client has been asked to retract the foreskin for examination of the glans, he is reminded to

Table 21-1

Developmental changes in the appearance of the male genital organs

Developmental time	Appearance		
	Pubic hair	**Penis**	**Testes and scrotum**
Stage 1 Sexual maturity	None except for fine body hair as on the abdomen	Size proportional to body size as in childhood	Size proportional to body size as in childhood
Stage 2 Sexual maturity	Sparce, long, slightly pigmented, thin hair at the base of the penis	Slight enlargement	Enlargement of testes and scrotum; reddened pigmentation; texture more prominent
Stage 3 Sexual maturity	Darkens, becomes more coarse and curly; growth extends over symphysis	Elongation	Enlargement continues

Illustrations adapted from Tanner JM: Growth at adolescence, ed 2, Oxford, 1962, Blackwell Scientific Publications.

Continued

Table 21-1

Developmental changes in the appearance of the male genital organs—*cont'd*

Developmental time	Appearance		
	Pubic hair	**Penis**	**Testes and scrotum**
Stage 4 Sexual maturity	Continues to darken, thicken, and become coarser and more curly; growth extends laterally, superiorly, and inferiorly.	Breadth and length increase; glans develops	Enlargement continues; skin pigmentation darkens
Stage 5 Sexual maturity	Adult distribution and appearance; growth extends to inner thighs, umbilicus, and anus and is abundant.	Adult appearance	Adult appearance
Elderly clients	Hair sparce and gray	Decrease in size	Testes hang low in scrotum; scrotum appears pendulous

return the foreskin to its usual position after the glans is inspected. The client is next asked to compress the glans anteroposteriorly. This opens the distal end of the urethra for inspection. The examiner observes for evidence of neoplastic lesions or inflammatory processes.

If any discharge is present, a smear and culture for gonorrhea are obtained (see Chapter 22 on assessment of the female genitalia and procedures for smears and cultures). If the client has reported a discharge, he is

requested to strip the penis from the base to the urethra; if a discharge is present, a culture should then be made.

The procedure for stripping the penis is as follows: the client grasps the base of the penis with the thumb and fingers—thumb at the front and fingers behind. Applying a moderate amount of consistent pressure, he moves the thumb and fingers slowly from the base to the tip of the penis.

Among the more common penile lesions are syph-

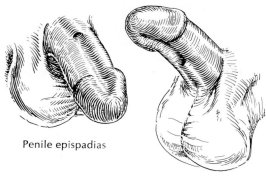

Penile epispadias

Penile hypospadias

Figure 21-5

Malpositioning of the urethral meatus.

ilitic chancre, condylomata acuminata, and cancer. The syphilitic chancre is the primary lesion of syphilis. It begins as a single papule that eventually erodes into an oval or round red ulcer with an indurated base that discharges serous material. It is usually painless.

Condylomata acuminata are wart-appearing growths. They are caused by a venereal infection and may be seen occurring singly or in multiple, cauliflower like patches.

Carcinoma of the penis occurs most frequently on the glans and on the inner lip of the prepuce. It may appear dry and scaly, ulcerated, or nodular. It is usually painless.

The urethral meatus should appear pink and slit-like and should be positioned rather centrally on the glans. When the distal urethral ostium occurs on the ventral corona or at a more proximal and ventral site on the penis or perineum, the condition is called hypospadias (Fig. 21-5). A similar malpositioning of the urethral meatus in the dorsal area is called epispadias.

When hyposadias or epispadias is noted, the location of the urethral meatus should be described as precisely as possible. Hypospadias can be classified as being glandular, penile, penoscrotal, or perineal, Epispadias can be classified as being glandular, penile, or complete. Glandular refers to a location somewhere between the normal position and the junction of the glans with the body of the penis. Penile refers to a location on the penile shaft. Penoscrotal hypospadias indicates a positioning of the meatus along the anterior margin of the scrotum. Hypospadias is described as perineal when the urethral orifice is on the perineum. In the latter condition, the scrotum is bifid. Epispadias is described as complete when the urethral orifice is located anterior to and off the penis.

The prepuce, if present, should be easily retractable from the glans and returnable to its original posi-

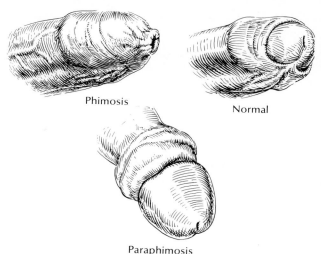

Phimosis

Normal

Paraphimosis

Figure 21-6

Phimosis, normal retraction of prepuce, and paraphimosis.

tion. Phimosis exists when retraction cannot occur (Fig. 21-6). This condition presents problems with cleanliness and prevents observation of the glans and interior surfaces of the prepuce. If the foreskin has been partially retracted but has impinged on the penis, so that it cannot be returned to its usual position, the condition is called paraphimosis.

The penile shaft should be carefully palpated with the thumb and the first two fingers of the examining hand. The penis should feel smooth and semifirm. The overlying skin appears slightly wrinkled and feels slightly movable over the underlying structures. Swelling, nodules, and induration are noted as possibly abnormal findings. Occasionally, hard, nontender subcutaneous plaques are palpated on the dorsomedial surface. The client with this condition, called Peyronie's disease, may report penile bending with erection and painful intercourse.

Scrotum

The client is instructed to hold the penis out of the way, and the examiner observes the general size, superficial appearance, and symmetry of the scrotum. The scrotum normally appears asymmetric because the left testis is generally lower than the right testis. Also, the tone of the dartos muscle determines the size of the scrotum; it contracts when the area is cold and relaxes when the area is warm. In advanced age, the dartos muscle is somewhat atonic and the scrotum may appear pendulous.

The scrotal skin is more darkly pigmented than that of the rest of the body. When the scrotal skin is being observed, its rugated surface should be spread. Also, the examiner should remember to inspect the posterior and posterolateral and anterior and anterolateral skin areas. A common abnormality, occurring as a single lesion or as multiple lesions, is that of sebaceous cysts. These are firm, yellow to white, nontender cutaneous lesions measuring up to 1 cm in diameter.

The scrotum can be edematous, and palpation may produce pitting. This may occur in any condition that causes edema in the lower trunk, for example, cardiovascular disease.

The contents of each half of the scrotal sac are palpated. Both testes should be present in the scrotum at birth; if not present, their location should be determined by retracing their course of descent back into the abdomen.

Both testes are palpated simultaneously between the thumb and the first two fingers. Their consistency, size, shape, and response to pressure are determined. They should be smooth, homogeneous in consistency, regular, equal in size, freely movable, and slightly sensitive to compression.

Next, each epididymis is palpated. The epididymides are located in the posterolateral area of the testes in 93% of the male population. In approximately 7% they are in the anterolateral or anterior areas. They are palpated, and their size, shape, consistency, and tenderness are noted. They should feel smooth, discrete, larger cephalad, and nontender. Then each of the spermatic cords is palpated by bilaterally grasping each between the thumb and the forefinger, starting at the base of the epididymis and continuing to the inguinal canal. The vas deferentia feel like smooth cords and are movable; the arteries, veins, lymph vessels, and nerves feel like indefinite threads along the side of the vas.

If swelling, irregularity, or nodularity is noted in the scrotum, attempts are made to transilluminate it by darkening the room and placing a lit flashlight behind the scrotal contents. Transillumination is a red glow. Serous fluid will transilluminate; tissue and blood will not. The more commonly occurring abnormalities of the scrotum are described and illustrated in Table 21-2.

All scrotal masses should be described by their placement, size, shape, consistency, and tenderness and by whether they transilluminate.

Prostate Gland

With an ambulatory client it is most satisfactory to execute the rectal and prostate examination with the client standing, hips flexed, toes pointed toward each other, and upper body resting on the examining table. This position flattens the buttocks, deters gluteal contraction, and makes the anus and rectum more accessible to eval-

uation. A debilitated client may be examined in the left lateral or lithotomy position. In the left lateral position he is reminded to flex his right knee and hip and to have his buttocks close to the edge of the examining table. The general procedure for the anal and rectal examination is described in Chapters 16 and 17 on assessment of the abdomen and rectosigmoid region. The general rectal examination is performed first; then the prostate gland and seminal vesicles are palpated (see Fig. 21-4). The pad of the index finger is used for palpation. The prostate gland is located on the anterior rectal wall but should not be protruding into the rectal lumen.

Prostatic enlargement is protrusion of the prostate gland into the rectal lumen and is commonly described in grades:

Grade I: Encroaches less than 1 cm into the rectal lumen
Grade II: Encroaches 1 to 2 cm into the rectal lumen
Grade III: Encroaches 2 to 3 cm into the rectal lumen
Grade IV: Encroaches more than 3 cm into the rectal lumen

The gland should be approximately 3 cm long, symmetric, movable, and of a rubbery (like a pencil eraser) consistency. Its median sulcus normally can be felt. The lateral margins of the prostate gland should be discrete, and a moderate degree of mobility can be noted when the tip of the index finger is hooked over the upper border of the gland and the gland is pulled down. The proximal portions of the seminal vesicles can sometimes be palpated as corrugated structures above the lateral to the midpoint of the gland. Normally they are too soft to be palpated. The examiner should attempt to examine all available surfaces of the prostate gland and seminal vesicles. Significant abnormalities of the prostate gland or seminal vesicles include protrusion into the rectal lumen; hard, nodular areas; bogginess; tenderness; and asymmetry (see box below).

A hard, single or multiple lesion on a firm and fixed prostate gland may indicate cancer. The initial le-

---

Assessment of Prostate Gland and Seminal Vesicles

The examiner should mentally consider the following questions about these structures:
Surface: Smooth or nodular?
Consistency: Rubbery, hard, boggy, soft, or fluctuant?
Shape: Rounded or flat?
Size: Normal, enlarged, or atrophied?
Sensitivity: Tender or not?
Movability: Movable or fixed?

Table 21-2

Description of scrotal abnormalities

Abnormality	Definition/causation	Basis for diagnosis
Hydrocele	An accumulation of serous fluid between the visceral and parietal layers of the tunica vaginalis	Transilluminates; fingers can get above the mass
Scrotal hernia	A hernia within the scrotum	Bowel sounds auscultated; does not transilluminate; fingers cannot get above the mass
Varicocele	Abnormal dilatation and tortuosity of the veins of the pampiniform plexus; often described as a "bag of worms" in the scrotum*	Complaints of a dragging sensation or dull pain in the scrotal area; feels like a soft bag of worms; collapses when the scrotum is elevated and increases when the scrotum is dependent; more commonly present on the left side; usually appears at puberty
Spermatocele	An epididymal cyst resulting from a partial obstruction of the spermatic tubules*	Transilluminates; round mass, feels like a third testis; painless

---

*Betesh S, editor: Diseases of the urinary tract and male genital organs, Geneva, 1974, Council for Internal Organizations for Medical Sciences, pp 86-90.
Continued

Table 21-2

Description of scrotal abnormalities—*cont'd*

Abnormality	Definition/causation	Basis for diagnosis
Epididymal mass or nodularity	May be a result of benign or malignant neoplasms, syphilis, or tuberculosis	Nodules are not tender; in tuberculosis lesions, vas deferens often feels beaded
Epididymitis	An inflammation of the epididymis, usually resulting from *Escherichia coli*, *Neisseria gonorrhoeae*, or *Mycobacterium tuberculosis* organisms*	Spermatic cord often thickened and indurated; pain relieved by elevation
Torsion of the spermatic cord	Axial rotation or volvulus of the spermatic cord, resulting in infarction of the testicle	Elevated mass; pain not relieved by further elevation; more common in childhood or adolescence; history of extreme pain and tenderness of the testis, followed by hyperemic swelling and hydrocele
Testicular tumor	Multiple causes	Usually not painful; hydroceles may develop as a result of a tumor—if a testis cannot be palpated, fluid may need to be aspirated so that the testis can be accurately evaluated.

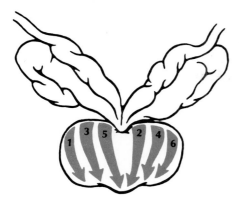

Figure 21-7

Prostatic massage. The arrows indicate the areas of the prostate that are massaged and the sequence and direction of the massage. It is important that all areas of the prostate available to the palpating fingers be massaged.

sion of carcinoma is frequently on the posterior lobe and can be easily identified during the rectal examination. A soft, symmetric, boggy, nontender prostate gland may indicate benign prostatic hypertrophy, a condition very common in men over 50 years of age. In the later stages of this condition, the median sulcus may be obliterated. A boggy, fluctuant, or tender prostate gland may indicate acute or chronic prostatitis.

The prostate gland can be massaged centrally from its lateral edges to force secretions into the urethra. The method of prostate massage is indicated in Fig. 21-7. The prostate is stroked from its distal to proximal areas using the order of strokes indicated in the figure. Secretion at the urethral opening can be examined and cultured.

SCROTAL SELF-EXAMINATION

Testicular self-examination is a means of early identification of scrotal cancer. Malignant scrotal tumors are the most common neoplasms in men aged 20 to 34. In addition to age, the following are risk factors for scrotal cancer: (1) history of undescended testes; (2) white race; (3) history of maternal use of oral contraceptives or diethylstibestrol during early pregnancy; (4) history of maternal abdominal or pelvic x-ray examination during pregnancy; (5) higher social class; and (6) never married or late marriage.

The health-oriented practitioner should assess the male client's level of knowledge about testicular self-examination, reinforce the importance of a monthly self-examination, and provide instruction for the examination. The following outline can be used for the health teaching along with pictures of the anatomy of the male genitalia:

1. Examine the testicles once a month.

2. Do the self-examination following a shower or warm bath when the testes are descended and accessible for palpation.
3. Hold the scrotum in the palms of the hands.
4. Use the thumbs and the index and middle fingers for examination with the thumbs on top and the fingers on the underside of the scrotum.
5. Roll the contents of the scrotum between your thumbs and fingers. The normal testicle is about 1½ to 2 in long. It feels smooth, rubbery, and firm but not hard. The epididymis is the storage tube found behind each testicle. Each should feel soft and spongy and sometimes slightly tender. The spermatic cords extend from the bottom of the epididymides and up into the pelvis. They should feel like smooth, firm tubes.
6. The examination should not be painful unless the pressure is too hard or there is some problem. A small amount of tenderness may be noticed during the palpation of the testes and epididymides and is normal.
7. Any lump or change in texture, whether painful or not, should be reported to and assessed by a health care provider as soon as possible.

Inguinal Area: Assessment for Hernias

If a client has an inguinal or groin area hernia, he (or she) will probably complain of a swelling or bulging in that area, especially during abdominal straining. All clients should be screened for inguinal and femoral hernias, even if they do not complain of groin swelling, as part of the routine physical examination.

No special equipment is needed for the examination. Some examiners may want to wear rubber gloves.

ANATOMY

The following is a review of the anatomy of the inguinal area (Fig. 21-8).

The inguinal (Poupart's) ligament extends from the anterosuperior spine of the ilium to the pubic tubercle. The inguinal canal is a flattened tunnel between two layers of abdominal muscle, measuring approximately 4 to 6 cm in the adult. Its internal ring is located 1 to 2 cm above the midpoint of the inguinal ligament. The spermatic cord traverses through this internal ring, passes through the canal, exists the canal at its external (subcutaneous) ring, and then moves up and over the inguinal ligament and into the scrotum.

Hesselbach's triangle is the region superior to the inguinal canal, medial to the inferior epigastric artery, and lateral to the margin of the rectus muscle.

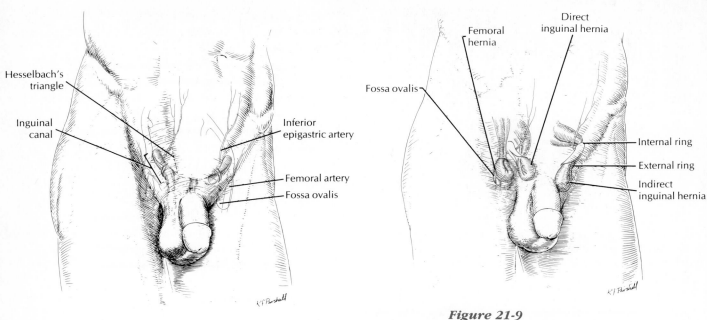

Figure 21-8

Superficial anatomy of the anterior pelvic area.

Figure 21-9

Three common pelvic area hernias.

The femoral canal is a potential space just inferior to the inguinal ligament and 3 cm medial and parallel to the femoral artery. If the examiner's right hand is placed on the client's right anterior thigh with the index finger over the femoral artery, the femoral canal will be under the ring finger.

The three main types of pelvic area hernias are shown in Fig. 21-9. In the *indirect inguinal hernia,* the hernial sac enters the internal inguinal canal, and its tip is located somewhere in the inguinal canal or beyond the canal. In men, indirect inguinal hernias may descend into the scrotum. The *direct inguinal hernia* emerges directly from behind and through the external inguinal ring. The *femoral hernia* emerges through the femoral ring, the femoral canal, and the fossa ovalis.

The three main types of hernias are compared in Table 21-3.

EXAMINATION

Inspection and palpation are the techniques used. Whenever possible, the examination for hernias is performed with the client standing. However, if the client is debilitated or especially tense, the examination may be performed while the client is lying down on a flat surface.

First, the areas of inguinal and femoral hernias are exposed and observed with the client at rest and while the client holds his breath and exerts abdominal pressure with the diaphragm. Straining is preferred to coughing

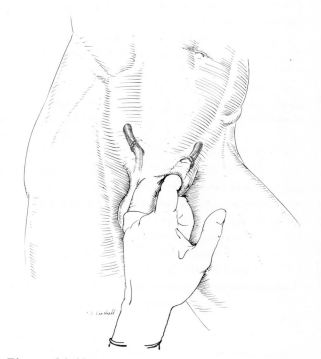

Figure 21-10

Examination of a male client for indirect inguinal hernia.

Table 21-3

Comparison of inguinal and femoral hernias

| | Inguinal hernia | | Femoral hernia |
	Indirect	Direct	
Course	Sac emerges through the internal inguinal ring, lateral to the inferior epigastric artery; can remain in the canal, exit the external ring, or pass into the scrotum	Sac emerges directly from behind and through the external inguinal ring; located in the region of Hesselbach's triangle	Sac emerges through the femoral ring, the femoral canal, and the fossa ovalis; observed lateral to the femoral vein
Incidence	More common in infants under 1 year and in young men 16 to 20 years; more common in men than in women at a ratio of approximately 4:1, 60% of all hernias	Most often observed in men over 40 years of age; rarer than the indirect hernia	Less common than inguinal hernias; seldom seen in children; more common in women; 4% of all hernias
Cause	Congenital or acquired	Congenital weakness exacerbated by (1) lifting, (2) atrophy of abdominal muscles, (3) ascites, (4) chronic cough, or (5) obesity	Acquired; may be caused by (1) stooping frequently, (2) increased abdominal pressure, or (3) loss of muscle substance
Clinical symptoms and signs	Soft swelling in the region of the internal inguinal ring— swelling increases when client stands or strains, is sometimes reduced when client reclines; pain during straining	Abdominal bulge in the area of Hesselbach's triangle, usually in the area of the internal ring; usually painless; easily reduced when client reclines; rarely enters scrotum	Right side more commonly affected; pain may be severe; strangulation frequent; sac may extend into the scrotum, into the labium, or along the saphenous vein

because a more sustained pressure is elicited. Sometimes the impulse of coughing can be confused with the impulse of a hernia. Often, small hernias in women and children are more easily observed than felt because of the fatty tissue in the area.

The examiner palpates for a direct inguinal hernia by placing two fingers over each external inguinal ring and instructing the client to bear down. The presence of a hernia will produce a palpable bulge in the area.

To determine the presence of an indirect inguinal hernia, the client is asked to flex the ipsilateral knee slightly while the examiner attempts to direct his index or little finger into the path of the inguinal canal. When the finger has traversed as far as possible, the client is asked to strain. A hernia will be felt as a mass of tissue meeting the finger and then withdrawing. The left index

or little finger, hand with palm side out, is used to examine the client's left side. The right hand in turn is used for the client's right side. In women, the canal is narrow, and the finger cannot be inserted far, if at all. In men, the finger invaginates scrotal skin into the inguinal canal (Fig. 21-10).

In both men and women, each fossa ovalis area is palpated while the client is straining. The femoral hernia will be felt as a soft tumor at the fossa, below the inguinal ligament and lateral to the pubic tubercle.

Occasionally, the client may complain of the symptoms of hernia, but none can be palpated. In such cases a load test is suggested. The client lifts a heavy object while the inguinal area is being observed. A previously unobserved bulge may become prominent.

Health History
Male Genitalia

NOTE: A yes response to any question *must* be further investigated. Use the following indicators throughout the assessment: (1) onset (specific date, sudden or gradual), (2) duration, (3) frequency, (4) precipitating factors, (5) aggravating or alleviating factors, (6) treatment received, and (7) outcome.

Present status

1. Do you have penile discharge?
   a. Description: color, amount, odor, pain as burning, fever
2. Do you do scrotal self-exams?
   a. Frequency
3. Do you have sexual difficulties?
   a. Description: pain, difficulty obtaining or maintaining an erection, premature ejaculation
4. Do you have an infertility problem?
   a. Description: type, cause

Past history

1. Have you had any changes in urination?
   a. Description: frequency, small amounts, difficulty starting stream, changes in urine color or odor, pain or burning
2. Have you had a penile lesion?
   a. Appearance
   b. Discharge
   c. Associated symptoms: pain, burning, or itching, fever
3. Have you ever had a scrotal mass, swelling, or tenderness?
   a. Description: soft, firm, moveable, painful

4. Have you or a sexual partner had a sexually transmitted disease?
   a. Type
5. Have you had reproductive or hernia surgery?
   a. Type
   b. When performed
   c. Residual effects
6. Have you had groin or scrotum swelling?
   a. Pain or tenderness
   b. Size or character change
   c. Reducibility

Associated conditions

1. Do you have diabetes?
2. Did you have or were you exposed to mumps after puberty?

Family history

1. Do any male family members have cancer of the prostate?
2. Have any male family members had infertility problems?

Sample assessment record

Client states swelling of the scrotum started 2 weeks ago, States there is no pain, yet clothes are uncomfortable, an athletic support alleviates some discomfort. No previous swelling noted. Unable to identify any precipitating factors. Denies discharge, changes in urination, and lesions. Has had no reproductive or hernia surgery. Denies exposure to infectious processes. Denies familial prostate cancer.

BIBLIOGRAPHY

Blesch KS: Health beliefs about testicular cancer and self-examination among professional men, Oncol Nurs Forum 13, 29-33, 1986.

Bodner H: Diagnostic and therapeutic aids in urology, Springfield, Ill, 1974, Charles C Thomas, Publishers.

Brandes D, editor: Male accessory sex organs, New York, 1974, Academic Press.

Btesh S, editor: Disease of the urinary tract and male genital organs, Geneva, 1974, Council for International Organizations for Medical Sciences.

Calman CH: Atlas of hernia repair, St Louis, 1966, The CV Mosby Co.

Haggerty BJ: Prevention and differential of scrotal cancer, Nurse Pract 8:45, 1983.

Harrison JH and others: Campbell's urology, Philadelphia, 1978, WB Saunders Co.

Johnson DE, editor: Testicular tumors, ed 2, Flushing, NY, 1976, Medical Examination Publishing Co.

Maingot R, editor: Abdominal operation, ed 8, Norwalk, Conn, 1985, Appleton-Century-Crofts.

Marty PJ, McDermott RJ: Teaching about testicular cancer and testicular self-examination, J School Health 53:351-356, 1983.

Ostwald SK and Rothenberger J: Development of a testicular self-examination program for college men, J Am Coll Health 33:234-239, 1985.

Ravitch MM: Repairs of hernias, Chicago, 1969, Year Book Medical Publishers.

Scott R, editor: Current controversies in urologic management, Philadelphia, 1972, WB Saunders Co.

Smith DR: General urology, Los Altos, Calif, 1981, Lange Medical Publications.

Stanford J: Testicular self-examination, Prof Nurse 1:132-133, 1986.

Stanford J: Testicular self-examination: teaching, learning and practice by nurses, J Adv Nurs 12:13-19, 1986.

Thornhill JA and others: Public awareness of testicular cancer and the value of self-examination, Br Med J 293:480-481, 1986.

Wallis LA, Tardiff K, and Deane K: Evaluation of teaching programs for male and female genital examinations, J Med Educ 58:664-666, 1983.

Zornow DH and Landes RR: Scrotal palpation, Am Fam Physician 23:150, 1981.

22

Assessment of the female genitalia

OBJECTIVES

Upon successful review of this chapter, learners will be able to:

- Describe anatomy and physiology of female genitalia throughout the life span

- Outline history relevant to assessment of female genitalia

- State related rationale and demonstrate assessment of female genitalia, including client positioning, inspection, speculum procedures, and palpation techniques

- Recognize anatomical findings of bimanual vaginal and rectovaginal examinations

- Recognize common appearances and lesions of the vulva, vagina, and cervix

- Describe procedures used for smears and cultures

Female Genitalia

Most female clients perceive the examination of their reproductive organs as being different from the examination of other body parts. Past admonitions of "do not touch" and "keep it covered" have created a population of anatomically unaware and sometimes inappropriately "modest" women who are often unnecessarily difficult to examine. Most practitioners believe that a great amount of information about a female client can be obtained by examining the genital area and performing screening tests; but because of their experience with the fearful and tense reactions of many clients, practitioners have sometimes routinely omitted the examination of the genital organs or have referred their clients to gynecologic specialists for routine examinations.

One cause of the female client's tenseness during an examination of the genital area may be fear of discovery. During the history the practitioner investigates areas of anatomic and physiologic function and dysfunction. The review of systems on all clients should include a sexual history. If this portion of the history is accomplished skillfully and if the client has been cooperative, she should not be apprehensive about the possible discovery of sexual "secrets."

Other causes of tenseness during the pelvic examination include fear of discovery of disease and the memory of previous, uncomfortable pelvic examinations.

Also, many clients are not knowledgeable regarding the anatomy of the pelvic area. The practitioner should determine the client's need for basic information regarding the structure of the genital organs and provide this instruction before the pelvic examination, along with a demonstration of the instruments and an explanation of the procedure. The client should be shown the speculum and the mechanism used to open and close it. The client

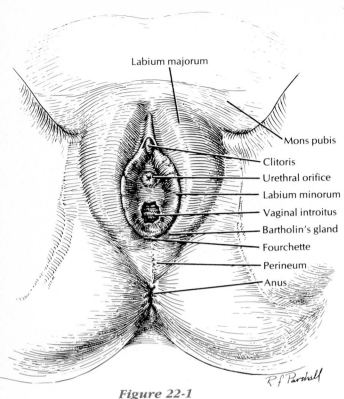

Labium majorum

Mons pubis

Clitoris

Urethral orifice

Labium minorum

Vaginal introitus

Bartholin's gland

Fourchette

Perineum

Anus

R.P.Parshall

Figure 22-1

Female external genitalia.

should be advised regarding the clicking sounds normally made by a speculum as it is opened and closed. If a relatively short amount of time were taken to inform and orient all female clients at their first examination, practitioners and clients would reap the benefits of enhanced mutual cooperation.

Teaching the client a relaxation technique will often make an examination shorter or even possible. One relaxation technique that has been successful is the following: the client is instructed to place her hands on her chest at about the level of the diaphragm, breathe deeply and slowly through her mouth, concentrate on the rhythm of breathing, and relax all body muscles with each exhalation. The tense client is apt to hold her breath and tighten. Even the coached client may forget and hold her breath; a gentle reminder, advising her to keep breathing, usually enables the client to maintain relaxation. This technique is particularly helpful in the adolescent or virginal client, whose introitus may be especially small.

Another relaxation or, more specifically, distraction technique that has been used by some practitioners is the placement of a sign or mobile above the examining table. Clients appreciate having something to look at, and their attention is constructively diverted from the examiner's activities.

For most clients it is distressing to attempt to con-

verse while in a lithotomy position. Most clients appreciate an explanation and reassurance from the examiner but prefer not to have to respond to questions until they are again upright and at eye level with the examiner. Questioning a client during the pelvic examination is apt to make her tense.

Environmental conditions are also important in enhancing cooperation during examination of the genital area. The environment and the client should be warm. The examining area should be private and safe from unexpected intrusion. The room, the examiner's hands, and all materials touching the client should be warm.

ANATOMY AND PHYSIOLOGY

External Genitalia

The external female genitalia are termed the vulva or pudendum (Fig. 22-1). The symphysis pubis is covered by a pad of fat called the mons pubis or mons veneris. In the postpubertal female the mons is covered by a patch of coarse, curly hair that extends to the lower abdomen. The abdominal portion of the female escutcheon is flat and forms the base of an inverted triangle of hair.

The labia majora are two bilobate folds of adipose tissue extending from the mons to the perineum. After puberty, their outer surfaces are covered with hair and their inner surfaces are smooth and hairless. The labia minora are two folds of skin that are thinner and darker than the labia majora. The labia minora lie within the labia majora and extend from the clitoris to the fourchette. Anteriorly, each labium minus divides into a medial and a lateral part. The lateral parts join posteriorly to form the prepuce of the clitoris, and the medial parts join anterior to the clitoris to form the frenulum of the clitoris. The clitoris is composed of erectile tissue, homologous to the corpora cavernosa of the penis. Its body is normally about 2.5 cm long; the length of its visible portion is 2 cm or less.

The vestibule is the boat-shaped anatomic region between the labia minora. It contains the urethral and vaginal orifices. The urethral orifice is located approximately 2.5 cm posterior to the clitoris and is visualized as an irregular, vertical slit. The vaginal orifice, or introitus, lies immediately behind the urethral orifice and can be observed as a thin vertical slit or as a large orifice with irregular skin edges, depending on the condition of the hymen. The hymen is a membranous, annular, or crescentic fold at the vaginal opening. When unperforated, it is usually a continuous membrane but on occasion may be cribriform. After perforation small rounded fragments of hymen attach to the introital margins; these are called hymenal caruncles.

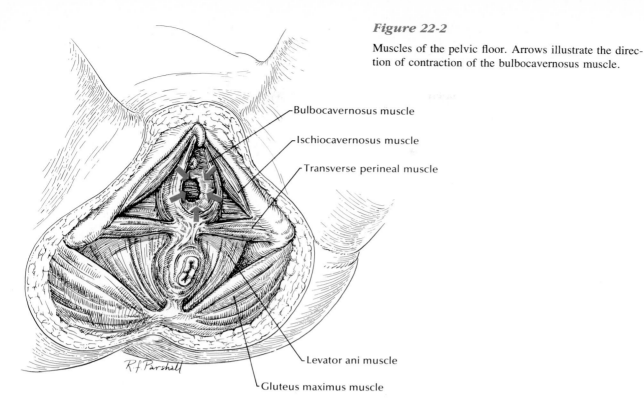

Figure 22-2

Muscles of the pelvic floor. Arrows illustrate the direction of contraction of the bulbocavernosus muscle.

The ducts of two types of glands open on the vulva. Skene's glands are multiple, tiny organs located in the paraurethral area. Their ducts, numbering approximately 6 to 31, lie inside and just outside of the urethral orifice and are usually not visible. These ducts open laterally and slightly posterior to the urethral orifice in approximately the 5 and 7 o'clock positions; the urethral orifice is the center of the clock. Bartholin's glands are small, ovoid organs located lateral and slightly posterior to the vaginal orifice, partially behind the bulb of the vestibule. Their ducts are approximately 2 cm long and open in the groove between the labia minora and the hymen in approximately the 5 and 7 o'clock positions. These ducts are also usually not visible.

The perineum consists of the tissues between the introitus and the anus.

The pelvic floor consists of a group of muscles attached to points on the bony pelvis (Fig. 22-2). These muscles form a suspended sling that assists in holding the pelvic contents in place. The muscles are pierced by the urethral, vaginal, and rectal orifices and function both passively as a pelvic support and actively in voluntary contraction of the vaginal and anal orifices.

Internal Genitalia

Fig. 22-3 illustrates the internal genitalia.

The vagina is a pink, transversely rugated, collapsed tube that in the adult is approximately 9 cm long posteriorly and 6 to 7 cm long anteriorly. It inclines

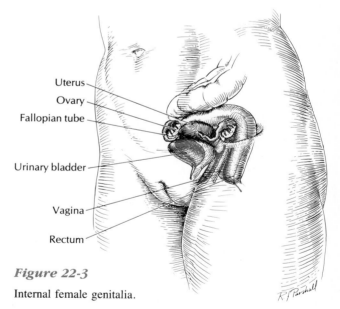

Figure 22-3

Internal female genitalia.

posteriorly at approximately a 45-degree angle with the vertical plane of the body. The vagina is highly dilatable, especially in its superior portion and anteroposterior dimension. When collapsed, it is roughly H shaped in transverse section. Superiorly and usually anteriorly, the vagina is pierced by the uterine cervix. The recess between the portion of the vagina adjacent to the cervix and the cervix is called the vaginal fornix. Although it is actually continuous, the fornix is anatomically divided into anterior, posterior, and lateral fornices.

The uterus is an inverted, pear-shaped, muscular organ that is flattened anteroposteriorly. It is usually found inclined forward 45 degrees from the vertical plane of the erect body and is approximately 5.5 to 8 cm long, 3.5 to 4 cm wide, and 2 to 2.5 cm thick. The uterus of the parous client may be normally enlarged an additional 2 to 3 cm in any of the three dimensions. The uterus is divided into two main parts: the body and the cervix. The body in turn is composed of three parts: the fundus, the prominence above the insertion of the fallopian tubes; the body, or main portion, of the uterus; and the isthmus, the constricted lower portion of the uterus, which is adjacent to the cervix. The cervix extends from the isthmus and into the vagina.

The uterine cavity communicates with the vagina through an ostium, the cervical os. The os is a small, depressed, circular opening in the nulliparous client. In women who have borne children the os is enlarged and irregularly shaped. The position of the uterus is not fixed; it is a relatively movable organ. The uterus may be anteverted, anteflexed, retroverted, or retroflexed in position; or it may be in midposition. (See Table 22-2 for illustration of these positions.) In the normal adult with an empty bladder the uterus is usually anteverted and slightly anteflexed in position.

The ovaries are a pair of oval organs; each is approximately 3 cm long, 2 cm wide, and 1 cm thick. They are usually located near the lateral pelvic wall, at the level of the anterosuperior iliac spine. The two fallopian tubes insert in the upper portion of the uterus, are supported loosely by the broad ligament, and run laterally to the ovaries. Each tube is approximately 10 cm long.

The uterus, ovaries, and tubes are supported by four pairs of ligaments: the cardinal, uterosacral, round, and broad ligaments (Fig. 22-4).

The rectouterine pouch, or Douglas' cul-de-sac, is a deep recess formed by the peritoneum as it passes over the intestinal surface of the rectum. It is the lowest point in the abdominal cavity.

EXAMINATION

Preparation

Clients should be advised not to douche during the 24 hours preceding the pelvic examination and reminded to empty their bladders immediately before the examination.

Materials (see box on p. 551) needed for the examination should be assembled and readily available before the client is put in the lithotomy position.

Some clients have difficulty assuming the lithotomy position, especially moving their buttocks sufficiently downward to the edge of the table. The practi-

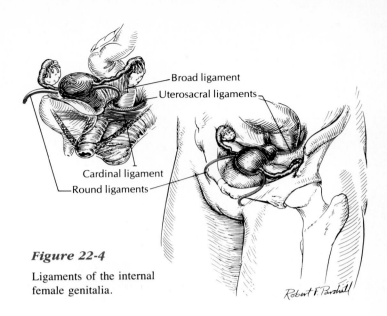

Figure 22-4

Ligaments of the internal female genitalia.

tioner can assist the client (see the box on p. 551) by asking the client to raise her buttocks (while the client is lying on the table with heels in the stirrups) and by guiding the client's buttocks downward from a position at the client's side or from a position at the foot of the table. Clients usually feel more comfortable wearing shoes when their feet are in the stirrups, rather than supporting their weight with bare heels against the hard, cold stirrups.

Components of the Examination

The regional examination of the female genital system consists of (1) the abdominal examination, (2) inspection of the external genitalia, (3) palpation of the external genitalia, (4) the speculum examination, (5) obtaining specimens, (6) the bimanual vaginal examination, and (7) the rectovaginal examination.

The client and the examiner assume several positions for the examination. For the abdominal examination, the client is lying on the examination table and the examiner is facing the client's right side. For the inspection and palpation of the external genitalia and the speculum examination, the client is in the lithotomy position and the examiner is seated on a stool, facing the client's genitalia. For the bimanual examination and the rectovaginal examination, the client remains in the lithotomy position and the examiner is standing.

The abdominal examination is discussed in Chapter 16 on assessment of the abdomen. The examination of the female genital system should be preceded by a thorough examination of the abdomen.

It is recommended that the examiner wear two gloves for the genital area examination. This will allow

Examination Materials

Materials needed for the examination minimally include:
- Rubber gloves
- Speculums of various sizes
- Culture plates for gonorrhea screening
- Glass slides
- Glass cover slides
- Ayre spatulas
- Sterile cotton swabs
- Lubricant on a piece of paper or gauze*
- Cotton balls
- Sponge forceps
- Cytology fixative
- Source of light
- Hand mirror

*An amount of lubricant, sufficient for the examination, should be placed on a piece of paper or gauze. The examiner should avoid handling the whole tube of lubricant during the examination, since it might be contaminated during handling and become a source of infection between clients.

for a thorough external examination and complete spreading of the labia and also will protect subsequent clients from the possible transfer of infection.

Inspection of the external genitalia

The examiner is seated on a stool, facing the external genitalia. First, the skin and hair distribution are observed. Hair distribution should be approximately shaped as an inverse triangle. Some abdominal hair is normal and may be hereditary. Male hair distribution patterns in women are abnormal.

In the adolescent client, sexual maturity is assessed by observation of breast growth and pubic hair growth. Table 22-1 outlines and illustrates sexual maturity ratings for the appearance of the female genitalia. Along with changes in pubic hair, the following also occur:

1. Increase in prominence in labia majora
2. Enlargement of the labia minora
3. Increase in size of the clitoris
4. Increase in elasticity of vaginal tissue
5. Enlargement of vagina and ovaries

The total skin area is inspected for lesions and parasites. The gloved fingers of one hand are used to spread the hair and labia so that all skin surfaces can be adequately visualized. Although the client knows she will be touched, she may startle when the fingers are placed on the genitalia for the initiation of the palpation. In an anxious client, touching the client's inner thigh with the back of a hand might prevent excess tensing of pelvic muscles.

Assisting the Client into the Lithotomy Position

1. Instruct the client to lie down on the examination table and assist her to put her heels (with shoes on) into the stirrups and to stabilize them.
2. Retract the end of the table if it is still extended.
3. Assist the woman to bring her buttocks to the very edge of the table. Gentle guidance by the examiner or advising the woman to feel for and aim for the end of the table herself are useful mechanisms of assistance.
4. Redrape the client so that the knees and symphysis pubis are covered. Depress the drape between the knees so that the examiner can view the client face to face during the examination.

The labia are flat in childhood and atrophic in old age. Estrogen influences fat deposition, which causes a round, full appearance of the labia. The labia majora of the nulliparous client will be in close approximation covering the labia minora and the vestibule area. After a vaginal delivery, the labia may appear slightly shriveled and gaping. They appear reasonably symmetric.

The skin of the vulvar area is a slightly darker pigment than the skin of the rest of the body. The mucous membranes are normally dark pink in color and moist in appearance.

Common abnormalities of the skin and labia include parasites, skin lesions of all types, areas of leukoplakia, varicosities, hyperpigmentation, erythema, depigmentation, and swelling. Leukoplakia appears as white, adherent patches on the skin; it may be likened to spots of dried white paint.

The clitoris is examined for size; the visible portion of the clitoris should not exceed 2 cm in length and 1 cm in width. The area of the clitoris particularly is a common site for chancres of syphilis in the younger client and for cancerous lesions in the older client.

The urethral orifice normally appears slitlike or stellate and is of the same color as the membranes surrounding it. The openings of the paraurethral (Skene's) glands are not usually visible. Erythema or a polyp located in this area or a discharge from the urethra or gland ducts is abnormal.

The examiner next observes the area of Bartholin's glands and their ducts for swelling, erythema, duct enlargement, or discharge. The presence of any of these conditions is abnormal.

The perineum is inspected for evidence of an episiotomy and its healing. The anus is also inspected at this time (see Chapter 16 on assessment of the abdomen).

Table 22-1

Developmental changes in the general appearance of female genitalia

Developmental stage	Description	Developmental stage	Description
Stage 1 sexual maturity (preadolescence)	No pubic hair, except for fine body hair	Stage 4 sexual maturity	Texture and curl of pubic hair as in adult but not as thick and not spread over the thighs (usually seen between ages 13 and 14)
Stage 2 sexual maturity	Sparse growth of long, slightly pigmented, fine pubic hair, which is slightly curly and located along the labia (usually seen at ages 11 to 12)	Stage 5 sexual maturity	Adult appearance in quality and quantity of pubic hair; growth is spread onto the inner aspect of the upper thighs
Stage 3 sexual maturity	Pubic hair becomes darker, curlier, and spreads over the symphysis (usually seen at ages 12 to 13)	Elderly	Pubic hair is thin, sparse, brittle, and gray

Palpation of the external genitalia

One gloved hand is used to spread the labia open while the other hand is used to palpate generally the labia major and labia minora. The labia should feel soft, and the texture should be homogeneous. Any areas of observed abnormality below the skin surface are palpated to determine the size, shape, consistency, and tenderness of any mass or lesion.

The index finger and the middle finger are inserted into the vagina. First, the urethra and area of Skene's duct openings are gently milked from about the level of 4 cm in on the anterior vaginal wall down to the orifice (Fig. 22-5). This procedure should not normally cause pain or discharge. If a discharge is present, a specimen is inoculated onto a Thayer-Martin culture plate. Then the area of Bartholin's glands and their ducts are palpated for swelling or tenderness (Fig. 22-6). Normally Bartholin's glands are not palpable.

While the examiner's fingers are in the vagina, several maneuvers are performed to assess the integrity

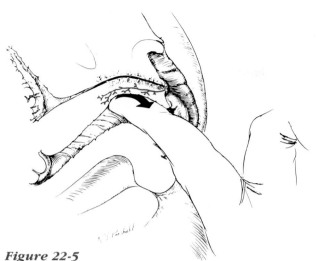

Figure 22-5

Palpation of Skene's glands.

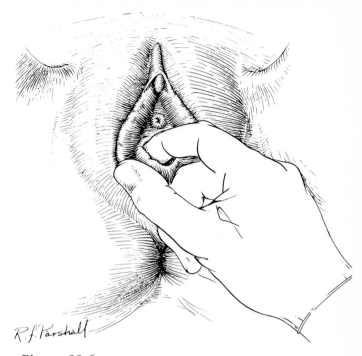

R.f.Parshall

Figure 22-6

Palpation of Bartholin's glands.

of the pelvic musculature. First, the perineal area is palpated between the fingers inside the vagina and the thumb of that same hand. In the nulliparous client the perineum is felt as a firm, muscular body. After an episiotomy has healed, the perineum feels thinner and more rigid because of scarring. If this area is very thin and if the palpating fingers can almost approximate, the client should be questioned again about bowel or sexual problems.

The client is then asked to constrict her vaginal orifice around the examiner's fingers while they are placed in the vagina. A nulliparous client will demonstrate a high degree of tone; a multiparous client, less tone.

In the third maneuver the index and middle fingers remain in the vagina; they are spread laterally, and the client is asked to push down against them. The presence of urinary stress incontinence, cystocele, rectocele, enterocele, or uterine prolapse can be observed if present.

Cystocele is the prolapse into the vagina of the anterior vaginal wall and the bladder. Clinically, a pouching would be seen on the anterior wall as the client strains.

Rectocele is the prolapse into the vagina of the posterior vaginal wall and the rectum. Clinically, a pouching would be seen on the posterior wall as the client strains.

Enterocele is a hernia of the pouch of Douglas into the vagina. Clinically, a bulge would be seen emerging from the posterior fornix. If this is observed, the client should be additionally examined by assessing the effect of straining (1) during the speculum examination with the inserted speculum, half opened, three fourths of its length into the vagina; and (2) during the bimanual examination with the intravaginal fingers in the posterior fornix.

There are three degrees of *uterine prolapse*. In first-degree prolapse, the cervix appears at the introitus when the client strains. In second-degree prolapse, the cervix is outside of the introitus when the client strains. In third-degree prolapse, the whole uterus is outside the introitus and the vagina is essentially turned inside out when the client strains.

Speculum examination

The examiner will have obtained clues regarding the most appropriate type and size of speculum to use in the speculum examination through the history and inspection of the external genitalia. There are two basic types of speculums, the Graves speculum and the Pederson speculum (Fig. 22-7 and see the box on p. 554). The Graves speculum is one of the most commonly used in examination of the adult female client. It is available in lengths varying from 3½ to 5 in and in widths from ¾ to 1½ in. The Pederson speculum is both narrower and flatter than the Graves speculum and is used with virgins, nulliparous clients, or clients whose vaginal orifices have contracted postmenopausally.

A metal speculum should be warmed before insertion. An effective way to do this is by running warm water over it. Lubricant is bacteriostatic and also distorts cells on Papanicolaou (Pap) smears; thus, it cannot be used if a culture or smear is to be obtained. The warm

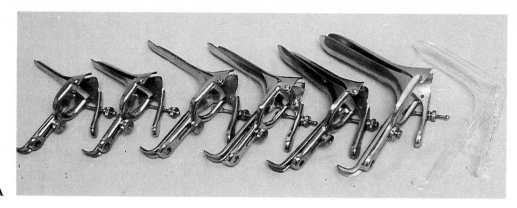

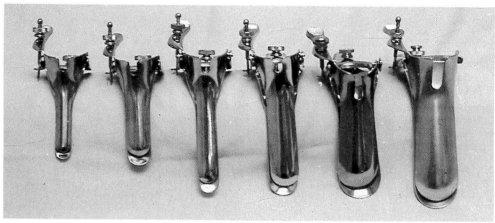

Figure 22-7

Vaginal specula. From left to right. **A,** Short-billed pediatric, pediatric, small Pederson, Pederson, small Graves, large Graves, plastic Graves. **B,** Short-billed pediatric, pediatric, small Pederson, Pederson, small Graves, large Graves.
(From Seidel HM and others: Mosby's guide to physical examination, St Louis, 1987, The CV Mosby Co.)

About Speculums

A vaginal speculum consists of two blades, a handle, and some mechanism to open the distal end of the blades. Vaginal speculums may be reusable metal or disposable plastic and are available in two basic types and a variety of sizes within each of the types. The Graves speculum is the commonly used type; the Pederson speculum, with flatter and narrower blades than the Graves, is used for women with narrow vaginal openings.

Metal and plastic specula operate somewhat differently, although both have levers that, when depressed, open the distal ends of the blades; mechanisms that allow for separation of the proximal ends of the blades; and locking mechanisms. Metal speculums have two positioning devices: depression of the lever opens the distal end of the blades, and fixing of the screw on the lever locks the blades open at that point. In addition, the opening at the proximal ends of the blades can be widened and locked open by loosening and then refitting a plate attached to both the handle of the speculum and the upper blade.

The distal and proximal blade-opening mechanisms are connected in the plastic speculum. As the plastic lever is depressed in the plastic speculum, the distal end of the blades open; if the lever is fully dpressed and then pushed upward on the handle, the proximal ends of the blades also open. The lever fixes automatically into grooves on the handle of the speculum. The clicking sound of the plastic speculum is loud and sharp and is perceived as alarming to some clients, who think that the speculum is breaking inside of them. Anticipatory warning about the sound of the plastic mechanism is advised.

Because each type of speculum operates differently, the beginning examiner should spend some time practicing with the mechanisms apart from actual examinations and before use with clients.

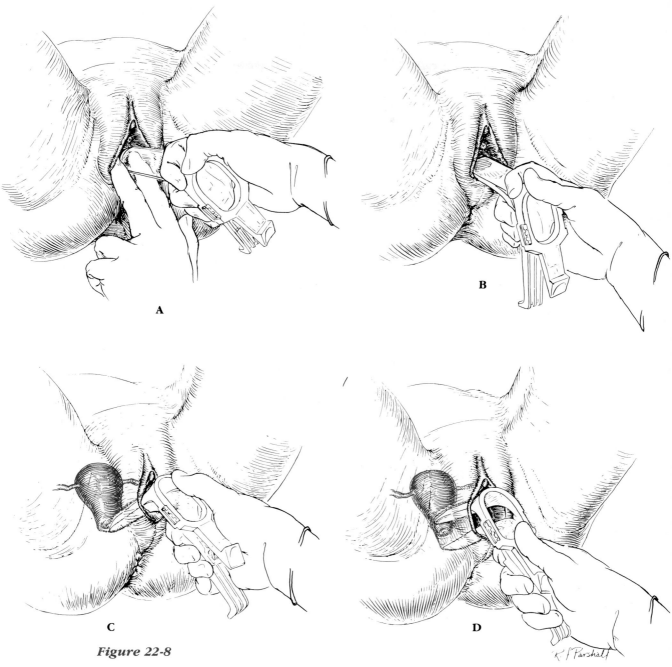

Figure 22-8

Procedure for vaginal examination. **A,** Opening of the introitus. **B,** Oblique insertion of the speculum. **C,** Final insertion of the speculum. **D,** Opening of the speculum blades.

water also assists in lubricating both the metal and plastic speculums and may be used if cultures and smears are to be taken.

The index finger and middle finger of one hand are placed 1 in into the vagina. The fingers are then spread, and pressure is exerted toward the posterior vaginal wall. The client is advised that she will feel intravaginal pressure. The speculum is held in the opposite hand with the blades between the index and middle fin-

gers. The client is asked to bear down. This maneuver helps to additionally open the vaginal orifice and to relax perineal muscles (Fig. 22-8).

The speculum blades are inserted obliquely, taking advantage of the H configuration of the relaxed vagina (Fig. 22-8, *B*). They are inserted at a plane parallel to the examining table until the end of the speculum has reached the tips of the fingers in the vagina.

The speculum is then rotated to a transverse position, and the plane is altered in adaptation to the plane of the vagina, approximately one of a 45-degree angle with the examining table (Fig. 22-8, *C*). The intravaginal fingers are simultaneously withdrawn, and the speculum is inserted until it touches the end of the vagina. The lever of the speculum is then depressed; this opens the blades and allows visualization. Ideally, the cervix is seen between the blades (Fig. 22-8, *D*). Sometimes, however, especially for the beginning examiner, it is not. In such cases the speculum is either anterior (usually the situation) or posterior to the cervix. If this occurs, the speculum is withdrawn halfway and reinserted in a different plane. After the entire cervix is in view of the examiner, the depressed lever is fixed in an open position.

If the client is tense and is resisting insertion of the speculum, the examiner should not withdraw the speculum but stop the insertion and leave the speculum in its position, remind the client to use relaxation techniques, and continue the examination when relaxation has occurred.

The appearance of the normal cervix has already been described. The cervix is observed for color, position, size, projection into the vaginal vault, shape, general symmetry, surface characteristics, shape and patency of the os, and discharge:

1. *Color:* The cervix is normally pale after menopause and cyanotic in pregnancy. Cyanosis can occur with any condition that causes systemic hypoxia or regional venous congestion. Hyperemia may indicate inflammation. An additional cause of pallor is anemia.
2. *Position:* A cervix projecting more deeply than 3 cm into the vaginal vault may indicate uterine prolapse. A cervix situated on a lateral vaginal wall may indicate tumor or adhesion of a superior structure.
3. *Size:* A cervix larger than 4 cm in diameter is hypertrophied, and the presence of inflammation or tumor should be considered.
4. *Surface characteristics:* Lesions and polyps are commonly seen on the cervix and require more than visual assessment to determine if a pathologic condition exists. Any irregularity or nodularity of the cervical surface should be considered possibly abnormal (Fig. 22-9). One relatively benign condition is the presence of nabothian cysts, which appear as smooth, round, small (less than 1 cm in diameter) yellow lesions. Nabothian cysts are caused by obstruction of the cervical gland ducts.

When the squamocolumnar junction is on the ectocervix, the columnar epithelium will appear as a red, relatively symmetric circle around the os. This condition may be a normal variation of the placement of the squamocolumnar junction or may be caused by the separation

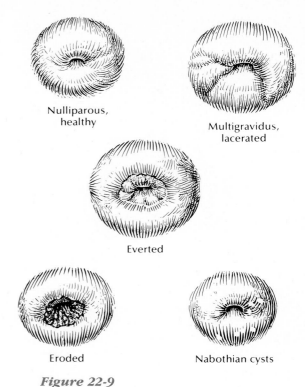

Figure 22-9

Common appearances and lesions of the cervix.

by speculum blades of a cervix whose external os has been altered and enlarged by childbirth. This condition is termed *eversion* or *ectropion*. Erosions appear similar to eversions but are usually irregular, rough, and friable. Erosions frequently indicate a pathologic condition and require further assessment and treatment. Because of the occasional presence of the squamocolumnar junction on the ectocervix, the differential assessment of normal cervix from abnormal cervix using inspection alone is impossible.

Diffuse punctate hemorrhages, colloquially termed "strawberry spots," are occasionally observed in association with trichomonal infections.

5. *Discharge:* The character of the normal cervical mucus varies in the menstrual cycle. It is always odorless and nonirritating. Its color and consistency may vary from clear to white and from thin to thick and stringy. Colored or purulent discharges exuding from the os or present in the area of the cervix are probably abnormal.

6. *Shape of the os:* The cervical os of the nulliparous client is small and evenly round. The cervical os of a parous client shows the effects of the stretching and laceration of childbirth and is irregular in shape.

Many clients have not seen their cervices. The client should be asked if she wishes to see her cervix.

This visualization can easily be accomplished through the use of a hand mirror.

After the cervix is inspected, a Pap smear, culture for gonorrhea, and hanging drop specimen may be obtained if indicated. The procedures for these are described at the end of this chapter. The vagina is then inspected. This is done during speculum insertion, while the speculum is open, and during its removal. The color and condition of the vaginal mucosa and the color, odor, consistency, and appearance of vaginal secretions are noted. Pallor, cyanosis, and hyperemia may be present for the same reasons as described for the cervix. Leukoplakia may also occur on vaginal mucosa.

As with cervical discharge, vaginal discharge is normally odorless, nonirritating, thin or mucoid, and clear or cloudy. Also, the presence of some whitish, creamy material is normal. Any other vaginal discharge should be described according to its color, odor, consistency, amount, and appearance. Three basic types of vaginal infections produce observable discharge: monilial infections, characterized by thick, white, curdy exudates that appear as adherent patches and free discharge; trichomonal infections, characterized by a profuse watery, gray or green, frothy, odorous discharge; and bacterial infections, characterized by an odorous, gray, homogeneous discharge of moderate amount.

After the inspection of the vaginal area, the speculum is slowly withdrawn. As it is withdrawn, the nut, or catch, is loosened and the lever is again controlled by the thumb. The blades are slowly closed as they are removed, and the speculum is carefully rotated so that all areas of vaginal tissue are inspected. As the blades are closed, caution is taken to prevent pinching of tissue or the catching of hairs in the blades.

The speculum is inspected for odors and is either discarded (plastic) or placed in a soaking solution (metal).

Bimanual vaginal examination

The purpose of the bimanual examination is the palpation of the pelvic contents between the examiner's two hands (Figs. 22-10 and 22-11). Examiners vary in their preference of the placement of the dominant, more sensitive hand. The beginning examiner should attempt alternating hands for examinations and then decide on a routine that is most workable.

The client remains in the lithotomy position. The examiner stands between the client's legs. The vaginal examining hand assumes the obstetric position: index and middle fingers extended and together, thumb abducted, and fourth and little fingers folded on the palm of the hand. The vaginal examining fingers are lubricated. The

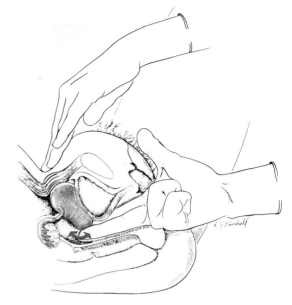

Figure 22-10

Bimanual palpation of the uterus.

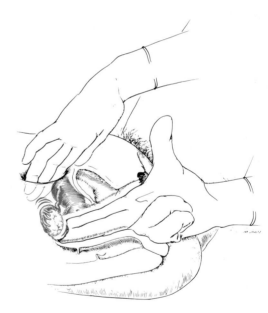

Figure 22-11

Bimanual palpation of the adnexa.

labia are spread with the thumb and index finger of the opposite hand. The lubricated fingers are inserted into the vagina with the palmar surface of the hand directed toward the anterior vaginal wall. The examiner should always palpate with the palmar surface of the fingers rather than with the less sensitive tips or backs. In the case of a young or old client with a small and narrow vagina, the examination may be performed with one intravaginal finger. The other hand is placed on the abdomen. This hand will be used to press the abdominal and pelvic contacts toward the intravaginal hand. Movement of both hands should be slow and firm. For the examiner to palpate adequately, the client must be relaxed. If the client becomes tense, the procedure is stopped and the client is helped to relax; however, the examiner's hands remain in position.

The cervix is located and assessed for size, contour, surface characteristics, consistency, position, patency of the os, and mobility. The palmar surfaces of both fingers are used to completely palpate the cervix and fornices. A fingertip is gently placed into the external os to assess its patency. It is determined on which vaginal wall the cervix is placed and if the cervix is approxi-

mately midline. The fingers are placed in the lateral fornices, and the cervix is wagged, or moved back and forth, between the fingers for approximately 1 to 2 cm in each direction. The cervix and uterus should be freely movable and should move without tenderness. An immobile or tender cervix and uterus are abnormal.

The surface of the cervix is normally smooth. Nabothian cysts, tumors, or lesions will make it feel nodular or irregular. The consistency of the cervix is firm and slightly resilient and feels analogous to the tip of the nose. The cervix softens in pregnancy and hardens with tumors. The cervix is normally located on the anterior wall in the midline or on the posterior wall. A laterally displaced cervix may indicate tumor or adhesion. The

---

Table 22-2

Findings in bimanual vaginal and rectovaginal examination

| Position of uterus | Bimanual | |
	Position of the cervix	Body and fundus
Anteverted	Anterior vaginal wall	Palpable by one hand on the abdomen and the fingers of the other in the vagina
Midposition	The apex of the vagina	May not be palpable

external os in the nonpregnant client should admit a finger for about ¼ in. It should be open and firm. A stenosed external os is abnormal.

The size, shape, surface characteristics, consistency, position, mobility, and tenderness of the uterine body and fundus are assessed. First it is useful to determine the position of the uterus because techniques used to assess the uterine body and fundus will vary with the uterine position in the client (Table 22-2). The uterus is in one of the three basic positions: anteversion, midposition, or retroversion. Version in this context indicates deflection, specifically the relationship of the long axis of the uterus to the long axis of the body. If the axis of the uterus is deflected anteriorly, the uterus is said to be anteverted; if the uterus is deflected posteriorly, the uterus is said to be retroverted; and if the long axis of the uterus is roughly parallel to that of the total body, the uterus is in mid-position. When the long axis of the uterus is not straight but is bent on itself, the uterus is said to be flexed. Thus, the anteverted or retroverted uterus can be flexed, or bent on itself, to produce two additional variations of position: anteflexion and retroflexion.

The position of the cervix provides the examiner with clues of the uterine position. A cervix on the anterior wall may indicate an antepositioned or retroflexed uterus; a centrally located cervix probably indicates a uterus in midposition; and a cervix on the posterior vaginal wall implies a uterus in retroposition.

Anterior and posterior portion of uterus	Rectovaginal	
	Cervix	Body and fundus
Palpable as the uterus is rotated even more anteriorly	Palpable through the rectovaginal septum	Not palpable by fingers in the rectum
May not be palpable	Posterior portion felt through the rectovaginal septum	May not be palpable

Continued

Table 22-2

Findings in bimanual vaginal and rectovaginal examination—*cont'd*

| Position of uterus | Bimanual | |
	Position of the cervix	Body and fundus
Retroverted	Posterior vaginal wall	Not palpable
Anteflexed	Anterior vaginal wall or apex	Easily palpable; angulation of the isthmus may be felt in the anterior fornix
Retroflexed	Anterior or posterior vaginal wall or apex	Not palpable

| Anterior and posterior portion of uterus | Rectovaginal | |
	Cervix	Body and fundus
Posterior portion may be palpable by fingers in the posterior fornix	May not be palpable by fingers in the rectum	Body easily palpable by fingers in the rectum; fundus may not be palpable
Easily palpable	Same as anteverted	Same as anteverted
Not palpable	Palpable through the rectovaginal septum	Angulation palpable; body and fundus easily palpable

Approximately 85% of uteri are in anteposition; therefore, palpation is first attempted anteriorly. The intravaginal fingers are placed in the anterior fornix. The hand on the abdomen is placed flat on the midline and in a position approximately halfway between the symphysis pubis and the umbilicus. This hand acts as a resistance against which the pelvic organs are palpated by the intravaginal fingers. The fingers in the anterior fornix gently lift the tissues against the hand on the abdomen. If the uterus is in anteposition, it will be palpated between the hands. If the uterus is not palpated anteriorly, the fingers are placed in the posterior fornix and again raised forward toward the hand on the abdomen. If the uterus is in retroversion, only the isthmus will be felt between the hands and the corpus may be felt with the backs of the intravaginal fingers. A retroverted uterus is felt best during the rectovaginal examination.

If the uterus is identified as being in anteposition or midposition, an attempt is made to palpate all its anterior and posterior surfaces by maneuvering its position and by "walking up" its surface with the intravaginal fingers. After the uterus is palpated, the adnexal areas are examined. The structures in these areas are of a size, consistency, and position that they may not be specifically palpated. If the examiner has appropriately examined the area and no masses larger than the normal-size ovaries are identified, it is assumed that no masses are present.

Each of the adnexal areas, left and right, is palpated. The index and middle finger of the intravaginal hand are placed in one of the lateral fornices; the hand on the abdomen is placed on the ipsilateral iliac crest; and the hands are brought together and moved in an inferior and medial direction, allowing the tissues lying between the two hands to slip between them (see Fig. 22-11). The hand on the abdomen acts as resistance, and the intravaginal hand palpates the organs between the hands. Frequently, no specific organ is palpated in this maneuver. If normal ovaries are palpated, they are smooth, firm, slightly flattened, ovoid, and no larger than 4 to 6 cm in their largest dimension. Ovaries of prepubertal girls or postmenopausal women are normally smaller than 4 cm in their largest dimension. The ovaries are sensitive to touch but are not tender. They are highly movable and will easily slip between the palpating hands.

Normal fallopian tubes are not palpable. One clue to an ectopic pregnancy is the presence of arterial pulses in the adnexal areas.

Cordlike structures that are sometimes palpable are round ligaments.

Rectovaginal examination

The rectovaginal examination is uncomfortable for most women; however, because it enables examination not pos-

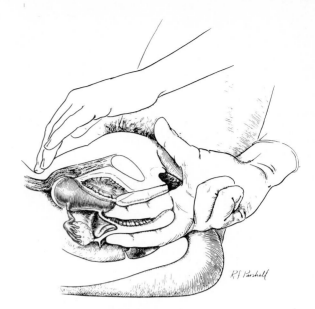

Figure 22-12

Rectovaginal palpation.

sible through the vaginal examination alone, it is recommended in all complete vaginal examinations. The rectovaginal examination allows for greater depth (1 in higher) than the vaginal examination and enables assessment of the posterior portion of the uterus and pelvic cavity. Because the examination is uncomfortable, the client should be prepared for it by instruction regarding its purpose and anticipatory guidance about the possible feeling of urgency for bowel movement.

After the vaginal examination is completed, the intravaginal hand is withdrawn, the glove on the internal examining hand is changed to prevent the possible transfer of infection from the vagina into the rectum, and the index and middle fingers are lubricated. The client is advised that the next procedure is the last part of the pelvic examination and is reminded to cooperate by relaxing the muscles. Next, the client is asked to bear down. Then, the index finger is placed into the vagina and is placed in the posterior fornix of the cervix, and the middle finger is placed into the rectum. Both fingers are inserted as far as possible. The other hand is placed above the symphysis, as for the vaginal examination, and depressed to enable the rectal finger to palpate the posterior portion of the uterus.

The uterine position is confirmed by the rectal examination. If the uterus is retroverted, its body and fundus are now palpated. In addition, the adnexal areas are reassessed. The procedure is the same as that described with the vaginal examination (Fig. 22-12).

The area of the rectovaginal septum and cul-de-sac is palpated. The rectovaginal septum should be palpated as a firm, thin, smooth, pliable structure. The pos-

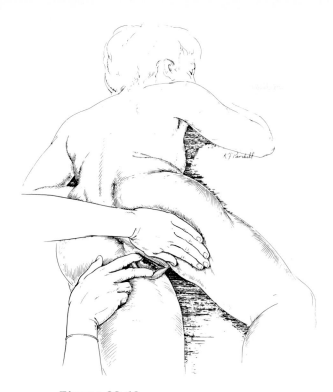

Figure 22-13

Left lateral position for genital examination.

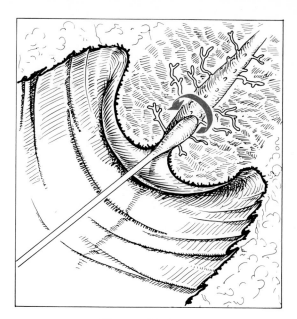

Figure 22-14

Endocervical smear.

terior cul-de-sac is a potential space. The normal pelvic organs are palpated through it. Often, abnormal masses and normal ovaries are discovered in the cul-de-sac.

Uterosacral ligaments may be palpable.

The rectal examination is completed (see Chapter 17 on assessment of the anus and rectosigmoid region), and the client is helped to sit up.

Because of the amount of lubricant used in the examination, the client will feel somewhat sticky. The examiner should provide her with disposable materials to clean herself and allow her to dress partially or completely (depending on the structure of the examination). Often the pelvic and rectal examinations are the very last portions of the physical assessment, and complete dressing occurs before consultation.

Examination of Clients Who Are Unable to Assume the Lithotomy Position

The lithotomy position is the optimum one for a pelvic examination. However, it may be difficult for a very ill or debilitated client to assume and maintain a lithotomy position. An alternative position for the female genital examination is a left lateral or Sims' position (Fig. 22-13). The client's buttocks should be close to the edge of the examining table as safety allows. The right leg is positioned on top of or over the left leg and bent and abducted. The examiner stands behind and at the side

of the client. All the examination procedures described previously in this chapter can be performed with the client in this position.

Procedures for Smears and Cultures

CERVICAL PAPANICOLAOU SMEAR

The client is in the lithotomy position, and the speculum has been inserted. All materials listed earlier in the chapter are assembled. If a cervical mucus plug is present, it can be removed with a cotton ball held with forceps. There are many variations among laboratories regarding the areas from which cell samples are to be obtained, the mixing of cells from two or more areas, and the fixing of cells. One procedure is described here. However, variations are acceptable, and the practitioner should consult with the cytopathologist reading the smears for locally recommended procedures.

Endocervical Smear

Fig. 22-14 illustrates the procedure for an endocervical smear:

1. A sterile applicator is inserted approximately 0.5 cm into the cervical os. It is rotated 360 degrees and left in 10 to 20 seconds to ensure saturation.
2. The endocervical smear is spread on a slide labeled "endocervix." The swab is rotated so that all sampled areas are smeared on the slide. The smear should not contain thick areas that would be difficult to visualize microscopically. The slide is immediately fixed by a spray fix or immersion into a fixative solution.

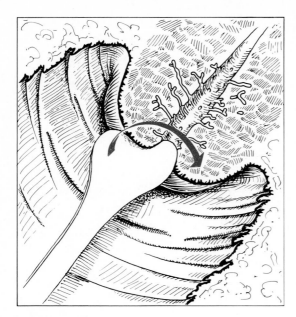

Figure 22-15

Cervical smear.

Cervical Smear

Fig. 22-15 illustrates the procedure for a cervical smear:
1. The larger humped end of the Ayre spatula is inserted into the cervical os so that the cervix fits comfortably into the groove created by the two humps. With moderate pressure, the spatula is rotated 360 degrees, scraping the entire cervical surface and the squamo-columnar junction.
2. The material from both sides of the spatula is spread on a slide marked "cervix."
3. The slide is fixed immediately.

Vaginal Pool Smear

1. With the paddle or handle end of the Ayre spatula, the area of the posterior cervical fornix is scraped.
2. The material on the spatula is spread in the area marked "vaginal pool."
3. The slide is fixed immediately by spraying or immersion into a fixative solution.

GONORRHEAL CULTURE

The female client is in the lithotomy position with a speculum inserted. If there is a history of oral intercourse, an oropharyngeal culture may be indicated also.

Endocervical Culture

1. A specimen from the endocervical canal is obtained with a sterile cotton applicator. The technique is the same as that described for the Pap smear.

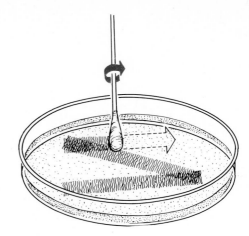

Figure 22-16

Inoculation of the Thayer-Martin culture.

2. The Thayer-Martin culture plate is inoculated. With the medium at room temperature, the swab is rolled in a large Z pattern on the culture plate; the swab is simultaneously rotated as it is creating the Z so that all swab surfaces will be inoculated (Fig. 22-16).
3. The culture plate is incubated within 15 minutes of its inoculation in a warm, anaerobic environment. The culture plate is placed medium side up in a candle jar, the candle is lit, the cover of the jar is tightly secured, and the jar is left in a warm area until specimens can be placed in an incubator. In some clinics the inoculation is immediately cross-streaked with a sterile

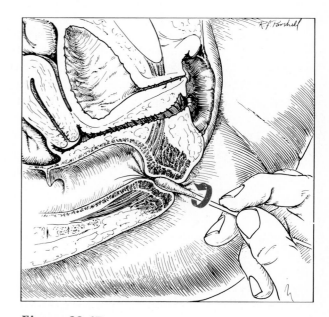

Figure 22-17

Anal smear.

wire loop. Usually, however, this is done in the laboratory, not in the examining room.

Anal Culture

Fig. 22-17 illustrates the procedure for an anal culture:
1. A sterile cotton-tipped applicator is inserted into the anal canal. The applicator is rotated 360 degrees and moved from side to side. It is left in for 10 to 30 seconds to allow for absorption of secretion and organisms. If the swab contains feces, it is discarded and another specimen taken.

2. The culture plate is inoculated and incubated as described previously, using a separate culture plate.

Oropharyngeal Culture

1. A specimen of secretion from the oropharynx is obtained with a sterile swab.
2. The medium is inoculated and incubated as described for endocervical specimens.

Health History
Female Genitalia

NOTE: A yes response to any question *must* be further investigated. Use the following indicators throughout the assessment: (1) onset (specific date, sudden or gradual), (2) duration, (3) frequency, (4) precipitating factors, (5) aggravating or alleviating factors, (6) treatment received, and (7) outcome.

Present status

1. When was your last pap smear?
   a. Date
   b. Results
2. Have your menses stopped?
   a. At what age
   b. Associated symptoms: sweating, hot flushes, mood swings
3. Do you have lower abdominal pain?
   a. Location
   b. Description: sharp, dull, aching, burning, knifelike, fullness
   c. Intensity: intolerable, tolerable
   d. Associated symptoms: malaise, nausea, vomiting, constipation
4. Are your menses regular or irregular?
   a. Time frame: be specific
5. Do you have symptoms associated with your menses?
   a. Description: pain, cramping, distention, weight gain, irritability, mood swings
6. What is the amount of menses flow?
   a. Number of pads or tampons used
7. Do you have a vaginal discharge?
   a. Description: consistency, amount, color, itching
8. Do you use oral contraceptives?
   a. Type
   b. How long used

Past history

1. At what age did your menses start?
2. Have you had any reproductive surgery?
   a. Type

b. When performed
   c. Residual effects
3. Have you had any pregnancies?
   a. Number
   b. Number of viable children
4. Have you had any miscarriages?
   a. Number
   b. At what stage
5. Have you or a sexual partner had a sexually transmitted disease?
   a. Type: gonorrhea, syphillis, herpes, hepatitis, AIDS, clymedia, condoloma

Associated conditions

1. Do you have diabetes?
2. Do you have endometriosis?

Family history

1. Do you have family history of reproductive problems?
   a. Obstetrical problems
   b. Reproductive organ cancer
   c. Endometriosis
2. Is there a family history of diabetes?

Sample assessment record

Client complains of constant, dull, aching pain in lower abdomen and lower back and of feeling tired and weak. Discomfort began 5 to 6 weeks ago following a 100° fever. No noted alleviating or aggravating factors. Menses began at age 13. Denies change in menses which are regular (every 30 days) with moderate flow (uses total of seven tampons in 3 days). Has had foul smelling vaginal discharge for last 4 weeks. Has had no pregnancies or miscarriages. Has used oral contraceptives for last 4 years. Denies exposure to any sexually transmitted diseases. Denies diabetes and has no family history of reproductive cancers or diabetes.

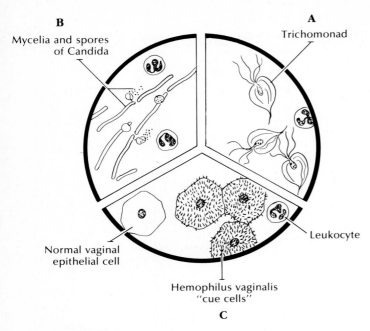

B
Mycelia and spores
of Candida

A
Trichomonad

Normal vaginal
epithelial cell

Leukocyte

Hemophilus vaginalis
"cue cells"

C

Figure 22-18

Microscopic appearance of vaginal microorganisms. **A,** *Trichomonas.* **B,** Mycelia and spores. **C,** Epithelial cells stippled by *Hemophilus vaginalis* bacteria.

SMEARS FOR VAGINAL INFECTIONS

1. A specimen of vaginal secretions is obtained directly from the vagina or from material in the inferior speculum blade. For *Trichomonas vaginalis,* the secretions are mixed with a drop of normal saline solution on a glass slide. For *Candida albicans,* the secretions are mixed with a drop of 10% potassium hydroxide solution on a slide. For *Hemophilus vaginalis,* the secretions are not mixed with any solution.

2. A cover glass is placed on the slide.

3. The slide is immediately observed under a microscope (Fig. 22-18). If positive for *T. vaginalis,* trichomonads will be seen. These are single-cell flagellates about the size of a white blood cell. If positive for *C. albicans,* mycelia and spores are seen. If positive for *H. vaginalis,* characteristic "cue cells" are seen.

BIBLIOGRAPHY

Droegemueller W, Herbst AL, Mishell DR, and Stenchever MA: Comprehensive gynecology, St Louis, 1987, The CV Mosby Co.

Fogel CI and Woods NF: Health care of women: a nursing perspective, St Louis, 1981, The CV Mosby Co.

Garrey MM and others: Obstetrics illustrated, ed 3, Edinburgh, 1980, Churchill Livingstone.

Howkins J and Hudson CN: Shaw's textbook of operative gynecology, Edinburgh, 1983, Churchill Livingstone.

Hughes EC, editor: Obstetric-gynecologic terminology, Philadelphia, 1972, WB Saunders Co.

Kistner RW: Gynecology: principles and practice, ed 4, Chicago, 1986, Year Book Medical Publishers.

Novak ER, Jones GS, and Jones HW, Jr: Textbook of gynecology, ed 10, Baltimore, 1981, Williams & Wilkins.

Olsson HM and Gullberg MT: Role of the woman patient and fear of the pelvic examination, West J Nurs Res 9:357-367, 1987.

Tanner JM: Growth of adolescence, ed 2, Oxford, 1962, Blackwell Scientific Publications.

Tunnadine P: The role of genital examination in psychosexual medicine, Clin Obstet Gynecol 7:283, 1980.

U.S. Department of Health, Education, and Welfare: Criteria and techniques for the diagnosis of gonorrhea, Atlanta, 1974, U.S. Public Health Service.

Wallis LA, Tardiff K, and Deane K: Evaluation of teaching programs for male and female genital examinations, J Med Ed 8:664-666, 1983.

Willson RJ, Carrington ER, and Ledger WJ: Obstetrics and gynecology, ed 7, St Louis, 1983, The CV Mosby Co.

Worth AM, Dougherty MC, and McKey PL: Development and testing of the circumvaginal rating scale, Nurs Res 35:166-168, 1986.

III
Health Assessment
Across the Life Span

23

Assessment of the pregnant client

OBJECTIVES

Upon successful review of this chapter, learners will be able to:

- Describe anatomic and physiologic changes that occur in normal pregnancy

- Outline factors important to a reproductive history

- Delineate prenatal risk factors

- Recognize physical signs of pregnancy associated with each stage of fetal development

- State related rationale and demonstrate prenatal assessment, including five procedures essential to each prenatal visit

- Delineate usual findings of abdominal inspection, measurement, palpation, and auscultation, including
  Fundal characteristics
  Fetal characteristics
  Fetal heart tones and uterine souffle

- Delineate measurement techniques for the bony pelvis, including usual findings and common variations

In this chapter the physical changes that occur in normal pregnancy are presented, as well as the adaptation of the health history and the physical examination for the pregnant client. The student practitioner should either know or review the performance of the female genital examination presented in Chapter 22 because it is a component of the assessment of the prenatal client. That assessment procedure will not be repeated here except as the examination or findings may change in pregnancy.

PHYSICAL CHANGES IN PREGNANCY

Hormonal Changes

All the physiologic changes of pregnancy are directly or indirectly initiated by the hormones produced by the fetal chorionic tissues and placenta. In early pregnancy, the fetal trophoblast produces large amounts of human chorionic gonadotropic hormone (HCG) that provides the basis for biologic pregnancy testing. HCG is present in detectable amounts by immunologic tests 8 to 10 days after conception.

Large amounts of estrogens and progesterone are produced during pregnancy. Estriol, an estrogen, is produced in large amounts during middle and late pregnancy. Estriol is the basis for biologic tests of placental and fetal well-being because a well-functioning placenta, a healthy fetus, and intact fetal circulation are prerequisites for the continuous production of this hormone. The estrogens and progesterone maintain the decidua of pregnancy and cause the growth and hyperemia of the uterus, other pelvic organs, and the breasts.

The thyroid gland is enlarged in over 50% of prenatal clients as a result of hyperplasia of glandular tissue, new follicle formation, and increased vascularity. The basal metabolic rate is increased largely because of increased growth and oxygen consumption by the pregnant uterus, the fetus, and the placenta.

Uterine, Cervical, and Vaginal Changes

Changes in the uterus include the development of the decidua, hypertrophy of muscle cells, increased vascularity, formation of the lower uterine segment, and softening of the cervix. The overall size of the uterus increases 5 to 6 times, the weight increases about 20 times, and the capacity increases from approximately 2 to 5000 ml.

Hormones supply the initial stimulus for uterine hypertrophy. During the first 6 to 8 weeks of pregnancy, the uterus will increase in size whether the pregnancy is uterine or extrauterine. In early pregnancy, the uterus is a pelvic organ and only internally palpable. At about 10 to 12 weeks' gestation the growing uterus is double its nonpregnant size and reaches the top of the symphysis, where it is palpable abdominally. The uterine fundus is about halfway between the symphysis and umbilicus at about 16 weeks and is at the umbilicus at about 20 to 22 weeks' gestation. After the 20th week, the average upward growth of the uterus is about 3.75 cm per month. At approximately 36 weeks' gestation, the uterus reaches the xiphisternum. In the last month of pregnancy, the fundus of the uterus may drop several centimeters if the fetal head descends deeply into the pelvis.

The position of the uterus changes during gestation. In early gestation an exaggerated anteflexion is common. As the uterus ascends into the abdomen, a slight dextrorotation develops. The uterus changes from a flattened pear shape to a globular shape in early pregnancy. This globular shape continues until approximately 20 to 24 weeks, when a definite ovoid shape develops and continues until delivery.

In about the sixth to eighth week of gestation, the uterine isthmus becomes softened and easily compressible, so that the cervix, on palpation, seems almost detached from the uterine fundus. At about the eighth week of gestation, the entire uterus softens.

During pregnancy the uterus contracts intermittently. These painless contractions, called Braxton Hicks contractions, begin in early pregnancy and are first noted by the client and examiner at about 24 weeks' gestation. They can be stimulated by palpation of the uterus. If a contraction occurs during abdominal examination, the examiner should wait until the contraction ends to continue palpation and subsequently palpate more gently.

Three major changes occur in the cervix: (1) hypertrophy of the glands in the cervical canal, (2) softening of the cervix, and (3) bluish discoloration. These changes begin early in pregnancy—at about the sixth week of gestation. Because of changes in the cervical epithelium, commonly a portion of the squamous epithelium is replaced by an outward extension of the columnar epithe-lium, producing an observable cervical ectropion or eversion of the cervical canal. This condition usually persists throughout pregnancy but disappears soon after.

The increase in pelvic vascularity causes a bluish discoloration of the cervix, vagina, and vulva at about 6 to 8 weeks. In addition, the vaginal mucosa thickens, the connective tissue becomes less dense, and the muscular areas hypertrophy. These changes are reflected in palpatory findings of softening and relaxation. The hypertrophied glands secrete more mucus; the total vaginal discharge is increased and is more acid in reaction.

Breast Changes

Breast changes begin at about the eighth week of pregnancy with enlargement of the breasts. Shortly afterward, the nipples become larger and more erectile, the areolae become more darkly pigmented, and the sebaceous glands (Montgomery's tubercles) in the areolae hypertrophy. Sometimes an irregular secondary areola develops, extending from the primary areola. Hypertrophy of the breasts often causes a slight tenderness. In women with well-developed axillary breast tissue, the hypertrophy may produce symptomatic lumps in the armpits. Colostrum can be expressed from the breast at about the 24th week of pregnancy. The colostrum appears clear and yellowish at first, but it becomes cloudy later.

Stretching of the skin on the breast may produce striae, and increased vascular supply may visibly engorge superficial breast veins.

Abdominal Changes

The muscles of the abdominal wall stretch to accommodate the growing uterus, and the umbilicus becomes flattened or protrudes. The rapid stretching of abdominal skin may cause the formation of striae gravidarum, which appear pink or red during pregnancy and become silvery white after delivery. In the third trimester of pregnancy, the rectus abdominis muscles are under considerable stress, and their tone is diminished. A wide, permanent separation of these muscles, called diastasis recti abdominis, may occur. This condition allows abdominal contents to protrude in the midline of the abdomen.

In pregnancy, peristaltic activity is reduced, resulting in decreased bowel sounds. Smooth muscle relaxation or atony contributes to a variety of changes in gastrointestinal function. These include a high incidence of pregnancy-associated nausea and vomiting, heartburn, and constipation. In addition, the increased regional blood flow to the pelvis and venous pressure contribute to hemorrhoids—a source of discomfort in late pregnancy. Nausea and vomiting should not persist beyond the third month, but heartburn, constipation, and hemorrhoids are more characteristic and troublesome in late pregnancy.

Less frequently noted gastrointestinal symptoms include ptyalism or excessive salivation, and pica, a craving for substances of little or no food value. Pica is often an expression of the folkways of some cultural groups and is a common concern when it interferes with good nutrition.

The enlarging uterus displaces the colon laterally, upward, and posteriorly. This changes the anatomic situation of the appendix, and signs of appendicitis during pregnancy are not localized in McBumey's area of the right lower quadrant.

Skin, Mucous Membrane, and Hair Changes

The melanocytes in all portions of the skin are extremely active in pregnancy. There is a tendency toward generalized darkening of all skin, especially in skin hyperpigmented in the nonpregnant state. In some women a brownish black pigmented streak may appear in the midline of the abdomen. This line of pigmentation is called the linea nigra. Some women develop a dark, pigmented configuration on the face that has been characteristically called the "mask of pregnancy," or chloasma. Scars and moles may also darken during pregnancy from the influence of melanocyte-stimulating hormone (MSH). Palmar erythema and spider nevi on the face and upper trunk may accompany pregnancy.

Many women observe hypertrophy of gums or epulis resulting from hormones and increased vascularity.

The hair of pregnant women may straighten and change in oiliness. Some women experience hair loss, especially in frontal and parietal areas. Occasionally, increases in facial and abdominal hair resulting from increased androgen and corticotropic hormone are noted.

Cardiovascular System Changes

Many changes—too numerous to discuss adequately here—occur in the maternal circulatory system during pregnancy. Several of those changes that alter physical examination findings are mentioned.

Blood volume is increased up to 45% and cardiac output is increased up to 30% in pregnancy compared with the prepregnant state. Blood volume and cardiac output changes contribute to auscultatory changes common in pregnancy. Heart sounds are accentuated, and a low-grade systolic murmur (usually grade II) is often noted.

As pregnancy advances, the heart is displaced upward and laterally. The point of *maximum impulse* (PMI) or apical impulse is displaced to a point 1 to 1.5 cm

lateral to that of the nonpregnant client. The pulse rate increases about 10 beats per minute more than prepregnancy rates and palpitations may be noticed during pregnancy. The blood pressure is unchanged or sometimes decreased in the second trimester.

There is a progesterone-induced generalized relaxation of the smooth muscle, arteriolar dilatation, and increased capacity of the vascular compartment. Systolic blood pressure remains the same or slightly lower during mid-pregnancy. There is no change in venous pressure in the upper body, but venous pressure increases in the lower extremities when the woman is supine, sitting, or standing. This predisposes the woman to varicosities of the legs and vulva and to edema.

Respiratory System Changes

During pregnancy, tidal volume increases and there is a slight increase in respiratory rate. Alveolar ventilation is increased, and a more efficient exchange of lung gases occurs in the alveoli. Oxygen consumption rises by almost 20%, and plasma carbon dioxide content is decreased.

As the uterus enlarges, the thoracic cage and diaphragm are pushed upward and the thorax is widened at the base. A change in respiration from abdominal to costal may be noted on physical examination. Also, dyspnea is a common complaint, especially in the last trimester, and deep respirations and sighing may be more frequent.

The tissue of the respiratory tract and nasopharynx manifests hyperemia and edema. This may contribute to engorgement of the turbinates, nasal stuffiness, and mouth breathing. Some women note increased nasal and sinus secretion and nosebleeds. Vocal cord edema may cause voice changes. Increased vascularity of the tympanic membranes and blockage of the eustachian tubes may contribute to decreased hearing, a sense of fullness in the ears, or earaches.

Musculoskeletal System Changes

The pelvic joints exhibit slight relaxation in pregnancy resulting from some unknown mechanism. This relaxation is maximum from about the seventh month onward. Because the gravid uterus has caused the pregnant client's weight to be thrust forward, the muscles of the spine are used to achieve a temporary new balance. The pregnant woman throws her shoulders back and straightens her head and neck. The lower vertebral column is hyperextended.

The musculoskeletal changes are often reflected in postural and gait changes, lower backache, and fatigue.

Often the pregnant woman's gait is described as waddling.

PRENATAL HEALTH HISTORY

The health history is important in pregnancy because information derived from the history assists the practitioner in differentiating the client who is essentially normal and who will be expected to deliver a full-term, healthy baby from the high-risk expectant mother whose pregnancy is likely to affect her own health negatively or who may not deliver a full-term or healthy baby. High-risk clients are given special care in most health care systems. The early identification and referral of the high-risk client enable the special program to achieve maximum benefit for the mother and baby.

The health history for the obstetric client follows the same basic protocol as that presented for all adults in Chapter 5. However, in prenatal care, the following areas of history-taking should receive special and complete attention:

  I. Age
 II. Race
III. Marital status
IV. Parity

A four-number code with the abbreviation T-P-A-L is often used to summarize parity information.

First digit = number of full-term births (T)

Second digit = number of preterm births, i.e., those between 21 and 37 weeks gestation (P)

Third digit = number of abortions, i.e., those terminated at or before the 20th week of gestation (A)

Fourth digit = number of living children (L)

Thus, for example, the parity of 2-1-1-3 indicates that the client has three living children, two of whom were delivered after full-term gestation and one of whom was premature, and has had one abortion.

An alternate method of indicating parity is a two-digit code. The first digit indicates gravity, defined as the total number of pregnancies. The second digit indicates gravity, the number of live births.

 V. Past obstetric history, including the following for each pregnancy:
   A. Date of delivery
   B. Duration of gestation
   C. Significant problems
   D. Manner in which labor started, specifically whether labor was spontaneous or induced; if induced, the reason for induction should be noted. Abortion should be described as being spontaneous (S) or induced (I).
   E. Length of labor
   F. Complications of labor
   G. Presentation of infant at delivery
   H. Type of delivery—vaginal or cesarean; if cesarean, the reason
   I. Type of anesthesia used at delivery
   J. Condition of infant(s) at birth and birth weight
   K. Postpartum problems, especially infections, hemorrhage, or thrombophlebitis
   L. Problems of the infant, especially jaundice, respiratory distress, infection, or congenital anomalies
   M. Type of infant feeding
   N. Current health of child
VI. Present obstetric history
   A. Last normal menstrual period (LNMP)
      An important task during the prenatal history is estimation of the expected date of confinement (EDC). Because the exact date of conception is unknown for the majority of prenatal clients, the EDC is calculated according to the first day of the last normal menstrual period (LNMP). The EDC is determined by counting backwards 3 calendar months from the LNMP and adding 7 days (Nägele's rule). The year, of course, may change. For example, if the LNMP were 10-15-84, the EDC would be 7-22-85. If the client has a history of irregular menses, the EDC would be more accurately estimated by physical examination than by using the LNMP. Critical features that aid in determination or validation of the EDC are the date of quickening, when the mother first notices fetal movement (at about 18 weeks), and the time at which the fetal heart tones can be auscultated (at about 20 weeks' gestation). Because of the variation that characterizes these events, ultrasonic measurement of fetal size and growth is being used more frequently to "date" pregnancy and assess fetal growth, along with measurement of the progressive enlargement of the uterus.
   B. Symptoms of pregnancy
   C. Feelings about pregnancy, especially determination if pregnancy was planned or unplanned
   D. Bleeding since last normal menstrual period
   E. Date when fetal movements were first felt
   F. Fetal exposure to infections, radiation, and drugs
VII. Current and past medical and gynecologic history
   A. Urinary and venereal infections
   B. Bacterial and viral infections during pregnancy
   C. Diabetes
   D. Hypertension

E. Heart disease

F. Endocrine disorders

G. Anemia

H. Genital tract history, especially:
   1. Anomaly
   2. Cervical incompetence
   3. Myomas
   4. Contracted pelvis
   5. Ovarian mass
   6. Vaginal infections
   7. Surgery
   8. Abnormal Pap test results
   9. Use of hormones (e.g., birth control pills)
   10. Menstrual history and functioning
   11. Endometriosis

I. Medication history

J. Habitual use of alcohol, tobacco, or mood-altering drugs

VIII. Family history

Features of the family history that have special significance in pregnancy include diabetes, renal or hematologic disorders, hypertension, multiple pregnancy, and congenital defects or retardation. It is important to learn if the primigravida's mother had preeclampsia or high blood pressure during pregnancies, especially if she convulsed.

IX. Emotional, psychological, and developmental status.

Pregnancy is an important developmental event in a woman's life. The developmental tasks of pregnancy are incorporation, differentiation, and, eventually, separation from the fetus. These tasks roughly coincide with the three trimesters of pregnancy.

During the first trimester, the gravida is involved with the process of accepting the fetus as a fact and a part of her body. Most women initially experience some ambivalence about their pregnancy with a resultant increase in anxiety. Many body changes occur that cause increased somatic awareness and inward focus. Relationships with key persons, especially the baby's father and the gravida's mother, become especially important. Unresolved feelings and conflicts undergo reexamination. Feelings of dependency and vulnerability occur and can be additional causes of anxiety.

In the second trimester, the fetus develops a separate identity. The gravida has had some time to become accustomed to her bodily changes and often feels better because the nausea has ceased. The baby's movements are an important event, confirming the presence of the fetus and reminding the woman of the independence of the fetal move-

ments from her control. She begins to daydream about the baby and their future. Worries about the possibility of producing an abnormal baby are common.

In the last trimester of pregnancy, the gravida prepares her separation from the fetus and entrance into a new relationship with the newborn. This time is occupied with preparatory activities such as attending parents' classes and buying clothing and equipment for the newborn. Concerns about labor and delivery and physical discomforts of late pregnancy contribute to the woman's readiness for separation from the fetus and movement to the tasks of parenthood.

X. Social, economic, and cultural status

Because pregnancy and birth are important events in the development of any family and because the quality of the family affects the infant's health, the circumstances relating to the pregnancy and the family environment must be assessed. The following are several important areas of exploration in the social history.

A. Client's desire for and feelings about this pregnancy

B. Feelings of significant others regarding this pregnancy

C. Client's personal and culturally derived health beliefs about pregnancy

D. Client's knowledge regarding pregnancy and parenting

E. Amount of support and assistance provided by family and significant others

F. Economic burdens imposed on client or family by pregnancy

G. Condition of the family's physical and emotional environment

PRENATAL RISK FACTORS

The following is a list of factors that have been associated with increased morbidity and mortality of mothers and infants. Special note should be taken of these factors during the health history interview and its recording:

Maternal characteristics

Age: less than 18 or over 40
Poverty
Single
Family disorganization
Conflict about pregnancy
Height less than 5 ft
Weight less than 100 lb
Inadequate diet
Low education level

Reproductive history

More than one previous abortion
Perinatal death
Infant less than 2500 g
Infant over 4000 g
Infant with isoimmunization or ABO incompatibility
Infant with major congenital or perinatal disease
Uterine anomaly
Myomas
Ovarian masses

Medical problems

Hypertension
Renal disease
Diabetes mellitus
Heart disease
Sickle cell disease
Anemia
Pulmonary disease
Endocrine disorder
Addiction to tobacco, alcohol, or drugs

Present pregnancy

Bleeding
Premature rupture of membranes

Anemia
No prenatal care
Preeclampsia or eclampsia
Hydramnios
Multiple pregnancy
Breech, transverse, or abnormal fetal position
Low or excessive weight gain
Hypertension (blood pressure greater than 140/90, a 30 mm Hg systolic increase, or a 15 mm Hg diastolic increase)
Abnormal fasting blood sugar
Rh-negative sensitized
Exposure to teratogens
Viral infections
Syphilis
Bacterial infections
Protozoal infections
Postmaturity

Sometimes a scoring system is used to estimate the level or extent of risk for maternal or fetal illness or prematurity. Table 23-1 presents a mechanism for quantifying the risk of a prenatal client using data collected through the history. Local populations may require adaptation of the content of the scoring mechanism or the weighting of factors. However, such a summarization of

Table 23-1

Rating scale of prenatal risk factors

			Factors	
Score	Socioeconomic	Past history	Habits	Current pregnancy
1	2 children at home	1st trimester abortion × 1 <1 years since last birth	Work outside home	Unusual fatigue
2	<20 years >40 years Single parent	1st trimester abortion × 2	>10 cigarettes/day >6 cups coffee/day	< 12 lb weight by 32 weeks Albuminuria Hypertension Bacteriuria
3	Low socioeconomic status Malnourished Less than 5 ft Less than 100 lb	1st trimester abortion × 3	Unusual anxiety Heavy work Long tiring trip Long commuting distance	Breech at 32 weeks Weight loss of 2 kg Head engaged before 34 wk Febrile illness Leiomyomas
4	Less than 18 years	Pyelonephritis		Uterine bleeding after 12 wk Effacement or dilatation of cervix before 36 wk Uterine irritability
5		Uterine anomaly 2nd trimester abortion DES exposure		Placenta previa Hydramnios
10		Premature delivery Repeated 2nd trimester abortion		Twins Abdominal surgery

Adapted from Zuspan FP and Quilligan EJ: Practical manual of obstetric care, St Louis, 1982, The CV Mosby Co.
Total score is computed by adding the scores for the total set of factors present for given client. 0 to 5 points, minimal risk; 6 to 9 points, moderate risk; >10 points, high risk.

risk factors is usually helpful in the care of individuals and a total clinic population.

PHYSICAL ASSESSMENT DURING PREGNANCY

General Physical Examination

A complete physical examination should be made on the first prenatal visit because (1) the examination may reveal problems that need special or immediate attention and (2) initial data serve as a baseline against which changes later in pregnancy can be compared. The initial, general physical examination of the prenatal client is the same as that for other clients, except for special emphasis on the diagnosis of pregnancy, the assessment of pelvic adequacy, and the assessment of fetal growth and well-being.

A number of nonreproductive system signs may be normally altered in pregnancy. Such alterations of physical findings are listed in the box below.

Diagnosis of Pregnancy

Pregnancy is diagnosed from the history of subjective symptoms noticed by the woman together with objective signs noted by the examiner. In addition, laboratory tests are especially helpful in confirming early pregnancy.

Traditionally, the signs and symptoms of pregnancy have been categorized as presumptive symptoms, probable signs, and positive signs.

Presumptive symptoms are those concerns that the prenatal client identifies in the present illness and chief complaint portions of the history and several additional general physical signs. They include the subjective data that may have led the client to seek confirmation of pregnancy. Presumptive symptoms include (1) absence of menses 10 or more days after the expected date of onset, (2) morning nausea or appetite change, (3) frequent urination, (4) soreness or a tingling sensation in the breasts, (5) Braxton Hicks contractions, (6) quickening, (7) abdominal enlargement, and (8) bluish discoloration of the vagina.

The following are probable signs of pregnancy: (1) progressive enlargement of the uterus, (2) softening of the uterine isthmus (Hegar's sign), (3) asymmetric, soft enlargement of one uterine cornu (Piskacek's sign), (4) bluish or cyanotic color of the cervix and upper vagina (Chadwick's sign), (5) softening of the cervix (Goodell's sign), (6) internal ballottement, (7) palpation of fetal parts, and (8) positive test results for HCG in urine or serum. These signs are termed "probable" because clinical conditions other than pregnancy can cause any of these signs. However, if they occur together, a strong case can be made for pregnancy.

Physical Findings Altered in Pregnancy

Respiratory system

Change in breathing from abdominal to costal
Shortening and widening at the base of the thoracic cage
Elevation of the diaphragm
Increase in respiratory rate

Cardiovascular system

Displacement of the apical impulse laterally 1 to 1.5 cm
Grade II systolic murmur
Increase in pulse rate
Slight fall in blood pressure in the second trimester

Musculoskeletal system

Slight instability of pelvis
Alteration of standing posture and gait to compensate for gravid uterus

Abdominal region

Contour changes because of gravid uterus
Striae gravidarum
Decrease in muscle tone
Linea nigra
Reduced peristaltic activity

Skin and mucous membranes

Chloasma
Linea nigra
Hyperpigmentation of skin and bony prominences
Palmar erythema
Spider nevi on face and upper trunk
Striae gravidarum on breasts and abdomen
Gum hypertrophy

Breasts

Enlargement
Large, erect nipples
Darkening of areolar pigment
Development of a secondary areola
Hypertrophy of sebaceous glands in the areola
Formation of colostrum
Tenderness on palpation
Striae gravidarum
Engorgement of superficial veins

Other alterations

Straightening of hair
Loss of hair over frontal and parietal regions
Enlarged thyroid

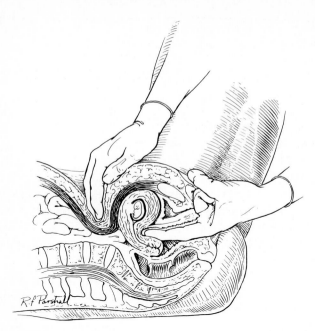

Figure 23-1

Hegar's sign, softening of the lower uterine segment.

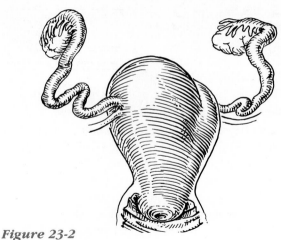

Figure 23-2

Piskacek's sign, asymmetric enlargement of the uterine fundus.

In pregnancy, uterine enlargement can be noted on pelvic examination about 6 to 8 weeks after the last normal menses. The uterus first enlarges in the pelvis, and by 12 weeks' gestation it can be palpated abdominally just above the symphysis pubis. In addition to enlarging, the uterus becomes globular and then ovoid.

The uterus softens in pregnancy because of increased vascularity. The isthmus of the uterus is the first part to soften. At about 6 to 8 weeks' gestation, the softened isthmus produces a dramatic palpatory finding. On palpation, the enlarged, globular uterus feels almost detached from the still not completely softened cervix because the isthmus feels so indistinct (Fig. 23-1). This phenomenon is called Hegar's sign. By 7 or 8 weeks the cervix and uterus can be easily flexed at their junction (McDonald's sign).

Cyanosis of the cervix is noted on speculum examination as early as 6 to 8 weeks' gestation and results from the increased vascularity in the area.

Often uterine enlargement does not progress symmetrically. Rather, the area of placental development enlarges more rapidly. This produces a palpatory asymmetric enlargement of one uterine cornu, called Piskacek's sign (Fig. 23-2).

Immunologic tests for the presence of HCG are commonly used to assist in the diagnosis of pregnancy. The commonly used immunologic tests are the hemagglutination inhibition test and the latex agglutination test. These tests depend on an antigen-antibody reaction be-

tween HCG and an antiserum obtained from rabbits immunized against this antigen. These tests are available for use by both health professionals and women themselves and are very sensitive. Most commercial tests use standardized anti-HCG rabbit serum and dead cells or standardized latex particles coated with HCG. Anti-HCG serum is mixed first with a sample of the client's urine, then HCG-coated red blood cells or particles are added. The lack of agglutination is a positive test because urine containing HCG has neutralized the HCG antibodies. If the urine sample contains no HCG, agglutination would occur, indicating a negative test for pregnancy.

Pregnancy tests based on the presence of HCG in the urine can be reliably made from 2 weeks after the first missed menses through 16 weeks' gestation. During this time, the production of HCG is at its peak.

The positive signs of pregnancy are those that prove the presence of a fetus: (1) documentation of a fetal heartbeat by auscultation; electrocardiogram, or Doppler instrument; (2) palpation of active fetal movements; and (3) radiologic or ultrasonographic demonstration of fetal parts. Ultrasonographic techniques can demonstrate the presence of a gestational sac as early as the sixth week of gestation. Doppler instruments can detect a fetal heartbeat as early as 10 to 12 weeks.

Currently, clinical diagnosis of pregnancy depends more on the probable signs than on the presumptive symptoms and positive signs of pregnancy. However, with new developments in immunologic blood testing, radioimmunoassay, and more available ultrasonographical technology, the methods of pregnancy diagnosis may change.

The radioimmunoassay test that is specific for the B subunit of the HCG molecule at very low concentrations is also considered a positive test for pregnancy.

Table 23-2

The physical signs of pregnancy and corresponding stage of fetal development

Sign	Approximate gestation (weeks since last menses)		Fetal development
Amenorrhea.	2	0-4	Fertilization occurs.
			Blastocyst implants.
			Placental circulation established.
			Organogenesis initiated.
			Development of nervous system and vital organs initiated.
			Anatomic structures and systems are in rudimentary form.
			Size: 0.25 in by fourth week.
Softening of cervix (Goodell's sign).	4-6		
Softening of cervicouterine junction (Ladin's sign).	5-6	5-8	All major organs in rudimentary form.
Gestational sac may be noted by ultrasonography.	6		Fingers are present.
Compressibility of the lower uterine segment (Hegar's sign).	6-8		Ears and eyes are formed.
Dilatation of breast veins.			Heart complete and functioning.
Pulsation of uterine arteries in lateral fornices (Oslander's sign).			Development of muscles is initiated. Size: 1.25 in by eighth week.
Flexing of fundus of cervix (McDonald's sign).	7-8		
Asymmetrical softening and enlarging of uterus (Piskacek's sign).			
Uterus changes from pear to globular shape.			
Bluish coloration of the vagina and cervix (Chadwick's sign).	8-12	9-12	Organs forming and growing. Swallowing and sucking reflexes present.
Detection of fetal heart beat with a Doppler instrument.	10-12		Body movements increase. Size: 3 in, 0.5 oz by 12th week.
Uterus palpable just above symphysis pubis.	12	13-16	Circulatory system is established.
Ballottement of fetus possible by abdominal and vaginal examination.	16		Size: 6 in, 4 oz by 16th week.
Uterus palpable halfway between symphysis and umbilicus.			
Fetal movements noted by mother (quickening).	16-20	17-20	Rapid growth.
Pigment change may occur.			Size: 8 in, 8 ounces by 20th week.
Uterine fundus at lower border of umbilicus.	20	21-24	Meconium present in intestines.
Fetal heart beat auscultated with fetoscope.			Size: 11 in, 1-1.5 lb by 24th week.
Fetus palpable.	24		
Mother begins to notice Braxton Hicks contractions.	24-26	25-28	Nervous system can control breathing and temperature.
Uterus changes from globular to ovoid shape.			Size: 12 in, 2-3 lb by 28th week.
Fetus easily palpable, very mobile, and may be found in any lie, presentation, or position.	28	29-32	Fat deposits under skin. Size: 13 in, 3-5 lb by 32nd week.
Uterus is approximately half the distance from the umbilicus to the xiphoid.			
Fetus usually lies longitudinally with a vertex presentation.	32	33-36	Primitive reflexes are present. Size: 14 in, 5-6 lb by 36th week.
Uterine fundus is approximately two thirds the distance betwen the umbilicus and the xiphoid.			
Uterine fundus is just below the xiphoid.	34		
Vertex presentation may engage in the pelvis.	36-40	37-40	Less active because of crowding. Size: 19-21 in, 6-8 lb by 40th week.

With this test there is no cross-reaction with luteinizing hormone as with other immunologic tests, and thus it is more accurate for HCG itself.

The timetable for physical signs of pregnancy is presented in Table 23-2. Table 23-2 also includes an outline of fetal development during pregnancy. During prenatal assessments, both the mother and the developing fetus are being examined.

PRENATAL EXAMINATIONS

After the initial assessment, the prenatal client is examined at regular intervals. Reexamination schedules vary for clients, but the schedule includes examination approximately every 3 to 4 weeks during the first 28 weeks of pregnancy, then every 2 to 3 weeks until 36 weeks, and weekly thereafter.

At each prenatal revisit, the following parameters are usually assessed:
1. Weight
2. Blood pressure
3. Urine screening for glucose and albumin
4. Determination if edema is present
5. Abdominal assessment
   a. Determination of uterine growth
   b. Determination of fetal presentation and position
   c. Measurement of fetal heart rate

Weight Gain

Optimum weight gain during pregnancy based on the lowest rate of complications and low birthweight infants is 24 to 27.5 lb (a wider range is 20 to 30 lbs). High prepregnancy weight correlates significantly with an increased risk of preeclampsia. Women with low prepregnancy weight who gain little weight during pregnancy are more likely to have low birth weight babies (i.e., babies weighing 2500 g or less). Sudden weight gain, especially in the third trimester, usually means fluid retention and is evaluated in conjunction with maternal blood pressure. Apart from this transient cause of weight gain, many women tend to add to their body fat stores during pregnancy, and this weight gain may not be entirely lost after delivery. The gain in weight should occur gradually, averaging 1½ to 2 lbs per month during the first 24 weeks and ½ to 1 lb a week during the remainder of pregnancy.

Blood Pressure

Mean systolic blood pressure and mean diastolic blood pressure are essentially unchanged during pregnancy except, as indicated, for a mild and transient decrease during the middle trimester. Hypertension, however, contributes significantly to prenatal morbidity and mortality,

and pregnancy-induced hypertension is a disease peculiar to pregnancy. This disorder typically develops after the 24th week of pregnancy and is characterized by the following:
1. A systolic blood pressure of at least 140 mm Hg or a rise of 30 mm Hg or more above the usual level in two readings 6 hours apart
2. A diastolic pressure of 90 mm Hg or more or a rise of 15 mm Hg above the usual level in two readings 6 hours apart
3. Proteinuria
4. Edema of the face or hands

Clinicians have described what has come to be known as the Roll Over Test to detect gravidas who are likely to develop hypertension in late pregnancy. Such women have an increased vascular reactivity and have lost their resistance to vasopressor substances that characterize normal pregnancy. This sensitivity or vascular reactivity is exhibited by an increase of 20 mm Hg in diastolic pressure when a woman of 28 to 32 weeks' gestation turns from her side to her back. This increase is termed a positive Roll Over Test, and such a woman requires closer monitoring of her blood pressure during the latter portion of her pregnancy because she is much more likely to develop the classic signs and symptoms of preeclampsia.

Assessment of Edema and the Extremities

Ankle swelling and edema of the lower extremities occur in two thirds of women in late pregnancy. Women notice this swelling later in the day after standing for some time. Sodium and water retention caused by steroid hormones, an increased hydrophilic property of intracellular connective tissue, and increased venous pressure in the lower extremities during pregnancy contribute to this edema. Assessment includes palpation of the ankles and pretibial areas to determine the extent of the edema and observation for hand, face, or generalized edema. Generalized edema may be manifested by pitting in the sacral area or by the appearance of a depression on the gravid abdomen from the rim of the fetoscope after it has been pressed against the abdomen to auscultate the fetal heart rate.

In addition to assessment for edema formation, examination of the legs includes inspection for varicose veins and dorsiflexion of the foot with the legs extended to check for Homans' sign and thrombophlebitis. In the presence of an elevated or a borderline elevated blood pressure, deep tendon reflexes are assessed. Hyperreflexia and clonus, combined with other signs, can indicate preeclampsia.

Leg cramps during pregnancy may accompany extension of the foot and sudden shortening of leg muscles.

This may be caused by an elevation of serum phosphorus with a diet that includes a large quantity of milk.

A variety of discomforts and sensations in the legs are attributed to compression of nerves from the pressure of the enlarging uterus. This includes numbness in the lateral femoral area, resulting from compression of that nerve beneath the inguinal ligament. Medial thigh sensation may result from the compression of the obturator nerve against the side walls of the pelvis. Periodic numbness of the fingers is reported to occur in at least 5% of gravidas. This is apparently caused by a brachial plexus traction syndrome from drooping shoulders. This drooping is associated with the increased weight of the breasts as pregnancy advances. Movement of fingers may be impaired by compression of the median nerve in the arm and hand caused by physiologic changes in fascia, tendons, and connective tissue during pregnancy. This is known as carpal tunnel syndrome and is characterized by a paroxysm of pain, numbness, tingling, or burning in the sides of the hands and fingers—particularly the thumb, second, and third fingers and the side of the fifth finger.

Abdominal Examination

As pregnancy progresses, the uterus enlarges steadily. The height of the uterine fundus serves as a rough guide to fetal gestation and overall fetal growth. Fig. 23-3 displays the expected fundal height at various gestational ages. At the 12th week of pregnancy, the fundus is palpable just above the symphysis. At 16 weeks, the fundus is approximately halfway between the symphysis and umbilicus. At the 20th gestational week, the fundus usually reaches the lower border of the umbilicus. After the 20th week, the uterus increases in height at approximately 3.75 cm per month or around 1 cm per week until weeks 34 to 36, when the fundus almost reaches the xiphoid. Then, in approximately 65% of gravidas, the fetal head drops further into the pelvis with lightening. If this occurs, the fundal measurement at 36 weeks may be greater than that later in pregnancy.

Unless the fetal head drops into the pelvis, the fundal height between weeks 37 and 40 will stay the same. During this period the fetus is enlarging, but the amount of amniotic fluid decreases.

The abdominal examination consists of the following components:
1. Inspection
2. Measurement of fundal height
3. Assessment of the fetal position
   a. Fundal palpation
   b. Lateral palpation
   c. Pawlik palpation
4. Auscultation of fetal heart rate.

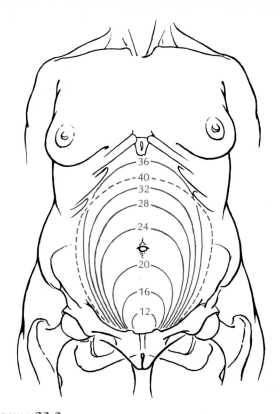

Figure 23-3

Approximate levels of the uterine fundus at various gestational points. Numbers indicate weeks of gestation.

Inspection

In addition to the observations the practitioner makes when observing the abdomen (e.g., skin and scars), for the pregnant client, the examiner also observes the size and configuration of the enlarging uterus.

Normally, the uterine size should relate to the estimated gestational age. Any discrepancy between observed size and estimated gestational age should be further explored. A uterus larger than expected may indicate incorrect gestational age estimation or multiple pregnancy; a smaller uterus may indicate a poorly growing fetus or gestational miscalculation.

Observation of the abdomen may provide the first clues to fetal presentation and position. Asymmetric appearance or distention in width versus longitudinal enlargement may suggest a transverse or oblique fetal lie that can be verified by palpation. After about week 28 fetal movements may be seen.

Measurement of fundal height

The uterus is palpated to determine the top, or height, of the fundus. The examiner stands at the right side of the supine client. The palmar surface of the examiner's

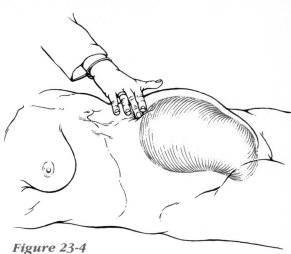

Figure 23-4

Palpation to determine height of the uterine fundus.

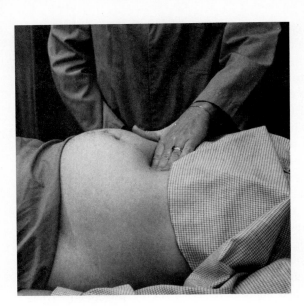

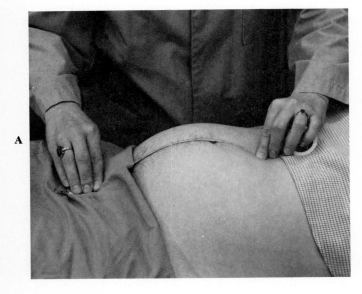

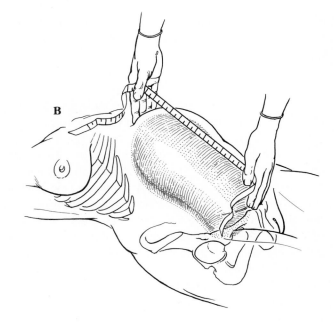

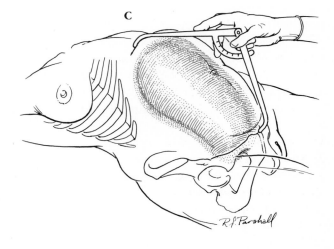

Figure 23-5

Various methods of measuring height of the fundus. **A,** Measurement accounting for some of the fundal curve. **B,** Measurement avoiding the fundal curve. **C,** Measurement using obstetric calipers. This method also avoids measuring the fundal curve.

left hand is placed approximately 3 to 4 cm above where the fundal apex is expected to be located in the midline of the abdomen. This hand palpates downward in small progressive steps until the examiner can differentiate between the softness of the abdomen generally and the firm, round fundal edge (Fig. 23-4). The use of only the palmar surface of the middle finger of the examining hand can assist in locating the precise level of fundal height.

When the fundal edge is located, its distance from

A

B

C

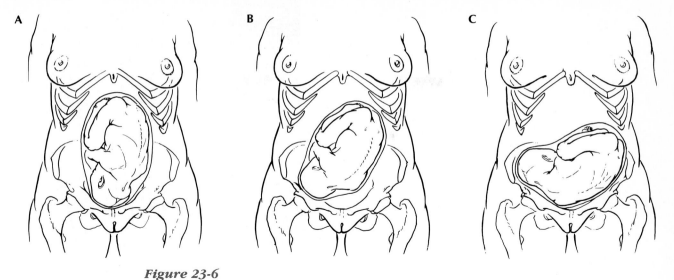

Figure 23-6

Examples of fetal lie. **A,** Longitudinal lie. **B,** Oblique lie. **C,** Transverse lie.

the symphysis is estimated. When the fundus is below the umbilicus, the measurement in centimeters above the symphysis or below the umbilicus can be estimated or measured with a measuring tape.

When the fundus is above the umbilicus, measurement with a measuring tape is recommended. The examiner places the zero point of the tape at the top of the symphysis and measures the distance to the top of the fundus (Fig. 23-5). Various methods exist for estimating fundal height. Methods that avoid measurement of the fundal curve and abdominal adipose tissue are more accurate estimations of actual fundal growth. The practitioner should choose one method and use it consistently. This measurement is approximate, and estimates of fundal height measurement may vary 1 to 2 cm among examiners. However, measurement is more reliable than visual estimation beyond 20 weeks and, if it is practiced consistently by one examiner, should provide an excellent picture of fetal growth with each visit.

Assessment of fetal position

The examiner next palpates the abdomen to determine fetal lie, presentation, position, attitude, and size.

The lie is the relationship of the long axis of the fetus to the long axis of the uterus. The lie can be longitudinal, oblique, or transverse (Fig. 23-6).

The presentation of the fetus is that fetal part that is most dependent. The presentation can be vertex, brow, face, shoulder, or breech (Fig. 23-7).

The position is the relationship of a specified part of the fetal presentation, the denominator, to a particular part of the maternal pelvis (Fig. 23-8). The denominator in a vertex presentation is the occiput (O); in a breech

presentation, it is the sacrum (S); and in a face presentation, it is the mentum (M), that is, the chin. The position is standardly abbreviated according to the left or right of the pelvis, the denominator, and the pelvic portion as follows:

Side of pelvis	Denominator	Pelvic portion
L = Left	O = Occiput	A = Anterior
R = Right	S = Sacrum	P = Posterior
	M = Mentum	L = Lateral
		T = Transverse

For example, if the occiput were closest to the left anterior portion of the pelvis, the fetal position would be LOA.

The fetal attitude is the relationship of the fetal head and limbs to its body (Fig. 23-9). The fetus may be fully flexed, poorly flexed, or extended. When the fetus is fully flexed, the spine is flexed, the head is flexed on the chest, and the arms and legs are crossed over the chest and abdomen.

Engagement is said to have occurred when both the biparietal and suboccipitobregmatic diameters of the fetal head have passed into the inlet of the pelvis (Fig. 23-10). When this has occurred, the fetal head can be felt at the level of the ischial spines on vaginal palpation.

Determination of fetal lie, presentation, position, attitude, and size is accomplished by abdominal palpation. The abdomen is systematically palpated using Leopold's maneuvers in the four sequential steps, as follows:

1. Fundal palpation
2. Lateral palpation
3. Pawlik palpation
4. Deep pelvic palpation

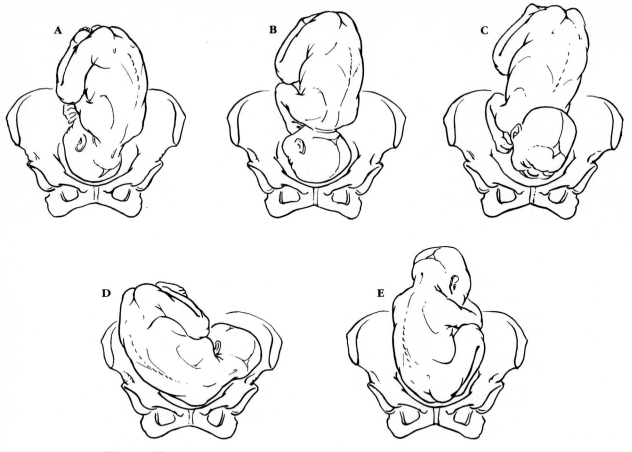

Figure 23-7

Examples of fetal presentation, **A,** Vertex. **B,** Brow. **C,** Face. **D,** Shoulder. **E,** Breech.

Figure 23-8

Examples of fetal position.

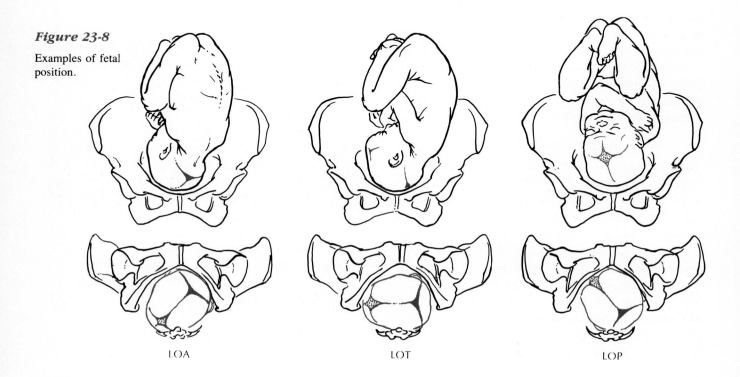

LOA   LOT   LOP

A
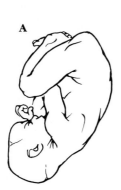

B
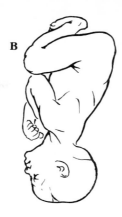

C
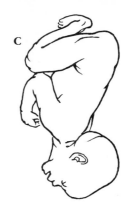

Figure 23-9

Fetal attitude. **A,** Fully flexed. **B,** Poorly flexed. **C,** Extended.

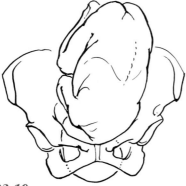

A
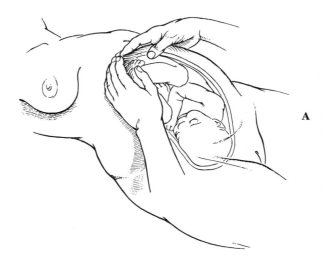

Figure 23-10

Engagement. Both the biparietal and suboccipitobregmatic diameters of the fetal head have passed into the inlet of the pelvis.

Leopold's maneuvers are usually not especially productive until 26 to 28 weeks' gestation, when the fetus is large enough for its parts to be differentiated through abdominal and uterine structures.

For this examination the client is supine. Elevation of the client's knees may assist in decreasing tension of the abdominal muscles and making the examination more comfortable for the client.

Fundal palpation. The examiner stands at the client's right side, facing her head, and places the palmar surface of both hands on the uterine fundus to determine what part of the fetus is occupying the fundus (Fig. 23-11). Leopold's first maneuver, the method of determining the location of the top of the fundus, has already been described. Usually the buttocks of the fetus will be in the fundus and be felt as a soft, irregular, and slightly movable mass. The lower limbs are felt adjacent to the buttocks. If the head is in the fundus, it is felt as smooth, round, hard, and ballottable. The groove of the neck is felt between the trunk and the upper limbs. The head is freely movable in contrast to the buttocks, which can only move sideways and with the trunk.

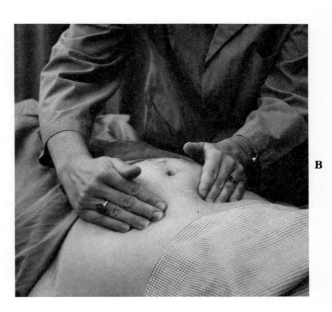

B

Figure 23-11

Palpation to determine the contents of the uterine fundus.

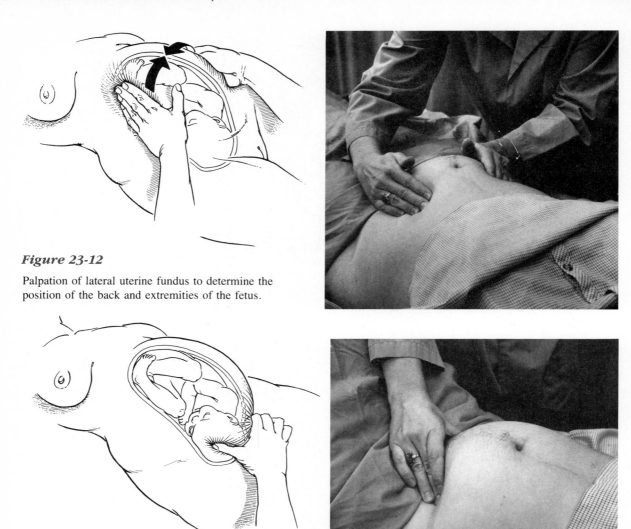

Figure 23-12

Palpation of lateral uterine fundus to determine the position of the back and extremities of the fetus.

Figure 23-13

Pawlik palpation to determine fetal presenting part.

Lateral palpation.   For Leopold's second maneuver (Fig. 23-12), the examiner, while still facing the client's head, moves both hands to either side of the uterus to determine which side the fetal back is on. The examiner supports the fetus with one hand while the other hand palpates the fetus. The examiner then reverses the procedure to palpate each side of the uterus. The fetal back is felt as a continuous, smooth, firm object, whereas the fetal limbs, or small parts, are felt as small, irregular, sometimes moving objects. On each side, the examiner palpates the flank to the midline, making special note of the edge of the fetal back as a landmark in determining the fetal position.

Pawlik palpation.   This procedure is done with the right hand only to determine what fetal part lies over the pelvic inlet. The right hand is placed over the symphysis so that the fingers are on the left side of the uterus

and the thumb is on the right side (Fig. 23-13). The hand should be approximately around the fetal presenting part, usually the head. The presenting part is gently palpated to determine its form and consistency and grasped and gently moved sideways to determine its movability. This palpation confirms impressions about the presenting part and determines if the presenting part (if the fetal head) might be engaged. If the fetal head is movable above the symphysis, it is not engaged. If the head is not movable, it may be engaged. Engagement can only be confirmed by pelvic examination to determine if the biparietal diameter of the fetal head is level with the ischial spines.

Deep pelvic palpation.   The examiner changes position (Fig. 23-14). The examiner remains on the right side of the client but is turned and facing the woman's feet. A hand is placed on each side of the uterus near the pelvic brim. The client is asked to take a deep breath and

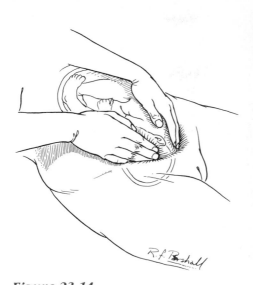
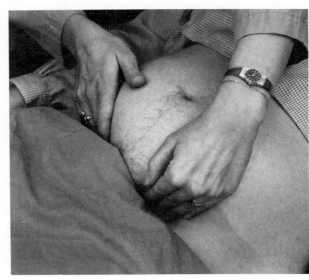

Figure 23-14

Deep pelvic palpation to determine fetal attitude and descent.

to exhale slowly. As she does, the examining fingers are allowed to sink deeply above the pubic bones to palpate the presenting part and to determine which side the cephalic prominence is on. If the presenting part is the head, the location of the cephalic prominence, that is, the forehead, assists in determining the fetus' position and attitude. If the head is flexed, the occiput lies deeper in the pelvis, is flatter, and is less defined than the forehead, which is more prominent and on the same side as the small parts. If the head is not well flexed, the cephalic and occipital prominences will be palpated at the same level, and the occipital portion may feel more prominent and is on the same side as the back.

Throughout these maneuvers the examiner assesses the congruence of the size of the fetus with the gestational age.

In summary to this section on abdominal assessment, a series of questions the examiner mentally asks about each client are listed with an indication of the procedures that assist in answering the questions.

Question	Methods of obtaining evidence to answer the question
What is the fetal lie?	Abdominal inspection Lateral abdominal palpation
What is the fetal presentation?	Fundal palpation Pawlik palpation Deep pelvic palpation
What is the fetal position?	Lateral palpation Deep pelvic palpation
What is the fetal attitude?	Deep pelvic palpation
Is the fetal growth congruent with gestational age?	Fundal height measurement All Leopold's maneuvers

Auscultation

The fetal heart rate is an indicator of fetal health status and is monitored throughout pregnancy. Auscultation of the fetal heart rate is accomplished by use of a special stethoscope, or fetoscope, or a Doppler instrument. With the Doppler instrument, the fetal heart rate can be monitored after about 10 weeks' gestation. Using a fetoscope, the examiner can first hear the fetal heart rate between the 16th and 20th weeks of gestation.

The use of the fetoscope is demonstrated in Fig. 23-15. The fetal heart rate is rapid and soft. The use of a fetoscope avoids noises produced by fingers on the stethoscope and makes use of the benefits of both air and bone conduction. The bell of an ordinary stethoscope can be used but is less effective than a fetoscope in listening to fetal heartbeats, especially around 20 weeks.

The fetal heart rate is normally between 120 and 160 beats per minute, and the heartbeats resemble a watch tick heard through a pillow. They are best heard through the fetal back. When the fetus is large enough for its position to be determined, the bell of the fetoscope or the Doppler head is placed at the back of the fetal thorax. When the fetus is under 20 weeks' gestation, the heart rate is often best heard at the midline, just above the pubic hairline.

The fetal heart rate is counted for at least 15 seconds and is recorded in number of beats per minute. The fetal heart rate is normally much faster than the maternal heart rate and thus can usually be well differentiated from it. Moreover, the fetal and maternal heart rates are not synchronous, and the maternal rate can be differentiated by palpating the mother's pulse while auscultating the abdomen.

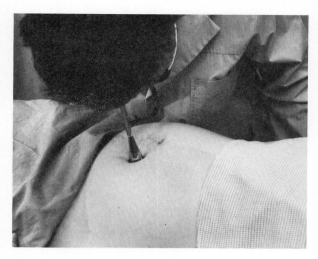

Figure 23-15

Use of the fetoscope to auscultate the fetal heartbeat.

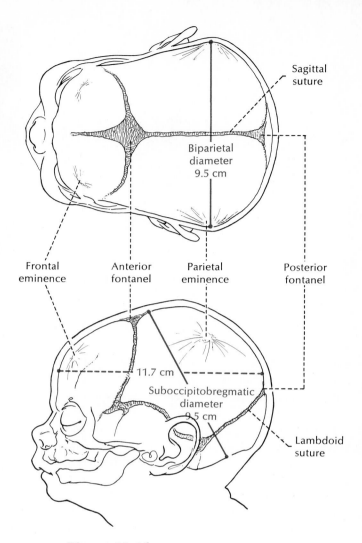

Figure 23-16

Various diameters of the fetal head at term.

Blood rushing through the placenta can be heard as a uterine souffle. The uterine souffle is a soft, blowing sound synchronous with the maternal pulse. The intensity of the souffle has been interpreted as an indicator of uterine blood flow and placental function. A loud uterine souffle has been associated with high urinary estriol levels and a soft or absent souffle with lower estriol levels. Thus, a soft or absent uterine souffle may indicate poor uterine blood flow and placental function, particularly in late pregnancy.

EXAMINATION OF THE BONY PELVIS

The purpose of the examination of the bony pelvis is to determine if the pelvic cavity is large enough to allow for passage of a full-term infant. This examination is performed on the initial prenatal evaluation and need not be repeated if the pelvis is of adequate size. However, if findings indicate that the pelvis is of borderline adequacy or if the examination could not be done on the initial visit because of client tenseness and subsequent muscular contraction, the examination should be repeated between 32 to 36 weeks' gestation. In the third trimester of pregnancy, there is a relaxation of pelvic joints and ligaments, and the client is more accustomed to examination. Thus, the examination of the bony pelvis can be more thoroughly and accurately accomplished then.

The examination of the bony pelvis is done not so much to diagnose the type of pelvis but to determine its configuration and size. Because the examiner does not have direct access to the bony structures and because the bones are covered with variable amounts of soft tissue, estimates are approximate. Precise bony pelvis measure-

ments can be determined using roentgenogram examination. However, roentgenogram examinations are not needed or indicated for the vast majority of prenatal clients.

The assessment of the bony pelvis must be put in the perspective of the capacity needed to accommodate a full-term fetus. When the head of a full-term fetus is well flexed, the two largest presenting diameters are the biparietal and the suboccipitobregmatic, each measuring approximately 9.5 cm (Fig. 23-16).

The pelvis consists of four bones: the two innominate bones, the sacrum, and the coccyx. Each innominate bone consists of three bones that fuse after puberty. These three bones are the ilium, the ischium, and the os pubis (Fig. 23-17). The innominate bones form the anterior and lateral portions of the pelvis.

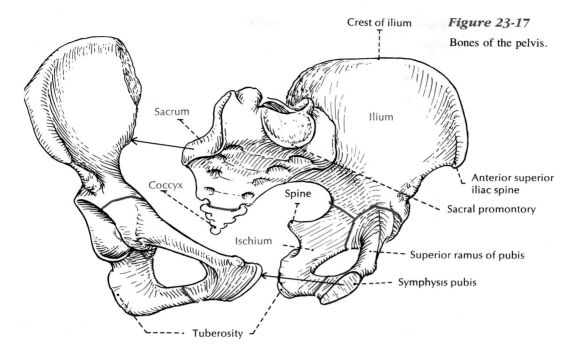

Crest of ilium

Figure 23-17

Bones of the pelvis.

Sacrum

Ilium

Coccyx

Spine

Anterior superior
iliac spine

Sacral promontory

Ischium

Superior ramus of pubis

Symphysis pubis

Tuberosity

The sacrum and coccyx form the posterior portion of the pelvis. The sacrum is composed of five fused vertebrae. Its upper anterior portion is termed the sacral promontory, which forms the posterior margin of the pelvic brim. The coccyx is composed of three to five fused vertebrae and articulates with the sacrum.

The pelvis is divided by the brim into two parts: the false pelvis and the true pelvis. The false pelvis is that part above the brim and is of no obstetric interest.

The true pelvis is that portion of the pelvis that includes the brim and the area below. The true pelvis is divided into three parts: the inlet or brim, the mid-pelvis or cavity, and the outlet. The inlet is formed anteriorly by the upper margins of the pubic bones, laterally by the iliopectineal lines, and posteriorly by the anterior upper margin of the sacrum, the sacral promontory. The cavity is formed anteriorly by the posterior aspect of the symphysis pubis, laterally by the inner surfaces of the ischial and iliac bones, and posteriorly by the anterior surface of the sacrum. The outlet is diamond-shaped and is formed anteriorly by the inferior rami of the pubic and ischial bones, laterally by the ischial tuberosities, and posteriorly by the inferior edge of the sacrum, if the coccyx is movable.

Each of the pelvic portions can be imagined as a series of planes: the plane of the brim, or pelvic inlet; the planes of the mid-pelvis; and the plane of the outlet. These planes are illustrated in Fig. 23-18.

The plane of the inlet in an average female pelvis measures approximately 11 to 13 cm in the anteroposterior diameter and 13 to 14 cm in the transverse diameter.

The anteroposterior diameter of the inlet measured from the middle of the sacral promontory to the superior posterior margin of the symphysis pubis is called the true conjugate and is an important obstetric measurement. However, it cannot be assessed directly, except by radiographic methods. An estimate of the true conjugate is made by measuring the diagonal conjugate, which is the distance between the inferior border of the symphysis pubis and the sacral promontory. The diagonal conjugate is about 1 to 2 cm longer than the true conjugate, depending on the height and inclination of the symphysis. The clinical measurement of the diagonal conjugate, the most valuable single measurement of pelvic adequacy, will be discussed later in this section.

The mid-pelvis contains the planes of greatest and least pelvic dimensions. The plane of least pelvic dimensions is bounded by the junction of the fourth and fifth sacral vertebrae, the symphysis, and the ischial spines. The average dimensions of this plane are 12 cm (anteroposterior diameter) and 10.5 cm (transverse diameter). The transverse diameter is the distance between the ischial spines.

The pelvic outlet is composed of two triangular planes, having a common base in the most inferior portion of the transverse diameter between the ischial tuberosities. The obstetric anteroposterior diameter of the outlet is the distance between the inferior edge of the symphysis pubis and the edge of the sacrum, if the coccyx is movable. This measurement is usually 11.5 cm.

The transverse diameter of the outlet is the distance between the inner surfaces of the ischial tuberosities

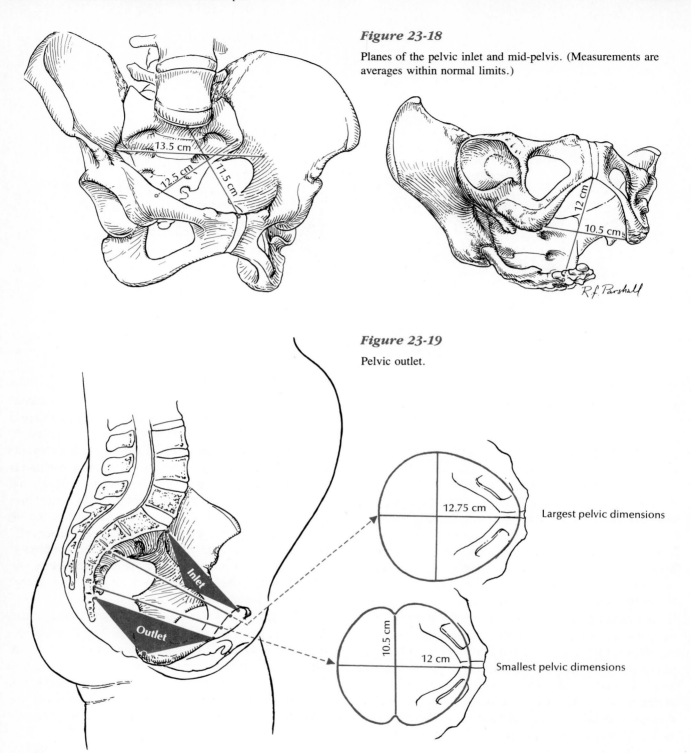

Figure 23-18

Planes of the pelvic inlet and mid-pelvis. (Measurements are averages within normal limits.)

Figure 23-19

Pelvic outlet.

and usually measures about 11 cm (Fig. 23-19).

Although there is a characteristic shape of the adult female pelvis that is different from the characteristically male pelvis, a female client may have any one of four types of human pelves or a mixture of these types. In addition, the shape of the pelvis may have been distorted congenitally or by disease.

The four basic pelvic types as classified by Caldwell and colleagues (1939) are (1) gynecoid, (2) android, (3) anthropoid, and (4) platypelloid.

The typical female pelvis is the gynecoid pelvis, which is found in approximately 40% to 50% of adult women. This pelvis is characterized by a rounded inlet, except for a slight projection of the sacral promontory;

a deep posterior half made possible by a wide sacrosciatic notch and concave sacrum, and a wide anterior half made possible by a wide, subpubic angle.

The android pelvis is found in approximately 15% to 20% of adult women. This pelvic type is roughly wedge- or heart-shaped with the transverse diameter of the inlet approximately equal to the anteroposterior diameter but with the widest transverse diameter located closer to the sacrum. Other characteristics of the android pelvis include the following:
1. Narrow subpubic arch
2. Convergent side walls
3. Large encroaching spines
4. Short sacrosciatic notch and sacrospinous ligament
5. Short interspinous diameter
6. Straight sacrum
7. Short intertuberous diameter

The anthropoid pelvis has an elongated anteroposterior diameter and is found in approximately 25% to 35% of women. It is characterized by the following:
1. Narrow subpubic arch
2. Prominent ischial spines
3. Wide sacrosciatic notch and long sacrospinous ligaments
4. Deeply curved sacrum

The platypelloid pelvis has a flattened anteroposterior dimension with a relative widening of the transverse diameter. This pelvic type is seen in approximately 5% of women. The platypelloid pelvis is characterized by the following:
1. Wide subpubic arch
2. Flat ischial spines
3. Wide sacrosciatic notch and long sacrospinous ligaments
4. Straight sacrum

The various dimensions of the four basic pelvic types are compared and contrasted in Fig. 23-20. Pure pelvic types are unusual; most pelves are admixtures of two pelvic types, with the characteristics of one type predominating.

The examination of the bony pelvis can be uncomfortable for the client, and it should be done after the internal examination of the soft pelvic organs. Therefore, preparation of the client should include explanation of the procedure, the client's emptying of her bladder, and instructions on relaxation.

A routine standard procedure is recommended for the bony pelvis examination, beginning with examination of the anterior pelvis, proceeding to lateral examination on one side, comparing the initially examined side with the opposite side, and concluding with examination of the posterior and inferior portions.

The following bony pelvis parts and landmarks are especially important in examining the pelvis:

1. Subpubic arch
2. Symphysis pubis
3. Side walls
4. Ischial spines
5. Sacrosciatic notch
6. Sacrum
7. Coccyx
8. Sacral promontory
9. Ischial tuberosities

The width of the subpubic arch is palpated, and its angle is estimated. Normally both examining fingers should fit comfortably in the arch, which optimally forms an angle measuring slightly more than a right angle (i.e., a 90-degree angle) (Fig. 23-21).

The length and inclination of the symphysis pubis are estimated by sweeping the examining fingers under the symphysis (Fig. 23-22). Also, the examiner palpates the retropubic curve of the forepelvis and envisions its configuration. Measurement difficulties created by a large amount of soft tissue in the area and reliability with slope measurements preclude a precise estimation of the length and inclination of the symphysis. The examiner essentially screens for an unusually long or steeply inclined symphysis pubis and for an angular rather than a rounded forepelvis.

Next, the right or left lateral pelvic area is examined. First, the side walls are palpated to determine if they are straight, convergent, or divergent. The splay of the side walls can be assessed by following a line from the point of origin of the widest transverse diameter of the inlet downward to the inner aspect of the tuberosity. Another method for assessing the side walls is to place the examining fingers on the base of the ischial spine as a landmark and then to palpate above and below the landmark to determine inclination.

The ischial spine and sacrospinous ligament are examined. The spine is assessed as being blunt, prominent, or encroaching. The sacrosciatic notch is outlined with palpating fingers, if possible, and its width is determined in centimeters or finger breadths. Often the examiner cannot trace the entire notch, and the sacrospinous ligament is useful in estimating the width of the notch (Fig. 23-23).

The other side of the pelvis is then examined in the manner previously described to determine overall pelvic symmetry. The examiner should attempt to do this part of the examination with the palm of the hand up, rather than rotating the hand so that the palm is down.

The interspinous diameter is an important obstetric measurement. This diameter is estimated by moving the examining fingers in a straight line from one spine across to the other (Fig. 23-24). The hand may need to be pronated for this estimation. The estimate is calculated

Brim, spines   Sacrosciatic notch   Subpubic angle

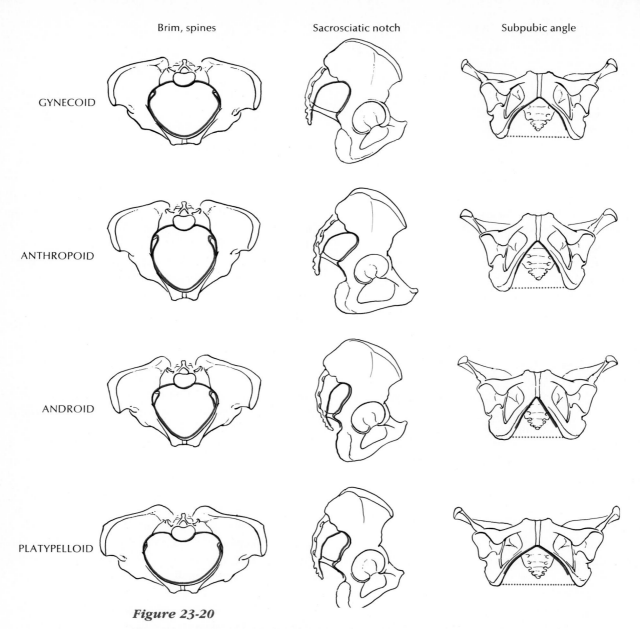

GYNECOID

ANTHROPOID

ANDROID

PLATYPELLOID

Figure 23-20

Comparisons and contrasts of various portions of the four basic pelvic types.

in centimeters. The usual measurement is 10.5 cm. Special calipers are available to measure the interspinous diameter, but these are not often used in clinical practice.

Next the sacrum and coccyx are examined. The fingers are swept down the sacrum, noting whether it is straight, curved, or hollow and if its inclination is forward or backward. The coccyx is examined gently because it may be tender on movement. The coccyx is gently pressed backward to determine if it is movable or fixed. Its tilt is noted as anterior or posterior.

The diagonal conjugate is assessed last because this assessment can be uncomfortable for the client. A moderate amount of constant pressure is needed to de-

press the perineum adequately. Pressure is better exerted by the examiner's body than by the hand and forearm only. It is recommended that the examiner place the foot (the one on the same side as the examining hand) on a stool and the elbow of the examining arm on the thigh or hip. The needed pressure is then applied and controlled by the trunk of the examiner's body. For this examination, the fingers and wrist should form a straight line with the forearm.

The examiner locates the sacrum with the examining fingers and, with the middle finger, "walks" up the sacrum until the promontory is reached or until the examiner can no longer reach the sacrum. The point where

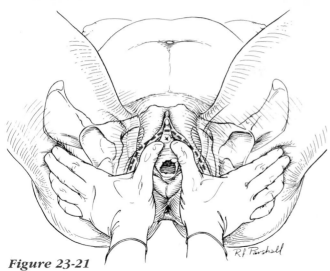

Figure 23-21

Method of estimating the angle of the subpubic arch.

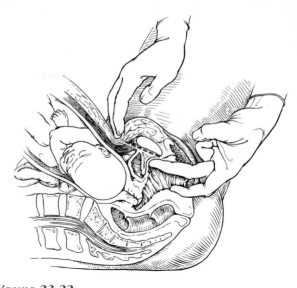

Figure 23-22

Estimation of the length and inclination of the symphysis pubis.

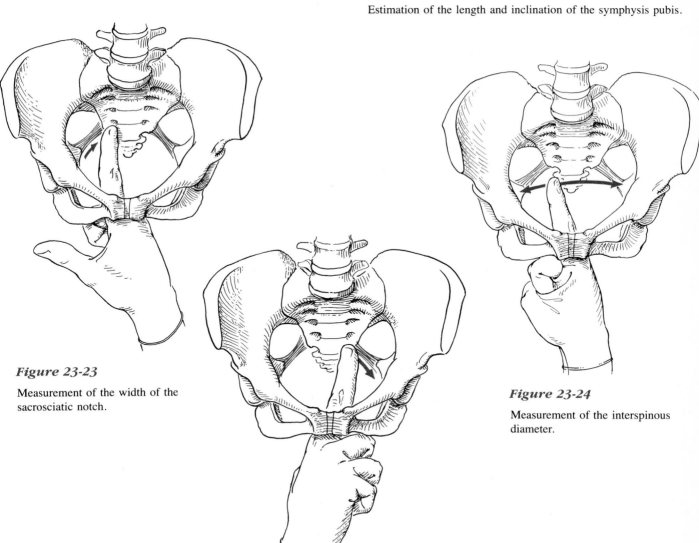

Figure 23-23

Measurement of the width of the sacrosciatic notch.

Figure 23-24

Measurement of the interspinous diameter.

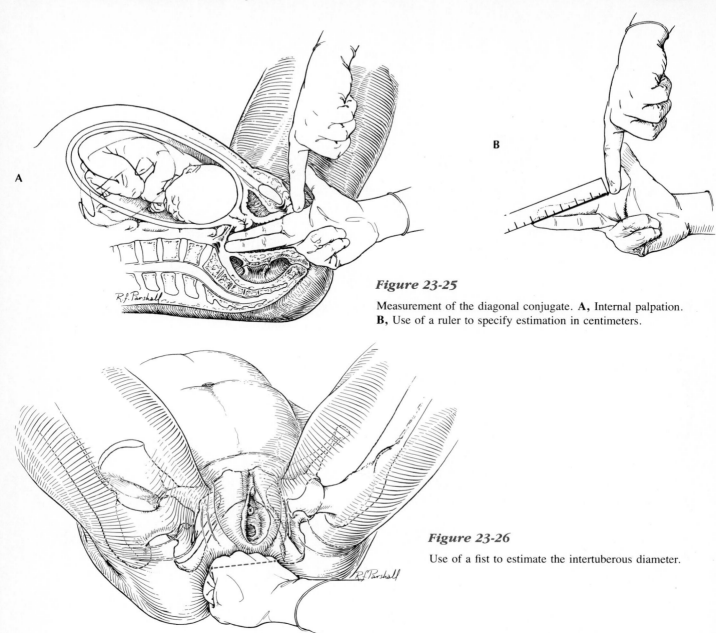

Figure 23-25

Measurement of the diagonal conjugate. **A,** Internal palpation. **B,** Use of a ruler to specify estimation in centimeters.

Figure 23-26

Use of a fist to estimate the intertuberous diameter.

the client's symphysis touches the examiner's hand is marked with the thumb of the opposite hand, and the distance is measured in centimeters by a rule (Fig. 23-25). In obstetric examining rooms, a ruler is often fixed to the wall for this measurement.

Often, the examiner will not reach the sacral promontory. The examiner should become familiar with the "reach" of the examining fingers and record the findings as greater than (>) the centimeters of this reach. Normally the diagonal conjugate is greater than 12.5 cm.

The examining hand is withdrawn from the vagina, and the intertuberous diameter is measured. Using both thumbs, the examiner externally traces the descending rami down to the tuberosities. The examiner then makes a fist and attempts to insert the fist between the tuberosities to measure the transverse diameter of an outlet (Fig. 23-26). The intertuberous diameter is usually 10 to 11 cm. Again, the examiner knows the span of his or her own fist and estimates the intertuberous diameter accordingly.

An instrument called the Thom's pelvimeter can be used to measure the intertuberous diameter (Fig. 23-27). This instrument has two arches that are held against the tuberosities by the examiner's thumbs. The precise intertuberous diameter can be determined by calibrations on the instrument's midportion.

In summary, the areas of bony pelvic examination and the assessment descriptors for these areas are noted as follows:

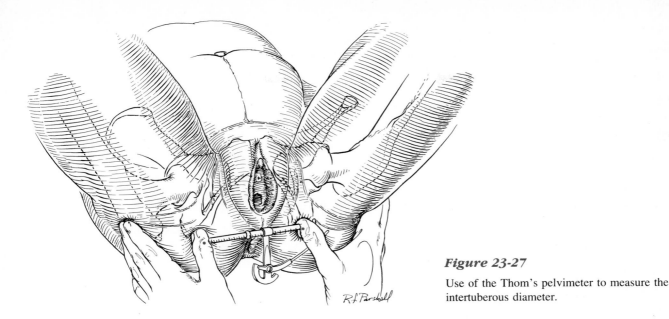

Figure 23-27

Use of the Thom's pelvimeter to measure the intertuberous diameter.

Sequence of areas of bony pelvic examination	*Assessment descriptors*
1. Subpubic arch	Less than 90 degrees; more than 90 degrees
2. Side walls	Parallel; convergent; divergent
3. Ischial spines	Size: small; average; large Prominence: blunt; prominent; encroaching
4. Sacrosciatic notch Sacrospinous ligament	Estimated width or length in centimeters or finger breadths (usual length 3 to 4 cm)
5. Opposite pelvic side	Symmetric; asymmetric
6. Interspinous diameter	Estimated length in centimeters (usual length 10.5 cm)
7. Sacrum	Concave; straight; convex
8. Coccyx	Position: straight; projects anteriorly; projects posteriorly Movability: movable; fixed
9. Diagonal conjugate	Actual length or length greater than the measurement the examiner can reach (usual length 12.5 cm)
10. Intertuberous diameter	Actual length in centimeters if Thom's pelvimeter is used or an estimated length using a closed fist (usual length 10 to 11 cm)

BIBLIOGRAPHY

Aladjem S, editor: Obstetrical practice, St Louis, 1980, The CV Mosby Co.

American College of Obstetricians and Gynecologists: Standards for obstetric-gynecologic services, ed 5, Washington, DC, 1982, The College.

Bailey RE: Mayes' midwifery: a textbook for midwives, ed 9, London, 1976, Cassell & Collier Macmillan Ltd.

Caldwell WE, Moloy HC, and Swenson PC: The use of the roentgen ray in obstetrics: anatomical variations in the female pelvis and their classification according to morphology, Am J Roentgenol 41:505, 1939.

Fogel CI and Woods NF: Health care of women: a nursing perspective, St Louis, 1981, The CV Mosby Co.

Gant NF and others: A clinical test for predicting the development of acute hypertension in pregnancy, Am J Obstet Gynecol 120:1, 1974.

Hickman MA: Midwifery, Oxford, 1985, Blackwell Scientific Publications, Ltd.

Humenick SS: Analysis of current assessment strategies in the health care of young children and childbearing families, East Norwalk, Conn, 1982, Appleton-Century-Crofts.

Martin LL: Health care of women, Philadelphia, 1978, JB Lippincott Co.

Niswander KR: Obstetrics: essentials of clinical practice, ed 2, Boston, 1981, Little, Brown & Co.

Page EW, Willee CA, and Villee DB: Human reproduction: the core content of reproductive and perinatal medicine, ed 3, Philadelphia, 1978, WB Saunders Co.

Oxhorn H and Oxhorn-Foote W: Human labor and birth, Norwalk, Conn, 1986, Appleton-Century-Crofts.

Suonio S, Saarikoski S, Raty E, and Vohlonen I: Clinical assessment of the pelvic cavity and outlet, Arch Gynecol 329:11-16, 1986.

Tucker S: Pocket guide to fetal monitoring, St Louis, 1988, The CV Mosby Co.

Willson JR, Carrington ER, and Ledger WJ: Obstetrics and gynecology, ed 7, St Louis, 1983, The CV Mosby Co.

Zuspan FP and Quilligan EJ: Practical manual of obstetric care, St Louis, 1982, The CV Mosby Co.

24

Assessment of the pediatric client

OBJECTIVES

Upon successful review of this chapter, learners will be able to:

- Describe guidelines used to assess health during infancy, childhood, and adolescence
- Outline history relevant to a pediatric client, including
  Family data
  Prenatal, birth, and postnatal data
  Developmental and behavioral data
  Nutritional data
  Health information, including usual habits, immunization, illness, and allergy data
  Health risks, including depression and suicide data
- Recognize sociocultural and psychological data pertinent to the health of pediatric clients
- Identify methods for facilitating interview and physical examination of pediatric clients
- State related rationale and demonstrate assessment of pediatric clients, including
  Developmental milestones
  Growth measurements
  Vital signs
  Inspection, palpation, percussion, and auscultation techniques of body systems
  Reflexes and nerves
- Recognize usual findings, common variations, and characteristics suggesting pathology

Pediatric care is, to a large extent, health care aimed at promoting the health of the child and preventing illness and disability through early identification of problems.

The examination of the child is ideally carried out over an extended time in a planned sequential pattern. The dynamic changes that occur in the child's normal growth and development require the practitioner to assess carefully the increments in growth; the changes in physiologic function; and the development of *cognitive,* social, and motor skills of the child during each examination.

It is by comparing the individual child's current growth achievements and parameters of health with that found in previous examinations and with other normal, healthy children that the health of the child is determined. The child should be seen more frequently during infancy, when growth changes are most rapid and dramatic, and then at less frequent intervals throughout the childhood years.

The examination of the child also considers the environment in which the child lives and the parental concerns in child-rearing. The adults responsible for the child's care often have concerns about the child's development and about their own ability to manage. They need respect, support, and guidance that encourages them to express the concerns they may have and to discuss their needs and the needs of the child. The mother is usually the person most familiar with the child and the child's care and is the one most likely to detect changes, both normal and abnormal, that go unnoticed by others, including the health care practitioner. The practitioner should also be alert to any signs of stress between the mother and child. A mother who is concerned, anxious, or angry about a child's behavior or physical condition may be showing evidence of stress that can interfere with the mother-child relationship and ultimately with the child's development. Therefore, consideration is given to the needs of the mother or other adults caring for the child as well as to those of the child.

The practitioner should always demonstrate respect for both the child and the parent, be willing to listen to problems, and help in finding adequate solutions. Both the child and the parent will be sensitive to the practitioner's attitudes and will respond according to their impressions.

In essence, the examiner must be sensitive to the child as a growing, developing human being who is ever changing.

This chapter includes a discussion of the approaches to the child and the parent and some of the techniques used in obtaining health information and in assessing the child's health. In addition, some of the physical differences between the child and the adult are discussed.

It is not possible to include a survey of all the components of child development that are assessed. The reader is referred to standard pediatric texts and Chapter 2 for assistance in understanding the parameters of normal development and health of children.

GUIDELINES FOR HEALTH SUPERVISION

Guidelines prepared by the Committee on Practice and Ambulatory Medicine (1981) and approved by the Executive Committee of the American Academy of Pediatrics (1982) suggest the schedule of care shown in Table 24-1 for the care of children who are receiving competent parenting, have no manifestations of any important health problems, and are growing and developing in a satisfactory fashion. Circumstances that may indicate the need for additional visits, as outlined in the 1977 edition of the Standards of Child Health Care of the American Academy of Pediatrics, include the following:

1. Firstborn or adopted children or those not with natural parents
2. Parents with a particular need for education and guidance
3. Disadvantaged social or economic environment
4. The presence or possibility of perinatal disorders (such as prematurity, low birth weight, *congenital* defects, or familial diseases)
5. Acquired illness or previously identified disease or problems

THE PEDIATRIC HISTORY

The pediatric history provides the opportunity to interview both the child and the parent to gather information about the child's health, development, relationships with others, and care. It also provides the opportunity for the child to become acquainted with the practitioner before being examined. The pediatric history is an adaptation of the model used for an adult history. It also incorporates areas uniquely pertinent to the child, such as the history of the mother's health during the pregnancy and the history of birth and the neonatal period.

Cultural differences and individual parental differences influence the care of the infant and child and will be revealed in the history of the child's care. Needless to say, these differences should be respected and careful judgments made in regard to counseling.

The informant for the history may be a parent, a relative, a caretaker, or the child. The interviewer should identify the informant and indicate the reliability of the information obtained. It is common for the child, even the young child, to participate in the interview and to volunteer useful information. The information gained from the child should be indicated as such in the history.

The health history described in Chapter 5 is adapted for the pediatric client with some changes in the format. The history of development and the nutritional data are placed before the review of systems, since the data obtained are usually critical to the present health status of the infant or child:

1. Biographical information
2. Chief complaint or client's request for care
3. Present illness or present health status
4. Past history
5. Developmental data
6. Nutritional data
7. Family history
8. Review of systems
   a. Physical systems
   b. Sociologic system
   c. Psychological system

Demographic Data

The information obtained in this category is essentially the same as for the adult client.

Chief Complaint or Client's Request for Care

The chief complaint (CC) statement gives the reason for making the visit and should be in the words of the informant. Children are seen most frequently for health care, and the CC statement may indicate a visit for routine health care rather than for the treatment of a health problem. An example would be "It is time for his checkup," or "well baby check."

Table 24-1

Guidelines for health supervision

Age[2]	Infancy						Early childhood				
	By 1 mo.	2 mos.	4 mos.	6 mos.	9 mos.	12 mos.	15 mos.	18 mos.	24 mos.	3 yrs.	4 yrs.
History											
Initial/Interval	●	●	●	●	●	●	●	●	●	●	●
Measurements											
Height and Weight	●	●	●	●	●	●	●	●	●	●	●
Head Circumference	●	●	●	●	●	●					
Blood Pressure										●	●
Sensory Screening											
Vision	S	S	S	S	S	S	S	S	S	S	○
Hearing	S	S	S	S	S	S	S	S	S	S	○
Devel./Behav. Assessment[4]	●	●	●	●	●	●	●	●	●	●	●
Physical Examination[5]	●	●	●	●	●	●	●	●	●	●	●
Procedures[6]											
Hered./Metabolic[7] Screening	●										
Immunization[8]		●	●	●			●	●	●		
Tuberculin Test[9]	←————————————————————→ ●						←————————————————————→		●		
Hematocrit or Hemoglobin[10]	←————————————————→ ●						←————————————————→		●		
Urinalysis[11]	←————————————→ ●						←————————————→		●		
Anticipatory Guidance[12]	●	●	●	●	●	●	●	●	●	●	●
Initial Dental Referral[13]										●	

Source: From The American Academy of Pediatrics Committee on Psychosocial Aspects of Child and Family Health, 1988.

1. Adolescent related issues (e.g., psychosocial, emotional, substance usage, and reproductive health) may necessitate more frequent health supervision.
2. If a child comes under care for the first time at any point on the schedule, or if any items are not accomplished at the suggested age, the schedule should be brought up to date at the earliest possible time.
3. At these points, history may suffice; if problem suggested, a standard testing method should be employed.
4. By history and appropriate physical examination; if suspicious, by specific objective developmental testing.
5. At each visit, a complete physical examination is essential, with infant totally unclothed, older child undressed and suitably draped.
6. These may be modified, depending upon entry point into schedule and individual need.
7. Metabolic screening (e.g., thyroid, PKU, galactosemia) should be done according to state law.
8. Schedule(s) per Report of Committee on Infectious Disease, *1986 Red Book*.
9. For low risk groups, the Committee on Infectious Diseases recommends the following options: (1) no routine testing or (2) testing at three times–infancy, preschool, and adolescence. For high risk groups, annual TB skin testing is recommended.

Present Illness or Present Health Status

The present illness (PI) section incorporates the same categories of information obtained in the adult health history and includes a statement about the usual health, a description of the chronologic story, any relevant family history, negative information, and a disability assessment. The following is an example of a history of the present illness of a child brought to the examiner for health care:

This 7-year-old, white female, who is in the second grade of the urban Elementary School, was brought to clinic by her mother for an annual physical examination. She has been in good health except for approximately four colds since her visit 1 year ago. The child, Debbie, stated that she enjoys school

Age[2]	Late childhood					Adolescence[1]			
	5 yrs.	6 yrs.	8 yrs.	10 yrs.	12 yrs.	14 yrs.	16 yrs.	18 yrs.	20 + yrs.
History									
Initial/Interval	●	●	●	●	●	●	●	●	●
Measurements									
Height and Weight	●	●	●	●	●	●	●	●	●
Head Circumference									
Blood Pressure	●	●	●	●	●	●	●	●	●
Sensory Screening									
Vision	○	○	○	S	○	○	S	○	○
Hearing	○	S[3]	S[3]	S[3]	○	S	S	○	S
Devel./Behav. Assessment[4]	●	●	●	●	●	●	●	●	●
Physical Examination[5]	●	●	●	●	●	●	●	●	●
Procedures[6]									
Hered./Metabolic[7] Screening						●			
Immunization	●								
Tuberculin Test[9]						←————	●	————→	
Hematocrit or Hemoglobin[10]		←————	●	————→		←————	●	————→	
Urinalysis[11]		←————	●	————→		←————	●	————→	
Anticipatory Guidance[12]	●	●	●	●	●	●	●	●	●
Initial Dental Referral[13]									

10. Present medical evidence suggests the need for reevaluation of the frequency and timing of hemoglobin or hematocrit tests. One determination is therefore suggested during each time period. Performance of additional tests is left to the individual practice experience.

11. Present medical evidence suggests the need for reevaluation of the frequency and timing of urinalysis. One determination is therefore suggested during each time period. Performance of additional tests is left to the individual practice experience.

12. Appropriate discussion and counselling should be an integral part of each visit for care.

13. Subsequent examinations as prescribed by dentist.

N.B.: **Special chemical, immunologic, and endocrine testing** are usually carried out upon specific indications. Testing other than newborn (e.g., inborn errors of metabolism, sickle disease, lead) are discretionary with the physician.

Key: ● = to be performed; S = subjective, by history;
○ = objective, by a standard testing method.

but thinks her teacher "is too hard sometimes." Her mother indicated that all school reports are good and that Debbie has many friends in school and the neighborhood and has recently started "sleeping over" with her girl friends. The only problem that the mother expressed was in regard to dental care. Debbie has two small cavities, which were found on her visit to the dentist 2 months ago, and the mother is questioning the value of having "baby teeth filled." Debbie has complained of a toothache on only one occasion, just before the visit to the dentist. The pain was relieved by giving aspirin, 5 grains.

The PI description in this example is that of a child in good health who is functioning well. The negative information concerning the dental caries gives information that the dental caries are not interfering with the child's ability to function but that further consideration is necessary to prevent a more serious problem for the child. An attempt should be made to learn the reason for deciding not to continue dental care. The mother may be seeking assurance that she is right in not making a plan

Table 24-2

The Apgar scoring system for newborns

Clinical sign	Assigned score		
	0	1	2
Heart rate	Absent	100	100
Respiratory effort	Apnea	Slow and irregular	Immediate, strong
Muscle tone	Flaccid	Some flexion of arms and legs	Active movement
Reflex irritability*	No response	Grimace or cry	Crying vigorously
Color	Pale, blue	Body pink, extremities blue	Pink all over

*Reaction when soft rubber catheter is inserted into the external nares.
A score of 8 to 10 is excellent, 4 to 7 guarded, and 0 to 3 critical.

for dental care, or she may be seeking information that the experience will not be difficult for the child and should be planned. Whatever the outcome, information and support must be given to help the child and the parent reach a more appropriate decision.

Past History

The past history of infants, young children, and any child with a possible developmental deficiency should include the following information:

1. Prenatal history
   a. Health of the mother while pregnant with this child
   b. Mother's feelings about the pregnancy
   c. Amount of prenatal care, and when initiated
   d. History of complications (excessive weight gain, hypertension, vaginal bleeding, nausea and vomiting, urinary problems, or infections such as rubella, cytomegalovirus (CMV), or venereal disease)
   e. Medications or drugs prescribed or used during pregnancy
   f. Use of alcohol and cigarettes during pregnancy
2. Birth history
   a. Date of birth
   b. Hospital where child was born
   c. Duration of the pregnancy
   d. Parity of the mother
   e. Nature and duration of the labor
   f. Type of delivery
   g. Use of sedation or anesthesia
   h. Birth weight of the baby
   i. State of the infant at birth and use of any *special* procedures
   j. Apgar score, if known (Table 24-2)
3. Postnatal history
   a. Any problems during first days of life (including

skin color, bleeding, seizures, respiratory distress, congenital anomalies or birth injuries, difficulty in sucking, rashes, or poor weight gain during the first days and weeks after birth)
   b. Age of infant at discharge from hospital after birth
4. Past illnesses
   a. Childhood illnesses (including communicable diseases)
   b. Injuries
   c. Hospitalizations
   d. Operations
   e. Other major illnesses
   f. Frequency of infections
5. Allergies
   a. Environmental
   b. Ingestion
   c. Drug
   d. Other
6. Immunizations (including booster inoculations) (Tables 24-3 and 24-4)
7. Habits
   a. Alcohol
   b. Tobacco
   c. Drugs
   d. Coffee, tea
8. Medications taken regularly
   a. By practitioner's prescription
   b. By self-prescription

Developmental Data

The assessment of the development of the child is discussed in Chapter 2. The history of the child's development is a component of that assessment and should provide clues that indicate when a more formal assessment is indicated. The initial history should include the following:

Table 24-3

Recommended schedule for active immunization of normal infants and children

Recommended age	Immunization(s)	Comments
2 mo	DTP,[1] OPV[2]	Can be initiated as early as 2 wk of age in areas of high endemicity or during epidemics
4 mo	DTP, OPV	2-mo interval desired for OPV to avoid interference from previous dose
6 mo	DTP (OPV)	OPV is optional (may be given in areas with increased risk of poliovirus exposure)
12 mo	DTP,[4,5] OVP[5]	
15 mo	Measles, Mumps, Rubella (MMR)[3]	MMR preferred to individual vaccines; tuberculin testing may be done (see Tuberculosis)
18 mo	Hib[6]	
4-6 yr[7]	DTP, OPV	At or before school entry
14-16 yr	Td[8]	Repeat every 10 yr throughout life

[1]DTP—Diphtheria and tetanus toxoids with pertussis vaccine.
[2]OPV—Oral, poliovirus vaccine contains attenuated poliovirus types 1, 2, and 3.
[3]MMR—Live measles, mumps, and rubella viruses in a combined vaccine (see text for discussion of single vaccines versus combination).
[4]Should be given 6 to 12 months after the third dose.
[5]May be given simultaneously with MMR at 15 months of age.
[6]*Haemophilus* influenza b conjugate vaccine (Hib) should be given at 18 months.
[7]Up to the seventh birthday.
[8]Td—Adult tetanus toxoid (full dose) and diphtheria toxoid (reduced dose) in combination.

1. The age at which the child attained specific developmental achievements
   a. Held head erect
   b. Rolled over
   c. Sat alone
   d. Walked alone
   e. Said first words
   f. Used sentences
   g. Controlled feces
   h. Learned urinary continence
2. A comparison of this child's development with siblings or other children the same age (Table 24-5). An

Table 24-4

Recommended immunization schedules for children not immunized in first year of life

Recommended time	Immunization(s)	Comments
Less than 7 years old		
First visit	DTP, OPV, MMR	MMR if child ≥15 mo old; tuberculin testing may be done (see Tuberculosis)
Interval after first visit		
1 mo	Hib*	For children 24-60 mo
2 mo	DTP, OPV	
4 mo	DTP, (OPV)	OPV is optional (may be given in areas with increased risk of poliovirus exposure
10-16 mo	DTP, OPV	OPV is not given if third dose was given earlier
Age 4-6 yr (at or before school entry)	DTP, OPV	DTP is not necessary if the fourth dose was given after the fourth birthday; OPV is not necessary if recommended OPV dose at 10-16 mo following first visit was given after the fourth birthday
Age 14-16 yr	Td	Repeat every 10 yr throughout life
7 years old and older		
First visit	Td, OPV, MMR	
Interval after first visit		
2 mo	Td, OPV	
8-14 mo	Td, OPV	
Age 14-16 yr	Td	Repeat ever 10 yr throughout life

Haemophilus influenza b conjugate vaccine.

example of a tool used to assess development (the Denver) is also shown (Fig. 24-1).
3. Any periods of decreased or increased growth
4. Questions regarding school achievement are included in the review of systems but may be appropriate to incorporate into the developmental assessment if early delays have been noted.

Table 24-5

Developmental/behavioral milestones

Age	Expectations	Age	Expectations
Newborn	Demonstrate the newborn's ability to fix and follow a human face and alert toward a human voice.	6 months, cont'd	Turns to sounds that originate from out of his immediate sight and changes his activity
	Observe for		Shows signs of stranger anxiety; appears able, on the basis of facial and body gestures, to distinguish between angry and friendly voice patterns
	Consolability		
	Self-quieting		
	Cuddlesomeness		Laughs, squeals, takes the initiative in vocalizing and babbling at others; blows bubbles; imitates such things as a cough, a "raspberry"; may play at making sounds while alone or with others
	Tendency to startle		
1 month	At this age the typical infant:		
	Raises her head slightly when lying prone.		
	Fixes on a face or object and follows movement with her eyes.	9 months	At this age the typical child:
2 months	At this age the typical child:		Sits well
	Holds his head temporarily erect but unsteadily when held upright, until 3 months of age		Crawls, creeps on her hands, hitches on her bottom
			Pulls to a stand; cruises and has parachute reflex
	Grasps a rattle when placed in his hand		Uses inferior pincher grasp; pokes with the index finger
	Holds a rattle briefly		Finger-feeds partially
	Exhibits a social smile—an important developmental milestone		Imitates vocalizations; demonstrates monosyllabic and possibly polysyllabic babbling (e.g., may say "dada" or "mama" in a nonspecific way)
	Coos; reciprocally vocalizes		
	Regards one's face when it is in his direct line of vision; begins to distinguish and respond more to his parents than to others		Responds to her own name, to questions such as "Where is mama or dada?", or to familiar objects when named
	Responds to loud sounds		Understands a few words: "no-no," "bye-bye"
4 months	At this age the typical child:		Enjoys social games with adults, such as peek-a-boo and pat-a-cake
	Holds her head high and raises her body on her hands when lying prone		Reacts to strangers with soberness, anxiety, or even fear
	Maintains steady head control when held upright, no head lag when pulled to sit		Has a concept of object permanence; retrieves a toy hidden by a cloth
	Rolls from prone to supine position	12 months	At this age the typical child:
	Opens hands while at rest; can play with hands, hold a rattle		Pulls to stand; cruises; walks with support; may take a few steps alone
	Looks at a mobile and activates her arms		Shows a precise pincer grasp; points; bangs two blocks together; can put one object inside another
	Follows parent(s) and objects with her eyes through a 180° range		May say one to three meaningful words besides using "mama" and "dada" correctly; imitates vocalization
	Initiates social contact by smiling, cooing, laughing, squealing; may be displeased or cry when a parent moves away		
	Recognizes preparations for feeding and is able to wait a short time		Has a concept of object permanence (eg, looks for a dropped or hidden object)
6 months	At this age the typical child:		Plays social games (e.g., peek-a-boo, pat-a-cake, so-big); waves bye-bye
	Rolls over		May cooperate in dressing and in feeding himself; uses a cup
	Shows no head lag when pulled to a sitting position		
	Sits with support or leans forward on his hands when placed in a sitting position; begins to demonstrate the right- and left-side parachute reflex	15 months	At this age the typical child:
			Walks alone, stops and starts, stoops, explores
	Bears some weight on the lower extremities		Self-feeds with fingers; drinks well from a cup
	Reaches for and grasps objects; by the end of six months, transfers objects from hand to hand		Has a three- to six-word vocabulary; uses jargon and gestures
	May be able to hold his own bottle to feed		Scribbles spontaneously
	Looks at and may approach tiny objects with a raking movement		Points to one or two body parts on request; understands simple commands
	Plays with his feet		Pats a picture in a book and attends to a story being read

From American Academy of Pediatrics: Guidelines for Health Supervision II, Chicago, 1988, The Asssociation.

Table 24-5

Developmental/behavioral milestones—*cont'd*

Age	Expectations	Age	Expectations
15 months, cont'd	Indicates wants by pulling, pointing, grunting, or vocalizing Stacks two blocks Gives and takes a toy Hugs	3 years	At this age the typical child: Jumps in place, kicks a ball, balances and stands briefly on one foot Pedals a tricycle Alternates feet when ascending stairs Opens doors Builds a tower of nine cubes; imitates a bridge made of three cubes Demonstrates speech that is mostly intelligible (The child who fails to speak in sentences or whose speech is unintelligible to strangers should be referred for speech, language, and hearing evaluation.) Knows his name, age, and sex May comprehend "cold," "tired," "hungry," and may understand the prepositions "on" and "under"; differentiates "bigger" and "smaller"; can convey the use of a ball, scissors, key, and pencil Copies a circle, may imitate a cross, and begins to visually discriminate colors Describes action in picture books Puts on some clothing and shoes Feeds himself
18 months	At this age the typical child: Walks fast, may run stiffly, walks up stairs with one hand held, walks backwards, sits in a small chair, climbs into an adult chair, kicks and throws a ball Stacks three or four blocks; may place rings on a cone, then dump them and try again Turns single pages in book or magazine; looks selectively at pictures and names some objects Uses a vocabulary of 4 to 10 words with specificity; may combine two-word phrases; understands and follows some simple directions; may voice two or more wants; shows an imitative vocabulary greater than his vocabulary of spontaneously used words; identifies (points to) some body parts on request Pulls a toy Feeds himself, uses a spoon appropriately, holds and drinks from a cup adequately Imitates a crayon stroke on paper May dump a raisin from a bottle without previous demonstration Holds and "loves" a doll or stuffed animal; may use a household-type toy (e.g., toy telephone) functionally Puckers lips and kisses parent on the cheek		
24 months	At this age the typical child: Climbs and descends steps alone, one step at a time, holding the stair rail or the parent's hand Opens doors, climbs on furniture, uses a spoon and cup well, kicks a ball, throws overhand Stacks five or six cubes and aligns two or three blocks after demonstration May have a vocabulary of at least 20 words, although language development shows great variability at this age; makes two-word phrases with pronouns; refers to herself by name. (If speech is unintelligible or delayed, consider referral for developmental assessment including speech and hearing evaluations.) Responds to two-part verbal commands Spontaneously makes or imitates horizontal and circular strokes with a crayon Shows interest in bowel and bladder control Enjoys imitating adults Shows interest in helping the parent dress her; washes and dries hands Uses a toy appropriately (e.g., hammers pegs in a cobbler's bench)	4 years	At this age the typical child: Alternates feet when descending stairs, hops, jumps forward, can stand on one foot for 3 to 5 seconds Climbs a ladder Rides a tricycle Can walk on tiptoes Holds and uses a pencil with good control Builds a tower of ten or more cubes Has the ability to cut and paste Engages in conversational give-and-take Asks why, when, how, and inquires about the meaning of words May name three or four primary colors Counts from 1 to 5; can sing a song Enjoys jokes Washes and dries hands and brushes teeth Dresses and undresses with supervision except for handling laces and buttons, if allowed sufficient time to dress; may begin to be selective about clothes Initiates dramatic make-believe and dressing-up play in which the child assumes a specific role Is imaginative and intensely curious Has formed gender identification Copies a cross and a circle Draws a person with two to three parts Enjoys the companionship of other children, plays cooperatively, and shows interest in other children's bodies Meets the challenges of kindergarten class

Continued

Table 24-5

Developmental/behavioral milestones—*cont'd*

Age	Expectations	Age	Expectations
5 years	At this age the typical child: Skips, walks on tiptoes, broad jumps Can cut and paste Names four or five colors and can identify coins Tells a simple story and knows several nursery rhymes Defines at least one word (e.g., "ball," "shoe," "chair," "table," "dog") Dresses and undresses without supervision Copies a triangle from an illustration Recognizes most letters of the alphabet Draws a person with a head, body, arms, and legs Begins to understand right and wrong, fair and unfair Engages in dramatic make-believe and dressing-up play, in which the child assumes a specific role; engages in domestic role-playing Enjoys the companionship of other children; plays cooperatively Has formed gender identification ("Are you a boy or a girl?")	6 years, cont'd 8 years 10 years	Counts up to 10, prints her first name, prints numbers up to 10 Knows right from left Draws a person with six body parts, with the figure depicted wearing clothing At this age the typical child: Can tell time (although this may be a nine-year achievement) Can read for pleasure and use a library card Has a sense of humor ("Do you know any good jokes? What's your favorite joke?") Is concerned about rules and good (fair) vs. bad (unfair) Cares for room and belongings; can take responsibility for home chores At this age, the child may be expected to: Display self-confidence with a sense of mastery and pride in school and extracurricular activities Make a few friends and participate in group activities Understand and comply with most rules at home and at school Assume reasonable responsibility for health, school work, and chores
6 years	At this age the typical child: Bounces a ball four to six times, throws and catches Skates Rides a bicycle Ties her shoelaces		

Nutritional Data

The questions regarding nutrition will vary depending on the child's age. The information obtained for the infant, who is growing rapidly, is usually more detailed and specific than the history obtained for the older child.

I. Early infancy
   A. The type of feeding (breast-feeding, commercial formula, or home-prepared formula)
   B. Frequency of feedings
   C. Amount consumed with each feeding and during a 24-hour period
   D. Any changes in feeding (such as from breast-feeding to bottle feeding and time of change)
   E. Any problems observed with feeding (such as colic or spitting)
   F. How long does mother plan to continue breast-feeding or bottle feeding
   G. Vitamin, iron, or fluoride supplements (including the name of the preparation, when it was started, the amount given, and the method of administration)
   H. Solid foods (including the type—commercially prepared or home prepared, the amount given,

how they are given—by spoon or in bottle, and the frequency)
   I. Water (including the amount given, frequency offered, given plain or with a sweetener)
   J. Infant's appetite and reaction to eating
      If the infant is breast-feeding, additional questions about the mother must be asked:
      1. How the mother cares for her breasts
      2. Her program of daily exercise, rest, diet, and fluid intake
      3. Medications being taken (specify name, frequency, purpose, and effectiveness) (The boxed material on p. 605 provides a list of drugs known to be excreted in human milk and to have side effects in breast-fed infants.)
      4. The mother's feelings about breast-feeding
      5. The support she receives from family members
         If the infant is receiving bottle feedings, it is important to learn if he or she is held for all feedings. The baby who receives a bottle of milk or juice at bedtime or naptime to be used in much the same way as a pacifier is

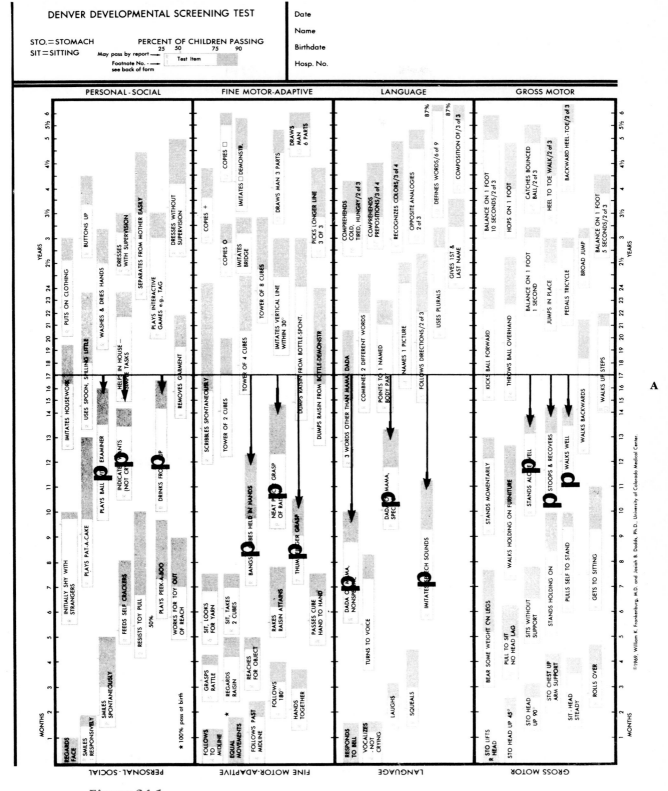

Figure 24-1

A, Denver developmental screening test (DDST).
(**A,** From Frankenberg WK, Sciarillo W, and Burgess O: J Pediatr 99:995-999, 1981.)

Continued

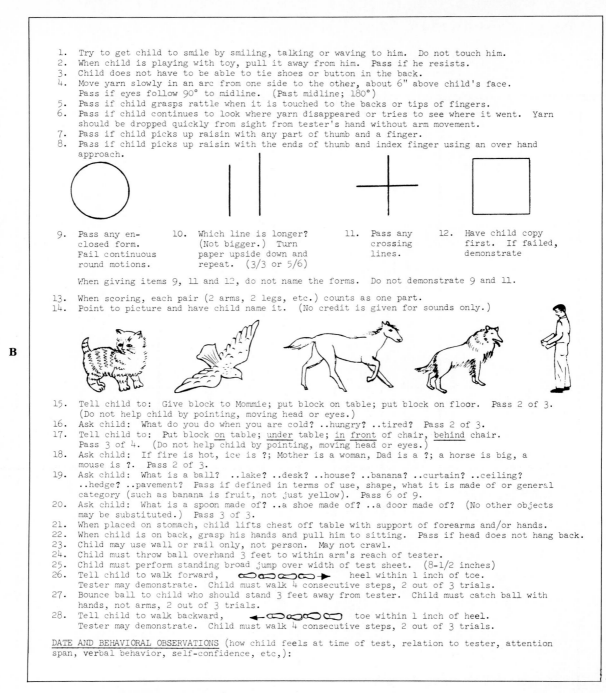

1. Try to get child to smile by smiling, talking or waving to him. Do not touch him.
2. When child is playing with toy, pull it away from him. Pass if he resists.
3. Child does not have to be able to tie shoes or button in the back.
4. Move yarn slowly in an arc from one side to the other, about 6" above child's face.
    Pass if eyes follow 90° to midline. (Past midline; 180°)
5. Pass if child grasps rattle when it is touched to the backs or tips of fingers.
6. Pass if child continues to look where yarn disappeared or tries to see where it went. Yarn
    should be dropped quickly from sight from tester's hand without arm movement.
7. Pass if child picks up raisin with any part of thumb and a finger.
8. Pass if child picks up raisin with the ends of thumb and index finger using an over hand
    approach.

| 9. Pass any en-closed form. Fail continuous round motions. | 10. Which line is longer? (Not bigger.) Turn paper upside down and repeat. (3/3 or 5/6) | 11. Pass any crossing lines. | 12. Have child copy first. If failed, demonstrate |

When giving items 9, 11 and 12, do not name the forms. Do not demonstrate 9 and 11.

13. When scoring, each pair (2 arms, 2 legs, etc.) counts as one part.
14. Point to picture and have child name it. (No credit is given for sounds only.)

15. Tell child to: Give block to Mommie; put block on table; put block on floor. Pass 2 of 3.
    (Do not help child by pointing, moving head or eyes.)
16. Ask child: What do you do when you are cold? ..hungry? ..tired? Pass 2 of 3.
17. Tell child to: Put block on table; under table; in front of chair, behind chair.
    Pass 3 of 4. (Do not help child by pointing, moving head or eyes.)
18. Ask child: If fire is hot, ice is ?; Mother is a woman, Dad is a ?; a horse is big, a
    mouse is ?. Pass 2 of 3.
19. Ask child: What is a ball? ..lake? ..desk? ..house? ..banana? ..curtain? ..ceiling?
    ..hedge? ..pavement? Pass if defined in terms of use, shape, what it is made of or general
    category (such as banana is fruit, not just yellow). Pass 6 of 9.
20. Ask child: What is a spoon made of? ..a shoe made of? ..a door made of? (No other objects
    may be substituted.) Pass 3 of 3.
21. When placed on stomach, child lifts chest off table with support of forearms and/or hands.
22. When child is on back, grasp his hands and pull him to sitting. Pass if head does not hang back.
23. Child may use wall or rail only, not person. May not crawl.
24. Child must throw ball overhand 3 feet to within arm's reach of tester.
25. Child must perform standing broad jump over width of test sheet. (8-1/2 inches)
26. Tell child to walk forward,   heel within 1 inch of toe.
    Tester may demonstrate. Child must walk 4 consecutive steps, 2 out of 3 trials.
27. Bounce ball to child who should stand 3 feet away from tester. Child must catch ball with
    hands, not arms, 2 out of 3 trials.
28. Tell child to walk backward,   toe within 1 inch of heel.
    Tester may demonstrate. Child must walk 4 consecutive steps, 2 out of 3 trials.

DATE AND BEHAVIORAL OBSERVATIONS (how child feels at time of test, relation to tester, attention
span, verbal behavior, self-confidence, etc,):

Figure 24-1, cont'd

B, Directions for Denver developmental screening test.

(**B,** Courtesy Frankenberg WK and Jacobs JB: University of Colorado Medical Center, 1969.)

at risk for dental caries and destruction of the anterior maxillary teeth referred to as "baby bottle syndrome" (Fig. 24-2).

II. Later infancy (6 to 18 months)

The infant during this period is beginning to vigorously manipulate the body and the environment. In addition to the questions outlined for the period of early infancy, questions regarding the baby's developing skills should be included:

A. Has the baby started using a cup, finger feeding, or using a spoon?

B. Does he receive coarser foods as junior foods or table foods?

Examples of Medicants, Foods, and Sundries That Are Excreted in Breast Milk and That May Be Contraindicated During Breast-feeding*

Analgesics
    Codeine in habituated doses
    Heroin in habituated doses
    Meperidine in habituated doses
    Morphine in habituated doses
    Propoxyphene in IV
    Sodium salicylate in high doses
Antihistamines
Antimicrobials
    Ampicillin
    Chloramphenicol
    Metronidazole
    Penicillin
    Sulfonamides
    Tetracyclines
Depressants
    Barbiturates
        Long-acting, hypnotic doses
        Short-acting, hypnotic doses
    Others
        Alcohol
        Bromides, hypnotic doses
        Chloral hydrate
        Diazepam
        Reserpine
Diuretics
    Hydrochlorothiazide, chlorothiazide

Hormonal compounds
    Iodides
    Oral contraceptives
    Pregnane beta-diol
    Propylthiouracil
    Thyroid
Anthraquinone derivatives
    Cascara
    Danthron
Social drugs (legal)
    Caffeine
    Tobacco
Social drugs (illegal)
    Cocaine and other abuse drugs: stimulants, depressants, narcotics, psychedelics in high doses
Miscellaneous
    Amethopterin
    Anticoagulants, oral
    Cimetidine
    Cyclophosphamide
    DDT
    Ergotrate maleate
    Fluorides
    Foods: white navy beans, corn, egg white, chocolate, unripe fruit, pickles, peanuts, cottonseed, and wheat
    Gold salts
    Radiopharmaceuticals

Data from Levin R: In Herfindal ET and Hirschman J, editors: Clinical pharmacy and therapeutics, Baltimore, 1975, Williams & Wilkins; and from Committee on Drugs: Pediatrics 72:375, 1983.
*Refer questions to physician.

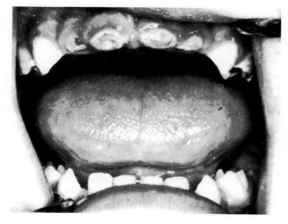

Figure 24-2

Nursing bottle caries in a 20-month-old child. There is extensive carious involvement of maxillary primary incisors and first molars. (From McDonald RE and Avery DR: Dentistry for the child and adolescent, ed 3, St Louis, 1978, The CV Mosby Co.)

    C. How does the mother feel about the infant's developing independent feeding behaviors?

III. Preschool, school age children, and adolescents
Nutritional assessment is discussed in Chapter 3, Nutritional Assessment. The *24-hour recall method* and the *dietary history method* are described and are appropriate for obtaining information about the diet and eating habits of the child. A sample form for gathering nutritional data is included at the end of Chapter 3.

Family History

The family history of the child is similar to the history obtained for the adult client as described in Chapter 5, The Health History. It includes the health and age of the grandparents, maternal and paternal aunts and uncles, parents, and siblings and the age at death and cause of death for deceased relatives. In addition, the pediatric family history should include information about miscarriages and stillbirths.

The information outlined in the family history or in the form of a family tree is used to identify any illnesses or problems that may have implications for the child's future health and current health. The family tree is similar to the pedigree used in a genetic study, which allows a study of the patterns of distribution of genetic traits in kindred people. When the information obtained in the family history reveals suspected genetic problems, the child and parents can be referred to a specialist in genetics for diagnosis and counseling.

Fig. 24-3 illustrates a family tree for a pediatric client.

Review of Systems

The review of systems is essentially the same as that carried out in the adult history (see Chapter 5) except for age-appropriate modifications. The format remains the same.

Physical systems

General (additional questions)
> Recent and significant gain or loss of weight, failure to gain weight appropriate for age, or failure to increase in height
> *Changes in behavior* such as increased crying, irritability, nervousness, or withdrawal or changes in sleep patterns. These questions are usually found under the review of the central nervous system (CNS) in the adult history. However, behavior changes in children may represent the first symptoms of a problem in any physical system or may indicate psychosocial problems including abuse and neglect.

Night sweats, fatigability

Skin (additional questions)
> Birthmarks, rashes

Eyes (additional questions)
> Strabismus, discharge

Mouth and throat (additional questions)
> Age of eruption of teeth
> Cleft lip or cleft palate
> Number of teeth at 1 year
> Thrush

Neck and nodes (additional questions)
> Limitation of movement, enlarged nodes

Breasts (deletions and additional questions)
> Questions about breast development should be addressed to the preadolescent and the adolescent boy or girl.
> Questions about individual concerns regarding breast development, such as comparisons made with peers

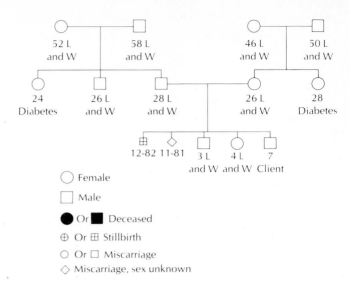

Figure 24-3

The family tree used in a pediatric history.

or the unequal development of the breasts, should be asked.
> Self-breast examination should be taught once breast buds begin to develop.

Respiratory and cardiovascular systems (additional questions) Stridor, wheezing, history of heart murmur
> Reduced exercise tolerance—does child play as actively as other children or curtail strenuous exercise?

Gastrointestinal system
> Abdominal pain, constipation

Genital system (deletions and additional questions)
Male
> Questions about the development of the secondary sex characteristics should be addressed to the preadolescent and adolescent male client:
> Increase in size of testes
> Appearance of pubic hair
> Appearance of hair on face and body
> Appearance of axillary hair
> Questions about individual concerns regarding sexual development should be asked.
> Delete the question about impotence until it is determined that the young man is sexually active.

Female
> Questions about development of the secondary sex characteristics should be addressed to the preadolescent and the adolescent female client:
> Appearance of pubic hair
> Appearance of axillary hair
> Onset of menses
> Questions about individual concerns regarding sexual development should be asked.

Delete the questions about menses until menarche has occurred. Determine if periods are painful.

Delete the questions about obstetric history until it is determined that the girl is sexually active.

Delete the question about Pap tests until the girl is 15 years of age unless it is determined that the girl less than 15 years is sexually active or was exposed to DES (diethylstilbestrol) before birth and has begun to menstruate.

Both sexes

Questions about sexual activity and venereal disease should be asked once the child is about 10 years old. The reason questions must be asked should be explained.

Extremities and musculoskeletal system (additional questions)

"Growing pains"

Postural deformities or changes

Changes in gait

Injuries to muscles or joints

Central nervous system

Ability to concentrate, hyperactivity, headaches

Additional information about this system will be obtained in the developmental history and social history.

Sociologic system

1. Relationship with family and significant others
   a. Client's position in the family, natural child or adopted (addition)
   b. Person(s) with whom client lives
   c. Persons with whom client relates (who is the primary caretaker, arrangements for babysitters, does the child have special friends)
   d. Recent family crises or changes (should include history of parental divorce, separation, or remarriage)
2. Environment
   a. Home (Heated? Adequate hot water? Number of rooms, toilets, cooking facilities? Where does child play?)
   b. Neighborhood
   c. Work (school)
   d. Recent changes in environment
   e. To what degree are cultural practices observed?
3. Occupational history (if appropriate)
   a. Jobs held
   b. Satisfaction with present and past employment
   c. Current place of employment
4. Economic status and resources
   a. Parents' occupations and source of income
   b. Parents' perception of adequacy or inadequacy of income
   c. Effect of child's illness on parents' economic status
5. Educational level
   a. Name of child's school
   b. Current grade level, has child ever been held back
   c. Judgment of intellect relative to age (parent may be asked to make this judgment by asking how this child performs compared with siblings or to other children the same age)
6. Daily profile
   a. Sleep, rest, activity patterns
   b. Social activities (play activities)
   c. Special weekend activities
   d. Recent changes in daily activities
   e. Parental concerns and management of any specific behavior such as masturbation, thumb sucking, temper tantrums, or bed-wetting
7. Patterns of health care
   a. Private and public primary care agencies
   b. Dental care
   c. Preventive care
   d. Emergency care

Psychological system

The outline for the psychological system review provided in Chapter 5, The Health History, is appropriate for use with the child and parent. The assessment includes the parent and the child because it will be the parent who is primarily responsible for the child's care during the childhood years. The adolescent child will be more responsible for self-care but will continue to need direction and support from an informed, understanding parent.

The Adolescent Interview

When assessing the adolescent client (children aged 11 years and older), the nurse must explore some additional areas. These include depression and suicide potential, involvement with drugs and alcohol, and sexuality. Table 24-6 and the boxes on p. 609 will give the nurse ideas of what to cover and how to get the most information. Inform teens that all they share will be kept confidential unless they or someone else are in danger of physical harm. At the same time, encourage teens to talk with their parents about these issues.

THE PHYSICAL EXAMINATION

The physical examination provides the opportunity to obtain objective information about the child and may have greater importance than the history when the parents are

Table 24-6

Opening lines, good and bad

	Poor	Better	Reason
Home	Tell me about mom and dad	Where do you live, and who lives there with you?	Parent(s) may have died or left the home. Open-ended question enables one to collect "environmental" as well as personal history
Education	How are you doing in school?	What are you good at in school? What is hard for you? What grades do you get?	Poor questions can be answered "okay." Good questions ask for information about strengths and weaknesses and allow for quantification/objectification
Activities	Do you have any activities outside of school?	What do you do for fun? What things do you do with friends? What do you do with your free time?	Good questions are open-ended and allow patient to express himself
Drugs	Do you do drugs?	Many young people experiment with drugs, alcohol, or cigarettes. Have you or your friends ever tried them? What have you tried?	Good question is an expression of concern with specific follow-up. With younger teens, it is best to begin by asking about friends
Sexuality	Have you ever had sex? Tell me about your boyfriend/girlfriend	Have you ever had a sexual relationship with anyone? Most young people become interested in sexual relationships at your age. Have you had any with boys, girls, or both? Tell me about your sex life	What does the term "have sex" really mean to teenagers? Asking only about heterosexual relationships closes doors at once

From Goldenring JM and Cohen E: Getting into adolescent heads, Contemp Pediatr 5:75-86, 1988.

poor historians and the child is too young to communicate.

The physical examination of the infant or child varies according to the primary purpose of the visit. Three types of examinations might be performed. The first is the screening of a healthy child. This examination is usually complete but does not go into any great depth with a particular organ system. The second is the evaluation of a chief complaint, and a more intensive examination of a particular area may be in order. The third is the follow-up examination of a complaint or disease that has been under treatment, and the focus is usually on one or two organ systems. Sometimes these three types of examinations are combined, particularly when it is the child's first visit and he or she is in need of a screening examination and a careful evaluation of a chief complaint.

Performance of the physical examination of the infant or child also varies according to the child's age, development, and behavior and the type of setting in which the care is being provided. If consideration is not given to the child's age and development, it is likely that the examination will be incomplete. The practitioner must understand the physical differences and development expected according to the child's age. If the child is fearful or fatigued, the practitioner will be more selective, when possible, in performing the examination.

When carrying out a pediatric examination, the examiner should keep in mind that each visit for health care is a learning experience for the child and the parent(s). The experience may result in increased confidence in themselves and others, or they may experience feelings of failure and distrust in the people who care for them. Thus, it is most productive to provide opportunities to develop positive relationships during the visits for routine health care. It also is important to remember that any separation of the child from the parent may provoke anxiety in both and may increase their level of fear and distrust. Therefore it is important to encourage parents to participate in the examination to support their child. The older child may be able to participate more freely without the parent present. Most parents will recognize the child's need to develop independence and encourage the child to participate alone. Finally, it is important to prepare the child and parent for any new or painful procedures. An appreciation for the feelings of children and parents will make them more cooperative.

The performance of the physical examination of a child must be organized and systematic. There are,

The HEADS Psychosocial Interview for Adolescents

Home

Who lives with patient? Where?
Own room?
What are relationships like at home?
What do parents and relatives do for a living?
Ever institutionalized? Incarcerated?
Recent moves? Running away?
New people in home environment?

Education and employment

School/grade performance—Any recent changes? Any dramatic past changes?
Favorite subjects—worst subjects? (include grades)
Any years repeated/classes failed?
Suspension, termination, dropping out?
Future education/employment plans/goals?
Any current or past employment?
Relations with teachers, employers—school/work attendance?
Recent change of schools—number of schools in last four years?

Activities

With peers (what do you do for fun? where and when?)
With family or clubs?

Sports—regular exercise?
Church attendance, clubs, projects?
Hobbies—other home activities?
Reading for fun—what?
TV—how much weekly—favorite shows?
Favorite music?
Does patient have car, use seat belts?
History of arrests—acting-out—crime?

Drugs

Use by peers? Use by patient? (include alcohol/tobacco)
Use by family members? (include alcohol/tobacco)
Amounts, frequency, patterns of use/abuse, and car use while intoxicated?
Source—how paid for?

Sexuality

Orientation?
Degree and types of sexual experience and acts?
Number of partners?
Masturbation? (Normalize)
History of pregnancy/abortion?
Sexually transmitted diseases—knowledge and prevention?
Contraception? Frequency of use?
Comfort with sexual activity, enjoyment/pleasure obtained?
History of sexual/physical abuse.

From Goldenring JM and Cohen E: Getting into adolescent heads, Contemp Pediatr 5:75-86, 1988.

Suicide Risk/Depression Screening

1. Sleep disorders (usually induction problems; also early/frequent waking or greatly increased sleep and complaints of increasing fatigue)
2. Appetite/eating behavior change
3. Feelings of "boredom"
4. Emotional outbursts and highly impulsive behavior
5. History of withdrawal/isolation
6. Hopeless/helpless feelings
7. History of past suicide attempts, depression, psychological counseling
8. History of No. 7 in family or peers
9. History of drug/alcohol abuse, acting-out/crime, recent change in school performance
10. History of recurrent serious "accidents"
11. Psychosomatic symptomatology
12. Suicidal ideation (including significant current and past losses)
13. Decreased affect on interview, avoidance of eye contact—depression posturing
14. Preoccupation with death (clothing, music, media, art)

From Goldenring JM and Cohen E: Getting into adolescent heads, Contemp Pediatr 5:75-86, 1988.

however, differences between an adult and a pediatric examination. The practitioner performs distressing parts of the examination at the end, if it is believed the child will be unable to cooperate. An example would be the ear, nose, and throat examination. The order of the examination may be altered to accommodate the individual child's behavior, for example, listening to the heart and lungs early in the examination before crying starts or becomes more vigorous. A good idea is to start the examination of a child with a body part that is least likely to interfere with developing a sense of trust and confidence, for example, inspection of the hands and feet.

Approach to the Child

Little difficulty is encountered in the performance of the physical examination of the infant in the first 6 months of life, since the infant has little fear of strangers. The infant can be distracted by the parent or the examiner with repetitive vocal sounds and smiles. However, the examination of the ears and mouth may cause distress and should be the last part of the examination. It is wise to take advantage of the opportunities that are offered. If the infant is quiet or sleepy, it is best to start with the auscultation of the chest and to do so while the caretaker is still holding the infant. If the infant is playful and active, it is easier to start with the extremities and wait for a quieter moment to examine the chest.

During the last half of the first year of life, the infant experiences an increasing fear of strangers; thus, it is often profitable to conduct the entire examination while the infant is held on the parent's lap. Even under the best of circumstances, it may not be possible to create a situation that is ideal; the infant may remain resistant throughout the examination. This requires the examiner to be efficient in carrying out the examination in the least amount of time and with minimum restraint of the infant. The parent often experiences discomfort or embarrassment because of the infant's behavior and needs reassurance that the infant is behaving normally. The situation is ideal for helping the parent understand normal development and the needs of the infant at this age.

The child from 1 to 3 years of age is a challenge to even the most experienced examiner. The child is learning to use the body and to manipulate and experiment with all aspects of the environment. Any restraint in the pursuit of desired activities may be seen by the child as an interference, resulting in unhappiness or frustration for the child. The child at this age is getting lots of pleasure from recently acquired skills such as walking and talking and enjoys the new ability to manipulate objects such as doors and wastebaskets. At the same time, the child is still unsure of strangers and needs the parent's presence to feel safe. The 2- or 3-year-old child may be charming and cooperative or difficult to examine; whichever the case, the examiner is required to make many modifications in the organization of the examination. The child may be examined in a standing position with the examiner in a seated position or on the parent's lap. The child usually does not like to have all clothing removed at one time but will often cooperate if only one article of clothing is removed at a time as the examination is carried out. The child also needs the opportunity to handle and use the examining instruments. He or she may enjoy doing this but may also reject the offer if it is too fear-provoking. Despite the difficulties in examining the child of this age, the child's ability to relate more positively at each subsequent visit can be rewarding and profitable for the examiner.

The child at 3 or 4 years of age is usually able to understand and cooperate during the examination. He or she is anxious to please and is usually a delightful participant. This child has better control of feelings and behavior than the younger child but may still lose control if fear is great. The child should receive recognition for efforts to participate, so that self-image is enhanced. This

child especially enjoys trying out the examiner's equipment and will very likely demonstrate new learning in future play activities; this is a way to incorporate the role of the examiner and master fears (Fig. 24-4). Again, it may be helpful to permit the child to remain on the caretaker's lap.

The school-age child may be approached in much the same way as the adult. He or she is usually curious and interested and benefits from explanations on what is going to be done. This child wants to perform well and will usually cooperate but may have concerns about his or her body and feel threatened by the examination. The child should be encouraged to ask questions. Modesty should be respected and attempts made to conduct the examination with as little exposure as possible.

The adolescent is not easy to anticipate as behaviors are not predictable. He or she may be angry and hostile or charming and self-confident. The adolescent is primarily concerned about himself or herself and carries the egocentric belief that others are as preoccupied with his or her behavior and appearance as he or she is. The adolescent is likely to anticipate the responses of other people based on self-beliefs, self-criticism, and self-admiration. The adolescent self-consciously plays to an audience because he or she believes self-behaviors, thoughts, and appearance are important to many people. Despite this egocentric view, the adolescent will be sensitive to a nonjudgmental examiner who encourages relevant conversation. He or she may not be able to do this during the first visit, but if the experience is worthwhile to him, the adolescent may reveal more of these concerns at a later visit. He or she usually needs an opportunity to talk with the examiner alone. This can sometimes be arranged early in the interview with the parents and adolescent during an explanation of what will happen during the visit. The adolescent can be asked if he or she would agree to being examined without the parent present to provide the opportunity to ask private questions. The nurse can inform the parent that it is the policy to examine children aged 12 and older alone so that the parent does not feel offended. It can be explained that both the parent and the adolescent are needed for the history to make it as complete as possible. It will also be necessary to discuss plans with both of them together after the examination. This young person is self-conscious and easily embarrassed and should be gowned during the examination and given complete privacy when dressing and undressing.

Methods of Restraint

There are occasions when the physical examination involves an uncooperative child. The practitioner may need

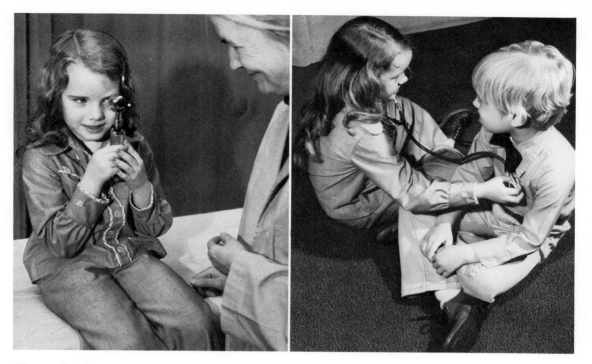

Figure 24-4

The child enjoys trying out the examiner's equipment.

to use one or more of a variety of safe child-restraint methods. Clinical experience and knowledge of the child's behavior during previous visits will aid the practitioner in choosing a safe restraint method. When restraint is necessary, the procedure should be carried out as quickly as possible and without criticism of the child.

One of the most common restraints used during the examination of the infant or young child when examining the ears, nose, and mouth is done with the aid of the parent or another adult. The child is placed in the supine position with the arms extended and held alongside the head by the assisting adult (Fig. 24-5). Occasionally an older child cannot cooperate, and the same method is used with a second adult assistant holding the child's legs.

Another method for the older child is sometimes called the "hug." The child sits on the parent's lap with the legs to the side and one arm tucked under the parent's arm while the parent holds the child's other arm securely. Greater immobility of the child can be obtained by having the parent place the child's legs between his or her own (Fig. 24-6).

The parent may be uncomfortable about assisting with a restraint, and another adult may be asked to help. However, the child will feel less threatened if the parent holds him.

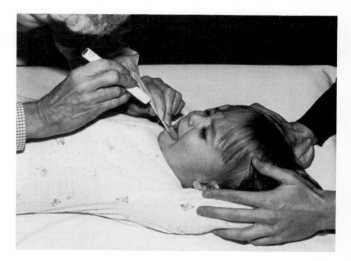

Figure 24-5

Restraint of the young infant with the parent assisting.

Measurements

The measurements of the temperature, pulse rate, respiratory rate, blood pressure, height, and weight are part of the physical examination of the child. In addition, the measurements of the head circumference are noted for the child under 3 years of age. The comparison of the physical measurements of a child with those of other healthy children over time makes it possible to determine

Figure 24-6

Restraint of the older child using the "hug" and leg restraint.

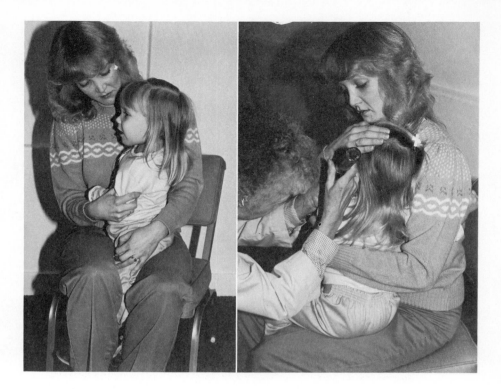

if the child is progressing within normal parameters or if there are significant deviations.

Assessment of vital signs

Temperature.   The three body areas commonly used for obtaining temperature measurements—the mouth, the axilla, and the rectum—are discussed in Chapter 7, General Assessment, Including Vital Signs. The method used is determined by the child's ability to cooperate and the health status.

A rectal temperature is often the method used during the first few years of a child's life. The main drawback is the danger of perforation of the rectum in the young infant and the increased discomfort for the young child, who experiences this as an intrusive procedure. It should not be used with children who cannot tolerate this kind of stimulus to the CNS, as is the case with some children who have epilepsy. A safe restraint method for taking a rectal temperature of a young infant is to lay the child face down on the parent's lap or on a padded table. The adult should place the left forearm firmly across the child's hip area, so that the child cannot raise the buttocks off the adult's lap or the table. The practitioner uses the thumb and forefinger of the nondominant hand to separate the buttocks, and then the dominant hand is free to gently insert the lubricated thermometer. The infant's rectum is quite short; therefore the thermometer should be inserted only a short distance. Three considerations that may be used to determine sufficient entry include noting that the

column of mercury is rising steadily, inserting no more than ½ in., and observing a decrease in the child's effort to push against the thermometer. It is normal for the child to push against the thermometer as the rectal sphincter muscles contract in response to the stimulus. The practitioner waits until the sphincter relaxes before continuing to insert. The thermometer is held firmly enough to keep the child from pushing it out. Care must be taken to hold the thermometer firmly but not to push it in further. Also, the child must be held securely to prevent jerking and pushing the thermometer further into the rectum.

Obtaining an oral temperature reading is usually reserved for children who are 5 to 6 years of age and older. The child must be able to understand not to bite on the glass thermometer and to keep the mouth closed during the procedure. Sometimes the child's health condition interferes with being able to use this method, for example, mouth breathing or limited intellectual functioning.

An axillary temperature can be obtained on any child and reduces the risk of injury and is less intrusive. It can be done when the child objects to the rectal temperature and the oral temperature is not appropriate. The thermometer is placed in the axilla and the arm held close to the body. The child can be restrained by using the "hug" if necessary.

Temperature regulation is less exact in children than adults. The rectal temperature is normally higher in infants and younger children, and the average tempera-

Table 24-7

Average heart rate for infants and children at rest

Age	Average rate
Birth	140
1st mo	130
1-6 mo	130
6-12 mo	115
1-2 yr	110
2-4 yr	105
6-10 yr	95
10-14 yr	85
14-18 yr	82

Table 24-8

Amplitude, quality of the heart rate, and site, as they relate to differential diagnosis of heart dysfunction in young infants and children

Amplitude, quality, site	Cardiac dysfunction
Narrow, thready	Congestive heart failure
	Severe aortic stenosis
Bounding	Patent ductus arteriosus
	Aortic regurgitation
Pulsation in suprasternal notch	Aortic insufficiency
	Patent ductus arteriosus
	Coarctation of the aorta
Palpable thrill in suprasternal notch	Aortic stenosis
	Valvular pulmonary stenosis
	Coarctation of the aorta, occasionally patent ductus arteriosus

Data from Kempe CH, and others: Current pediatric diagnosis and treatment, ed 5, Los Altos, 1978, Lange Medical Publications.

Table 24-9

Variations in respiration with age

Age	Rate/minute
Premature	40-90
Newborn	30-80
1 yr	20-40
2 yr	20-30
3 yr	20-30
5 yr	20-25
10 yr	17-22
15 yr	15-20
20 yr	15-20

Data from Lowrey GH: Growth and development of children, Chicago, 1978, Year Book Medical Publications, Inc.

ture is above 99° F (37.2° C) until age 3 years. The increase in temperature with even a minor infection is usually greater in infants and young children than in adults. However, young infants with a severe infection may have a normal or subnormal temperature.

Pulse and respiration. Apprehension, crying, and physical activity, as well as the examination procedure itself, can alter a child's heart and respiratory rates. Thus, it is desirable to take these measurements while the child is at rest, either sleeping or lying quietly. If the child has been active, the measurement is delayed until the child has relaxed about 5 to 10 minutes.

The child's pulse is to be examined for rate, rhythm, quality, and amplitude, just as in an adult. Auscultation of the heart—measuring the apical pulse—is the most easily obtained pulse in a young infant. The average heart rate of the infant at birth is 140 beats per minute. At 2 years of age the child's heart has adjusted downward to 110. At 10 years the rate is 85, and by the time the child reaches age 18, the pulse may be observed to have lowered to 82. A child, usually an adolescent, who engages in exercise regularly, such as swimming laps, may exhibit a much slower rate, that is, in the 60s.

Table 24-7 lists the average heart rates for children from birth to 18 years. Heart rhythm in children is not always regular. Often it reflects the phasic action of the heart in relation to the respiratory cycle. This is called sinus arrhythmia, and it is considered normal in children.

Palpation of the brachial and the femoral pulses is an essential step in the examination of the young infant. Irregularities often are the first signs of serious heart dysfunction. The amplitude and time of appearance of the femoral pulse are expected to equal those of the brachial pulse. Absence or weakness of the femoral pulse alerts the examiner to the possibility of coarctation of the aorta in the young infant. Table 24-8 compares some

differences in amplitude, quality, and site and how they may relate to the differential diagnosis of heart disorders in children.

The respiratory rate may be obtained by inspection or auscultation. The average range of normal respirations is 30 to 80 per minute in the newborn period compared with 20 to 30 in the 2-year-old. By 10 years of age the rate has adjusted to 17 to 22, and by age 20 it averages 15 to 20 respirations per minute. Table 24-9 exhibits variations in respiration with age.

Blood pressure. The levels of systolic and diastolic blood pressure gradually increase during childhood, and there is normally a considerable variation in a child's pressure. The systolic pressure of the child may be raised by crying, vigorous exercise, or anxiety. It is therefore appropriate to choose a time when the child is quiet and comfortable to obtain this measurement.

The National Task Force on Blood Pressure Control in Children has recommended that children 3 years or older should have their blood pressure measured annually as part of their regular health care. The child of this age is usually able to cooperate when the procedure for obtaining a blood pressure measurement is explained. The blood pressure of the child under 3 years of age is not routinely measured unless there are indications of underlying problems such as renal or cardiac disease.

The most common method of measuring the blood pressure of the child is still auscultation using a mercury or aneroid sphygmomanometer. The selection of the cuff size and the method of measuring the blood pressure are described in Chapter 7, General Assessment, Including Vital Signs. Pediatric cuffs can be obtained in several sizes for newborns, infants, and children. A pediatric stethoscope with a small diaphragm is also essential when measuring the blood pressure of a young child. The systolic pressure is recorded as that point at which the Korotkoff sounds are initially heard. The diastolic pressure is recorded for the point at which the fourth phase Korotkoff sound is heard, when the sound first becomes muffled. In young children the fourth and fifth sounds frequently occur simultaneously, and sometimes the Korotkoff sounds are heard all the way to zero.

The Doppler instrument, although relatively expensive, is useful with young infants and children. The Doppler measures systolic blood pressure, which is the first sound heard. The reliability for accurate diastolic pressure measurement has not yet been documented.

The flush method is used with the young infant or child when a Doppler is not available and provides only a measure of mean pressure. This method is described in Chapter 7, General Assessment, Including Vital Signs.

The blood pressure measurements obtained should be recorded on appropriate blood pressure charts such as those developed by the Second National Task Force on Blood Pressure Control in Children (Table 24-10) that were based on studies supported by the National Heart, Lung and Blood Institute. They allow the examiner to record the blood pressure measurements in serial fashion, determine how this child compares with other children the same age, and observe a trend or pattern for this child over time. A diagnosis of hypertension can only be made after taking serial readings (see boxed material).

Growth measurements

The routine measurement of growth is a screening procedure rather than a diagnostic procedure yet can provide clues to serious health problems. Growth is a continuous process that must be evaluated over time. Successive, serial measurements plotted on a standardized growth chart provide objective information about the individual child's rate and pattern of growth compared with the general population. The information obtained is useful in providing reassurance to parents and professionals re-

---

Tips for Taking Children's Blood Pressures

1. Child should be seated. Pressure should be taken routinely in the right arm held at heart level.
2. Do not press too hard with the stethoscope.
3. If no pediatric cuff is available, use an adult cuff around the child's thigh and place stethoscope over the popliteal area (behind knee) to hear Korotkoff sounds. This measurement averages about 10 mm Hg higher than blood pressure taken in the arm.
4. A child with abnormally high serial readings should be referred to a physician.
5. Significant hypertension is blood pressure persistently between the 95th and 99th percentile for age and sex.
6. Severe hypertension is blood pressure persistently at or above the 99th percentile for age and sex.

Table 24-10

Classification of hypertension by age group

Age group	Significant hypertension (mm Hg)	Severe hypertension (mm Hg)
Newborns	Systolic BP $\geq$96	Systolic BP $\geq$106
(7 d) (8-30 d)	Systolic BP $\geq$104	Systolic BP $\geq$110
Infants	Systolic BP $\geq$112	Systolic BP $\geq$118
(<2 yr)	Diastolic BP $\geq$74	Diastolic BP $\geq$82
Children	Systolic BP $\geq$116	Systolic BP $\geq$124
(3-5 yr)	Diastolic BP $\geq$76	Diastolic BP $\geq$84
Children	Systolic BP $\geq$122	Systolic BP $\geq$130
(6-9 yr)	Diastolic BP $\geq$78	Diastolic BP $\geq$86
Children	Systolic BP $\geq$126	Systolic BP $\geq$134
(10-12 yr)	Diastolic BP $\geq$82	Diastolic BP $\geq$90
Adolescents	Systolic BP $\geq$136	Systolic BP $\geq$144
(13-15 yr)	Diastolic BP $\geq$86	Diastolic BP $\geq$92
Adolescents	Systolic BP $\geq$142	Systolic BP $\geq$150
(16-18 yr)	Diastolic BP $\geq$92	Diastolic BP $\geq$98

Reprinted with permission from the Report of the Second Task Force on Blood Pressure Control in Children—1987, Pediatrics 79:1-25, 1987.

garding the child who is growing normally, assessing the nutritional status of the child, and identifying the child who may have abnormalities affecting the various growth parameters. Examples of abnormalities that could impair growth include growth hormone deficiency, inflammatory bowel disease, and cardiac and renal disorders.

The three parameters of growth routinely measured during each examination of the child under 3 years of age are recumbent length, body weight, and head circumference. For the child over 3 years of age it is sufficient to obtain standing height and weight measurements only. Assessment of body segments, skinfold thickness, bone age, and dentition may be used for further study of body growth but are not usually included in the routine physical examination.

The growth charts published by the National Center for Health Statistics (NCHS) in 1976 should be used to record growth measurements. They are based on large, nationally representative samples of children. Two groups of charts were developed from the data: the first for the age interval from birth to 36 months and the second for the interval from 2 to 18 years. There are actually 14 charts. The charts for infants (birth to 36 months) include graphs for head circumference, recumbent length by age, weight by age, and weight by length for both boys and girls. The charts for children 2 to 18 years include graphs for stature (standing height) by age, weight by age, and weight by stature of prepubescent children for both boys and girls.

The appropriate use of the charts requires that the measurements be done in the same way the reference measurements were done. For instance, standing height or stature should not be recorded on the birth to 36 months chart, since the infant will appear shorter than if recumbent length had been plotted. For the youngest children recumbent length is greater than stature by almost 1 in. For greater accuracy it is suggested that children be-

tween 2 and 3 years of age be measured supine and weighed on the infant scale according to the reference measures for the birth to 36 months chart. However, there are always exceptions, and 2- to 3-year-old children will be measured in a standing position. See the Tips box below.

Length or height. Recumbent length (birth to 3 years) is measured in the supine position with the legs extended. When measuring length, the procedure is facilitated by having two people participate. The parent is usually available and interested in providing this assistance. If a measuring board is used, the infant's head is placed against the fixed headboard and held in the midline by the parent while the examiner gently pushes on the knees until the legs are fully extended and both heels are firmly touching the movable footboard (Fig. 24-7). If a measuring device is not available, the same procedure is followed placing the child on a paper-covered, flat surface and marking the paper at the top of the child's head and at the bottom of the heels. The child is then removed, and the distance between the two points is measured.

Standing height or stature (2 to 18 years) is measured with the shoes off. The child is asked to stand as tall as possible and look straight ahead so that the top of the head is parallel with the ceiling. The feet should be together, and the shoulders, buttocks, and heels should be touching the wall without any flexion of the knees. A block, squared at right angles against the wall or measuring board, is brought to the top of the child's head (Fig. 24-8). When a measuring device is not available, a mark can be made on the wall at the top of the child's head and the distance from the floor measured.

Weight. Appropriately sized beam scales with nondetachable weights should be used. Two scales are suggested: one for infants and small children that measures weights to the nearest 0.5 oz or 10 g and one for older children and adults that measures weights to the

---

Tips for Using Pediatric Growth Charts

Age- and sex-specific growth charts are readily available from the major formula manufacturers and from the makers of growth hormone. They have been standardized using data from thousands of children so that comparison may be made. Proper documentation of height and weight onto growth charts is as important as proper assessment. On the sample growth chart (Fig. 24-10) note that crossed lines are drawn with a straight edge to ensure that the child's age and measurements are recorded exactly. If the child is 9 years and 9 months old, the vertical line will be drawn in a different place than if the child is 9 years and 2 months old. This can make a big difference

as to which percentile the child's height, weight, or head circumference falls into.

If a child is born prematurely, it is important to use the "corrected age" on growth charts and developmental assessments until the child is 2½ years old. To calculate "corrected age," simply subtract the number of weeks the child was born prematurely from the child's chronologic age. EXAMPLE: One would expect a 15-month-old child born 6 weeks prematurely to be in the same growth and developmental range of normal as a 13-month-old.

Figure 24-7

Recumbent length measured.

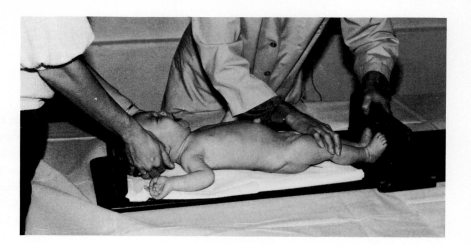

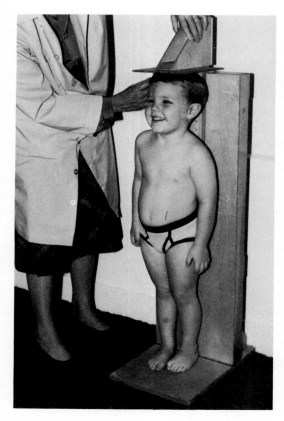

Figure 24-8

Measurement of stature (standing height).

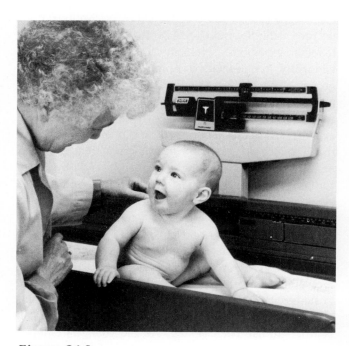

Figure 24-9

Weighing the young infant.

nearest 0.25 lb or 100 g. Before weighing the child, the scale should be checked to determine if it is balanced. The weights are returned to the zero setting, and balance is observed to rest in the middle.

Infants (up to 3 years) are weighed naked on the infant scale (Fig. 24-9). Older children (2 to 18 years) are weighed on the upright adult scale dressed only in underpants or a light gown.

Head circumference.   The head circumference is measured during each examination between birth and 3 years of age. A nonstretchable tape measure is passed over the most prominent part of the occiput and just above the supraorbital ridges. The average head circumference at birth is 35 cm (14 in) and by age 2 has increased to 49 cm (19.2 in). The head circumference is an important measure to obtain because it is related to intracranial volume and allows an estimation of the rate of growth of the brain. Sequential measurements are plotted on the appropriate NCHS growth chart. Any discrepancy or deviation should be checked. The conditions of microcephaly and hydrocephaly are considered.

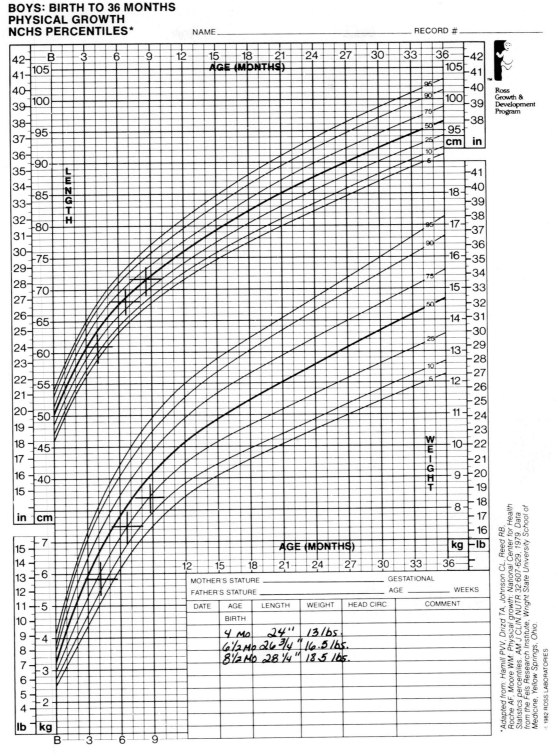

BOYS: BIRTH TO 36 MONTHS
PHYSICAL GROWTH
NCHS PERCENTILES*

NAME _____ RECORD # _____

DATE	AGE	LENGTH	WEIGHT	HEAD CIRC	COMMENT
	BIRTH				
	4 MO	24"	13 lbs.		
	6½ Mo	26 ¾"	16.5 lbs.		
	8½ Mo	28 ¼"	18.5 lbs.		

MOTHER'S STATURE _____ GESTATIONAL
FATHER'S STATURE _____ AGE _____ WEEKS

*Adapted from: Hamill PVV, Drizd TA, Johnson CL, Reed RB, Roche AF, Moore WM. Physical growth: National Center for Health Statistics percentiles. AM J CLIN NUTR 32:607-629, 1979. Data from the Fels Research Institute, Wright State University School of Medicine, Yellow Springs, Ohio.
© 1982 ROSS LABORATORIES

Ross
Growth &
Development
Program

Figure 24-10

Sample National Health Center growth chart.
(Courtesy Ross Laboratories.)

It is also important to measure the head circumference of the child who is suspected of having a neurologic problem or a developmental delay, regardless of age.

Chest circumference. The measurement of the circumference of the chest at delivery and in early infancy has become significant in that it may indicate birth injury, congenital anomalies, or system dysfunction, for example, cardiac enlargement. Otherwise, measuring the chest circumference on a regular basis after the first 9 months of life is unnecessary. Exceptions to this might include observed body disproportion or malformation of the thoracic cage. The chest circumference of the child is measured by placing a nonstretchable cloth tape measure at the level of the nipple, with the child in a supine position. Measurement is made midway between inspiration and expiration.

Growth curves of the body as a whole and of the three types of tissue—lymphoid, neural, and genital—demonstrate the age ranges when children are expected to exhibit growth spurts.

Areas of Assessment
General inspection

The survey or general inspection is discussed in Chapter 7, General Assessment, Including Vital Signs. The general inspection of the child includes the many observations described in Chapter 7. The examiner also must keep in mind those physical and behavioral characteristics that are expected for the individual child at the present chronologic age. Chapter 2, Psychosocial Assessment, describes normal physical and behavioral changes that occur during the child's development.

Some of the physical changes to be observed are the normal changes in facies, posture, and body contour; changes in gait; and the development of secondary sex characteristics. The criteria for assessing pubertal status developed by Tanner are useful in describing the child's stage of pubertal development (Figs. 24-11 to 24-14).

Observations are made regarding the child's development during the examination, and the findings may indicate that a more formal assessment is indicated.

The child's behavior is also observed and de-

Development	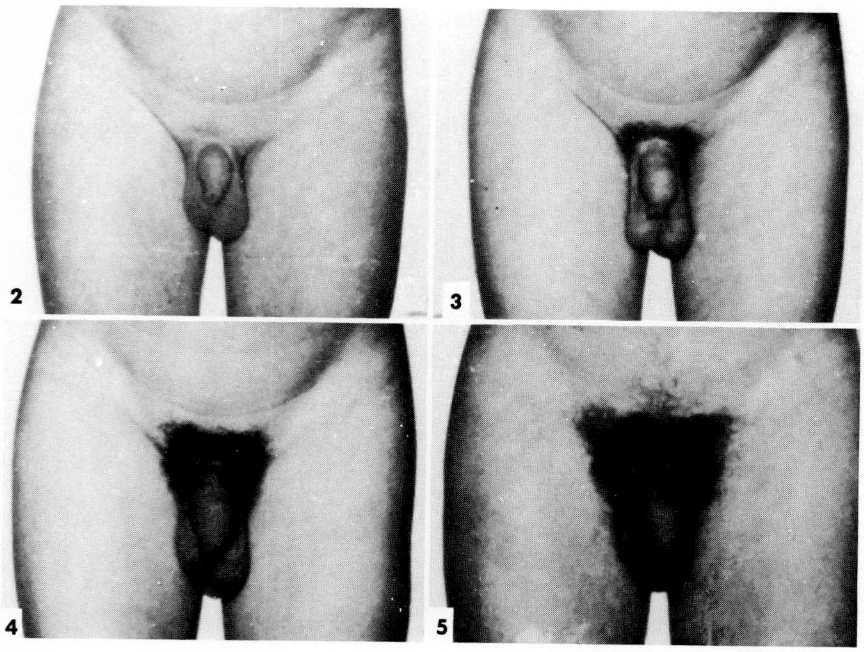	Stage	Description
		1	None; preadolescent
		2	Scant, long, slightly pigmented
		3	Darker, starting to curl small amount
		4	Resembles adult, but less quantity; coarse, curly
		5	Adult distribution, spread to medial surface of thighs

Figure 24-11

Pubic hair development in males.
(From Tanner JM: Growth of adolescence, ed 2, Oxford, 1962, Blackwell Scientific Publications.)

scribed. Is this a quiet, shy child or an active, restless child? Is this child comfortable during the visit, or anxious and afraid? Does the child respond to the parent or other adults in an appropriate way? Each child is a unique being, and it is a challenge to observe and record a description of any child's behavior. It is also necessary to keep in mind that the behavior seen during a visit for health care may not be typical for that child.

Skin

The examination of the skin provides valuable information about the general health of the child and evidence of specific skin problems. The skin of the entire body

should be noted at each examination. The normal condition of the skin changes with age, and it is helpful to become familiar with those changes seen in children.

The skin of the newborn is soft and smooth and appears almost transparent. The superficial vessels are prominent, giving the skin its red color. A mild degree of jaundice is present after the second or third day in normal infants; if the jaundice is severe or occurs in the first 24 hours, however, the examiner should consider the presence of a serious problem. Small papular patches, called nevus flammeus, may be present over the occiput, forehead, and upper eyelids in the newborn period and usually disappear by the end of the first year of life. The

Development	Stage	Description
	1	Penis, testes, and scrotum preadolescent
	2	Enlargement of scrotum and testes, texture alteration; scrotal sac reddens; penis usually does not enlarge
	3	Further growth of testes and scrotum; penis enlarges and becomes longer
	4	Continued growth of testes and scrotum; scrotum becomes darker; penis becomes longer; glans and breadth increase in size
	5	Adult in size and shape

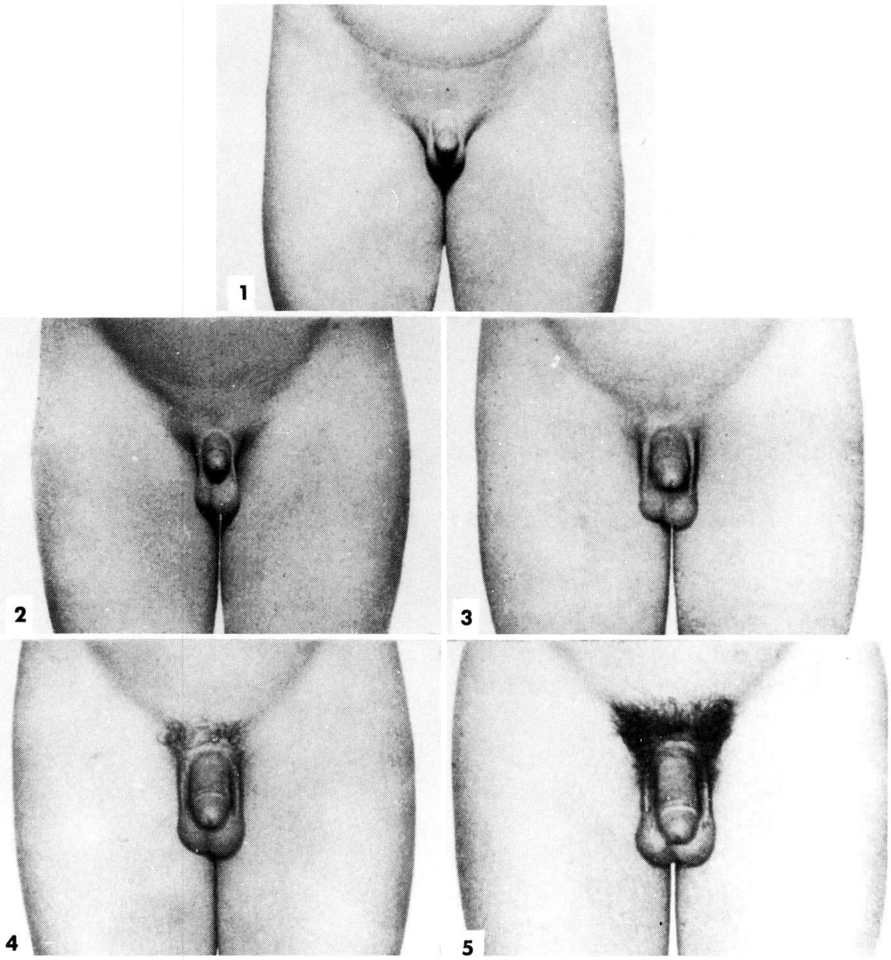

Figure 24-12

Penis and testes/scrotum development in males.
(From Tanner JM: Growth of adolescence, ed 2, Oxford, 1962, Blackwell Scientific Publications.)

Development		Stage	Description
		1	None; preadolescent
		2	Sparse, lightly pigmented, straight along medial border of labia
		3	Darker, beginning to curl, increased amount
		4	Coarse, curly, abundant amount but less than adult
		5	Adult female triangle, spread to medial surface of thighs

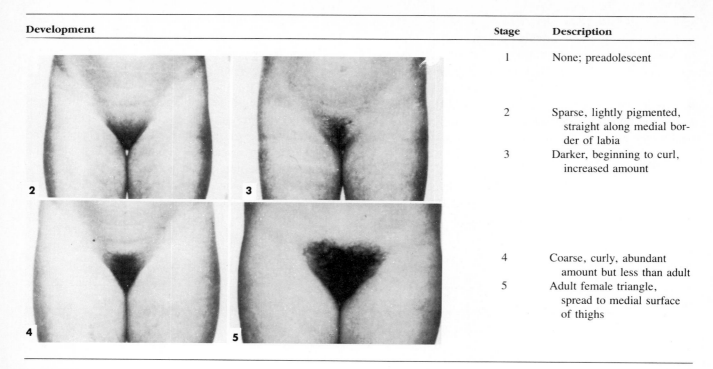

Figure 24-13

Pubic hair development in females.
(From Tanner JM: Growth of adolescence, ed 2, Oxford, 1962, Blackwell Scientific Publications.)

nose and cheeks are frequently covered by small white papules caused by plugging of the sebaceous glands during the neonatal period. Both sweat and sebaceous glands are present in the newborn but do not function until the second month of life. Some desquamation is common during the first weeks and varies in individual babies. Mongolian spots, which are blue, irregularly shaped flat areas, are found in the sacral and buttocks area of some infants, usually those who have more darkly pigmented skin. These usually disappear by the end of the first or second year but occasionally persist for a longer time. There is a considerable amount of fine hair, called lanugo, over the body of the newborn, which is lost during the first weeks of life. The nails of the full-term newborn are well formed and firm in contrast to those of the premature infant, which are imperfectly formed.

During the first year of life there is a continuing increase in the proportion of subcutaneous fat, and raw areas resulting from skin rubbing against skin are more prevalent in young obese infants. This is called intertrigo. During the second year of life there is a decrease in the proportion of subcutaneous fat, and intertrigo is less common. Skin turgor is a good indicator of hydration status.

After the first year of life the normal child shows little changes in the skin until the onset of puberty, when there is considerable development of both sweat and sebaceous glands. Associated with the development of the sebaceous glands is acne vulgaris, which is so common in its mildest forms that it is sometimes considered a normal physiologic change. Early evidence of acne is the occasional comedo, or blackhead, on the nose and chin. At age 13 or 14, papules and small pustules may begin to appear, and by age 16 many children will have recovered completely. There are also changes in the amount and distribution of hair. Hair growth becomes heavier; the appearance of pubic, axillary, and most of the more prominent body hair is influenced by sexual development during adolescence.

Lymph nodes

Lymph nodes in children have the same distribution as that found in adults, but the nodes are usually more prominent until puberty. The amount of lymphoid tissue is considerable at birth and increases steadily until after puberty. It is common to find shotty, discrete, movable, small, nontender nodes in the occipital, postauricular, anterior and posterior cervical, parotid, submaxillary, sublingual, axillary, epitrochlear, and inguinal areas in the normal healthy child. Lymph nodes are examined during the examination of each part of the body.

Stage	Breast development	Development description

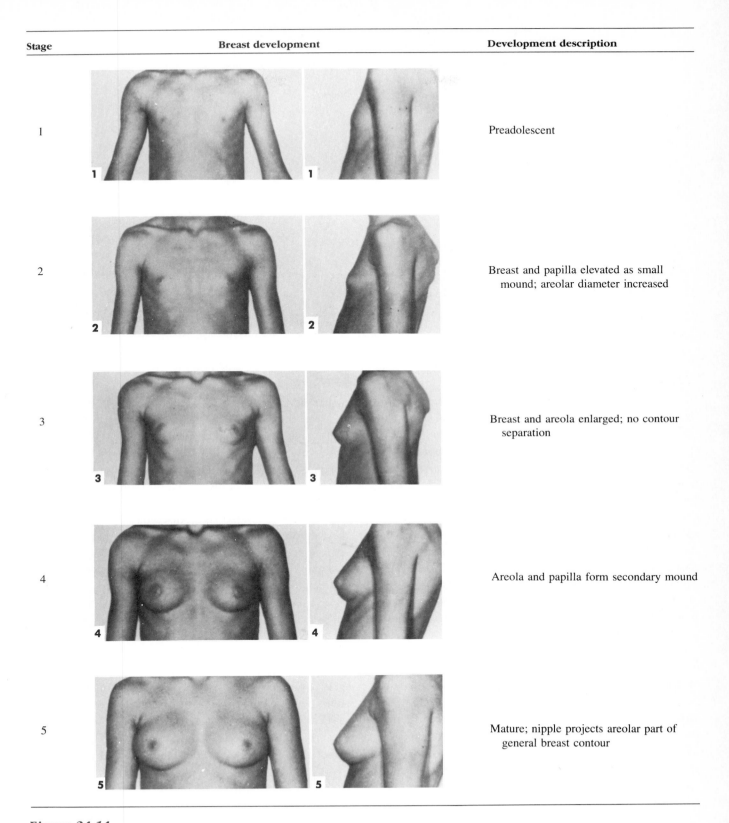

Stage 1 — Preadolescent

Stage 2 — Breast and papilla elevated as small mound; areolar diameter increased

Stage 3 — Breast and areola enlarged; no contour separation

Stage 4 — Areola and papilla form secondary mound

Stage 5 — Mature; nipple projects areolar part of general breast contour

Figure 24-14

Maturational sequence in girls.
(From Tanner JM: Growth of adolescence, ed 2, Oxford, 1962, Blackwell Scientific Publications.)

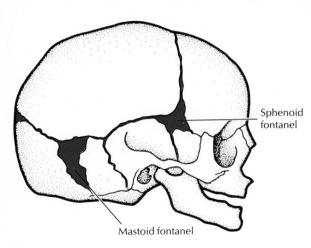

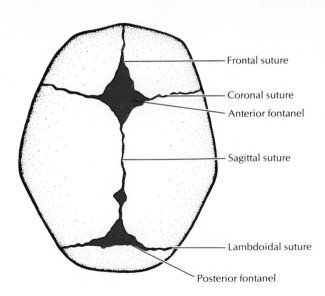

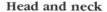

Figure 24-15

Skull bones of the infant, showing fontanels and sutures.

Head and neck

The shape of the newborn infant's head is often asymmetric as a result of the molding that occurs during the passage through the birth canal, and it may be a few days or weeks before the normal shape is restored. The newborn has a skull that molds easily because the bones of the cranium are not fused, which allows some overlapping of the bones. Trauma may result in caput succedaneum or cephalohematoma. *Caput succedaneum* is an edematous swelling of the superficial tissues of the scalp manifested by a generalized soft swelling not bounded by suture lines. This is temporary and is usually resolved within the first few days of life. *Cephalohematoma* occurs as a result of bleeding into the periosteum and results in swelling that does not cross the suture line. Most cephalohematomas are absorbed within 2 weeks to 3 months. Flattening of the head is often seen in normal children but can also indicate problems such as mental retardation or rickets.

The sutures of the skull are palpated and can usually be felt as ridges until the age of 6 months. The fontanels are palpated during each examination of the infant and young child to determine the size, shape, and presence of any tenseness or bulging. Normally, the posterior fontanel closes by 2 months of age and the anterior fontanel closes by the end of the second year (Fig. 24-15). Tenseness or bulging of the fontanels is most easily detected when the child is in a sitting position and should be assessed when the child is quiet. Bulging of the fontanels may be depressed when the infant is dehydrated or malnourished. Early closure or delayed closure of the fontanels should be noted. Early closure may result from microcephaly and delayed closure from prolonged intracranial pressure.

The importance of measuring the head circumference of the child up to 3 years of age has already been discussed.

Transillumination of the skull is a useful procedure in the initial examination of the infant and for any infant with an abnormal head size. Transillumination is carried out in a completely darkened room with an ordinary flashlight equipped with a rubber adaptor. The light is placed against the infant's head. If the cerebrum is absent or greatly thinned, as from increased intracranial pressure, the entire cranium lights up. Often, defects transilluminate in a more limited way. Auscultation of the skull may reveal bruits, which are commonly found in normal children up to 4 years of age. After the age of 4, bruits are evidence of problems such as aneurysms or increased intracranial pressure.

The young infant's scalp is inspected for evidence of crusting, which often results from a seborrheic dermatitis.

The shape of the face is inspected. A facial paralysis is most easily observed when the child cries or smiles and the asymmetry is increased. An abnormal or unusual facies may indicate a chromosomal abnormality such as Down's syndrome.

The frontal and maxillary sinuses should be percussed by the direct method and palpated in the child over 2 or 3 years of age. Until that age the sinuses are too small and poorly developed for percussion or palpation (Fig. 24-16).

The submaxillary and sublingual glands are palpated in the same way as in the adult examination. Local swelling of the parotid gland is most easily determined by observing the child in the sitting position with the head raised and the neck extended and by noting any

A　　　　　　B　　　　　　C　　　　　　D

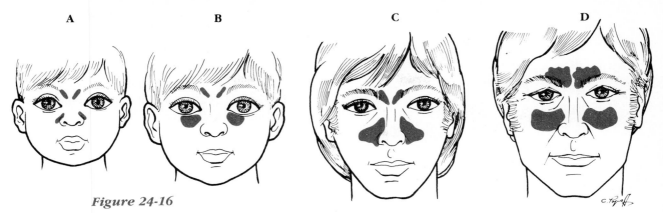

Figure 24-16

Development of the frontal and maxillary sinuses. **A,** Early infancy. **B,** Early childhood. **C,** Adolescence. **D,** Adulthood.

swelling below the angle of the jaw. The swollen parotid gland may be felt by palpating downward from the zygomatic arch. Unilateral or bilateral swelling of the parotid gland usually indicates mumps.

　　The neck is examined with the child lying flat on the back. The size of the neck is noted. The neck of the infant normally is short; it lengthens at about 3 or 4 years of age. The lymph nodes are palpated, as are the thyroid gland and trachea. The sternocleidomastoid muscle is carefully palpated. A mass on the lower third of the muscle may indicate a congenital torticollis. Finally, the mobility of the neck is determined by lifting the child's head and turning it from side to side. Any resistance to flexion may indicate meningeal irritation.

Eyes

The examination of the eyes is most easily accomplished when the child is able to cooperate. The school-age child is able to participate, and the examination is carried out as described in Chapter 10 on assessment of the eyes. The infant and young child are much more of a challenge to the examiner.

　　Visual function at birth is limited but improves as the structures develop. Vision may be grossly tested in the very young infant by noting the pupillary response to light; this is one of the most primitive visual functions and is normally found in the newborn. The blink reflex is also present in normal newborns and young infants. The infant will blink the eyes when a bright light is introduced. It is important to make sure the infant has a red reflex in each eye. A white reflex could indicate cataract or retinoblastoma.

　　At 5 or 6 weeks of age the child should be able to fixate and give some evidence of following a bright toy or light. At 3 or 4 months of age the infant begins to reach for objects at different distances. At 6 to 7 months

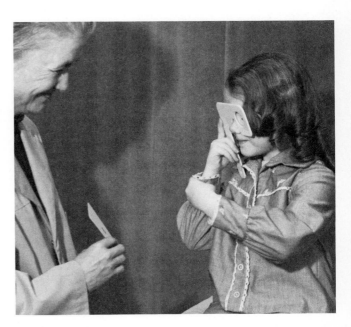

Figure 24-17

Preparing the child for participation in testing of visual acuity.

of age, the infant can have a funduscopic examination performed. For children 3 to 6 years of age Snellen's E chart can be used. The child is asked to hold the fingers in the same direction as the fingers of the E (Fig. 24-17). The young child is normally farsighted and does not achieve visual acuity of 20/20 until the age of 7 years.

　　Tests for strabismus (squint, cross-eye), which is an imbalance of the extraocular muscles, are important because strabismus can lead to amblyopia exanopsia (lazy eye), a functional loss of vision in one eye that occurs when there is a disconjugate fixation. Early recognition is essential to restore binocular vision, since the prognosis for a successful outcome for the child over 6 years of age is poor. An easy method for detecting strabismus is

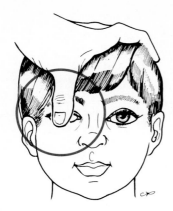

Figure 24-18

Modification of the cover test for testing young children for strabismus.

the observation of a bright light reflected off the corneas. The reflection of the light should come from approximately the same part of the eye, and any deviation should be noted. Another test to assess muscle imbalance is the cover-uncover test described in Chapter 10. This test can be used with older children and, in some instances, with younger children. A modification of the cover test that may be successful with the younger child is accomplished by the examiner's placing the palm of the hand on top of the child's head and extending the thumb down over one eye without touching it (Fig. 24-18). As the vision of the one eye is obstructed by the examiner's thumb, the other eye is observed for movement. Then the examiner lifts the thumb, and the recently covered eye is observed for movement. A slight jerking movement of the eye as it is uncovered indicates strabismus. The test is repeated for the other eye. Transient strabismus is frequently seen during the first months of life; if it persists beyond 6 months of age, however, or becomes fixed at an earlier age, the child should be referred to an ophthalmologist.

Extraocular movements can be tested during the first weeks of life, as soon as the child is able to demonstrate following movement. The visual fields can also be at least partially examined in infants and young children by having the child sit on the parent's lap with the head in the midline and one eye covered. As the light or bright object is brought into the visual field, the child will look at it or reach for it.

Inspection of the outermost structures of the eyes is done in the same way as in the adult examination. The ophthalmoscopic examination depends on the child's ability to cooperate and on the examiner's efficiency in observing as much as possible in a limited time. Attempts to restrain the child and force the eyes to remain open prove unsuccessful. If possible, the child's attention

should be directed toward an object or light while the examiner approaches without touching the child. The appearance of the red reflex alone is important information for ruling out opacities of the cornea and lens and cataracts. The use of the ophthalmoscope to observe the red reflex should be attempted at each examination of the infant beginning in the first weeks of life.

Ears

Examination of the ears is often difficult but is important because the immature structure of the young child's ears makes them more prone to infection.

The external ear and the posterior mastoid areas are inspected and palpated for any obvious deformities. The position and size of the ears are noted. Normally the top of the ear is on a horizontal line with the inner and outer canthus of the eye.

Next, the otoscope is used. This examination becomes more difficult as the child grows older, and it is usually helpful to spend some time preparing the child by letting him or her see the light and by inserting the speculum gently for only a few seconds and then removing it to assure the child that discomfort will be minimal. When it is necessary to use restraint, the child should be held firmly by the parent. Before the otoscope is inserted, the meatus is inspected for evidence of a foreign body or external otitis. In infancy and early childhood the auditory canal is directed upward, and the pinna should be pulled downward to aid in visualization (Fig. 24-19). The otoscope is held so that the hand holding it rests firmly on the head, and the top of the speculum is inserted only ¼ or ½ in into the canal to avoid any unnecessary discomfort (Fig. 24-20). Before the drum is examined, the canal should be carefully examined for evidence of furuncles or redness.

If the canal is filled with cerumen, it may occasionally be necessary to remove the cerumen by irrigation or curettage. The irrigation procedure is unpleasant, may cause vomiting, and is not done unless necessary. It is never done if a perforation of the tympanic membrane is suspected. It is inadvisable to clean the wax out with a curet unless the examiner is skillful. The procedure may cause pain and bleeding and result in increased crying, which only increases the redness of the membrane. Flexible, plastic curets are now available and seem easier for many children to tolerate. Often the cerumen that is not dry but is fairly soft will move during the examination. Visualization of the membrane then becomes possible without any special procedures to remove the cerumen. It is important to avoid discomfort so that the child will not become conditioned to expect pain with future ear examinations.

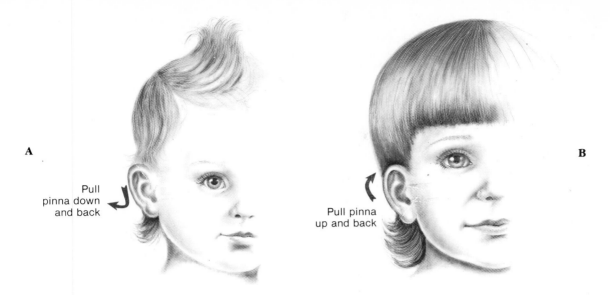

A

B

Pull
pinna down
and back

Pull pinna
up and back

Figure 24-19

Positioning of eardrum in infant, **A,** and child over 3 years of age, **B.**
(From Whaley L and Wong D: Essentials of pediatric nursing, ed 3, St Louis, 1989, The CV Mosby Co.)

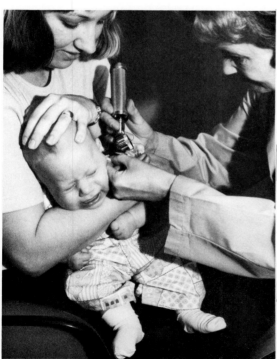

Figure 24-20

Examination of the child's ear may be facilitated if the child is
held on the parent's lap or placed in the supine position with
restraint. Note the pinna is pulled downward. Remember that the
tympanic membrane will become reddened in a child who has been
crying.

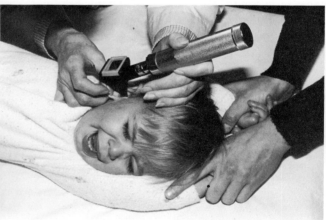

The hearing is estimated. In the infant, it can be
tested by asking an assistant to stand behind the child
and make a noise, such as a hand slap, several inches
away from the ear while the examiner observes the child
for an eye blink. This is often inaccurate, since the child
may be responding to air movement. In the young child,
hearing can be grossly tested with the whispered voice.
The examiner stands behind the child and whispers the
child's name. The child will usually turn when hearing
the name.

See boxed material on pneumotoscopy on p. 626.

Nose

Purulent secretions are common with any nasal infection,
including the common upper respiratory infection. Children with redness, discharge, and crusting on the outer

---

Pneumotoscopy: An Important Technique in Pediatrics

Pneumotoscopy is an important technique to learn especially when working with children. It involves blowing air into the ear canal (either with a rubber squeeze bulb as shown or by gently blowing or sucking with the end of the rubber tube in the examiner's mouth). The normal tympanic membrane will move in and out as positive and negative pressures are applied. In the presence of infection there is fluid behind the tympanic membrane and therefore a decrease in mobility when pressure is applied.

---

edges of the alar may have a beta-hemolytic streptococcal infection. Watery nasal secretions may indicate foreign bodies, the common cold, or an allergy.

Any unusual shape of the nose is noted, as well as flaring of the nostrils and the character and amount of discharge.

Examination of the septum, turbinates, and vestibule is accomplished by pushing the tip of the nose upward with the thumb of the left hand and shining a light into the naris. A speculum is usually not necessary; it might cause the child to be apprehensive.

Mouth and oropharynx

This area can be examined last, since this examination is often fear-provoking to the child. However, it is helpful to some children to do this examination first. The child who is anticipating discomfort may be relieved to have it accomplished and can then cooperate with the rest of the examination. This approach requires the examiner to have knowledge about the individual child's behavior and responses.

The procedures are the same as in the adult examination; however, there are differences from adults in the findings. The number of deciduous and permanent teeth and the pattern of eruption are determined by the child's age and development. There are 20 deciduous teeth, and their eruption is completed by the age of 2½ years. The first permanent molar and lower incisor erupt at 6 years of age (Fig. 24-21). The tonsils are normally larger in children than in adults and usually extend beyond the palatine arch until the age of 11 or 12 years. The palate is inspected for a cleft. A bifid uvula may indicate a submucous cleft palate (a cleft covered by membrane), which cannot be identified by inspection alone.

Chest

The examination of the chest begins with an inspection of the general shape and circumference. In infancy the chest is almost round; the anteroposterior diameter is as great as the transverse diameter. The circumference is normally the same as or slightly less than the head circumference until age 2 years. Respiratory activity is abdominal and does not become primarily thoracic until age 7 years. Little intercostal motion is seen in infants and young children. Therefore, if intercostal motion is seen in the young child, lung disease may be suspected.

Palpation may be carried out and tactile fremitus evaluated while the child is crying.

Percussion of the chest may be done directly or

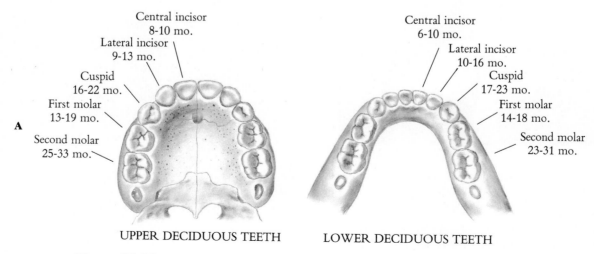

Figure 24-21

A, Dentition of deciduous teeth and their sequence of eruption.
(From Seidel HM and others: Mosby's guide to physical examination, St Louis, 1987, The CV Mosby Co.)

by the indirect method; the chest is normally more resonant than in the adult.

Breath sounds will seem much louder because of the thinness of the chest wall and are almost all bronchovesicular (Fig. 24-22).

Heart

A quiet child and environment are necessary for accurate assessment of the heart. It is a good idea to make this the first part of the examination. The examination of the cardiovascular system, as described in Chapter 15, applies to the examination of the child, but some cardiac findings of normal children are not considered normal in adults.

The pulse rate found in children of different ages is discussed earlier in this chapter. The palpation of pulses in all the extremities is a part of the cardiovascular examination; the pulses in the lower extremities, especially the femoral pulses, are of special importance in children. Their absence or diminution may indicate coarctation of the aorta.

During infancy the heart is more nearly horizontal and has a larger diameter in comparison with the total diameter of the chest than it does in the adult (Fig. 24-23). The apex is one or two intercostal spaces above that considered normal for the adult. Therefore, the apical impulse in young children is normally felt in the fourth intercostal space just to the left of the mid-clavicular line.

This location changes gradually, and by 7 years of age the apical impulse is normally found in the fifth intercostal space at the mid-clavicular line.

Sinus arrhythmia is a normal finding in infants and children. The degree of arrhythmia is less in the young infant and greatest in the adolescent.

The heart sounds are louder because of the thinness of the chest wall. They are also of a higher pitch and shorter duration than those of the normal adult. A splitting of the second heart sound can be heard in the second left intercostal space in most infants and children. The split normally widens with inspiration. A third heart sound is present in about one third of all children and is best heard at the apex.

Many children have murmurs without heart disease, and the significance of a murmur may be difficult to determine. Innocent murmurs are characteristically systolic in timing, are grade 1 or 2 in intensity, have a soft, blowing quality, and are not transmitted to other areas. It is not always possible to determine whether the murmur is innocent or pathologic by auscultation alone, although murmurs of grade 3 or louder usually indicate heart disease. A venous hum is commonly found in children. It is a continuous, low-pitched sound originating in the internal jugular vein and is heard either above or below the clavicles. It is accentuated in the upright position and disappears when the child is lying down. Because it is not pathologically significant, it should be

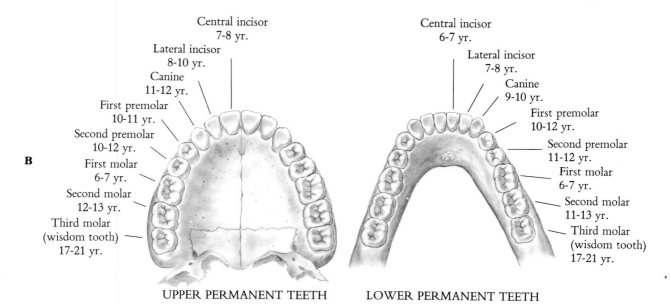

B

UPPER PERMANENT TEETH   LOWER PERMANENT TEETH

Figure 24-21, cont'd

B, Dentition of permanent teeth and their sequence of eruption.
(From Seidel HM and others: Mosby's guide to physical examination, St Louis, 1987, The CV Mosby Co.)

Figure 24-22

Auscultation of breath sounds is most easily
accomplished when the child is comfortable.

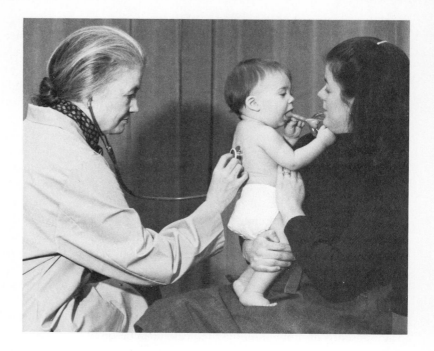

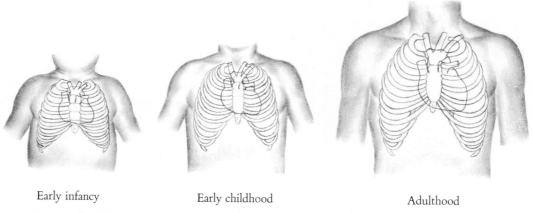

Early infancy   Early childhood   Adulthood

Figure 24-23

Position of heart at various ages.
(From Seidel HM and others: Mosby's guide to physical examination, St Louis, 1987, The CV Mosby Co.)

differentiated from a murmur. Any murmur that is symptomatic (i.e., accompanied by chest pains or palpitations) should be referred to a physician.

Abdomen

The abdomen is somewhat easier to examine in the child than in the adult, because of the less well-developed abdominal wall. To win the child's cooperation, several approaches may be helpful; for example, a bottle may be offered to the infant, or the young child may be more comfortable and relaxed if examined while sitting on the parent's lap. Each examiner will find the approaches that are most productive in a particular situation (Fig. 24-24). See Tips box opposite.

Tips on Abdominal Assessment

In a relaxed child the abdomen is somewhat easier to examine than in the adult because the abdominal wall is less well developed and (usually) less adipose tissue. If a child's muscles become tense, however, the task becomes quite difficult.

Many children become anxious or very ticklish during this part of the examination. To help the child relax make sure he or she keeps the knees bent while lying on the back, and have the child keep a hand over yours as you palpate. The practitioner can also have the child's hand under the examining fingers during palpation.

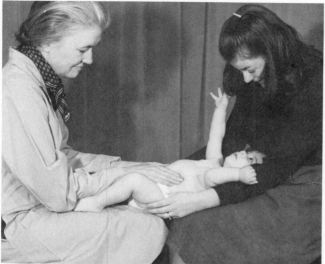

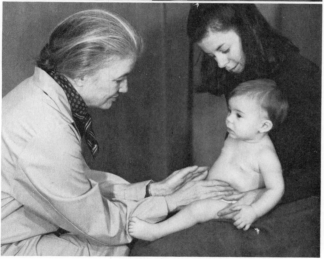

Figure 24-24

Modification in approach to the examination of the abdomen of the young child.

The order of the abdominal examination procedures for the young child may be changed to avoid introducing the stethoscope and using percussion until after the child has experienced procedures that appear less threatening. First, the abdomen is inspected. The abdomen is larger than the chest in children under 4 years of age and appears "pot bellied" in both supine and sitting positions. The child up to 13 years of age will have a "pot belly" in the standing position. This normal shape must be differentiated from the real distention that is caused by enlargement of organs or the presence of tumors, cysts, or ascites. A depressed abdomen may result from dehydration or malnutrition. Respirations are largely abdominal in children up to 7 years of age. Any splinting or loss of movement may indicate peritonitis, appendicitis, or other acute problems. The umbilicus is

normally closed, but umbilical hernias are common in white children up to 2 years of age and for longer periods in black children. The abdomen is also observed for peristaltic waves (indicating pyloric stenosis) and dilated veins (indicating liver disease).

Auscultation of the abdomen is carried out in the same manner as described in the examination of the adult. It is done before palpation.

Palpation is carried out in the same way as in the examination of the adult except for the modifications in approach and in the positions of the child. Light palpation enables the examiner to determine the tenseness of the abdominal muscles, the presence of superficial masses, and the presence of tenderness. The child is often not able to pinpoint the area of tenderness, and only by watching the facial expressions can the examiner determine the point of maximum tenderness. The liver is generally palpable 1 to 2 cm below the right costal margin during the first year of life. If it extends more than 2 cm below the costal margin, further investigation is warranted. The spleen is normally palpable 1 to 2 cm below the left costal margin in the first weeks of life. Any increase in size should be noted and any evidence of tenderness may indicate serious blood dyscrasias or other problems. Tissue turgor is also determined by grasping a few inches of skin and subcutaneous tissue over the abdomen, pulling it up, and then quickly releasing it. If the creases formed do not disappear immediately, dehydration is present. Deep palpation is done in all four quadrants by single-handed or bimanual methods. The inguinal and femoral regions are palpated for hernias, lymph nodes, and femoral pulses.

Finally, percussion may be useful in obtaining the boundaries of the liver, spleen, and any tumors.

Genitalia

The examination of the genitalia of both male and female children is usually carried out by inspection and palpation.

Male genitalia.   In the male child there are two primary areas to be examined: the penis and the scrotum. The foreskin of the penis is examined first. The foreskin of the uncircumcised infant is normally tight for the first 2 or 3 months of life and does not retract easily. If the tightness persists beyond this period, it is called a phimosis and should be observed to determine if there is any interference with urination. Any retraction of the foreskin should be done carefully, since the delicate membranes attached to the foreskin may be easily torn and result in adhesions. Next, the meatus is examined to determine its position and the presence of any ulceration. The meatus is normally located at the tip of the shaft. An abnormal location of the meatus on the ventral surface

Figure 24-25

Palpation of the scrotum to determine if the testes are descended.

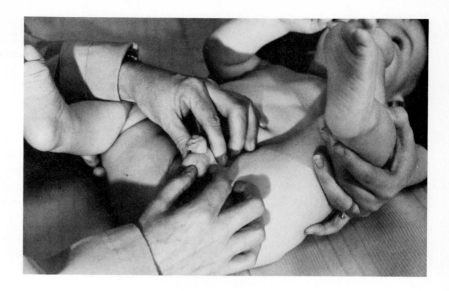

is called a hypospadias; an abnormal location on the dorsal surface is called an epispadias.

The scrotum is inspected for evidence of enlargement. An enlarged scrotum may be indicative of a hernia or hydrocele. The scrotum is also palpated to determine if the testes are descended (Fig. 24-25). The examiner's index finger is used to block the inguinal canal and is gently pushed toward the scrotum. The finger and thumb of the opposite hand are used to palpate the scrotum and grasp the testes as they are pushed downward into the scrotum. If the testes cannot be easily palpated in an older boy, he should sit in a chair with his legs apart, his heels on the seat of the chair, and his arms around his knees. This procedure interrupts the cremasteric reflex and creates pressure by flexing abdomen and thigh. The testes are felt as a soft mass about 1 cm in diameter and are normally descended if they can be palpated in the scrotum even if retraction into the inguinal canal occurs immediately. In an infant, palpate the testes as soon as the diaper is removed, before retraction occurs from the cold room air.

Female genitalia. The genitalia of the female child is inspected by separating the labia majora between the thumb and forefinger to expose the labia minora, urethral meatus, and vaginal orifice. The young infant can be held in a supine position on the mother's lap with the knees held in a flexed position and separated. The examiner sits facing the mother and child. Urethral discharges are pathologic and indicate infection somewhere in the urinary tract. A bloody vaginal discharge during the first month of life is normal but not common. Purulent or mucoid vaginal discharges indicate infection or a foreign body. The labia and clitoris are inspected for any abnormality in size or for evidence of adhesion or infec-

tion. The vaginal area is inspected but not usually palpated. An imperforate hymen may be noted if there is fluid behind it.

The vaginal examination is usually omitted for the child. If there are concerns or symptoms that require this examination, the child is referred to a gynecologist or experienced clinician.

Musculoskeletal system

The skeleton of the infant and young child is made up largely of cartilaginous tissues, which accounts for the relative softness and malleability of the bones. It is also the reason that many defects identified early in life can be corrected with more ease than in later years.

Much of the examination is done while watching the child or while playing with the child. The younger child or infant is not able to understand directions, and much of the examination is done by helping the child passively go through range-of-motion movements. An older child will be able to follow directions, and a routine musculoskeletal examination can be completed.

The neck, extremities, hips, and spine are inspected for symmetry, increased or decreased mobility, and anatomic defects.

The newborn at rest assumes the position maintained in utero and the feet are rarely straight. They are usually held in the varus (with the forefoot turned in) or valgus (with the forefoot turned out) position and simulate the clubfoot. To determine whether this is a true abnormality or a transient position, the examiner can scratch the outside border and the inside border of the foot. The normal foot will usually assume a right angle position with the leg. If this is a fixed deformity or it is difficult

Table 24-11

Four primary deformities of the foot in relation to the position of the heel, forefoot, and/or toes

Primary deformity	Heel	Forefoot	Toes
Varus	Inverted	Adducted inverted (sole in)	
Valgus	Everted	Abducted everted (sole out)	
Equinus	Plantar flexed		At level lower than heel
Calcaneus	Dorsiflexed		At level higher than heel
Combinations			
Equinovarus	Plantar flexed inverted	Adducted inverted (sole in)	At level lower than heel
Equinovalgus	Plantar flexed everted	Abducted everted (sole out)	At level lower than heel
Calcaneovarus	Dorsiflexed inverted	Adducted inverted (sole in)	At level higher than heel
Calcaneovalgus	Dorsiflexed everted	Abducted everted (sole out)	At level higher than heel

Data from Swanger R: Common problems of toddlers and preschoolers, lecture, 1972.

to bring the foot to the neutral position, the infant should be referred for an orthopedic evaluation (Table 24-11 and boxed material on p. 632).

Infants generally have bowlegs until 12 to 18 months. When they begin walking, their gait is wide based, and some children tend to evert their feet so that they bear weight on the inner aspects of the feet. This is normal. The young child also has a fat pad under the arch of the foot and may appear flat-footed until about 3 to 4 years of age. The child's bow-legged appearance changes as the gait improves, and then the child becomes mildly knock-kneed. The normal configuration of the legs develops by age 6 or 7.

Intoeing may result from metatarsus varus (forefoot turned in), from medial tibial torsion where the entire foot turns in while the knee remains straight, or from medial femoral torsion when the entire leg turns in with the foot and knee turned medially (Fig. 24-26). As mentioned earlier, the child who has intoeing as a result of a fixed deformity of the forefoot that cannot be corrected to neutral should be referred for orthopedic care. The problems of medial tibial torsion and medial femoral torsion are more cosmetic than functional and usually disappear by age 4 or 5 years.

The hips should be examined for congenital dislocation or subluxation at every routine visit during the first year of life. Congenital dislocation means that the head of the femur is found outside the acetabulum, and relocation may or may not be possible. *Subluxation* means the capsule is lax enough to allow the femoral head to be displaced but not dislocated. Clinical signs of an abnormal hip may be asymmetry of the skinfolds, creases on the dorsal surfaces, and an apparent leg length inequality (Fig. 24-27). However, these signs may not be apparent in the young infant who has a hip susceptible

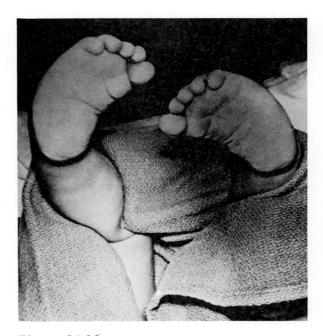

Figure 24-26

Marked metatarsus varus.
(Courtesy Mead Johnson & Co., Evansville, Ind, 1971.)

to dislocation rather than a dislocated hip. The examination of the hips is done with the infant in the supine position. The hips and knees are flexed, then *abducted* fully. In the newborn each thigh should abduct to almost 90 degrees (Fig. 24-28). Any limitation in the abduction of either or both hips may indicate dislocation.

To check the stability of the individual hip, the long finger of the examiner is placed over the greater trochanter (Fig. 24-24) with the thumb placed medially. The thigh is *adducted* while still in the flexed position,

Orthopedic Disorders Common to Various Age Groups of Children

Neonate

Oligohydramnios
  Compressed face
  Limb deformities
  Thoracic compression
  Lung hypoplasia
Prolonged breech position
Dislocation of hip
Deformations of knee
Hyperextension of knee
Dislocation of knee
Foot deformities
  Calcaneovalgus
  Metatarsus adductus
  Equinovarus
  Overlapping toes
Craniofacies
  Compressed face
    Molding of calvaria
    Mandibular asymmetry
  Torticollis
Dislocated hip(s)
Postural scoliosis

Preschooler

Postural-orthopedic abnormalities of the foot
Abnormalities of the toenail
Disorders of the skin
Deviations in gait
Poor foot hygiene
Inadequate footgear

School-age child

Idiopathic adolescent scoliosis
Other types of scoliosis
Kyphosis
Lordosis
Alignment problems of lower extremity
Juvenile arthritis
Athletic injuries
  Unstable knee
  Upper extremity, elbow clean
  Epiphyseal injuries

Young adult

Disabling low back pain
Osteoarthritis
Athletic injuries
  Jogging-related injuries

and pressure is applied along the long axis of the femur in the direction of the posterior lip of the acetabulum. As dislocation occurs, the click of exit is felt (Barlow's test). A similar click or "clunk" is felt when the maneuver is reversed and the head of the femur slips back into the joint (Ortolani maneuver). When lateral movement of the head of the femur is felt without dislocation, the hip is subluxed. Most dislocated hips in the newborn will relocate. However, an unstable hip may become fixed in the dislocated position during the first weeks of life and the Ortolani maneuver cannot replace the head. Dislocated hips can resolve spontaneously, but there is no way to be sure this will happen. The infant suspected of having a dislocation should be referred to an orthopedist without delay, since treatment is far more effective at an early age.

All children should have their spines examined during each health visit. In the young infant and child, a tuft of hair or small dimple usually toward the distal portion of the spine but which may be found anywhere from the coccyx to the skull may indicate an underlying spina bifida or may only be a superficial anomaly. If a dimple is seen, the interior and depth should be noted. These often indicate a dermoid cyst, which may become a site of infection. The young infant and child should be examined for a congenital scoliosis, whereas the child of 10 years or older should be examined for an idiopathic scoliosis. The method of examination is the same as for the adult (Fig. 24-29). The shoulders are observed for symmetry in the standing position. The child is asked to bend the shoulders forward with the arms hanging freely

Figure 24-27

Examination of the hips. **A,** Normal gluteal folds.
B, Abnormal gluteal folds.

(Courtesy Mead Johnson & Co., Evansville, Ind, 1972.)

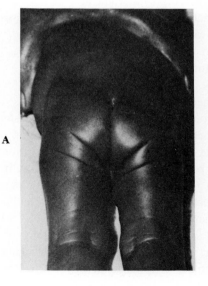
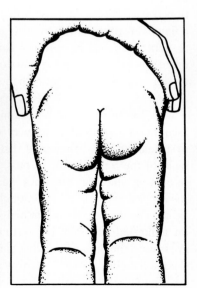

A   B

Figure 24-28

Examination of the hips for dislocation.

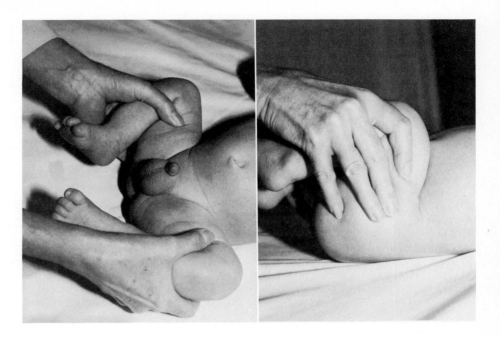

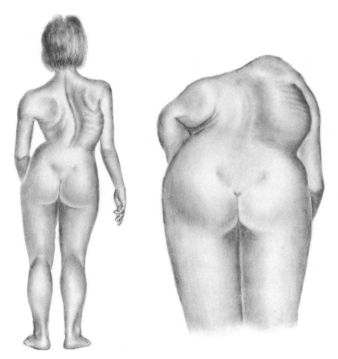

Figure 24-29

Scoliosis, lateral curvature of the spine.
(From Seidel HM and others: Mosby's guide to physical examination,
St Louis, 1987, The CV Mosby Co.)

and the head down. In this position any prominence of one side of the rib cage can be seen. The young infant can be examined in a sitting position while bending the child forward on the examiner's hand. If a scoliosis is suspected, the child should be referred to an orthopedist.

Athletic injuries are becoming more common with the increase in organized sports activities for preadolescents and adolescents. The growing child is at risk for epiphyseal fractures where the least resistance to stress is found. Stress fractures of the tibia or femur occur frequently, and the child complains of pain in the proximal region of the tibia or distal portion of the femur. A painful knee may be a dislocation of the patella. The history of the child's recent activities will give some indication of the kind of injury sustained. An evaluation by an orthopedist is indicated.

Neurologic system

The formal neurologic examination of the infant or child must be adapted to the age of the individual, but at all times a complete examination consists of an assessment of the cranial nerves and special senses, the motor system, coordination and cerebellar function, sensation, and both superficial and deep reflexes. In children under 2 years of age, the neurologic assessment is closely related to the increasing myelinization and maturation of the neural system. In this age group, the degree of maturation can only be estimated rather than quantified.

In the newborn, infant, and child over 2 years, the primary mode of examination is one of observation and inspection. This is usually reinforced by palpation and passive manipulation.

Observation of the child in the natural state and then with purposeful stimulation is often the examiner's most valuable tool. This is the best opportunity to determine how the child's overall function and behavior meet age-related norms. Seven areas can be observed:

Table 24-12

Primitive reflexes routinely evaluated: procedure for examination, expected findings, time of appearance and disappearance

Reflex (appearance)	Procedure and findings
Palmar grasp (birth)	Making sure the infant's head is in midline, touch the palm of the infant's hand from the ulnar side (opposite the thumb). Note the strong grasp of your finger. Sucking facilitates the grasp. It should be strongest between 1 and 2 months of age and disappear by 3 months (Fig. 24-30, *A*).
Plantar grasp (birth)	Touch the plantar surface of the infant's feet at the base of the toes. The toes should curl downward. It should be strong up to 8 months of age (Fig. 24-30, *B*).
Moro (birth)	With the infant supported in semisitting position, allow the head and trunk to drop back to a 30-degree angle. Observe symmetric abduction and extension of the arms, fingers fan out and thumb and index finger form a C. The arms then adduct in an embracing motion followed by relaxed flexion. The legs may follow a similar pattern of response. The reflex diminishes in strength by 3 to 4 months and disappears by 6 months (Fig. 24-30, *C*).
Placing (4 days of age)	Hold the infant upright under its arms next to a table or chair. Touch the dorsal side of the foot to the table or chair edge. Observe flexion of the hips and knees and lifting of the foot as if stepping up on the table. Age of disappearance varies (Fig. 24-30, *D*).
Stepping (between birth and 8 weeks)	Hold the infant upright under the arms and allow the soles of the feet to touch the surface of the table. Observe for alternate flexion and extension of the legs, simulating walking. It disappears before voluntary walking (Fig. 24-30, *E*).
Tonic neck or "fencing" (by 2 to 3 months)	With the infant lying supine and relaxed or sleeping, turn its head to one side so the jaw is over the shoulder. Observe for extension of the arm and leg on the side to which the head is turned and for flexion of the opposite arm and leg. Turn the infant's head to the other side, observing the reversal of the extremities' posture. This reflex diminishes at 3 to 4 months of age and disappears by 6 months. Be concerned if the infant never exhibits the reflex or seems locked in the fencing position. This reflex must disappear before the infant can roll over or bring its hand to its face (Fig. 24-30, *F*).

From Seidel HM and others: Mosby's guide to physical examination, St Louis, 1987, The CV Mosby Co.

symmetry of spontaneous movements, appearance, positioning, posture, movement of extremities, seizure activity, and the infant's responsiveness to the parents and environment.

A good tool for assessing neurologic status in an infant and young child is the Denver Developmental Screening Test (see Fig. 24-1). Gross and fine motor skills, language skills, and social skills provide clues to neurologic status when the child is compared with other children the same age.

Because the neurologic system affects every other system, it is necessary to integrate the neurologic examination. For example, changes in the pigmentation of the skin, lesions of the skin, masses in the abdomen, abnormal size and shape of the head, gaps and protrusions in the spinal column, and limited range of motion can all reflect a disease, lesion, or injury to the nervous system. In addition, because a child is going through an intense period of development that is in part related to the increasing myelinization and maturation of the neural system, a meticulous look at the child's developmental progress is required. The quality, pitch, loudness, and

duration of a child's cry; drowsiness; irritability; and social, adaptive, language, and motor skills are all measures of how well the neurologic system is functioning.

The automatic infant reflexes that are normal at birth and disappear around 4 months of age, as voluntary control begins to develop, include the Moro reflex, the palmar grasp reflex, and the rooting reflex. Absence of these reflexes at birth may indicate a severe problem of the CNS. Persistence of these reflexes may be equally serious.

Babinski's reflex is normally present in the newborn and disappears by the age of 12 to 24 months. Table 24-12 describes several reflexes found in full term infants. Fig. 24-30 illustrates them.

Children 2 years of age or older can be examined with many of the same methods used with an adult. Only the conversation, directions, and developmental tasks are altered to be more suitable to the child's interests and knowledge level. In a child of this age, more specific examination is possible, including auditory testing, funduscopic examination, and stereogenesis testing. Assessment can be expanded to observe the quantity and

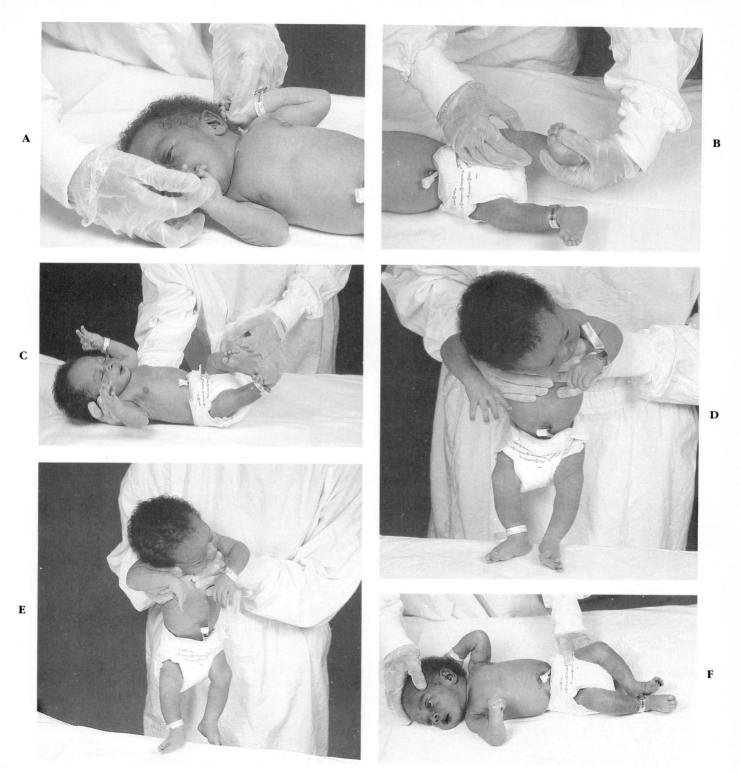

Figure 24-30

Elicitation of the primitive reflex. **A,** Palmar grasp. **B,** Plantar grasp. **C,** Moro reflex. **D,** Placing reflex. **E,** Stepping reflex. **F,** Tonic neck reflex. This illustration shows proper positioning of the head and neck, but this infant is too young for the reflex to be present.

(From Seidel HM and others: Mosby's guide to physical examination, St Louis, 1987, The CV Mosby Co.)

Table 24-13

Testing procedures and expected behaviors for indirect cranial nerve evaluation in newborns and infants

Cranial nerves	Procedures and observations
CN II, III, IV, and VI	Optical blink reflex: shine a light at the infant's open eyes. Observe the quick closure of the eyes and dorsal flexion of the infant's head. No response may indicate poor light perception. Gazes intensely at close object or face. Focuses on and tracks an object with its eyes. Doll's eye maneuver: see CN VIII.
CN V	Rooting reflex: touch one corner of the infant's mouth. The infant should open its mouth and turn its head in the direction of stimulation. If the infant has been recently fed, minimal or no response is expected. Sucking reflex: place your finger in the infant's mouth, feeling the sucking action. The tongue should push up against your finger with a fairly good rate. Note the pressure, strength, and pattern of sucking.
CN VII	Observe the infant's facial expression when crying. Note the infant's ability to wrinkle its forehead and the symmetry of the smile.
CN VIII	Acoustic blink reflex: loudly clap your hands about 30 cm from the infant's head; avoid producing an air current. Note the blink in response to the sound. No response after 2-3 days of age may indicate hearing problems. Infant will habituate to repeated testing. Moves eyes in direction of sound. Freezes position with high-pitched sound. Doll's eye maneuver: hold the infant under the axilla in an upright position, head held steady, facing you. Rotate the infant first in one direction and then in the other. The infant's eyes should turn in the direction of rotation and then the opposite direction when rotation stops. If the eyes do not move in the expected direction, suspect a vestibular problem or eye muscle paralysis.
CN IX and X	Swallowing and gag reflex.
CN XII	Coordinated sucking and swallowing ability. Pinch infant's nose; mouth will open and tip of tongue will rise in a midline position.

From Seidel HM and others: Mosby's guide to physical examination, St Louis, 1987, The CV Mosby Co.

Table 24-14

Cranial nerve examination procedures for young children

Cranial nerves	Procedures and observations
CN II	If the child cooperates, the Snellen E or Picture Chart may be used to test vision. Visual fields may be tested, but the child may need the head immobilized.
CN III, IV, and VI	Have the child follow an object with the eyes, immobilizing the head if necessary. Attempt to move the object through the cardinal points of gaze.
CN V	Observe the child chewing a cookie or cracker, noting bilateral jaw strength. Touch the child's forehead and cheeks with cotton and watch the child bat it away.
CN VII	Observe the child's face when smiling, frowning, and crying. Ask the child to show the teeth. Demonstrate puffed cheeks and ask the child to imitate.
CN VIII	Observe the child turn to sounds such as a bell or whisper. Whisper a commonly used word behind the child's back and have the child repeat the word. Perform audiometric testing.
CN IX and X	Elicit gag reflex
CN XI and XII	Instruct older child to stick out the tougue and shrug the shoulders or raise the arms.

From Seidel HM and others: Mosby's guide to physical examination, St Louis, 1987, The CV Mosby Co.

quality of spontaneous voluntary motor activity, the ease in performing voluntary movements, lateral dominance, spontaneous drawing, articulation of sounds, and language acquisition. Also, the examiner notes the child's auditory discrimination, memory, reading, speech, and calculation skills. Lastly the child can be tested for awareness of body parts, spatial orientation, and emotional lability.

In a child of any age, if the examiner suspects meningeal irritation during an illness episode, he or she must note the presence of paradoxical irritability, Kernig's sign, or Brudzinski's signs. In paradoxical irritability, the child is not easily comforted when held by the parent, contrary to usual behavior. To elicit Kernig's sign, the examiner has the child lie on the table, face up, with the leg bent at the knee. The examiner then attempts to extend the hip by raising the knee. If pain and resistance are encountered, the maneuver is positive for meningeal irritation. Brudzinski's sign is obtained by having the child lie supine on a table; the examiner proceeds to bend the neck gently. If the child's knees flex spontaneously, this sign is positive. Tables 24-13 and 24-14 give detailed information on techniques for evaluating cranial nerve function in infants and young children.

• • •

A good working knowledge of growth and development will help the nurse successfully assess pediatric patients.

BIBLIOGRAPHY

American Academy of Pediatrics: Report of the Committee on Infectious Diseases, Evanston, Ill, 1988, The Academy.

American Academy of Pediatrics: Guidelines for health supervision II, ed 2, Elk Grove Village, Ill, 1988, The Academy.

Asher M: Orthopedic screening, Pediatr Clin North Am 24:713, 1977.

Behrman RE and Vaughn VC, III: Nelson's textbook of pediatrics, ed 12, Philadelphia, 1982, WB Saunders Co.

Britton CV: Blood pressure measurement and hypertension in children, Pediatr Nurs 7:13-17, 1981.

Brook CGD: Growth assessment in childhood and adolescence, Boston, 1982, Blackwell Scientific Publications, Inc.

Goldenring JM and Cohen E: Getting into adolescent heads, Contemp Pediatr 5:75-86, 1988.

Haddock N: Blood pressure monitoring in neonates, Matern Child Nurs J 5:131, 1980.

Kempe CH and others: Current pediatric diagnosis and treatment, ed 5, Los Altos, 1978, Lange Medical Publications.

Lowrey GH: Growth and development of children, Chicago, 1978, Year Book Medical Publishers, Inc.

McKusick VA: Human genetics, ed 6, Englewood Cliffs, NJ, 1985, Prentice-Hall, Inc.

National Heart, Lung and Blood Institute: Report of task force on blood pressure control in children, Pediatrics 59(suppl):803, 1977.

Schwartz and others: Principles and practice of clinical pediatrics, Chicago, 1987, Year Book Medical Publishers, Inc.

Seidel HM and others: Mosby's guide to physical examination, St Louis, 1987, The CV Mosby Co.

Stangler SR, Huber CJ, and Routh DK: Screening growth and development of preschool children, New York, 1980, McGraw-Hill Book Co.

Tanner JM: Growth of adolescence, ed 2, Oxford, 1962, Blackwell Scientific Publications, Inc.

U.S. Department of Health, Education and Welfare: NCHS growth curves for children birth to 18 years, Hyattsville, Md, Nov, 1977, National Center for Health Statistics.

Valadian I and Porter D: Assessing physical growth and development, Boston, 1977, Little, Brown & Co.

Whaley LF and Wong DL: Nursing care of infants and children, ed 3, St Louis, 1987, The CV Mosby Co.

Zitelli B and Davis H: Atlas of pediatric physical diagnosis, New York, 1987, Gower Medical Publishing Ltd.

Assessment of the aging client

OBJECTIVES

Upon successful review of this chapter, learners will be able to:

- Describe physical and psychosocial changes that occur with age
- Outline history relevant to an aging client, including
  Present symptoms or illness
  Mental state and cognitive functioning
  Medication data
  Psychosocial information
  Sexual data
  Self-care and functional status
- State related rationale and demonstrate assessment of aging clients, including
  Nutritional status
  Visual, hearing, smell, and taste abilities
  Mouth and dental conditions
  Reflex and nerve status
  Examination sequence, inspection, palpation, percussion, and auscultation techniques of body systems
- Recognize usual findings in the aging client and characteristics suggesting pathology

The number of persons in the United States who are over 65 years of age is 25 million or 11% of the population. By the year 2000, the size of this group is expected to reach 52 million, nearly half of whom will be 75 years of age or older. Thus, it is increasingly important to understand age-related changes of body structure and function and to recognize common medical and social pathologic states that may occur in older persons.

THE INTERVIEW

The social use of the age 65 as the demarcation point between middle age and old age had its origin in Bismarck's laws. This is the time designated for retirement from work and for the eligibility for funds and services designated for the aged. Gerontologists have classified old age into two groups:
1. *Early old age or later maturity:* 65 to 74
2. *Advanced old age:* 75 and older
    Although the use of specific years has been useful for governmental and social agency purposes, it has served to prejudice the public and health personnel, so that all the changes attributable to the aged, both ill and well, are expected to be present in each aged client.
    Maximum life span for humans is approximately 110 years. The mean life span or life expectancy was 46 years in 1900. Considerable improvement in life expectancy has resulted primarily from prevention of premature deaths in persons under the age of 50. The life expectancy has not changed significantly in the United States over the past 20 years (Fig. 25-1). However, the life expectancy is predicted to reach 85 years by the year 2020.
    Both black and white women outlive their respective male counterparts, so that women make up more

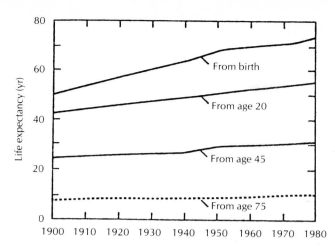

Figure 25-1

Life expectancy changes in the United States between 1900 and 1980 showing that life expectancy at birth has increased by 28 years, whereas at age 75 it has increased by only 3 years. (From Fries JF: N Engl J Med 303:130, 1980. Reprinted, by permission of The New England Journal of Medicine.)

than 55% of the elderly population. There are five times as many widows as widowers over age 65. There are 150 older women for every 100 older men. In the over 75 age group, the ratio is 180 women for every 100 men. It has been documented that approximately 35% of women and 15% of elderly men are alone. Only 5% of the elderly are institutionalized.

The number of elderly individuals in the United States is increasing. Medicare and other health care insurance plans have enabled older persons to obtain more health care. However, most health care provided older persons is curative rather than preventive.

Two general thoughts should be borne in mind by the practitioner in examining the older individual. On the one hand, advancing years are not necessarily equated with disease. Thus, the practitioner should not expect all older clients to be ill. On the other hand, when one problem is identified, others must be suspected, since multiple disease is the primary characteristic of health problems in the elderly. In addition, the differentiation of the client's major problem may be complicated by decreases of acuity in the sensory processes, so that clearly defined symptoms may not be reported.

Although a representative of the U.S. Census Bureau has declared that most of the elderly in the United States are poor, uneducated, and generally unemployed, it is important to remember that many clients are educated and gainfully employed. A 1975 study showed that only 2% of white people had no formal schooling and 19% had 1 to 7 years. Among black persons, 12% had no

schooling and 50% had 1 to 7 years. Approximately 16.3% of persons aged 65 years and older are at or below the poverty line.

The usual age for retirement in the United States is 62 years (and even younger in dangerous occupations), but it has been shown that 42% of individuals between 70 and 74 years of age and 19% of those between 75 and 79 years of age are still working for pay. Often, however, forced retirement means retirement from a valued job to a less satisfying form of work, such as caretaker or watchman, which this society values little and therefore allots to the elderly.

For those not working, retirement may be fraught with financial worries, particularly if the client has been stretching his or her income to the limit during the working years or for other reasons has been unable to establish any savings. Thus, one of the problems of the elderly in the United States (except those 70 or older) is earning money to meet the costs of living without jeopardizing their qualifications for Social Security benefits. Most of the cost-of-living estimates indicate that governmental support to the elderly is not sufficient for total support. Few states have enacted legislation that will allow the elderly the option of seeking work without risking the loss of Social Security payment.

Although the more affluent may not experience the problems related to the curtailment of monetary supply, they may experience an even more universal feeling. This is the feeling of loss or demoralization associated with aging. This society has devalued the elderly by making them ineligible for many highly valued activities that are reserved for younger members. The aging person is considered appropriate for menial, boring, and low-paying jobs. In addition, the elderly are frequently rejected in a real or imagined sense by younger relatives and acquaintances.

The presence of emotional illness has been estimated to be as high as 20% in the otherwise well population over 65 years of age and 40% in those with physical illness. Thus, particularly in assessment of the elderly, consideration must be given to both the psychological and the social, as well as to the physical, aspects of the client's development. One must also bear in mind that a problem associated with one of these functional areas may well lead to a disturbance in one or both of the other two.

The examiner must have examined his or her own view of "old" before examining the aging client. The self-examination would have the purpose of moving to an objective appraisal of each unique elderly person uncolored by the examiner's culture and experience.

THE HEALTH HISTORY   •

Identifying the major presenting symptom or sign may be difficult in the elderly client. Some slowly progressing diseases such as chronic infections and malignancies may be manifested only by loss of interest in social activities, disregard of personal hygiene, fatigue, or loss of weight. Confusion may be the only indicator of infection, dehydration, cardiac failure, or stroke.

Obtaining an accurate history from elderly clients may be difficult. Frequently, they attribute problems to the aging process and ignore important signs and symptoms. The data that they are able to provide may be vague and nonspecific. It may be necessary to devote a good deal more time and patience to get an adequate history from the aging client. Difficulties in obtaining information may be related to auditory or visual sensory loss, impaired cognition, fear of the possible consequences of the evaluation, or poor physical endurance.

The loss of auditory acuity is the most common sensory loss among aging individuals and may seriously impede history taking. The examiner should face the client so that the client can clearly see lips and eyes. Simple, direct questions should be used. Since shouting obscures the consonants and only amplifies vowels, this process should be avoided. In instances where the client is totally deaf, it may be necessary to have the client fill out a written health questionnaire. Only the most pertinent responses should be pursued in writing, since this process is quite exhausting. Further data can be collected at a subsequent interview.

One of the common fallacies of thinking that must be avoided by the examiner of aging clients is that general intelligence declines as a function of advancing years. Although some of the older correlation studies would seem to support this conclusion, more recent controlled studies deny this phenomenon. Thus the examiner should interact with the aging client with respect for both the intelligence and the experience the client's years have granted him or her.

As with any individual, learning that involves the unlearning of previously held information is the most difficult type of learning for the older client. Because of the greater number of learning years, the elderly client may have a good deal to unlearn during the acquisition of most new information. Thus, difficulties for the aging person in learning new tasks may be understood. When disorders of memory or learning ability are apparent, the examiner should be alert to the necessity of repeating questions, instructions, and explanations. Directions should be given in simple phrases and in words familiar to the older client. It may be necessary to obtain information from a relative or an individual who has spent a good deal of time with the client. The testimony of persons who have been with the client at home may be particularly valuable in answering questions concerning changes in behavior or symptoms that the client may have experienced.

Previous medical records should be sought to help validate current historical data, to fill in gaps in current data, to eliminate duplication of diagnostic testing and expense to the patient, to identify previously tried but unsuccessful treatment regimens, and to identify previous efforts in client education.

Mental State

Depression

The incidence of depression increases with age. Some authors suggest the rate of depression among the elderly is as great as 14%. The high incidence of depression in the elderly may result from multiple loss, unresolved interpersonal conflicts, or inadequate mastery of developmental challenges. (See assessment of cognitive function on p. 641.)

Depression may be viewed as an affective expression of a state of hopelessness. Thus, the focus of assessment is the identification of the client's feelings of despair, pessimism, or hopelessness. The classification of signs and symptoms falls into one of three different conditions: (1) a feeling tone or prevailing mood, (2) a syndrome that is a cluster of signs and symptoms, or (3) a group of expressive disorders.

The depressed person may discuss feeling depressed, sad, blue, hopeless, low, "down in the dumps," or irritable. The client describes or acts out a loss of interest or pleasure in usual work or leisure activities. At least four of the following conditions must be present to define the client as depressed: (1) decline in appetite or excessive eating—significant weight loss or gain, (2) psychomotor agitation or slowing (retardation), (3) loss of energy or fatigue, (4) feeling of worthlessness, self-reproach, or inappropriate levels of guilt, (5) retardation of thinking or indecisiveness, and (6) recurrent thoughts of death or suicide attempt. The client who is depressed has no *delusions, hallucinations,* or bizarre behavior in periods between depressed behavior.

Dementia

The cognitive disorders previously described as "organic brain syndromes," "senile dementia," and "presenile dementia" are defined in the Diagnostic and Statistical Manual of Mental Disorders III-R (DSM-III-R) as dementia (American Psychiatric Association, 1987). The criteria for the diagnosis of dementia include (1) loss of intel-

---

Assessment of Cognitive Function

1. Orientation to person, time, and place
2. Ability to calculate numbers
3. Ability to identify objects
4. Ability to follow commands
5. Ability to write a sentence
6. Ability to copy a drawing
7. Ability to remember three objects after 5 minutes
8. Ability to respond appropriately to a judgment question
9. Ability to understand analogies and proverbs

Barriers to Psychiatric Care

1. Limited availability of psychiatric care in most communities
2. Resistance by psychiatrists to provide psychotherapy to the elderly
3. Stigma associated with mental health problems
4. Limited finances and health insurance coverage to pay for the service

---

lectual abilities of sufficient severity to interfere with social or occupational functioning, (2) memory impairment, and (3) one or more of the following—cognitive impairments in abstract thinking, judgment, or higher cortical function such as *agnosia* or *apraxia* or a personality change.

The incidence of dementia is 5% to 10% in the 65- to 79-year age group and 20% in those over 80 years of age. It is estimated that up to 50% of clients in nursing homes are demented. It has been demonstrated that 15% have dementia that is reversible and that 20% to 25% more can be functionally improved.

Delirium

Delirium is described in the *DSM-III-R* as the clouding of consciousness accompanied by an impaired ability to shift, focus, and sustain attention to environmental stimuli; disorientation; and memory impairment. Furthermore, at least two of the following behavioral changes must be present: (1) perceptual disturbances such as misinterpretations, illusions, or hallucinations; (2) incoherent speech; (3) disturbance of the sleep-wakefulness cycle, such as insomnia or daytime drowsiness; or (4) a change in psychomotor activity. The signs and symptoms appear over a short time, usually hours to days.

Drug History

It is particularly important to assess the medicines prescribed for the older client and those nonprescription medicines the client is choosing to ingest. In addition to a careful drug history taken at the initial interview, a periodic review of drug intake is important. It is very useful to ask the client or family member to bring to each visit all the medication the client has access to. Outdated medications can then be discarded, and duplicate medication can be combined in one container. Medications the patient should not be taking can be eliminated. Just as important as the drugs that are being used are those

that have been ordered by a physician and not taken. Some clients do not fill prescriptions. Others stop taking medicine because they feel better. Dispensing dates on the medication bottles should be checked against the number of pills left to assess accuracy of self-administration. With the product in hand, the action, side effects, and purpose for the medication usage can be reviewed with the client.

A simple and clearly written instruction sheet should be given to the elderly client whenever a medication change is made. Circle the most important item listed on the sheet so that if all else fails, perhaps the most important therapeutic change will be followed. It may also be important to advise the elderly client to use a plastic medication dispensing device to facilitate the ease of self-medication. Observe the client fill the dispenser during a visit to determine accuracy and to provide an opportunity for further instruction, if needed. Ask the elderly client to bring the filled dispensing kit from home and again check for accuracy.

Many of the drugs frequently prescribed for common medical problems pose a greater danger to the aged client than to the younger adult. When used by older adults, there is a higher incidence of gastrointestinal bleeding caused by aspirin and the nonsteroidal anti-inflammatory drugs; potassium depletion caused by diuretics; and a severe drop in standing blood pressure leading to falls caused by antidepressants.

The changes in reaction to drugs may be caused by diminished central nervous system (CNS) function, altered metabolism, and a reduction in elimination of drugs due to the functional decline of both the liver and the kidneys. In the management of older persons taking oral drugs, the following normal aging changes must be considered: (1) decreased absorption; (2) decreased protein binding of the drug, since liver proteins such as albumin are decreased; (3) altered metabolism of the drug, which may be related to diminished enzyme production; (4) decreased renal excretion; (5) change in distribution; and (6) variation in target sensitivity. The presence of side effects must carefully be monitored while the practitioner observes the client's response to therapy.

Frequently, *iatrogenic* illness is not identified, because practitioners do not recognize symptoms as drug induced, since they are part of the stereotype of old age: slowed reaction time, confusion, disorientation, loss of memory, tremors, loss of appetite, noncompliant behavior, or anxiety.

Psychosocial History

When caring for aging clients, it is important to collect data in the following areas:

1. Educational level: determine ability to read and write, languages spoken, and major language.
2. Job history: previous occupation, date retired, reason for retirement, satisfaction with retirement, and current job or volunteer work.
3. Marital history: number of marriages, duration, current status, significant other.
4. Family network: children's and relatives' ages; location, frequency, and type of contact.
5. Current living situation: a short description of its design and facilities; identification of all inhabitants including pets.
6. Income: source and adequacy to meet needs.
7. Type of health insurance(s).
8. Use of community services.
9. Safety measures: seat belt use, grab bars, adequate lighting, and smoke detectors are some examples. Questions regarding safety must be geared to each individual's potential safety needs.
10. Leisure activities, hobbies, and exercise.
11. Spiritual activity or source of strength and hope.
12. Description of a typical day.
13. Current stressors, coping patterns, and support systems.
14. Self-care: knowledge of health problems, a description of problem self-care management, and perceived difficulty with managing a self-care regimen.
15. Osteoporosis knowledge and prevention measures.
16. Satisfaction with life, views on aging, future plans, and health goals.

Functional Assessment

Elderly clients' ability to maintain an independent state depends on their ability to meet their basic physical and life management needs or to use community resources to help them compensate for deficits in these areas. The aging client should be questioned about bathing, grooming, dressing, toileting, feeding, mobility, and cooking as well as cleaning, laundry, telephone use, managing medication, shopping, home maintenance, and managing money. When older clients express deficits in any of these areas, they should be questioned about the management of their functional limitations. See Chapter 27.

PHYSICAL APPRAISAL

The approach to the physical examination in the elderly is essentially identical to that performed on a client of any age. However, special effort should be made to ensure comfort, avoid rushing, and prevent fatigue in the elderly client. The examiner may need to allow more time for response to requests such as a change of position. The examiner should note evidence of muscle weakness or lack of coordination so that the client who needs help in moving or turning can be assisted. Be attentive to elderly clients at all times so that they do not inadvertently fall off the examination table, and never leave an elderly client alone on the examination table.

Patience is the most helpful asset in dealing with the elderly. A hurried or annoyed manner may cause tension, such that the elderly client retreats or makes minimal attempts to comply with procedures. An aged client with an obvious physical disability such as blindness, gross joint abnormalities from rheumatoid arthritis, or hemiplegia from a stroke might welcome the examiner's asking what assistance is needed to facilitate the examination process. This helps to minimize the client's discomfort and embarrassment, allows the client to feel more self-sufficient, and reduces the client's sense of dependence on the examiner.

The sequence of areas assessed during the physical examination is important. The examiner might select a sequence that is followed consistently so that no areas of data collection are omitted (see the box on p. 643). Three quarters of the physical assessment of the elderly can be completed with the client sitting on the edge of the examination table. The integument is examined throughout the examination process. The gait can be assessed while the older client is walking to the examination room. If the client complains of a gait disturbance, a more detailed assessment of this area should be carried out. It should include a Romberg test, heel-toe and tandem walking, and an evaluation for proximal lower extremity muscle weakness. Proximal muscle weakness can be determined by observing whether the client can rise from a sitting position without pushing off with the arms or by asking the client to step up and sit on the examination table without help. If the client complains of *paresthesia* or a gait disturbance, sensation should then be evaluated. Diminished vibratory sensation in the elderly client is very common, but a decline in position sense, light touch, or

---

Physical Examination Sequence

Sitting

Posterior examination: thorax and chest, vertebral column, back musculature, cervical lymph nodes, position of the trachea, thyroid, and carotid pulses.

Anterior examination: peripheral pulses, reflexes and sensation, range of motion of the extremities, muscle tone and strength, cranial nerves, visual acuity, eyes, extraocular muscles, funduscopic examination, ears, nose, and mouth, submental and submaxillary lymph nodes, anterior thorax and chest, breasts, heart, and axillary lymph nodes.

Lying

Repeat the breast and heart examination, abdomen, femoral pulses, inguinal lymph nodes, external genitalia, pelvic (for women), rectal, and prostate (for men).

pain is abnormal, and further evaluation is warranted. Manual dexterity can be observed while the patient is undressing. During the routine musculoskeletal examination of the aged client, muscular stiffness and interruptions of fluid muscle movement at the elbow and wrist should be checked because of the increasing incidence of Parkinson's disease. A sensitive test to determine if the client has a hearing deficit is for the examiner to turn the head away while asking questions and notice if the client has difficulty comprehending what has been said. Several such observations should be enough for the examiner to recommend that the client have an audiogram.

The following review of examinations includes only those parameters that may differ in the aged client compared with the younger adult and includes a description of normal aging changes in the elderly client.

General Inspection

There is an average lifetime height loss of 2.9 cm for men and 4.9 cm for women. This change is attributed to the thinning of cartilage between bones. The decline in height begins at age 50. With loss of connective tissue, contours appear sharper and hollows are deeper, especially the orbits and axillae. Muscles appear more prominent. Because cartilage continues to be laid down in old age, the elderly client's ears and nose may be larger and appear more prominent in relation to the face. The earlobes elongate, as does the nose. Wrinkling and relaxation (sagging) of the skin are recognized as signs of the aging process, as are the loss of pigmentation and thinning of the hair. The skin may be the source of external clues that aging changes are occurring: gray hair, sagging skin folds, wrinkling, and lentigines. Some skin changes are

known to be associated with aging. The rate of cell turnover is decreased, the sebaceous glands decline in function, and eccrine sweat gland cells atrophy.

Connective Tissue Changes

As tissues age, collagen fibers increase in number and in size, and cross-linkage develops between fibers. As a result of these changes, the skin loses its elasticity and wrinkles. Joints become stiffened by an increase in fibrous tissue around them. Lungs lose elastic recoil. The costal cartilages become stiff. Loss of hydration from intervertebral disks results in shrinking of stature. The chambers of the heart are less distensible. The arteries become rigid, valves stiffen, and pacemaker cells may be replaced by collagen.

Histologic Changes

A gradual loss of cells has been documented in the aging individual. The cells that decline with age are those that are incapable of reproduction. The cells most affected are neurons and muscle cells.

Nutritional Changes

Some of the changes that accompany aging are known to play a role in nutrition. The basal metabolic rate decreases by about 20% between the ages of 20 and 90 years of age.

Although the gastrointestinal tract undergoes changes in secretion, there is no evidence that absorption of foodstuffs is compromised. However, there is evidence that the degree of absorption may change for certain dietary components. For instance, it is known that calcium absorption declines with aging and that fat digestion is less efficient.

Animal studies have provided supportive studies indicating that nutritional intervention modifies the aging process. Rats fed a lifelong calorie-restricted diet had lower serum cholesterol and a reduction in the aging of collagen and lived longer than those rats that were not fed a calorie-restricted diet. Other studies have indicated that calorie restriction delays the onset of certain diseases.

A reduction in the daily energy requirements is a well-documented change that accompanies aging. In men the energy expenditure declines by 21% from age 20 to age 74 and another 31% by age 99. It is posited that one third of the reduction in energy expenditure results from a decline in basal metabolism, whereas two thirds results from a decline in physical activity.

Body composition. Although total body weight tends to remain constant in aging, an age-related decline in lean body mass has been documented. The decline in lean body mass is accompanied by an increase in total fat. An overall reduction in organ size and weight has been reported for the following structures: liver (18%), lungs (11%), and kidneys (9%). The skeletal muscles incur a 40% loss of mass, and bone decreases 12% in men and 25% in women. There is a reduction in cell mass relative to body weight.

Metabolic function. Age-related changes are thought to occur in the processes of intermediary metabolism that may be related to a decline in enzyme production. There is an age-related increase in postprandial blood glucose levels, and studies have indicated that protein synthesis may be impaired as a function of aging.

Lipid metabolism. Increased serum lipid levels have been associated with aging. Serum cholesterol levels have been shown to increase through the age of 60 in women and 50 in men. Lipoprotein profiles reveal these changes.

Effect of alcoholism. The incidence of alcoholism in the elderly is significant. The U.S. population over 60 years of age has been shown to have a 2% to 10% rate of alcoholism, and the percentage of alcoholics admitted to hospitals is 20%. The possibility of alcohol abuse should be considered in the malnourished, older person. It has been demonstrated that 50% of alcohol abusers have some malabsorption of folate, vitamin A, thiamin, vitamin B_{12}, and fat. Malabsorption is thought to result from mucosal damage of the intestine, increased gastrointestinal motility, and inhibition of biliary and pancreatic secretion. There is also an increased incidence of osteoporosis in alcoholism.

Nutritional Assessment

Assessment should include data to indicate if the client is able to buy appropriate food to maintain nutrition. Since it is estimated that 15% to 20% of Americans over 65 years of age are at or near the poverty line, the amount of money appropriated for food may be less than adequate. Folate deficiency in the older American population is largely found in the lower socioeconomic groups. Many of the elderly live alone: 36% of elderly women and 15% of elderly men. Living alone has been shown to affect nutritional status.

Systematic analysis of nutritional status includes the following:

A. Twenty-four hour dietary recall
B. Number of servings per day of:
 1. Protein
 2. Vegetables
 3. Fruit
 4. Roughage
 5. Carbohydrates and starches
 6. Milk and other dairy products
 7. Salt
 8. Quantity of fluids
 9. Concentrated sweets
 10. Quantity of caffeine and alcoholic beverages
C. Laboratory tests such as complete blood count, total protein, albumin, and vitamin B_{12}, and folic acid.
D. Clinical evaluation

The recommendations for nutritional requirements in the elderly are estimated for the most part on data from studies done in young adults. Some protein requirement studies in the elderly have suggested that the recommendations for protein intake may not be sufficient to meet the protein needs of the majority of healthy elderly clients. Additional studies are needed to establish the requirements for other nutrients and to define the nutritional requirements for the elderly in various disease states that occur in this age group. The method of nutritional assessment based on norms for young or even middle-aged adults may not be appropriate for the elderly. The nutrients most frequently found lower than the recommended daily allowance (RDA) in the elderly are as follows:

1. Total calories
2. Calcium
3. Iron
4. Vitamin A
5. Thiamin
6. Folate

Mucous membranes, skin, and nails. The mucous membranes, skin, and nails may provide many clues to nutritional status in the elderly. Vitamin B_6 and riboflavin deficiency may be evident in examination of the mouth. *Glossitis, cheilosis*, angular *stomatitis*, and bleeding gums may be caused by lack of vitamin B.

Vitamin C deficiency. Indicators that the client has vitamin C deficiency include irregular hairs with broken ends, poor wound healing, and *ecchymoses* and *petechiae* of the skin. Gingival tissues become edematous and erythematous and ulcerate and bleed spontaneously due to defective collagen formation.

Vitamin A deficiency. Dermatitis or dry, "toadlike," and follicular hyperkeratoses are associated with vitamin A deficiency. The mucous membrane of the mouth is *hyperplastic* and *hyperkeratotic*.

Iron deficiency. Koilonychia (spoon nails) are associated with iron deficiency. Generalized pallor of the oral mucosa is a prominent sign. Localized papillary atrophy of the tongue can progress to total denudation. White spots on the nail may be related to zinc deficiency. Bands across the nails may reflect protein deficiency.

Tissue maintenance and repair. The synthesis of structural proteins and enzymes by cells depends

Figure 25-2

Arcus senilis around the periphery of the cornea (arrow). (From Steinberg FU, editor: Care of the geriatric patient in the tradition of CV Cowdry, ed 6, St Louis, 1983, The CV Mosby Co.)

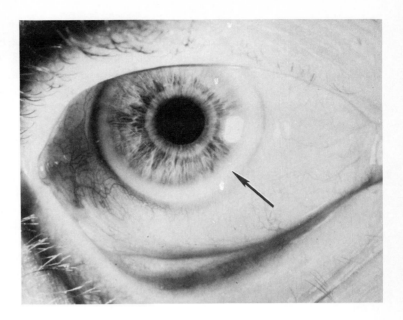

Table 25-1

Drug-vitamin relationships

Drug	Nutrient absorption interference
Aspirin	Vitamin C, folate
Tetracycline	Vitamin C
Cardiac glycosides	Riboflavin
Hydralazine	Vitamin B_6
Colchicine	Vitamin B_{12}
Biguanidines	Vitamin B_{12}

Table 25-2

Visual changes in the elderly

Visual function	Changes with aging
Lens transparency	Decreased, folate
Acuity	Decreased
Accommodation to far object	Improved
Accommodation to near object	Decreased
Astigmatism	Corneal shape more spherical
Adaptation (light to dark)	Reduced
Color vision	Decreased; pastels are discriminated less readily; color blindness is worse
Flicker adaption	Decreased
Peripheral vision	Decreased
Pupillary response	Decreased response to light changes; pupil smaller
Intraocular fluid reabsorption	Decreased; glaucoma more likely

on protein availability. In addition, immune competence is related to protein status.

Certain drugs interfere with vitamin use. The drug-vitamin relationships are explained in Table 25-1.

Head and Neck

Eyes

The loss of fat from the orbit causes a sunken appearance of the eyes and senile *ptosis*. Loss of neuromuscular stimulation and loss of control of the muscles of accommodation lead to a pupillary response that may be sluggish. The lacrimal glands decrease in tear production with aging, so the eyes may appear dry and lusterless. However, the lacrimal ducts may *stenose* and the lower lid sags so that tears flow onto the cheeks, giving the impression of increased tears. Other eye changes may include arcus senilis, scleral discolorations, and diminution of pupil size. *Arcus senilis* (Fig. 25-2) is the accumulation of a lipid substance on the cornea. It characteristically appears as a grayish arc or complete circle almost at the edge of the cornea. The cornea tends to cloud with age. Entropion and ectropion are not uncommon in the elderly. Table 25-2 lists the visual changes in the elderly person's eyes.

Vision

The amount the eye can alter its refractive power in focusing on a far object and a near object is called the amplitude of accommodation. When the ciliary muscle is relaxed (in viewing objects at a distance), the lens is flattened. Contraction of the ciliary muscle (in viewing near objects) causes the muscle to shorten, and the tension on the capsule is relieved, allowing a near object to come into focus on the retina.

The amplitude of accommodation decreases progessively with age, a condition known as presbyopia. The reduction in near vision results from loss of elastic properties of the capsule, hardening or sclerosis of the lens substance, and weakening of the ciliary muscle.

Loss of elasticity and transparency of the lens cause vision changes, requiring many aging individuals to wear corrective lenses. Normal changes in the eye may predicate changes in the eyeglasses every 3 to 5 years. The examiner should assess visual acuity with the client wearing glasses and determine how long it has been since the client last had an ophthalmologic examination.

Peripheral vision is diminished in the aged. In addition, there is a decrease in the rate of dark adaptation. *Sclerotic* changes in the iris result in a small (miotic) and somewhat fixed pupil. Restriction of upward movement occurs with age. The aged person may have to tip the head back further and further to look up. An elevation in the threshold for visible light perception has been noted, along with a loss of visual acuity in dim lighting. The number of vitreous floaters increases with age. Glau-coma and cataracts are other problems frequently associated with aging. When attempting to check the lens for opacities or when evaluating the anterior structures of the eye, set the ophthalmoscope on black diopter 10 or 12. Look closely at the cup-disc ratio when trying to assess for signs of glaucoma, optic atrophy, or occlusion of the retinal artery. The clue to an abnormally large cup is the disappearance of the smallest blood vessels near the edge of the disc.

In the aged client, the ophthalmoscopic examination reveals mildly narrowed vessels, granular pigment in the macula, and a loss of bright macular and foveal reflexes. The fundus itself lacks luster and may appear more yellow.

Changes in the macular area lead to a loss of central vision in the elderly. Macular degeneration (Fig. 25-3) is not uncommon and is a leading cause of blindness in this age group. Since there is an increase in pathologic conditions of the eye in the elderly, routine ophthalmologic examinations should be encouraged.

Ears

Outer ear.   Aging changes begin to appear in the outer ear between 30 and 50 years of age. The skin becomes dry and less resilient, and connective tissue is lost. Hair growth may be noted along the periphery of the helix, anthelix, and tragus of the pinna. The hairs are coarse and wirelike. The pinna increases in both length and width during the process of aging. The skin of the ears may be dry, and the earlobes may be elongated. The

Figure 25-3

The macula shows the "mottled" appearance of depigmentation and hyperpigmentation of the senile macular degeneration.
(From Steinberg FU, editor: Care of the geriatric patient in the tradition of CV Cowdry, ed 6, St Louis, 1983, The CV Mosby Co.)

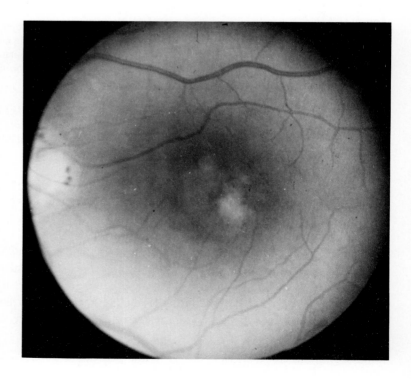

ear wax is drier among older persons, and there is a decrease in the wax-producing ceruminous glands.

Middle ear. The eardrum is more translucent and rigid. Calcification of ligaments and ossification and fixation of the middle ear bones have been described.

Inner ear. A degeneration of hair cells beginning in the basal part of the cochlea and extending to the apex is associated with old-age deafness. The damage is associated with the organ of Corti. Typically the lesion is confined to a few millimeters of the basal position. The reason for the loss of sensory cells is not clear.

Atrophic changes and stiffness of the basilar membrane and modifications in middle ear mechanics may also account for aging changes in hearing.

Central mechanism of presbycusis. The characteristic of the aging central auditory system is that the brain of the older person receives the impulse (hears) but does not understand the words.

Most elderly persons have more hearing difficulties than do younger adults. Over half the persons in the United States with bilateral hearing losses are 65 years or older. Hearing loss in the elderly is most frequently the result of presbycusis or *otosclerosis*. Presbycusis is the loss in perception of auditory stimuli that accompanies degenerative changes of the neural structures of the inner ear or the auditory nerve, or both. It is the most common auditory disorder in the entire population. The first symptom is the loss of high-frequency tones. Threshold increases for auditory perception at all frequencies for pure tone. The rate of impaired hearing loss (defined as elevated thresholds in the traditional "speech" frequencies— 500, 1000, and 2000 Hz) increases sharply after age 64 to include 25% of the population at age 75.

A mild loss of speech frequency noises may pose little problem for the older person when listening to normal, well-articulated conversation spoken in a quiet room. However, when speech is masked by environmental noise or when the talker delivers the message at a rate greater than 160 words per minute, the higher frequencies have a more important role, and loss of speech frequencies causes functional problems.

Otosclerosis is a common condition. This generally results in fixation of the foot-plate of the stapes in the oval window; occasionally, however, the otosclerotic process may affect the cochlea, resulting in a neural deafness.

Hearing loss, which affects almost all elderly people, may have severe psychological effects resulting from social isolation. Since cerumen impaction is so common, assess elderly clients for this problem before sending them for an audiogram. This process will avoid expense to the client and embarrassment to the practitioner. The practitioner should be knowledgable and skilled in carrying out an ear lavage.

Nose

The sense of smell is markedly diminished in the older adult because of a decrease of olfactory nerve fibers and atrophy of the remaining fibers.

Mouth

Atrophy of the papillae of the lateral edges of the tongue is common in persons past age 45. There is a decline in the number of papilla and in the number of taste buds per papilla. One of the indications of loss of taste perception is that the elderly must be exposed to 11 times the concentration of sugar required by younger clients to sense sweetness. All taste modalities (sweet, salty, sour, bitter) decline with age. However, sweet and salty tastes are lost first.

Examination of the mouth. Oral changes that accompany normal aging include tooth loss, a decrease in secretion of saliva, atrophy of the oral mucosa, atrophy of the muscles of mastication, and loss of acuity of taste.

Referral to dentist. Elderly persons have more unmet dental needs and make fewer visits to the dentist than any other age group in the United States. Tooth loss increases with age. Approximately 20% of individuals in the 45- to 64-year-old age group are edentulous; by age 65, 50% have no teeth, and the value reaches 60% for those older than 75 years. Tooth loss is not a normal aging process; older persons lose teeth because they have dental disease. (See the box below.) The condition that most frequently leads to tooth loss is periodontal disease. There are several conditions that, when recognized in the elderly client, would necessitate referral of the client to a dentist. Halitosis is a common problem that generally indicates infection and necrosis of tissues of the mouth, sinuses, or gastrointestinal tract or degeneration of debris from mastication of food. In most cases oral infection involves caries or periodontal disease. The elderly person may be unable to chew normally because of painful, diseased teeth or gums or malocclusion. Poorly fitting

---

Review of Dental Hygiene

1. Review the type of dental care products used for cleansing the teeth or dentures.
2. Question the client about the frequency and technique used for brushing and flossing the teeth.
3. Question the client about the frequency of receiving dental care and encourage dental cleaning every 6 months.

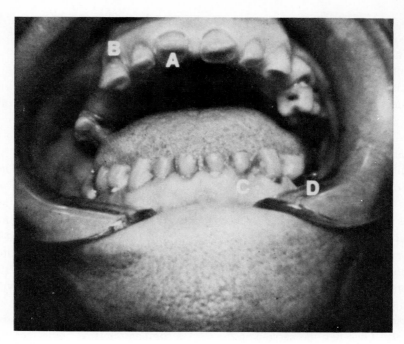

Figure 25-4

The aging dentition: *A*, attrition; *B*, abrasion; *C*, erosion; *D*, cervical caries.
(From Steinberg FU, editor: Care of the geriatric patient in the tradition of CV Cowdry, ed 6, St Louis, 1983, The CV Mosby Co.)

dentures can also interfere with chewing. Areas of friction are often fiery red (Fig. 25-4). Oral cancer may present as an asymptomatic red or white lesion. Conditions appropriate for dental referral include the following:
1. Halitosis
2. Abnormal chewing
3. Infection
4. Lesions; red, white, ulcerated
5. Bleeding gums
6. Dental caries
7. Loose teeth
8. Poorly fitting dentures

Other changes. Saliva does not decrease as a function of aging. Healthy persons who are not taking medications that inhibit salivary secretion have no decline in production of saliva. However, dry mouth, called xerostomia, may be caused by ingestion of anticholinergic drugs, which are commonly taken by older persons. Some classes of drugs known to cause xerostomia are antidepressants, antihistamines, antihypertensives, antineoplastics, antispasmodics, decongestants, tranquilizers, and diuretics.

Tissue changes in the mouth that occur with aging are thought to predispose the client to a variety of oral disease. Tissue resistance to infection is lowered. Atrophy of the oral mucosa increases the opportunity for irritation, trauma, and infection.

Breasts

The amount of fat in breasts increases in most women, whereas glandular tissues atrophy. As a rule, the general size remains the same. However, the breasts change in consistency and shape and are often described as pendulous (elongated) or flaccid. Because of the diminution of connective tissue, the presence of breast lesions is detected earlier than in the younger adult. The detection of a lump in the elderly woman is of greater significance because cystic mastitis is not common past the menopausal years. Careful examination of the breasts is imperative because of the high incidence of breast cancer between 55 and 73 years of age, and a yearly mammogram is recommended.

Respiratory System

With aging there is an advancing *kyphosis* associated with changes in cartilage, osteoporosis, and vertebral collapse; a calcification of the vertebral cartilages, resulting in reduced mobility of the ribs; and an increase in the anteroposterior diameter of the chest. Thus, the chest wall is less compliant, and the strength of muscle contraction is diminished.

The intra-alveolar septa degenerate with aging, resulting in coalesced or large alveoli and widening of the alveolar ducts and bronchioles. With aging the lung loses elasticity, and therefore less force is required to stretch it. The lung becomes more compliant. Lung mass decreases by 21% between 60 and 90 years of age due to loss of alveolar parenchyma.

Tracheal deviation in the elderly may be the result of upper dorsal scoliosis.

Maximum breathing capacity, forced vital capacity, and inspiratory reserve volume are known to decline with age, whereas functional residual capacity increases. Since there is a smaller force working against the elastic forces of the chest wall, the breaths taken by the elderly client are not as deep as those taken by the younger client. Furthermore, there is a loss of diffusion capacity, or the passage of oxygen from the environment into the pulmonary capillaries, and of carbon dioxide from the pulmonary capillaries to the external side of the alveolus. For identical pulmonary blood flow rates, an 80-year-old client gets one third as much oxygen into the cardiovascular system as a 20-year-old.

Although the number of alveoli remains constant in the healthy aging person, the alveoli become smaller and more shallow, reducing the alveolar surface. The alveolar ducts apparently increase in size. Vital capacity is reduced.

The lung loses elasticity with aging. Less force is required to stretch a unit amount; the lung becomes more compliant. The lung does not resume its resting shape as readily after having been stretched, and deflation is incomplete. A significant degree of alveolar dilatation occurs, the so-called senile emphysema.

The small airways without cartilaginous support are kept open by the effect of the elastic tissue surrounding them and by the subatmospheric intrapleural pressure. The loss of elastic recoil with age reduces the stability of small airways, leading to a tendency for these airways to close, particularly in the lower, dependent portions of the lung. *Collagen* is present in high concentration in the lung and contributes to maintaining the form of the lung. The amount of collagen is markedly reduced with aging.

Cilia are decreased from the airways of older persons, and the strength of contraction of those remaining is decreased. Thus, the mucus elevator is less effective in removing particulate material. The alveolar macrophages are less efficient in phagocytosis.

The elderly client with cardiac disease more frequently gives a chief complaint of fatigue rather than of shortness of breath. The elderly client with known respiratory disease who has marked fatigue that has been present for only a short time is frequently found to be suffering an acute respiratory system infectious process. Cough is the most frequent symptom of pulmonary congestion (see the box opposite).

Cardiovascular System

Cardiovascular disease is the most common problem in the elderly and the principal cause of death.

The resting heart rate and stroke volume at maximum load decline in the elderly, along with the cardiac output. The heart rate returns to the resting state more slowly following a challenge in the elderly. The heart also becomes less distensible as collagen increases.

The electrocardiogram (ECG) reveals a decrease in the amplitude of the QRS complex and lengthening of the PR, QRS, and QT intervals.

The effective strength of blood vessels is decreased as connective tissue replaces smooth muscle cells, and fibroconnective tissue deposits have been observed.

Elasticity is also decreased as elastic fibers fragment. The proximal arteries tend to thin and dilate as aging progresses, whereas the peripheral arterial walls become thicker and dilate less readily.

Baroreceptor sensitivity is known to be blunted with age. Normal sinus rhythm is 70 to 75 beats per minute but may vary from 60 to 80 in the elderly person. Premature contraction or extrasystole can result from irritable foci anywhere in the heart. The elderly may have three to four extrasystoles per minute. It is considered pathologic when ten or more extrasystoles per minute occur.

The older individual's response to maximum exercise is not as great as that of the younger adult for either cardiac output or heart rate. The older person develops a greater increase in systolic blood pressure than does a young adult performing the same amount of physical work. Cardiac valves stiffen and hypertrophy with age.

Changes that have been observed in the aged heart include (1) decreased strength of contraction, (2) decreased cardiac output, (3) decreased speed and force of contraction, (4) decreased stroke volume, (5) decreased *ventricular ejection fraction,* (6) decreased left ventricular diastolic compliance and filling, and (7) increased impedance to left ventricular ejection.

Because of the compromises in function in the old heart, sudden physical and emotional stresses may result

---

Respiratory Hygiene

An ineffective cough mechanism in the elderly leads to mucus plugs and increased potential for developing a serious respiratory infection. Drinking six to eight glasses of water a day serves as a cheap and effective expectorant to help prevent this problem.

in cardiac arrhythmias, heart failure, and sudden death in the elderly.

Inspection and auscultation of the neck may provide valuable data. Heart disease and congestive heart failure should be suspected when the neck veins are distended in a client reclining at a 45-degree angle in bed.

Auscultation of the neck over the carotid arteries may reveal bruits. A bruit may disappear as occlusion of a vessel reaches 50% or more.

Precordial palpation in the elderly is influenced by the changes in the shape of the chest. Clients with chronic obstructive pulmonary disease may have no detectable cardiac impulse because of the increased anteroposterior diameter of the chest.

The most common murmur in the elderly client is functional aortic, systolic murmur caused by dilatation of the aortic annulus and ascending aorta and thickening, deformity, or slight calcification of aortic leaflets. The murmur is of low intensity, peaks early in systole, and is short. The murmur is best heard at the right base. Diastolic murmurs are always abnormal. The second heart sound is usually split.

Fourth heart sounds (S_4) are commonly heard in the elderly (94%) and are thought to be caused by decreased compliance of the left ventricle, which is contracting against an increased impedance.

Congestive heart failure and arrhythmias are generally associated with one or more cardiovascular pathologic conditions. The most frequent causes of congestive heart failure and arrhythmia are (1) arteriosclerotic heart disease, (2) valvular disease (degenerative calcific changes in the mitral or aortic valve), (3) hypertension, and (4) myocardial infarction.

A common complaint that is elicited from the elderly client with a cardiovascular disorder is substernal pain or respiratory distress following rapid walking, climbing stairs, or other exertion. On the other hand, cardiac pain as a result of myocardial infarction may be slight or absent. Silent or painless myocardial infarctions may occur in which sudden fatigue or breathlessness may be the only presenting sign. Dyspnea, orthopnea, dizziness, and syncope are symptoms that alert the interviewer to focus on detection of other indications of cardiovascular disease. Dyspnea is commonly the predominant complaint in cardiovascular disease. Exertional dyspnea may be more prominent than chest pain or pressure as a symptom of angina. Myocardial infarction is more often characterized by dyspnea or exacerbation of stable congestive heart failure than by chronic chest pain.

Kyphoscoliosis, frequently seen in the aging individual, may cause a downward dislocation of the cardiac apex, so that its location loses diagnostic significance.

The National High Blood Pressure Coordinating Committee (1979) indicated a systolic measurement of 160 mm Hg and a diastolic measurement of 95 mm Hg as the pressures at which drug treatment should begin, and this standard holds true today. Systolic blood pressures increase with age in both sexes. It has been shown that while systolic pressures continue to rise with each decade in adulthood, diastolic pressures tend to plateau after 40 or 50 years of age.

Hypertensive individuals die prematurely. Actuarial studies indicate that increased cardiovascular morbidity and mortality accompany even slightly raised systolic or diastolic blood pressures.

A progressive rigidity of the aorta and its branches occurs with aging. Some of the processes that have been associated with this rigidity include deposition of a collagen matrix, fracturing and uncoiling of elastic fibers and the deposition of collagen and calcium within the media, thickening, and atheromatous changes in the intima.

Baroreceptor insensitivity has also been documented as a part of the aging process. The decline of the moment-to-moment adjustment of variation in pressure also results in alterations in blood pressure. The most evident change may be orthostatic hypotension (10% incidence in the elderly) as the postural reflexes become less sensitive.

Examination for hypertension should include two or more measurements of blood pressure with the client both sitting and standing. The funduscopic examination for this condition focuses on determining the presence of arteriolar narrowing, arteriovenous crossing changes, hemorrhage, and exudates. Auscultation for carotid and abdominal vessel bruits is aimed at determining a diastolic component, since a systolic bruit in the abdomen of older clients is common. The neurologic examination is aimed at detecting indicators of focal deficits.

Dizziness, blackouts, or syncope seen in the elderly may be the result of marked aortic stenosis but may also result from impaired carotid flow. Fainting also occurs when cardiac output is not increased in response to exertion and also with marked vasodilation of skeletal muscle beds.

Data from phonocardiographic studies show that murmurs are present in 60% or more of aging clients. The most common is a soft systolic ejection murmur heard at the base of the heart as a result of sclerotic changes at the bases of the cusps of the aortic valve.

Pulses. The arteries are felt more readily in the elderly because of a loss of adjacent connective tissue and increased hardness of the arteries resulting from arteriosclerosis and atherosclerosis.

Edema. Edema is frequently observed in the elderly and is often wrongly attributed to congestive heart failure. In cardiac disease with left ventricular failure, symptoms of pulmonary congestion generally predominate rather than edema. Peripheral edema is frequently the result of chronic venous insufficiency of hypoproteinemia.

Blood

Anemia. Both hemoglobin and red blood cell (RBC) counts are slightly lower in the elderly than in younger people. The decreased half-life of the RBC in the elderly is believed to result from a decrease in the enzyme function of the RBC. The number of hematopoietic cells is decreased in the elderly, whereas the fat content of the bone marrow is increased.

Causes of anemia in the elderly have been classified as (1) decreased hematopoiesis related to malnutrition; (2) blood loss resulting from chronic bleeding; and (3) increased blood destruction caused by infection, a malignancy, or drug use. Iron deficiency anemia occurs more frequently in the elderly than in the young.

Leukopenia with a decline in leukocyte function has been observed in the elderly.

Leukemia. Acute myelogenous leukemia is most commonly seen in individuals more than 40 years of age.

Abdomen

Since there is a general loss of fibroconnective tissue and muscle wasting in the elderly, the abdominal wall of the elderly client will be slacker and thinner, making palpation simpler and ostensibly more accurate than in the younger individual. This does not hold true if the older client is extremely obese.

Abdominal wall rigidity is not as common a sign of peritoneal irritation in the elderly client as it is in the younger individual.

In an acute abdominal emergency, the elderly client generally complains less of discomfort than would the younger person with a similar condition.

Gastrointestinal function. Gastric acid secretion has been shown to decline with advancing age. Decreases in the production of both hydrochloric acid and digestive enzymes have been measured and may explain the elderly client's complaints of anorexia and difficulty in digesting meals.

The elderly have a higher incidence of gastrointestinal disorders. Older individuals have increased esophageal spasms and contraction and weaker activity of the lower esophageal sphincter. Gastric acid secretion is impaired. Atrophic gastritis is more common. A de-

cline in motility of the gastrointestinal system has been noted. The reduction in colonic motility may result in a number of dysfunctions, including constipation.

Constipation is a frequent complaint. However, although a decline in the motility of the gastrointestinal tract has been proved to occur with advancing years, it has been shown that 90% of individuals over 60 years of age have at least one bowel movement a day.

Gastrointestinal bleeding in the older client. The percentage of clients with upper gastrointestinal bleeding was 48% in 1970. The mortality for persons with upper gastrointestinal bleeding is 7% to 10%.

Biliary disease in the aging client. Biliary disease affects 15% to 20% of all adults, and the incidence rises steadily with age. It is estimated that 35% to 80% of elderly persons have gallstones by age 75, with a 2:1 ratio of women to men. Approximately 40% of clients with gallstones have no symptoms.

Colorectal cancer. The incidence of colon cancer begins to rise significantly at age 40 to 45. Approximately 116,000 cases of colorectal cancer are detected in the United States each year. Colon cancer discovered before symptoms develop is usually localized in the bowel wall, and the 5-year survival rate is greater than 85%. Most colon cancer originates from neoplastic polyps.

Liver. Liver weight is known to decrease with advancing age, and a decrease in the number of liver cells has been documented. No alteration in liver function tests has been noted. Impaired metabolism of some drugs occurs with aging.

Endocrine System

Antidiuretic hormone (ADH). In the human, the maximum achievable urine osmolality decreases with increasing age. The decrease in maximum urine-concentrating ability is also related to diminished ability of the kidney cells of the distal convoluted tubules and collecting ducts to respond to ADH and the decreased glomerular filtration rate that occurs with age. The development of dilutional hyponatremia following the stress of surgery in the elderly led to the theory that there is a disturbance in the release of ADH.

Thyroid gland. Recent studies indicate a modest (not exceeding 15%) decrease of thyroxine (T_4) occurs with advancing age in healthy individuals, as well as an increase in thyroid-stimulating hormone (TSH). The basal metabolic rate is known to decrease with age, but this is related to a reduction in muscle mass. The prevalence of thyroid nodules may increase with age.

The diagnosis of hyperthyroidism and hypothyroidism is more difficult in the elderly. The older person is more likely to have signs and symptoms indicating involvement of only one system, such as heart disease with congestive failure.

Pancreas. Adult-onset diabetes mellitus is observed to have a high incidence among the elderly. Most individuals are managed successfully with diet alone or with diet and oral hypoglycemics. Few require insulin. If insulin is needed, the elderly client is said to be insulin-requiring, not insulin-dependent; insulin dependency refers to a complete deficiency of insulin, as seen only in juvenile diabetes.

There is some evidence that accelerated aging accompanies the diabetic state. A more rapid rate of cell death of the endothelial cells in capillaries results in microangiopathy. The thickening of the capillary basement membrane observed in most aged subjects occurs more rapidly in diabetics.

Glucose tolerance. The ability to metabolize a glucose load is influenced by a client's age, activity, and diet. Aging is known as one of the most important factors influencing performance on glucose tolerance testing. The 1- and 2-hour glucose values progressively rise at the rate of 10 mg/dl for each decade beyond age 50. A decrease in tissue sensitivity to insulin is the major factor responsible for the diminution in glucose tolerance. Failure to correct the glucose tolerance test for age would result in as many as 70% of the clients above the age of 70 being labeled diabetic.

A further compromise of ability of older persons to metabolize glucose is related to inactivity. The effect of inactivity is to diminish tissue sensitivity to insulin. The glucose tolerance test results may also be affected by use of diuretics.

Genitourinary System

Because of the decreased cardiac output, blood flow to the kidneys and glomerular filtration rate are markedly diminished in the aged, leading to a loss of kidney function.

Structural changes in the kidneys result in aging changes in renal function. There is a gradual decline in renal plasma flow (RPF), in glomerular filtration rate (GFR), and in renal tubular resorptive capacity.

There is reduced renal excretion of many substances. In day-to-day activities the changes produce no signs or symptoms. The danger to the elderly client is that the aging kidneys fail to respond effectively to rapid or massive changes in fluid and electrolyte balance.

The glomerular filtration rate decreases from 120 ml per 1.73 m^2 (body surface) in young adults to 80 ml

per 1.73 m^2 in the elderly person. A more precise study of creatinine clearance indicates the values are normal to the mid-40s and then decline at the rate of 8 ml per minute per 1.73 m^2 per decade.

The two most common signs of genitourinary dysfunction in the elderly are nocturnal frequency of micturition and incontinence of urine. In the elderly male client, frequency of micturition accompanied by problems in initiating and ending the stream and a decrease in the force of the stream are generally the result of prostatic enlargement.

Incontinence in the elderly client is a symptom; it does not result from a natural aging process. Incontinence is an involuntary loss of urine with or without warning and sensation. Incontinence has been classified as stress, urge, overflow, or functional.

Stress incontinence is the involuntary loss of urine from the urethra that occurs with coughing, laughing, lifting, or standing up suddenly. These activities increase intra-abdominal and intravesicular pressure so that the sphincter mechanism is overwhelmed. Stress incontinence occurs most frequently in women. The amount of urine that is lost involuntarily may vary from a few drops to amounts so great that the individual wears diapers.

Relaxation of the perineal muscles in the elderly female client leads to stress incontinence. For the most part, female incontinence results from the loss of the urethrovesical angle with inferior displacement of the bladder base into the pelvis. When the bladder neck remains in the young adult position high behind the symphysis pubis, an increase in intra-abdominal pressure is transmitted to the urethra rather than to the bladder neck. Stress incontinence may also be caused by urethral dysfunction. This type of stress incontinence results from a loss of urethral tone and thickness at the bladder neck, leading to leakage.

Urge incontinence is the result of the inability to suppress the urge to void. Uninhibited bladder contractions may be the result of a local condition such as a urinary tract infection, bladder stones, or bladder cancer. When the urethra becomes obstructed by the prostate or a urethral tumor, the bladder distention that results causes bladder wall irritability and bladder contractions. The muscle spasm that occurs from these conditions may be strong enough to overcome cortical control. Clients who have had a stroke may not have adequate cortical control, and for some of the elderly, this problem is *idiopathic* and leads to urge incontinence. This type of incontinence usually results in the loss of large amounts of urine.

Overflow incontinence results from a large urinary residual that alters the functional capacity of the bladder, causing frequent leakage of small amounts of urine. This

Table 25-3

Changes noted in the four phases of intercourse in the aging female client

Phase	Alteration
Excitement	Delay in production of vaginal secretion and lubrication
Plateau	Reduction in expansion, both in length and width, of vagina
	Uterus does not elevate into false pelvis as much as in younger women
	Labia majora flaccid—do not elevate and flatten against perineum
	Labia minora do not undergo sex color change from pink to burgundy or become congested
	Clitoral size decreases after 60 years of age
Orgasm	Shorter than in younger women
Resolution	Occurs more rapidly

Table 25-4

Changes noted in the four phases of intercourse in the aging male client

Phase	Alteration
Excitement	Slower increment in excitement; sex flush less in duration and intensity; involuntary spasms diminished; longer time required to obtain erection; less testicular elevation and scrotal sac vasocongestion in erection
Plateau	Longer duration; increase in penile diameter due to less preejaculatory fluid emission
Orgasm	Shorter duration; fewer contractions in expulsion of semen bolus
Resolution (refractory)	Lasts 12 to 24 hours compared with 2 minutes in the younger client; loss of erection (return of penis to flaccid state) may take a few seconds compared with minutes or hours in the younger client

condition may result from urethral obstruction, a neurologic pathologic condition due to diabetes, or from fecal impaction (one of the most common causes of urinary incontinence).

Functional incontinence results from clients' inability to maintain balance in front of the toilet, raise and lower themselves from the toilet seat, undo garments, or ambulate at all or in time to get to the toilet before leakage occurs. The client may not remember where the toilet is or not have the judgment to use the toilet on a regular basis. Environmental factors affect a client's ability to use the toilet. Availability and location of toilet facilities may be a problem, as well as response by people to the client's request for assistance to the toilet.

Reproductive Status

Female client.   Since the cells of the reproductive tract and the breasts are estrogen-dependent, both for growth and for function, the decline of estrogen production starting at menopause is responsible for many changes observed in these tissues in elderly female clients.

The uterus is diminished in size because of a loss of myometrial fibers; the uterine mucosa is normally thin and atrophic. The cervix is also decreased in size. The vagina of the eldery client is observed to be narrower and shorter because of an increase in the amount of submucosal connective tissue. The vaginal epithelium atrophies, and the surface appears thin and pale. Because of the fragility of the mucosa, it is easily traumatized, and

special attention should be devoted to observing for erosion, ulcerations, and adhesions. Change gloves between the pelvic and the rectal examinations. Friable atrophic vaginal tissue in the elderly female may contaminate the examining glove with a few RBCs and give a false-positive hemoccult from the rectal examination. Changes noted during intercourse are shown in Table 25-3.

Male client.   Although the decline of testosterone production in the male client occurs at a later time in life than that of estrogen in the female client, clinically observable signs and symptoms do accompany the decline in production of this reproductive hormone.

The client may report a decline in sexual energy. During the act of intercourse, physiologic reactions are less intense and reactions are slowed (Table 25-4).

There is a gradual decline in strength of the muscles associated with the act of intercourse. The testes decrease in size and are less firm on palpation. The result of this degenerative change is a decrease in production of spermatozoa. The prostate gland is enlarged, and secretion is impaired. The seminal fluid is reduced in amount and viscosity.

These changes do not necessarily mean a decrease in libido or a loss in the sense of satisfaction from the sex act. A frequency of intercourse of one or two times per week in most men over 60 has been reported. The level of sexual activity, although generally in decline, parallels the amount of activity the client engaged in as a younger person.

Musculoskeletal System

Although muscle mass is known to decline progressively with age, loss of strength is not necessarily the result. The practitioner may use the opportunity afforded by the examination session to determine if the aging client is exercising. The client is queried concerning planned exercise during recreation and the amount of activity experienced through work.

Osteoarthritic changes in the joints are almost universally observed in the elderly. Proliferative changes in the spine cause bony overgrowths called *osteophytes*. Osteoarthritic bony overgrowths involving the distal finger joints are termed *Heberden's nodes*. Bouchard's nodes are overgrowths involving the proximal joints.

Muscle mass is subject to a 30% loss between the ages of 30 and 80. Muscles are hypotonic and atrophic. Muscle contours are less evident and add to a sagging appearance of the soft tissue.

A stooped posture and reduction in arm swing is the description of the overall motor changes that progressively develop with aging. The elderly client's posture and movements are much like those seen in parkinsonism. Some older persons assume a posture of mild generalized flexion accompanied by some rigidity and poverty of movement. Movement of the arms may be limited on ambulation and contribute to unsteady gait. Flexion of the knees and hips may displace the weight forward and further contribute to *festinating* gait.

Osteoporosis is a pathophysiologic condition characterized by increased mobilization of calcium from the bones. It results in a reduction in total skeletal mass and increased fragility of the bones. Bone loss in women is approximately 25%, whereas the decrement in men is 12%. Osteoporosis predisposes the elderly to fractures and is a major cause of morbidity and mortality in the elderly; osteoporosis is associated with 80% of clients with hip fractures. It is known that 20% of the elderly persons who sustain hip fractures die within 3 months.

Kyphosis in the elderly client may be the first indication of osteoporosis. The client may complain of sudden pain along the vertebrae; this may signal the occurrence of a vertebral fracture.

Skin

The skin of elderly people appears thin and translucent. Atrophy of the epidermal structures results from the degeneration of collagen and elastin. In addition there is a loss of subcutaneous fat and increased vascular fragility. There is a loss of skin turgor over the extremities, and, therefore, the skin of the forehead is recommended for the pinch-fold test for dehydration. The elderly have less scalp, axillary, and pubic hair, and the hair of the eye-

brows and other facial hair in women becomes coarse.

Since eccrine sweat gland and sebaceous gland production is diminished, the skin is dry and flaky. As a result of the decline in *melanophore* activity, the skin appears pale. Nail growth slows.

Skin changes are not necessarily associated with a specific period in the individual's life. However, skin disease is estimated to affect 65% of the population over 65 years of age. Aging changes of the skin are influenced by many factors, such as heredity, changes in the connective and epithelial tissues, endocrine alterations, and inadequate nutrition as a result of vascular changes. Excessive exposure to the sun and extremes of weather are known to accelerate the changes characteristic of aging.

The appearance of senile white skin has been described as wrinkled, dry, and inelastic. In many cases the skin takes on a yellowish hue and resembles parchment. Aging changes in black skin occur at a later age than in white skin.

For many persons, wrinkling of the skin is the hallmark of aging. In those cultures where age is respected, wrinkling of the skin may be symbolic of character and status. In youth-oriented countries such as the United States, a good deal of time and money may be invested in preventing wrinkles. Wrinkling is first apparent on the skin of the face and neck, since the tissues contain a rich meshwork of collagen and elastic fibers.

Telangiectasias are visible, dilated blood vessels. As the dermis thins, there is a loss of support for blood vessel walls, resulting in dilation. The dermal thinning also makes the dilated vessels more visible. The visible vessels have been called "broken blood vessels," "venous stars," and "spider nevi" and are bright red, very fine, linear, stellate, or punctate.

Senile lentigines, seborrheic keratoses, and angiomas appear more often in clients over 40 and must be distinguished from malignant lesions.

Senile lentigines are flat, tan to brown macules often as large as 1 or 2 cm that appear on the dorsal surface of the hand and other areas of sun-exposed skin of middle-aged and older clients.

Seborrheic keratoses are benign hyperplastic warty lesions of the skin. The borders are irregular, and the surface is scaly. The lesions have been described as having a "pasted-on" appearance. The early lesion is yellowish to tan, but the pigmentation increases over time to dark brown or black. The lesions appear with greatest frequency on the face, shoulders, and trunk. Large seborrheic keratoses are not common before the seventh or eighth decade. Although the lesions are benign, some clients desire their removal for cosmetic reasons.

Actinic keratoses (Fig. 25-5) are lesions that ap-

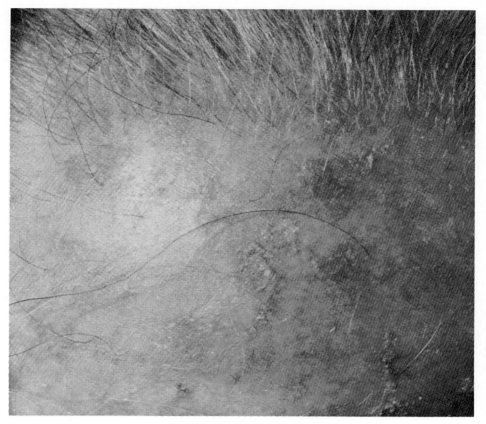

Figure 25-5

Actinic keratosis. Extensive involvement of the forehead.
(From Stewart WD, Danto JL, and Maddin S: Dermatology: the diagnosis and treatment of cutaneous disorders,
ed 4, St Louis, 1978, The CV Mosby Co.)

pear on sun-exposed areas of the skin at about age 50. The most common sites are the face, ears, and dorsal surfaces of the arms and hands. The lesions are pink to slightly red with indistinct borders and are considered premalignant.

Cherry angiomas are caused by proliferation and dilation of the superficial capillaries of the skin. The lesions are bright red, soft, and dome-shaped with a diameter of 1 ml or more. Trauma resulting in extravasation from the capillaries or clotting in the vessels may cause the lesions to appear bluish black. Although cherry angiomas may be observed early in adulthood, they are most numerous after 40 years of age. The lesions are benign.

A decrease in elastic and connective tissue, which becomes more marked with aging, is evident in examination of the skin. There is a decrease in collagen, and that which remains becomes rigid. The skin appears thinner, caused by a loss of dermis and subcutaneous fat, particularly over the backs of the hands. Because of the loss of elastic fibers, the skin, when pinched between the examiner's thumb and finger takes a good deal longer to return to its natural shape. Sebaceous and sweat glands are less active. Thus, the client may complain of "dry skin," particularly over the extremities where circulation is less effective.

In addition, hair growth often becomes scanty or absent as the peripheral circulation is compromised. This is particularly evident over the dorsum of the feet and lower legs. Along with the general thinning of the hair that is characteristic of the aging phenomenon, the elderly suffer a loss of scalp hair. In women the hairs appear finer or sparser, or both. There is also a general thinning of pubic and axillary hair, whereas the hairs of the nostrils, ears, and eyebrows are coarser and bristlelike. Nails grow more slowly in the elderly. They develop longitudinal striations and tend to split and peel off in layers.

Pruritus, or itching, is a common symptom of aging skin. The itching may be related to the drying of the aging skin, but the examiner must be alert to other symptoms and signs of systemic disease also associated with pruritus, such as liver disease, diabetes, kidney disease, thyroid disorders, and cancer.

In examination of the skin, the examiner should be particularly alert to the presence of ecchymoses, since the presence of a bruise may indicate a recent injury. The client may have forgotten the injury or may have been unaware of it because of the decrease in sensory perception. Bruising from senile purpura is common, especially over the forearm.

Pigment may be deposited as melanotic freckles (lentigines), although overall the skin may be paler. Cells lose their capacity to spread out melanin. Vitiligo, areas of skin lacking pigment, may be localized or generalized in distribution; this hypopigmentation tends to increase with age. Vitiligo is thought to be an autoimmune phenomenon. Be alert for skin cancer (see the box opposite).

Cutaneous tags are a common skin change seen in the elderly. The lesions are soft, flesh colored, and pedunculated and vary from a pinhead to a pea (1 to 3 mm). They are most commonly noted on the vertical and lateral surfaces of the neck and in the axillary area. The lesions have no clinical significance and can be ignored, unless the client frequently injures them with clothing or jewelry or if they are disturbing from a cosmetic point of view.

Nervous System

After age 50, brain cells are thought to decrease in number at a rate of about 1% per year. However, because of the immense number of reserve cells involved, no clinical signs may be observed.

Conduction velocity in some nerves is known to decline with age. The startle response takes twice as long in some aged clients. The speed of conduction of nerve impulses decreases 10% over the age span of 30 to 90 years.

Since the tactile sense is known to be blunted, more intense clues may be used to test this sensory modality. The aged need stronger signals (greater amplitude) to detect vibration; as with other sensory phenomena, this is probably the result of decline of CNS function.

The assessment of sensory abilities is particularly important in effectively advising modifications of the client's living quarters to increase sensory input and to avoid serious accidents.

Although the response to deep tendon reflex testing is decreased or absent in some elderly clients, all reflexes may be elicited in the healthy elderly adult. As a rule of progression, reflexes are preserved in the arms

---

Skin Cancers

Carefully examine the following areas for skin cancer in the elderly:
- Neck
- Ears
- Face, especially above the eyebrows and cheek bones
- Forearms and hands
- Legs (years ago, many women wore skirts while working in the field)

---

but lost in the lower legs at first. Muscle strength deteriorates less rapidly than coordination.

Achilles reflexes (ankle jerks) may diminish and disappear in some cases. The plantar reflex may be difficult to elicit. The superficial reflexes such as the abdominal reflexes may disappear.

Immune Response

The thymus gland undergoes a process of involution that begins at sexual maturity and is complete by 45 to 50 years of age. Thymic hormones play a role in the differentiation of lymphocytes. The hormones decline as the number of thymic cells does; thymic hormones can no longer be detected in humans older than 60 years of age.

Autoantibodies to smooth muscle, lymphocytes, gastric parietal cells, immunoglobulin, and thyroglobulin have been found with increased frequency in older humans. It has been suggested that autoantibodies and circulating immune complexes contribute to the pathologic changes that occur with aging. The response of elderly persons to foreign antigens decreases with age. Furthermore, the antibody response is maintained for a shorter time.

Infections in the Elderly

Some bacterial pathogens such as gram-negative bacilli are more likely to occur in older clients than in young adults. On the other hand, some pathogens are less likely to affect the elderly.

The elderly person may have altered signs and symptoms to a given pathogen from the young adult. Older clients with pneumonia are less likely to complain of cough, and elderly clients with meningitis often deny a stiff neck. Sometimes the client ignores the symptoms of infection, believing that they are signs of other conditions of aging.

Both the incidence and mortality from many bacterial infections are higher in the elderly. The effectiveness of the immune system declines with age, and the older person is more likely to have predisposing illnesses.

Bacterial pneumonia has become a major cause of morbidity and mortality in the older client. The elderly client with pneumonia is more likely to develop bacteremia and complications. The pneumonia of the elderly has been described as latent, without chills or cough. Lethargy may be the first sign of pneumonia. Pneumococcal infection frequently results in death.

The incidence of and mortality from bacterial meningitis is increasing in the aged. Bacterial infection may spread from the urinary tract, the lung, the ear (in otitis media), or an infected sinus.

Delay in making a diagnosis has resulted from attributing changes in mental status to senility or psychosis, stroke, and cerebral anoxia.

Bacterial endocarditis has become more common in the elderly population. Bacterial endocarditis is caused by streptococci and staphylococci in 25% to 80% of cases of endocarditis in the elderly. The signs and symptoms of malaise, anorexia, weight loss, and neurologic findings are often attributed to other diseases.

The elderly have a higher incidence of urinary tract infections than do younger adults. The incidence is 3% in men aged 65 to 70; this rises to 20% after age 70. In women, the urinary tract infection rate is 20% after age 65 and 23% to 50% after age 80. The incidence for both sexes increases markedly among the institutionalized elderly.

Most older persons with urinary tract infections are asymptomatic. Urinary tract symptoms such as dysuria or frequency occur less frequently. Change in cognitive function, loss of appetite, and loss of urine control are more common presentations of this problem in the elderly.

Influenza is common among the elderly. Approximately 70% of the deaths caused by pneumonia and influenza occur in persons older than 65, and 95% of those persons have underlying chronic disease. Clients with pneumonia and cardiovascular disease are at greatest risk.

The symptoms of influenza are usually more prolonged and severe in the elderly but are of the typical respiratory and generalized nature.

Herpes zoster is a disease that occurs primarily in the older adult. Both the severity of the infection and the neuralgia that follows the eruption of vesicles increase with age.

Immunizations
Baseline PPD/*Candida* Tetanus booster, every 8 to 10 years Pneumovac—once in a lifetime Influenza—yearly in late fall

Immunization Status

Tetanus has a high incidence in the elderly. When questioned, the elderly client frequently reports never having been immunized against tetanus. Pneumovac immunization should be given to all elderly clients. Their *autoimmune* systems will more effectively produce antibodies to this dreaded infection if it is received during their 60s. All aged clients should have a baseline purified protein derivative (PPD) test in their database. When a PPD is placed on a client's arm, a *Candida* dose should be placed on the opposite arm as a control. If the arm with the *Candida* does not become erythematous, then a negative PPD should be considered a possible false-negative test. The box above lists immunizations the elderly should have.

Temperature Regulation

An absent or diminished febrile response is frequently observed in elderly clients. The assessment of a low body temperature (35°C [96.9°F] or lower) occurs more frequently among the elderly than other age groups. Since temperature control is poorly controlled in the elderly, they should be warned about the hazards of hypothermia and hyperthermia. In cold weather, the indoor temperature should be kept at 70 degrees. The elderly should wear multiple layers of lightweight clothing, eat frequent small meals, and drink warm liquids throughout the day. During hot weather the elderly should avoid going outdoors during the heat of the day, avoid strenuous activity, and wear lightweight clothing. They should also eat light meals, drink cool liquids, and during extreme conditions take tepid baths.

Variability in Aging

There is considerable support for the idea that the rate of aging, like the rate of growth, may vary between individuals and that a person may age more rapidly in some parts of the body than others. Whether an individual is aging faster than chronologic agemates or whether the changes are the result of the aging process alone or of disease cannot yet be determined.

BIBLIOGRAPHY

American Psychiatric Association: Diagnosis and statistical manual of mental disorders, ed 3 rev, Washington, DC, 1987, The Association.

Berman N: Geriatric cardiology, Lexington, Mass, 1982, DC Heath & Co.

Borkan GA and Norris AH: Assessment of biological age using a profile of physical parameters, Gerontology 35:177, 1980.

Brocklehurst JC: Textbook of geriatric medicine and gerontology, ed 3, Edinburgh, 1985, Churchill Livingstone, Inc.

Burnside I: Nursing and the aged, ed 3, New York, 1988, McGraw-Hill Book Co.

Busse EW and Pfeiffer E, editors: Behavior and adaptation in late life, ed 2, Boston, 1977, Little, Brown & Co.

Butler RN and Lewis MI: Aging and mental health, ed 3, St Louis, 1982, The CV Mosby Co.

Carnevali DL and Patrick M: Nursing management for the elderly, ed 2, Philadelphia, 1986, JB Lippincott Co.

Delafuente JC and Stewart RB, editors: Therapeutics in the elderly, Baltimore, 1988, Williams & Wilkins.

Elkowitz EB: Geriatric medicine for the primary care practitioner, New York, 1981, Springer Publishing Co, Inc.

Matteson MA and McConnell ES: Gerontological nursing: concepts and practice, Philadelphia, 1988, WB Saunders Co.

McCue JD, editor: Medical care of the elderly, Lexington, Mass, 1983, DC Heath & Co.

National High Blood Pressure Coordinating Committee, Washington, DC, September 1979, US Government Printing Office.

Pitt B: Psychogeriatrics: an introduction to the psychiatry of old age, New York, 1982, Churchill Livingstone, Inc.

Reichel W, editor: Clinical aspects of aging, ed 3, Baltimore, 1988, Williams & Wilkins.

Roe D: Geriatric nutrition, Englewood Cliffs, NJ, 1983, Prentice-Hall Inc.

Rossman I: Clinical geriatrics, ed 3, Philadelphia, 1986, JB Lippincott Co.

Schrier RW: Clinical internal medicine in the aged, Philadelphia, 1982, WB Saunders Co.

Steinberg FU: Cowdry's care of the geriatric patient, ed 6, St Louis, 1983, The CV Mosby Co.

Health Assessment of
Special Populations

26

Cultural considerations in health assessment

OBJECTIVES

Upon successful review of this chapter, learners will be able to:

- Describe reasons why cultural data should be incorporated into a health assessment

- Define the following terms
  Culture and subculture
  Race, ethnicity, and minority group
  Customs and rituals
  Values and norms
  Cultural paradigms
  Enculturation and aculturation
  Cultural determinism
  Ethnocentrism and ethnoscience
  Disease, illness, and sickness

- Appraise the following cultural variables
  Diet and nutritional status
  Socioeconomic status
  Perceptions of pain
  Family structure and roles

- Use the following categories to contrast differences in various groups of people living in North America
  Language and general life-style characteristics
  Health beliefs
  Health practices
  Family characteristics
  Culturally specific data

- Outline questions relevant to a cultural assessment

The information provided in this book enables nurses to perform a comprehensive assessment for virtually any clients whom they are likely to encounter. In addition to a comprehensive approach to the physical examination, this book has presented special considerations and techniques appropriate for clients of all age groups and some frequently encountered special populations. Along the way, the text has emphasized documentation of the client's health history, psychosocial issues related to systems and groups, and an awareness of the family and environmental considerations within which individuals exist in both health and illness. That is the meaning of holistic health assessment, an approach that belongs uniquely to nursing. A truly holistic assessment, however, cannot ignore the critical cultural considerations that are an essential dimension in every client.

This chapter first presents the rationale for cultural considerations as part of the health assessment. It then briefly defines major terms related to culture. Emphasis is then placed on certain broad variables the nurse is likely to encounter when performing health assessments on members of various cultural groups. Finally, the specific considerations characteristic of the prevalent cultural groups in North America are presented.

NURSING AND CULTURE

More than half of all health problems are the result of behavior and life-style. If the goal of nursing is to promote health while respecting individual value systems and life-styles, it is clear that nurses must understand culture-based health behavior. Cultural beliefs and personal characteristics determine health behavior in individuals and families.

Nurses as a group reflect the cultural mix of society in general. In North America, the majority of nurses hold values, beliefs, and attitudes typical of the dominant middle class. In addition, nurses belong to a separate culture as members of the health care team. When two people of differing cultural backgrounds interact, significant communication barriers may arise unless one of the persons is willing and able to recognize and adapt to the other's values. To care for others, nurses must be able to accept a wide diversity of beliefs, practices, and ideas about health and illness, including many that differ from their own.

Acceptance of alternate beliefs about health and illness can be more difficult for nurses than one might initially assume. As health care professionals educated in and exposed to the established health care system, nurses share certain values, attitudes, and beliefs about health and illness that they may not consciously think about. These ways of thinking have been shaped by more than 2000 years of Western thought broadly known as Hippocratic medicine. Modern health care is based on rational, scientific, biomedical principles directed toward solving human health problems. As part of the dominant culture, the health care culture is interwoven with established social, religious, political, and economic systems. Certain aspects of the health care culture, such as nurse-physician relationships and physician-patient relationships, are governed by a broadly shared set of customs and protocols.

The cultural beliefs of some clients may conflict with the cultural beliefs shared by most nurses. Nurses cannot hope to plan meaningful health care for their clients without at least understanding their health beliefs. That is why it is necessary to perform a sensitive cultural assessment. A thorough assessment of the cultural aspects of a client's life-style, health beliefs, and health practices will enhance the nurse's decision making and clinical judgment during provision of care.

TERMINOLOGY ASSOCIATED WITH CULTURAL CONSIDERATIONS

Culture is a complex, integrated system that includes knowledge, beliefs, skills, art, morals, law, customs, and any other *acquired* habits and capabilities of a group of people. Culture is characterized by being learned, shared, adapted to the environment, and subject to change. As a learned set of traits, culture is transmitted from one generation to the next by both formal education and imitation.

Subculture is a group of persons within a culture with one or more shared traits. These include age, socioeconomic status, race, ethnic origin, education, and occupation. There are literally thousands of subcultures within a culture, and everyone is a member of several.

Although subcultures have an identity uniquely their own, they are also related to the culture in certain ways. Major subcultural groups in the United States include Afro-Americans (11.7%), Hispanics (6.4%), Asian Americans (1.5%), and American Indians (0.6%). In Canada, major subcultures include French Canadians (27%) and Natives (2%).

Race refers to the classification of human beings on the basis of such physical characteristics as skin pigmentation, head form, or stature. The recognized races are Caucasian, Negroid, and Mongoloid.

Ethnic groups share such traits as a common national or regional origin and linguistic, ancestral, and physical characteristics. Within the major North American subcultures, distinct ethnic groups include African, Haitian, or Dominican (Black); Mexican, Cuban, or Puerto Rican (Hispanic); and Japanese, Chinese, Filipino, Korean, Vietnamese, Guamian, or Samoan (Asian).

Minority group is a frequently misunderstood term. More normative than descriptive, it refers to any group that receives different and unequal treatment from others in the larger group or society and whose members see themselves as victims of discrimination. This is an important concept for nurses to understand, since many people in our society are discriminated against, and discrimination takes place in the health care system. However, an individual's membership in a minority group is unrelated to the individual's cultural affiliations, and this distinction has an important bearing on cultural assessment.

Customs refers to the learned behaviors shared by and associated with a particular cultural group.

Rituals are highly structured patterns of behavior characteristic of cultural groups. They are prescribed ways to define basic human activities within a cultural context. Rituals may govern a group's approach to communication, traditions, taboos, religion, trade, means of travel, sexual activities, or recreation.

Values and norms are judgments that cultural groups apply to behavior. Values are universal to all cultures and define the desirable or undesirable state of affairs within a culture. Norms provide direction for applying values and are the rules that govern human behavior. Cultural norms set limits. Members of a culture are rewarded or punished as they conform or deviate from them. Norms perform a number of important functions. They influence a person's perception of others. They direct a person's responses to situations and to others. They provide a basis for self-evaluation. They provide a foundation for forming opinions. They motivate behavior, and they give meaning to life and self-esteem. Values and norms exert a very powerful influence over an individual's beliefs, attitudes, and practices, and the nurse must explore the client's value system to gain an appreciation for health-related behavior.

Cultural paradigms encompass abstract explanations used by groups to account for major life events. The term is synonymous with the idea of world view. The three dominant cultural paradigms are magicoreligious, holistic, and scientific. This concept is crucial to health care professionals because all beliefs and values regarding health are derived from a person's basic world view. Aspects of all three world views can be identified in most cultures, but one view usually predominates. The magicoreligious paradigm proffers a mystical cause-and-effect relationship between health and illness. The holistic paradigm provides the basis for a sense of balance and harmony between humans and the larger environment. The scientific view defines health as the absence of disease symptoms.

Enculturation is the process of acquiring one's cultural identity as it is transmitted by the previous generation. The *degree* of enculturation is important to assess before planning care, especially if the nurse anticipates that the client would obtain health benefits by modifying some culturally based aspect of health beliefs, attitudes, or practices.

Aculturation refers to the process of adapting to a culture different from the one a person was enculturated in. Since North America is a continent of immigrants, nurses frequently encounter clients undergoing aculturation. Since culture is a learned group of traits, it is possible for an individual to acquire a new cultural identity. Again, it is necessary for the nurse to assess the *degree* of aculturation to predict the client's inclination to comply with a desirable modification in health care beliefs, attitudes, or practices. When a client is undergoing aculturation, the nurse can play a significant role in teaching the sort of acquired health behavior the client is already attempting to learn.

Cultural determinism is simply a term for conveying the notion that a person's behavior is *determined* by cultural beliefs. The concept is central to cultural assessment because the nurse must understand it to formulate client goals. A goal is something the client, not the nurse, wants to achieve. A goal therefore must take into account the client's culturally determined behavior, or else the nurse cannot expect client compliance.

Ethnocentrism is the tendency to view people unconsciously by using one's group and one's own customs as the standard for all judgments. A nurse with this tendency will gather data only selectively in accordance with personal standards, values, and judgments and will

not be able to see what the patient has to offer or the different ways in which the patient views the world. This bias will limit the data that are gathered and distort their interpretation.

Ethnoscience refers to a systematic study of the way of life of a designated cultural group to obtain an accurate account of the people's behavior and how they perceive and interpret their universe. An ethnoscience approach includes the various ethnic groups' views on health and illness. This chapter takes an ethnoscience approach to cultural assessment because it presents the beliefs of cultural groups as they relate to health and illness.

Disease, illness, and sickness are frequently used, and misused, similar terms. The distinctions among them are important to cultural assessment. *Disease* is a medical term, arising from the dominant, scientifically based health care subculture. It refers to a pathologic process within human structure and function. *Illness* is a subjective term clients may use to describe the symptoms of discomfort. *Sickness,* on the other hand, is a personal state of illness with distinct social dimensions. Depending on the norms within any given culture, role behaviors are modified when a person becomes sick. These modified role behaviors are an important aspect of cultural assessment.

MAJOR VARIABLES IN CULTURAL ASSESSMENT

Diet and Nutrition

Anthropologists have shown that cultural groups differ in their dietary beliefs and practices, but this is obvious to anyone who associates particular foods with specific ethnic groups. The development of national cuisines is a complex process related to the availability of certain kinds of food, the price of food, the efficiency of its distribution, the subjective preferences of taste and spices, and patterns of trade and commerce. Food preferred by groups living relatively closer to the equator, where the climate is warmer, are hotter and spicier than those preferred by groups living in higher latitudes in more temperate climates. The variety of foods available in industrialized countries is greater than that in Third World countries. Moreover, quite apart from its nutritional value, food carries a range of symbolic meanings. Food that is popular in one society may be rigorously forbidden in another. Food, and the social aspects of eating it, plays a central role in daily life. Consequently, nurses must appreciate that dietary beliefs and practices are notoriously difficult to change, even if they interfere with adequate nutrition.

It is therefore essential to understand the ways in

which various cultures view their food, and the ways food is classified, before attempting to change nutrition practices. Food is usually classified into definitions of (1) what is edible and what is not, (2) what is sacred and what is profane, (3) the ways food is grouped, (4) food as medicine, and (5) social food.

By referring to the dominant culture in North America, with which most nurses are familiar, one can see how these classifications are made. Rancid butter is not normally considered edible in our culture, yet it is a standard condiment in tea in many central Asian regions. By the same token, food commonly eaten in North America, such as pork rinds, would be considered repulsive in some other cultures. Snails and eel, for instance, are considered delicacies by some people but inedible by others.

In the United States and Canada, industrialized countries peopled with immigrants, few foods are generally considered profane. But among specific religious groups, some examples of sacred and profane foods are quite familiar. Many Jews will not eat pork, whereas many Catholics will not eat meat on Fridays. Apart from religious-based sanctions, many people are vegetarians, while other groups eschew highly processed foods.

In our culture, food is classified into four main groups—dairy, grains, meat, and fruits and vegetables. Many people regard food in terms of its use by the body—protein, fat, and starch and carbohydrates. We live in a culture strongly influenced by science, and the biochemistry of food is part of our general fund of knowledge. The staples in the diets of a great many North Americans are meat and potatoes, something sweet for dessert, salads, soups, and fruit juices, all reflecting the conception of a healthy diet as one containing a balance of the food groups widely recognized and accepted as healthy. In other cultures, standard dishes might include pastas or rice, sausage, or bread.

Medicinal qualities are ascribed to various foods, rightly or wrongly, across the world. North Americans have their own widely shared beliefs associating food with medicine. Apples keep doctors away. Honey and lemon help reduce congestion. Fish is brain food. Citrus fruits protect one from colds. Oats unclog arteries.

Finally, all cultures tend to associate foods with social occasions unique to their cultures. There are occasions that seem to demand wine and occasions that seem to demand hot chocolate. Certain foods are eaten at baseball games, while other foods are eaten as family traditions on various holidays.

Other cultures are no different from the dominant culture in these broad aspects of food. Only the foods that carry strong cultural preferences or taboos vary from one culture to another.

Socioeconomic Status

Virtually all cultures are stratified. That is, they contain the range of socioeconomic classes. When members of a cultural group can be called a minority group, however, which is defined as a group receiving unequal treatment from the dominant group, socioeconomic characteristics can have implications for health and health care.

Public health research shows that people in lower socioeconomic groups have the highest rates of death and disease resulting from virtually every health problem. Thus, although it is incorrect to speak of "a culture of poverty," it is true that socioeconomic status is an important predictor of health and disease. Because of the way health care systems are structured, particularly in the United States, people in poverty make less use of the health care system, and their choice of providers, as well as their criterion for seeking health care, is different from the frequency and criterion associated with more affluent citizens. Therefore, an awareness of a client's economic status has implications for care.

Pain

Pain is among the most common symptoms found in clinical practice, yet it is not purely a neurophysiologic response. Pain is influenced by social, psychological, and cultural factors.

Culture influences both pain intensity and pain tolerance. Culture determines a person's attitudes toward pain and beliefs about it. Emotions associated with the context in which pain is experienced can have a powerful effect on how pain is felt. There are cases where soldiers are wounded in battle and do not realize it until afterward. In some cultures, meditation or religious trances dissipate the sensation of pain, such as the firewalkers of Sri Lanka, who are apparently oblivious to the expected intensity of the pain they experience. Other cultures value the ability to withstand pain without complaint or physical manifestations, as in the case of certain American Indian and African tribes, who demonstrate their adulthood by withstanding painful stimuli.

It is difficult to separate the ability to withstand pain that is culturally determined from that mediated by neurologic mechanisms. Nurses often encounter the so-called placebo effect, in which an inactive drug relieves suffering. A simple *belief* in the effectiveness of the placebo can release endorphins in the brain, actually providing physiologic pain relief.

Culture also determines when pain is abnormal, requiring medical attention and treatment. The extent to which pain is considered a normal part of life also affects a person's willingness to withstand it. Studies show, for instance, that Polish women are for more able to accept the pain associated with childbirth than their American counterparts, who have greater access to anesthesia during labor.

Each culture has its own language of distress, which includes facial expressions, changes in activity, sounds, and words used to describe feeling. These norms determine acceptable ways pain is expressed to others. For example, Italian-Americans dramatize their pain as a means of allaying anxiety and dissipating the pain. Irish-Americans, by contrast, are more reticent about their bodily complaints.

Pain is a subjective sensation that has physiologic, cultural, and emotional components. The actual cause or intensity of pain is difficult to assess. In treating it, the nurse must remember that it is the client's experience of pain, as the client feels it, that determines how it must be treated. However, cultural considerations that affect a client's ability or willingness to report pain as a sign of illness, as well as inclination to seek treatment, must be carefully assessed because of these implications for the person's actual degree of illness.

Family

Attitudes toward family structure and family roles and relationships have been traditionally mediated by cultural considerations. However, over the past 20 years, cultural differences related to families, once a defining characteristic of different cultural groups, are rapidly being obliterated. Our society has become highly mobile and more integrated, tearing down barriers that once kept family norms intact within subcultures. The media have focused our attention on alternate family arrangements and practices, making them more familiar and thus acceptable.

Twenty years ago, the concept of the nuclear family was predominant. Typically, young men and women married someone who was raised within 25 miles of them. People married people with whom they shared cultural or group affiliations. Couples tended to share the same race, religion, and socioeconomic status. They had children, and the mother provided child care while the father earned the income. They tended to stay married for life, and they tried to transmit these values to their children. This, however, has proved a losing battle. Because of mass communication, easy access to cheap and fast transportation, and economic changes promoting urbanization, today's young people often move far away from their parents. More young people attend college and use this opportunity to migrate elsewhere. Far from the daily influences of their families, new group affiliations develop, based on common interests, education, and jobs. There has been an increased incidence and even acceptance of divorce, dual-income families, single-parent families, teenage parents, and involvement of fathers in

child care. The nuclear family is not nearly as prevalent now, and neither are culturally mediated family practices that used to distinguish one cultural group from another.

This is not to say that cultural differences in attitudes toward family structure and role no longer exist. Rather, they cannot be taken for granted. The nurse therefore cannot make any assumptions about the relationship between family and culture and must take a value-free approach to assessing family dimensions, which can be so important to one's health and well-being.

A neutral starting point in assessing the client's family is to determine the family structure. A simple family tree or family diagram, sometimes called a genogram, establishes who the members of the family are and how the client fits in. Since many individuals live so far apart from their natural families and often feel only a weak bond with them, it is often important to extend the genogram concept to a broader tool known as an ecogram. This tool maps the network of the client's significant others, including friends, neighbors, peers, and associates who may be more important to the client's health and well being than are actual family members.

Once the structure is clear, roles and relationships can be explored to determine whom the client is attached to and how the dynamics of various relationships work. Relationships, both within families and in broader associations, can be close or distant, dependent or hostile. In each relationship, the sharing of power and decision making, as well as approaches to problem solving, can vary widely. Communication patterns can be observed, and the willingness to express feelings and offer support can be assessed. Individuality may be submerged or fostered. Many tools exist to provide for an orderly assessment of these roles and functions. A familiar one is the Family APGAR (see the box on p. 666).

Despite the rapid obliteration of family structure and function neatly associated with distinct cultural groups, it is important to be aware that for many individuals, cultural considerations remain very important. Family practices associated with individual cultural groups are pointed out below as various cultural groups are discussed.

THE NORTH AMERICAN CULTURE

Significant cultural differences exist between the societies of Canada and the United States. These differences are very important to the citizens of both countries as they seek to maintain their unique national identities in the face of broader economic ties, mass communication, and more interaction. Canadians are very acutely aware of these differences because the population of Canada is approximately one tenth that of the United States, and the danger of assimilation by their more populous south-

---

Family APGAR

Definition

Adaptation is the use of intrafamilial and extrafamilial resources for problem-solving when family equilibrium is stressed during a crisis.

Partnership is the sharing of decision-making and nurturing responsibilities by family members.

Growth is the physical and emotional maturation and self-fulfillment that is achieved by family members through mutual support and guidance.

Affection is the caring or loving relationship that exists among family members.

Resolve is the commitment to devote time to other members of the family for physical and emotional nurturing. It also usually involves a decision to share wealth and space.

Functions measured by the Family APGAR

How resources are shared, or the degree to which a member is satisfied with the assistance received when family resources are needed.

How decisions are shared, or the member's satisfaction with mutuality in family communication and problem-solving.

How nurturing is shared, or the member's satisfaction with the freedom available within the family to change roles and attain physical and emotional growth or maturation.

How emotional experiences are shared, or the member's satisfaction with the intimacy and emotional interaction that exists in the family.

How time (and space and money) is shared, or the member's satisfaction with the time commitment that has been made to the family by its members.

Relevant open-ended questions

How have family members aided each other in time of need?

In what way have family members received help or assistance from friends and community agencies?

How do family members communicate with each other about such matters as vacations, finances, medical care, large purchases, and personal problems?

How have family members changed during the past years? How has this change been accepted by family members?

In what ways have family members aided each other in growing or developing independent life-styles?

How have family members reacted to your desires for change?

How have members of your family responded to emotional expressions such as affection, love, sorrow, or anger?

How do members of your family share time, space, and money?

Modified from Smilkstein G: The Family APGAR: a proposal for a family function test and its use by physicians, J Fam Pract 6:1231-1239, 1978.

---

ern neighbor as economic barriers disappear is real. Moreover, Canada is composed of two dominant cultural groups separated by language, geography, and politics, whereas differences in cultures in the United States are more diffuse.

Nevertheless, broadly speaking, the two nations share a common history, geography, economic system, language, religion, and ethnic origin, and it is possible to make some generalizations about elements of a shared culture. In fact, it is the tradition of individualism, shared by citizens of both Canada and the United States, that will help to preserve the national identity of each country even as social and economic differences recede.

North Americans share a unique heritage of pioneering frontier people, immigrants seeking freedom, economic opportunity, and self-determination. The work ethic, borrowed from the many Protestant groups but shared by North Americans of all religions, has fostered a continent of people who work hard, take responsibility for making their own way in the world, and survive in the face of hardship. The culture places a high value on resourcefulness and lowers barriers to social mobility. As a result, the citizens of North America are an optimistic people, adaptable to change, who believe that their children can inherit a society that is better than the one they were born into.

In recent years, North Americans have become less aggressively independent and have developed closer group associations. This trend reflects our greater mobility, the weakening of family ties, and our increasing social and economic interdependence.

Health Care in North America

North Americans place a high premium on their health. They pay a large percentage of their national wealth for health care, and in recent years they have devoted more energy and resources to preventive health care through proper diet, more exercise, and the avoidance of health hazards. Canadians spend about 7% of their gross national product on health care, and Americans spend about 9%. Both nations are highly stratified free-enterprise systems. Consequently, affluent people buy a great deal of health care, while those in the lower socioeconomic groups have far more restricted access to quality health care. Still, the federal governments of both countries devote upward of 40% of their budgets to health care–related costs.

Two common measures of national health are infant mortality and longevity. Although both countries rank very high in longevity, Canada and the United States rank only eighth and eighteenth, respectively, among the nations of the world in infant mortality. Although progress has been made in birth control, spread of infectious diseases, and better nutrition, both countries suffer from restricted access to wellness-oriented health care, inconsistent prenatal care, and a similar set of social problems. These social problems are more widespread in the United States, resulting in a much higher prevalence of very-low-birth-weight infants, accounting for the higher infant mortality in the United States.

ASSESSMENT CONSIDERATIONS FOR MAJOR CULTURAL GROUPS IN NORTH AMERICA
Chinese
General characteristics. North Americans of Chinese descent have played an important role in opening the western frontier of both Canada and the United States. As long as the political climate in China remains in turmoil, and in anticipation of the reversion of Hong Kong to the People's Republic of China in 1997, the immigration of Chinese people to North America will continue and accelerate. North Americans of Chinese descent are already well represented among health care professionals, and their influence on health care in North America will increase over the coming decade. More than most ethnic groups, they have maintained their unique cultural traditions and identity. Most major cities in North America include enclaves of Chinese people who maintain their language, traditional occupations, social ties, and cultural beliefs, including those related to health care.

Health beliefs. The Chinese believe in a holistic cultural paradigm or world view, in which health is an expression of balance, often referred to as yin and yang. Health is highly valued, as is the human body. Health is evidence of a good balance in relation to the environment, and one's body represents a gift from one's parents, a physical relationship with one's past and family, and the literal embodiment of cultural ties. Illness is thus seen as imbalance, and emphasis is placed on the role of blood and energy and their deficiencies in explaining disease.

Health practices. Since the Chinese conceive of recovery from illness as the restoration of balance, certain practices involving the application of heat to the skin or the careful mixture of hot and cold foods are common remedies for illness. The reliance on herbs reflects similar beliefs, and a spiritual component of recovery is stronger among the Chinese than among most groups. The use of acupuncture, although not well understood in the context of scientific Western medical knowledge, is a common modality, proved effective over centuries of practice. Nurses must guard against ethnocentric biases against acupuncture and regard it as part of the total treatment plan when it is used. Monosodium glutamate is a favorite condiment in the Chinese diet,

and its use should be assessed within the context of specific disorders and diet therapies.

Family assessment. Traditional Chinese families are patriarchal, and elders are respected members who play an important role. Extended families are common, so information developed from family members can be quite important during the assessment. In some cases, elders may even speak for younger clients, who often defer to their elders. The Chinese are reticent and seldom complain about their illnes or express emotions. Even children often act more like adults. During the assessment, it is important to observe the importance of roles played by family members and carefully explore symptoms. Unlike many groups, Chinese often express a lack of comprehension by smiling, so it is important to verify responses to questions.

Other considerations. The Chinese are genetically predisposed to alpha thalassemia and adult lactose intolerance. Perhaps in response to the frequency of lactose intolerance, Chinese children are often breast-fed for 4 or 5 years. The Chinese are rather sensitive to pain, although they may try to conceal their expression of it, and the use of acupuncture may be therapeutic. They are so respectful of their bodies that they may resist surgery or invasive techniques, and they may be squeamish about having blood taken. Religious Chinese often believe in reincarnation. Thus, they may resist invasive procedures. Their belief also alters their attitude toward death and dying, which is frequently seen as a natural, necessary, transitional phase of life. Many older Chinese associate hospitals with places to die and may resist hospitalization.

Japanese
General characteristics. The influence of the Japanese on our society has grown enormously in the years since World War II. They are an adaptive, practical people who have been able to integrate within the dominant culture, working in occupations that reflect all walks of life. Because of the rapid westernization of Japan after centuries of traditional, highly stratified and religious culture, the Japanese possess a complex mixture of eastern and western thought and sets of traits.

Health beliefs. Health beliefs can vary widely among North Americans of Japanese descent, depending on their degree of aculturation. Traditional Japanese may hold health beliefs influenced by Chinese and Korean beliefs in balance and harmony. Those who believe in Shintoism regard disease as the result of evil outside influences, perhaps manifested by contact with impure substances. However, more aculturated Japanese subscribe to the dominant western scientific theory of health and illness.

Health practices.   Like the Chinese, many Japanese practice acupuncture, herbal cures, and use of hot and cold food and compresses to restore the balance characteristic of good health. Unlike the Chinese, Japanese will readily consent to the removal of a diseased part. Their pragmatism manifests itself in good preventive health care, and the health of Japanese children is a source of great pride to Japanese parents.

Family assessment.   The bond of family is quite strong among the Japanese. Although gregarious people, they tend to keep problems within the family unit. Japanese children are often indulged and encouraged to act like children until they reach school age, at which time a very high value is placed on achievement and self-control. It is not uncommon, for instance, for a Japanese child who is ill to be sent to school anyway, so important is education in the lives of the Japanese. Elders are venerated, and Japanese families regard care for older family members as a point of family responsibility and honor.

Other considerations.   Japanese whose native language is not English are eager to learn it. Still, older people and recent immigrants who cannot speak or write English well can often read and understand it very well. Like the Chinese, the Japanese are reserved and may not express discomfort, making accurate pain assessment important. Although the Japanese are patient people, they are also acutely aware of time and regard it as a precious resource not to be wasted. Consequently, they can be expected to be punctual for appointments and economical in their use of time.

Vietnamese

General characteristics.   The most recent wave of immigrants to North America, the Vietnamese share with most other groups of new immigrants the characteristics of industry, strong family bonds, and the formation of ethnic communities. Although most Vietnamese are becoming successful through hard work, many have experienced extreme culture shock. The language barrier is significant. The transition from a rural agrarian society to a western urban life-style has been difficult. Many Vietnamese have experienced extreme hardship, losses, and privation. They are not yet well integrated into the mainstream of society, and some have been subjected to discrimination.

Health beliefs.   Coming from a society imbued with a combination of animism and Buddhism, the Vietnamese share with the Chinese a holistic world view in which health is regarded as a balance between yin and yang. There is an element of fatalism and predestination in their world view that sometimes leads them to accept disease without seeking health care. By the same token,

good health is often seen as the result of the accumulation of good deeds performed by one's ancestors.

Health practices.   The Vietnamese have shown themselves reluctant, in general, to seek health care. Disease, when it occurs, seems inevitable. Often, the period of illness is simply waited out without intervention as something to be endured. The family accepts responsibility for caring for a sick relative, and a spiritualist, such as a fortune teller or priest, is often preferred over a physician. Certain diets are often used to treat disease.

Family assessment.   For the Vietnamese, the individual is less important than the family. Males have more status than females, elders are respected, and children, who are highly prized, are taught to be obedient. Several generations of a family typically live together, and the family may be the only social network a person has.

Other considerations.   The language barrier is a serious obstacle for most Vietnamese, many of whom are very recent immigrants. Besides being unable to ask questions of the nurse performing the assessment, the Vietnamese may view asking questions as disrespectful. Since they may be distrustful of the health care provider, and since their reluctance to seek medical help often means that a serious illness has developed, the communication problems are serious and must be overcome. The Vietnamese are a polite people who may avoid eye contact out of deference and may seek to avoid conflict or disagreement. They may be indirect in expressing their feelings, since they do not express emotions easily. In addition to propriety, their status is important to them. A relaxed view of time may cause them to be late or early for appointments. Because of the extreme stress many Vietnamese have undergone and continue to experience, assessing for depression is especially important.

Blacks

General characteristics.   Because of the rapid assimilation of blacks into the middle class, many sociologists are predicting the emergence of two distinct classes of blacks in North America. Blacks who have been able to take advantage of the opportunities now open to them, after years of discrimination and privation, have been able to leave segregated inner-city neighborhoods, taking with them the commerce, churches, and professional services that once provided the lifeblood of these communities, and leaving behind an "underclass" of blacks in desperate poverty, subjected to continuing discrimination, crime, and lack of economic opportunity. This has resulted not only in a worsening situation for the blacks left out of the mainstream of society but also caused considerable distress for middle-class blacks, whose exodus has contributed inadvertently to the further deterioration of inner-city black neighborhoods. Although our society is gradually becoming more integrated, especially in schools and workplaces, housing patterns have remained pointedly segregated, even among middle-class blacks. Discrimination in housing still exists, but a strong cultural bond has drawn many economically successful blacks together in more affluent communities where elements of black culture have been carefully transplanted.

Health beliefs. The bifurcation of black society has led to a divergence in health beliefs. As blacks are integrated into the dominant culture, differences in health beliefs begin to disappear. However, traditional beliefs are still common. Most notably, there is a persistent belief that serious diseases can be avoided, a sense of denial that often results in postponing medical attention. Many traditional blacks believe in evil influences, such as witchcraft or voodoo, beliefs especially prevalent among ethnic blacks from the Caribbean and African countries. Fundamentalist blacks may ascribe disease to the will of God.

Health practices. Traditional blacks may use folk remedies or consult spiritualists. Spiritualists may include a figure called an "old lady," who often prescribes herbal treatments, or a "root doctor," who prescribes similar treatments. The black minister is traditionally a respected figure in the community, and he may be consulted on health matters. Prayer is commonly used, and home remedies are traditions in many families. Blacks frequently postpone medical evaluation. This is commonly related to the feeling that serious illness can be avoided, but it also has as much to do with the restricted access to health care that many poor blacks must endure.

Family assessment. Although family relationships can take many different forms, with different groups of relatives living with one another and many instances of single parent and stepfamilies, blacks place a high value on family. This loyalty to family manifests itself in ambition and a belief in hard work for the good of the group.

Other considerations. Since many blacks deny health problems until they are too serious to be denied, a careful assessment is often required. Blacks also typically fail to seek health care either because they are poor and cannot afford it or else they have been treated callously during past visits and thus are reluctant to subject themselves to further insensitivity. Blacks expect to be treated with dignity and respect and may insist on this more than other groups. Because of their long history of discrimination, they may be suspicious of health care providers and alert for any signs of discrimination. Blacks

may even "test" health care workers to satisfy themselves that they will be treated fairly. Take a direct, open approach. Be alert for diseases and disorders seen more frequently in blacks, including sickle cell anemia, plumbism, and hypertension. Be ready to develop strategies to help the client overcome any degree of denial he or she may be experiencing.

Hispanics

General characteristics. Hispanic is a term used to include Spanish-speaking residents of the United States and Canada whose national origin is Mexican, Central or South American, or Puerto Rican. It subsumes the terms Mexican-American, Latino, Chicano, or Raza-Latino. Hispanics occupy all socioeconomic strata, but many live in poverty as migrant workers or inner-city residents.

Health beliefs. Many Hispanics are religious, with Catholicism the dominant religion. Their health beliefs have strong magicoreligious overtones. Illness may be conceived of as a punishment from God in the form of supernatural forces. There is also an element of imbalances involving heat and cold or wet and dry. Conversely, health is viewed as a gift from God for good behavior and as a balance among good diet, hard work, and prayer. The wearing of religious medals, amulets, and relics is common as a means of practicing health.

Health practices. Like many cultural groups, Hispanics often turn to alternate health care providers, including healers called Curandero or Curandera, who use herb and folk remedies. Often rituals, prayers, and visits to shrines are performed, and the regular health care system may be used only as a last resort.

Family assessment. Families are male dominated, with women and children serving subservient roles. Family life is home centered with strong family attachments. Frequently, the entire family goes as a group on household errands. Children are viewed as gifts of God and highly prized.

Other considerations. Language is sometimes a barrier, although most Hispanics speak at least some English, and there is usually a family member who can translate for a non-English-speaking client. Family issues are kept private, and discussion among family members in the presence of a nurse may be held in Spanish. Hispanics are modest and prize privacy. They may be reluctant to disrobe for an examination, and their modesty may even contribute to their failure to seek medical care. Hispanics have a relaxed concept of time and may be late for appointments. Many are fearful of hospitals and regard them as a place to die.

Health History
Culture

Self-assessment questions (Questions the nurse should answer)

How do I feel toward people of cultural groups different from my own?

What are my attitudes toward poor people?

How do I feel and react when I cannot understand my client's language?

How accepting am I of different life-styles, health practices, diets, family relationships, and beliefs?

How well do I listen?

General questions

Age? (What year were you born?)

What do you consider your race?

In what country were you born? If born in another country, when did you come here? If born in this country, in what country were your parents born?

What language(s) do you speak? If more than one, what is your primary language, and what do you speak at home? Do you need an interpreter to understand my questions?

Do you work? If so, doing what? How many hours? What is your level of income? Do you have any supplemental income? If you do not work, where do you get money? If you get money from another person, what is your relationship with that person?

What leisure and recreational activities do you pursue?

Are you taking any medications?

Health beliefs

What is your religion?

Do you believe God has an influence on your health?

Do you believe that religious practices can influence your state of health?

Do you use prayer or meditation to try to influence your health?

What do you think causes illnesses?

Can you identify anything in your environment that may influence your health?

What do you do when you feel sick? Who do you go to? Do you do anything to treat yourself?

What is the best thing about being sick? (Try to determine secondary gains, if any.)

What is your attitude toward the health care system?

How do you think I can help you?

Health behaviors

Have you ever been hospitalized?

What practices do you use to maintain your health?

What kinds of food do you eat?

Do you smoke?

Do you wear seat belts?

Do you use any drugs?

Do you drink alcohol? If so, what kind, how much, and how often?

What would you do to feel better about yourself? Lose or gain weight? Change specific behavior? Get or change jobs? Spend more or less time on certain activities?

What do you do to reduce stress?

Have you ever hit anyone or used violence?

Have you ever been a victim of violence, abuse, or neglect?

Who takes care of you at home when you are sick?

Family assessment

Are you married? If so, for how long?

Who lives at your house, and what is your relationship to them?

Do you have any children? If so, what are their ages and genders?

What other relatives are you close to?

What is your role in your family?

Whom are you closest to in your family?

How important is your family in your life?

Native Americans

General characteristics. There are well over 100 tribes of Native Americans living in the United States and Canada, so generalizations are difficult to make. It would be useful for the nurse to ask clients about the beliefs and practices unique to the particular group. Nevertheless, a large percentage of Native Americans live on reservations, and poverty, joblessness, alcoholism, and poor health care practices are characteristic of many such people.

Health beliefs. Theology, medicine, and health are strongly interrelated concepts in all tribes. Illness is believed to have a supernatural component and is often viewed as a punishment for violating a taboo or offending God. Consequently, many rituals are performed to safeguard health. Fear of witchcraft or malevolent gods and forces, believed to cause disease, is common.

Health practices. Native Americans may be reluctant to make use of the established health care system, preferring instead to consult tribal medicine men. Such figures may be seen simply as altruistic and wise or as magical. Some are seen as having the power to cure, while others are seen as only having the power to diagnose. Many of those believed invested with magical powers are seen as capable of inflicting harm as well as providing cures.

Family assessment. Elders are accorded more respect than they are by most other cultural groups. Extended families are common.

Other considerations. The concept of time is very present oriented, so appointments may be a concept alien to many. Hospitals are seen as places to go in cases of disease, and they may not be used for prenatal care or preventive purposes. High accident rates and health problems related to alcohol abuse, depression, and obesity are common.

BIBLIOGRAPHY

American Nurses Association: Cultural diversity in the nursing curriculum: a guide for implementation (ANA #G-171:11), Kansas City, American Nurses Association, 1986.

American Nurses Association: Nursing: a social policy statement, Kansas City, American Nurses Association, 1980.

Boyle JS and Andrews MM: Transcultural concepts in nursing care, Boston, Little, Brown & Co, 1989.

Bureau of the Census: General population characteristics. I. United States summary, 1980 census of population, vol 1, Washington, DC, US Government Printing Office.

Char EL: The Chinese American. In Clark AL, editor: Culture and childrearing, Philadelphia, 1981, FA Davis Co.

Chen-Louie T: Nursing care of Chinese American patients. In Orque MS, Bloch B, and Monrroy LSA: Ethnic nursing care, St Louis, 1983, The CV Mosby Co.

Chow E: Cultural health traditions: Asian perspectives. In Branch MF and Paxton PP, editors: Providing safe nursing care for ethnic people of color, New York, 1976, Appleton-Century-Crofts.

Clark M: Community nursing: health care for today and tomorrow, Reston, VA, Reston Publishing Co.

Ehling MB: The Mexican American (El Chicano). In Clark AL, editor: Culture and childrearing, Philadelphia, 1981, FA Davis Co.

Greathouse B and Miller VG: The black American. In Clark AL, editor: Culture and childrearing, Philadelphia, 1981, FA Davis Co.

Halleran C: Nursing beyond national boundaries: the 21st century, Nurse Outlook 36:72-74, 1988.

Hanlon JJ and Pickett GT: Public health: administration and practice, ed 8, St Louis, 1984, The CV Mosby Co.

Hartog J and Hartog EA: Cultural aspects of health and illness behavior in hospitals, West J Med 139:911-916, 1983.

Hashizume and Takano: Nursing care of Japanese American patients. In Oroque MS, Bloch B, and Monrroy LSA, editors: Ethnic nursing care, a multicultural approach, St Louis, 1983, The CV Mosby Co.

Hautman MA: Folk health and illness beliefs, Nurse Pract 4:4, 1979.

Health Resources and Service Administration: Health status of minorities and low income groups, DHHS pub. no. HRS-P-DV 85-1, Washington, DC, 1985, US Government Printing Office.

Healthy people: the Surgeon General's report on health promotion and disease prevention. HEW no. 79-55071, Washington, DC, 1979, US Public Health Service.

Heckler M: Report of the secretary's task force on black and minority health, vols I to VIII, DHHS, Washington, DC, 1985, US Government Printing Office.

Helman C: Culture, health and illness, London, 1984, John Wright and Sons.

Henderson G and Primeaux M: Transcultural health care, Menlo Park, CA, 1981, Addison-Wesley.

Holland WR: Mexican American medical beliefs: science or magic? In Martinez RA, editor: Hispanic culture and health care, St Louis, 1978, The CV Mosby Co.

Holland S and Sweeney E: Vietnamese children and families: the impact of culture, Washington, DC, 1985, Association for Care of Children's Health.

Hollingsworth AO, Brown LP, and Brooten DA: The refugees and childbearing: what to expect, RN 43:45-48, 1980.

Jacques G: Cultural traditions: a black perspective. In Branch MF and Paxton PP: Providing safe nursing care for ethnic people of color, New York, 1976, Appleton-Century-Crofts.

Joe V: A new lifestyle in a new land, Can Nurse 7:6-10, 1981.

Kileumura A and Kitano H: Interracial marriage: a picture of the Japanese Americans, J Soc Issues 29:67-81, 1973.

Kleinman A, Eisenberg L, and Good B: Clinical lessons from anthropologic and cross cultural research, Ann Intern Med 88:251-258, 1978.

Kleinman A, Eisenberg L, and Good B: Culture, illness and care: clinical lessons from anthropologic and cross-cultural research. Ann Intern Med 88:251-258, 1976.

Klucklhohn F: Dominant and variant value orientations. In Brink PJ, editor: Transcultural nursing: a book of readings, Englewood Cliffs, NJ, 1976, Prentice-Hall.

Kwok AWH: Culture conflict: a study of the problems of Chinese immigrant adolescents in Canada, Can Nurs 78:32-34, 1982.

Lacay G: The Puerto Rican in mainland America. In Clark AL, editor: Culture and childrearing, Philadelphia, 1981, FA Davis Co.

Landy D: Medical systems in transcultural perspective. In Landy D, editor: Culture, disease, and healing: studies in medical anthropology, New York, 1977, Macmillan Co.

Leininger MM: Qualitative research methods in nursing, New York, 1985, Grune & Stratton.

Leininger MM: Transcultural nursing: concepts, theories and practices, New York, 1978, John Wiley & Sons.

Lewis G: Cultural influences on illness behavior, a medical anthropological approach. In Eisenberg L and Kleinman A, editors: The relevance of social science for medicine, Dordrecht, 1981, Reidel.

Logan MH: Selected references on the hot-cold theory of disease, Med Anthropol News 6:8-14, 1975.

Lopez-Bushnell FKL: Broken prenatal appointments among Spanish speaking women, unpublished master's thesis, New Haven, 1972, Yale University.

Noble GP: Social considerations in northern health care, Can Nurs 74:16, 18, 1978.

Orque MS, Bloch B, and Monrroy LSA: Ethnic nursing care, a multicultural approach, St Louis, 1983, The CV Mosby Co.

Overfield T: Biological variation: concepts from physical anthropology. In Henderson G and Primeaux M, editors: Transcultural health care, Menlo Park, CA, 1981, Addison-Wesley.

Pender NJ: Health promotion in nursing practice, Norwalk, CT, 1987, Appleton-Lang.

Rubel J: The epidemiology of folk illness: susto in Hispanic America. In Sandy D, editor: Culture, disease and healing: studies in medical anthropology, New York, 1977, Macmillan Co.

Smith LS: Ethnic differences in knowledge of sexually transmitted diseases in North American Black and Mexican-American migrant farmworkers, Res Nurs Health 11:51-58, 1988.

Snow LF: Folk medical beliefs and their implications for the care of patients: a review based on studies of black Americans. In Henderson G and Primeaux M, editors: Transcultural health care, Menlo Park, CA, 1974, Addison-Wesley.

Snow LF and Johnson SM: Folklore, food, female reproductive cycle, Ecol Food Nut 7:41-49, 1978.

Sodetani-Shibata AE: The Japanese American. In Clark AL, editor: Culture and childrearing, Philadelphia, 1981, FA Davis Co.

Spector R: Sociocultural influences on children's health. In Scipien G, Barnard M, Chard M, et al, Comprehensive pediatric nursing, ed 3, New York, 1986, McGraw-Hill.

Syme SL: Social determinants of disease, Ann Clin Res 19:44-52, 1987.

Thierderman SB: Ethnocentrism: a barrier to effective health care, Nurse Prac 11:53-59, 1986.

Zbrowoski: Cultural components in response to pain, Sociol Issues 8:16-30, 1952.

Zola IK: Culture and symptoms: an analysis of patients presenting complaints, Am Sociol Rev 31:615-630, 1966.

chapter

27

Functional assessment

OBJECTIVES

Upon successful review of this chapter, learners will be able to:

- Describe rationale for including functional data in health assessment

- Define terms, variables, and parameters used for functional assessment

- Contrast pros and cons of various functional assessment tools

- Recognize uses of the following functional assessment tools
    Katz ADL Index
    PULSES Profile
    Barthel Index
    Instrumental ADL Scale
    Physical Self-Maintenance Scale (PSMS)
    Functional Activities Questionnaire (FAQ)
    Rapid Disability Rating Scale
    Functional Status Rating System
    Functional Independence Measure (FIM) and FIM Expanded
- Recognize sources of additional functional assessment tools

RATIONALE FOR INCLUDING FUNCTIONAL ASSESSMENT IN A COMPREHENSIVE OR FOCUSED HEALTH ASSESSMENT

The various components of the physical examination and health history provide some indication of the health of an individual's body systems and data about the relationship of the individual with the environment, defined broadly. For most clients, the data also implicitly provide information about the individual's self-care and overall functional abilities. For special populations, specifically the elderly and handicapped, the traditional components of the health assessment may be insufficient in providing adequate information regarding the client's capability and actual performance, i.e., a functional assessment. This chapter presents and discusses several approaches to measure functional assessment and guidelines to incorporate a functional assessment into the routine health assessment.

In practice with a given client group, a practitioner may choose to use standardized tools for all clients or to integrate functional assessment questions and techniques into the routine health assessment as needed. Advantages as well as disadvantages are noted with either method. Because standardized tools are devised to yield comparable numerical scores, they are useful in situations where information must be summarized for communication across systems and providers or when patient, program, or other outcome evaluation is desired for general planning or discharge planning purposes for individuals or client groups. However, standardized tools are often not fully applicable across all elderly and handicapped groups and may include items not relevant for specific clients or client groups.

Functional assessment parameters, chosen for individual clients, can be integrated into the client's health assessment. Such integration can be effective if the approach to the health history and physical examination is highly individualized and there is sufficient time to add items. However, the difficulty in obtaining reliable data in vulnerable populations may serve to foster neglect in obtaining functional assessment information that could influence choice and scope of intervention.

Pinholt and colleagues (1987) compared the sensitivity and specificity of routine assessments and comprehensive functional assessment instruments. They found that physicians and nurses could identify severe impairments with routine approaches, but more prevalent and less prominent impairments were poorly recognized. The authors recommended the use of functional assessment instruments to detect moderate impairments, especially those remediable through early intervention.

DEFINITIONS AND ORIENTATION TO KEY TERMS

Several conceptual definitions are useful in reading this chapter and other literature in the area of functional assessment. The following definitions have been developed by the World Health Organization (WHO) (1980) to standardize terminology and facilitate communication in this area:

Impairment: An impairment is any loss or abnormality of psychological, physiological, or anatomical structure or function. An impairment is independent of its etiology and does not necessarily mean that a disease is still present. An example of an impairment is loss of a limb.
Disability: A disability is any restriction or lack of ability to perform an activity in the manner or within the range considered normal for a person of the same age and similar circumstances. A disability may be temporary or permanent and can occur in any component of human functioning. Different impairments may result in similar disabilities, and the same impairments do not necessarily result in similar disabilities. Not all impairments result in disability. An example of a disability is inability to climb stairs.
Handicap: A handicap is a disadvantage for a given individual, resulting from an impairment or a disability, that limits or prevents the fulfillment of a role that is normal for that individual. A handicap is characterized by a difference between what an individual appears to be able to do and the expectations of the particular group of which he is a member. The state of being handicapped is strongly influenced by existing societal values.
Functional Status: Functional status refers to the normal or characteristic performance of the individual. Functional status can be conceptualized into four categories:

Physical function: sensory-motor performance.
Mental function: intellectual, cognitive, or reasoning capabilities of the individual.
Emotional function: affect and effectiveness in coping psychologically with life stresses.
Social function: performance of social roles or obligations.

The following additional definitions are derived from legislative practice (NH Rev Stat Ann §§ 464-A:2 [VII], [XI] [1983]. Cited in Nolan, 1984, p. 213):

Incapacity means a legal, not a medical, disability and shall be measured by functional limitations. It shall be construed to mean or refer to any person who has suffered, is suffering, or is likely to suffer substantial harm due to an inability to provide for his personal needs for food, clothing, shelter, health care or safety or an inability to manage his or her property or financial affairs.
Functional limitations means behavior or conditions in an individual which impair his or her ability to participate in and perform minimal activities of daily living that secure and maintain proper food, clothing, shelter, health care or safety for himself or herself.

The following models by Granger and colleagues (1987), based on the work of Nagi (1975) and of Wood (1975), provide insight into the relationships among disease, impairment, and handicap.

Nagi Model
Pathologic condition → Impairment → Functional limitations → Disability

Wood Model
Disease or
disorder →   Impairment →   Disability →   Handicap
(Intrinsic) → (Exteriorized) → (Objectified) → (Socialized)

FUNCTIONAL ASSESSMENT VARIABLES

Functional assessment tools include measurement of various types of variables. Most tools contain some combination of self-care and mobility items and, occasionally, other variables. The following is a list of general categories of activities measured in functional assessment tools:

Self-Care

Basic Activities of Daily Living (ADL)
Grooming and personal hygiene
Skin care management
Bathing
Dressing and undressing
Managing brace or prosthesis
Toileting
Eating and feeding

Instrumental Activities of Daily Living (IADL)
Personal financial management
Managing business affairs
Shopping
Cooking
Preparing balanced meals
Problem-solving skills
Managing medications

Mobility

Capability of upper and lower extremities
Body movement
Bed activities: turning, sitting, shifting
Transfer: between bed and wheelchair, wheelchair and chair, chair and toilet
Wheelchair skills
Walking on level surface
Ascending and descending stairs
Travel

Other Functional-Related Issues

Medical condition
Amount of medical supervision needed
Continence—bowels and bladder
Speech

Communication
Reading
Auditory comprehension
Language expression (verbal)
Language expression (gestural)
Writing (motor)
Written language expression

Senses
Hearing
Vision

Mental capability
Orientation
Understanding
Communication
Reading
Writing
Attention span
Memory
Judgment and reasoning
Ability to play games and work on hobbies
Awareness of current events
Ability to comprehend movies and books
Memory of appointments and commemorations
Ability to manage travel instructions

Resources
Significant others
Social support
Social interaction

Behavior problems
Presence of emotional or psychiatric disorders
Amount of supervision required
Cooperation
Depression

The practitioner interested in measuring functional assessment through integration into the basic history and physical examination could choose a set of areas for exploration from the above list and devise appropriate questions to obtain the information as indicated and appropriate.

The practitioner choosing to use a standardized tool for a given population should first determine the

variables of primary interest and then match those variables with items on extant tools. The practitioner examining potential screening and assessment tools should not only examine the content of the items but also the scope of measurement, i.e., to determine if certain functional disability exists only or the extent to which the functions are enabled through human or mechanical assistance also. Desirable characteristics of a functional assessment tool include the following:

1. *Applicability:* appropriate for the client population.
2. *Continuity:* applicable to client population across phases of treatment.
3. *Ease in administration:* ability to be administered by various health care professionals.
4. *Efficiency:* balance between comprehensiveness and time required for administration.
5. *Reliability:* demonstration of good test-retest and interrater reliability.
6. *Validity:* findings consistent with other assessment data.
7. *Sensitivity:* ability to differentiate among clients and a given client during various stages of treatment.

Numerous tools have been developed to measure functional status. Only a subset of extant tools are presented in this chapter. Tools presented in this chapter were selected on the basis of their perceived applicability to a health assessment framework. Criteria for selection include length of the tool, broad applicability to the elderly or the handicapped, ability to complement the usual components of a history and physical examination, ease of administration, and published data about the tool's conceptual bases, validity, reliability, usability, and quality.

ISSUES RELATED TO THE ADMINISTRATION OF TOOLS

The functional assessment tools in this chapter are generally designed to be administered by health care professionals. Sometimes the care provider may wish the client or client caregiver to self-administer the tools, for example, after hospital discharge and between clinic visits. However, findings from various studies, comparing client self-report with professional and caregiver assessments, indicate that type of rater may influence scores. McGinnis and others (1986) compared the use of a modified Barthel Index by clients and health care professionals. Findings indicated that assessments were significantly different between groups, with providers rating clients higher in abilities at a time immediately before discharge.

Rubenstein and others (1984) compared the ratings of hospitalized elderly by various groups using three instruments: the Lawton Personal Self-Maintenance Scale

(PSMS), the Instrumental Activities of Daily Living Scale (IADL), and the Katz Activities of Daily Living Scale (ADL). Comparisons of ratings by the clients themselves, the clients' nurses, and clients' significant others revealed that the PSMS scores by clients were significantly higher than those of significant others, that the clients' IADL scores were significantly higher than scores by the nurses and the significant others, and that client scores for the ADL were significantly higher than the nurses' scores. The authors concluded that clients may tend to overestimate their abilities and that significant others may underestimate clients' functional abilities compared with professional nursing assessments.

Another issue regarding functional assessment is the relative reliability of various forms of client self-report. Spiegel and associates (1985) observed that clients with arthritis are more willing to admit difficulties with self-care activities in a self-administered questionnaire than in a personal interview.

PREPARATION FOR THE FUNCTIONAL ASSESSMENT

The functional assessment can be done at any time during the routine health assessment. However, it is probably most logically done at the end of the history and before the examination. Findings may provide guidance for particular follow-up during the physical examination.

No special equipment is needed for the functional assessment; most of the approaches require only interview and observation. However, the practitioner should be prepared to verify responses to various questions as needed. For example, the practitioner may ask the client to demonstrate operation of a wheelchair or ability to climb stairs.

SPECIFIC FUNCTIONAL ASSESSMENT TOOLS

This section of the chapter presents a number of standardized functional assessment tools that may be useful with populations commonly seen in ambulatory and long-term care settings. The tools were selected for their broad applicability to client groups, ease of administration, and fit within a comprehensive health assessment. Numerous other tools exist, and the reader is referred to McDowell and Newell (1987) or Rothstein (1985) for additional information about the tools presented in this chapter and for information about additional tools designed for special populations and for research applications.

Katz ADL Index (Revised Version 1976)

The original Katz ADL (activities of daily living) tool was among the earliest tools to standardize the assessment of functional assessment. Both the original and revised

versions focus on several basic activities of daily living and are very easy to administer and score (Katz and associates, 1963; Katz and Akpom, 1976). The revised version of the Katz ADL Index (see the box on p. 677) measures self-care and mobility, specifically the following activities:

- Bathing
- Dressing
- Toileting
- Transfer
- Continence
- Feeding

Each activity is rated as 1 or 0, 1 indicating performance of the activity without human help and 0 indicating performance of the activity with human assistance or that the activity is not performed at all. The scores form an ordinal or Guttman scale as noted on the top portion of the ADL box on p. 677.

The original Katz tool has been adapted for scoring by a Likert-type scale, using a scale range of 0 to 3 (0, complete independence; 1, use of a devise; 2, use of human assistance; 3, complete dependence). There is no category for clients who use both a devise and human assistance. The scores are added to obtain an overall score. A community-based version of the Katz adds items of walking and grooming but excludes continence.

The reliability and validity of the tool have been evaluated and have been judged as good (Brorsson and Asberg, 1984).

The Katz tool is a general measure of self-care and a very limited measure of mobility and is probably most applicable with populations in which a level of disability is assumed or already established, e.g., individuals with chronic illnesses. It is short and very easy to administer; therefore, a version could be easily included on a printed history form. Its scoring approaches allow for comparison of a given individual over time or compilation across client groups.

PULSES Profile

The PULSES Profile, developed by Moskowitz and McCann (1957), was originally designed to assess the functional independence of chronically ill, elderly persons. The PULSES instrument (Table 27-1) measures impairment, and the title of the tool is an acronym for its assessment components:

P = Physical condition
U = Upper limb functioning
L = Lower limb functioning
S = Sensory components
E = Excretory function
S = Support factors

The Index of Independence in Activities of Daily Living: Scoring and Definitions

The index of Independence in Activities of Daily Living is based on an evaluation of the functional independence or dependence of patients in bathing, dressing, going to toilet, transferring, continence, and feeding. Specific definitions of functional independence and dependence appear below the index.

    A—Independent in feeding, continence, transferring, going to toilet, dressing and bathing.
    B—Independent in all but one of these functions.
    C—Independent in all but bathing and one additional function.
    D—Independent in all but bathing, dressing, and one additional function.
    E—Independent in all but bathing, dressing, going to toilet, and one additional function.
    F—Independent in all but bathing, dressing, going to toilet, transferring, and one additional function.
    G—Dependent in all six functions.
    Other—Dependent in at least two functions, but not classifiable as C, D, E, or F.

Independence means without supervision, direction, or active personal assistance, except as specifically noted below. This is based on actual status and not on ability. A patient who refuses to perform a function is considered as not performing the function, even though he is deemed able.

Bathing (sponge, shower or tub)

Independent: assistance only in bathing a single part (as back or disabled extremity) or bathes self completely
Dependent: assistance in bathing more than one part of body; assistance in getting in or out of tub or does not bathe self

Dressing

Independent: gets clothes from closets and drawers; puts on clothes, outer garments, braces; manages fasteners; act of tying shoes
    is excluded
Dependent: does not dress self or remains partly undressed

Going to toilet

Independent: gets to toilet; gets on and off toilet; arranges clothes; cleans organs of excretion; (may manage own bedpan used at
    night only and may or may not be using mechanical supports)
Dependent: uses bedpan or commode or receives assistance in getting to and using toilet

Transfer

Independent: moves in and out of bed independently and moves in and out of chair independently (may or may not be using
    mechanical supports)
Dependent: assistance in moving in or out of bed and/or chair; does not perform one or more transfers

Continence

Independent: urination and defecation entirely self-controlled
Dependent: partial or total incontinence in urination or defecation; partial or total control by enemas, catheters, or regulated use of
    urinals and/or bedpans

Feeding

Independent: gets food from plate or its equivalent into mouth; (precutting of meat and preparation of food, as buttering bread, are
    excluded from evaluation)
Dependent: assistance in act of feeding (see above); does not eat at all or parenteral feeding

Adapted from Katz S, Downs TD, Cash HR, and Grotz R: The index of independence in activities of daily living, progress in development of the index of ADL, Gerontologist, 10:23, 1970.

Each dimension is scored using an ordinal scale from 1 to 4, with 1 representing essential intactness and 4 representing total dependence. The six categories are equally weighted, and the scores are summed to produce a total score ranging from 6 to 24. Scores over 12 imply serious impairment, and scores over 16 usually reflect severe disability.

The reliability and validity evidence for the scale has been reviewed by several authors (McDowell and Newell, 1987; Jette, 1985) and has been assessed as acceptable.

The main limitations of the tool are the general focus on a broad array of categories and redundancy with items commonly measured in a routine history and physical examination. The instrument was designed for use in a rehabilitation setting and is probably most applicable

Table 27-1

The PULSES profile

	P **Physical condition** Cardiovascular pulmonary and other visceral disorders	**U** **Upper extremities** Shoulder girdles, cervical and upper dorsal spine	**L** **Lower extremities** Pelvis, lower dorsal and lumbosacral spine	**S** **Sensory function** Vision hearing speech	**E** **Excretory functions** Bowel and bladder	**S** **Social and mental status** Emotional and psychiatric disorders
NORMAL	1 Health maintenance	1 Complete function	1 Complete function	1 Complete function	1 Continent	1 Compatible with age
MILD	2 Occasional medical supervision	2 No assistance required	2 Fully ambulatory despite some loss of function	2 No appreciable functional impairment	2 Occasional stress incontinence or nocturia	2 No supervision required
MODERATELY SEVERE	3 Frequent medical supervision	3 Some assistance necessary	3 Limited ambulation	3 Appreciable bilateral loss or complete unilateral loss of vision or hearing. Incomplete aphasia	3 Periodic incontinence or retention	3 Some supervision necessary
SEVERE	4 Total care Bed or chair confined	4 Nursing care	4 Confined to wheelchair or bed	4 Total blindness Total deafness Global aphasia or aphonia	4 Total incontinence or retention (including catheter and colostomy)	4 Complete care in psychiatric facility

Adapted from McDowell I and Newell C: The presentation of the PULSES profile as published in Functional disability and handicap, *Measuring health: a guide to rating scales and questionnaires,* New York, 1987, Oxford University Press, pp 46-47.

P. *Physical* conditon including diseases of the viscera (cardiovascular, pulmonary, gastrointestinal, urologic, and endocrine) and cerebral disorders which are not enumerated in the lettered categories below.
   1. No gross abnormalities considering the age of the individual.
   2. Minor abnormalities not requiring frequent medical or nursing supervision.
   3. Moderately severe abnormalities requiring frequent medical or nursing supervision yet still permitting ambulation.
   4. Severe abnormalities requiring constant medical or nursing supervision confining individual to bed or wheelchair.
U. *Upper* extremities including shoulder girdle, cervical and upper dorsal spine.
   1. No gross abnormalities considering the age of the individual.
   2. Minor abnormalities with fairly good range of motion and function.
   3. Moderately severe abnormalities but permitting the performance of daily needs to a limited extent.
   4. Severe abnormalities requiring constant nursing care.
L. *Lower* extremities including the pelvis, lower dorsal and lumbosacral spine.
   1. No gross abnormalities considering the age of the individual.
   2. Minor abnormalities with a fairly good range of motion and function.
   3. Moderately severe abnormalities permitting limited ambulation.
   4. Severe abnormalities confining the individual to bed or wheelchair.
S. *Sensory* components relating to speech, vision, and hearing.
   1. No gross abnormalities considering the age of the individual.
   2. Minor deviations insufficient to cause any appreciable functional impairment.
   3. Moderate deviations sufficient to cause appreciable functional impairment.
   4. Severe deviations causing complete loss of hearing, vision or speech.
E. *Excretory* function, i.e., bowel and bladder control.
   1. Complete control.
   2. Occasional stress incontinence or nocturia.
   3. Periodic bowel and bladder incontinence or retention alternating with control.
   4. Total incontinence, either bowel or bladder.
S. *Mental and emotional status.*
   1. No deviations considering the age of the individual.
   2. Minor deviations in mood, temperament and personality not impairing environmental adjustment.
   3. Moderately severe variations requiring some supervision.
   4. Severe variations requiring complete supervision.

in situations where changes in levels of impairment are anticipated.

Barthel Index

The Barthel Index (BI) (Mahoney and Barthel, 1965; Granger, 1982) (Table 27-2) is a weighted index for assessing dependence in various items of self-care, mobility, and continence. The original scale contained 10 items that were scored with a weighted ratings of 15, 10, 5, or 0, depending on the amount of help needed to perform the function. Total scores range from 0 (total dependence) to 100 (total independence) and were intended to indicate the amount of assistance a client requires. A score of 60 indicates the threshold between independence and dependence; a score of 40 or below indicates severe dependence; and a score of 20 or below reflects total dependence in self-care and mobility.

The test-retest reliability and interrater agreements have been reported as 0.89% and 95%, respectively (Granger and associates, 1979).

The original BI was modified by Fortinsky and associates (1981) (Table 27-3). The modified BI contains 15 items and the following changes: two items of dressing (i.e., upper and lower body) rather than one general item;

Table 27-2

Original Barthel Index

	With help	Independent
1. Feeding (if food needs to be cut up = help)	5	10
2. Moving from wheelchair to bed and return (includes sitting up in bed)	5-10	15
3. Personal toilet (wash face, comb hair, shave, clean teeth)	0	5
4. Getting on and off toilet (handling clothes, wipe, flush)	5	10
5. Bathe self	0	5
6. Walking on level surface (or if unable to walk, propel a wheelchair)	10	15
	0[a]	5[a]
7. Ascend and descend stairs	5	10
8. Dressing (includes tying shoes, fastening fasteners)	5	10
9. Controlling bowels	5	10
10. Controlling bladder	5	10

From Mahoney FI and Barthel DW: Functional evaluation: the Barthel index, Maryland State Med J 14:61, 1965.
[a]Score only if unable to walk.

Instructions for scoring the Barthel Index (Note: A score of zero is given when the patient cannot meet the defined criterion):

1. Feeding
   10 = Independent. The patient can feed himself a meal from a tray or table when someone puts the food within his reach. He must put on an assistive device if this is needed, cut up the food, use salt and pepper, spread butter, etc. He must accomplish this in a reasonable time.
   5 = Some help is necessary (when cutting up food, etc., as listed above).

2. Moving from wheelchair to bed and return
   15 = Independent in all phases of this activity. Patient can safely approach the bed in his wheelchair, lock brakes, lift footrests, move safely to bed, lie down, come to a sitting position on the side of the bed, change the position of the wheelchair, if necessary, to transfer back into it safely, and return to the wheelchair.
   10 = Either some minimal help is needed in some step of this activity or the patient needs to be reminded or supervised for safety of one or more parts of this activity.
   5 = Patient can come to a sitting position without the help of a second person but needs to be lifted out of bed, or if he transfers with a great deal of help.

3. Doing personal toilet
   5 = Patient can wash hands and face, comb hair, clean teeth, and shave. He may use any kind of razor but must put in blade or plug in razor without help as well as get it from drawer or cabinet. Female patients must put on own make-up, if used, but need not braid or style hair.

4. Getting on and off toilet
   10 = Patient is able to get on and off toilet, fasten and unfasten clothes, prevent soiling of clothes, and use toilet paper without help. He may use a wall bar or other stable object of support if needed. If it is necessary to use a bed pan instead of a toilet, he must be able to place it on a chair, empty it, and clean it.
   5 = Patient needs help because of imbalance or in handling clothes or in using toilet paper.

5. Bathing self
   5 = Patient may use a bathtub, a shower, or take a complete sponge bath. He must be able to do all the steps involved in whichever method is employed without another person being present.

Continued

Instructions for scoring the Barthel Index—cont'd

6. Walking on a level surface

   15 = Patient can walk at least 50 yards without help or supervision. He may wear braces or prostheses and use crutches, canes, or a walkerette but not a rolling walker. He must be able to lock and unlock braces if used, assume the standing position and sit down, get the necessary mechanical aides into position for use, and dispose of them when he sits. (Putting on and taking off braces is scored under dressing.)

   10 = Patient needs help or supervision in any of the above but can walk at least 50 yards with a little help.

6a. Propelling a wheelchair

   5 = If a patient cannot ambulate but can propel a wheelchair independently. He must be able to go around corners, turn around, maneuver the chair to a table, bed, toilet, etc. He must be able to push a chair at least 50 yards. Do not score this item if the patient gets score for walking.

7. Ascending and descending stairs

   10 = Patient is able to go up and down a flight of stairs safely without help or supervision. He may and should use handrails, canes, or crutches when needed. He must be able to carry canes or crutches as he ascends or descends stairs.

   5 = Patient needs help with supervision of any one of the above items.

8. Dressing and undressing (Women need not be scored on use of a brassiere or girdle unless these are prescribed garments.)

   10 = Patient is able to put on and remove and fasten all clothing, and tie shoe laces (unless it is necessary to use adaptations for this). The activity includes putting on and removing and fastening corset or braces when these are prescribed. Such special clothing as suspenders, loafer shoes, dresses that open down the front may be used when necessary.

   5 = Patient needs help in putting on and removing or fastening any clothing. He must do at least half the work himself. He must accomplish this in a reasonable time.

9. Continence of bowels

   10 = Patient is able to control his bowels and have no accidents. He can use a suppository or take an enema when necessary (as for spinal cord injury patients who have had bowel training).

   5 = Patient needs help in using a suppository or taking an enema or has occasional accidents.

10. Controlling bladder

   10 = Patient is able to control his bladder day and night. Spinal cord injury patients who wear an external device and leg bag must put them on independently, clean and empty bag, and stay dry day and night.

   5 = Patient has occasional accidents or cannot wait for the bed pan or get to the toilet in time or needs help with an external device.

Table 27-3

Modified Barthel Index scoring

Independent		Dependent			Independent		Dependent		
I **Intact**	**II** **Limited**	**III** **Helper**	**IV** **Null**		**I** **Intact**	**II** **Limited**	**III** **Helper**	**IV** **Null**	
10	5	0	0	Drink from cup/feed from dish	15	15	7	0	Transfer, chair
5	5	3	0	Dress upper body	6	5	3	0	Transfer, toilet
5	5	2	0	Dress lower body	1	1	0	0	Transfer, tub or shower
0	0	−2		Don brace or prosthesis	15	15	10	0	Walk on level 50 yards or more
5	5	0	0	Grooming	10	10	5	0	Up and down stairs for one flight or more
4	4	0	0	Wash or bathe	15	5	0	0	Wheelchair/50 yards—only if not walking
10	10	5	0	Bladder continence					
10	10	5	0	Bowel continence					
4	4	2	0	Care of perineum/clothing at toilet					

Adapted from the presentation of the Modified Barthel Index in Fortinsky RH, Granger CV, and Seltzer GB: The use of functional assessment in understanding home care needs, Med Care 19:489, 1981.

addition of items for use (brace or prosthesis), transfer to toilet, transfer to tub or shower; and differentiation of the walking and wheelchair propelling items.

Advantages of the BI include its widespread use, the clarity of scoring, and completeness of the set of items.

Instrumental ADL Scale

The Instrumental ADL Scale (Lawton, 1972) (see the box on p. 681) measures behaviors that are more cognitively and less directly physically oriented than the other self-care scales. The tool has eight items measuring ability to use a telephone, shop, prepare food, keep

---

The Instrumental Activities of Daily Living Scale

A. Ability to use telephone
   1. Operates telephone on own initiative—looks up and dials numbers, etc.
   2. Dials well-known numbers.
   3. Answers telephone but does not dial.
   4. Does not use telephone at all.
B. Shopping
   1. Takes care of all shopping needs independently.
   2. Shops independently for small purchases.
   3. Must be accompanied on any shopping trip.
   4. Completely unable to shop.
C. Food preparation
   1. Plans, prepares, and serves adequate meals independently.
   2. Prepares adequate meals if supplied with ingredients.
   3. Heats and serves prepared meals, or prepares meals but does not maintain adequate diet.
   4. Needs to have meals prepared and served.
D. Housekeeping
   1. Maintains house alone or with occasional assistance.
   2. Performs light daily tasks such as dishwashing, bed-making.
   3. Performs light daily tasks but cannot maintain acceptable level of cleanliness.
   4. Needs help with all home maintenance tasks.
   5. Does not participate in any housekeeping tasks.
E. Laundry
   1. Does personal laundry completely.
   2. Launders small items—rinses socks, stockings, etc.
   3. All laundry must be done by others.

F. Mode of transportation
   1. Travels independently on public transportation or drives own car.
   2. Arranges own travel by taxi but does not otherwise use public transportation.
   3. Travels on public transportation when assisted or accompanied by another.
   4. Travel limited to taxi or automobile with assistance of another.
   5. Does not travel at all.
G. Responsibility for own medications
   1. Is responsible for taking medications in correct dosages at correct time.
   2. Takes responsibility if medications are prepared in advance in separate dosages.
   3. Is not capable of dispensing own medications.
H. Ability to handle finances
   1. Manages financial matters independently (budgets, write checks, pay rent, bills, go to bank), collect and keep track of income.
   2. Manages day-to-day purchases but needs help with banking, major purchases, etc.
   3. Incapable of handling money.

From Brody E and Lawton M Powell: Philadelphia Geriatric Center, 5301 Old York Road, Philadelphia, PA 19141.

---

house, do laundry, use public transportation, take responsibility for one's medications, and handle finances. Each item is scored on a 3-, 4-, or 5-point scale reflecting the amount of assistance used or limitation in performance of the activity.

The Instrumental ADL Scale expands the concept of self-care beyond specific and basic physical ability by measuring performance in the usual household maintenance activities. This scale could be used with community-based populations and individuals whose mobility is compromised or who are at risk of progressive debilitation, e.g., the frail elderly.

The Physical Self-Maintenance Scale

The Physical Self-Maintenance Scale (PSMS) (also known as the Lawton and Brody Scale, 1969) (see the box on p. 682) includes six items of self-care and mobility that are rated using an unique Guttman scale for each item. The six items are toileting (including continence), feeding, dressing, grooming, physical ambulation, and

bathing. Two scoring methods may be used: a count of the number of items for which disability is noted, or a severity scale summing the response codes for each item, resulting in a summary score ranging from 6 to 30.

This tool demonstrates good reliability and validity (McDowell and Newell, 1987). The scale is probably most applicable to homebound or institutionalized populations. It is easily and rapidly administered.

The Functional Activities Questionnaire

The Functional Activities Questionnaire (FAQ) (Pfeffer and associates, 1984) (see the box on pp. 683-684) is a screening tool for assessing independence in daily activities and was designed to measure universal skills among older adults. The FAQ is completed by the client's significant other and consists of ten items relating to tasks necessary for independent living. For each activity, four levels ranging from dependence (score = 3) to independence (score = 0) are rated. For activities not usually done by the client, the respondent specifies whether the

---

The Physical Self-Maintenance Scale

A. Toilet
  1. Cares for self at toilet completely, no incontinence.
  2. Needs to be reminded, or needs help in cleaning self, or has rare (weekly at most) accidents.
  3. Soiling or wetting while asleep more than once a week.
  4. Soiling or wetting while awake more than once a week.
  5. No control of bowels or bladder.

B. Feeding
  1. Eats without assistance.
  2. Eats with minor assistance at meal times and/or with special preparation of food, or help in cleaning up after meals.
  3. Feeds self with moderate assistance and is untidy.
  4. Requires extensive assistance for all meals.
  5. Does not feed self at all and resists efforts of others to feed him.

C. Dressing
  1. Dresses, undresses and selects clothes from own wardrobe.
  2. Dresses and undresses self, with minor assistance.
  3. Needs moderate assistance in dressing or selection of clothes.
  4. Needs major assistance in dressing but cooperates with efforts of others to help.
  5. Completely unable to dress self and resists efforts of others to help.

D. Grooming (neatness, hair, nails, hands, face, clothing)
  1. Always neatly dressed, well-groomed, without assistance.
  2. Grooms self adequately with occasional minor assistance, e.g., shaving.
  3. Needs moderate and regular assistance or supervision in grooming.
  4. Needs total grooming care, but can remain well-groomed after help from others.
  5. Actively negates all efforts of others to maintain grooming.

E. Physical Ambulation
  1. Goes about grounds or city.
  2. Ambulates within residence or about one block distant.
  3. Ambulates with assistance of (check one) a ( ) another person, b ( ) railing, c ( ) cane, d ( ) walker, e ( ) wheelchair.
      1 _____ Gets in and out without help.
      2 _____ Needs help in getting in and out.
  4. Sits unsupported in chair or wheelchair, but cannot propel self without help.
  5. Bedridden more than half the time.

F. Bathing
  1. Bathes self (tub, shower, sponge bath) without help.
  2. Bathes self with help in getting in and out of tub.
  3. Washes face and hands only, but cannot bathe rest of body.
  4. Does not wash self but is cooperative with those who bathe him.
  5. Does not try to wash self and resists efforts to keep him clean.

Adapted from the presentation of the Physical Self-Maintenance scale in Lawton MP and Brody EM. Assessment of older people: self-maintaining and instrumental activities of daily living, Gerontologist 9-180, 1969.

---

person would be unable to undertake the task if requested (score = 1). The total score is the sum of individual items, with higher scores reflecting greater dependency.

The authors of the FAQ are in the process of revising and testing a new version of this tool that includes the addition of four items on activities of daily living and one item on initiative.

The evidence regarding validity and reliability of the original tool has been reviewed by McDowell and Newell (1987), who concluded that the initial findings were very promising.

Linn Rapid Disability Rating Scale

The Rapid Disability Rating Scale-2 (Linn and Linn, 1982) (Table 27-4) is an 18-item global disability scale measuring assistance needed with activities of daily living, disability, and special problems according to the assistance required, degree of disability, or degree of special problems. Each item is briefly defined and has options of four scale points. The total scores range from 18 to 72, with higher values indicating greater disability.

The scale demonstrates high reliability in use (McDowell and Newell, 1987; Rothstein, 1985), and the initial results of validity examination are positive.

This tool contains several items that would be included in the routine health assessment, e.g., hearing, sight, diet, medication, and may be most appropriate for screening situations.

The Functional Status Rating System

The Functional Status Rating System tool (Forer, 1981) (see the box on p. 686) measures the amount of assistance needed in self-care and mobility and the amount of impairment in communication, psychosocial adjustment, and cognitive function. It is unusually comprehensive for a functional assessment tool, covering 30 items under five topics. Although the tool may in small part duplicate portions of the health assessment, most of the items would measure new assessment factors.

The Functional Activities Questionnaire

Activities questionnaire to be completed by spouse, child, close friend or relative of the participant.

Instructions: The following pages list ten common activities. *For each activity,* please read all choices, then choose the *one* statement which best describes the *current* ability of the participant. Answers should apply to *that persons's* abilities, not your own. Please check off a choice for *each* activity; do not skip any.

1. Writing checks, paying bills, balancing checkbook, keeping financial records
   _____ A. Someone has recently taken over this activity completely or almost completely.
   _____ B. Requires frequent advice or assistance from others (e.g., relatives, friends, business associates, banker), which was *not previously necessary.*
   _____ C. Does without any advice or assistance, but more difficult than used to be or less good job.
   _____ D. Does without any difficulty or advice.
   _____ E. Never did and would find quite difficult to start now.
   _____ F. Didn't do regularly but can do normally now with a little practice if they have to.

2. Making out insurance or Social Security forms, handling business affairs or papers, assembling tax records
   _____ A. Someone has recently taken over this activity completely or almost completely, and that someone did not used to do any or as much.
   _____ B. Requires more frequent advice or more assistance from others than in the past.
   _____ C. Does without any more advice or assistance than used to, but finds more difficult or does less good job than in the past.
   _____ D. Does without any difficulty or advice.
   _____ E. Never did and would find quite difficult to start now, even with practice.
   _____ F. Didn't do routinely, but can do normally now should they have to.

3. Shopping alone for clothes, household necessities, and groceries
   _____ A. Someone has recently taken over this activity completely or almost completely.
   _____ B. Requires frequent advice or assistance from others.
   _____ C. Does without advice or assistance, but finds more difficult than used to or does less good job.
   _____ D. Does without any difficulty or advice.
   _____ E. Never did and would find quite difficult to start now.
   _____ F. Didn't do routinely but can do normally now should they have to.

4. Playing a game of skill such as bridge, other card games or chess or working on a hobby such as painting, photography, woodwork, stamp collecting
   _____ A. Hardly ever does now or has great difficulty.
   _____ B. Requires advice, or others have to make allowances.
   _____ C. Does without advice, or assistance, but more difficult or less skillful than used to be.
   _____ D. Does without any difficulty or advice.
   _____ E. Never did and would find quite difficult to start now.
   _____ F. Didn't do regularly, but can do normally now should they have to.

5. Heat the water, make a cup of coffee or tea, and turn off the stove
   _____ A. Someone else has recently taken over this activity completely, or almost completely.
   _____ B. Requires advice or has frequent problems (for example, burns pots, forgets to turn off stove).
   _____ C. Does without advice or assistance but occasional problems.
   _____ D. Does without any difficulty or advice.
   _____ E. Never did and would find quite difficult to start now.
   _____ F. Didn't usually, but can do normally now, should they have to.

6. Prepare a balanced meal (e.g., meat, chicken or fish, vegetables, dessert)
   _____ A. Someone else has recently taken over this activity completely or almost completely.
   _____ B. Requires frequent advise or has frequent problems (for example, burns pots, forgets how to make a given dish).
   _____ C. Does without much advice or assistance, but more difficult (for example, switched to TV dinners most of the time because of difficulty).
   _____ D. Does without any difficulty or advice.
   _____ E. Never did and would find quite difficult to do now even after a little practice.
   _____ F. Didn't do regularly, but can do normally now should they have to.

7. Keep track of current events, either in the neighborhood or nationally
   _____ A. Pays no attention to, or doesn't remember outside happenings.
   _____ B. Some idea about *major* events (for example, comments on presidential election, major events in the news or major sporting events).
   _____ C. Somewhat less attention to, or knowledge of, current events than formerly.
   _____ D. As aware of current events as ever was.
   _____ E. Never paid much attention to current events, and would find quite difficult to start now.
   _____ F. Never paid much attention, but can do as well as anyone now when they try.

Adapted from the presentation of the Functional activities questionnaire in McDowell I and Newell C: Functional disability and handicap. Measuring health: A guide to rating scales and questionnaires. New York, 1987, Oxford University Press, pp. 86-87.

Continued

The Functional Activities Questionnaire—cont'd

8. Pay attention to, understand, and discuss the plot or theme of a one hour television program; get something out of a book or magazine
   - _____ A. Doesn't remember, or seems confused by, what they have watched or read.
   - _____ B. Aware of the *general idea,* characters, or nature while they watch or read, but may *not recall* later; may *not grasp theme* or have opinion about what they saw.
   - _____ C. Less attention, or less memory than before, less likely to catch humor, points which are made quickly, or subtle points.
   - _____ D. Grasps as quickly as ever.
   - _____ E. Never paid much attention to or commented on T.V., never read much and would probably find very difficult to start now.
   - _____ F. Never read or watch T.V. much, but read or watch as much as ever and get as much out of it as ever.

9. Remember appointments, plans, household tasks, car repairs, family occasions (such as birthdays or anniversaries), holidays, medications
   - _____ A. Someone else has recently taken this over.
   - _____ B. Has to be reminded some of the time (more than in the past or more than most people).

- _____ C. Manages without reminders but has to rely heavily on notes, calendars, schemes.
- _____ D. Remembers appointments, plans, occasions, etc. as well as they ever did.
- _____ E. Never had to keep track of appointments, medications or family occasions, and would probably find very difficult to start now.
- _____ F. Didn't have to keep track of these things in the past, but can do as well as anyone when they try.

10. Travel out of neighborhood: driving, walking, arranging to take or change buses and trains, planes
   - _____ A. Someone else has taken this over completely or almost completely.
   - _____ B. Can get around in own neighborhood but gets lost out of neighborhood.
   - _____ C. Has more problems getting around than used to (for example, occasionally lost, loss of confidence, can't find car, etc) but usually OK.
   - _____ D. Gets around as well as ever.
   - _____ E. Rarely did much driving or had to get around alone and would find quite difficult to learn bus routes or make similar arrangements now.
   - _____ F. Didn't have to get around alone much in past, but can do as well as ever when has to.

The amount of currently available psychometric information available about the tool is limited.

Functional Independence Measure (FIM) and FIM Expanded

A recent innovation in the field of rehabilitation medicine is the development of a uniform, national data system for functional assessment. This standardized database would establish a uniform language and set of definitions for communicating disability and rehabilitation information. Toward this end the major researchers in the field have developed the minimum data set for the field, the Functional Independence Measure (FIM) tool. The FIM tool measures 18 items in the categories of self-care, mobility, locomotion, communication, and social cognition measured on a seven-point scale. The seven-point rating scale is designed to assess the patient's level or degree of independence, the amount of assistance required, use of adaptive or assistive devices, and the percentage of a given task completed successfully. The FIM requires 15 to 20 minutes for administration and can be administered by a variety of health care professionals.

The FIM has been expanded to a 29-item scale, titled the Functional Assessment Measures (FAM), by

the staff of the Santa Clara Medical Center (see the box on pp. 687-700). The expanded tool uses the same rating scheme and requires 20 to 25 minutes for administration. Both the FIM and its expanded version, the FAM, are likely to replace most of the other tools listed in this chapter in the field of rehabilitation medicine in the future. The new tools have clearly been built on the content of the older tools, and the possibility of uniformity across systems holds promise for enhancing communication and knowledge.

ADDITIONAL TOOLS

The Kenny Self-Care Evaluation

This tool is an elaborate measure of functional performance including bed activities, transfers, locomotion, dressing, personal hygiene, bowel and bladder assistance needs, and feeding (see Iverson, Silberg, Steven, and Schoening, 1973). This tool has been used primarily in rehabilitation settings.

Modified ADL Index

This tool includes 15 basic ADL and two instrumental ADL items rated on a 3-point scale (see Sheikh and others, 1979).

Table 27-4

The Rapid Disability Rating Scale-2

Directions: Rate what the person *does* to reflect current behavior, Circle one of the four choices for each item. Consider rating with any aids or prostheses normally used. None = completely independent or normal behavior. Total = that person cannot, will not or may not (because of medical restriction) perform a behavior or has the most severe form of disability or problem.

Assistance with activities of daily living

Eating	None	A little	A lot	Spoon-feed: intravenous tube
Walking (with cane or walker if used)	None	A little	A lot	Does not walk
Mobility (going outside and getting about with wheelchair, etc., if used)	None	A little	A lot	Is housebound
Bathing (include getting supplies, supervising)	None	A little	A lot	Must be bathed
Dressing (include help in selecting clothes)	None	A little	A lot	Must be dressed
Toileting (include help with clothes, cleaning, or help with ostomy, catheter)	None	A little	A lot	Uses bedpan or unable to care for ostomy/catheter
Grooming (shaving for men, hairdressing for women, nails, teeth)	None	A little	A lot	Must be groomed
Adaptive tasks (managing money/possessions; telephoning; buying newspaper, toilet articles, snacks)	None	A little	A lot	Cannot manage

Degree of disability

Communication (expressing self)	None	A little	A lot	Does not communicate
Hearing (with aid if used)	None	A little	A lot	Does not seem to hear
Sight (with glasses, if used)	None	A little	A lot	Does not see
Diet (deviation from normal)	None	A little	A lot	Fed by intravenous tube
In bed during day (ordered or self-initiated)	None	A little (<3 hrs)	A lot	Most/all of time
Incontinence (urine/feces, with catheter or prosthesis, if used)	None	Sometimes	Frequently (weekly +)	Does not control
Medication	None	Sometimes	Daily, taken orally	Daily: injection: (+ oral if used)

Degree of special problems

Mental confusion	None	A little	A lot	Extreme
Uncooperativeness (combats efforts to help with care)	None	A little	A lot	Extreme
Depression	None	A little	A lot	Extreme

Adapted from the presentation of the Rapid Disability Rating Scale-2 as published in Linn MW and Linn BS: The rapid disability rating scale-2, J Am Geriatr Soc 30:380, 1982.

Functional Assessment Tool for Alzheimer's-Type Dementia (FAST)

This tool is an ordinal measure (from normality to severe dementia of the Alzheimer's type) of daily activities for clients with dementia (see Reisberg, Ferris, and Franssen, 1985).

Comprehensive Assessment and Referral Evaluation (CARE)

This tool is an extensive (143 to 1500 items in various versions), broad tool measuring the medical, psychiatric, nutritional, economic, and social problems of the elderly (see Gurland, 1977, 1984 and Teresi, 1984).

Text continued on p. 700.

The Functional Status Rating System

Functional status in self-care

A. *Eating/feeding:* Management of all aspects of setting up and eating food (including cutting of meat) with or without adaptive equipment.
B. *Personal hygiene:* Includes set up, oral care, washing face and hands with a wash cloth, hair grooming, shaving, and makeup.
C. *Toileting:* Includes management of clothing and cleanliness.
D. *Bathing:* Includes entire body bathing (tub, shower, or bed bath).
E. *Bowel management:* Able to insert suppository and/or perform manual evacuation, aware of need to defecate, has sphincter muscle control.
F. *Bladder management:* Able to manage equipment necessary for bladder evacuation (may include intermittent catheterization).
G. *Skin management:* Performance of skin care program, regular inspection, prevention of pressure sores, rashes, or irritations.
H. *Bed activities:* Includes turning, coming to a sitting position, scooting, and maintenance of balance.
I. *Dressing:* Includes performance of total body dressing except tying shoes, with or without adaptive equipment (also includes application of orthosis & prosthesis).

Functional status in mobility

A. *Transfers:* Includes the management of all aspects of transfers to and from bed, mat, toilet, tub/shower, wheelchair, with or without adaptive equipment.
B. *Wheelchair skills:* Includes management of brakes, leg rests, maneuvering and propelling through and over doorway thresholds.
C. *Ambulation:* Includes coming to a standing position and walking short to moderate distances on level surfaces with or without equipment.
D. *Stairs and environmental surfaces:* Includes climbing stairs, curbs, ramps or environmental terrain.
E. *Community mobility:* Ability to manage transportation.

Functional status in communication

A. *Understanding spoken language*
B. *Reading comprehension*

C. *Language expression (non-speech/alternative methods):* Includes pointing, gestures, manual communication boards, electronic systems.
D. *Language expression (verbal):* Includes grammar, syntax, & appropriateness of language.
E. *Speech intelligibility*
F. *Written communication (motor)*
G. *Written language expression:* Includes spelling, vocabulary, punctuation, syntax, grammar, and completeness of written response.

Functional status in psychosocial adjustment

A. *Emotional adjustment:* Includes frequency and severity of depression, anxiety, frustration, lability, unresponsiveness, agitation, interference with progress in therapies, motivation, ability to cope with and take responsiblity for emotional behavior.
B. *Family/significant others/environment:* Includes frequency of chronic problems or conflicts in patient's relationships, interference with progress in therapies, ability and willingness to provide for patient's specific needs after discharge, and to promote patient's recovery and independence.
C. *Adjustment to limitations:* Includes denial/awareness, acceptance of limitations, willingness to learn new ways of functioning, compensating, taking appropriate safety precautions, and realistic expectations for long-term recovery.
D. *Social adjustment:* Includes frequency & limitation of social contacts, responsiveness in one to one & group situations, appropriateness of behavior in relationships, and spontaneity of interactions.

Functional status in cognitive function

A. *Attention span:* Includes distractability, level of alertness and responsiveness, ability to concentrate on a task, ability to follow directions, immediate recall as the structure, difficulty and length of the task varies.
B. *Orientation*
C. *Judgment reasoning*
D. *Memory:* Includes short- and long-term.
E. *Problem-solving*

Summary of rating scales

Self-care and mobility items

1.0 = Unable—totally dependent
1.5 = Maximum assistance of 1 or 2 people
2.0 = Moderate assistance
2.5 = Minimal assistance
3.0 = Standby assistance
3.5 = Supervised
4.0 = Independent

Communication, psychosocial and cognitive function items

1.0 = Extremely severe
1.5 = Severe
2.0 = Moderately severe
2.5 = Moderate impairment
3.0 = Mild impairment
3.5 = Minimal impairment
4.0 = No impairment

Adapted from the presentation of the Functional Status Rating System as published in McDowell C and Newell C: Functional disablity and handicap. Measuring health: A guide to rating scales and questionnaires. New York, 1987, Oxford University Press, pp 69-70, 1987.

Functional Assessment Measures (FAM)

The 7-point Rating Scale is as follows:

Independent   Another person is not required for the activity (NO HELPER).

7   **Complete Independence**—All of the tasks described as making up the activity are typically performed safely without modification, assistive devices, or aids and within reasonable time.

6   **Modified Independence**—Activity requires any one or more of the following: An assistive device, more than reasonable time, or there are safety (risk) considerations.

Dependent   Another person is required for either supervision or physical assistance in order for the activity to be performed, or it is not performed (REQUIRES HELPER).
MODIFIED DEPENDENCE—The subject expends half (50%) or more of the effort. The levels of assistance required are:

5   **Supervision or Setup**—Subject requires no more help than standby, cuing or coaxing, without physical contact. Or, helper sets up needed items or applies orthoses.

4   **Minimal Contact Assistance**—With physical contact the subject requires no more help than touching, and subject expends 75% or more of the effort.

3   **Moderate Assistance**—Subject requires more help than touching, or expends half (50%) or more (up to 75%) of the effort.
COMPLETE DEPENDENCE—The subject expends less than half (less than 50%) of the effort, maximal or total assistance is required, or the activity is not performed. The levels of assistance required are:

2   **Maximal Assistance**—Subject expends less than 50% of the effort, but at least 25%.

1   **Total Assistance**—Subject expends less than 25% of the effort.
Each item is operationally defined in terms of these 7 levels on the following pages.

Self care items

1. FEEDING   Includes use of suitable utensils to bring food to mouth, chewing and swallowing, once meal is appropriately prepared. Opening containers, cutting meat, buttering bread and pouring liquids are *not* included as they are often part of meal preparation.

No helper

7   **Complete Independence**—Eats from a dish and drinks from a cup or glass presented in the customary manner on a table or a tray. Uses ordinary knife, fork, spoon.

6   **Modified Independence**—Uses an adaptive or assistive device such as a straw, spork, rocking knife or requires more than a reasonable time to eat.

Helper

5   **Supervision or Setup**—Requires supervision (e.g., standby, cuing, or coaxing) or setup (application of orthoses).

4   **Minimal Contact Assistance**—Subject performs 75% or more of feeding tasks.

3   **Moderate Assistance**—Performs 50% to 74% of feeding tasks.

2   **Maximal Assistance**—Performs 25% to 49% of feeding tasks. Or, the individual does not eat or drink full meals by mouth, but relies in part on other means of alimentation, such as parenteral or gastrostomy feedings, then he/she administers the feedings him/her self.

1   **Total Assistance**—Performs less than 25% of feeding tasks. Or, the individual does not eat or drink full meals by mouth but must rely in part on other means of alimentation, such as parenteral or gastrostomy feedings, and does not administer the feedings him/herself.

2. GROOMING   Includes oral care, hair grooming, washing hands and face, and either shaving or applying makeup.

No helper

7   **Complete Independence**—Cleans teeth or dentures, combs or brushes hair, washes hands and face, shaves or applies makeup, including all preparations.

6   **Modified Independence**—Uses specialized equipment or takes more than a reasonable time, or there are safety considerations.

Functional Assessment Measures (FAM)—cont'd

2. GROOMING—cont'd

Helper

5   **Supervision or Setup**—Requires supervision (e.g., standby, cuing, or coaxing) or setup (application of orthoses, setting out specialized grooming equipment, and initial preparation such as apply toothpaste to brush, opening makeup containers).

4   **Minimal Contact Assistance**—Subject performs 75% of grooming tasks.

3   **Moderate Assistance**—Performs 50% to 74% of grooming tasks.

2   **Maximal Assistance**—Performs 25% to 49% of grooming tasks.

1   **Total Assistance**—Performs less than 25% of grooming tasks.

3. BATHING   Includes bathing the body from the neck down (excluding the back), either tub, shower or sponge/bed bath.

No helper

7   **Complete Independence**—Bathes and dries the body.

6   **Modified Independence**—Uses specialized equipment or takes more than a reasonable time or there are safely considerations.

Helper

5   **Supervision or Setup**—Requires supervision (e.g., standby, or cuing or coaxing) or setup (setting out specialized bathing equipment, and initial preparation such as preparing the water or washing materials).

4   **Minimal Contact Assistance**—Subject performs 75% or more of bathing tasks.

3   **Moderate Assistance**—Performs 50% to 74% of bathing tasks.

2   **Maximal Assistance**—Performs 25% to 49% of bathing tasks.

1   **Total Assistance**—Performs less than 25% of bathing tasks.

4. DRESSING— UPPER BODY   Includes dressing above the waist as well as donning and removing prosthesis or orthosis when applicable.

No helper

7   **Complete Independence**—Dresses and undresses including obtaining clothes from their customary places such as drawers and closets; manages bra, pull-over garment, and front-opening garment; manages zippers, buttons, and snaps; dons and removes prosthesis or orthosis when applicable.

6   **Modified Independence**—Uses special adaptive closure such as velcro, or assistive device, or takes more than a reasonable time.

Helper

5   **Supervision or Setup**—Requires supervision (e.g., standby, cuing, or coaxing) or setup (application or orthoses, setting out clothes or specialized dressing equipment).

4   **Minimal Contact Assistance**—Subject performs 75% or more of dressing tasks.

3   **Moderate Assistance**—Performs 50% to 74% of dressing tasks.

2   **Maximal Assistance**—Performs 25% to 49% of dressing tasks.

1   **Total Assistance**—Performs less than 25% of dressing tasks, or is not dressed.

Functional Assessment Measures (FAM) — *cont'd*

---

5. DRESSING— LOWER BODY   Includes dressing from the waist down as well as donning or removing prosthesis or orthosis when applicable.

No helper

7	**Complete Independence**—Dresses and undresses including obtaining clothes from their customary places such as drawers and closets; manages underpants, slacks, skirt, belt, stockings, and shoes; manages zippers, buttons, and snaps; dons and removes prosthesis or orthosis when applicable.
6	**Modified Independence**—Uses special adaptive closure such as velcro, or assistive device, or takes more than a reasonable time.

Helper

5	**Supervision or Setup**—Requires supervision (e.g., standby, cuing, or coaxing) or setup (application or orthoses, setting out clothes or specialized dressing equipment).
4	**Minimal Contact Assistance**—Subject performs 75% or more of dressing tasks.
2	**Maximal Assistance**—Performs 25% to 49% of dressing tasks.
1	**Total Assistance**—Performs less than 25% of dressing tasks, or is not dressed.

6. TOILETING   Includes maintaining perineal hygiene and adjusting clothing after toileting.

No helper

7	**Complete Independence**—Cleanses self after voiding or bowel movement; puts on sanitary napkins/inserts tampons; adjusts clothing after using toilet.
6	**Modified Independence**—Uses specialized equipment or takes more than reasonable time or there are safety considerations.

Helper

5	**Supervision or Setup**—Requires supervision (e.g., standby, cuing, or coaxing) or setup (application of adaptive devices or opening packages).
4	**Minimal Contact Assistance**—Performs 75% or more of toileting tasks.
3	**Moderate Assistance**—Performs 50% to 74% of toileting tasks.
2	**Maximal Assistance**—Performs 25% to 49% of toileting tasks.
1	**Total Assistance**—Performs less than 25% of toileting tasks.

Comment: If subject requires assistance with sanitary napkins (usually 3-5 days per month) level of assistance is 5, supervision or setup.

7. SWALLOWING   Ability to safely eat a regular diet by mouth.

Helper

7	**Complete Independence**—Able to eat a regular diet of choice in a reasonable period of time.
6	**Modified Independence**—Able to eat a regular diet by mouth. May require excessive time for eating. May require assistive devices or multiple swallows to clear food.

No helper

5	**Supervision** (Modified Dependence)—Able to take all nourishment by mouth. May need modified diet. Supervision required for cueing, coaxing. May need assistance with food choices.
4	**Minimal Assistance** (Modified Dependence)—Able to take primary nourishment by mouth. May require diet restrictions. Minimal assistance required to monitor speed and amount of food intake. Subject performs 75% of the activity.
3	**Maximal Assistance** (Modified Dependence)—Able to take some nourishment by mouth. May require diet restrictions and modifications. May require moderate assistance to monitor speed and amount of food intake. Subject performs 50-74% of the activity.
2	**Maximal Assistance** (Dependent)—Unable to receive adequate nourishment via oral feedings. Tube feedings provide primary nutrition. Oral feedings are limited and require maximal assistance. Subject performs 25-49% of the activity.
1	**Unable** to take anything by mouth. Nutrition is *provided via tube feedings*.

Continued

Functional Assessment Measures (FAM)—cont'd

Sphincter control

8. BLADDER MANAGE-MENT

Includes complete intentional control of urinary bladder and use of equipment or agents necessary for bladder control.

No helper

7   **Complete Independence**—Controls bladder completely and intentionally and is never incontinent.

6   **Modified Independence**—Requires a catheter, urinary collecting device, or urinary diversion or uses medication for control; if catheter is used, the individual instills or irrigates catheter without assistance; cleans, sterilizes, and sets up the equipment for irrigation without assistance. If the individual uses a device, he/she assembles and applies condom drainage or an ileal appliance without assistance of another person; empties, puts on, removes, and cleans leg bag or empties and cleans ileal appliance bag. No accidents.

Helper

5   **Supervision or Setup**—Requires supervision (e.g., standby, cuing, or coaxing) or setup of catheterization equipment to maintain a satisfactory voiding pattern or to maintain an external device; or because of the lapse of time to get to bed pan or the toilet the individual may have occasional bladder accidents, but less often than *monthly*.

4   **Minimal Contact Assistance**—Requires minimal contact assistance to maintain an external device; the individual performs 75% or more of bladder management tasks; or may have occasional bladder accidents, but less often than *weekly*.

3   **Moderate Assistance**—Requires moderate assistance to maintain an external device; the individual performs 50% to 74% of bladder management tasks; or may have occasional bladder accidents, but less often than *daily*.

2   **Maximal Assistance**—Despite assistance, the individual is wet on a frequent or almost daily basis, necessitating wearing diapers or other absorbent pads, whether or not a catheter or ostomy device is in place. The individual performs 25% to 49% of bladder management tasks.

1   **Total Assistance**—Despite assistance, the individual is wet on a frequent or almost daily basis, necessitating wearing diapers or other absorbent pads, whether or not a catheter or ostomy device is in place. The individual performs less than 25% of bladder management tasks.

Comment: The functional goal of bladder management is to open the bladder sphincter only when that is needed and to keep it closed the rest of the time. This may require devices, drugs or assistance in some individuals. This item, therefore, deals with two variables: 1) level of success in bladder management and 2) level of assistance required. Usually the two follow each other. E.g., when there are more accidents usually more assistance is required. However, should the two levels not be exactly the same, always record the *lower* level.

9. BOWEL MANAGE-MENT

Includes complete intentional control of bowel movement and use of equipment or agents necessary for bowel control.

No helper

7   **Complete Independence**—Controls bowels completely and intentionally and is never incontinent.

6   **Modified Independence**—Uses digital stimulation or stool softeners, suppositories, laxatives, or enemas on a regular basis, or uses other medications for control. If the individual has a colostomy, he/she maintains it. No accidents.

Functional Assessment Measures (FAM) — *cont'd*

9. BOWEL MANAGEMENT — *cont'd*

Helper

5   **Supervision or Setup**—Requires supervision (e.g., standby, cuing, or coaxing) or setup of equipment necessary for the individual to maintain a satisfactory excretion pattern or to maintain an ostomy device; or the individual may have occasional bowel accidents, but less often than *monthly*.

4   **Minimal Contact Assistance**—Requires minimal contact assistance to maintain a satisfactory excretion pattern by using suppositories or enemas or an external device; the individual performs 75% or more of bowel management tasks; or may have occasional bowel accidents, but less often than *weekly*.

3   **Moderate Assistance**—Requires moderate assistance to maintain a satisfactory excretory pattern by using such means as suppositories or enemas or to maintain an external device; the individual performs 50% to 74% of bowel management tasks; or may have occasional bowel accidents, but less often than *daily*.

2   **Maximal Assistance**—Despite assistance, the individual is soiled on a frequent or almost daily basis, necessitating wearing diapers or other absorbent pads, whether or not an ostomy device is in place. The individual performs 25% to 49% of bowel management tasks.

1   **Total Assistance**—Despite assistance, the individual is soiled on a frequent or almost daily basis, necessitating wearing diapers or other absorbent pads, whether or not an ostomy device is in place. The individual performs less than 25% of bowel management tasks.

Comment: The functional goal of bowel management is to open the anal sphincter only when that is needed and to keep it closed the rest of the time. This may require devices, drugs or assistance in some individuals. This item, therefore, deals with two variables: 1) level of success in bowel management and 2) level of assistance required. Usually the two follow each other. E.g., when there are more accidents usually more assistance is required. However, should the two levels not be exactly the same, always record the *lower* level.

Mobility items

10. TRANSFERS: BED, CHAIR, WHEELCHAIR   Includes all aspects of transferring to and from bed, chair, or wheelchair, or coming to a standing position, if walking is the typical mode of locomotion.

No helper

7   **Complete Independence**—If *walking*, approaches, sits down and gets up to a standing position from a regular chair; transfers from bed to chair. Performs safely.
If in a wheelchair, approaches a bed or chair, locks brakes, lifts foot rests, removes arm rests if necessary, and performs either a standing pivot or sliding transfer and returns. Performs safely.
Modified Independence—Uses adaptive or assistance device such as a sliding board, a list, grab bars, or special seat or chair or brace or crutches; takes more than reasonable time or there are safety considerations.

Helper

5   **Supervision or Setup**—Requires supervision (e.g., standby, cuing, or coaxing) or setup (positioning sliding board, moving foot rests, etc.)
4   **Minimal Contact Assistance**—Subject performs 75% or more of transferring tasks.
3   **Moderate Assistance**—Performs 50% to 74% of transferring tasks.
2   **Maximal Assistance**—Performs 25% to 49% of transferring tasks.
1   **Total Assistance**—Performs less than 25% of transferring tasks.

Continued

Functional Assessment Measures (FAM)—*cont'd*

11. TRANSFERS: TOILET   Includes getting on and off a toilet.

No belper

7   **Complete Independence**—*If walking*, approaches, sits down on and gets up from a standard toilet. Performs safely.
If in a wheelchair, approaches toilet, locks brakes, lifts foot rests, removes arm rests if necessary and does either a standing pivot or sliding transfer and returns. Performs safely.

6   **Modified Independence**—Uses adaptive or assistive device such as a sliding board, a lift, grab bars, or special seat; takes more than reasonable time or there are safety considerations.

Helper

5   **Supervision or Setup**—Requires supervision (e.g., standby, cuing, or coaxing) or setup (positioning sliding board, moving foot rests, etc).

4   **Minimal Contact Assistance**—Subject performs 75% or more of transferring tasks.

3   **Moderate Assistance**—Performs 50% to 74% of transferring tasks.

2   **Maximal Assistance**—Performsf 25% to 49% of transferring tasks.

1   **Total Assistance**—Performs less than 25% of transferring tasks.

12. TRANSFERS: TUB OR SHOWER   Includes getting into and out of a tub or shower stall.

No belper

7   **Complete Independence**—*If walking*, approaches, enters and leaves a tub or shower stall. Performs safely.
If in a wheelchair, approaches tub or shower, locks brakes, lifts foot rests, removes arm rests if necessary and does either a standing pivot or sliding transfer and returns. Performs safely.

6   **Modified Independence**—Uses adaptive or assistive device such as a sliding board, a lift, grab bars, or special seat; takes more than reasonable time or there are safety considerations.

Helper

5   **Supervision or Setup**—Requires supervision (e.g., standby, cuing, or coaxing) or setup (positioning sliding board, moving foot rests, etc).

4   **Minimal Contact Assistance**—Subject performs 75% or more of transferring tasks.

3   **Moderate Assistance**—Performs 50% to 74% of transferring tasks.

2   **Maximal Assistance**—Performs 25% to 49% of transferring tasks.

1   **Total Assistance**—Performs less than 25% of transferring tasks.

13. CAR TRANSFERS   The activity includes approaching the car, managing the car door and lock, getting on or off the car seat and managing the seat belt. If a wheelchair is used for mobility, the activity includes loading and unloading the wheelchair.

7   **Complete Independence**—The patient is able to complete the activity without assistive devices, or aids, and within a reasonable amount of time.

6   **Modified Independence**—The patient requires an assistive device or aid, requires more than a reasonable amount of time or there is a safety risk in completing the activity.

5   **Supervision** (Modified Dependence)—The patient requires cueing, but no physical assistance, to complete the activity.

4   **Minimal Assistance** (Modified Dependence)—The patient performs at least 75% of the activity, requiring contact assistance with less than 25% of the activity.

3   **Moderate Assistance** (Modified Dependence)—The patient performs 50-75% of the activity, requiring more than contact guard with 25-50% of the activity.

2   **Maximal Assistance** (Complete Dependence)—The patient performs only 25-50% of the activity and requires heavy assistance for 50-75% of the activity.

1   **Total Assistance** (Complete Dependence)—The patient performs less than 25% of the activity and requires heavy assistance for more than 75% of the activity.

Functional Assessment Measures (FAM)—*cont'd*

LOCOMOTION

14. WALKING/WHEEL-CHAIR

Includes walking, once in a standing position, or using a wheelchair, once in a seated position, indoors.

Check most frequent mode of locomotion. If both are about equal, check W *and* C.

( ) W = *Walking*   ( ) C = wheel*c*hair

No belper

7   **Complete Independence**—*Walks* with a minimum of *150* feet without assistive devices. Does not use a wheelchair. Performs safely.

6   **Modified Independence**—*Walks* with a minimum of *150* feet but uses a brace (orthosis) or prosthesis on leg, special adaptive shoes, cane, crutches, or walkerette; takes more than reasonable time or there are safety considerations.

If not walking, operates manual or electric wheelchair independently for a minimum of *150* feet; turns around; maneuvers the chair to a table, bed, toilet; negotiates at least a 3 percent grade; maneuvers on rugs and over door sills.

Helper

5   **Supervision or Setup**—*If walking*, requires standby supervision, cuing or coaxing to goal minimum of *150* feet, *or* walks independently only short distances (a minimum of *50* feet).

If not walking, requires standby supervision, cuing, or coaxing to go a minimum of *150* feet in wheelchair, *or* operates manual or electric wheelchair independently only short distances (a minimum of *50* feet).

4   **Minimal Contact Assistance**—Subject performs 75% or more of locomotion effort to go a minimum of *150* feet.

3   **Moderate Assistance**—Performs 50% to 74% of locomotion effort to go a minimum of *150* feet.

2   **Maximal Assistance**—Performs 25% to 49% of locomotion effort to go a minimum of *50* feet. Requires assistance of one person only.

1   **Total Assistance**—Performs less than 25% of effort, or requires assistance of two people, or does not walk or wheel a minimum of *50* feet.

Comment: There are several ways to estimate percent of effort. For instance, a disabled individual who can walk *unassisted* for 75 feet (that is 50% (½) of the 150 feet) then requires assistance for the remaining 75 feet, would be at level 4 if steadying was required, or level 3 if full support of one person was required the rest of the way.

15. STAIRS

Goes up and down 12 to 14 stairs (one flight) indoors.

No belper

7   **Complete Independence**—Goes up and down at least one flight of stairs without any type of handrail or support. Performs safely.

6   **Modified Independence**—Goes up and down at least one flight of stairs using side support or handrail, cane, or portable supports; takes more than reasonable time or there are safety considerations.

Helper

5   **Supervision or Setup**—Requires standby supervision, cuing, or coaxing to go up and down one flight.

4   **Minimal Contact Assistance**—Performs 75% or more of stair climbing effort.

3   **Moderate Assistance**—Performs 50% to 74% of stair climbing effort.

2   **Maximal Assistance**—Performs 25% to 49% of stair climbing effort. Requires the assistance of one person only.

1   **Total Assistance**—Performs less than 25% of the effort or requires the assistance of two people, or does not not go up and down one flight of stairs, or is carried.

Comment: Note that 6 steps equals 25% (¼) of 12 steps up and down (24 total steps).

Continued

Functional Assessment Measures (FAM)—*cont'd*

---

16. COMMUNITY
    MOBILITY

Ability to manage transportation including planning a route, time management, paying fares, and anticipating access barriers (excluding car transfers).

No helper

7   **Complete Independence**—The patient independently uses public transportation (bus, van or taxi) or is able to drive a car.

6   **Modified Independence**—The patient uses adaptive devices to drive, must keep trips to a short distance due to needed rest periods; or there are safety considerations in using public transportation.

Helper

5   **Supervision** (Modified Dependence)—The patient requires cueing to use public transportation or ride in a car.

4   **Minimal Assistance** (Modified Dependence)—The patient is able to use public transportation or rides in a car, but needs assistance for up to 25% of the activity.

3   **Moderate Assistance** (Modified Dependence)—The patient uses public transportation or rides in a car, but needs assistance for 25-50% of the activity.

2   **Maximal Assistance** (Complete Dependence)—The patient may use public transportation or ride in a car but needs assistance for 50-75% of the activity.

1   **Total Assistance** (Complete Dependence)—The patient is unable to use public transportation or ride in a car without heavy assistance for more than 75% of the activity.

Communication items

17. COMPREHENSION

Includes comprehension of either auditory or visual communication. *This* means, understanding linguistic information by the spoken or written word.

   Check and evaluate the most usual mode of comprehension. If both are about equally used, check A *and* V.

( ) A = Auditory   ( ) V = Visual

No helper

7   **Complete Independence**—Understands spoken or written directions (such as three-step commands) or conversation that is complex or abstract; comprehends either spoken or written native language.

6   **Modified Independence**—Understands spoken or written directions (such as three-step commands) or conversation that is complex or abstract with mild difficulty. May require a hearing or visual aid, other assistive device, or extra time to understand the information.

Helper

5   **Standby Prompting**—Understands conversation or reading material about every day situations more than 90% of the time. Requires prompting less than 10% of the time.

4   **Minimal Prompting**—Understands conversation or reading material about every day situations 75% to 90% of the time.

3   **Moderate Prompting**—Understands conversation or reading material about every day situations 50% to 74% of the time.

2   **Maximal Prompting**—Understands conversation or reading material about every day situations 25% to 49% of the time. Needs prompting more than half the time.

1   **Total Assistance**—Understands conversation or reading material about every day situations less than 25% of the time or does not understand or may not respond appropriately or consistently despite assistance.

Functional Assessment Measures (FAM) —*cont'd*

---

18. EXPRESSION

Includes clear expression of verbal or non-verbal language. This means expressing linguistic information verbally or graphically with appropriate and accurate meaning and grammar.

Check and evaluate the most usual mode of expression. If both are about equally used, check V *and* N.

( ) V = Verbal   ( ) N = Non-verbal

No helper

7   **Complete Independence**—Expresses complex or abstract ideas intelligibly and fluently, verbally or non-verbally, including either signing or writing.

6   **Modified Independence**—Expresses complex or abstract ideas with mild difficulty. May require an augmentative communication device or system.

Helper

5   **Standby Prompting**—Expresses basic needs and ideas about every day situations more than 90% of the time. Requires prompting less than 10% of the time.

4   **Minimal Prompting**—Expresses basic needs and ideas about every day situations 75% to 90% of the time.

3   **Moderate Prompting**—Expresses basic needs and ideas about every day situations 50% to 74% of the time.

2   **Maximal Prompting**—Expresses basic needs and ideas 25% to 49% of the time. Needs prompting more than half the time.

1   **Total Assistance**—Expresses basic needs and ideas less than 25% of the time or does not express basic needs appropriately or consistently despite assistance.

19. READING

7   **Complete Independence**—Completely able to read and understand complex, lengthy paragraphs (newspapers, books, etc).

6   **Modified Independence**—Able to read and understand complex sentences or short paragraphs. May demonstrate reduced speed or retention problems.

5   **Standby Prompting**—Able to read and understand short, simple sentences but shows increased difficulty with length or complexity.

4   **Minimal Prompting**—Able to recognize single words and familiar short phrases.

3   **Moderate Prompting**—Able to recognize letters, objects, forms, etc. Able to match words to pictures (under 50% accuracy).

2   **Maximal Prompting**—Able to match identical objects, forms, letters (under 50% accuracy) but may require cues.

1   **Total Assistance**—Unable to consistently match or recognize identical letters, objects or forms.

20. WRITING

7   **Complete Independence**—Able to write with complete average accuracy in spelling, grammar, syntax, punctuation, and completeness.

6   **Modified Independence**—Able to accurately write sentences and form short paragraphs. May have occasional spelling or grammatical errors.

5   **Standby Prompting**—Able to write phrases or simple sentences. Evidences spelling, grammar, syntax errors.

4   **Minimal Prompting**—Able to write simple words, occasional phrases to express ideas. Spelling errors and reduced legibility are evident.

3   **Moderate Prompting**—Able to write name (cueing may be required) and some familiar words. Legibility is poor.

2   **Maximal Prompting**—Able to write some letters spontaneously. Able to trace or copy letters and numbers.

1   **Total Assistance**—Unable to copy letters or simple shapes.

Continued

Functional Assessment Measures (FAM)—*cont'd*

21. SPEECH INTELLIGIBILITY

7   **Complete Independence**—Able to converse with well articulated, well modulated articulation and voice. No difficulty understanding what is being said.

6   **Modified Independence**—Evidence of minor sound distortions but generally adequate intelligibility. Speaking rate may be reduced.

5   **Standby Prompting**—Speech intelligibility is always reduced. Articulation is consistently distorted. May attempt self-corrections.

4   **Minimal Prompting**—Able to intelligibly produce single words and simple phrases. General conversation intelligibility.

3   **Moderate Prompting**—Can produce single syllable words with adequate intelligibility. Listener burden evident for sentences or longer verbalization.

2   **Maximal Prompting**—Can produce vowels, some consonants. Can imitate some single words but productions may require listener guessing.

1   **Total Assistance**—No intelligible speech.

Psychosocial adjustment items

22. SOCIAL INTERACTION   Includes skills related to getting along and participating with others in therapeutic and social situations. It represents how one deals with one's own needs and the needs of others.

7   **Complete Independence**—Interacts appropriately with staff, other patients, and family members (e.g., controls temper, accepts criticism, is aware that words and actions have an impact on others).

6   **Modified Independence**—Interacts with staff, other patients, and family members in structured situations or modified environments.

Helper

5   **Supervision**—Requires supervision (e.g., standby, cuing, or coaxing) only under stressful or unfamiliar conditions, but no more than 10% of the time.

4   **Minimal Direction**—Interacts appropriately 75% to 90% of the time.

3   **Moderate Direction**—Interacts appropriately 50% to 74% of the time.

2   **Maximal Direction**—Interacts appropriately 24% to 49% of the time. May need restraint occasionally.

1   **Total Assistance**—Interacts appropriately less than 25% of the time. May need restraint continuously.

Examples of socially inappropriate behaviors: temper tantrums, loud, foul, or abusive language, excessive laughing, crying, physical attack.

23. EMOTIONAL ADJUSTMENT   Includes frequency and severity of depression, anxiety, frustration, lability, unresponsiveness, agitation, interference with progress in therapies and/or homelife, ability to cope with and take responsibility for emotional behavior.

7   **Complete Independence**—Patient rarely exhibits depression, anxiety, frustration, lability and/or agitation and is effectively able to control this behavior reflecting self responsibility and involvement in treatment and homelife.

6   **Modified Independence**—Patient may exhibit occassional but minimal depression, anxiety, frustration, lability and/or agitation. Coping skills are adequate to keep distress within manageable limits. Behavior does not interfere with progress in therapies and/or homelife.

5   **Supervision**—Patient exhibits occassional and mild depression, anxiety, frustration, lability and/or agitation. Patient has assumed responsibility for most of this behavior and is learning to cope with his/her condition. This behavior does not significantly interfere with progress in therapies.

4   **Minimal Direction**—Patient exhibits frequent and moderate depression, anxiety, frustration, lability and/or agitation. Patient is assuming more responsibility for this behavior and it interferes with progress in therapies and/or homelife less than 25% of the time.

Functional Assessment Measures (FAM)—*cont'd*

---

23. EMOTIONAL ADJUSTMENT—cont'd

3   **Moderate Direction**—Patient exhibits frequent and moderate depression, anxiety, frustration, lability and/or agitation. Patient is beginning to assume responsibility for some behavior but this behavior still interferes with progress in therapies and/or homelife 25-50% of the time.

2   **Maximal Direction**—Patient exhibits constant and severe depression, anxiety, frustration, lability and/or agitation. Patient is rarely able to control this behavior and this behavior interferes with progress in therapies and/or homelife 50-75% of the time.

1   **Total Assistance**—Patient exhibits constant and severe depression, anxiety, frustration, lability, unresponsiveness, and/or agitation. Patient is unaware and unable to control this behavior which continually interferes with progress in therapies and/or homelife more than 75% of the time.

24. ADJUSTMENT TO LIMITATIONS   Includes denial/awareness, acceptance of limitations, willingness to learn new ways of functioning, compensating, taking appropriate safely precautions, and realistic expectations for long term recovery.

7   **Complete Independence**—Patient demonstrates ability to compensate for limitations which are the result of the patient's disease or injury, exercises safe judgement in ADL's, and has realistic expectations for long term recovery.

6   **Modified Independence**—Patient may have some denial of physical, emotional or social limitations, but this denial does not interfere with progress in therapy and/or homelife. Patient compensates for most of these limitations and has learned new ways of functioning. Patient may have some unrealistic expectations for long term recovery. Patient exercises safe judgement in ADL's most of the time.

5   **Supervision**—Patient's denial of physical, emotional and social limitations interferes with progress in therapies less than 25% of the time. Patient is beginning to compensate for some of these limitations and is willing to learn new ways of functioning. Patient may still have unrealistic expectations for long term recovery. Patient exercises safe judgement in ADL's 75% of the time.

4   **Minimal Direction**—Patient's denial of limitations interferes with progress in therapies and/or homelife 25-50% of the time. Patient resists compensating for limitations and learning new ways of functioning.

3   **Moderate Direction**—Patient may have some awareness of physical, emotional, or social limitations which are the result of the patient's disease or injury. Denial of limitations interferes with progress in therapies and/or homelife 50-75% of the time.

2   **Maximal Direction**—Patient may have limited awareness of physical, emotional, or social limitations which are the result of the patient's injury or disease. Denial of limitations interferes with progress in therapies and/or homelife 75-100% of the time.

1   **Total Assistance**—Patient has no awareness of physical, emotional or social limitations which are the result of the patient's disease or injury. Patient's denial of these limitations continually interferes with progress in therapies and/or homelife.

Continued

Functional Assessment Measures (FAM)—cont'd

25. VOCATIONAL RE-ENTRY	The term employed as used in this scale represents a job in one or more of the following categories:
	• in the regular workforce
	• in a sheltered workshop
	• as a student
	• as a homemaker
	• as a community service volunteer
	Score to be assessed on the basis of a combination of the above if patient is involved in more than one activity.
7	**Complete Independence**—Patient is successfully employed full time.
6	**Modified Independence**—Patient is employed part time, with an adjusted workload, requires an assistive device, requires more than a reasonable time to do the job, or there are safety consideration.
5	**Supervision**—Patient is involved in a retraining program to develop necessary skills for employment (i.e., vocational retraining, O.T. for homemaking training) and requires supervision.
4	**Minimal Assistance**—Patient is involved in a retraining program and requires minimal assistance.
3	**Moderate Assistance**—Patient is involved in a retraining program and requires moderate assistance.
2	**Maximal Assistance**—Patient is able to participate in a retraining program on a limited basis, has made the necessary contacts but has not actively enrolled and requires maximal assistance with job related tasks.
1	**Total Assistance**—Patient is unable to regain employment or develop necessary employment skills and requires total assistance.

Cognitive function items

26. PROBLEM SOLVING	Includes skills related to solving problems of daily living. This means making reasonable, safe, and prudent decisions regarding financial, social and personal affairs and initiating, sequencing and self-correcting tasks and activities to solve the problems.

No helper

7	**Complete Independence**—Consistently makes appropriate decisions, initiates and carries out a sequence of steps to solve problem until task is completed, and self-corrects if errors are made.
6	**Modified Independence**—Has some difficulty deciding, initiating, sequencing, or self-correcting in unfamiliar situations.

Helper

5	**Supervision or Setup**—Requires supervision (e.g., cuing, or coaxing) to solve problems only under stressful or unfamiliar conditions, but no more than 10% of the time.
4	**Minimal Contact Assistance**—Solves problems 75% to 90% of the time.
3	**Moderate Assistance**—Solves problems 50% to 74% of the time.
2	**Maximal Assistance**—Solves problems 25% to 49% of the time. Needs direction more than half the time.
1	**Total Assistance**—Solves problems less than 25% of the time or does not effectively solve problems.

Examples: Adapting to a change in hospital schedule. Getting food into the house either by shopping or arranging to have food or meals brought in.

Functional Assessment Measures (FAM)—*cont'd*

---

27. MEMORY   Includes skills related to awareness in performing daily activities in an institutional or community setting. It includes ability to store and retrieve information, particularly verbal and visual. A deficit in memory impairs learning as well as performance of tasks.

No helper

7   **Complete Independence**—Recognizes people frequently encountered and remembers daily routines; executes requests of others without need for repetition.

6   **Modified Independence**—Has some difficulty recognizing people, remembering daily routines and requests of others. May use self-initiated or environmental cues, prompts or aids.

Helper

5   **Supervision**—Requires prompting (e.g., cuing, or coaxing) only under stressful or unfamiliar conditions, but no more than 10% of the time.

4   **Minimal Prompting**—Recognizes and remembers 75% to 90% of the time.

3   **Moderate Prompting**—Recognizes and remembers 50% to 74% of the time.

2   **Maximal Prompting**—Recognizes and remembers 25% to 49% of the time. Needs prompting more than half the time.

1   **Total Assistance**—Recognizes and remembers less than 25% of the time or does not effectively recognize and remember.

28. ORIENTATION   Includes consistent orientation to person, place, time and situation.

7   **Complete Independence**—Completely oriented to person, place, time and situation 100% of the time without cues.

6   **Modified Independence**—Patient may require more than a reasonable amount of time but without cues.

5   **Supervision**—Patient requires cueing less than 25% of the time.

4   **Minimal Prompting**—Patient requires minimal assistance and is oriented 75% of the time.

3   **Moderate Prompting**—Patient requires moderate assistance and is oriented 50-75% of the time.

2   **Maximal**—Patient requires maximal assistance and is oriented 25-50% of the time.

1   **Total Assistance**—Patient is consistently disoriented to person, place, time and situation. Total assistance is required. Patient is oriented less than 25% of the time.

29. ATTENTION SPAN   Includes distractibility, level of alertness and responsiveness, ability to concentrate on a task, ability to follow directions, immediate recall as the structure, difficulty and length of task varies.

7   **Complete Independence**—Patient is able to concentrate on complex tasks for one hour or more without structure. Patient can independently initiate and complete most tasks.

6   **Modified Independence**—Patient is able to concentrate on more complex tasks for longer periods of time (30 to 40 minutes), but still requires some structure. Patient may be distracted occassionally but can resume the task. Patient is able to immediately recall most past activities.

5   **Supervision**—Patient exhibits differentiated and purposeful responses to environmental stimuli 75-100% of the time. Selected attention to tasks may be impaired especially with difficult or unstructured tasks, but is now functional for common daily activities (20 to 30 minutes). Patient is mildly distractible and immediate recall is somewhat impaired.

Continued

Functional Assessment Measures (FAM)—*cont'd*

---

29. ATTENTION SPAN—cont'd

4   **Minimal Direction**—Patient exhibits differentiated and purposeful responses to environmental stimuli 50-75% of the time. Patient appears alert and is able to respond to simple commands fairly consistently. As the difficulty or length of the task increases, patient is more easily distracted and requires frequent structure or redirection back to the task. Patient is able to concentrate on simple tasks for 10 to 20 minutes. Patient's immediate recall of activities is limited.

3   **Moderate Direction**—Patient's attention span is easily aroused and patient exhibits differentiated and purposeful responses to environmental stimuli 25-50% of the time. Patient is able to concentrate on simple tasks for less than 10 minutes. Patient is able to follow one or two step directions, but as the difficulty and length of the task increase, patient is more easily distracted and responses are delayed. Frequent cues may be necessary to maintain patient's attention.

2   **Maximal Direction**—Patient inconsistently exhibits differentiated and purposeful responses to environmental stimuli. Patient may be able to concentrate on simple tasks, follow one step directions for short periods of time with delayed responses. Continuous cues may be necessary to maintain patient's attention for short periods of time (one to two minutes).

1   **Total Assistance**—Patient exhibits non-purposeful and undifferentiated responses to environmental stimuli. Patient is unable to concentrate on a task or follow directions, and is easily and continually distracted.

The Self-Care Assessment Schedule (SCAS)

This self-administered questionnaire is designed to be used with psychiatric clients, measuring the frequency of ten self-care behaviors (see Barnes and Benjamin, 1987 and Benjamin and Barnes, 1987). Behaviors measured are up and dressed before 10 AM; self-maintenance of tidy hair and appearance; bath or shower without assistance; prepared a meal; lay on a bed between 10 AM and 4 PM; dressed without assistance; being outside of home; eaten a meal in bed; shopping; and cleaned or tidied home.

SUMMARY

Use of an organized functional assessment is recommended for all clients whose daily activities may be affected by impairments or disabilities: The elderly and the handicapped are the more obvious examples of such groups. The literature has shown that health care providers often do superficial assessments of this area and may not appreciate the client's capabilities or limitations. This lack of appreciation may cause inappropriate treatment, lack of support, and neglect of problems that may be treatable.

The approaches and tools presented in this chapter have some use across the range of settings and circumstances in which health assessments are done. Because the functional assessment is not commonly a component of the health assessment, a standardized approach across practitioners does not exist for general populations. Therefore, the practitioner is advised to explore the measurement options and to select and use, as indicated, a tool that is most applicable and useful.

Functional Assessment Worksheet

Rating Scale: 7 Complete Independence (Timely, safely)
                  6 Modified Independence (Extra time, device)
                  5 Supervision
                  4 Minimal Assist (subject 75% of task)
                  3 Moderate Assist (50-74% of task)
                  2 Maximal Assist (25-49% of task)
                  1 Total Assist (subject 25% of task)

Self-care items

   1. Feeding   Adm _____ Goal _____ D/C _____ F/U _____
   2. Grooming   Adm _____ Goal _____ D/C _____ F/U _____
   3. Bathing Technique _____   Adm _____ Goal _____ D/C _____ F/U _____
   4. Dressing Upper Body   Adm _____ Goal _____ D/C _____ F/U _____
   5. Dressing Lower Body   Adm _____ Goal _____ D/C _____ F/U _____
   6. Toileting   Adm _____ Goal _____ D/C _____ F/U _____
* 7. Swallowing   Adm _____ Goal _____ D/C _____ F/U _____

Sphincter control

   8. Bladder Management   Adm _____ Goal _____ D/C _____ F/U _____
   9. Bowel Management   Adm _____ Goal _____ D/C _____ F/U _____

Mobility items
Transfers technique _____

  10. Bed, Chair, Wheelchair   Adm _____ Goal _____ D/C _____ F/U _____
  11. Toilet   Adm _____ Goal _____ D/C _____ F/U _____
  12. Tub or Shower   Adm _____ Goal _____ D/C _____ F/U _____
*13. Car Transfers   Adm _____ Goal _____ D/C _____ F/U _____

Locomotion

  14. Walking/Wheelchair   Adm _____ Goal _____ D/C _____ F/U _____
  15. Stairs   Adm _____ Goal _____ D/C _____ F/U _____
*16. Community Mobility   Adm _____ Goal _____ D/C _____ F/U _____

Communication items

  17. Comprehension   Adm _____ Goal _____ D/C _____ F/U _____
  18. Expression   Adm _____ Goal _____ D/C _____ F/U _____
*19. Reading   Adm _____ Goal _____ D/C _____ F/U _____
*20. Writing   Adm _____ Goal _____ D/C _____ F/U _____
*21. Speech Intelligibility   Adm _____ Goal _____ D/C _____ F/U _____

Psychosocial adjustment items

  22. Social Interaction   Adm _____ Goal _____ D/C _____ F/U _____
*23. Emotional Adjustment   Adm _____ Goal _____ D/C _____ F/U _____
*24. Adjustment to Limitations   Adm _____ Goal _____ D/C _____ F/U _____
*25. Vocational Re-entry   D/C _____ F/U _____

Cognitive function

  26. Problem Solving   Adm _____ Goal _____ D/C _____ F/U _____
  27. Memory   Adm _____ Goal _____ D/C _____ F/U _____
*28. Orientation   Adm _____ Goal _____ D/C _____ F/U _____
*29. Attention   Adm _____ Goal _____ D/C _____ F/U _____

---

*Added to the FIM (Functional Independent Measure) tool. D/C = at discharge; F/U = at follow-up.

BIBLIOGRAPHY

Barnes D and Benjamin S: The self-care assessment schedule (SCAS)—I. The purpose and construction of a new assessment of self care behaviors, J Psychosom Res 31:191-202, 1987.

Barnes D and Benjamin S: The self-care assessment schedule (SCAS)—II. Reliability and validity, J Psychosom Res 31:203-214, 1987.

Boies AH: Activities of daily living, Home Healthcare Nurse 5:40-41, 1987.

Bower FN and Patterson J: A theory-based nursing assessment of the aged, Top Clin Nurs 8:22-32, 1984.

Brorsson B and Asberg KH: Katz index of independence in ADL: Reliability and validity in short-term care, Scand J Rehabil Med 16:125-132, 1984.

Buchanan B: Functional assessment: Measurement with the Barthel Index and PULSES profile, Home Healthcare Nurse 4:11-17, 1986.

Forer SK: Revised functional status rating instrument, Glendale, Calif: 1981, Rehabilitation Institute, Glendale Adventist Medical Center.

Fortinsky RH, Granger GB, and Seltzer GB: The use of functional assessment in understanding home care needs, Med Care 19:489-497, 1981.

Fuhrer M, editor: Rehabilitation outcomes: analysis and measurement, Baltimore, 1987, Brookes.

Golden RR, Teresi JA, and Gurland BJ: Development of indicator scales for the comprehensive assessment and referral evaluation (CARE) interview schedule, J Gerontol 39:138-146, 1984.

Granger CV: Health accounting-functional assessment of the long-term patient. In Kottke FJ, Stillwell GK, and Lehmann JF, editors: Krusen's handbook of physical medicine and rehabilitation, ed 3, Philadelphia, 1982, WB Saunders Co.

Granger CV, Albrecht GL, and Hamilton BB: Outcome of comprehensive medical rehabilitation: measurement by PULSES profile and the Barthel Index, Arch Phys Med Rehabil 60:145-154, 1979.

Granger CV and Gresham G, editors: Functional assessment in rehabilitation medicine, Baltimore, 1984, Williams & Wilkins.

Granger CV, Hamilton BB, Keith RA and others: Advances in functional assessment for medical rehabilitation, Topics Clin Rehabil 1:59-74, 1986.

Granger CV, Seltzer GB, and Fishbein CF: Primary care of the functionally disabled: assessment and management, Philadelphia, 1987, JB Lippincott Co.

Gulick EE: The self-assessment of health among the chronically ill, Top Clin Nurs 8:74-82, 1986.

Gurland B, Kuriansky J, Sharpe L and others: The comprehensive assessment and referral evaluation (CARE)—rationale, development and reliability, Int J Aging Human Develop 8:9-42, 1977.

Gurland B, Golden RR, Teresi JA, and Challop J: The SHORT-CARE: an efficient instrument for the assessment of depression, dementia, and disability, J Gerontol 39:166-169, 1984.

Gurland BJ and Wilder DE: The CARE interview revisited: Development of an efficient systematic clinical assessment, J Gerontol 39:129-137, 1984.

Hamilton GG, Granger CV, Sherwin FS and others: A uniform national data system for medical rehabilitation. In Fuhrer MJ, editor: Rehabilitation outcomes: analysis and measurement, Baltimore, 1987, Brookes, pp 137-147.

Hertanu JS, Demopoulos JT, Yang WC and others: Stroke rehabilitation: correlation and prognostic value of computerized to-mography and sequential functional assessments, Arch Phys Med Rehabil 65:505-508, 1984.

Iverson IA, Silberg NE, Stever RC, and Schoening HA: The revised Kenny self-care evaluation: a numerical measure of independence in activities of daily living, Minneapolis, 1973, Sister Kenny Institute.

Jacelon CS: The Barthel index and other indices of functional ability, Rehab Nurs 11:9-11, 1986.

Jette AM: State of the art in functional status assessment. In Rothstein JM: Measurement in physical therapy, New York, 1985, Churchill Livingstone, pp 137-168.

Katz S and Akpom CA: Index of ADL, Med Care 14:116-118, 1976.

Katz S, Ford AB, Moskowitz RW and others: Studies of illness in the aged. The index of ADL: a standardized measure of biological and psychosocial function, JAMA 185:914-919, 1963.

Keith RA: Functional assessment measures in medical rehabilitation: Current status, Arch Phys Med Rehabil 65:74-78, 1984.

Keith RA, Granger CV, Hamilton BB, and Sherwin FS: The functional independence measure: a new tool for rehabilitation. In Eisenberg MG and Grzesiak RC, editors: Advances in clinical rehabilitation, Vol 1, New York, 1987, Spring, pp 6-18.

Lawton MP: Assessing the competence of older people. In Kent D, Kastenbaum R, and Sherwood S, editors: Research planning and action for the elderly, New York, 1972, Behavioral Publications.

Lawton MP and Brody EM: Assessment of older people: Self-maintaining and instrumental activities of daily living, Gerontologist 9:180, 1969.

Linn MW and Linn BS: The rapid disability rating scale-2, J Am Geriatr Soc 30:378-382, 1982.

Mahoney FI and Barthel DW: Functional evaluation: the Barthel index, Maryland State Med J 14:61, 1965.

McDowell I and Newell C: Measuring health: a guide to rating scales and questionnaires, New York, 1987, Oxford University Press.

McGinnis GE, Seward ML, DeJong G, and Osberg JS: Program evaluation of physical medicine and rehabilitation departments using self-report Barthel, Arch Phys Med Rehabil 67:123-125, 1986.

Moskowitz E and McCann CB: Classification of disability in the chronically ill and aging, J Chronic Dis 5:342-346, 1957.

Moskowitz E: PULSES Profile in retrospect, Arch Phys Rehabil 66:647-648, 1985.

Nagi S: Disability, concepts and prevalence. Unpublished paper presented at the First Mary Switzer Memorial Seminar, Cleveland, Ohio, May 1975.

Ninos M and Makohon R: Functional assessment of the patient, Geriatric Nurs 6:139-142, 1985.

Nolan BS: Functional evaluation of the elderly in guardianship proceedings, Law, Medicine and Healthcare, 12:210-218, 1984.

O'Toole DM, Goldberg RT, and Ryan B: Functional changes in vascular amputee patients: Evaluation by Barthel, PULSES profile and ESCROW scale, Arch Phys Med Rehabil 66:508-511, 1985.

Pfeffer RI, Kurosaki TT, Chance JM and others: Index in older adults: reliability, validity, and measurement of change over time, Am J Epidemiol 120:922-935, 1984.

Pinholt EM, Kroenke K, Hanley JF and others: Functional assessment of the elderly: a comparison of standard instruments with clinical judgment, Arch Int Med 147:484-488, 1987.

Reisberg B, Ferris SH, and Franssen E: An ordinal functional assessment tool for Alzheimer's type dementia, Hospital Community Psychiatr 36:593-595, 1985.

Rothstein JM: Measurement in physical therapy, New York, 1985, Churchill Livingstone.

Rubenstein LZ, Schairer C, Weiland GD, and Kane R: Systematic biases in functional status assessment of elderly adults: Effects of different data sources, J Gerontol 39:686-691, 1984.

Sheikh K, Smith DS, Meade TW and others: Repeatability and validity of a modified Activities of Daily Living (ADL) index in studies of chronic disability, Int Rehab Med 1:51, 1979.

Spiegel JS, Hirshfield MS, and Spiegel TM: Evaluation self-care activities: Comparison of a self-reported questionnaire with an occupational therapist interview, Br J Rheumatol 24:357-361, 1985.

Teresi JA, Golden RR, and Gurland BJ: Concurrent and predictive validity of indicator scales developed for the comprehensive assessment and referral evaluation interview schedule, J Gerontol 39:158-165, 1984.

Teresi JA, Golden RR and others: Construct validity of indicator scales developed from the comprehensive assessment and referral evaluation interview schedule, J Gerontol 39:147-157, 1984.

Wood P: Classification of impairments and handicaps, Geneva, 1975, World Health Organization.

World Health Organization: International classification of impairments, disabilities, and handicaps, Geneva, 1980, The Organization.

Using Health Assessment Data

28

Integration of the physical assessment and documentation

OBJECTIVES

Upon successful review of this chapter, learners will be able to:

- List equipment and supplies generally needed for a complete physical examination

- Prepare clients for a complete physical examination

- Outline and perform procedures of a complete physical examination

- Record concise findings from a complete physical examination

- Use guidelines to adapt examination techniques that accommodate individual client needs

This chapter discusses two issues relating to the complete physical assessment: the performance of an integrated, screening physical examination and the recording of the physical examination.

PERFORMANCE OF INTEGRATED SCREENING PHYSICAL EXAMINATION

After practicing and acquiring proficiency in the performance of regional examinations, the student is advised to develop a procedure for performing an integrated physical examination. In actual practice, the examiner will perform complete regional examinations, such as in acute care settings, as well as complete examinations, such as in health maintenance or screening situations.

In developing a personal routine for a complete examination, the student should consider factors of efficiency and client comfort. If procedures are performed systematically and efficiently, time is conserved and the examiner is less likely to forget a procedure or a part of the body than if the examination were performed haphazardly.

Clients who are ill or debilitated lose energy quickly. Developing a system of examination that requires the fewest number of client position changes will enhance acceptability and decrease the number of examinations and portions of examinations that must be deferred because of client intolerance.

The manner in which the examiner conducts the physical examination can enhance or compromise rapport developed during the history-taking interview. A disorganized examiner who leaves the room to obtain missing equipment, who runs around the examination table several times in a short period, or who has the client change positions frequently may lose the client's confidence.

Equipment and Supplies

The equipment and supplies generally needed for a complete physical examination include the following:

Cotton balls
Cotton swabs
Flashlight
Gauze
Marking pencil
Materials to test pain and light touch sensation
Measuring tape
Nasal speculum
Odoriferous substances
Ophthalmoscope
Otoscope
Printed material for visual acuity and comprehension examination
Reflex hammer
Rubber gloves
Ruler
Snellen's eye chart
Sphygmomanometer
Stethoscope with diaphram and bell heads
Substances for taste sensation evaluation
Thermometer
Tongue blades
Tuning forks
Watch with a second hand

If a pelvic or a rectal examination is to be done, the following equipment and supplies are also needed:

Lubricant
Materials to process vaginal secretions or specimens for laboratory examination
Materials to examine fecal material for occult blood
Mirror
Vaginal speculums

The outline presented here is a suggested procedure for performing the physical examination. It is intended as a guide for the beginning practitioner for use in practice sessions. In actual client care situations, this outline may require adaption because of the client's age or disability, examination protocols and priorities of the care agency, or examiner preference.

The suggested procedure is organized to avoid excessive movement of the client or examiner. Examination of body systems is integrated into the examination of body regions. A list of equipment and supplies is given in the box on above.

The physical examination should occur in a comfortable room that allows for privacy and a reasonable amount of space for client and examiner movement (see the box opposite). The needed equipment in the examination room includes the following:

Examining table
Desk with two chairs
Stool
Examination lamp
Stand or counter to hold supplies
Scale
Sink

Outline for Examination

I. Client enters examination room and initiates encounter; examiner observes client.
   A. Observe general appearance.
      1. Observe skin color.
      2. Observe appearance.
      3. Observe facial expression.
      4. Assess state of nutrition.
   B. Observe stature.
      1. Assess symmetry.
      2. Observe posture.
      3. Assess body build.
      4. Observe gait.
   C. Observe demeanor.
      1. Observe composure.
      2. Observe speech.
      3. Assess mental status.
      4. Assess disposition.
II. Measurements are taken.
   A. Measure weight.
   B. Measure height.
   C. Take temperature.
III. *Client* is sitting on the bed or examination table, head and shoulders uncovered. *Examiner* is facing client (Fig. 28-1).
   A. Observe generally.
   B. Observe and palpate upper extremities.
      1. Examine skin (color, temperature, vascularity, lesions, hydration, turgor, texture, edema, masses), muscle mass, and skeletal configuration.
      2. Examine nails (color and condition).
   C. Assess pulses (radial and brachial).
   D. Measure blood pressure (both arms).
   E. Measure respiration.

Preparation for the Examination

- Orient client to the examination
- Have client empty bladder
- Check for availability of needed materials
- Have client undress and put on gown

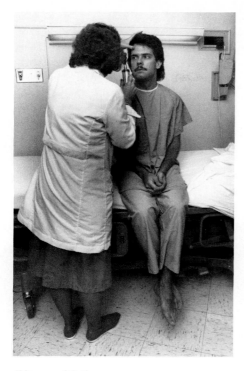

Figure 28-1

Client seated; examiner facing client.

F. Examine head.
   1. Observe configuration of skull.
   2. Observe scalp, face, and hair.
   3. Palpate head, face, and hair.
   4. Palpate paranasal sinus areas.
G. Examine eyes.
   1. Measure visual acuity (cranial nerve [CN] II).
   2. Assess visual fields (CN II).
   3. Determine alignment of eyes (perform cover test and light reflex).
   4. Test extraocular movements (CN III, CN IV, CN VI).
   5. Observe eyebrows, eyelids, conjunctiva, cornea, sclera, iris, and palpebral fissures.
   6. Palpate lacrimal organs.
   7. Test pupillary responses (light and accommodation).
   8. Perform ophthalmoscopic examination of lens, media, and retina (CN II).
H. Examine ears.
   1. Inspect auricle.
   2. Palpate auricle.
   3. Perform otoscopic examination. (Inspect canals and drums.)
   4. Determine auditory acuity (CN VIII).
   5. Perform Weber's and Rinne tests.

I. Examine nose.
   1. Determine patency of each nostril.
   2. Test for olfaction (CN I).
   3. Determine position of septum.
   4. Inspect mucosa, septum, and turbinates with nasal speculum.
J. Examine mouth and pharynx.
   1. Inspect lips, total buccal mucosa, teeth, gums, tongue, sublingual area, roof of mouth, tonsillar area, and pharynx.
   2. Test glossopharyngeal nerve (CN IX) and vagus nerve (CN X) ("ah" and gag reflex).
   3. Test hypoglossal nerve (CN XII) (tongue movement).
   4. Test taste (CN VII).
K. Complete examination of cranial nerves.
   1. Test trigeminal nerve (CN V) (jaw clenching, lateral jaw movements, corneal reflex, pain, and light touch to face).
   2. Test facial nerve (CN VII). (Client raises eyebrows, shows teeth, puffs cheeks, keeps eyes closed against resistance.)
   3. Test spinal accessory nerve (CN XI) (trapezius and sternocleidomastoid muscles).
L. Palpate temporomandibular joint.
M. Observe range of motion of the head and neck.
N. Palpate nodes (preauricular, posterior auricular, occipital, tonsillar, submaxillary, submental, anterior cervical, posterior cervical, supraclavicular, and infraclavicular nodes).
O. Palpate carotid arteries.
P. Palpate thyroid gland.
Q. Palpate for position of trachea.
R. Auscultate carotid arteries and thyroid gland.
IV. *Client* is sitting on the bed or examining table, total chest uncovered if male, breasts covered if female (Fig. 28-2). *Examiner* is standing behind client.
A. Examine back.
   1. Inspect spine.
   2. Palpate spine.
   3. Inspect skin and thoracic configuration.
   4. Palpate muscles and bones.
   5. Palpate costovertebral area, asking client about tenderness.
B. Examine lungs (apices and lateral and posterior areas). NOTE: Apical, posterior, and lateral lung regions can usually be examined from a position behind client.
   1. Observe respiration and total thorax.
   2. Palpate for thoracic expansion and tactile fremitus.
   3. Percuss systematically.
   4. Determine diaphragmatic excursion.

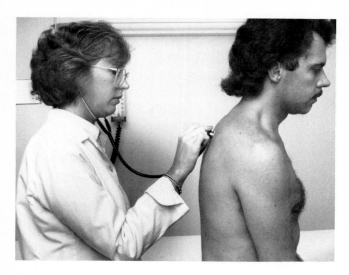

Figure 28-2

Client seated; examiner behind client.

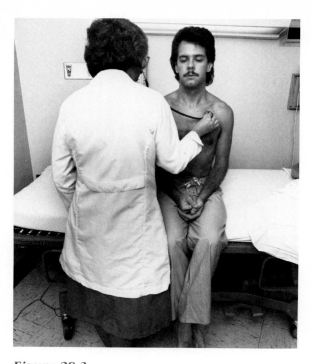

Figure 28-3

Client seated (uncovered to waist); examiner facing client.

5. Auscultate systematically.
6. Auscultate for vocal fremitus.
V. *Client* is sitting on the bed or examining table, uncovered to the waist. *Examiner* is facing client (Fig. 28-3).
   A. Examine breasts.
      1. Observe breasts with client's arms and hands at the side; above the head; and pressed into the hips, eliciting pectoral contraction.
      2. Observe breasts with client leaning forward.
      3. Ask client about lesions; if present, palpate them.
      4. If large breasts, perform a bimanual examination.
   B. Palpate axillary nodes.
   C. Examine lungs (anterior areas).
      1. Inspect configuration and skin.
      2. Palpate for tactile fremitus.
      3. Percuss lungs systematically.
      4. Auscultate lungs systematically.
   D. Examine heart.
      1. Inspect precordium.
      2. Palpate precordium.
      3. Auscultate precordium.
      4. Observe external jugular vein and internal jugular pulsations.
VI. *Client* is supine. *Examiner* is at the right side of client (Fig. 28-4).
   A. Examine breasts.
      1. Palpate breasts systematically.
      2. Attempt to express secretion from the nipples.

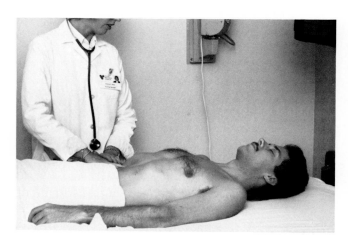

Figure 28-4

Client lying on back; examiner at client's right side.

   B. Examine heart.
      1. Inspect precordium.
      2. Palpate precordium.
      3. Auscultate precordium.
      4. Observe jugular venous pulses and pressures (elevate client to 45 degrees if possible).
   C. Measure blood pressure (both arms).
   D. Examine abdomen.
      1. Inspect abdomen.
      2. Auscultate bowel sounds, aorta, renal arteries, and femoral arteries.

3. Percuss and measure liver.
4. Percuss spleen.
5. Palpate liver, spleen, inguinal and femoral node and hernia areas, general abdomen, and femoral pulses systematically.
6. Test abdominal reflexes.

E. Examine genitals of male client.
1. Inspect penis, uretheral opening, and scrotum.
2. Palpate scrotal contents.

F. Examine lower extremities.
1. Inspect skin, hair distribution, muscle mass, and skeletal configuration.
2. Palpate for temperature, texture, edema, popliteal pulses, posterior tibial pulses, and dorsal pedal pulses.
3. Test range of motion.
4. Test strength.
5. Test sensation (pain, light touch, and vibration).
6. Test position sense.

VII. *Client* is sitting on the bed or examining table. *Examiner* is standing in front of client (Fig. 28-5).
A. Assess neural system.
1. Elicit deep tendon reflexes (biceps, triceps, brachioradialis, patellar, and Achilles reflexes).
2. Test for Babinski's reflex.
3. Test for coordination of upper and lower extremities.

B. Test upper extremities for strength, range of motion sensation, vibration, and position.

VIII. *Client* is standing. *Examiner* is standing next to client (Fig. 28-6).
A. Examine spine.
1. Observe with client bending over.
2. Test for range of motion.

B. Assess neural system.
1. Observe gait.
2. Perform Romberg test.
3. Observe heel and toe walks.

C. Test for inguinal and femoral hernias.

IX. *Female client* is in lithotomy position, genital area uncovered. *Examiner* is sitting, facing the genital area.
A. Examine genitalia.
1. Inspect genitalia.
2. Palpate external genital area.
3. Perform speculum examination.
4. Take smears and cultures.
5. Perform bimanual vaginal examination.

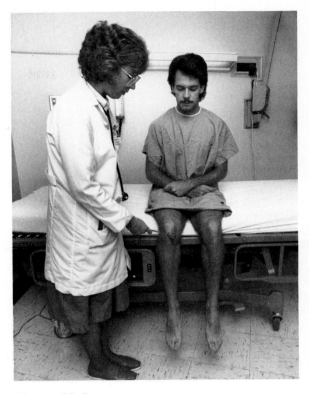

Figure 28-5

Client seated; examiner facing client.

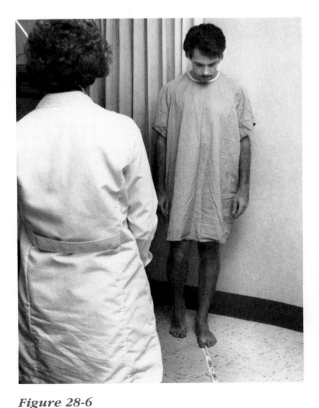

Figure 28-6

Client standing; examiner standing.

B. Examine rectum: perform bimanual rectovaginal examination.

X. *Male client* is standing and leaning over examination table.
  A. Examine rectum.
  B. Palpate rectum.
  C. Palpate prostrate.
  D. Palpate seminal vesicles.

RECORDING OF THE PHYSICAL EXAMINATION

In recording the physical examination, the practitioner is continuously attempting to achieve a balance between conciseness and comprehensiveness. The record should describe what was seen, heard, palpated, and percussed. Whenever appropriate, the exact description is written; evaluations such as "normal," "good," or "poor" are avoided or used judiciously. Too frequently, a major system, such as the cardiovascular system, is described in one word, "normal." This description does not indicate what components of that system were assessed or the examiner's parameters of normal.

Conciseness is achieved through the use of outlines, phrases, and abbreviations. Grammar is sacrificed, and only essential words are written. Often it is helpful to use a form for recording the physical examination. A form provides an outline into which data can be entered. Forms serve as reminders for completeness. They also save time. And, if they are systematically used by all the members of a health care system, they are extremely useful as indexes for rapid information retrieval.

As recommended in the recording of the history (see Chapter 5 on the health history), the beginning practitioner should overrecord and include all findings from the examination. With increased skill and discrimination regarding the significance of findings, the practitioner will be able to weed out the irrelevant information and consolidate the significant data.

Table 28-1 is a guideline designed to assist the beginning recorder (see also the box below). The first column indicates the body systems or regions that are

Text continued on p. 717.

Guidelines for Recording the Physical Examination

- Be complete
- Be concise
- Be specific
- Avoid using the terms "negative," "normal," and "good"
- Use agreed-on and understood abbreviations

Table 28-1

Areas and examples of recording for the physical examination

Area of examination	Descriptions usually recorded	Descriptions recorded in detail if abnormalities are present (partial listing only)	Examples of recording

Vital signs	Temperature: oral or rectal
	Pulse
	Respiration
	Blood pressure: both arms in at least two positions (lying and sitting recommended)
	Weight: indicate if client is clothed or unclothed
	Height: without shoes
		Blood pressure in standing position and in both thighs	T: 98.6°F (oral)
			P: 76/min—strong and regular: R: 16/min
			BP:
			  Lying: R, 110/70/60; L, 112/68/60
			  Sitting: R, 116/74/67; L, 120/76/65
			Wt: 130 lb, unclothed
			Ht: 5 ft 3 in

General health	Appearance as relative to chronologic age Apparent state of health Awareness Personal appearance Emotional status Nutritional status Affect Response Cooperation	Handshake Speech Respiratory difficulties Gross deformity Movements Unusual behavior	Slightly obese, alert, white male who looks younger than his stated age of 45. Moves without difficulty; no gross abnormalities apparent. Appears healthy and in no acute distress; is neatly dressed, responsive, and cooperative. Responds appropriately; smiles frequently.

Table 28-1

Areas and examples of recording for the physical examination—*cont'd*

Area of examination	Descriptions usually recorded	Descriptions recorded in detail if abnormalities are present (partial listing only)	Examples of recording
Skin and mucous membranes	Color Edema Moisture Temperature Texture Turgor	Discharge Drainage Lesions: distribution, type, configuration Superficial vascularity Mobility Thickness	*Skin:* Uniformly brown in color; soft, warm, moist, elastic, of normal thickness. No edema or lesions. *Mucous membranes:* Pink, moist, slightly pale.
Nails	Color of beds Texture	Lesions Abnormalities in size or shape Presence of clubbing	Nail beds pink, texture hard, no clubbing.
Hair and scalp	Quantity Distribution Color Texture	Lesions Parasites	*Hair:* Normal male distribution; thick, curly; black color with graying at temples. *Scalp:* Clean, no lesions.
Cranium	Contour Tenderness	Lesions	Normocephalic, no tenderness.
Face	Symmetry Movements Sinuses CN V CN VII	Tenderness Edema Lesions Parotid gland	Symmetric at rest and with movement. Jaw muscles strong, no crepitations or limitation in movement of temporomandibular joint. Sinus areas not tender. Sensory: pain and light touch intact.
Eyes	Visual acuity Visual fields Alignment of eyes Alignment of eyelids Movement of eyelids Conjunctiva Sclera Cornea Anterior chamber Iris Pupils: size, shape, symmetry, reflexes (PERRLA may be used for "Pupils, equally round, react to light and accommodation") Lens Lacrimal apparatus Ophthalmologic examination (disc, vessels, retina, macular areas)	Eyebrows Tonometry Lesions Exophthalmia	Vision (distant with glasses): R, 20/40; L, 20/30; can read newspaper at 18 in. Visual fields full. Alignment: no deviation with cover test; light reflex equal; palpebral fissure normal. Extraocular movements: bilaterally intact; no nystagmus, ptosis, lid lag. Conjunctiva: clear, slightly injected around area of R inner canthus. Sclera: white. Cornea: clear, arcus senilis, R eye. Anterior chamber: not narrowed. Iris: blue, round. Pupils: PERRLA. Lens: clear. Funduscopic examination: normal veins and arteries; disc round, margins well defined, color yellowish pink; macular areas normal; no arteriolovenous (AV) nicking, hemorrhages, or exudates. Lacrimal system: no swelling or discharge. Corneal reflex: present.

Continued

Table 28-1

Areas and examples of recording for the physical examination—*cont'd*

Area of examination	Descriptions usually recorded	Descriptions recorded in detail if abnormalities are present (partial listing only)	Examples of recording
Ears	Auricle Canal Otoscopic examination (color, presence of landmarks) Rinne and Weber's tests	Position Discharge Pathologic alterations present on otoscopic examination Lesions Mastoid tenderness General tenderness	Auricle: no lesions, canal clean. Otoscopic examination: drum intact color gray, landmarks and light reflex present. Hearing: finger rub heard in both ears at 3 ft. Rinne and Weber's tests: equal laterization, AC 2× > BC.
Nose	Patency of each nostril Olfaction Turbinates and mucous membranes	External nose Vestibule Transillumination of sinuses	Nostrils patent, odors identified. Septum: slightly deviated to R. Turbinates and membranes: pink, moist, no discharge.
Oral cavity	Buccal mucosa Gums Teeth (decayed, missing, filled) Floor of mouth Hard and soft palate Tonsillar areas Posterior pharyngeal wall Taste Tongue position and movement	Breath odor Lips Lesions Laryngoscopic examination Palpation of mouth Parotid duct	Membranes: pink and moist, no lesions. Gums: no edema or inflammation. Teeth: 3D, 1M, 10F (approximately). Palate: intact, moves symmetrically with phonation, gag reflex present. Tonsils: present, not enlarged. Pharynx: pink and clean. Tongue: strong, midline, moves symmetrically. Taste: able to differentiate sweet and sour.
Neck	Movements: rotation and lateral bend Symmetry Thyroid gland Tracheal position Glands and nodes	Postural alignment Tenderness Tone of muscles Lesions Masses	Rull ROM, strong symmetrically, thyroid not palpable, trachea midline, no enlargement of head and neck regional nodes.
Breasts	Axillary nodes Supraclavicular nodes Infraclavicular nodes Breasts: observation and palpation Nipples and areolar areas Discharge Masses	Retraction Dimpling	No nodes palpable—axillary, infraclavicular, or supraclavicular; no masses, retraction, or discharge; L breast slightly larger than R breast, otherwise symmetrical at rest and with movement. Nipples symmetrically positioned.
Chest and respiratory system	Shape of thorax Symmetry of thorax Respiratory movements Respiratory excursion Palpation: tactile fremitus, tenderness, masses Percussion notes Diaphragmatic excursion and level Auscultation: breath sounds, adventitious sounds	Adventitious sounds Deformity Use of accessory muscles of respiration Vocal fremitus Egophony, bronchophony, whispered pectoriloquy	Thorax oval, AP diameter < lateral diameter; symmetrical at rest and with movements; excursion normal; tactile fremitus equal bilaterally; no masses or tenderness; percussion tones resonant, diaphragmatic excursion 5 cm bilaterally between T10 and T12; vesicular breath sounds bilaterally; no adventitious sounds.

Table 28-1

Areas and examples of recording for the physical examination—*cont'd*

Area of examination	Descriptions usually recorded	Descriptions recorded in detail if abnormalities are present (partial listing only)	Examples of recording
Central cardio-vascular system	Position in which the heart was examined; lying, sitting, left lateral, recumbent Inspection: bulging depression, pulsation (precordial and juxta-precordial) Palpation: thrusts, heaves, thrills, friction rubs Point of PMI Auscultation: rate and rhythm, character of S_1, character of S_2, comparison of S_1 in aortic and pulmonic areas, comparison of S_1 and S_2 in major auscultatory areas, presence or absence of extra sounds—if present, description	Murmur or extra sound: whether systolic or diastolic; intensity; pitch; quality; site of maximum transmission; effect of position, respiration, and exercise; radiation	Examined in sitting and lying positions; no abnormal pulsations or lifts observed; PMI in the 5th ICS, slightly medial to the LMCL; no abnormal pulsations palpated. Apical pulse: 72, regular; S_1 single sound; S_2 splits with inspiration; A_2 is louder than P_2, S_1 heard loudest at apex, S_2 heard loudest at base; no murmurs or other sounds.
Arterial pulses	Radial pulse: rate, rhythm; consistency and tenderness of arterial wall Amplitude and character of peripheral pulses: superficial temporal, brachial, femoral, popliteal, posterior tibial, dorsal pedal Carotid pulses: equality, amplitude, thrills, bruits	Any abnormality: analysis of type	Radial pulse: bilaterally equal, regular, strong; no tenderness or thickening of vessels; 76/min. Peripheral pulses: *Right* *Left* Temporal As above As above Brachial As above As above Femoral As above As above Popliteal Not felt Not felt Posterior tibial As above As above Dorsal pedal As above As above Carotid pulses: equal, strong, no bruits.
Venous pulses and pressures	Jugular venous pulsations, presence of waves a, c, and v Venous pressure: distention present at 45 degrees	Hepatojugular reflex Analysis of jugular venous waves	Jugular venous pressure, 5 cm with client at 45 degrees; venous a and v waves present, a wave strongest.

Abdomen	Inspection: scars, size, shape, symmetry, muscular development, bulging, movements
	Auscultation: peristaltic sounds—present or absent; vascular bruits—present or absent
	Palpation
	  Masses
	  Tenderness (local, referred, rebound), tone of musculature
	  Liver: size, contour, character of edge, consistency, tenderness
	  Kidney (indicate if palpable or not)
	  Costovertebral area: tenderness
	Percussion: liver size at MCL, spleen, masses
		Diastasis
		Distention
		Mass or bulging: specific description
		Palpable spleen: indication of size, surface contour, splenic notch, consistency, tenderness, mobility
		Palpable kidney: indication of location, size, shape, consistency
		Distention of urinary bladder
		Fluid wave
		Flank dullness
		Shifting dullness
		Aorta
		Gallbladder
			Healed scar RLQ (appendectomy); slightly obese, protuberant; symmetrical, no bulging; normal bowel sounds, no bruits; no abnormal movements, symmetric; no masses; no tenderness; liver 11 cm in RMCL; no CVA tenderness; no organs palpated; muscle tone lax.
			Area of midline diastasis: 6 cm × 2 cm inferior and superior to the umbilicus.
			
			3 cm

Continued

Table 28-1

Areas and examples of recording for the physical examination—*cont'd*

Area of examination	Descriptions usually recorded	Descriptions recorded in detail if abnormalities are present (partial listing only)	Examples of recording

Neural system	Orientation
	Intellectual performance
	Emotional status
	Insight
	Memory
	Cranial nerves
	Coordination
	Sensory: touch, pain, position, vibration
	Babinski's sign
	Romberg test
		Thought content
		Speech
		Sensory: hot, cold, two-point discrimination
		Stereognosis
		Involuntary movements
			Alert, oriented ×3; mood appropriate and stable; remote and recent memory intact; several calculations by 6 accurate; insight normal; cranial nerves all intact, examined and recorded in head and neck regions; all movement coordinated; able to perform rapid coordinated movements with upper and lower extremities.
			
			Reflexes (0-4+)
			  0 = absent
			  + (or 1+) = decreased
			  + + (or 2+) = normal
			  + + + (or 3+) = hyperactive
			  + + + + (or 4+) = clonus
			Sensory: light touch, pain, and vibration to face, trunk, and extremities normal and symmetric; walks with coordination, able to maintain standing position with eyes closed.

Extremities and musculoskeletal system	Both upper and lower extremities: general assessments—size, shape, mass, symmetry, hair distribution, color; temperature; edema; varicosities; tenderness; epitrochlear lymph nodes Bones and joints: range of motion, tenderness, gait Muscles: size, symmetry, strength, tone, tenderness, consistency Back: posture, tenderness; movement—extension, lateral bend, rotation	Lesions Deformities Color and temperature changes on elevation and dependency Homans' sign Redness Heat Swelling Deformity Crepitations Contractures Muscle spasms Tenderness Atrophy Hypertrophy	Muscular development and mass normal for age; arms and legs symmetric; skin warm, soft, neither moist nor dry; normal male hair growth on arms, legs, and feet; no edema, varicosities, or tenderness; no nodes palpated; joints nontender, not swollen; normal ROM; muscle tone and strength normal bilaterally; back—full ROM; no tenderness or deformities.

Table 28-1

Areas and examples of recording for the physical examination—*cont'd*

Area of examination	Descriptions usually recorded	Descriptions recorded in detail if abnormalities are present (partial listing only)	Examples of recording
Rectal area	Anal area Skin Hemorrhoids Sphincter tone Rectum Tumors Stool color Occult blood	Lesions Fissures Pilonidal sinus Condition of perineal body Tenderness Proctoscopic examination	Skin clean, no lesions; sphincter tone good; no hemorrhoids or masses noted; stools brown, guaiac negative.
Inguinal area	Hernia: inguinal, femoral Nodes	Size, shape, consistency, tenderness, reducability of hernia or nodes	Hernias not present; no enlargement of nodes noted.
Male genitalia	Penis: condition of prepuce, skin Scrotum: size, skin, testes, epididymides, spermatic cords Prostate gland: size, shape, symmetry, consistency, tenderness Seminal vesicles: size, shape, consistency	Scars Lesions Structural alterations Masses Swelling Nodules	Penis: circumsized, clean, no lesions. Scrotum and contents: normal size, no masses or tumors noted. Prostate and inferior portions of seminal vesicles: palpated, normal consistency, nontender. Prostate: not enlarged, rubbery, not tender. Seminal vesicles: soft, not nodular.
Female genitalia	External: hair distribution; labia; Bartholin's glands, urethral meatus, Skene's glands (BUS); hymen; introitus Vaginal observation: presence or absence of rectocele, urethrocele, cystocele; tissue; discharge (smears or cultures taken); cervix Bimanual examination: cervix, uterus, adnexa Rectovaginal examination; uterus, cul-de-sac, septum	Lesions Tumors Prolapses	Normal female hair distribution; no lesions or masses. BUS: no tenderness, redness, or discharge. Hymen: present in caruncles. Labia: approximate, intact. Introital tone: good; no prolapses; no scars, perineum thick. Vagina: pink, discharge—small amount, thin, clean nonodorous. Cervix: pink, nulliparous, firm, not tender, movable, midline. Uterus: pear-shaped, movable, normal size, firm, no masses. Tubes: not palpable. Ovaries: palpable, movable, not tender, approximately 2 × 3 × 2 cm; smooth surface, no lesions, firm consistency. Rectovaginal septum: thick and firm; no masses palpated in rectum or cul-de-sac.

examined. The second column contains a list of the areas of recording. These areas should be described for all clients. The third column is a partial list of areas to be recorded if abnormalities are identified in the examination of that system. The fourth column contains examples of recording for each body system or area. The examples

of recording do not relate to one client; therefore, column four should not be read as an example of the composite physical examination of one client. A sample worksheet for recording a physical examination can be found on pp. 718-723.

Worksheet for Recording a Physical Examination

Vital signs

Temperature _____ Respiration _____ BP   (L)   Arm   (R)

                                                                   _____ Supine _____

                                                                    _____ Sitting _____

                                                                    _____ Standing _____

Height _____ Weight _____ (Stripped or clothed)

General

Skin, hair, nails, mucous membranes

Head

Scalp _____

Face _____

(CNs V and VII) _____

_____

Sinus areas _____

Nodes _____

Cranium _____

Eyes

Visual acuity _____

Visual fields _____

Ocular movements (CNs III, IV, and VI) _____

Corneal light reflex _____

Lids, lacrimal organs _____

Conjunctiva, sclera _____

Cornea (CN V) _____

Lens and media _____

Pupils: Pupillary reflexes (CN III) _____

    Light, direct and consensual _____

    Near point _____

Fundi (CN II) _____

Intraocular pressure _____

Worksheet for Recording a Physical Examination—*cont'd*

Ears

External structures _____

Canal _____

Tympanic membranes _____

Hearing (CN VIII) _____

Nose

Septum _____

Mucous membranes _____

Patency _____

Olfactory sense (CN I) _____

Oral cavity

Lips _____

Mucous membranes _____

Gums _____

Teeth _____

Palates and uvula (CNs IX and X) _____

Tonsillar areas _____

Tongue (CN XII) _____

Floor _____

Voice _____

Breath _____

Taste (CN VII) _____

Neck

General structure _____

Trachea _____

Thyroid _____

Nodes _____

Muscles (CN XI) _____

Continued

Worksheet for Recording a Physical Examination—cont'd

Breasts and area nodes

_____

_____

Chest, respiratory system

Chest shape _____

Type of respiration _____

Expansion _____

Fremitus _____

General palpation _____

Percussion _____

_____ Diaphragmatic excursion: (R) _____ cm (L) _____ cm

Breath sounds _____

_____

_____

Adventitious sounds _____

_____

Cardiovascular system

Rate and rhythm: Rapid (palpation) _____

Apical (auscultation) _____

Precordium: Inspection _____

Palpation _____

Auscultation _____

S_1 _____

S_2 _____

S_3 _____

S_4 _____

Extra sounds _____

Murmur(s): Systolic _____

Diastolic _____

Worksheet for Recording a Physical Examination—*cont'd*

Cardiovascular system—cont'd

Carotid arteries _____

Jugular venous pulse and pressure _____

_____

Description of peripheral pulses

Brachial	Radial	Femoral	Popliteal	Dorsal pedal	Post. tibial

R _____

L _____

Abdomen and inguinal areas

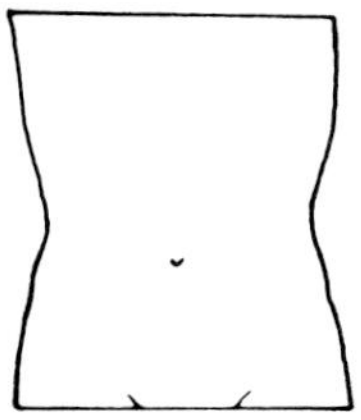

Contour, tone _____

Scars, marks _____

Auscultation _____

_____

Liver _____ Span _____ cm at RMCL

Spleen _____

Kidneys _____ CVA tenderness _____

Bladder _____

Hernias _____

Masses _____

Palpation _____

_____

Percussion _____

_____

Genitalia and area nodes

_____

_____

_____

Continued

Worksheet for Recording a Physical Examination—*cont'd*

Rectal examination

Musculoskeletal system

Gait _____

Deformities _____

Joint evaluation _____

_____

Muscle strength _____

_____

Muscle mass _____

Range of motion _____

Spine

Contour _____

Position _____

Motion _____

_____

Nervous system

Mental status _____

Language _____

Cranial nerves (summarize) _____

Motor: Coordination: Upper extremities _____

Lower extremities _____

Involuntary movements _____

Worksheet for Recording a Physical Examination—*cont'd*

Deep tendon reflexes:

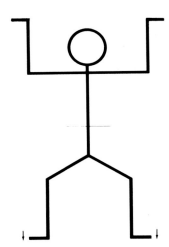

Note: +s denote finger jerks, brachioradialis, biceps, triceps, reflexes, 4-quadrant abdominal scratch reflexes, patellar Achilles reflexes, and plantar reflexes. Abdominal reflexes are recorded as 0 or +. Scale: 0-4 (+ + + +); normal = 2 (+ +).

Sensory

Light touch _____

Pain (pinprick) _____

Vibration _____

Position _____

29

Decision making

OBJECTIVES

Upon successful review of this chapter, learners will be able to:

- Delineate four steps of the decision-making process
- Describe theory-based guidelines to problem solving, including differences between a medically oriented body systems approach and a nursing focus
- List the nine human response patterns of the Unitary Person Framework
- Explain how the North American Nursing Diagnosis Association's (NANDA's) Taxonomy I helps to guide assessment and decision making
- Describe the relationship between nursing diagnoses and defining characteristics
- Explain how Taxonomy I is used to investigate specific assessment findings
- Explain how decision making and nursing diagnoses relate to the nursing process

The preceding chapters have focused on teaching effective methods of assessment. The purpose of performing an assessment is to collect data. But why collect data? The answer seems obvious. The practitioner collects data to assist in formulating some conclusion regarding the client's health status. To reach this conclusion, or diagnosis, the clinician uses a process known as diagnostic reasoning, or decision making. This chapter will discuss the process of decision making and its relationship to nursing process and diagnosis. In addition, some methods for facilitating decision making will be presented.

THE DECISION-MAKING PROCESS

Many investigators have studied how physicians diagnose illness. By comparison, there have been few studies concerning nursing decision making. However, some of the research that has been done suggests that physicians and nurses use similar decision-making processes. This conclusion seems reasonable, since it has been suggested that both tradition and necessity require nurses to make both medical and nursing judgments.

Researchers have found that there are four major steps in the medical diagnostic reasoning or decision-making process. These steps are listed in Table 29-1.

Cue Recognition

In the first phase of decision making, the practitioner must recognize that a *cue* is significant. A cue is merely a fact or piece of information. It can consist of either subjective or objective data. For example, a subjective cue might be the client's statement, "I feel nervous." In contrast, an objective cue might be the observation that the client has a hand tremor.

Table 29–1

Stages of diagnostic reasoning or decision making

Stage	Example
Attending to cues (cue recognition)	Look at client's face—notice cyanosis as abnormal
Formulating hypotheses (hypothesis formulation)	Client is experiencing impaired gas exchange
Collecting data to test the hypotheses (hypothesis testing)	Arterial blood gas result: pH 7.32, pCO$_2$ 55, pO$_2$ 65. The client appears restless and confused. Weak cough effort
Evaluating hypotheses (hypothesis evaluation)	Do enough data exist to confirm the diagnosis of impaired gas exchange? If yes, then diagnosis is made. Impaired gas exchange related to . . .

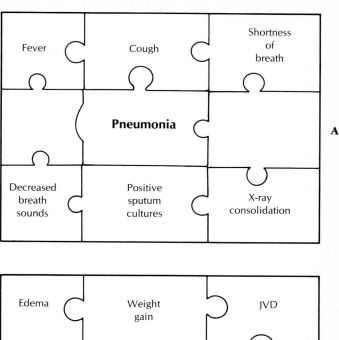

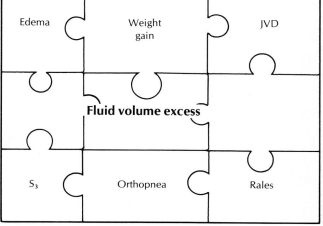

Figure 29-1

Cue association puzzle. **A,** Medical diagnosis. **B,** Nursing diagnosis.

Whether a cue is considered significant depends on the practitioner's ability to distinguish between normal and abnormal behavior, physical characteristics, and diagnostic findings. This ability, in turn, depends on the clinician's knowledge base and expertise. The subtleness of the cue also affects the practitioner's ability to recognize important data. A knowledgeable and experienced practitioner, for example, might note the slight pallor of a client's nail beds and consider the diagnosis of anemia. In contrast, an inexperienced student might not even notice the subtle change in nail-bed color.

In summary, the first phase of decision making, *cue recognition,* serves a function similar to that of a car's fuel filter. During the health assessment, the practitioner receives thousands of pieces of information. This process is similar to filling the gas tank and starting the car. Next, the clinician begins to sort the data, keeping some pieces of information and ignoring others. The data that are ignored or considered to be insignificant are like the dirt that remains caught in the fuel filter. The remaining data or cues are similar to the filtered gasoline because they serve as a more efficient resource for the next step in the process, "the running of the engine."

Hypothesis Formulation

During the second phase of decision making the practitioner decides on tentative explanations for the cues recognized in the previous step. This phase is often referred to as *hypothesis formulation.* Before making any tentative conclusions, the clinician must first cluster or link some or all of the collected cues and determine any emerging patterns. One cue, in isolation, is rarely enough to suggest a particular hypothesis or diagnosis. Rather, the existence of several cues that are usually or always associated with one or more specific problems helps indicate tentative conclusions for further investigation. The process of finding associations between cues similar to working a jigsaw puzzle (Fig. 29-1).

As in the first phase, a clinician's knowledge and expertise strongly affect the decision-making process. In this instance, the practitioner's knowledge base influences the interpretation and relative importance of the remaining cues. Often the novice jumps to early and erroneous conclusions caused by misinterpreting or focusing on one cue. As practitioners gain knowledge and experience, they build associations between cues and

Table 29–2

General strategies for hypothesis testing

Approach	Explanation	Example
Cue-based	Explore each aspect of initial cues until all facets are covered	Facial cyanosis—mucous membranes, ears, skin color
Hypothesis-driven	Investigate the defining characteristics to confirm their presence or absence	Hypoxia? Hypercapnea? Restlessness? Somnulence? Confusion? Irritability? Inability to move secretions?
Systematic	Review body systems	Start with respiratory system, then move to cardiovascular system, then investigate neurologic system, etc.
Hit and miss	No recognizable strategy	Ask client when last bowel movement took place.

Table 29–3

Hypothesis testing strategies used by experts

Strategy	Explanation
Confirmation	Seek data to confirm hypothesis
Elimination	Eliminate hypothesis based on absence of key signs and symptoms (defining characteristics)
Discrimination	Investigate defining characteristics that separate diagnoses with similar signs and symptoms; i.e., look for those characteristics that are different
Exploration	Consider investigation of diagnoses with similar manifestations

clinical situations. These associations enable the clinician to cluster cues into meaningful groups and formulate hypotheses.

The formulation of hypotheses or tentative conclusions helps focus further data collection efforts on a manageable group of possibilities. However, one must be careful not to limit further investigation to only one hypothesis, since the likelihood of an accurate final diagnosis increases when several explanations are considered.

To continue with the automobile analogy, hypothesis formulation is like harnessing the energy released as the filtered gasoline is ignited. The hypotheses generated during this phase help to turn the gears of the decision-making process and propel the practitioner toward a final conclusion.

Hypothesis Testing

During the third stage of diagnostic reasoning, the practitioner focuses on gathering data to support or reject the previously generated hypotheses. This phase is called *hypothesis testing*. Many different data collection strat-

egies are used by clinicians during this stage. These methods of continued inquiry are listed in Table 29-2 and 29-3. One or more of these techniques may be appropriate for a given clinical situation. In addition, the practitioner may be more comfortable using some methods than others. The use of familiar strategies can often facilitate this phase of decision making.

Hypothesis testing is similar to deciding which route to take when driving an automobile. There may be many routes to choose from, and some may be shorter than others. Some may also be more difficult than others with more opportunities for making wrong turns. It is up to the practitioner to steer the car in the right direction through knowledge and expertise.

As with driving, there may be road hazards as the practitioner continues the decision-making process. For example, the clinician might direct investigation toward a favored hypothesis or prematurely accept or reject a possible explanation. In addition, the practitioner can be influenced by biases concerning hypotheses (Table 29-4).

Hypothesis Evaluation

Once the clinician is satisfied that all reasonable explanations for the initial set of cues have been thoroughly investigated, each hypothesis must be evaluated in light of the new evidence that has been collected and a final diagnosis or conclusion reached (Fig. 29-2). This process requires synthesis of all data that have been collected, since information that was obtained to refute one hypothesis may support another. Careful recording of data as it is collected is crucial. Failure to document assessment data fully increases the possibility that information

Table 29–4

Biases affecting diagnosis

Bias	Explanation
Frequency of occurence	If the diagnosis being considered has been made frequently, it has a higher probability of being chosen.
Recency of experience	If the clinician has made the considered diagnosis in the recent past, the clinician may be more familiar with this diagnosis than with other related diagnoses.
Profoundness of memory	Vivid impressions of cases in which a certain diagnosis was made can influence decision making in favor of this diagnosis.

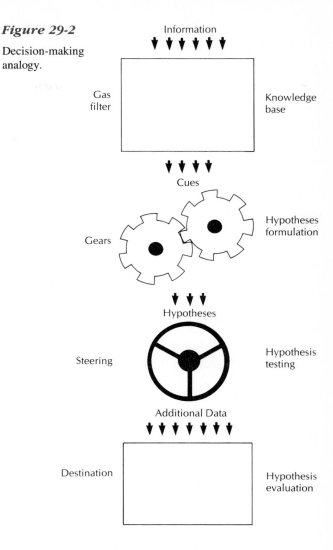

Figure 29-2

Decision-making analogy.

necessary for the hypothesis evaluation process will be inadvertently lost or forgotten. Missing data, in turn, can lead to erroneous conclusions. Chapter 28 contains an example of one form that can be used to record data during the assessment process. Another data collection form with a very different format will be discussed later in this chapter.

During the final phase of decision making, *hypothesis evaluation,* the practitioner usually determines which explanation has the most supporting data and chooses this hypothesis as the diagnosis. In some cases, however, the clinician can only eliminate hypotheses until only the one with the highest probability remains.

THE INFLUENCE OF THEORETICAL FRAMEWORKS OF DECISION MAKING

Although nurses and physicians seem to use the same general decision-making process, the conclusions reached by these two groups of professionals are quite different. The reason for this difference stems from each profession's distinct focus of concern.

Medical and Nursing Concerns

The focus of medicine, and physicians, is the diagnosis of disease and its causes. The knowledge base physicians use is derived, in part, from cell and germ theories. As a result, physicians concentrate their investigations on cellular and tissue abnormalities and on the etiologies of these derangements.

In contrast, nursing's primary focus is the diagnosis of *human responses* to actual or potential health problems. These health problems may not be disease states. For nurses, assessment centers on the client's physical, psychological, and spiritual reactions to illness and the environment. There are many theoretical frameworks nurses use to explain these phenomena. Some examples are Roy's adaptation model, Orem's self-care deficit model, and the unitary person framework proposed by the North American Nursing Diagnosis Association (NANDA).

The Benefits of Theory-Based Decision Making

Using a theoretical framework to guide assessment and decision making is beneficial because it helps organize knowledge and provides direction for further investigation of initial cues. A framework also provides practitioners with specific terminology, which facilitates more effective communication between members of the same discipline. NANDA has been instrumental in striving to provide nursing with a common language to communicate nursing findings and a common framework to explain the phenomena observed by nurses. The language provided by NANDA consists of *nursing diagnoses*. These diagnoses have been arranged in a meaningful pattern, called Taxonomy I, based on the tenets of the unitary person framework.

The Unitary Person Framework

According to the unitary person framework, a person is an open system. This system interacts with the environment and develops into an increasingly more complex and unique being through a process called *negentropy*. Health is a form of exchange with the environment that promotes negentropy. Further, an individual's health status is manifested by observable phenomena that can be classified into *nine human response patterns* (see the box below). Judgments regarding the health of the unitary person are based on data collected from these nine human response patterns. These judgments are *nursing diagnoses*.

Taxonomy I—A Nursing Classification System

As mentioned previously, Taxonomy I is a nursing diagnosis classification system based on the unitary person framework. Taxonomy I, like other classification systems, is arranged in a hierarchy from the general to the specific. The most general concept of the system is the

unitary person. A slightly more specific concept concerning the unitary person is health. Health, in turn, is determined by functioning within the nine human response patterns. These nine patterns act as the major categories for Taxonomy I. The next level of this system consists of nursing diagnoses and other subcategory headings that have been determined to be related to a particular pattern by NANDA's Taxonomy Committee. The boxed material on p. 729 shows the accepted diagnoses arranged according to the nine human response patterns of the unitary person framework and Taxonomy I. The subcategories that were added to Taxonomy I to enhance the clarity of its structure do not appear in this list.

In Taxonomy I, the first level of diagnoses and headings under the response patterns are broad and can be further defined. For example, "Altered Elimination" can be further specified as either bowel or urinary. "Altered Elimination: Bowel" can then be further broken down into the diagnoses of Constipation, Diarrhea, or Incontinence. Occasionally, diagnoses such as these can be made even more specific, for example, Colonic Constipation (Fig. 29-3).

The nursing diagnosis levels are also specifed by diagnostic qualifiers that were defined and approved by NANDA (see the box below). At the finest level of specificity, nursing diagnoses have been defined and deter-

---

> ### *Nine Human Response Patterns of the Unitary Person Framework*
>
> *Exchanging:* a human response pattern involving mutual giving and receiving
>
> *Communicating:* a human response pattern involving sending messages
>
> *Relating:* a human response pattern involving establishing bonds
>
> *Valuing:* a human response pattern involving the assigning of relative worth
>
> *Choosing:* a human response pattern involving the selection of alternatives
>
> *Moving:* a human response pattern involving activity
>
> *Perceiving:* a human response pattern involving the reception of information
>
> *Knowing:* a human response pattern involving the meaning associated with information
>
> *Feeling:* a human response pattern involving the subjective awareness of information

From the North American Nursing Diagnosis Association, St Louis, 1986.

> ### *Nanda Diagnosis Qualifiers*
>
> **Category 1**
>
> Actual: existing at the present moment; existing in reality
> Potential: can, but has not yet, come into being; possible
>
> **Category 2**
>
> Ineffective: not producing the desired effect; not capable of performing satisfactorily
> Decreased: smaller, lessened; diminished; lesser in size, amount, or degree
> Increased: greater in size, amount or degree; larger, enlarged
> Impaired: made worse, weakened; damaged, reduced, deteriorated
> Depleted: emptied wholly or partially; exhausted of
> Deficient: inadequate in amount, quality, or degree; defective; not sufficient; incomplete
> Excessive: characterized by an amount or quantity that is greater than necessary, desirable, or usable
> Dysfunctional: abnormal; impaired or incompletely functioning
> Disturbed: agitated, interrupted, interfered with
> Acute: severe but of short duration
> Chronic: lasting a long time; recurring; habitual; constant
> Intermittent: stopping and starting again at intervals; periodic; cyclic

From the North American Nursing Diagnosis Association, St Louis, 1986.

Classification of Nursing Diagnoses by Human Response Patterns
(NANDA Taxonomy 1—Revised)

Exchanging

Altered nutrition: more than body requirements
Altered nutrition: less than body requirements
Altered nutrition: potential for more than body requirements
Potential for infection
Potential altered body temperature
Hypothermia
Hyperthermia
Ineffective thermoregulation
Dysreflexia
Constipation
Perceived constipation
Colonic constipation
Diarrhea
Bowel incontinence
Altered patterns of urinary elimination
Stress incontinence
Reflex incontinence
Urge incontinence
Functional incontinence
Total incontinence
Urinary retention
Altered (specify type) tissue perfusion (renal, cerebral, cardio-
    pulmonary, gastrointestinal, peripheral)
Fluid volume excess
Fluid volume deficit (1)
Fluid volume deficit (2)
Potential fluid volume deficit
Decreased cardiac output
Impaired gas exchange
Ineffective airway clearance
Ineffective breathing pattern
Potential for injury
Potential for suffocation
Potential for poisoning
Potential for trauma
Potential for aspiration
Potential for disuse syndrome
Impaired tissue integrity
Altered oral mucous membrane
Impaired skin integrity
Potential impaired skin integrity

Communicating

Impaired verbal communication

Relating

Impaired social interaction
Social isolation
Altered role performance
Altered parenting
Potential altered parenting
Sexual dysfunction
Altered family processes
Parental role conflict
Altered sexuality patterns

Valuing

Spiritual distress (distress of the human spirit)

Choosing

Ineffective individual coping
Impaired adjustment
Defensive coping
Ineffective denial
Ineffective family coping: disabling
Ineffective family coping: compromised
Family coping: potential for growth
Noncompliance (specify)
Decisional conflict (specify)
Health-seeking behaviors (specify)

Moving

Impaired physical mobility
Activity intolerance
Fatigue
Potential activity intolerance
Sleep pattern disturbance
Diversional activity deficit
Impaired home maintenance management
Altered health maintenance
Feeding self-care deficit
Impaired swallowing
Ineffective breastfeeding
Bathing/hygiene self-care deficit
Dressing/grooming self-care deficit
Toileting self-care deficit
Altered growth and development

Perceiving

Body image disturbance
Self-esteem disturbance
Chronic low self-esteem
Situational low self-esteem
Personal identity disturbance
Sensory/perceptual alterations (specify) (visual, auditory, kin-
    esthetic, gustatory, tactile, olfactory)
Unilateral neglect
Hopelessness
Powerlessness

Knowing

Knowledge deficit (specify)
Altered thought processes

Feeling

Pain
Chronic pain
Dysfunctional grieving
Anticipatory grieving
Potential for violence: self-directed or directed at others
Post-trauma response
Rape-trauma syndrome
Rape-trauma syndrome: compound reaction
Rape-trauma syndrome: silent reaction
Anxiety
Fear

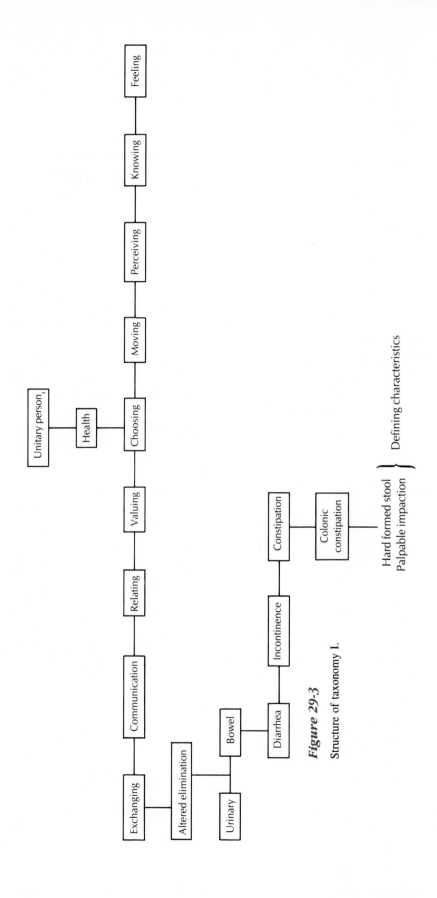

Figure 29-3

Structure of taxonomy I.

termined to have certain signs and symptoms called *defining characteristics*. It is these defining characteristics that most often serve as cues for decision making.

The predictive relationships between defining characteristics and nursing diagnoses are not perfect. These relationships are initially based on the observations of experienced clinicians who propose new nursing diagnoses. Much research is currently being conducted to validate the defining characteristics of the diagnoses accepted by NANDA. Although the association of a cluster of signs and symptoms with a nursing diagnosis may be very strong, no single group of characteristics will ever absolutely indicate a particular nursing diagnosis.

Because the task of determining nursing diagnoses and refining the taxonomy is currently unfinished, there are some gaps in the structure of Taxonomy I. As more nursing diagnoses are developed, defined, and verified, the taxonomy will continue to be refined. This, in turn, will make the nursing diagnosis process easier.

USING A CLASSIFICATION SYSTEM TO FACILITATE DECISION MAKING

Classification systems such as Taxonomy I serve as road maps for diagnostic reasoning. From any given location in the classification scheme, a practitioner can investigate in the direction of either a more general or a more specific conclusion, whichever is appropriate for the situation.

Body Systems Approach

One classification system frequently used in physical assessment is the body systems approach. Using the medically oriented body systems approach, a clinician might choose to evaluate the gastrointestinal system. This is a general category that consists of several organs and tissues. After choosing the system to be assessed, the practitioner focuses on evaluating the functioning of the various organs and tissues. When an abnormal finding occurs, the clinician then searches for additional signs and symptoms known to be associated with this finding. Based on which signs and symptoms are found, the practitioner makes a differential diagnosis.

The body systems approach can also be used to move from a specific complaint or finding to an evaluation of the functioning of one or more systems. For example, a practitioner investigating tachycardia might first search for other cardiac-related signs and symptoms such as an enlarged heart seen on x-ray study or jugular venous distention. However, if the clinician does not encounter these findings but observes that the client has exophthalmos, appears flushed, and has an elevated body temperature, the diagnostician might then turn attention to assessing the endocrine system for other data to confirm the tentative medical diagnosis of hyperthyroidism or a nursing diagnosis of hyperthermia.

Nurses, as well as physicians, have traditionally used the body systems approach to assessment. However, this approach does not facilitate the formulation of nursing diagnosis. To ease the process of making nursing diagnoses, nurses must employ a nursing theory–based approach to assessment and decision making.

The Taxonomy I Approach

As mentioned earlier, Taxonomy I is a classification system based on a nursing framework. Like the body systems classification scheme, Taxonomy I can also be used to guide decision-making activities. As in the body systems approach, a practitioner using the Taxonomy I approach can start from a general response pattern and assess for signs and symptoms of diagnoses that belong to that particular pattern. For example, the clinician wishing to evaluate the Exchanging Pattern might start by assessing the client's elimination, since "Altered Elimination" is one diagnosis found in this pattern. The practitioner must then decide which type of elimination to evaluate first, bowel or urinary. The clinician choosing to assess bowel elimination must then look for signs and symptoms of diarrhea, constipation, or incontinence. If the defining characteristics for one of these disorders exists, a nursing diagnosis can be made.

A practitioner can also use Taxonomy I to investigate a specific finding, such as an abdomen that is firm to palpation. Other cues may be associated with this finding, for example, the client's complaint of a feeling of abdominal fullness. Based on these cues, the practitioner makes a tentative diagnosis of constipation. The clinician will then test this diagnosis by searching for the presence of its other defining characteristics. If several of these signs and symptoms are present, the diagnosis of "Constipation" can be made.

Using the Taxonomy I method of assessment and decision making may be difficult at first, since nurses traditionally have not been taught to organize their thinking in this manner. One method of facilitating the transition to nursing theory–based assessment and diagnosis is to use a data collection form that is organized according to a particular nursing theory. An example of one such tool, based on the unitary person framework and organized according to Taxonomy I, appears in Figure 29-4.

In this data collection form, the order of the human response patterns, as they appear in Taxonomy I, was changed in this tool to allow interview data to be collected before physiologic data were collected. Within each human response pattern section, items called *variables*

Text continued on p. 737.

MEDICAL-SURGICAL ASSESSMENT TOOL

Name _Mrs. S.R._ _____ Age _34_ Sex _F_ _____
Address _444 Fourth Avenue, Seattle Washington_ ___ Telephone _555-4444_ _____
Significant other _Husband; Mr. R._ _____ Telephone _Same_ _____
Date of admission _27 August_ ____ Medical diagnosis _R/O Inoperative Shunt vs Gastric Ulcer_
Allergies _Erythromycin (causes nausea & vomiting)_ _____

Nursing Diagnosis
(Potential or Altered)

COMMUNICATING ▪ A pattern involving sending messages
English (circle): (read), (write), (understand)   Communication
Other languages _Nonfluent – German_ _____   Verbal
Tracheostomy _Ø_ _____ Speech impaired _Ø_ _____   Nonverbal
Alternate form of communication _Ø_
Speech therapy consultant: yes (no)   Date sent _____

VALUING ▪ A pattern involving the assigning of relative worth
Religious preference _Catholic, Byzantine_ _____   Spiritual state
Important religious practices _"Prayer – it's a little support"_   Distress
Cultural orientation _"Born & brought up in Tacoma, Washington_   Despair
Cultural practices _"Nothing specific"_
Ministry consultant: yes (no)   Date sent _____

RELATING ▪ A pattern involving establishing bonds
Role
Marital status _Married 5 years_ _____   Role performance
Age & health of significant other _34 yrs., excellent health_   Parenting
_____   Sexual dysfunction
Number of children _1_ Ages _5 months, girl (Mary)_   Work
Role in home _"Housewife now" (medically retired army officer)_   Family
Financial support _Husband's income & military disability pay_   Social/leisure
Occupation _Husband – realtor, patient was finance officer_
  Job satisfaction/concerns _Prior to illness, enjoyed job_   Family processes
Sexual relationships (satisfactory/unsatisfactory) _(see concerns)_   Sexuality patterns
  Physical difficulties/effects of illness on relationship _Exhausted, (R) arm_
spasticity
  Sexual habits _↓ Intercourse, one partner_
  Sexual concerns or problems _"Has not had sexual intimacy with_
husband for over a year, it's not a problem or a necessity at this point"

Socialization
Relationships with others _"Most relationships are strong"_   Impaired social interaction
  Patient's description _"Fine, not a lot of friends but good ones"_
  Significant others' descriptions _—_
  Staff observations _Quiet, keeps to herself, slightly introverted_
Problems verbalized _None_
Verbalizes feelings of being alone _No_   Social isolation
Attributed to _—_   Social withdrawal

Figure 29-4

Medical-surgical assessment tool.
(From Guzzetta CE and others: Clinical assessment tools for use with nursing diagnoses, St Louis, 1989, The CV Mosby Co.)

KNOWING ▪ A pattern involving the meaning associated with information

Current health problems *↑ NAUSEA & VOMITING OVER LAST FEW WEEKS*

Current medications *TYLENOL #3, 1-2 TABS, PO, PRN FOR HEADACHE*

Previous illnesses/hospitalizations/surgeries *① RESECTION OF MENINGIOMA, ② SHUNT REVISION x3, ③ HOSPITALIZATION x6 FOR HYPEREMESIS ④ C-SECTION c̄ DAUGHTER*

History of the following: Patient   Family Member   (Knowledge deficit)

	Patient	Family Member
Anemia/blood dyscrasias	∅	∅
Cancer	∅	*MOTHER—UTERINE CA*
Diabetes	∅	∅
Heart disease	∅	∅
Hypertension	∅	∅
Peripheral vascular	∅	∅
Kidney disease	∅	∅
Stroke	∅	∅
Tuberculosis	∅	∅
Alcohol/substance use	∅	∅
Smoking	∅	∅
Other		*BOTH PARENTS HAVE ULCERS*

Perception/knowledge of illness/tests/surgery *KNOWLEDGABLE CONCERNING SHUNT REVISIONS, UNDERSTANDS THE NEED FOR SHUNT TO WORK CORRECTLY. QUESTIONS CAUSE OF CONTINUED NAUSEA & VOMITING*

Expectations of therapy *EVALUATE NAUSEA & VOMITING, CORRECT PROBLEM SOURCE (i.e., SHUNT)*

Misconceptions *FEELS NAUSEA & VOMITING CAN ONLY BE RELATED TO INOPERATIVE SHUNT*

Readiness to learn *ASKING APPROPRIATE QUESTIONS, APPEARS READY TO LEARN*

  Requesting information concerning *NOTHING AT THIS TIME*

  Educational level *COLLEGE — BS*   (POTENTIAL)

  Learning impeded by *WHEN SHUNT WAS NOT WORKING — THOUGHT PROCESSES ARE SLOWER, MORE CONFUSED*   (Thought processes)

Orientation

  Level of alertness *FULLY ALERT AT THIS TIME*   Orientation

  Orientation: Person *YES*   Place *YES*   Time *YES*   Confused

  Appropriate behavior/communication *YES*

Memory   *PARTIAL*

  Memory intact:(yes)/no   Recent *YES*   Remote *USUALLY*   Memory

FEELING ▪ A pattern involving the subjective awareness of information

Comfort

  Pain/discomfort:(yes)/no

    Onset *1-2 HRS. AFTER MEALS*   Duration *VARIES*   Comfort

    Location *UPPER ABDOMEN MAINLY*   Pain/chronic

    Intensity *BURNING/GASEOUS PRESSURE (7)*   Radiation *—*   (Pain/acute)

    Associated factors *HEAD & NECK PAIN WHICH IS DULL IN NATURE*   Discomfort

    Aggravating factors *MOVEMENT*

    Alleviating factors *SOMETIMES FOOD OR LIQUID, TYLENOL #3 FOR HEADACHE*

Emotional Integrity/States

  Recent stressful life events *"BIRTH OF BABY AT 8 MONTHS BY C-SECTION & REMOVAL OF BRAIN TUMOR SAME DAY*   Grieving / Anxiety

  Verbalizes feelings of: *"FEAR & GUILT"*   (Fear)

    Source *"RECURRENT TUMORS & NOT CARING FOR HER CHILD"*   Anger

  Physical manifestations *PATIENT DOES NOT FEEL NAUSEA & VOMITING MAY BE RELATED TO THESE EVENTS.*   (Guilt) / Shame / Sadness

Figure 29-4, cont'd

Continued

MOVING ▪ A pattern involving activity

Activity   History of physical disability *YES, FOLLOWING BRAIN SURGERY*   (Impaired physical mobility)
          Use of device (cane, walker, artificial limb) *4-POINT CANE*   Activity intolerance
          Limitations in daily activities *FULL RANGE OF MOTION, DECREASED*
          COORDINATION, (R) ARM JERKS
          Verbal report of fatigue or (weakness) *"MY BODY IS ALWAYS WEAK."*

          Exercise habits *WALK, SWIM*
          Physical therapy consultant: (yes)/no   Date sent *27 AUGUST*

Rest
     Sleep environment: Hours slept/night ___*8*___   Feels rested: (yes)/no   Sleep pattern disturbances
          Sleeps alone: yes/(no) *C̄ HUSBAND* Temperature *"NORMAL ROOM"*   Hypersomnia
          Position preference *"EITHER SIDE"*   Insomnia
          Naps during the day *OCCASIONALLY*   Nightmares
          Other ___—___
     Sleep aids (pillows, meds, food) *NONE*
     Difficulty falling/remaining asleep *No*

Recreation
     Leisure activities *"READ A LOT"*   Deficit in diversional activity
     Social activities *"HAVE COMPANY OVER — OCCASIONALLY WE DINE OUT"*

Environmental Maintenance
     Home maintenance management   Impaired home maintenance
          Size & arrangement of home (stairs, bathroom) *2 FLOORS, LARGE HOME*   management
          _____ Safety needs *STAIRS C̄ ASSISTANCE*   Safety hazards
          Housekeeping responsibilities *"I DO VERY LITTLE. WE HIRED A HOUSE-*
          KEEPER v MY PARENTS HELP. MY HUSBAND CARES FOR THE BABY, COOKS, DOES IT ALL."
          Social services consultant: (yes)/no   Date sent *27 AUGUST*
          (DISCHARGE NEEDS v CHILD CARE
Health Maintenance
     Health insurance *MILITARY*
     Regular physical checkups *"THEY ARE DONE WITH MY CT SCANS."*

Self-Care
     Ability to perform ADLs: Independent _____ Dependent ___✓___   (Self-care)
     Specific deficits *PT. RIGHT HANDED; FINE MOTOR SKILLS, COORDINATION*   Feeding
     v CONTROL DECREASED. ATAXIC   Bathing/hygiene
     Discharge planning needs *LEARNING ADAPTATIONS TO COMPENSATE*   Dressing/grooming
     FOR CURRENT LOSSES v DECREASES (PT. CONSULT SENT AS ABOVE)   Toileting
     Community health nurse consultant: yes/(no)   Date sent _____

PERCEIVING ▪ A pattern involving the reception of information
Self-Concept
     Presenting appearance *NEAT, NO MAKE-UP, DOES NOT WEAR WIG OR SCARF OVER HEAD.*
     Patient's description of self *"IT'S AMAZING WHAT YOU CAN DO WITH NO HAIR."* Body image
     Effects of illness/surgery *"I'D LIKE TO SEE WHAT I LOOK LIKE MORE*   Self-esteem
     OFTEN, BUT NO ONE OFFERS ME A MIRROR."   Personal identity

Meaningfulness
     Verbalizes hopelessness *"IT'S NOT HOPELESS YET"*   Hopelessness
     Perceived/verbalized loss of control *YES — "THE THOUGHT OF GOING IN*   (Powerlessness)
     AGAIN MAKES ME SICK."
     Nonverbal cues *NEGATIVE (LEFT TO RIGHT) SHAKING OF HEAD*

Figure 29-4, cont'd

Sensory/Perception
History of restrictive environment ___*No*___   Sensory perception
Vision impaired ___*No*___ Glasses ___*No*___   Visual
Auditory impaired ___*No*___ Hearing aid ___*No*___   Auditory
Kinesthetic impaired ___*YES —ATAXIC*___   (Kinesthetic)
Reflexes grossly intact ___(R) *SIDE= HYPERREFLEXIA*___

EXCHANGING ▪ A pattern involving mutual giving and receiving
Circulation
Cerebral   Cerebral tissue perfusion
   Neurologic changes/symptoms ___*WORD/THOUGHT SEARCH ALTERED*___
___*"I MUST STOP TO GROPE FOR CORRECT WORDS"*___
   Pupils: Left 2 3 4 (5) 6 mm   Right 2 3 4 (5) 6 mm
       Reaction: Brisk ___*R/L*___ Sluggish _____ Nonreactive _____
   Verbal response ___*APPROPRIATE*___
   Motor response ___*ALTERED BALANCE, JERKING (R) ARM*___
Cardiac   Cardiopulmonary tissue
   Pacemaker (brand, frequency, mode) ___—___   perfusion
   Heart rate rhythm ___*78, STRONG RHYTHMIC*___   Fluid volume
   Heart sounds/murmurs ___*S₁ S₂ NO MURMURS NOTED*___   Deficit
   Blood pressure: R ___*¹³⁰/₈₀*___ L ___*¹³⁰/₇₆*___ Position ___*SITTING*___   Excess
   Pulses ___*ALL PALPABLE, STRONG*___
   Skin temp ___*WARM*___ Color ___*PALE*___
   Capillary refill ___*< 2 SECONDS*___ Clubbing ___—___   Cardiac output
   Edema ___—___

Physical Integrity
Tissue integrity/location of changes: Impaired skin integrity
   Abrasions ___—___ Bruises ___*OLD IV SITES, BLOOD DRAWING*___   Impaired tissue integrity
   Burns ___∅___
   Lacerations ___∅___
   Lesions ___∅___ Petechiae ___∅___
   Pressure sores ___∅___
   Rashes ___∅___
   Stoma/ostomy ___∅___
   Surgical incision ___*ABDOMEN/C-SECTION; SCALP/SHUNT, TUMOR REMOVAL*___
   Surgical dressings ___∅___
   Turgor ___*FAIR, EVIDENCE OF DEHYDRATION*___
   Enterostomal therapy consult: yes/(no)   Date sent _____

Oxygenation
Thoracic examination: Barrel ___∅___ Scoliosis ___∅___   Ineffective airway clearance
   Other ___*NONE*___   Ineffective breathing patterns
Complaints of dyspnea ___∅___ Precipitated by ___∅___   Impaired gas exchange
Orthopnea ___∅___
Rate ___*16*___ Rhythm ___*EVEN*___ Depth ___*NORMAL*___
Labored/(unlabored) (circle)
Use of accessory muscles ___*NO*___
Chest expansion ___*SYMMETRICAL*___
Pursed lips ___*No*___ Nasal flaring ___*No*___
Cough: productive/nonproductive ___*No*___
Sputum: Color ___—___ Amount ___—___ Consistency ___—___
Splinting ___∅___ Breath sounds ___*CLEAR BILATERALLY*___
Arterial blood gases ___—___
Oxygen percent and device ___—___

Figure 29-4, cont'd

Continued

Physical Regulation

Immune   Infection

Lymph nodes enlarged *No*   Location —   Hyperthermia

WBC count *13,500*   Differential *NEUTROPHILS — 60%*   Hypothermia

PT —   PTT —   Platelets —   Body temperature

Temperature *98.8° F*   Route *ORALLY*   Ineffective thermoregulation

Nutrition   Nutrition

Eating patterns

Number of meals per day: Usual *3*   Current *3 SMALL*

Special diet *No*

Where eaten *HOME OR OCCASIONALLY OUT*

Food preferences/~~intolerances~~ *EASTERN EUROPEAN, FRUIT, CHICKEN LIVERS*

Food allergies *NONE*

Fluid intake *DECREASED c̄ NAUSEA & VOMITING*

Appetite changes *"NOT HUNGRY, USUALLY JUST NAUSEATED"*

Difficulty swallowing *∅*   Impaired swallowing

History of ulcers *YES, PARENTS* Heartburn *No*

Anorexia/nausea/vomiting *"YES — ALL THREE FOR A FEW WEEKS"*

Condition of mouth/throat *MOIST MUCOUS MEMBRANES, NO REDNESS,*   Oral mucous membrane

NO LESIONS; TONGUE DRY   ~~More~~/less than body

Height *5'10"*   Weight *117#*   Ideal body weight *150# (HAS ALWAYS* (requirements)

                                           BEEN BELOW)   (POTENTIAL)

Dietary consultant: yes/no   Date sent

Current therapy   Fluid volume

NPO *FOR TESTING* NG suction —   Deficit

Enteral nutrition —   TPN —   Excess

IV fluids —

Labs (place * by abnormal values)

Hemoglobin *11g/dl**   Hematocrit *35%**   RBC —

Na *150 mEq/L**   K *3.2 mEq/L**   CL *90 mEq/L**   Glucose *110 mg/dl*

Cholesterol *180 mg/dl*   Triglycerides *94 mg/dl*   Fasting *No*

Total protein *8.8g/dl**   Albumin *5.4g/dl**   Iron *70 µg/dl*

Elimination

Gastrointestinal/bowel   Bowel elimination

Usual bowel habits *ONCE A DAY, "NO PROBLEMS IF I EXERCISE."*   (Constipation) (POTENTIAL)

Alterations from normal *SLIGHTLY HARDER STOOL*   Stoma/ostomy: yes/(no)   Diarrhea

Remedies used *NONE*   Incontinence

Abdominal physical examination *ABDOMEN SLIGHTLY TYMPANIC*   Gastrointestinal tissue

                                                             perfusion

Liver: Enlarged *∅*   Ascites *∅*

Occult blood test —

Renal/urinary   Urinary elimination

Usual urinary patterns *SEVERAL TIMES A DAY*   Incontinence

Alteration from normal *SMALLER AMOUNTS*   Stoma/ostomy: yes/(no)   Retention

Urine: Color *DK. YELLOW* Odor *STRONG*   Catheter —

Urine output: 24 hour —   Average hourly *20 cc*   Renal tissue perfusion

Bladder distention *ABSENT*

Genitalia

External genitalia examination *WITHIN NORMAL LIMITS*

Male: Prostate problems *N/A*

Female: LMP *LAST YEAR*   Vaginal discharge *∅*   Menstrual patterns

           Unusual vaginal bleeding *NO MENSES SINCE ILLNESS BEGAN*   Premenstrual syndrome

Figure 29-4, cont'd

CHOOSING ■ A pattern involving the selection of alternatives
Coping

Patient's usual problem-solving methods *"THINK THROUGH — DEAL c̄* ⬭ *(Ineffective individual coping)*
PROBLEMS AS THEY COME"   Ineffective family coping

Family's usual problem-solving methods *"WE TALK, ARGUE, & EVENTUALLY*
RESOLVE"

Patient's method of dealing with stress *"HOLD IT IN AND DO NOTHING"*

Family's method of dealing with stress *"MOM, DAD, & HUSBAND ARE PATIENT*
& WAIT IT OUT — THEY SEEM TO HANDLE IT WELL."

Patient's affect *INAPPROPRIATE*

Physical manifestations *SMILING INAPPROPRIATELY THROUGHOUT ASSESSMENT*

Support systems available *HUSBAND, BOTH PARENTS IN AREA*

Participation

Compliance with past/current health regimens *COMPLIANT IN PAST,* Noncompliance
COOPERATIVE TODAY.

Willingness to comply with future health care regimen *AGREES TO FOLLOW* Ineffective participation
MEDICAL/HEALTH CARE REGIMEN

Judgment

Decision-making ability   Judgment
  Patient's perspective *"BEFORE SURGERY IT WAS SOUND, NOT SURE NOW."* Indecisiveness
  Others' perspectives *APPROPRIATE, BUT QUESTIONABLE.*

Prioritized nursing diagnosis/problem list

1. *GUILT RELATED TO PHYSICAL DIFFICULTIES WHICH DECREASE PTS. INVOLVEMENT IN CHILD*
2. *KNOWLEDGE DEFICIT RELATED TO MISCONCEPTION OF NAUSEA & VOMITING ETIOLOGY, CARE.*
3. *INEFFECTIVE INDIVIDUAL COPING RELATED TO GUILT & FEAR WHICH MANIFEST AS NAUSEA →*
4. *ALTERED COMFORT RELATED TO ABDOMINAL PAIN.   VOMITING.*
5. _____

Signature *Stelia Bunton, Maj, AN*   Date *27 AUGUST, 2000 HOURS*

Figure 29-4, cont'd

focus assessment on determining the presence or absence of defining characteristics for the nursing diagnoses that belong to the response pattern being evaluated. In this way, the assessment tool itself assists in clustering cues.

The tool also provides the practitioner with tentative hypotheses, in the form of nursing diagnoses. These diagnoses are found in the right-hand column directly across from assessment variables that might yield the appropriate defining characteristics. As the clinician discovers abnormal findings for variables, he or she can circle the diagnosis in the right-hand column. Circling the diagnosis does not mean that the diagnosis exists; it merely indicates a tentative diagnosis that merits further evaluation.

Some signs and symptoms can indicate a variety of diagnoses. To avoid continued repetition of the same variables in several response patterns, the variables have been arranged with the diagnoses that is most likely to

result from the recorded findings. Because the variables are not repeated with every appropriate diagnosis, it is necessary to synthesize all the data once the assessment has been completed to determine if defining characteristics for a circled tentative diagnosis appear in other response patterns. This is the hypothesis evaluation stage of using this tool. If enough defining characteristics for one or more nursing diagnoses are found during the evaluation process, the diagnoses can then be prioritized and written at the end of the tool.

As one can see, the organization of this assessment form guides the user through the stages of the decision-making process. In addition, because the tool is based on the theoretical framework associated with nursing diagnosis, it facilitates the formulation of nursing diagnoses. Thus, the tool can be very useful to individuals who are learning decision making or who are experiencing difficulty in deriving nursing diagnoses from another assessment format.

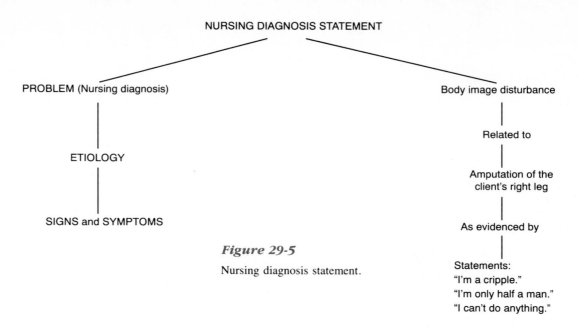

Figure 29-5

Nursing diagnosis statement.

DECISION MAKING AND THE NURSING PROCESS

Assessment and Decision Making

The nursing process consists of four phases: assessment, planning, implementation, and evaluation. According to Yura and Walsh, assessment, the first stage of this process, begins with history taking and ends with the determination of actual or potential nursing diagnoses. This definition implies that some form of decision making has occurred.

Looking at assessment from a decision-making viewpoint, one finds that assessment occurs before and during the decision-making process. During the initial phase of decision making, the practitioner performs a cursory initial assessment for significant cues. This initial assessment can be as simple as eliciting the client's presenting complaint and making some general observations concerning the client's appearance. Once the initial cues are clustered and tentative hypotheses are formulated, a second, more focused assessment is performed. Thus, assessment and decision making are intertwined.

Nursing Diagnoses and Decision Making

The culmination of nursing assessment and decision making is the formulation of nursing diagnoses. According to NANDA's recommendations, a nursing diagnosis should be stated in a problem-etiology-signs and symptoms (P-E-S) format. This format also conveniently summarizes the key decision-making factors or defining characteristics that led to the final diagnosis (Fig. 29-5).

When nursing diagnoses are recorded in this manner, any nurse reading the diagnostic statement will be able to determine how this decision was reached. In ad-

dition, nursing diagnoses written in P-E-S format provide clues concerning possible nursing interventions by indicating which defining characteristics are present and therefore require intervention. In this way, nursing diagnoses can also assist in the planning phase of the nursing process. For example, the diagnosis in Fig. 29-5 suggests planning interventions that would allow the client to ventilate feelings regarding the loss of a leg. Another suggested intervention would be fostering the client's independence by encouraging self-care and personal decision making.

SUMMARY

In conclusion, decision making is an integral part of the nursing process. All four phases of the decision-making process occur during nursing assessment. The end product of nursing assessment and decision making is nursing diagnoses. If nurses use a nursing framework to guide assessment and decision making, the formulation of nursing diagnoses will be facilitated. In addition, if identified nursing diagnoses are written in the P-E-S format, they will contribute useful information for the rest of the nursing process.

BIBLIOGRAPHY

American Nurses' Association: Nursing: a social policy statement, Kansas City, 1980, The Association.

Brennan PF and Romano CA: Computers and nursing diagnosis: issues in implementation, Nurs Clin North Am 22:935, 1987.

Carnevali DL and others: Diagnostic reasoning in nursing, Philadelphia, 1984, JB Lippincott Co.

Ciafrani KL: The influence of amounts and relevance of data on identifying health problems. In Kim MJ, McFarland GK, and

McLane A, editors: Classification of nursing diagnoses: proceedings of the fifth national conference, St Louis, 1984, The CV Mosby Co.

Ekwo EE: An analysis of the problem-solving process of third year medical students. In Proceedings of the 16th annual conference on research in medical education, Washington, DC, 1977, Association of American Medical Colleges.

Elstein A and others: Method and theory in the study of medical inquiry, J Med Educ 47:85, 1972.

Elstein A and others: Medical problem-solving: analysis of clinical reasoning, Cambridge, Mass, 1978, Harvard University.

Gordon M: Implementation of nursing diagnoses: an overview, Nurs Clin North Am 22:875, 1987.

Guzzetta CE, Bunton SD, Prinkey LA and others: Unitary person assessment tool: easing problems with nursing diagnoses, Focus Crit Care 15:12, 1988.

Guzzetta CE, Bunton SD, Prinkey LA and others: Clinical assessment tools for use with nursing diagnoses, St Louis, 1989, The CV Mosby Co.

Guzzetta CE and Kinney MR: Mastering the transition from medical to nursing diagnosis. Prog Cardiovasc Nurs 1:41, 1986.

Kassirer JP and Gorry CA: Clinical problem-solving: a behavioral analysis, Ann Intern Med 89:245, 1978.

Kim MJ and Moritz DA, editors: Classification of nursing diagnoses: proceedings of the third and fourth national conferences, New York, 1982, McGraw-Hill Book Co.

Orem DE: Nursing: concepts of practice, ed 3, New York, 1985, McGraw-Hill Book Co.

Putzier DJ and others: Diagnostic reasoning in critical care nursing, Heart Lung 14:430, 1985.

Roy C: Framework for classification systems development: progress and issues. In Kim MJ, McFarland GK, and McLane AM, editors: Classification of nursing diagnoses: proceedings of the fifth national conference, St Louis, 1984, The CV Mosby Co.

Roy C: Introduction to nursing: an adaptation model, ed 2, Englewood Cliffs, NJ, 1984, Prentice-Hall.

Theile JE and others: An investigation of decision theory: what are the effects of teaching cue recognition? J Nurs Ed 25:319, 1986.

Vincent KG: The validation of a nursing diagnosis: a nurse consensus survey, Nurs Clin North Am 20:631, 1985.

Westfall UE and others: Activating clinical inferences: a component of diagnostic reasoning in nursing, Res Nurs Health 9:269, 1986.

Yura H and Walsh MB: The nursing process: assessing, planning, implementing, and evaluating, ed 4, New York, 1983, Appleton-Century-Crofts.

chapter

30

Clinical laboratory procedures

OBJECTIVES

Upon successful review of this chapter, learners will be able to:

- List five ways laboratory data augment health assessment
- Recognize usual values, deviations, and possible pathology associated with
  Electrolytes
  Blood gases
  Glucose
  Bilirubin and creatinine
  Blood urea nitrogen (BUN)
  Uric acid
  Plasma proteins
  Triglycerides, cholesterol, and phospholipids
  Enzymes
- Recognize usual values, deviations, and possible pathology associated with screening hematologic examinations, including
  Complete blood cell count (WBC and RBC)
  Microscopic examination (WBC differential)
  Platelet count
- Recognize usual findings, deviations, and possible pathology asociated with
  Serological tests
  Urinalysis
  Stool examination

The information obtained through the physical examination is augmented and in many cases verified through the judicious use of laboratory diagnostic procedures to provide a biochemical database for use in the analysis of the client's state of health.

The tests most frequently included in a screening workup are a blood chemistry profile, hematology screening, a serologic test for syphilis, urinalysis, a chest roentgenogram, the Papanicolaou (Pap) cytologic examination for cancer diagnosis, hormonal evaluation of ovarian function in women from puberty onward, a proctoscopic examination, and an electrocardiogram (ECG) for all persons older than 40 years of age.

Blood chemistry profiles characteristically include determinations of sodium, potassium, chloride, calcium, phosphorus, glucose, bilirubin, blood urea nitrogen (BUN), uric acid, total proteins, albumin, cholesterol, serum glutamic-oxaloacetic transaminase (AST), lactic dehydrogenase (LDH), and alkaline phosphatase.

The hematology screening examination includes a study of the red blood cell (RBC) count, hematocrit, hemoglobin, mean corpuscular volume (MCV), and mean corpuscular hemoglobin concentration (MCHC). The total white blood cell (WBC) count and a differential count based on morphologic types are also included.

Urinalysis is performed for analysis of specific gravity, pH, and the presence of glucose, protein, acetone, blood, and microscopic formed elements.

The procedure for the Pap smear is described in Chapter 22 on assessment of the female genitalia and procedures for smears and cultures.

The tables of normal ranges found in textbooks of clinical pathology should be considered as relative guidelines. The values are often those of medical or nursing student volunteers and laboratory technicians and thus are nonspecific as to sex and age.

Furthermore, values vary from one clinical laboratory to another even though the same procedure may be used in each laboratory.

There may be real differences in values observed in geographically separated population groups; for example, generally higher cholesterol values are observed in sample populations in San Francisco. Seasonal changes may also play a role; for example, uric acid levels are observed to be greater in winter than in other seasons.

When abnormal values are observed in test results, the examiner should review the interview data to determine if any circumstances in the client's life-style, environment, drug use, or state of nutrition or hydration may have influenced the value. For instance, an elevated protein-bound iodine (PBI) level and low resin-uptake value (triiodothyronine [T_3]) may indicate that the client has been taking oral contraceptives.

Posture is known to affect laboratory values. Blood albumin, total protein, hemoglobin, cholesterol, and calcium values are known to be higher in the client who has been standing for a long time.

Diet, alcohol, and stress may also alter laboratory values. Bilirubin and AST values have been shown to be elevated during fasting. High fat content in the diet will produce hyperlipidemia. High-protein meals may produce an increased BUN level. Most professionals are aware of the possibility of increased blood glucose values incurred as a result of a "carbohydrate binge." Alcohol consumption or alcoholic liver damage has been shown to result in increased levels of uric acid, glucose, calcium, phosphorus, LDH, AST, creatine phosphokinase (CK), alkaline phosphatase, and triglycerides, accompanied by a low PBI level and albumin-globulin (A/G) ratio.

The blood specimens collected from a dehydrated individual will show the values to be consistent with the more concentrated fluid. These include increased levels of sodium, potassium, chloride, calcium, phosporus, glucose, BUN, uric acid, cholesterol, total protein, globulin, LDH, AST, and creatinine.

The overhydrated client might be expected to have decreased concentrations of sodium, potassium, chloride, calcium, phosphorus, BUN, uric acid, albumin, total proteins, and cholesterol in the blood.

Improper handling of specimens may also result in erroneous test results. Test tubes that have been washed with detergent and poorly rinsed may cause spuriously elevated calcium, sodium, and potassium levels.

Possible applications of results of laboratory procedures include the following:
1. Provision of health assessment parameters of both a morphologic and biochemical nature that are unavailable through the health history and physical examination.
2. Confirmation of a biochemical state of health when physical examination findings are negative.
3. Provision of further information in the differential diagnosis of disease. For example, the client with easy fatigability, shortness of breath on exertion, dizziness on exercise, and pale buccal mucosa may have a diagnosis of anemia confirmed through the results of screening hematologic studies.
4. Provision of a gauge of the severity of disease. The degree of anemia that is disclosed may determine the therapeutic regimen for the client. The milder form of iron deficiency anemia may well be ameliorated in time through diet and rest, allowing the client's blood-forming organs to make up the deficit. Medication may be necessary for more severe involvement, and blood replacement by transfusion may be necessary for marked reduction in hemoglobin and RBCs.
5. Provision of biochemical clues that will indicate appropriate dosages of medication. A serum iron determination may be made for the client who is suspected of having iron deficiency anemia to substantiate the physical examination findings. The serum iron levels may be used to monitor the efficiency of the treatment regimen.

BLOOD CHEMISTRY PROFILE

Automated machines are available in many pathology laboratories for the purpose of performing chemistry tests. These machines commonly perform six to 24 determinations, using a single small sample of blood. Two types of machines are used. The first type is a discrete sample analyzer (DSA), which separates the sample into as many chambers as there are tests to be performed. Translated into the language of technician-performed testing, this means the sample is separated into an individual test tube for each ordered test. The second type is a continuous flow analyzer (CFA), which separates the sample within a single tubing into discrete sections through the use of bubbles. These sections pass through the tubing, stopping at specific sites for analysis. Some caution must be used with these machines to be certain that the tubing is thoroughly cleaned between samples.

Most of these machines provide a printout sheet that records the client's data against a range of normal for the particular instrument.

Blood chemistry tests are performed on venous samples that are obtained following a period of fasting (usually at least 6 hours).

Some of these machines provide test results at a rate of greater than 3000 per minute and thus provide significantly more data at less cost to the consumer.

In general, the machines are carefully self-calibrated and are more accurate than the results produced when humans do the testing.

One disadvantage to the practitioner and the client is that more data may be generated than is actually necessary to assess the client's health status.

Electrolytes

Some electrolytes that are routinely analyzed in a screening examination include sodium (Na^+), potassium (K^+), chloride (Cl^-), and carbon dioxide (CO_2) combining power.

Plasma is an aqueous solution (90% water) that contains approximately 1% electrolytes.

The distribution of electrolytes in the normal individual is represented by the following values:

Na^+ 136 to 142 mEq/L	Cl^- 95 to 103 mEq/L
K^+ 3.8 to 5 mEq/L	PO_4^{3-} 1.8 to 2.6 mEq/L
Ca^{2+} 4.5 to 5.3 mEq/L	SO_4^{2-} 0.2 to 1.3 mEq/L
Mg^{2+} 1.5 to 2.5 mEq/L	HCO_3^- 21 to 28 mEq/L
	Protein $\cong$ 17 mEq/L

The distribution of these ions in the plasma is compared with those of the interstitial and cellular fluids in Fig. 30-1.

Electrolytes are carefully controlled through a variety of physical and chemical mechanisms, so that the range of normal for each of these compartments is quite narrow.

Sodium

Sodium is the major cation of the body. It is the most abundant extracellular ion and as such plays a prominent role in the osmolality of the extracellular fluid. The ion is necessary to the resting potential of excitable cells. The intake of sodium in the average adult diet is 10 to 12 g, but the amount is variable.

The kidney plays the principal role in homeostasis of sodium in the body fluids. Aldosterone is secreted by the adrenal cortex as a result of the activation of the renin angiotensin system when the whole blood sodium concentration or blood volume is decreased or when the potassium concentration is increased. Adrenocorticotropic hormone (ACTH) directly stimulates the cells of the adrenal cortex. Thus, aldosterone is also secreted in times of stress. Aldosterone facilitates the reabsorption of sodium in the distal tubule of the kidney.

The concentration of the particles necessarily depends on the water content of the blood. Although the whole blood sodium content might stay constant, the concentration of the sodium ions will be greater when water stores are less in quantity.

Osmotic diuretic agents, such as mannitol and glucose, are known to carry out sodium with them. In some cases of acidemia, the concentration of SO_4^{2-}, Cl^-, PO_4^{3-}, and organic acids overwhelms the kidneys' capacity to secrete H^+ and NH_3 while exchanging Na^+. Thus, the ions are excreted in the urine with a fixed base, which is sodium for the most part. In conditions where potassium is lost from the cellular compartment, sodium replaces the ion. This situation may occur in acidosis or when the sodium-potassium pump is malfunctioning.

Serum sodium: normal values and deviations

Normal values: 136 to 142 mEq/L

Normal osmolality of the blood: 280 to 295 mOsm/L

Deviations	*Cause*
Hyponatremia	Dehydration with loss of electrolytes
	Sweating
	Diarrhea
	Burns
	Nasogastric tube
	Addison's disease
	Diuretics
	Mercurial
	Chlorothiazide
	Chronic renal insufficiency
	Chronic glomerulonephritis
	Pyelonephritis
	Starvation
	Diabetic acidosis
	Water retention or dilution
	Cirrhosis
	Congestive heart failure
	Renal insufficiency
	Excessive ingestion of water
	Overhydration with intravenous therapy
Hypernatremia (uncommon)	Deficient water intake
	Excessive water loss—lack of antidiuretic hormone (ADH)
	Cushing's disease
	Primary hyperaldosteronism

Potassium

Potassium is the most abundant intracellular cation; since the majority of potassium is found within the cells, the total body content of the ion cannot be measured readily. Furthermore, the relationship between intracellular potassium and serum potassium is a highly dynamic one. For instance, intracellular potassium readily leaves the cell in the event of serum potassium deficiency. Potassium ions compete with hydrogen ions for excretion by the kidney; potassium is excreted largely by this mechanism, although some may be lost in sweat and gastrointestinal secretions.

The importance of homeokinetic control of extra-

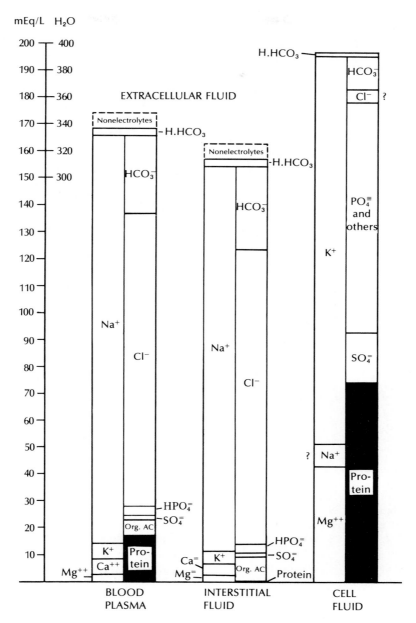

Figure 30-1

Electrolyte distribution in the fluid compartment of the body. The column of figures on the left (200, 190, 180, and so on) indicates amounts of cations or anions; the figures on the right (400, 380, 360, and so on) indicate the sum of cations and anions. Note that chloride and sodium values in cell fluid are questioned. It is probable that at least muscle intracellular fluid contains some sodium but no chloride.

(From Anthony CP and Thibodeau GA: Textbook of anatomy and physiology, ed 11, St Louis, 1983, The CV Mosby Co. Adapted from Mountcastle VB, editor: Medical physiology, vol 2, ed 14, St Louis, 1980, The CV Mosby Co.; after Gamble JL: Harvey Lect 42:247, 1946-1947.)

cellular potassium ions relate to the function of potassium in neuromuscular excitability. The resting membrane potential of the cells of these tissues is directly related to the ratio of intracellular potassium concentrations.

Serum potassium: normal values and deviations

Normal values: 3.8 to 5 mEq/L

Deviations	Cause	Possible effects
Hyperkalemia	↓ Excretion of K$^+$ Kidney disease Intestinal obstruction Addison's disease Hypoaldosteronism Iatrogenic K$^+$ replacement therapy Trauma Burns Diuretics such as spironolactone that cause ↓ K$^+$ excretion K$^+$ shift from tissues Muscle crush Acidosis	Changes in ECG; >8 mEq/L Widened P wave Symmetric peaking of T wave Widened QRS complex Depressed ST segment; >11 mEq/L Ventricular fibrillation Heart block in diastole Neuromuscular changes Flaccidity Muscle paralysis Numbness Tingling
Hypokalemia	↓ Ingestion of K$^+$ ↑ Excretion of K$^+$ Prolonged gastrointestinal suctioning Vomiting K$^+$ depleting diuretics Excessive administration of biocarbonate (K$^+$ enters the cells) Cirrhosis Cushing's disease Treatment with steroids Aldosteronism Excessive licorice intake Intravenous infusion of K$^+$ free fluids Fasting, starvation	Changes in ECG Flattening and inversion of T wave Prominent U wave Sagging of ST segment Muscle weakness Malaise Apathy Nausea and vomiting ↓ Reflexes ↓ Smooth muscle tone Distention Paralytic ileus ↓ Diastolic blood pressure Impairment of renal tubular function Polyuria

Chloride

Chloride is the major anion of the body and in general is found to behave in concert with sodium. More precisely, the chloride passively follows sodium in its transport through membranes. Chloride plays a prominent role in acid-base balance. In acidemia, Cl$^-$ concentration is increased, and thus more Cl$^-$ is associated with sodium. In alkalemia, more bicarbonate (HCO$^-_3$) is associated with sodium. Chloride deficit leads to increased reabsorption of bicarbonate in the distal tubules of the kidney and thereby leads to alkalemia. Since chloride is necessary to the synthesis of hydrochloric acid in the stomach, excessive loss of gastric secretions leads to alkalemia. Chloride is also lost from the intestinal tract in diarrhea or as a result of intestinal fistula. Chloride is excreted in the urine with cations in diuresis.

Serum chloride: normal values and deviations

Normal values: 95 to 103 mEq/L

Deviations	Cause	Possible effects
Hypochloremia	Hypokalemic alkalosis Ingestion of potassium compounds that do not contain chloride Potassium-sparing diuretics Excessive loss of gastric secretions Vomiting Nasogastric tube	Associated with ↓ K$^+$ and ↑ CO$_2$ combining power
Hyperchloremia (rare)	Diarrhea Iatrogenic Ammonium chloride ingestion	Fistulas

Calcium

Plasma calcium (Ca^{2+}) occurs in three forms. About half the calcium is bound to protein. Calcium in this form does not diffuse through the capillary wall. A second, nonionized, nondiffusable group of calcium compounds makes up approximately 5% of the plasma calcium. Somewhat less than half (45%) of the plasma calcium is ionized. This third form of calcium diffuses through the capillary membrane and is physiologically active.

The effects of calcium on skeletal and cardiac muscle, nerve tissue, and bone are due to the ionized calcium. The ionized calcium of the plasma is maintained within a fairly narrow range (±5%) as a result of the influence of parathyroid hormone (PTH) and thyrocalcitonin (TCT). PTH increases plasma ionized calcium by increasing absorption of calcium from the intestinal tract and reabsorption of calcium from the renal tubules of the kidney and by absorbing calcium salts from the bones through its action of osteoclasts. TCT lowers serum ionized calcium by increasing depositions of calcium in the bones through its influence on the osteoblasts.

Serum calcium: normal values and deviations

Normal values

Adults:
  Ionized: 4.2 to 5.2 mg/dl
  Total: 9 to 10.6 mg/dL
            4.5 to 5.3 mEq/l
Infants: 11 to 13 mg/dl

Deviations	Cause	Possible effects

Hypercalcemia	↑ PTH ⎫ Hyperpara-
	↓ TCT ⎭ thyroidism
	    (associated
	    with alka-
	    line phos-
	    phatase)
	↑ Vitamin D intake
	↑ Absorption of Ca^{2+}
	  in intestine
	↑ Reabsorption of
	  Ca^{2+} in renal tu-
	  bules
	Acidosis
	Paget's disease
	Destructive bone le-
	  sions
	Osteoporosis
	Immobilization
	Hypothyroidism
	Malignancy (associ-
	  ated with hyper-
	  gammaglobuline-
	  mia)
	↓ Urinary excretion
	Na^+ depletion
	Thiazide diuretics
		Polyuria; polydip-
		  sia
		↓ Neuromuscular
		  excitability
		Skeletal muscle
		  (↓ tone, weak-
		  ness, atrophy)
		Smooth muscle
		  (↓ tone, ob-
		  served in such
		  signs as nausea,
		  vomiting, and
		  constipation)
		Heart muscle
		Shortening of QT
		  interval of the
		  ECG
		Arteriovenous
		  block
		↓ Plasma phos-
		  phate
		Renal calculi
		  caused by pre-
		  cipitation of cal-
		  cium phosphate
		  $(Ca_3[PO_4]_2)$
		Alkalosis
		Ataxia
		Hyperreflexia

Hypocalcemia	↑ TCT ⎫ Hypopara-
	↓ PTH ⎭ thyroidism
	↓ Absorption of Ca^{2+}
	  from the gastroin-
	  testinal tract
	Steatorrhea
	Sprue
	Celiac disease
	Acute pancreatitis
	↓ Vitamin D (hypo-
	  vitaminosis)
	Hypoalbuminemia
	Pregnancy
	Diuretic ingestion
	Starvation
	↓ Magnesium
		↓ Neuromuscular
		  excitability (tet-
		  any)
		Prolongation of
		  the ST segment
		  of the ECG
		Osteomalacia in
		  adults
		Rickets in children

Phosphorus

The serum level of phosphate (PO_4^{3-}) generally bears a combination relationship with serum calcium concentra-

tion. Parathyroid hormone increases the amount of phosphate absorbed in the intestinal tract, since phosphate is absorbed when calcium is absorbed. The excretion of phosphate is accomplished largely by the kidney and is determined by the fact that phosphate is a threshold substance. Thus, the kidney regulates the serum phosphate level by secreting phosphate when the serum level exceeds 1 mMol/L and retaining phosphate when the serum concentration is less.

Serum phosphorus: normal values and deviations

Normal values

Adults: 3 to 4.5 mg/dl
           1.8 to 2.6 mEq/L
Children: 4 to 7 mg/dl
           2.3 to 4.1 mEq/L

Deviations	Cause	Possible effects

Hyperphos-
phatemia
	↑ TCT
	↑ Growth hormone
	↑ Ingestion of PO_4^{3-}
	Chronic glomerulo-
	  nephritis
	Sarcoidosis
		Associated with
		  ↓ BUN, creatinine
		Symptoms of hypocal-
		  cemia
		Associated with
		  ↓ gamma globulin

Hypophos-
phatemia
	↑ PTH
	↓ Ingestion of PO_4^{3-}
	Hyperinsulinism
		↓ ATP
		Symptoms of hyper-
		  calcemia
		Associated with indi-
		  cations of hypogly-
		  cemia

Magnesium

Magnesium (Mg^{2+}) influences muscular activity in much the same direction as does calcium. The ion appears to be necessary for the coenzyme activity in the metabolism of carbohydrate and protein.

Serum magnesium: normal values and deviations

Normal values: 1.5 to 2.5 mEq/L
                    1.8 to 3 mg/dl

Deviations	Cause	Possible effects

Hypermag-
nesemia
	↑ Ingestion of
	  Mg^{2+} (milk of
	  magnesia)
		↓ Neuromuscular ex-
		  citation
		↓ Muscle tone

Hypomag-
nesemia
	Malabsorption
	  syndrome
	Acute pancreatitis
		↑ Neuromuscular ex-
		  citation (tetany)
		Peripheral vasodila-
		  tation
		Arrhythmias

Gases and pH

The blood gases are not usually tested in the screening examination but may be indicated as necessary tests by clinical signs such as cyanosis or hyperventilation.

Oxygen

Tests for blood oxygen analysis are generally performed on arterial blood. The blood may be tested for oxygen content, hemoglobin saturation, and the gas tension (Pao_2, arterial blood; Pvo_2, venous blood). The oxygen content of the blood reflects the hemoglobin concentration. At standard temperature and pressure 1.34 ml of oxygen combines with 1 g of hemoglobin at full saturation. The oxygen saturation of hemoglobin is a comparison of the percentage of oxygen that is bound to hemoglobin with the total amount that it is possible for the hemoglobin to carry. The erythrocyte carries 98.5% of the oxygen in the blood bound to hemoglobin. Since the normal hemoglobin content of the adult male is 15 g/dl, the oxygen-carrying capacity is approximately 20 ml/dl of blood, or 20 vol%.

Blood oxygen: normal values and deviations

Normal values

	Arterial blood	Mixed venous blood
Content:	15 to 23 mg/dl	
Saturation:	94% to 100%	70% to 75%
Tension:	95 to 100 mm Hg	35 to 40 mm Hg

Deviations	Cause	Possible effects
Anoxic hypoxia	Inadequate environmental O_2 supply, such as occurs in high altitude (acute) Impaired respiratory exchange	Low Pao_2 Inadequate saturation of the arterial blood with oxygen Cyanosis ↑ Respiratory rate
Chronic hypoxia	Living at high altitude	↑ O_2 carrying capacity as RBCs increase
Anemic hypoxia	↓ Hemoglobin Competition for hemoglobin-binding sites (carbon monoxide poisoning)	↓ Saturation of hemoglobin possible
Stagnant hypoxia	↓ Circulatory function (failure to deliver O_2 to tissues) Cardiac failure Shock Peripheral impairment of flow (embolism)	Blood O_2 values may be normal
Histotoxic hypoxia	↓ Ability of cells to take up or use O_2, such as in poisoning	
Hyperoxia	Pure O_2 delivered at 1 atmosphere (766 mm Hg)	Bronchitis in 12 to 24 hours Fall in vital capacity in 60 hours Retrolental fibroplasia

At standard conditions arterial blood contains 0.3 ml of oxygen dissolved in 100 ml of plasma; this exerts a pressure of 100 mm Hg. The amount of oxygen combined with hemoglobin is decreased with an increase in temperature, acidity, and carbon dioxide tension ($Paco_2$, arterial blood; $Pvco_2$, venous blood).

Carbon dioxide

Carbon dioxide in the blood occurs in three forms: as bicarbonate, combined with protein (carbamino), and in simple solution. Carbon dioxide in an aqueous solution is in potential equilibrium with carbonic acid. The enzyme carbonic anhydrase is necessary to the catalysis of the equilibrium:

$$CO_2 + H_2O \rightleftharpoons H_2CO_3$$

The only test for carbon dioxide that is generally performed as part of the screening battery is the carbon dioxide–combining power, which measures the blood's buffering capacity. The sample is collected, and the serum is removed after clotting and centrifugation. The carbon dioxide tension of the serum is equilibrated to normal alveolar tensions of 40 mm Hg. The bicarbonate is converted to carbon dioxide by hydrolysis, and the gas that is given up is measured. Subtraction of the known amount of dissolved carbon dioxide in the blood gives a value that is essentially that of bicarbonate alone.

Normal $Paco_2$: 35 to 45 mm Hg
Normal $Pvco_2$: 41 to 55 mm Hg
Normal arterial whole blood HCO_3^-: 22 to 26 mEq/L
Normal venous whole blood HCO_3^-: 22 to 26 mEq/L

The base excess (BE) is a measure of alkaline substances in the blood. This includes bicarbonate and other bases in the blood.

Normal arterial BE: −2 to +2
Normal venous BE: −2 to +2

pH

Hydrogen ion concentration of the blood is reflected in the pH value. The degree of alkalinity or acidity of the body is important in that many enzymes are active only within narrow pH ranges. Furthermore, many other physiologic processes are pH dependent, notably respiration. Acidosis is the process whereby an individual develops acidemia, the accumulation of excess hydrogen ions in the blood—or decreased pH. The affected person is described as acidotic.

Alkalosis, on the other hand, is the process whereby alkalemia is incurred. Alkalemia may be defined as decreased hydrogen ion concentration in the blood—

or increased pH—and the individual may be described as alkalotic.

The Henderson-Hasselbalch equation describes pH relationships:

$$pH = pK + \log \frac{base}{acid}$$

pK is the dissociation constant (the ability to release hydrogen ions of the acid described). In the human being the bicarbonate ion is the most important buffering system, since the ion is present in large quantities. Thus, the equation may be written:

$$pH = 6.1 + \log \frac{HCO_3^-}{H_2CO_3}$$

The ratio $\dfrac{HCO_3^-}{H_2CO_3} = \dfrac{20}{1}$ in the normal person.

The bicarbonate ion is controlled by the lungs through the expiration of carbon dioxide and by the kidneys, which control excretion of bicarbonate and hydrogen ions.

Whole blood pH: normal values and deviations

Normal values

Arterial: 7.38 to 7.44 (7.40)
Venous: 7.30 to 7.41 (7.36)

Deviations

Acidemia (acidosis): pH < 7.35
Alkalemia (alkalosis): pH > 7.45

Glucose

Sucrose, lactose, and starches make up the majority of the carbohydrates ingested by humans. Slight amounts of alcohol, lactic acid, pyruvic acid, pectins, and dextrins are also consumed. These carbohydrates are hydrolyzed in the intestinal tract and broken down to the monosaccharides: glucose (80%), fructose (10%), and galactose (10%), in which form they are absorbed into the bloodstream.

Glucose is the principal form of fuel for cellular function; the liver can convert fructose and galactose to glucose so that all the absorbed sugars can be used. Fats and proteins may also be converted to glucose during fasting states or in times of increased glucose use, as in exercise. Glucose in excess of energy needs is converted to storage forms. The body can store about 100 g of glucose as glycogen. The majority of the remainder of glucose is converted to fat, but some is converted to amino acids.

The pancreatic hormones, insulin and glucagon, play a prominent role in glucose metabolism as well as in the metabolism of protein and lipid. Insulin is produced by the beta cells of the pancreas, and its secretion is primarily determined by the concentration of blood glucose. The secretion of insulin is increased by an increase from basal of blood glucose; it is decreased as the concentration of blood glucose becomes less than normal. Blood insulin values in excess of normal produce the following major changes in glucose metabolism: (1) the rate of glucose metabolism is increased by facilitating the transport of glucose into the cells through facilitated diffusion, (2) the process of glycogen storage is enhanced, (3) the process of glucose entry into fat cells is enhanced and fat storage increased, and (4) the process of glucose entry into muscle cells is enhanced.

On the other hand, a decrease of blood insulin is accompanied by (1) glycogenolysis, a breakdown of glycogen to glucose, and (2) glyconeogenesis, the manufacture of glucose by the liver from amino acids derived from protein stores and from glycerol derived from fat stores. These two processes are functions of glucagon.

Thus, blood glucose concentration in the fasting state is maintained within reasonably narrow limits. Blood glucose determination at any one time will provide data concerning the state of the body's metabolism for that specific point in the individual's daily cycle. However, the practitioner must bear in mind that the metabolic processes are determined by the state of nutrition and the energy expenditure. The normal individual, in dynamic equilibrium, will show remarkable variation throughout the day; the picture is even more complex in disease.

Care of specimens for blood glucose determination deserves special attention; glucose values for whole blood decrease 10 mg/dl per hour (at room temperature) unless a satisfactory preservative is employed. Fluoride is currently recognized as the most effective preservative.

Glucose analysis is accomplished by reducing and enzymatic methods. In both cases, a protein-free filtrate of the blood sample is tested. The reducing methods include the Folin-Wu and Somogyi-Nelson tests, both of which consist of color changes that occur in copper solutions. The enzymatic (glucose oxidase) tests measure hydrogen peroxide that is released during the enzymatic conversion of glucose to gluconic acid.

Blood glucose values are 120 to 130 mg/dl in mild hyperglycemia and greater than 500 mg/dl in marked hyperglycemia.

Blood glucose: normal values and deviations

Normal values

Serum or plasma: 70 to 110 mg/dl (Folin-Wu)
65 to 90 mg/dl (Somogyi-Nelson)
65 to 90 mg/dl (glucose oxidase)

Deviations	Cause	Possible effects
Hyperglycemia	Diabetes mellitus (most common cause) Pancreatic insufficiency Cushing's disease Treatment with steroids ↑ Catecholamines Pheochromocytoma Pancreatic neoplasm Hyperthyroidism (look for hydrocholesterolemia) Thiazide diuretics	Ketoacidosis Diuresis if >160 to 180 mg/1 bond ↓ CO_2 combining power >500 mg/dl
Hypoglycemia	Beta cell neoplasm (hyperinsulinism) Addison's disease Hypothyroidism Hepatocellular disease Starvation (late) Glycogen storage diseases	

A rising blood glucose concentration stimulates excessive insulin secretion in some individuals. Some amino acids (leucine) may also stimulate excessive beta cell secretion. Thus, glucose levels may be depleted as the insulin effects are manifested.

Two-hour postprandial glucose test.   The 2-hour postprandial glucose test consists of the serial collection of samples of blood glucose determination following a 100 g carbohydrate meal given to a client who has fasted for 12 hours. The following represent hyperglycemia results:

Time	Blood glucose determination
1 hour after meal	>170 mg/dl
2 hours after meal	>120 mg/dl

Glucose tolerance test.   The glucose tolerance test is performed in the fasting individual following the ingestion of 100 g of glucose; the blood glucose level rises 30 to 60 mg/dl above the fasting level by 30 minutes. By the end of an hour the blood glucose level begins to decline (20 to 50 mg/dl) and, after 2 to 3 hours, returns to the fasting level. Urine specimens are collected. Glucose does not appear in the urine of the normal individual during the course of the glucose tolerance test. The glucose tolerance test shows elevated values in the period following myocardial infarction.

Bilirubin

Bilirubin is a pigment mainly derived from the breakdown of heme in the hemoglobin of RBCs in Kupffer's cells of the reticuloendothelial system. The pigment has a golden hue and is the major pigment found in bile. Plasma containing the pigment enters the hepatic parenchymal cells and is enzymatically conjugated with glucuronic acid in preparation for excretion. The conjugated bilirubin is soluble in an aqueous medium and is actively excreted into the bile. A small amount of conjugated bilirubin is returned to the blood and accounts for the direct-reacting bilirubin found in the plasma of normal subjects. Because it passes through membranes, it may be detected in the urine.

Intestinal bacteria act on bilirubin to form urobilinogen. Since urobilinogen is highly soluble, it is readily reabsorbed through the intestinal mucosa into the blood and is for the most part recycled in the liver back to the intestine; some, however, is excreted in the urine.

Bilirubin is analyzed through its reaction (color change) with diazo reagents; this is the basis of van den Bergh's test. The conjugated form reacts expediently with the diazo reagents in aqueous solution and is called direct reacting. The unconjugated form must be treated with methyl alcohol for the reaction to occur and is called indirect reacting.

Bilirubin is called unconjugated, free, or indirect reacting before it is combined with glucuronic acid in the liver cell. It does not cross the membranes of the capillary or of the glomerular capsule. After combination with glucuronic acid in the hepatic cells, bilirubin is referred to as conjugated, glucuronide, or direct reacting. But the routine test gives only the total value.

The occurrence of jaundice (yellowish tint of the skin) represents the failure to remove or excrete the bilirubin. The skin may appear jaundiced when serum bilirubin levels are about three times the normal value. In most individuals pigmentation of the tissues is visible when serum bilirubin levels exceed 1.5 mg/dl.

Serum bilirubin: normal values and deviations
Normal values

Total: 0.1 to 1.2 mg/dl
Newborn total: 1 to 12 mg/dl

Deviations	Cause	Possible effects
Hyperbilirubinemia	Destruction of red cells Hemolytic diseases (↓ hemoglobin) Hemorrhage Hematoma Hepatic dysfunction	Jaundice

Deviations	Cause	
↑ Unconjugated bilirubin	Autoimmune disease Transfusion-initiated hemolysis Hemolytic diseases 　Sickle cell anemia 　Pernicious anemia Glucuronyl transferase deficiency (hemolytic disease of the newborn) Hemorrhage (bleeding into body cavities) Hematoma Impaired hepatic uptake of bile (infectious or toxic hepatitis)	Brain damage (22 mg/dl or more)
↑ Conjugated bilirubin	Impaired glucuronide excretion Hepatocellular disease (infectious, toxic, or autoimmune hepatitis) Cirrhosis Obstruction of biliary ducts Calculi Tumor Extrinsic pressure Cholangiolitis	"Regurgitation" of conjugated bilirubin back into the blood

Blood Urea Nitrogen

Urea is the end product of protein metabolism and is formed through deamination of amino acids in the liver. Urea is excreted by the kidneys.

Ingestion of protein does not cause a significant change in the BUN level. However, in the interest of accuracy this test is done in the fasting individual.

The severity of uremia is an indicator of the seriousness of renal involvement.

BUN: normal values and deviations

Normal values
Adults: 8 to 18 mg/dl
Children: 5 to 18 mg/dl
Normal values tend to be higher in men than in women.

Deviations	Cause
Increased BUN level of uremia	High protein intake Dehydration Protein catabolism Burns Intestinal obstruction Gastrointestinal hemorrhage

Deviations	Cause
	Renal disease 　Glomerulonephritis 　Pyelonephritis Prostatic hypertrophy
Decreased BUN level	↓ Protein ingestion Starvation Liver dysfunction Cirrhosis (loss of 80% to 85% hepatic function)

Creatinine

The metabolism of creatinine phosphate, a high-energy compound produced in skeletal muscle, results in the production of creatinine. The serum creatinine level does not vary markedly with diet or exercise and may be regarded as an indicator of total muscle mass.

Creatinine clearance by the kidney has been used as a measure of renal function. In addition to the serum creatinine level being fairly constant, creatinine clearance as a measure offers another advantage to the client in that an intravenous injection of the substance used in the clearance study is not needed. Renal plasma clearance of creatinine (C) is equal to the rate of creatinine excretion (UV) divided by the plasma concentration of creatinine (P):

$$C = \frac{UV}{P}$$

Since endogenous creatinine is fully filtered in the glomerulus and not reabsorbed by the tubules, its clearance is a useful clinical tool for estimation of the glomerular filtration rate (GFR). Thus, the removal of creatinine from the blood is a measure of renal efficiency. As renal function declines, the creatinine level rises.

Serum creatinine: Normal values and deviations
Normal values

Adults: 0.6 to 12 mg/dl
Normal values for men are slightly higher than for women.

Deviation	Cause	Possible effects
Hypercreatinemia	Renal disease (75% of nephrons are nonfunctional) Chronic glomerulonephritis Nephrosis Pyelonephritis Hyperthyroidism	Signs of renal failure

Uric Acid

Uric acid production is the final step in purine metabolism. Uric acid is not in stable solution at a normal human blood pH of 7.4. Uric acid is continuously produced in the human being and is excreted by the kidney. The quantity of uric acid found in the urine is about 10% of that which is filtered. Thus, it is obvious that uric acid is reabsorbed in the proximal tubules. It has been further shown that uric acid is secreted in the proximal tubules.

However, reabsorption overrides this process, and the plasma uric acid represents the balance of uric acid production and excretion.

Serum uric acid: normal values and deviation

Normal values

Women: 2 to 6.4 mg/dl
Men: 2.1 to 7.8 mg/dl
Children: 2.0-5.5 mg/dl

Deviation	Cause	Possible effects
Hyperuri- cemia (gout)	↑ Destruction of nucleic acid and purine products	Monosodium urate precipitate in joints (tophi)
	Chronic lymphocytic and granulocytic leukemia	Often associated with hyperlipidemia, atheromatosis
	Multiple myeloma	
	Chronic renal failure	Impaired clearance of uric acid
	Fasting	
	↑ Ingestion of Protein	
	↓ Excretion of uric acid	
	Gout	
	Fasting	
	Toxemia of pregnancy	
	Glomerulonephritis	
	Thiazide diuretics	
	Alpha-lipoprotein deficiency (Tangier disease)	
	Hypoparathyroidism	
	↑ Salicylate ingestion	
	Ethanol ingestion	

Monosodium urate deposits may occur in the presence of a normal serum uric acid value.

Hypouricemia is seldom observed unless the client is being treated with allopurinol, which depresses uric acid production.

Total proteins

Plasma proteins make up approximately 7% of the plasma volume. Albumin and globulin in the free state, as well as combined with lipid and carbohydrate substances, are the major plasma proteins. Through the application of zone electrophoresis and ultracentrifugation, the plasma proteins have been defined as albumin, the globulins

(alpha-1, alpha-2, beta-1, beta-2, and gamma), lipoproteins, and fibrinogen. Separation through centrifugation is possible because the sedimentation rate at high speeds is determined by molecular size and shape. Electrophoresis is the process of migration of charged particles in an electrolyte solution through which an electrical current is passed. The proteins move at various rates, depending on size, shape, and electrical charge. Immunoelectrophoresis separates the immune globulin fractions through a combination of electrophoresis and immunodiffusion.

The plasma proteins are large molecules that do not readily diffuse through the capillary membrane. The small amount of protein that does pass through the capillary wall is taken up by the lymphatic system and returned to the blood. It has been demonstrated that the plasma protein concentration exceeds that of the interstitial space nearly four times. Since the plasma proteins are the only dissolved substances in the plasma that do not pass through the capillary membrane, they are responsible for plasma oncotic pressure. Thus, proteins help to regulate intravascular volume. The plasma proteins also serve as buffers in acid-base balance and as binding and transporting agents for lipids, triglycerides, hormones, vitamins, calcium, and copper. In addition, they participate in blood coagulation. Furthermore, in the event the body tissues become depleted of protein, plasma proteins may be used for replenishment. The liver synthesizes nearly all of the plasma albumin and fibrinogen and about one half the globulins.

The rate of synthesis depends on the availability of amino acids in the plasma.

Normal plasma protein values

Total: 6 to 7.8 g/dl (60 to 18 g/L)
Albumin: 3.2 to 4.5 g/dl (32 to 45 g/L)
Globulins: 2.3 to 3.5 g/dl (23 to 35 g/L)
  Alpha-1 globulin 0.2 to 0.4 g/dl
  Alpha-2 globulin 0.5 to 0.9 g/dl
  Beta globulin   0.5 to 1.0 g/dl
  Gamma globulin   1.0 to 2.0 g/dl
Fibrinogen: 0.2 to 0.4 g/dl

Albumin

Normal plasma albumin, essentially all of which is synthesized in the liver, makes up 52% to 68% of the blood protein and is responsible for 80% of the oncotic pressure. Thyroxine, bilirubin, fatty acids, salicylates, barbiturates, and other drugs are bound and transported by albumin. Since the albumin molecule is small compared with other blood proteins, it is the plasma protein most frequently detected in the urine in the event of renal damage.

Serum albumin: normal values and deviation

Deviation	Cause
Hypoalbuminemia (2.5 g or less)	Chronic liver disease
	Protein malnutrition
	Malabsorption syndrome, especially of protein
	Nephrotic syndrome
	Chronic infection
	Acute stress

Serum albumin elevation is seldom encountered. The normal pregnant woman has decreased albumin levels that are progressive through delivery and do not return to normal until 8 weeks postpartum.

Globulins

The five globulin fractions serve as transport media or antibodies. Approximately 50% of the globulins are manufactured by the liver; the remainder are synthesized in the lymphatic tissue and other reticuloendothelial cells.

Alpha-1 globulins are known to bind or act as carriers for cortisol (transcortin), thyroxine (thyroxine-binding globulin), fats, lipids, and fat-soluble vitamins.

Alpha-2 globulins contain copper (ceruloplasmin); hemoglobin (haptoglobin); lipids; triglycerides; erythropoietin; glycoprotein; mucoprotein; prothrombin; angiotensinogen; and enzymes such as cholinesterase, lactic acid dehydrogenase, and alkaline phosphatase.

Beta globulins bind and transport heme (hemopexin) and iron (transferrin) and include lipid-soluble vitamins, hormones, glycerides, phospholipids, lipoprotein, cholesterol, fibrinogen, profibrinolysin, and complement components.

The gamma globulin fraction includes the immunoglobulins, or antibodies, and the cryoglobulins, or cold agglutinins.

Serum globulin: normal values and deviations

Deviations	Cause
Hyperglobulinemia	Hypergammaglobulinemia
	Hodgkin's disease
	Leukemia
	Myeloproliferative diseases (multiple myeloma)
	Chronic granulomatous infectious diseases (tuberculosis)
	Chronic hepatitis
	Collagen disease
	Sarcoidosis
Alteration in globulin fractions	
Absence of alpha-1 globulins	Alpha-1 (antitrypsin deficiency)
↓ Alpha-1 globulins	Nephrotic syndrome

Deviations	Cause
↑ Alpha-2 globulins	Stress situations
	Infection
	Injury
	Surgery
	Tissue necrosis
	Myocardial infarction
	Nephrotic syndrome
↑ Beta globulins	Pregnancy (third trimester)
	Associated with serum cholesterol
	Hypothyroidism
	Biliary cirrhosis
	Nephrosis
	Obstructive jaundice
	Hepatitis
↓ Gamma globulins	Hypogammaglobulinemia
	Nephrotic syndrome
	Lymphosarcoma
	Lymphocytic leukemia
	Multiple myeloma
↑ Gamma globulins	Infections
	Collagen diseases
	Hypersensitivity diseases
	Hodgkin's disease
	Malignant lymphoma
	Chronic lymphocytic leukemia
	Multiple myeloma
	Liver disease
	Hepatitis
	Cirrhosis
	Obstructive jaundice

Albumin-globulin ratio

In the normal client, the albumin is about double that of globulin.

Normal A/G ratio: 1.5:2.5

An A/G ratio of 2.5:3 strongly suggests chronic liver disease.

The levels of each of the globulins obtained from the electrophoretic zone patterns are more valuable data than the A/G ratio.

Fibrinogen

The bulk of fibrinogen is produced in the liver. Fibrinogen is the precursor of fibrin.

Serum fibrinogen: normal values and deviation
Normal values: 0.2 to 0.4 g/l

Deviation	Cause	Possible effects
Hypofibrinogenemia	Hepatic dysfunction	Disseminated intravascular coagulation

Lipids

Several lipid elements are present in the normal plasma: triglyceride, cholesterol, and phospholipid. They circulate as lipoproteins, which are macromolecular complexes of lipids and carrier proteins (apoproteins) that render them soluble in the aqueous media of the blood. The lipids that are transported in the blood are composed of exogenous triglycerides (glycerol esterified with fatty acids from ingested foods), endogenous triglycerides (manufactured by the liver), cholesterol, and phospholipids. All the serum lipoproteins contain these same substances and vary only in the amount of each substance and in the size of the molecule.

Exogenous triglycerides

Exogenous triglycerides are the major constituent of chylomicrons, the largest lipids; these lipids contain a lesser quantity of cholesterol (10%), phospholipids (7%), and protein (24%). Chylomicrons transport exogenous triglyceride following absorption from the small intestine to sites for use or storage.

The high triglyceride content results in a density less than water. Thus, the chylomicrons may rise to the top of blood that is left standing. The large size of the molecules results in light scattering, resulting in a turbid appearance of the plasma. The disappearance of chylomicrons from the blood depends on the presence of the enzyme lipoprotein lipase. The chylomicrons should return to basal levels within 6 hours following a fat-containing test meal. Chylomicrons are absent during fasting.

Since the chylomicron (and thus, triglyceride) level varies with dietary intake of fats, the most valuable data concerning lipid levels are obtained from testing done in the fasting state.

Endogenous triglycerides

Endogenous triglycerides are manufactured by the liver. Hepatic triglyceride synthesis appears to be independent of the sudden increase in dietary intake of fats but shows a relationship to the total ingestion of foodstuffs, particularly in regard to caloric value.

Endogenous triglycerides are transported to sites for use or storage in molecules that are less dense than chylomicrons; these molecules are called very low density (prebeta) lipoproteins (VLDLs). Endogenous triglycerides are the major constituent (55%) of these molecules; protein contributes a lesser amount (2% to 15%), and the remainder is made up of free and esterified cholesterol and phospholipids. Since chylomicrons are absent after a 6-hour fast, the majority of the circulating triglyceride is in the VLDL fraction.

Low-density lipoproteins (LDLs). Use and storage of triglycerides (exogenous and endogenous) are possible following release from the chylomicrons and VLDLs. The chylomicrons are cleared by the liver, whereas the VLDL remnants become an intermediate density called low-density (beta) lipoproteins (LDLs).

High-density lipoproteins (HDLs). The enzyme lecithin-cholesterol acyltransferase and high-density (alpha) lipoproteins (HDLs) are responsible for the clearance of cholesterol from peripheral tissues. The HDLs transport cellular cholesterol from the periphery to the liver. It has been suggested that less than normal levels of HDL may be responsible for ineffective cholesterol clearance from the cells. Since the cholesterol remains in the cell, the entry of LDL cholesterol would be inhibited, resulting in increased plasma levels of LDL.

Epidemiologic data as well as genetic and metabolic studies have served to associate LDL cholesterol directly to coronary artery disease, whereas an inverse relationship exists between HDL and coronary heart disease. Thus, HDL is the most positive indicator of the risk of coronary heart disease.

Lipoprotein phenotype	*Cholesterol*	*Triglyceride*	*Lipoprotein*
Type I		↑	Severe hyperchylomicronemia
Type IIa	↑		↑ LDL
Type IIb	↑	↑	↑ LDL and VLDL
Type III	↑	↑	↑ Remnants
Type IV		↑	↑ VLDL
Type V		↑	↑ Chylomicrons and VLDL

Lipoprotein phenotypes	*Genetic classification*	*Plasma lipoprotein elevation*
Type I	Familial lipoprotein lipase deficiency	Chylomicrons
Type IIa	Hypercholesterolemia (monogenic)	LDL
Type IIb	Hypercholesterolemia (polygenic)	LDL and VLDL
Type IIa, IIb, or IV	Familial hyperlipidemia (combined)	LDL and VLDL
Type III	Broad beta disease	Remnants
Type IV or V	Familial hypertriglyceridemia	VLDL

Familial lipoprotein lipase deficiency and familial hypertriglyceridemia have not been shown to be related to coronary artery disease. Monogenic hypercholesterolemia is the result of a defect in LDL uptake by peripheral cells. Affected individuals may have cutaneous xanthomas, xanthelasma, and retinal lipemia.

Laboratory tests of plasma lipids and lipoproteins include total cholesterol, total triglyceride, HDL, LDL, cholesterol/HDL ratio, phenotype determination, and centrifugation and separation.

Clinically significant hyperlipoproteinemia is said to exist with the following values:

Age of subject	Total plasma cholesterol	Plasma triglyceride
20 years	200 mg/dl	140 mg/dl
20 years	240 mg/dl	200 mg/dl

Phospholipids

Lecithin and sphingomyelin are the major serum phospholipids. Phospholipids are constituents of both HDLs and LDLs.

Normal serum phospholipid values: 150 to 375 mg/dl

Total serum lipids: normal values and deviations

Normal values: 350 to 800 mg/dl (adult)

Deviations	Cause	Predominant lipoprotein
Cholesterol: marked elevation; triglyceride: no change or elevation	↑ Ingestion of cholesterol	LDL (Type IIa)
Lipoprotein Cholesterol: elevation; triglyceride: no change or elevation	↑ Cholesterol manufacture by liver Obesity Hereditary ↓ LDL catabolism Hypothyroidism Hereditary	LDL (Type IIa) or LDL and VLDL (Type IIb)
	↓ Remnant removal Hypothyroidism Hereditary	Remnants (Type III) or VLDL and chylomicrons (Type V)
Cholesterol: no change or elevation; triglyceride: elevation	↑ Triglyceride synthesis Dietary intake (caloric) Alcohol Hyperinsulinism Obesity Corticosteroids	VLDL (Type IV) or VLDL and chylomicrons (Type V)

Deviations	Cause	Predominant lipoprotein
	Estrogen Hereditary ↓ Triglyceride clearance Insulin (diabetes) Hypothyroidism Renal failure Hereditary	VLDL (Type IV) or VLDL and chylomicrons (Type V)

Cholesterol

Exogenous cholesterol is absorbed from the small intestine into the lymph. Endogenous cholesterol is formed by all the cells of the body. Most of the endogenous cholesterol in the plasma is formed by the liver from acetate. It is the endogenous cholesterol that is measured in blood chemistry profiles. A control mechanism exists for these two processes, since endogenous cholesterol production is inhibited when cholesterol ingestion is increased. Cholesterol is present in the plasma primarily as LDLs. The LDL cholesterol is taken up by most peripheral tissues. This is a modified receptor process. In addition, most tissues are capable of cholesterol synthesis. Increased uptake of LDL inhibits cellular cholesterol production and decreased uptake results in increased cholesterol synthesis in the peripheral cells.

Cholesterol testing was the forerunner of serum lipid analysis and has served as a valuable but debatable tool for prediction of coronary artery disease caused by atheromatous or arteriosclerotic artery disease.

Because the liver esterifies cholesterol, the ratio of esterified to unesterified cholesterol may be considered an indication of liver function. The normal serum esterified cholesterol value ranges from 20% to 30%.

Obstruction of the biliary ducts is typified by an increased cholesterol level with a decrease in the amount of esterified cholesterol.

Serum cholesterol: normal values and deviations

Normal values: 150 to 250 mg/dl

Deviations	Cause	Possible effects
Hypercholesterolemia (marked: >400 mg/dl)	Liver disease Nephrotic stage of glomerulonephritis Familial hypercholesterolemia Hypothyroidism Pancreatic dysfunction Diabetes mellitus Obesity	Associated with ↑ alkaline phosphatase, ↑ bilirubin, ↑ BUN, ↑ creatinine

Deviations	*Cause*

Hypocholes-terolemia (significant: <150 mg/dl)	↓ Ingestion of cholesterol
	Malnutrition
	Fasting
	Liver disease
	Megaloblastic or hypochromic anemia
	↑ Estrogen
	↑ Thyroid hormone
	Hypermetabolic states
	   Fever
	   Exercise

Enzymes

Enzymes are individual molecules or aggregates of protein molecules occurring in globular form. Enzymes act as catalysts to biochemical reactions. If cells destroy an organ or tissue, the cytoplasmic enzymes are released into the plasma from the diseased cells. Enzymes are categorized by their functional effect. These groupings are called isoenzymes. Isoenzymes are enzymes with the same functional effect but with variations in configuration and physical characteristics. The isoenzyme content of many tissues and structures has been determined. There is sufficient variation in the enzyme content of the various organs that changes in the enzyme concentration in the blood may serve as an indicator of the site of disease. Electrophoresis may be used to separate these proteins. Serum enzyme determination results are also used to assess tissue rejection following transplantation procedures.

AST, serum LDH, and serum alkaline phosphatase determinations are included in most screening laboratory examinations. Enzyme determinations currently and commonly encountered in clinical practice are described in this section.

Serum glutamic-oxaloacetic transaminase (AST)

AST is found in many tissues. The transaminase enzymes catalyze the conversion of an amino acid to a keto acid; another keto acid is converted to an amino acid in the glycolytic cycle. This enzyme catalyzes conversions of glutamic and oxaloacetic acids. High tissue concentrations of AST have been demonstrated for the heart and liver, but appreciable amounts are found in RBCs, muscle, and kidney.

Colorimetric and spectrophotometric techniques are used in determining the serum concentration of these enzymes. Elevated levels of the enzyme may be identified 8 hours after tissue damage occurs. In the case of a single injury (such as myocardial infarction) that is not followed by further damage, the enzyme reaches a peak level in

24 to 36 hours and declines to basal levels in about 4 to 6 days.

The AST concentration is directly related to the degree of cellular damage.

AST: normal values and deviations

Normal values: 8 to 33 U/dl (Reitman-Frankel)
10 to 40 mU/ml (SMA 12/60)

Deviations	*Cause*

Elevation of AST values
   Elevation greater than 1000 U/ml (or more than 10 times normal)
	Myocardial infarction
	Hepatocellular disease
	   Infectious or toxic hepatitis
	   Severe liver necrosis

Elevation to 40 to 100 U/ml	Tachyarrhythmias Congestive heart failure Myocarditis Pericarditis Pulmonary infarction Cirrhosis Cholangitis Pancreatitis Metastatic liver disease Generalized infection (infectious mononucleosis) Trauma Shock Muscle disease Muscular dystrophy Dermatomyositis Skeletal muscle damage Generalized infection

Serum glutamic-pyruvic transaminase

Serum glutamic-pyruvic transaminase (ALT) catalyzes conversions between glutamic and pyruvic acid in the glycolytic pathway. The liver contains the highest concentration of ALT, but the enzyme is prominent in kidney, heart, and skeletal muscle. The pattern of release of ALT is similar to AST in cellular damage, although more damage than that necessary to elevate AST is generally present when ALT levels are increased.

Serum ALT: normal values and deviations

Normal values: 5 to 35 U/ml (Reitman-Frankel)

Deviations	*Cause*
Elevation of ALT values Marked elevation	Infectious or toxic hepatitis Infectious mononucleosis
Moderate elevation	Obstructive jaundice Postnecrotic cirrhosis
Slight elevation	Cirrhosis Myocardial infarction

Lactic dehydrogenase (LDH)

The tissue concentrations of LDH mimic those of AST. Furthermore, elevations in serum LDH levels correlate with the same conditions underlying increases in AST concentrations. LDH catalyzes the conversions between pyruvate and lactate in the glycolytic cycle. Following myocardial infarction, serum LDH levels increase five to six times in the first 48 hours and may remain elevated for 6 to 10 days. LDH has been separated into five isoenzymes, making it a sharper diagnostic tool. These isoenzymes may be separated by electrophoresis.

A variety of colorimetric tests are available for assessment of this serum enzyme concentration.

A hemolyzed blood specimen may give spuriously high values for LDH concentration in the serum, since the damaged RBCs give up LDH; this will be reflected in the concentration of the enzyme in the sample.

Since the 1970s, particular emphasis has been placed on the use of the isoenzymes of LDH. There are five isoenzymes of LDH, designated LDH_1 to LDH_5. Normally LDH_2 is greater than LDH_1 in the serum. However, the myocardium has an abundant LDH_1 content, and following myocardial infarction, the serum value of LDH_1 may exceed LDH_2. Thus, the LDH_1/LDH_2 ratio becomes greater; this is referred to as a reversed or flipped ratio. Increases in LDH_1 also occur in hemolytic states, hyperthyroidism, megaloblastic anemia, renal disease, and gastric malignancy.

Serum LDH: normal values and deviations

Normal values: 200 to 400 U/ml (Wroblewski)
100 to 225 mU/ml (SMA 12/60)

Deviations	Cause
Evaluation of LDH values	
Elevation greater than 1,400 Wroblewski units	Hemolytic disorders (marked hemolysis)
	Pernicious anemia
	Myocardial infarction
Elevation of 500 to 700 Wroblewski units	Chronic viral hepatitis
	Malignant neoplasms
	Liver
	Kidney
	Brain
	Skeletal muscle
	Heart
	Destruction of lung tissue
	Pulmonary emboli
	Pneumonia
	Destruction of renal tissue
	Infarction
	Infection
	Generalized viral infection

Alkaline phosphatase

Determinations of serum alkaline phosphatase levels are frequently used to determine the presence of liver and bone cell disease, since the enzyme has its greatest content in these two tissues. However, it is also found in significant concentrations in intestine, kidney, and placenta. The enzyme is thought to catalyze reactions in the process of bone matrix formation, because increased serum alkaline phosphatase levels correlate with osteoblastic activity. The isoenzymes from the liver, bone, intestine, kidney, and placenta can be separated by electrophoresis; thus, the source of the enzyme can be determined. Synthesis of alkaline phosphatase is thought to be small in the normal hepatic cell. The serum alkaline phosphatase level reflects placental function and may be used to monitor the progress of pregnancy.

A low alkaline phosphatase level may be associated with hypophosphatemia, hypothyroidism, or vitamin C deficiency.

Serum alkaline phosphatase: normal values and deviations

Normal values

Adults:	1.5 to 4.5 U/dl (Bodansky)
	4 to 13 U/dl (King-Armstrong)
	0.8 to 2.3 U/ml (Bessey-Lowry)
	30 to 100 mU/ml (SMA 12/60)
Children:	5 to 14 U/dl (Bodansky)
	3.4 to 9 U/ml (Bessey-Lowry)
	15 to 30 U/dl (King-Armstrong)
	(The level in children is about three times that of the adult.)

Deviations	Cause
Elevation of alkaline phosphatase values	
Marked elevation (15 U/dl or more—Bodansky)	Liver disease
	Obstructive disease
	Neoplasm
	Bone disease
	Paget's disease
	Sarcoma
	Metastatic carcinoma
Slight to moderate elevation (8 to 10 U/dl—Bodansky)	Liver disease
	Cholangitis
	Cirrhosis
	Hyperparathyroidism
	Osteomalacia
	Renal infarction, tissue rejection

Acid phosphatase

Acid phosphatase occurs in greatest amount in prostatic tissue. In the normal individual the enzyme is excreted in prostatic fluids. However, in prostatic metastatic carcinoma, the serum acid phosphatase level rises and thus becomes a tool in differential diagnosis.

Normal serum acid phosphatase values: 1 to 4 U/dl (King-Armstrong)

Creatine phosphokinase (CK)

CK catalyzes the phosphorylation of creatine by adenosine triphosphate (ATP). The greatest tissue content of CK is found in skeletal and cardiac muscle, although significant amounts occur in the brain. The serum CK level may be elevated as a result of intramuscular injection or following surgery and returns to basal levels in 24 to 48 hours. Since CK is not produced by the liver, elevated serum values of this enzyme may help eliminate liver disease in differential diagnosis.

Recent investigations have shown the usefulness of measuring the three isoenzymes of CK, designated as M, B, and MB. The M isoenzyme is present in skeletal and cardiac muscle, the B isoenzyme is found in the brain, and the MB isoenzyme is found in relatively high concentrations in the cardiac muscle but is also present in the skeletal muscle. The MB fraction has specific predictability in relation to myocardial infarction; it is typically the first enzyme detectable in abnormal concentration in serum following myocardial damage. The isoenzyme is first detectable 3 to 5 hours after infarction and reaches its peak in 12 to 24 hours, with a rapid decline to normal values in 24 to 48 hours.

CK–MB is also elevated in individuals with muscle trauma, polymyositis, muscular dystrophy, neuromuscular disease, pulmonary embolism, tachyarrhythmias, and unstable angina.

Serum CK: Normal values and deviation

Normal values: 5 to 75 mU/ml

Deviation	Cause

Elevation of serum CK values	Muscle disease
	  Duchenne's muscular
	    dystrophy (early)
	  Dermatomyositis
	  Polymyositis
	  Trauma
	Myocardial infarction
	Encephalitis
	Bacterial meningitis
	Cerebrovascular accident
	Hepatic coma
	Uremic coma
	Strenuous exercise
	Ingestion of salicylates

Aldolase

Aldolase catalyzes the splitting of fructose 1,6-diphosphate into glyceraldehyde phosphate and dihydroxyacetone phosphate. Aldolase occurs in greatest concentration in skeletal and heart muscle, but the liver contains a moderate amount, and all tissues contain some of the enzyme.

Serum aldolase: normal values and deviation

Normal values: 3 to 8 U/dl (Sibley-Lehninger)

Deviation	Cause

Elevation of serum aldolase values	Muscle disease
	  Progressive muscular
	    dystrophy
	  Dermatomyositis
	  Trichinosis
	Myocardial infarction
	Viral hepatitis
	Hepatic cellular necrosis
	Granulocytic leukemia
	Carcinomatosis

Amylase

Pancreatic amylase is synthesized in the pancreatic cells and secreted into the pancreatic ducts for transport to the duodenum, where it catalyzes the hydrolysis of starch and glycogen. Elevated serum amylase levels may be used to monitor damage to pancreatic cells. Although the salivary glands produce amylase, diseases of these cells do not affect the serum lipase level.

Serum amylase: normal values and deviation

Normal values: 60 to 150 U/dl (Somogyi)

Deviation	Cause
Elevation of serum amylase values	Acute pancreatitis

Lipase

Lipase is synthesized by the pancreatic cells and secreted into the pancreatic ducts for transport to the duodenum, where it catalyzes the hydrolysis of triglycerides to fatty acids. Elevation of serum lipase concentrations indicates damage to pancreatic cells. Serum lipase levels remain elevated longer following acute pancreatitis than do amylase levels.

Serum amylase: normal values and deviation

Normal values: 0 to 1.5 U/dl (Cherry-Crandall)

Deviation	Cause
Elevation of serum lipase values (lipasemia)	Acute pancreatitis

Cholinesterase

Cholinesterase (ChE) catalyzes the hydrolysis of acetylcholine and other cholinesters and has been classified as "true" cholinesterase or as pseudocholinesterase. True cholinesterase, or acetylcholinesterase, is more rapid in its action on acetylcholine and is found in greatest concentration in the brain and in RBCs. Pseudocholinesterase is found in plasma but not in the erythrocytes and is thought to be manufactured by the liver. Both of these enzymes are inactivated by organophosphates. Testing of acetylcholinesterase provides an indication of toxicity from insecticides containing these compounds.

Normal ChE (RBC) values: 0.65 to 1.00 pH units

Pseudocholinesterase (plasma): 0.5 to 1.3 pH units

SCREENING HEMATOLOGIC EXAMINATIONS

The hemogram, or complete blood cell count (CBC), includes the following determinations: RBC count, hematocrit (HCT), hemoglobin (Hgb), white blood cell (WBC) count, and differential WBC count. Other commonly performed hematologic examinations are determinations of the mean corpuscular volume (MCV), mean corpuscular hemoglobin (MCH), and mean corpuscular hemoglobin concentration (MCHC).

Red Blood Cells

RBC count

Erythropoiesis, the manufacture of RBCs, occurs in the bone marrow. Erythropoietin, a hormone produced by the kidney exposed to hypoxia, plays a prominent role in the control of erythropoiesis.

Electronic counting devices (such as the Coulter device) are faster and produce more accurate blood cell determinations than those of a technician counting the smear under a microscope.

Both anemias and polycythemias are classified as relative if they result from changes in plasma volume.

Red blood cells: normal counts and deviations

Normal counts

Men:	4.6 to 6.2 $\times$ $10^6/\mu l$
Women:	4.2 to 5.4 $\times$ $10^6/\mu l$

Deviations	Cause	Possible effects
Elevated RBC count (polycythemia)	Bone marrow hyperplasia (polycythemia vera)	Hyperviscosity of blood Tendency toward thrombosis Sluggish blood flow to tissues (tissue hypoxia) Hypervolemia Headache Tinnitus Dizziness Ruddy cyanosis
Decreased RBC count (anemia)	RBC production deficiency states Protein Iron Vitamin B_{12} Folic acid Toxicity (depressed bone marrow) Metabolites (urea, creatinine) Drugs (chloramphenicol) Ionizing radiation Hypothyroidism Hereditary (thalassemia)	Pallor Fatigue Rapid pulse Irritability Headache Dizziness Postural hypotension Menstrual irregularities Angina Shortness of breath

Hematocrit

The hematocrit examination is used to determine the volume-packed (centrifuged) RBCs in 100 ml of blood.

Normal hematocrit values

Men:	40% to 54%
Women:	38% to 47%

Hemoglobin

Hemoglobin consists of heme, a pigmented compound containing iron, and globin, a colorless protein. Hemoglobin binds with oxygen and carbon dioxide. The hemoglobin molecule binds oxygen and transports it to the periphery; it binds carbon dioxide as it is transported to the lung.

Normal hemoglobin values

Men:	13.5 to 18 g/dl
Women:	12.0 to 16 g/dl

Mean corpuscular volume

The MCV test measures RBCs in terms of individual volume. The value can be calculated through the use of the following formula:

$$MCV = \frac{HCT}{RBC}$$

The result is expressed in microcubic millimeters per blood cell.

Normal MCV: 80 to 94 μmm^3

This test is used to classify anemias as microcytic (RBC size smaller than normal), normocytic, or macrocytic (larger than normal).

Deviations	*Cause*
Microcytic anemia	Hypochromic
	Iron deficiency
	Thalassemia
	Chronic infections
	Chronic renal disease
	Malignancy
Normocytic anemia	Hypochromic
	Lead poisoning
	Chronic infection
	Chronic renal disease
	Malignancy
	Normochromic
	Hemorrhage
	Hemolytic anemia
	Bone marrow hypoplasia
	Splenomegaly
Macrocytic anemia	Normochromic
	Pernicious anemia
	Folic acid deficiency
	Hypothyroidism
	Hepatocellular disease

Mean corpuscular hemoglobin

The MCH examination measures the hemoglobin concentration weight of the individual RBCs. Expressed in picograms (micromicrograms), it can be calculated by dividing the hemoglobin in grams by the RBCs:

$$MCH = \frac{Hgb}{RBC}$$

The test allows the classification of anemia as hypochromic or normochromic.

Normal MCH values: 27 to 31 pg

Mean corpuscular hemoglobin concentration

The MCHC test measures the concentration of hemoglobin in grams per deciliter of RBCs. Expressed in percentages, it can be calculated using the following formula:

$$MCHC = \frac{Hgb\ (g)}{HCT}$$

Normal MCHC: 32% to 36%

An elevation of MCHC is seen only in hereditary spherocytosis.

Sedimentation rate

The erythrocyte sedimentation rate (ESR) is the speed with which RBCs settle in unclotted blood. The speed with which the RBCs settle depends on the concentration of the various plasma protein fractions and on the concentration of the RBCs. The cells settle out more rapidly when the plasma concentration is high and the RBC count is low. Increased concentration of fibrinogen or of the globulins speeds up the rate of sedimentation. The rate of settling is accelerated in many inflammatory conditions, in pregnancy, and in multiple myeloma. The sedimentation rate is decreased in sickle cell anemia; this may be caused by the abnormal shape and stickiness of the RBCs.

Normal ESR rate (Westergren)

Men under 50:	<15 mm/hr
Men over 50:	<20 mm/hr
Women under 50:	<20 mm/hr
Women over 50:	<30 mm/hr

Microscopic RBC examination

A stained smear of whole blood is examined microscopically to assess the morphologic characteristics of the RBCs.

Normal RBC: nonnucleated, biconcave disk, 7 to 8 μm in diameter; contains 95% hemoglobin

Nucleated RBCs may be observed in periods of marked erythropoiesis due to marrow stimulation. These immature cells are released from the marrow and are found in the circulating blood.

Reticulocytes. A reticulocyte is a precursor to the RBC, is larger than the normal RBC, and stains more with basic dye. The center does not appear pale, as does the normal RBC. In the normal individual 0.5% to 1.5%

reticulocytes are present in the circulating blood. During periods of accelerated erythropoiesis the number of reticulocytes in the general circulation increases. The reticulocyte count is generally elevated as a result of hemorrhage or hemolysis.

Nuclear fragments.   Structures that represent the degenerated nucleus of the erythroblast are seen as coarse dots, blue lines, and imperfect rings in the smear.

Basophilic stippling.   The term basophilic stippling refers to the presence of homogenous blue dots observed in RBCs treated with Wright's stain. This stippling may indicate thalassemia or toxic manifestations, resulting in abnormal hemoglobin production.

Siderotic granules.   Granules of iron-containing substances in addition to hemoglobin may be seen in some cells of smears of RBCs treated with Prussian blue dye. The cells are termed siderocytes and are increased in number following splenectomy and during the course of hemolytic anemias.

Heinz bodies.   The RBCs of the individual with glucose-6-phosphate dehydrogenase (G6PD) deficiency may contain inclusion bodies containing denatured hemoglobin called Heinz bodies, for example, in thalassemias.

Poikilocytosis.   A poikilocyte is an RBC of abnormal shape. Poikilocytosis refers to the presence of abnormally shaped RBCs in the blood. Leptocytes (target, or "Mexican hat," erythrocytes) are characterized by a central pigment bulls-eye area surrounded by a clear area, which is ringed by a hemoglobinated peripheral border. This type of erythrocyte is seen in the blood of individuals with hemoglobin C or A, or a combination of C and S. They are frequently seen in persons having thalassemia. Liver disease has been shown to be present in some individuals with demonstrated poikilocytosis. The sickle cell disease is characterized by long, crescent-shaped cells.

Anisocytosis.   Anisocytosis is the term used for blood that contains erythrocytes with excessive variations in size.

Platelets (thrombocytes).   Platelets may be seen in the microscopic examination of whole blood smears. The platelets are granular fragments of cytoplasm of megakaryocytes in the bone marrow. The platelets are largely phospholipids and polysaccharides. They are carriers for a variety of enzymes for clotting factors and serotonin. Thus, platelets play a major role in blood coagulation.

Thrombocytopathy refers to platelet cells of unusual size or shape.

Platelets: normal count and deviations

Normal count: 300,000/μl

Deviations	Cause
Thrombocytopenia	Bone marrow depression
Thrombocytosis	Polycythemia
	Splenectomy

WBC: normal counts and deviations

Normal counts: 4500 to 11,000/μl whole blood

Deviations	Cause
Elevated WBC count (leukocytosis)	Leukemia
	Bacterial infection
	Polycythemia (resulting from bone marrow stimulation)
Decreased WBC count (leukopenia)	Bone marrow depression
	Ionizing radiation
	Chloramphenicol
	Phenothiazines
	Sulfonamides
	Phenylbutazone
	Agranulocytosis
	Acute viral infection
	Acute alcohol ingestion

White Blood Cells

WBC count

The WBC count is the assessment of the number of WBCs (leukocytes) in 1 μl of whole blood. The WBCs function to protect the body against infectious disease. Neutrophils and monocytes destroy microorganisms by phagocytosis. Lymphocytes and plasma cells are thought to produce antibodies. Eosinophils play a role in allergy. Granulocytes, monocytes, and some lymphocytes are produced in the bone marrow; lymphocytes are produced in the lymph nodes and thymic tissue. Disease processes may result in changes within individual leukocyte groups, which may include morphological and functional changes and variations in total numbers. These alterations may provide valuable clues that can be used in differential diagnosis.

Differential WBC count

Six different types of WBCs have been identified in the blood: polymorphonuclear neutrophils (PMNs), polymorphonuclear eosinophils (PMEs), polymorphonuclear basophils (PMBs), monocytes, lymphocytes, and plasma cells. Platelets (thrombocytes) are particles of megakaryocytes.

Increased granulation of leukocytes may indicate toxicity reactions.

A shift to the left means that increased numbers of immature neutrophils are present in the specimen and that they are band forms rather than lobulations. Acute stress to the bone marrow and severe bacterial infection may cause the release of early granulocytes. Increased lobulation (3 to 6) or segmentation of neutrophils is often observed in association with vitamin B_{12} deficiency.

Mild to moderate leukocytosis associated with mild to moderate lymphocytosis is characteristic of chronic infections such as tuberculosis. In relative lymphocytosis, the total number of circulating lymphocytes remains constant, but the WBC count is low because of neutropenia. Relative lymphocytosis is normal between 4 months and 4 years of age.

Monocytosis may occur even with no increase in WBCs.

Abnormal white blood cells of diagnostic importance

Plasma cells. Plasma cells are not normally found in the circulating blood. The presence of plasma cells in the blood predicates the necessity to differentiate multiple myeloma, infectious mononucleosis, serum sickness, and rubella.

Downey cells. Downey cells are abnormal lymphocytes that differ from the normal cells in size, cytoplasmic structures (vacuolated, foamy), and immature chromatin pattern. These cells are observed in individuals with infectious mononucleosis, viral disease (hepatitis), and allergic states.

LE cell. The LE cell is a polymorphonuclear leukocyte, generally a neutrophil that contains an inclusion body. The inclusion body has been shown to be denatured nuclear protein that is being phagocytosed by the neutrophil. The LE cell, which can be induced in the laboratory in the presence of LE factor, is present in the blood of many individuals who have lupus erythematosus.

Differential WBC count: normal percentages and deviations

Normal differential count

Type of cell	Percentage of total WBC count	Range
Neutrophils (PMNs)	56%	50% to 70%
Eosinophils (PMEs)	2.7%	5% to 6%
Basophils (PMBs)	0.3%	0 to 1%
Lymphocytes	34%	20% to 40%
Monocytes		0 to 7%

Deviations	*Cause*
Neutrophilic leukocytosis	Bacterial infections
	Pneumonia
	Systemic infections
	Inflammatory disease
	Rheumatic fever
	Rheumatoid arthritis
	Pancreatitis
	Thyroiditis
	Carcinoma
	Trauma (tissue destruction)
	Burns
	Crush injury
	Stress
	Cold
	Heat
	Exercise
	Electroshock therapy
	Panic, fear, anxiety
	Increased catecholamines
	Increased corticosteroids
	Cushing's disease
	Acute gout
	Diabetes mellitus
	Lead poisoning
	Acute hemorrhage
	Hemolytic anemia
Neutrophilopenia	Acute viral infections
	Bone marrow disease
	Nutritional deficiency
	Vitamin B_{12}
	Folic acid
Basophilic leukocytosis	Myeloproliferative diseases
	Myelofibrosis
	Polycythemia vera
Basophilopenia	Anaphylactic reaction
Eosinophilic leukocytosis	Allergic manifestations
	Asthma
	Hay fever
	Parasitic infestations
	Roundworm
	Flukes
	Malignancy (Hodgkin's disease)
	Colitis
	Eosinophilic granulomatosis
	Eosinophilic leukemia
Lymphocytosis	Leukemia (80% to 90% of total WBCs)
	Infectious diseases
	Infectious mononucleosis
	Pertussis
	Viral infections with exanthema
	Measles
	Rubella
	Roseola
	Chickenpox
	Thyrotoxicosis
	Cushing's disease

Deviations	Cause
Monocytosis	Typhoid fever
	Tuberculosis
	Subacute bacterial endocarditis
	Malaria

DETECTION OF SYPHILIS (LUES)

Syphilis is the disease caused by the spirochete *Treponema pallidum*. The disease is described in terms of its early or late manifestations or in terms of primary, secondary, and tertiary stages. It is transmitted by intimate mucous membrane contact or in utero. The destructiveness of the organism is attributed to its invasiveness and the elaboration of a weak endotoxin. Immunity is established by a single infection. One to 4 months after contraction of syphilis, two distinct antibodies appear in the serum. The complement fixation and flocculation diagnostic tests are based on one of these, syphilitic reagin, which combines with certain tissue lipids. *T. pallidum* is sensitive to penicillin. Thus, detection provides an opportunity for curative intervention.

Immunologic Tests for Syphilis

The first serologic test for syphilis (STS) was devised by Wassermann and, along with Kolmer's modification that superseded it, was a complement fixation test. Wassermann used extract from a syphilitic liver that had as its reactive ingredient cardiolipin, which is found in many tissues and, is not actually specific for syphilis. Thus, it was fortuitous that the syphilitic reagin reacted with it. A lipoidal substance is found in spirochetes that is thought to be similar to the cardiolipin lipoprotein complex, which would explain the reaction.

The procedure for the complement fixation test involves first mixing the sample serum with cardiolipin reagent. The antigen-antibody reaction serves to bind the complement, removing it from the reaction. Sheep blood indicator is then added to the mixture. Hemolysis of the blood cells indicates the presence of free complement. If the cells do not hemolyze, complement is absent because of an earlier antigen-antibody reaction. False positive results may occur if the serum contains anticomplement activity.

The flocculation tests include the Venereal Disease Research Laboratory (VDRL), rapid plasma reagin (RPR), Kahn, Hinton, Kline, and Mazzini tests. These tests are performed by adding a suspension of cardiolipin antigen particles to the sample serum. If the syphilitic reagin (antibody) is present, it produces clumping, or flocculation. The reaction is quantitated by the degree of flocculation.

T. pallidum immobilization test

Nichols strain of pathogenic spirochetes can be cultured in rabbits. These spirochetes are incubated with the suspected serum for the *T. pallidum* immobilization (TPI) test. If the specific antibody is present, the spirochetes are immobilized. This reaction can be observed under the microscope. Other treponema spirochetes are known to give positive reactions to this test.

Reiter protein complement fixation test

The nonpathologic Reiter strain of spirochetes can be cultured in artificial media for the Reiter protein complement fixation (RPCF) test. Antigen has been prepared from this strain and used in a complement fixation technique.

Fluorescent treponemal antibody absorption test

In the fluorescent treponemal antibody absorption (FTA-ABS) test, nonspecific cross-reacting antibodies are absorbed from the suspected serum through the use of the Reiter treponema antigen. The remaining serum is incubated on a smear of killed Nichols spirochetes. Following this, a solution containing fluorescent antibodies produced against human globulins is exposed to the sample.

Accuracy of Test Results

The STS tests are reported to produce as many as 25% to 45% biologic false-postive (BFP) results. That is, many positive tests have been reported for individuals who definitely have not been exposed to or do not have syphilis. Further investigation has shown these individuals to have acute viral or bacterial infections, hypersensitivity reactions, or a recent vaccination; in some cases such individuals have been found to have chronic systemic illness, such as collagen disease, malaria, or tuberculosis.

Positive test results obtained from nonspecific methods may be confirmed with the FTA-ABS test, which yields positive results midway through or at the end of the primary stage. Thus, in screening procedures a flocculation STS test is done initially and is followed up with the more specific FTA-ABS test.

All tests for syphilis give positive results in the secondary stage.

Antibiotic therapy may cause tests for syphilis to be negative.

Darkfield Examination

Serous fluid exudate may be removed from a syphilitic lesion by pipet. *T. pallidum*, if present, may then be identified by darkfield microscopy. This provides positive identification of the spirochete and may be the earliest method of identification, since antibodies are not apparent until late in the primary stage.

URINALYSIS

The urine examined for screening purposes is generally a voided specimen collected without regard to circadian variation of the components; that is, it is voided at any time during the 24-hour period. More accuracy can be expected in electrolyte determination, and less likelihood of bacterial contamination can be expected if a midstream or clean-catch specimen is employed. Ideally, the urine is collected on the client's arising, following a period of 12 hours in which no fluids were taken. The urine should be tested within 2 hours following its collection; spurious results may be obtained if urine is allowed to stand for long periods at room temperature; the urine pH is greater, bacteria multiply, and leukocytes and casts are known to deteriorate.

The standard urinalysis includes description of appearance, determination of specific gravity, pH, glucose, protein ketones, and microscopic examination of urinary sediment.

Appearance

The normal color of urine is pale golden yellow. Diluted urine is even paler in hue. The color is only reported in the event of abnormality. Orange, red, and brown hues of the urine may be associated with porphyria, hemoglobinuria, urobilinuria, or bilirubinemia. Porphyria may be indicated by urine that becomes burgundy red on exposure to light.

Deviations	Cause
Orange hue	Bile
	Ingestion of phenazopyridine (Pyridium)
Red hue	Blood
	Porphyria
	Urates
	Ingestion of dihydroxyanthraquinone (Dorbane)
Brown hue	Blood (melanin may turn black on standing)

Specific Gravity

The specific gravity of the urine provides an indicator of the kidney's ability to concentrate urine. The test is reported as the ratio of the weight of the urine tested to the weight of water.

Normal specific gravity of the urine

1.016 to 1.022 (in states of euhydration)
1.001 to 1.035 (range of normal without reference to hydration)

Low values suggest renal tubular dysfunction. Concentrated urine is observed in ADH deficiency.

pH

pH of urine: normal pH and deviation

Normal pH: freshly voided urine is generally acidic, with a pH of 4.6 to 8

Deviation	Cause
Alkaline urine	Metabolic alkalemia (except hypokalemic chloremia)
	Proteus infections
	Aged specimen

Glucose

The presence of glucose is not a normal finding for urine. Although glucose is freely filtered by the renal glomerulus, it is fully reabsorbed by the tubules. Only when the blood glucose levels reach the tubular maximum (T_m) of glucose (320 mg/min) or plasma threshold of 160 to 190 mg/dl is the kidney unable to completely reabsorb it. Glycosuria may indicate that the individual has a low renal threshold for glucose. The most common cause, however, is the presence of diabetes mellitus. Occasionally after high carbohydrate intake, the blood glucose level may be high enough to allow spilling of glucose into the urine. Both reducing and enzymatic tests may be used to identify urinary glucose.

The practitioner may measure both blood and urinary glucose concentrations with dipsticks, chemically treated papers that change color on exposure to glucose. Color charts provided with the testing materials allow standard comparison and subsequent identification of the degree of glucose concentration of the tested body fluid.

Deviation	Cause
Glucosuria	Diabetes mellitus
	Increased intracranial pressure
	Cushing's disease
	Pheochromocytoma
	Pregnancy

Protein

Tests for the protein content in urine depend on the principle that protein precipitates in the presence of heat in acidic urine. Sulfosalicylic acid is the acid most frequently used for this purpose. The protein content is estimated from the density of the precipitate as follows:

Precipitate description	Value	Percent protein
Faintly cloudy	1+	
Cloudy but transparent	2+	0.1
Opaque with clumping	3+	0.2 to 0.3
Dense, solid gel	4+	0.5

Normally, very small amounts of protein appear in urine that are not detectable by routine methods. Even trace quantities are an indication that follow-up should be done. A 24-hour quantitation of the protein excreted by the kidneys may be done. In addition, an electrophoretic determination of the type of protein in the urine may be done. Albumin is the most frequently encountered protein, since its molecular size is smaller than that of the globulins or fibrinogen.

The urine specimen of women may be contaminated with vaginal secretions. In many agencies it has become routine to use a clean-catch urine collection technique to obviate this protein contamination.

Bence Jones protein is an abnormal protein that appears in the urine of individuals with multiple myeloma.

Urinary protein: normal excretion and deviation

Normal excretion: 0.1 g/24 hr

Deviation	Cause
Proteinuria	Pregnancy
	Strenuous physical exercise
	Orthostatism
	Fever
	Kidney disease
	Glomerulonephritis
	Nephrotic syndrome
	Neoplasm
	Infarction
	Postrenal infection

Acetone and Diacetic Acid (Ketone Bodies)

Ketones are products of fat metabolism and are increased in the blood during periods when increased fats are being used as fuel, such as in starvation, after glycogen stores have been depleted. In diabetes mellitus, the lack of insulin makes glucose relatively unavailable to the cells, so that fats are again metabolized in greater quantity. The blood ketones are increased more rapidly than they can be metabolized and are excreted in the urine. Acetone determinations are indicated whenever the urinary glucose test is positive or blood glucose is elevated.

The acetone level of urine may be tested with a chemically treated dipstick that changes color in the presence of ketone bodies. This is read against a standard scale provided with the test papers.

Microscopic Examination of Urinary Sediment

The normal urinary sediment may contain one or two RBCs as well as WBCs and an occasional cast. All other substances are considered pathologic.

Red blood cells. Since RBCs are too large to filter through the glomerulus, the presence of blood in the urine indicates bleeding within the genitourinary tract. Common causes are calculi, cystitis, neoplasm, tuberculosis, and glomerulonephritis.

White blood cells. WBCs may indicate infection in any part of the genitourinary tract. Glomerulonephritis is typified by the presence of WBCs, casts, and bacteria. As a rule, pyuria from the kidney is associated with proteinuria, whereas only very small amounts of protein are present in the urine of the individual with an infection of the lower urinary tract.

Casts. Gelled protein and cellular debris precipitated in the renal tubules and molded to the tubular lumen are called casts. Portions of these casts may break off and are found in the urine. The casts are hyaline, granular, or cellular. Epithelial casts are made up of columnar renal epithelium or round cells. The hyaline casts are almost transparent and consist of homogeneous protein. The granular casts are dark colored and a degenerated form of the hyaline casts. The tubular shape of the casts has led to the use of the term *cylindruria.*

Casts consisting of WBCs are typical of pyelonephritis and the exudative stage of acute glomerulonephritis. Casts containing RBCs may appear clear or yellow.

The depositon of amyloid substance in urinary casts makes them appear waxy.

Urine that contains hyaline casts and protein may indicate a nephrotic syndrome.

Crystals. The acidity or alkalinity of the urine determines the type of crystals that may be identified in it. A urine with low pH is characterized by calcium oxalate, cystine, uric acid, and urate crystals. Alkaline urine is most frequently associated with carbonate crystals and amorphous phosphates.

EXAMINATION OF THE STOOL

In most cases a stool specimen is obtained by asking the individual to defecate, but digital removal of feces from the rectum can be done to facilitate collection when time constraints so dictate. Frequently a laxative is recommended to soften the stool, particularly if the individual has given a history of constipation. Because chemical analyses are calculated on the basis of daily output, the entire stool is sent to the laboratory. The feces are analyzed for size, shape, consistency, and color.

The normal individual excretes 100 to 200 g of feces daily. The volume depends on the fluid content of the bowel. About 500 to 1000 ml of chyme (liquid stool) are delivered to the colon each day, but most of the water and electrolytes are reabsorbed, primarily in the proximal colon. Sodium is absorbed, and chloride follows passively. The gradient established results in absorption of water. In addition, bicarbonate ions are secreted by the colon, and an equal amount of chloride is absorbed. About one fourth of the stool is solid material, which consists of the undigested residue of food, intestinal mucus and epithelium, bacteria, fat, and waste materials from the blood.

The rapid passage of stool through the colon in diarrhea results in larger stools (by volume) containing more liquid. Diarrhea is generally caused by inflammation of the colon but may also result from malaborption syndromes.

A fecalith or stercolith is a dried, hardened fecal mass.

Color

The normal color of the stool is brown as a result of food pigments as well as the breakdown products of bilirubin. Bilirubin is converted to biliverdin (green bile) by intestinal bacteria and then to stercobilin (a brown substance). Increased motility of the stool in diarrhea may result in green stools because of the presence of biliverdin that was allowed insufficient time for bacterial conversion in the colon.

Melena is a black stool caused by gastrointestinal bleeding (more than 100 ml) high enough in the tract that it is partially digested. Bleeding of the lower gastrointestinal tract is observed as bright- to dark-red blood in the stool. The guaiac test for occult blood is described in Chapters 16 and 17 on assessing the abdomen and rectosigmoid region.

Deviations	*Cause*
Melena	Esophagitis
	Esophageal varices
	Hiatal hernia
	Gastritis
	Peptic ulcer
	Carcinoma
Presence of bright- to dark-red blood	Polyps of the colon
	Carcinoma of the colon
	Diverticulitis
	Colitis
	Hemorrhoids

Ingestion of iron or bismuth compounds may cause the stool to be green to black. Green vegetables ingested in excessive amounts may also turn the stool green. A dietary intake that contains a good deal of milk but is low in protein may result in a light-colored stool.

Odor

The odor of feces and flatus is the result of bacterial action and depends on the colonic bacterial flora and the type of food ingested.

The normal stool is 10% to 20% fat. An excessive amount of fat in the stool is termed *steatorrhea*. The stool may appear grossly oily. Steatorrhea may be the result of pancreatic or small bowel malabsorption problems or liver disease. Sudan stain is an iodine compound that colors fat droplets, rendering them visible under the microscope. Excessive fat loss in the stool may also be associated with deficiency of the fat-soluble vitamin D.

Quantitative evaluation of fecal fat content is sometimes performed. In the performance of this test, the amount of dietary fat is usually controlled at 100 g of fat per day. A 3-day stool collection containing more than 5 g or fat for each day is considered pathologic.

Microscopic examination

The stool may be examined under the microscope to identify ova and parasites. At least three separate specimens are examined, since one negative examination is not sufficient to rule out the infestation.

The presence of WBCs in the stool indicates an inflammation in the gastrointestinal tract.

BIBLIOGRAPHY

Bauer JD: Clinical laboratory methods, ed 10, St Louis, 1986, The CV Mosby Co.
Cromwell L and others: Medical instrumentation for health care, Englewood Cliffs, NJ, 1976, Prentice-Hall, Inc.
Eastham RD: Clinical hematology, ed 7, Baltimore, 1986, Williams & Wilkins.
French RM: Guide to diagnostic procedures, ed 7, New York, 1987, McGraw-Hill Book Co.
Henry JB: Todd-Sanford-Davidshon clinical diagnosis and management by laboratory methods, ed 3, Philadelphia, 1987, WB Saunders Co.
Pagana KD and Pagana TJ: Diagnostic testing and nursing implications, a case study approach, ed 3, St Louis, 1990, The CV Mosby Co.
Ravel R: Clinical laboratory medicine, ed 2, Chicago, 1973, Year Book Medical Publishers, Inc.
Skydell B and Crowder AS: Diagnostic procedures: a reference for health practitioners and a guide to patient counseling, Boston, 1975, Little, Brown and Co.
Tilkian SM and Conover MB: Clinical implications of laboratory tests, ed 4, St Louis, 1987, The CV Mosby Co.
Wallach J: Interpretation of diagnostic tests: a handbook synopsis of laboratory medicine, ed 2, Boston, 1974, Little, Brown & Co.
Widmann FK: Goodale's clinical interpretation of laboratory tests, ed 10, Philadelphia, 1985, FA Davis Co.

A

Tables of normal values

Abbreviations used in tables

<	= less than		mg	= milligram		ng	= nanogram	
>	= greater than		ml	= milliliter		pg	= picogram	
dl	= 100 ml		mM	= millimole		μEq	= microequivalent	
gm	= gram		mm Hg	= millimeters of mercury		μg	= microgram	
IU	= International Unit		mIU	= milliInternational Unit		μIU	= microInternational Unit	
kg	= kilogram		mOsm	= milliosmole		μl	= microliter	
L	= liter		mμ	= millimicron		μU	= microunit	
mEq	= milliequivalent							

Table A-1

Whole blood, serum, and plasma chemistry

Component	System	Typical reference intervals		
		Conventional units	Factor*	Recommended SI units†
Acetoacetic acid				
Qualitative	Serum	Negative	—	Negative
Quantitative	Serum	0.2-1.0 mg/dl	98	19.6-98.0 μmol/L
Acetone				
Qualitative	Serum	Negative	—	Negative
Quantitative	Serum	0.3-2.0 mg/dl	172	51.6-344.0 μmol/L
Albumin				
Quantatitive	Serum	3.2-4.5 g/dl (salt fractionation)	10	32-45 g/L
		3.2-5.6 g/dl (electrophoresis)		32-56 g/L
		3.8-5.0 g/dl (dye binding)		38-50 g/L
Alcohol, ethyl	Serum or whole blood	Negative—but presented as mg/dl	0.22	Negative—but presented as mmol/L

*Factor, Number factor (note that units are not presented).   *Continued*
† Value in SI units, Value in conventional units × factor.
‡ Usually not measured in blood (preferred specimen in urine, hair, or nails except in acute cases where gastric contents are used.)
☐ From Henry JB: Todd-Sanford-Davidsohn clinical diagnosis and management by laboratory methods, ed 3, Philadelphia, 1987, WB Saunders Co.

Table A-1

Whole blood, serum, and plasma chemistry—*cont'd*

| Component | System | Typical reference intervals | | |
		Conventional units	Factor	Recommended SI units
Aldolase	Serum			
	Adults	3-8 Sibley-Lehninger U/dl at 37° C	7.4	22-59 mU/L at 37° C
	Children	Approximately 2 times adult levels		Approximately 2 times adult levels
	Newborn	Approximately 4 times adult levels		Approximately 4 times adult levels
Alpha-amino acid nitrogen	Serum	3.6-7.0 mg/dl	0.714	2.6-5.0 mmol/L
Alpha-aminolevulinic acid	Serum	0.01-0.03 mg/dl	76.3	0.76-2.29 μmol/L
Ammonia	Plasma	20-120 μg/dl (diffusion)	0.554	11.1-67.0 μmol/L
		40-80 μg/dl (enzymatic method)		22.2-44.3 μmol/L
		12-48 μg/dl (resin method)		6.7-26.6 μmol/L
Amylase	Serum	60-160 Somogyi units/dl	1.85	111-296 U/L
Argininosuccinic lyase	Serum	0-4 U/dl	10	0-40 U/L
Arsenic‡	Whole blood	<7 μg/dl	0.13	<0.91 μmol/L
Ascorbic acid (vitamin C)	Plasma	0.6-1.6 mg/dl	56.8	34-91 μmol/L
	Whole blood	0.7-2.0 mg/dl		40-114 μmol/L
Barbiturates	Serum, plasma, or whole blood	Negative	—	Negative
Base excess	Whole blood			
	Male	−3.3 to +1.2 mEq/l	1	−3.3 to +1.2 mmol/L
	Female	−2.4 to +2.3 mEq/l		−2.4 to +2.3 mmol/L
Base, total	Serum	145-160 mEq/l	1	145-160 mmol/L
Bicarbonate	Plasma	21-28 mM	1	21-28 mmol/L
Bile acids	Serum	0.3-3.0 mg/dl	10	3.0-30.0 mg/L
Bilirubin	Serum			
Direct (conjugated)		Up to 0.3 mg/dl	17.1	Up to 5.1 μmol/L
Indirect (unconjugated)		0.1-1.0 mg/dl		1.7-17.1 μmol/L
Total		0.1-1.2 mg/dl		1.7-20.5 μmol/L
Newborns total		1-12 mg/dl		17.1-205.0 μmol/L
Blood gases				
pH	Whole blood	7.38-7.44 (arterial)	1	7.38-7.44
		7.36-7.41 (venous)		7.36-7.41
P_{CO_2}	Whole blood	35-40 mm Hg (arterial)	0.133	4.66-5.32 kPa
		40-45 mm Hg (venous)		5.32-5.99 kPa
P_{O_2}	Whole blood	95-100 mm Hg (arterial)	0.133	12.64-13.30 kPa
Bromide	Serum	0-5 mg/dl	0.125	0-0.63 mmol/L
BSP (Bromsulphalein) (5 mg/kg)	Serum	Less than 6% retention 45 min after injection	0.01	Fraction retention <0.06 at 45 min after dye injection
Calcium				
Ionized	Serum	4-4.8 mg/dl	0.25	1.0-1.2 mmol/L
		2.0-2.4 mEq/l	0.5	
		30-58% of total	0.01	0.30-0.58 of total
Total	Serum	9.2-11.0 mg/dl	0.25	2.3-2.8 mmol/L
		4.6-5.5 mEq/l	0.5	23-28 mmol/L
Carbon dioxide (CO_2 content)	Whole blood (arterial)	19-24 mM	1	19-24 mmol/L
	Plasma or serum (arterial)	21-28 mM		21-28 mmol/L

Table A-1

Whole blood, serum, and plasma chemistry—*cont'd*

| Component | System | Typical reference intervals | | |
		Conventional units	Factor	Recommended SI units
Carbon dioxide	Whole blood (venous)	22-26 mM	1	22-26 mmol/L
	Plasma or serum (venous)	24-30 mM		24-30 mmol/L
CO_2 combining power	Plasma or serum (venous)	24-30 mM	1	24-30 mmol/L
CO_2 partial pressure (PCO_2)	Whole blood (arterial)	35-40 mm Hg	0.133	4.66-5.32 kPa
	Whole blood (venous)	40-45 mm Hg		5.32-5.99 kPa
Carbonic acid (H_2CO_3)	Whole blood (arterial)	1.05-1.45 mM	1	1.05-1.45 mmol/L
	Whole blood (venous)	1.15-1.50 mM		1.15-1.50 mmol/L
	Plasma (venous)	1.02-1.38 mM		1.02-1.38 mmol/L
Carboxyhemoglobin (carbon monoxide hemoglobin)	Whole blood			Fraction hemoglobin saturated
	Suburban nonsmokers	<1.5% saturation of hemoglobin	0.01	<0.015
	Smokers	1.5-5.0% saturation		0.015-0.050
	Heavy smokers	5.0-9.0% saturation		0.050-0.090
Carotene, beta	Serum	40-200 μ/dl	0.0186	0.74-3.72 μmol/L
Ceruloplasmin	Serum	23-50 mg/dl	10	230-500 mg/L
Chloride	Serum	95-103 mEq/l	1	95-103 mmol/L
Cholesterol				
Total	Serum	150-250 mg/dl (varies with diet, sex, and age)	0.026	3.90-6.50 mmol/L
Esters	Serum	65-75% of total cholesterol	0.01	Fraction of total cholesterol: 0.65-0.75
Cholinesterase	Erythrocytes	0.65-1.3 pH units	1	0.65-1.3 units
(Pseudocholinesterase)	Plasma	0.5-1.3 pH units		0.5-1.3 units
		8-18 IU/l at 37° C	1	8-18 U/L at 37° C
Citrate	Serum or plasma	1.7-3.0 mg/dl	52	88-156 μmol/L
Copper	Serum, plasma			
Male		70-140 μg/dl	0.157	11.0-22.0 μmol/L
Female		80-155 μg/dl		12.6-24.3 μmol/L
Cortisol	Plasma			
8 AM–10 AM		5-23 μg/dl	27.6	138-635 nmol/L
4 PM–6 PM		3-13 μg/dl		83-359 nmol/L
Creatine as creatinine	Serum or plasma			
Male		0.1-0.4 mg/dl	76.3	7.6-30.5 μmol/L
Female		0.2-0.7 mg/dl	76.3	15.3-53.4 μmol/L
Creatine kinase (CK)	Serum			
Male		55-170 U/I at 37° C	1	55-170 U/L at 37° C
Female		30-135 U/I at 37° C	1	30-135 U/L at 37° C
Creatinine	Serum or plasma	0.6-1.2 mg/dl (adult)	88.4	53-106 μmol/L
		0.3-0.6 mg/dl (children <2 yr)		27-54 μmol/L
Creatinine clearance (endogenous)	Serum or plasma and urine			
Male		107-139 ml/min	0.0167	1.78-2.32 ml/s
Female		87-107 ml/min		1.45-1.79 ml/s
Cryoglobulins	Serum	Negative	—	Negative

Continued

Table A-1

Whole blood, serum, and plasma chemistry—*cont'd*

Component	System	Typical reference intervals		
		Conventional units	Factor	Recommended SI units
Electrophoresis, protein	Serum	Percent		Fraction of total protein
Albumin		52-65% of total protein	0.01	0.52-0.65
Alpha-1		2.5-5.0% of total protein	0.01	0.025-0.05
Alpha-2		7.0-13.0% of total protein	0.01	0.07-0.13
Beta		8.0-14.0% of total protein	0.01	0.08-0.14
Gamma		12.0-22.0% of total protein	0.01	0.12-0.22
		Concentration		
Albumin		3.2-5.6 mg/dl	10	32-56 g/L
Alpha-1		0.1-0.4 gm/dl		1-4 g/L
Alpha-2		0.4-1.2 gm/dl		4-12 g/L
Beta		0.5-1.1 gm/dl		5-11 g/L
Gamma		0.5-1.6 gm/dl		5-16 g/L
Fats, neutral (see Triglycerides)				
Fatty acids				
Total (free and esterified)	Serum	9-15 mM	1	9-15 mmol/L
Free (non-esterified)	Plasma	300-480 μEq/I	1	300-480 μmol/L
Ferritin	Serum			
Male		15-200 ng/ml		15-200 μg/L
Female		12-150 ng/ml		15-150 μg/L
Fibrinogen	Plasma	200-400 mg/dl	0.01	2.00-4.00 g/L
Fluoride	Whole blood	<0.05 mg/dl	0.53	<0.027 mmol/L
Folate	Serum	5-25 ng/ml (bioassay)	2.27	11-56 nmol/L
		>2.3 ng/ml (radioassay)		>5.2 nmol/L
	Erythrocytes	166-640 ng/ml (bioassay)		376-1452 nmol/L
		>140 ng/ml (radioassay)		>318 nmol/L
Galactose	Whole blood			
Adults		None	—	None
Children		<20 mg/dl	0.055	<1.1 mmol/L
Gamma globulin	Serum	0.5-1.6 gm/dl	10	5-16 g/L
Globulins, total	Serum	2.3-3.5 gm/dl	10	23-35 g/L
Glucose, fasting	Serum or plasma	70-110 mg/dl	0.055	3.85-6.05 mmol/L
	Whole blood	60-100 mg/dl		3.30-5.50 mmol/L
Glucose tolerance				
Oral	Serum or plasma			
Fasting		70-110 mg/dl	0.055	3.85-6.05 mmol/L
30 min		30-60 mg/dl above fasting		1.65-3.30 mmol/L above fasting
60 min		20-50 mg/dl above fasting		1.10-2.75 mmol/L above fasting
120 min		5-15 mg/dl above fasting		0.28-0.83 mmol/L above fasting
180 min		Fasting level or below		Fasting level or below
Intravenous	Serum or plasma			
Fasting		70-110 mg/dl		3.85-6.05 mmol/L
5 min		Maximum of 250 mg/dl		Maximum of 13.75 mmol/L
60 min		Significant decrease		Significant decrease
120 min		Below 120 mg/dl		Below 6.60 mmol/L
180 min		Fasting level		Fasting level
Glucose 6-phosphate dehydrogenase (G6PD)	Erythrocytes	250-500 units/10^6 cells	1	250-500 μ units/cell
		1200-2000 mIU/ml packed erythrocytes	1	1200-2000 U/L packed erythrocytes
γ-Glutamyl transferase	Serum	5-40 IU/I	1	5-40 U/L at 37° C
Glutathione	Whole blood	24-37 mg/dl	0.032	0.77-1.18 mmol/L

Table A-1

Whole blood, serum, and plasma chemistry—*cont'd*

Component	System	Conventional units	Factor	Recommended SI units
		Typical reference intervals		
Growth hormone	Serum	<10 ng/ml	1	<10 μg/L
Guanase	Serum	<3 nM/ml/min	1	<3 U/L at 37° C
Haptoglobin	Serum	60-270 mg/dl	0.01	0.6-2.7 g/L
Hemoglobin	Serum or plasma			
Qualitative		Negative	—	Negative
Quantitative		0.5-5.0 mg/dl	10	5-50 mg/L
	Whole blood			
Female		12.0-16.0 g/dl	10	1.86-2.48 mmol/L
Male		13.5-18.0 g/dl		2.09-2.79 mmol/L
α-Hydroxybutyrate dehydrogenase	Serum	140-350 U/ml	1	140-350 kU/L
17-Hydroxycorticosteriods	Plasma			
Male		7-19 μg/dl	10	70-190 μg/L
Female		9-21 μg/dl		9-21 μg/L
After 24 USP Units of ACTH				
IM		35-55 μg/dl		350-550 μg/L
Immunoglobulins	Serum			
IgG		800-1801 mg/dl	0.01	8.0-18.0 g/L
IgA		113-563 mg/dl		1.1-5.6 g/L
IgM		54-222 mg/dl		0.54-2.2 g/L
IgD		0.5-3.0 mg/dl	10	5.0-30 mg/L
IgE		0.01-0.04 mg/dl		0.1-0.4 mg/L
Insulin	Plasma			
Bioassay		11-240 μIU/ml	0.0417	0.46-10.00 μg/L
Radioimmunoassay		4-24 μIU/ml		0.17-1.00 μg/L
Insulin tolerance (0.1 unit/kg)	Serum			
Fasting		Glucose of 70-110 mg/dl	0.055	Glucose of 3.85-6.05 mmol/L
30 min		Fall to 50% of fasting level	0.01	Fall to 0.5 of fasting level
90 min		Fasting level		Fasting level
Iodine				
Butanol-extraction (BEI)	Serum	3.5-6.5 μg/dl	0.079	0.28-0.51 μmol/L
Protein bound (PBI)	Serum	4.0-8.0 μg/dl		0.32-0.63 μmol/L
Iron, total	Serum	60-150 μg/dl	0.179	11-27 μmol/L
Iron binding capacity	Serum	250-400 μg/dl	0.179	54-64 μmol/L
Iron saturation	Serum	20-55%	0.01	Fraction of total iron binding capacity: 0.20-0.55
Isocitric dehydrogenase	Serum	50-240 units/ml at 25° C (Wolfson-Williams Ashman)	0.0167	0.83-4.18 U/L at 25° C
Ketone bodies	Serum	Negative	—	Negative
17-Ketosteroids	Plasma	25-125 μg/dl	0.01	0.25-1.25 mg/L
Lactic acid (as lactate)	Whole blood			
Venous		5-20 mg/dl	0.111	0.6-2.2 mmol/L
Arterial		3-7 mg/dl		0.3-0.8 mmol/L

Continued

Table A-1

Whole blood, serum, and plasma chemistry—*cont'd*

| Component | System | Typical reference intervals | | |
		Conventional units	Factor*	Recommended SI units†
Lactate dehydrogenase (LDH)	Serum	(lactate → pyruvate) 80-120 units at 30° C	0.48	38-62 U/L at 30° C
		(pyruvate → lactate) 185-640 units at 30° C	0.48	90-310 U/L at 30° C
		(lactate → pyruvate) 100-190 U/I at 37° C	1	100-190 U/L at 37° C
Lactate dehydrogenase isoenzymes	Serum			Fraction of total LDH
LDH$_1$ (anode)		17-27%	0.01	0.17-0.27
LDH$_2$		27-37%		0.27-0.37
LDH$_3$		18-25%		0.18-0.25
LDH$_4$		3-8%		0.03-0.08
LDH$_5$ (cathode)		0-5%		0.00-0.05
Lactate dehydrogenase (heat stable)	Serum	30-60% of total	0.01	Fraction of total LDH: 0.30-0.60
Lactose tolerance	Serum	Serum glucose changes similar to glucose tolerance test	—	Serum glucose changes similar to glucose tolerance test
Lead	Whole blood	0-50 μg/dl	0.048	0-2.4 μmol/L
Leucine aminopeptidase (LAP)	Serum			
Male		80-200 U/ml (Goldbarg-Rutenberg)	0.24	19.2-48.0 U/L
Female		75-185 U/ml (Goldbarg-Rutenberg)		18.0-44.4 U/L
Lipase	Serum	0-1.5 U/ml (Cherry-Crandall)	278	0-417 U/L
		14-280 mIU/ml	1	14-280 U/L
Lipids, total	Serum	400-800 mg/dl	0.01	4.00-8.00 g/L
Cholesterol		150-250 mg/dl	0.026	3.9-6.5 mmol/L
Triglycerides		10-190 mg/dl	0.109	1.09-20.71 mmol/L
Phospholipids		150-380 mg/dl	0.01	1.50-380 g/L
Fatty acids (free)		9.0-15.0 mM/I	1	9.0-15.0 mmol/L
		300-480 μEq/I	0.01	300-480 μmol/L
Phospholipid phosphorus		8.0-11.0 mg/dl	0.323	2.58-3.55 mmol/L
Lithium	Serum	Negative	—	Negative
Therapeutic interval		0.5-1.4 mEq/I	1	0.5-1.4 mmol/L
Long-acting thyroid-stimulating hormone (LATS)	Serum	None	—	None
Luteinizing hormone (LH)	Serum			
Male		6-30 mIU/ml	0.23	1.4-6.9 mg/L
Female		Midcycle peak: 3 times baseline value		Midcycle peak: 3 times baseline value
		Premenopausal <30 mIU/ml		Premenopausal <5 times baseline value
		Postmenopausal >35 mIU/ml		Postmenopausal >5 times baseline value

Table A-1

Whole blood, serum, and plasma chemistry—*cont'd*

Component	System	Typical reference intervals		
		Conventional units	**Factor**	**Recommended SI units**
Macroglobulins, total	Serum	70-430 mg/dl	0.01	0.7-4.3 g/L
Magnesium	Serum	1.3-2.1 mEq/I	0.5	0.7-1.1 mmol/L
		1.8-3.0 mg/dl	0.41	0.7-1.1 mmol/L
Methemoglobin	Whole blood	0.024 g/dl	10	0.0-2.4 g/L
		<1% of total hemoglobin	0.01	Fraction of total hemoglobin: <0.01
Mucoprotein	Serum	80-200 mg/dl	0.01	0.8-2.0 g/L
Muramidase	Serum	4-13 mg/I		4-13 mg/L
Non-protein nitrogen (NPN)	Serum or plasma	20-35 mg/dl	0.714	14.3-25.0 mmol/L
	Whole blood	25-50 mg/dl		17.9-35.7 mmol/L
5'Nucleotidase	Serum	0-1.6 units at 37° C	1	0-1.6 units at 37° C
Ornithine carbamyl transferase	Serum	8-20 mIU/ml at 37° C	1	8-20 U/L at 37° C
Osmolality	Serum	280-295 mOsm/kg	1	280-295 mmol/L
Oxygen				
Pressure (Po₂)	Whole blood (arterial)	95-100 mm Hg	0.133	12.64-13.30 kPa
Content	Whole blood (arterial)	15-23 volume %	0.01	Volume fraction: 0.15-0.23
Saturation	Whole blood (arterial)	94-100%		0.94-1.00
pH	Whole blood (arterial)	7.38-7.44	1	7.38-7.44
	Whole blood (venous)	7.36-7.41		7.36-7.41
	Serum or plasma (venous)	7.35-7.45		7.35-7.45
Phenylalanine	Serum			
Adults		<3.0 mg/dl	0.061	<0.18 mmol/L
Newborns (term)		1.2-3.5 mg/dl		0.07-0.21 mmol/L
Phosphatase				
Acid phosphatase	Serum	0.13-0.63 U/I at 37° C (paranitrophenylphosphate)	16.67	2.2-10.5 U/L at 37° C
Alkaline phosphatase	Serum	20-90 IU/I at 30° C (paranitrophenylphosphate in AMP buffer)	1	20-90 U/L at 30° C
Phospholipid phosphorus	Serum	8-11 mg/dl	0.323	2.6-3.6 mmol/L
Phospholipids	Serum	150-380 mg/dl	0.01	1.50-3.80 g/L
Phosphorus, inorganic	Serum			
Adults		2.3-4.7 mg/dl	0.323	0.78-1.52 mmol/L
Children		4.0-7.0 mg/dl		1.29-2.26 mmol/L
Potassium	Plasma	3.8-5.0 mEq/I	1	3.8-5.0 mmol/L
Prolactin	Serum			
Female		1-25 ng/ml	1	1-25 μg/L
Male		1-20 ng/ml		1-20 μg/L
Proteins	Serum			
Total		6.0-7.8 g/dl	10	60-78 g/L
Albumin		3.2-4.5 g/dl		32-45 g/L
Globulin		2.3-3.5 g/dl		23-35 g/L
Protein fractionation		See electrophoresis		See electrophoresis
Protoporphyrin	Erythrocytes	15-50 μg/dl	0.018	0.27-0.90 μmol/L
Pyruvate	Whole blood	0.3-0.9 mg/dl	114	34-103 μmol/L

Continued

Table A-1

Whole blood, serum, and plasma chemistry—*cont'd*

| Component | System | Typical reference intervals | | |
		Conventional units	Factor	Recommended SI units
Salicylates	Serum	Negative	—	Negative
Therapeutic interval		15-30 mg/dl	0.072	1.44-1.80 mmol/L
		150-300 μg/ml	0.0072	1.08-2.16 mmol/L
Sodium	Plasma	135-142 mEq/I	1	136-142 mmol/L
Sulfate, inorganic	Serum	0.2-1.3 mEq/I	0.5	0.10-0.65 mmol/L
		0.9-6.0 mg/dl as SO_4	0.104	0.09-0.62 mmol/L as SO_4
Sulfhemoglobin	Whole blood	Negative	—	Negative
Sulfonamides	Serum or whole blood	Negative	—	Negative
Testosterone	Serum or plasma			
Male		300-1200 ng/dl	0.035	10.0-42.0 nmol/L
Female		30-95 ng/dl		1.1-3.3 nmol/L
Thiocyanate	Serum	Negative	—	Negative
Thyroid hormone tests	Serum			
a) Expressed as thyroxine				
T_4 by column		5.0-11.0 μg/dl	13.0	65-143 nmol/L
T_4 by competitive binding— Murphy-Pattee		6.0-11.8 μg/dl		78-153 nmol/L
T_4 RIA		5.5-12.5 μg/dl	13.0	72-163 nmol/L
Free T_4		0.9-2.3 ng/dl		12-30 pmol/L
b) Expressed as iodine				
T_4 by column		3.2-7.2 μg/dl	79.0	253-569 nmol/L
T_4 by competitive binding— Murphy-Pattee		3.9-7.7 μg/dl		308-608 nmol/L
Free T_4		0.6-1.5 ng/dl	79.0	47-119 pmol/L
T_3 resin uptake		25-38 relative % uptake	0.01	Relative uptake fraction: 0.25-0.38
Thyroxine-binding globulin (TBG)	Serum	10-26 μg/dl	10	100-260 μg/L
TSH	Serum	<10 μU/ml	1	<10^{-3}IU/L
Transferases				
Aspartate amino transferase (AST or SGOT)	Serum	10-40 U/ml (Karmen) at 25° C	0.48	8-29 U/L at 30° C
		16-60 U/ml (Karmen) at 30° C		8-33 U/L at 37° C
Alanine amino transferase (ALT or SGPT)	Serum	10-30 U/ml (Karmen) at 25° C	0.48	4-24 U/L at 30° C
		8-50 Y/ml (Karmen) at 30° C		4-36 U/L at 37° C
Gamma glutamyl transferase (GGT)		5-40 IU/I at 37° C	1	5.40 U/L at 37° C
Triglycerides	Serum	10-190 mg/dl	0.011	0.11-2.09 mmol/L
Urea nitrogen	Serum	8-23 mg/dl	0.357	2.9-8.2 mmol/L
Urea clearance	Serum and urine			
Maximum clearance		64-99 ml/min	0.0167	1.07-1.65 ml/s
Standard clearance		41-65 ml/min, or more than 75% of normal clearance		0.68-1.09 ml/s or more than 0.75 of normal clearnace

Table A-1

Whole blood, serum, and plasma chemistry—*cont'd*

| Component | System | Typical reference intervals | | |
		Conventional units	Factor*	Recommended SI units†
Uric acid	Serum			
Male		4.0-8.5 mg/dl	0.059	0.24-0.5 mmol/L
Female		2.7-7.3 mg/dl		0.16-0.43 mmol/L
Vitamin A	Serum	15-60 μg/dl	0.035	0.53-2.10 μmol/L
Vitamin A tolerance	Serum			
Fasting 3 hr or 6 hr after 5000 units		15-60 μg/dl	0.035	0.53-2.10 μmol/L
Vitamin A/kg 24 hrs				
		200-600 μg/dl		7.00-21.00 μmol/L
		Fasting values or slightly above		Fasting values or slightly above
Vitamin B$_{12}$	Serum	160-950 pg/ml	0.74	118-703 pmol/L
Unsaturated vitamin B$_{12}$ binding capacity	Serum	1000-2000 pg/ml	0.74	740-1480 pmol/L
Vitamin C	Plasma	0.6-1.6 mg/dl	56.8	34-91 μmol/L
Xylose absorption	Serum			
Normal		24-40 mg/dl between 1 and 2 hr	0.067	1.68-2.68 mmol/L between 1 and 2 h
In malabsorption		Maximum approximately 10 mg/dl		Maximum approximately 0.67 mmol/L
Dose: Adult		25 g D-xylose	0.067	0.167 mol D-xylose
Children		0.5 g/kg D-xylose		3.33 mmol/kg D-xylose
Zinc	Serum	50-150 μg/dl	0.153	7.65-22.95 μmol/L

Table A-2

Urine

| Component | Type of urine specimen | Typical reference intervals | | |
		Conventional units	Factor	Recommended SI units
Acetoacetic acid	Random	Negative	—	Negative
Acetone	Random	Negative	—	Negative
Addis count	12 hr collection	WBC and epithelial cells		
		1,800,000/12 hr	1	1.8×10^6/12 h
		RBC 500,000/12 hr	1	0.5×10^6/12 h
		Hyaline casts: 0-5000/12 hr	1	5.0×10^3/12 h
Albumin				
Qualitative	Random	Negative	—	Negative
Quantitative	24 hr	15-150 mg/24 hr	1	0.015-0.150 g/24 h
Aldosterone	24 hr	2-26 μg/24 hr	2.77	5.5-72.0 nmol/24 h
Alkapton bodies	Random	Negative	—	Negative
Alpha-amino acid nitrogen	24 hr	100-290 mg/24 hr	0.0714	7.14-20.71 mmol/24 h
δ-Aminolevulinic acid	Random			
Adult		0.1-0.6 mg/dl	76.3	7.6-45.8 μmol/L
Children		<0.5 mg/dl		<38.1 μmol/L
	24 hr	1.5-7.5 mg/24 hr	7.63	11.15-57.2 μmol/24 h

Continued

Table A-2

Urine—*cont'd*

Component	Type of urine specimen	Typical reference intervals		
		Conventional units	Factor	Recommended SI units
Ammonia nitrogen	24 hr	20-70 mEq/24 hr		
		500-1200 mg/24 hr	0.071	35.5-85.2 mmol/24 h
Amylase	2 hr	35-260 Somogyi units/hr	0.185	6.5-48.1 U/h
Arsenic	24 hr	<50 mg/I	0.013	<0.65 μmol/L
Ascorbic acid	Random	1-7 mg/dl	0.057	0.06-0.40 mmol/L
	24 hr	>50 mg/24 hr	0.0057	>0.29 mmol/24 h
Bence Jones protein	Random	Negative	—	Negative
Beryllium	24 hr	<0.05 μg/24 hr	111	<5.55 nmol/24 h
Bilirubin, qualitative	Random	Negative	—	Negative
Blood, occult	Random	Negative	—	Negative
Borate	24 hr	<2 mg/I	16	<32 μmol/L
Calcium				
Qualitative (Sulkow-itch)	Random	1+ turbidity	1	1+ turbidity
Quantitative	24 hr			
	Average diet	100-240 mg/24 hr	0.025	2.50-6.25 mmol/24 h
	Low calcium diet	<150 mg/24 hr		<3.75 mmol/24 h
	High calcium diet	240-300 mg/24 hr		6.25-7.50 mmol/24 h
Catecholamines	Random	0-14 μg/dl	10	0-140 μg/L
	24 hr	<100 μg/24 hr (varies with activity)	1	<100 μg/24 h
Epinephrine		<10 ng/24 hr	5.46	<55 nmol/24 h
Norepinephrine		<100 ng/24 hr	5.91	<590 nmol/24 h
Total free catechol-amines		4-126 μg/24 hr	1	4-126 μg/24 h
Total metanephrines		0.1-1.6 mg/24 hr	1	0.1-1.6 mg/24 h
Chloride	24 hr	140-250 mEq/24 hr	1	140-250 mmol/24 h
Concentration test (Fishberg)	Random—after fluid restriction			
Specific gravity		>1.025	1	>1.025
Osmolality		>850 mOsm/I	1	>850 mmol/L
Copper	24 hr	0-50 μg/24 hr	0.016	0-0.48 μmol/24 h
Coproporphyrin	Random			
	Adult	3-20 μg/dl	0.015	0.045-0.30 μmol/L
	24 hr			
	Adult	50-160 μg/24 hr	0.0015	0.075-0.24 μmol/24 h
	Children	0-80 μg/24 hr	0.0015	0.00-0.12 μmol/24 hr
Creatine	24 hr			
	Male	0-40 mg/24 hr	0.0076	0-0.30 mmol/24 h
	Female	0-100 mg/24 hr		0-0.76 mmol/24 h
		Higher in children and during pregnancy	—	Higher in children and during pregnancy
Creatinine	24 hr			
	Male	20-26 mg/kg/24 hr	0.0088	0.18-0.23 mmol/kg/24 h
		1.0-2.0 g/24 hr	8.8	8.8-17.6 mmol/24 h
	Female	14-22 mg/kg/24 hr	0.0088	0.12-0.19 mmol/kg/24 h
		0.8-1.8 g/24 hr	8.8	7.0-15.8 mmol/24 h
Cystine, qualitative	Random	Negative	—	Negative
Cystine and cysteine	24 hr	10-100 mg/24 hr	0.0083	0.08-0.83 mmol/24 h

Table A-2

Urine—*cont'd*

Component	Type of urine specimen	Typical reference intervals		
		Conventional units	Factor	Recommended SI units
Diacetic acid	Random	Negative	—	Negative
Epinephrine	24 hr	0-20 μg/24 hr	0.0055	0.00-0.11 μmol/24 h
Estrogens				
Total	24 hr			
Male		5-18 μg/24 hr	1	5-18 μg/24 h
Female				
Ovulation		28-100 μg/24 hr		28-80 μg/24 h
Luteal peak		22-80 μg/24 hr		22-105 μg/24h
At menses		4-25 μg/24 hr		4-25 μg/24 h
Pregnancy		Up to 45,000 μg/24 hr		Up to 45,000 μg/24 h
Postmeno-pausal		Up to 10 μg/24 hr		Up to 10 μg/24 h
Fractionated	24 hr, nonpreg-nant, midcycle			
Estrone (E^1)	—	2-25 μg/24 hr	3.7	7-93 nmol/24 h
Estradiol (E^2)	—	0-10 μg/24 hr	3.7	0.37 nmol/24 h
Estriol (E^3)	—	2-30 μg/24 hr	3.5	7-105 nmol/24 h
Fat, qualitative	Random	Negative	—	Negative
FIGLU (N-formiminoglu-tamic acid)	24 hr	<3 mg/24 hr	5.7	<17.0 μmol/24 h
	After 15 g of L-histidine	4 mg/8 hr	5.7	23.0 μmol/8 h
Fluoride	24 hr	<1 mg/24 hr	0.053	0.053 mmol/24 h
Follicle-stimulating hor-mone (FSH)	24hr			
Adult		6-50 Mouse uterine units (MUU)/24 hr	1	4-25 mIU/ml
Prepubertal		<10 MUU/24 hr	1	4-30 mIU/ml
Postmenopausal		>50 MUU/24 hr	1	40-50 mIU/ml
Midcycle		2× baseline		
Fructose	24 hr	30-65 mg/24 hr	0.0056	0.17-0.36 mmol/24 h
Glucose				
Qualitative	Random	Negative	—	Negative
Quantitative	24 hr			
Copper-reducing sub-stances		0.5-1.5 g/24 hr	1	0.5-1.5 g/24 h
Total sugars		Average 250 mg/24 hr	1	Average 250 mg/24 h
Glucose		Average 130 mg/24 hr	0.0056	Average 0.73 mmol/24 h
Gonadotropins, pituitary (FSH and LH)	24 hr	10-50 MUU/24 hr	1	10-50 IU/24 h
Etiocholanolone	24 hr			
Male		1.4-5.0 mg/24 hr	3.44	4.8-17.2 μmol/24 h
Female		0.8-4.0 mg/24 hr		2.8-13.8 μmol/24 h
Dehydroepiandrosterone	24hr			
Male		0.2-2.0 mg/24 hr	3.46	0.7-6.9 μmol/24 h
Female		0.2-1.8 mg/24 hr		0.7-6.2 μmol/24 h
11-Ketoandrosterone	24 hr			
Male		0.2-1.0 mg/24 hr	3.28	0.7-3.3 μmol/24 h
Female		0.2-0.8 mg/24 hr		0.7-2.6 μmol/24 h
11-Ketoetiocholanolone	24 hr			
Male		0.2-1.0 mg/24 hr	3.28	0.7-3.3 μmol/24 h
Female		0.2-0.8 mg/24hr		0.7-2.6 μmol/24 h

Continued

Table A-2

Urine—*cont'd*

Component	Type of urine specimen	Conventional units	Factor	Recommended SI units
		Typical reference intervals		
11-Hydroxyandrosterone	24 hr			
Male		0.1-0.8 mg/24 hr	3.26	0.3-2.6 μmol/24 h
Female		0.0-0.5 mg/24 hr		0.0-1.6 μmol/24 h
11-Hydroxyetiocholano-lone	24 hr			
Male		0.2-0.6 mg/24 hr	3.26	0.7-2.0 μmol/24 h
Female		0.1-1.1 mg/24 hr		0.3-3.6 μmol/24 h
Lactose	24 hr	14-40 mg/24 hr	2.9	41-116 μmol/24 h
Lead	24 hr	<100 μg/24 hr	0.0048	<0.48 μmol/24 h
Magnesium	24 hr	6.0-8.5 mEq/24 hr	0.5	3.0-4.3 mmol/24h
Melanin, qualitative	Random	Negative	—	Negative
3-Methoxy-4-hydroxy-mandelic acid (VMA)	24 hr			
Adults		1.5-7.5 mg/24 hr	5.05	7.6-37.9 μmol/24 h
Infants		83 μg/kg/24 hr	0.0051	0.4 μmol/kg/24 h
Mucin	24 hr	100-150 mg/24 hr	1	100-150 mg/24 h
Muramidase (lysozyme)	24 hr	1.3-36 mg/24 hr		1.3-36 mg/24 h
Myoglobin				
Qualitative	Random	Negative	—	Negative
Quantitative	24 hr	<4 mg/l	1	<4 mg/L
Osmolality	Random	500-800 mOsm/kg water	1	500-800 mmol/kg
Pentoses	24 hr	2-5 mg/kg/24 hr	1	2-5 mg/kg/24 h
pH	Random	4.6-8.0	1	4.6-8.0
Phenosulfonphthalein (PSP)	Urine timed after 6 mg PSP IV			Fraction dye excreted
15 min		20-50% dye excreted	0.01	0.2-0.5
30 min		16-24% dye excreted		0.16-0.24
60 min		9-17% dye excreted		0.09-0.17
120 min		3-10% dye excreted		0.03-0.10
Phenylpyruvic acid, qualitative	Random	Negative	—	Negative
Phosphorus	Random	0.9-1.3 g/24 hr	32	29-42 mmol/24 h
Porphobilinogen				
Qualitative	Random	Negative	—	Negative
Quantitative	24 hr	0-1.0 mg/24 hr	4.42	0-4.4 μmol/24 h
Potassium	24 hr	40-80 mEq/24 hr	1	40-80 mmol/24 h
Pregnancy tests	Concentrated morning specimen	Positive in normal pregnancies or with tumors producing chorionic gonadotropin	—	Positive in normal pregnancies or with tumors producing chorionic gonadotropin
Pregnanediol	24 hr			
Male		0-1.5 mg/24hr	3.12	0-4.7 μmol/24 h
Female		1-8 mg/24 hr		3-25 μmol/24 h
Peak		1 week after ovulation	—	1 week after ovulation
Pregancy		<50 mg/24 hr		156 μol/24 h
Children		Negative	—	Negative
Pregnanetriol	24 hr			
Male		0.4-2.4 mg/24 hr	2.97	1.2-7.1 μmol/24 h
Female		0.5-2.0 mg/24 hr		1.5-5.9 μmol/24 h
Children		Up to 1 mg/24hr		Up to 3 μmol/24 h
Protein, qualitative	Random	Negative	—	Negative
	24 hr	40-150 mg/24hr	1	40-150 mg/24 h

Table A-2

Urine—*cont'd*

Component	Type of urine specimen	Typical reference intervals		
		Conventional units	Factor	Recommended SI units
Reducing substances, total	24 hr	0.5-1.5 mg/24 hr	1	0.5-1.5 mg/24 h
Sodium	24 hr	75-200 mEq/24 hr	1	75-200 mmol/24 h
Solids, total	24 hr	55-70 g/24 hr	1	55-70 g/24h
		Decreases with age to 30 g/24 hr	—	Decreases with age to 30 g/24 h
Specific gravity	Random			Relative Density (U 20° C/water 20° C)
		1.016-1.022 (normal fluid intake)	1	1.016-1.022 (normal fluid intake)
		1.001-1.035 (range)		1.001-1.034 (range)
Sugars (exluding glucose)	Random	Negative	—	Negative
Titratable acidity	24 hr	20-50 mEq/24 hr	1	20-50 mmol/24 h
Urea nitrogen	24 hr	6-17 g/24 hr	0.0357	0.21-0.60 mol/24 h
Uric acid	24 hr	250-750 mg/24 hr	0.0059	1.48-4.43 mmol/24 h
Urobilinogen	2 hr	0.3-1.0 Ehrlich Units	—	
	24 hr	0.05-2.5 mg/24 hr or	1.69	0.09-4.23 μmol/24 h
		0.5-4.0 Ehrlich units/24 hr	—	
Uropepsin	Random	15-45 units/hr (Anson)	7.37	111-332 U/h
	24 hr	1500-5000 units/24 hr (Anson)		11-37 kU/h
Uroporphyrins				
Qualitative	Random	Negative	—	Negative
Quantitative	24 hr	10-30 μg/24 hr	0.0012	0.012-0.37 μmol/24 h
Vanillylmandelic acid (VMA)	24 hr	1.5-7.5 mg/24 hr	5.05	7.6-37.9 μmol/24 h
Volume, total	24 hr	600-1600 mg/24 hr	0.001	0.6-1.6 L/24 h
Zinc	24 hr	0.15-1.2 mg/24 hr	15.3	2.3-18.4 μmol/24 h

Table A-3

Synovial fluid

Component	Typical reference intervals		
	Conventional units	Factor	Recommended SI units
Blood-serum synovial fluid glucose difference	<10 mg/dl	0.055	<0.55 mmol/L
Differential cell count	Granulocytes <25% of nucleated cells	0.01	Granulocytes number fraction: <25% of nucleated cells
Fibrin clot	Absent	—	Absent
Mucin clot	Abundant	—	Abundant
Nucleated cell count	<200 cells/μl	10^6	<2 × 10^8 cells/L
Viscosity	High	—	High
Volume	<3.5 ml	0.001	<0.0035L

Table A-4

Seminal fluid

| Component | Typical reference intervals | | |
	Conventional units	Factor	Recommended SI units
Liquefaction	Within 20 min	1	Within 20 min
Sperm morphology	>70% normal mature spermatozoa	0.01	Number fraction: >0.7 normal, mature spermatozoa
Sperm motility	>60%	0.01	Number fraction: >0.6
pH	>7.0 (average 7.7)	1	>7.0 (average 7.7)
Sperm count	60-150 million/ml	10^3	$60\text{-}150 \times 10^9/L$
Volume	1.5-5.0 ml	0.001	0.0015-0.005L

Table A-5

Gastric fluid

| Component | Typical reference intervals | | |
	Conventional units	Factor	Recommended SI units
Fasting residual volume	20-100 ml	0.001	0.02-0.10L
pH	<2.0	1	<2.0
Basal acid output (BAO)	0-6 mEq/hr	1	0-6 mmol/h
Maximum acid output (MAO) (after histamine stimulation)	5-40 mEq/hr	1	5-40 mmol/h
BAO/MAO ratio	<0.4	1	<0.4

Table A-6

Hematology

| Component | Typical reference intervals | | |
	Conventional units	Factor	Recommended SI units
Red cell volume			
Male	20-36 ml/kg body weight	0.001	0.020-0.036 L/kg body weight
Female	19-31 ml/kg body weight	—	0.019-0.031 L/kg body weight
Plasma volume			
Male	25-42 ml/kg body weight	0.001	0.040-0.050 L/kg body weight
Female	28-45 ml/kg body weight	—	0.040-0.050 L/kg body weight
Coagulation and hemostatic tests			
Bleeding time			
Mielke template	2-8 minutes		2-8 min
Simplate	3-8 minutes		3-8 min
Antithrombin III			
Immunologic	21-30 mg/dL		210-310 mg/L
Functional	80-120%		0.8-1.2
Clot retraction	40-94% of serum extruded in 1 hour at 37° C		
Euglobulin clot lysis time	Clot lyses between 2 and 4 hours at 37° C		

Table A-6

Hematology—*cont'd*

Component	Typical reference intervals		
	Conventional units	Factor	Recommended SI units
Factor assays (procoagulant)	0.5-1.5 U/mL		0.5-1.5
Factor VIII antigen (Factor VIIIR:Ag; Laurell)	0.5-1.5 U/mL		0.5-1.5
Ristocetin cofactor (Factor VIIIR:RCoF)	0.5-1.5 U/mL		0.5-1.5
Factor XIII (screening test)	Clot insoluble in 5M urea at 24 hours		
Fibrinogen	200-400 mg/dL		2-4 g/dL
Fibrinogen split products	10 ug/mL		10 mg/L
Partial thromboplastin time (PTT)	Depends upon phospholipid reagent used, typically 60-85 seconds		
Activated PTT	Depends upon activator and phospholipid reagents used, typically 20-35 seconds		
Plasminogen			
Immunologic	10-20 mg/dL		100-200 mg/L
Functional	2.2-4.2 CTA U/mL*		
Prothrombin time	Depends upon thromboplastin reagent used, typically 9.5-12 seconds		
Thrombin time	Depends upon the concentration of thrombin reagent used, typically 20-29 seconds		
Whole blood clot lysis time	None in 24 hours		
Complete blood count (CBC)			
Hematocrit			
Male	40-54%	0.01	Volume fraction: 0.40-0.54
Female	38-47%		0.38-0.47%
Hemoglobin			
Male	13.5-18.0 g/dl	0.155	2.09-2.79 mmol/L
Female	12.0-16.0 g/dl		1.86-2.48 mmol/L
Red cell count			
Male	$4.6\text{-}6.2 \times 10^6/\mu l$	10^6	$4.6\text{-}6.2 \times 10^{12}/L$
Female	$4.2\text{-}5.4 \times 10^6/\mu l$		$4.2\text{-}5.4 \times 10^{12}/L$
White cell count	$4.5\text{-}11.0 \times 10^3/\mu l$	10^6	$4.5\text{-}11.0 \times 10^9/L$
Erythrocyte indices			
Mean corpuscular volume (MCV)	80-96 cu microns	1	80-96 fl
Mean corpuscular hemoglobin (MCH)	27-31 pg	1	27-31 pg
Mean corpuscular hemoglobin concentration (MCHC)	32-36%	0.01	Concentration fraction: 0.32-0.36

White blood cell differential (adult)	Mean percent	Range of absolute counts		Mean number fraction†	Range of absolute count
Segmented neutrophils	56%	1800-7000/μl	10^6	0.56	$1.8\text{-}7.8 \times 10^9/L$
Bands	3%	0-700/μl	10^6	0.03	$0\text{-}0.70 \times 10^9/L$
Eosinophils	2.7%	0-450/μl	10^6	0.027	$0\text{-}0.45 \times 10^9/L$
Basophils	0.3%	0-200/μl	10^6	0.003	$0\text{-}0.20 \times 10^9/L$
Lymphocytes	34%	1000-4800/μl	10^6	0.34	$1.0\text{-}4.8 \times 10^9/L$
Monocytes	4%	0-800/μl	10^6	0.04	$0\text{-}0.80 \times 10^9/L$
Hemoglobin A_2	1.5-3.5% of total hemoglobin		0.01	Mass fraction: 0.015-0.035 of total hemoglobin	
Hemoglobin F	<2%		0.01	Mass fraction: <0.02	

*CTA, Committee on Thrombotic Agents.

†All percentages are multiplied by 0.01 to give fraction.

Continued

Table A-6

Hematology—*cont'd*

Component	Typical reference intervals						
	Conventional units			Factor	Recommended SI units		
Osmotic fragility		*% Lysis*		%NaCl—171		*Lysed fraction*	
	% NaCl	*Fresh*	*24 hr at 37° C*	% Lysis—0.01	*NaCl mmol/L*	*Fresh*	*24 h at 37° C*
	0.2	—	95-100		34.2	—	0.95-1.00
	0.3	97-100	85-100		51.3	0.97-1.00	0.85-1.00
	0.35	90-99	75-100		59.8	9.90-0.99	0.75-1.00
	0.4	50-95	65-100		68.4	0.50-0.95	0.65-1.00
	0.45	5-45	55-95		77.0	0.05-0.45	0.55-0.95
	0.5	0-6	40-85		85.5	0-0.06	0.40-0.85
	0.55	0	15-70		94.1	0	0.15-0.70
	0.6	—	0-40		102.6	—	0-0.40
	0.65	—	0-10		111.2	—	0-0.10
	0.7	—	0-5		119.7	—	0-0.05
	0.75	—	0		128.3	—	0
Platelet count	150,000-400,000/μl			10^6	0.15-0.4 $\times$ 10^{12}/L		
Reticulocyte count	0.5-1.5%			0.01	Number fraction: 0.005-0.015		
	25,000-75,000 cells/μl			10^6	25-75 $\times$ 10^9/L		
Sedimentation rate (ESR) (Westergren)							
Men under 50 yrs	<50 mm/hr			1	<15 mm/h		
Men over 50 yrs	<20 mm/hr				<20 mm/h		
Women under 50 yrs	<20 mm/hr				<20 mm/h		
Women over 50 yrs	<30 mm/hr				<30 mm/h		
Viscosity	1.4-1.8 times water			1	1.4-1.8 times water		
Zeta sedimentation ratio	41-54%			0.01	Fraction: 0.41-0.54		

Table A-7

Amniotic fluid

Component	Typical reference intervals		
	Conventional units	Factor	Recommended SI units
Appearance			
Early gestation	Clear	—	Clear
Term	Clear or slightly opalescent	—	Clear or slightly opalescent
Albumin			
Early gestation	0.39 g/dl	10	3.9 g/L
Term	0.19 g/dl		1.9 g/L
Bilirubin			
Early gestation	<0.075 mg/dl	17.1	<1.28 μmol/L
Term	<0.025 mg/dl		<0.43 μmol/L
Chloride			
Early gestation	Approximately equal to serum chloride	—	Approximately equal to serum chloride
Term	Generally 1-3 mEq/l lower than serum chloride	1	Generally 1-3 mmol/L lower than serum chloride

Table A-7

Amniotic fluid—*cont'd*

Component	Typical reference intervals		
	Conventional units	Factor	Recommended SI units
Creatinine			
Early gestation	0.8-1.1 mg/dl	88.4	70.7-97.2 μmol/L
Term	1.8-4.0 mg/dl (generally > 2 mg/dl)		159.1-353.6 μmol/L (generally > 176.8 μmol/L)
Estriol			
Early gestation	<10 μg/dl	0.035	<0.35 μmol/L
Term	>60 μg/dl		>2.1 μmol/L
Lecithin/sphingomyelin		1	
Early (immature)	<1:1	1	<1:1
Term (mature)	>2:1	1	>2:1
Osmolality			
Early gestation	Approximately equal to serum osmolality	1	Approximately equal to serum osmolality
Term	230-270 mOsm/l	1	<230-270 mmol/L
P_{CO_2}			
Early gestation	33-55 mm Hg	0.133	4.39-7.32 kPa
Term	42-55 mm Hg (increases toward term)		5.95-7.32 kPa (increase toward term)
pH			
Early gestation	7.12-7.38	1	7.12-7.38
Term	6.91-7.43 (decreases toward term)		6.91-7.43
Protein, total			
Early gestation	0.60 ± 0.24 g/dl	10	6.0 ± 2.4 g/L
Term	0.26 ± 0.19 g/dl		2.6 ± 1.9 g/L
Sodium			
Early gestation	Approximately equal to serum sodium	—	Approximately equal to serum sodium
Term	7-10 mEq/l lower than serum sodium	1	7-10 mmol/L lower than serium sodium
Staining, cytologic			
Oil red O			Stained fraction
Early gestation	<10%	0.01	<0.1
Term	>50%		>0.5
Nile blue sulfate			Stained fraction
Early gestation	0	0.01	0
Term	>20%		>0.2
Urea			
Early gestation	18.0 ± 5.9 mg/dl	0.166	2.99 ± 0.98 mmol/L
Term	30.3 ± 11.4 mg/dl		5.03 ± 1.89 mmol/L
Uric acid			
Early gestation	3.72 ± 0.96 mg/dl	0.059	0.22 ± 0.06 mmol/L
Term	9.90 ± 2.23 mg/dl		0.58 ± 0.13 mmol/L
Volume			
Early gestation	450-1200 ml	0.001	0.45-1.2 L
Term	500-1400 ml (increases toward term)		0.5-1.4 L (increases toward term)

Table A-8

Cerebrospinal fluid

| Component | Typical reference intervals | | |
	Conventional units	Factor	Recommended SI units
Albumin	10-30 mg/dl	10	100-300 mg/L
Calcium	2.1-2.7 mEq/l	0.5	1.05-1.35 mmol/L
Cell count	0-5 cells/μl	10^6	$0-5 \times 10^6$/L
Chloride			
Adult	118-132 mEq/l	1	118-132 mmol/L
Glucose	50-80 mg/dl	0.055	2.75-4.40 mmol/L
Lactate dehydrogenase (LDH)	Approximately 10% of serum level	—	Activity fraction: approximately 0.1 of serum level
Protein			
Total CSF	15-45 mg/dl	10	150-450 mg/L
Ventricular fluid	5-15 mg/dl		50-150 mg/L
Protein electrophoresis			Fraction
Prealbumin	2-7%	0.01	0.02-0.07
Albumin	56-76%		0.56-0.76
Alpha-1 globulin	2-7%		0.02-0.07
Alpha-2 globulin	4-12%		0.04-0.12
Beta globulin	8-18%		0.08-0.18
Gamma globulin	3-12%		0.03-0.12
Xanthochromia	Negative	—	Negative

Table A-10

Selected pediatric reference values—*cont'd*

S-γ-Glutamyltransferase

Premature newborn:	56-233 U/L
Newborn-3 wks:	10-103 U/L
3 wks-3 mos:	4-111 U/L
1-5 yrs:	2-23 U/L
6-15 yrs:	2-23 U/L
16 yrs-adult:	2-35 U/L

S-Haptoglobin

Newborn:	detectable haptoglobin in only 10-20%
1 yr and older:	at adult values

S-Immunoglobulin IgG

0-5 wks:	7500-15,000 mg/L
6 mos:	1500-7000 mg/L
1 yr:	1400-10,300 mg/L
5 yr:	3700-15,000 mg/L
10 yrs:	4400-15,500 mg/L

S-Immunoglobulin IgA

0-5 wks:	none
6 mos:	200-1300 mg/L
1 yr:	200-130 mg/L
5 yrs:	300-2000 mg/L
10 yrs:	500-2300 mg/L

S-Phosphorus (inorganic)

	Pre-term	Full-term
Newborn:	1.8-2.6 mmol/L (56.0-80.0 mg/L)	1.6-2.5 mmol/L (50.0-78.0 mg/L)
6-10 days:	2.0-3.8 mmol/L (61-117 mg/L)	1.6-2.9 mmol/L (49-89 mg/L)
4 mos:	1.6-2.6 mmol/L (48-81 mg/L)	
1 yr:	1.25-2.1 mmol/L (39-60 mg/L)	
2-16 yrs:	0.9-1.5 mmol/L (26-50 mg/L)	

S-Potassium

Pre-term newborn:	4.5-7.2 mmol/L
Full-term newborn:	5.0-7.7 mmol/L
2 d-2 wks:	4.0-6.4 mmol/L
2 wks-3 mos:	4.0-6.2 mmol/L
3 mos-1 yr:	3.7-5.6 mmol/L
1-16 yrs:	3.6-5.2 mmol/L

S-Testosterone

Age	Male	Female
0-2 yrs:	0.14-1.28 nmol/L	0.24-0.62 nmol/L
2-4 yrs:	0.17-5.55 nmol/L	0.24-0.69 nmol/L
4-6 yrs:	0.28-1.39 nmol/L	0.35-0.69 nmol/L
6-8 yrs:	0.21-9.72 nmol/L	0.52-1.04 nmol/L
8-10 yrs:	0.31-1.74 nmol/L	0.69-1.39 nmol/L
10-12 yrs:	0.29-10.06 nmol/L	0.69-1.74 nmol/L
12-14 yrs:	0.17-26.37 nmol/L	1.04-2.43 nmol/L
14-16 yrs:	3.12-19.43 nmol/L	1.21-3.30 nmol/L
16-18 yrs:	9.02-25.33 nmol/L	1.39-3.30 nmol/L
18-20 yrs:	13.88-24.98 nmol/L	1.39-3.30 nmol/L
20-25 yrs:	11.80-38.86 nmol/L	1.39-3.30 nmol/L

S-Immunoglobulin IgM

0-5 wks:	less than 200 mg/L
6 mos:	300-600 mg/L
1 yr:	300-1600 mg/L
5 yrs:	200-2200 mg/L
10 yrs:	300-1700 mg/L

Inulin clearance

<1 mo:	29-88 ml/min per 1.73 m^2 of body surface
1-6 mos:	40-112 ml/min per 1.73 m^2 of body surface
6-12 mos:	62-121 ml/min per 1.73 m^2 of body surface
>1 yr:	78-164 ml/min per 1.73 m^2 of body surface

U-17 Ketosteroids

0-3 days:	0-0.5 mg/d
1-3 yrs:	<2.0 mg/d
3-6 yrs:	0.5-3.0 mg/d
6-9 yrs:	0.8-4.0 mg/d
10-12 yrs:	male: 0.7-6.0 mg/d
	female: 0.7-5.0 mg/d
Adolescent:	male: 3-15 mg/d
	female: 3-12 mg/d

S-Lactate dehydrogenase

1-3 days:	up to 2 × adult values

S-Thyroxine

1-3 days:	142-296 nmol/L (11-23 μg/dl)
1 wk-1 mo:	116-232 nmol/L (9-18 μg/dl)
1-4 mos:	97-212 nmol/L (7.5-16.5 μg/dl)
4-12 mos:	71-187 nmol/L (5.5-14.5 μg/dl)
1-6 yrs:	71-174 nmol/L (5.5-13.5 μg/dl)
6-10 yrs:	64-161 nmol/L (5.0-12.5 μg/dl)

appendix b

B

Desirable weights

Table B-1

1983 Metropolitan height and weight tables*

Men			
Height	**Small frame**	**Medium frame**	**Large frame**
5'2"	128-134	131-141	138-150
5'3"	130-136	133-143	140-153
5'4"	132-138	135-145	142-156
5'5"	134-140	137-148	144-160
5'6"	136-142	139-151	146-164
5'7"	138-145	142-154	149-168
5'8"	140-148	145-157	152-172
5'9"	142-151	148-160	155-176
5'10"	144-154	151-163	158-180
5'11"	146-157	154-166	161-184
6'0"	149-160	157-170	164-188
6'1"	152-164	160-174	168-192
6'2"	155-168	164-178	172-197
6'3"	158-172	167-182	176-202
6'4"	162-176	171-187	181-207

Women			
Height	**Small frame**	**Medium frame**	**Large frame**
4'10"	102-111	109-121	118-131
4'11"	103-113	111-123	120-134
5'0"	104-115	113-126	122-137
5'1"	106-118	115-129	125-140
5'2"	108-121	118-132	128-143
5'3"	111-124	121-135	131-147
5'4"	114-127	124-138	134-151
5'5"	117-130	127-141	137-155
5'6"	120-133	130-144	140-159
5'7"	123-136	133-147	143-163
5'8"	126-139	133-150	146-167
5'9"	129-142	139-153	149-170
5'10"	132-145	142-156	152-173
5'11"	135-148	145-159	155-176
6'0"	138-151	148-162	158-179

*Weight in pounds at ages 29-59 years according to build. In shoes and 3 pounds of indoor clothing for women and 5 pounds for men. (Sources: Society of Actuaries, Build Study, 1979, Chicago, 1980, Society of Actuaries and Association of Life Insurance Medical Directors of America, Metropolitan Life Insurance Co, NY, 1983.)

Table B-2

Optimal weights for men and women*

Height	Fogerty Center acceptable weight† in pounds		Range of acceptable weights‡ in pounds	
			25% under- to 5% overweight	15% under- to 5% overweight
	Men	Women	Men	Women
5 ft 0 in	—	95-125	—	106-131
5 2	—	102-131	—	111-138
5 4	120-149	108-137	112-156	118-145
5 6	126-157	114-145	119-166	122-152
5 8	133-166	121-153	125-175	129-160
5 10	141-175	129-161	132-185	135-167
6 0	149-184	137-171	140-195	142-175
6 2	157-194	—	148-207	—
6 4	165-204	—	156-218	—

*Height and weight in street clothing.
†Recommended by the Fogerty International Center Conference on Obesity, Washington, DC, October 1973; adapted from the Metropolitan Life Insurance desirable weight tables, adjusted for height and weight to street clothing. (Sims EAH. In Bray GA: Obesity in America, NIH pub. no. 79-359, Washington, DC, 1979, U.S. Department Health, Education and Welfare.)
‡From tables of the Build Study, 1979. Mortality rates equal to or less than the average, adjusted for age, were obtained in range of 25% underweight to 5% overweight for men and 15% underweight for women. (Build Study, 1979, Chicago, 1980, Society of Actuaries and Association of Life Insurance Medical Directors of America.)

Table B-3

Determination of frame size

METHOD 1*

Height is recorded without shoes on.
Wrist circumference is measured just distal to the styloid process at the wrist crease on the right arm using a tape measure.
The following formula is used:

$$r = \frac{\text{Height (cm)}}{\text{Wrist circumference (cm)}}$$

Frame size can be determined as follows:

	Males	Females
Small	r>10.4	r>11.0
Medium	r = 9.6–10.4	r = 10.1–11.0
Large	r<9.6	r<10.1

METHOD 2†

The patient's right arm is extended forward perpendicular to the body, with the arm bent so the angle at the elbow forms 90° with the fingers pointing up and the palm turned away from the body. The greatest breadth across the elbow joint is measured with a sliding caliper along the axis of the upper arm, on the two prominent bones on either side of the elbow. This is recorded as the elbow breadth. The following tables give the elbow breadth measurements for medium-framed men and women of various heights. Measurements lower than those listed indicate a small frame size; higher measurements indicate a large frame size.

	Height in 1″ heels	Elbow breadth
Men	5′2″ –5′3″	2½″–2⅞″
	5′4″ –5′7″	2⅝″–2⅞″
	5′8″ –5′11″	2¾″–3″
	6′0″ –6′3″	2¾″–3⅛″
	6′4″	2⅞″–3¼″
Women	4′10″–4′11″	2¼″–2½″
	5′0″ –5′3″	2¼″–2½″
	5′4″ –5′7″	2⅜″–2⅝″
	5′8″ –5′11″	2⅜″–2⅝″
	6′0″	2½″–2¾″

*Data from Grant JP: Handbook of total parenteral nutrition, Philadelphia, 1980, WB Saunders Co.
†Data from the Metropolitan Life Insurance Co, 1983.

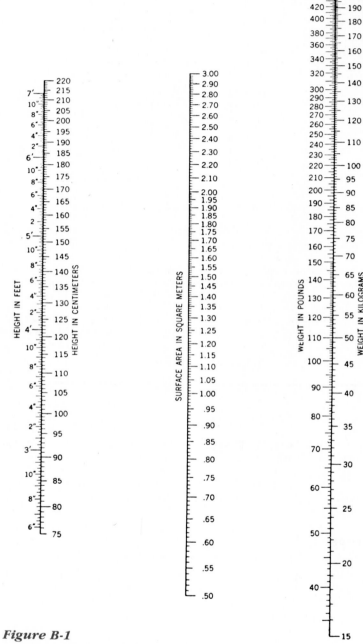

Figure B-1

Nomogram for the determination of body surface area of children and adults.
(From Boothby WM and Sandiford RB: Boston Med Surg J 185:337, 1921.)

Developmental assessment

Table C-1

Assessment of the newborn

Posture. Observed with infant quiet and in supine position. Score 0: Arms and legs extended; 1: Beginning of flexion of hips and knees, arms extended; 2: Stronger flexion of legs, arms extended; 3: Arms slightly flexed, legs flexed and abducted; 4: Full flexion of arms and legs.

Square window. The hand is flexed on the forearm between the thumb and index finger of the examiner. Enough pressure is applied to get as full a flexion as possible, and the angle between the hypothenar eminence and the ventral aspect of the forearm is measured and graded according to diagram. (Care is taken not to rotate the infant's wrist while doing this maneuver.)

Ankle dorsiflexion. The foot is dorsiflexed onto the anterior aspect of the leg, with the examiner's thumb on the sole of the foot and other fingers behind the leg. Enough pressure is applied to get as full flexion as possible, and the angle between the dorsum of the foot and the anterior aspect of the leg is measured.

Arm recoil. With the infant in the supine position the forearms are first flexed for 5 seconds, then fully extended by pulling on the hands, and then released. The sign is fully positive if the arms return briskly to full flexion (Score 2). If the arms return to incomplete flexion or the response is sluggish, it is graded as Score 1. If they remain extended or are only followed by random movements the score is 0.

Leg recoil. With the infant supine, the hips and knees are fully flexed for 5 seconds, then extended by traction on the feet, and released. A maximal response is one of full flexion of the hips and knees (Score 2). A partial flexion scores 1, and minimal or no movement scores 0.

Popliteal angle. With the infant supine and his pelvis flat on the examining couch, the thigh is held in the knee-chest position by the examiner's left index finger and thumb supporting the knee. The leg is then extended by gentle pressure from the examiner's right index finger behind the ankle and the popliteal angle is measured.

Heel to ear maneuver. With the baby supine, draw the baby's foot as near to the head as it will go without forcing it. Observe the distance between the foot and the head as well as the degree of extension at the knee. Note that the knee is left free and may draw down alongside the abdomen.

Scarf sign. With the baby supine, take the infant's hand and try to put it around the neck and as far posteriorly as possible around the opposite shoulder. Assist this manoeuver by lifting the elbow across the body. See how far the elbow will go across and grade according to illustrations. Score 0: Elbow reaches opposite axillary line; 1: Elbow between midline and opposite axillary line; 2: Elbow reaches midline; 3: Elbow will not reach midline.

Head lag. With the baby lying supine, grasp the hands (or the arms if a very small infant) and pull him slowly towards the sitting position. Observe the position of the head in relation to the trunk and grade accordingly. In a small infant the head may initially be supported by one hand. Score 0: Complete lag; 1: Partial head control; 2: Able to maintain head in line with body; 3: Brings head anterior to body.

Ventral suspension. The infant is suspended in the prone position, with examiner's hand under the infant's chest (one hand in a small infant, two in a large infant). Observe the degree of extension of the back and the amount of flexion of the arms and legs. Also note the relation of the head to the trunk.

If the score for an individual criterion differs on the two sides of the baby, take the mean.

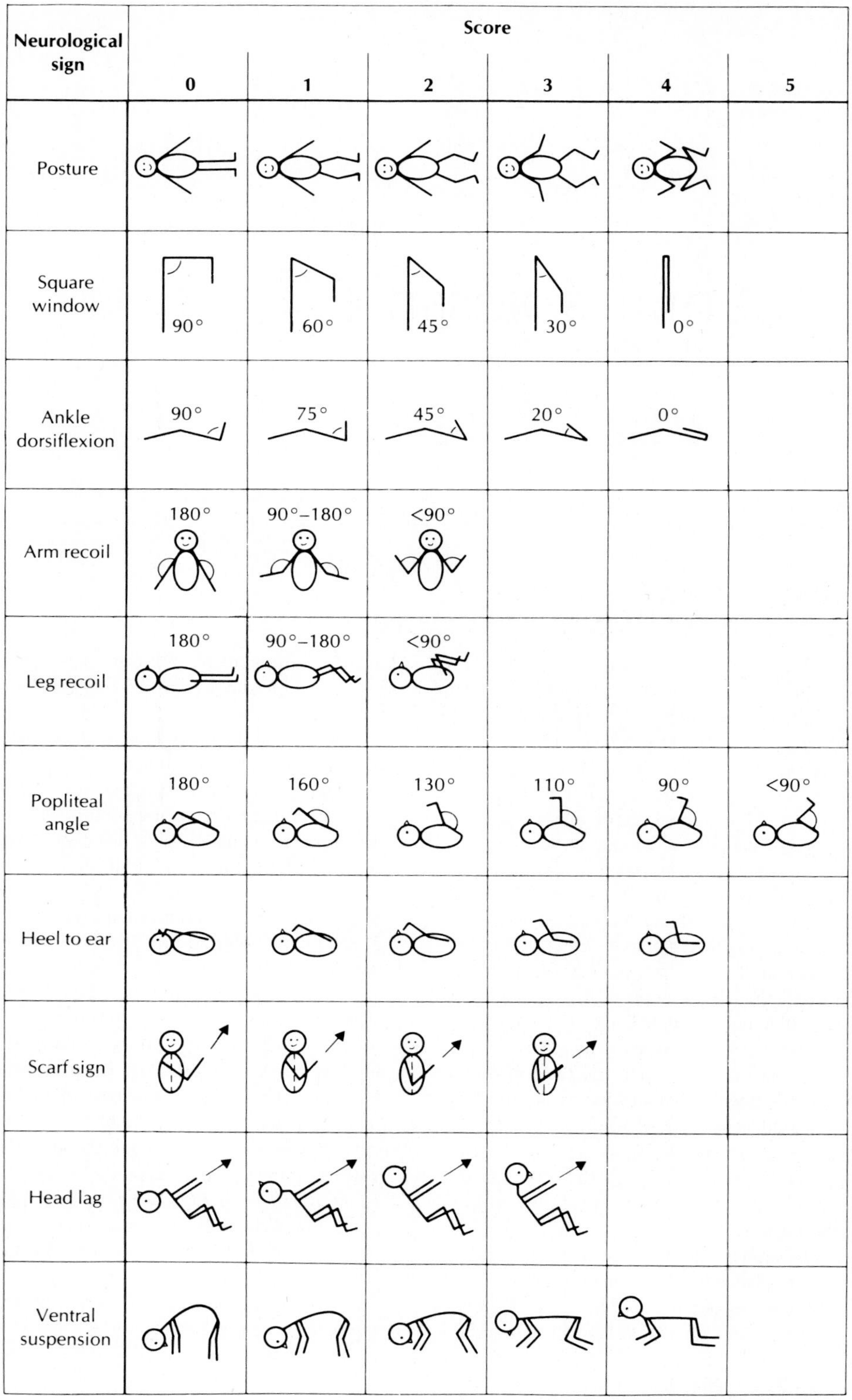

Neurological sign	Score					
	0	1	2	3	4	5
Posture						
Square window	90°	60°	45°	30°	0°	
Ankle dorsiflexion	90°	75°	45°	20°	0°	
Arm recoil	180°	90°–180°	<90°			
Leg recoil	180°	90°–180°	<90°			
Popliteal angle	180°	160°	130°	110°	90°	<90°
Heel to ear						
Scarf sign						
Head lag						
Ventral suspension						

Figure C-1

Neurologic criteria for assessment of gestational age in the newborn infant.
(From Dubowitz LMS, Dubowitz V, and Goldberg C: Clinical assessment of gestational age in the newborn infant, J Pediatr 77:4, 1970.)

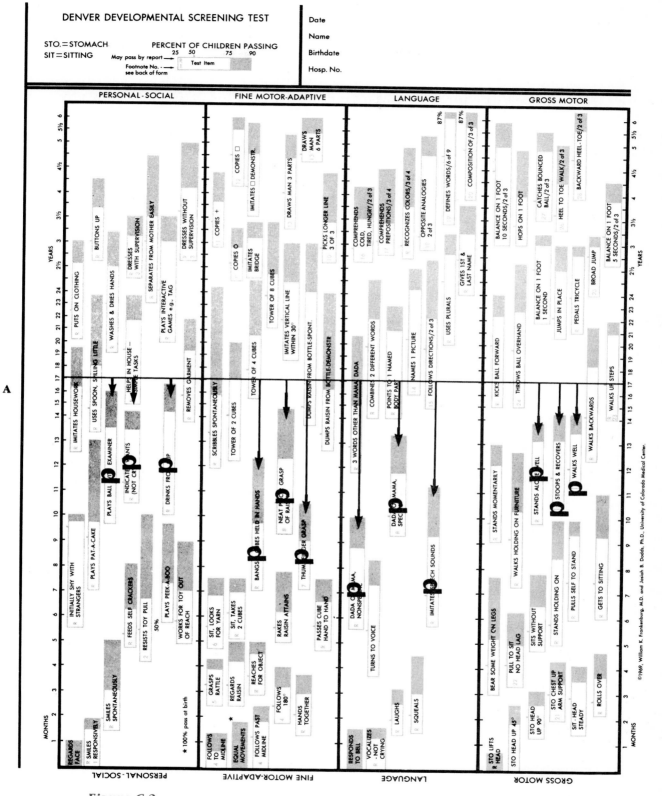

Figure C-2

A, Denver Developmental Screening Test (DDST). NOTE: P indicates those 12 items used in the abbreviated testing procedure to identify children with suspect test results who require full DDST.

Continued

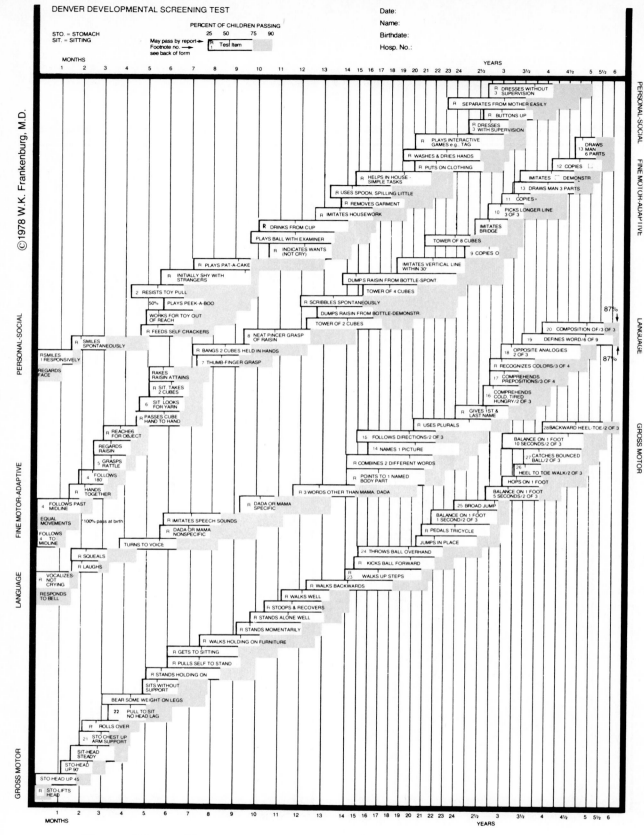

Figure C-2, cont'd

B, DDST revised (DDST-R). Resembling a growth curve, this form places items at lowest age level starting at bottom left and progresses upward to right with increasing age.

(**A** and **B,** from Frankenburg WK, Sciarillo W, and Burgess D: The newly abbreviated and revised Denver Developmental Screening Test, J Pediatr 99:995, 1981.)

```
                                    DATE
                                    NAME
          DIRECTIONS                BIRTHDATE
                                    HOSP. NO.
```

1. Try to get child to smile by smiling, talking or waving to him. Do not touch him.
2. When child is playing with toy, pull it away from him. Pass if he resists.
3. Child does not have to be able to tie shoes or button in the back.
4. Move yarn slowly in an arc from one side to the other, about 6" above child's face. Pass if eyes follow 90° to midline. (Past midline; 180°)
5. Pass if child grasps rattle when it is touched to the backs or tips of fingers.
6. Pass if child continues to look where yarn disappeared or tries to see where it went. Yarn should be dropped quickly from sight from tester's hand without arm movement.
7. Pass if child picks up raisin with any part of thumb and a finger.
8. Pass if child picks up raisin with the ends of thumb and index finger using an over hand approach.

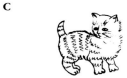 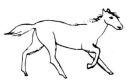

9. Pass any enclosed form. Fail continuous round motions.
10. Which line is longer? (Not bigger.) Turn paper upside down and repeat. (3/3 or 5/6)
11. Pass any crossing lines.
12. Have child copy first. If failed, demonstrate

       When giving items 9, 11 and 12, do not name the forms. Do not demonstrate 9 and 11.

13. When scoring, each pair (2 arms, 2 legs, etc.) counts as one part.
14. Point to picture and have child name it. (No credit is given for sounds only.)

C

  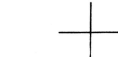

15. Tell child to: Give block to Mommie; put block on table; put block on floor. Pass 2 of 3. (Do not help child by pointing, moving head or eyes.)
16. Ask child: What do you do when you are cold? ..hungry? ..tired? Pass 2 of 3.
17. Tell child to: Put block on table; under table; in front of chair, behind chair. Pass 3 of 4. (Do not help child by pointing, moving head or eyes.)
18. Ask child: If fire is hot, ice is ?; Mother is a woman, Dad is a ?; a horse is big, a mouse is ?. Pass 2 of 3.
19. Ask child: What is a ball? ..lake? ..desk? ..house? ..banana? ..curtain? ..ceiling? ..hedge? ..pavement? Pass if defined in terms of use, shape, what it is made of or general category (such as banana is fruit, not just yellow). Pass 6 of 9.
20. Ask child: What is a spoon made of? ..a shoe made of? ..a door made of? (No other objects may be substituted.) Pass 3 of 3.
21. When placed on stomach, child lifts chest off table with support of forearms and/or hands.
22. When child is on back, grasp his hands and pull him to sitting. Pass if head does not hang back.
23. Child may use wall or rail only, not person. May not crawl.
24. Child must throw ball overhand 3 feet to within arm's reach of tester.
25. Child must perform standing broad jump over width of test sheet. (8-1/2 inches)
26. Tell child to walk forward, ⚬⚬⚬⚬➔ heel within 1 inch of toe. Tester may demonstrate. Child must walk 4 consecutive steps, 2 out of 3 trials.
27. Bounce ball to child who should stand 3 feet away from tester. Child must catch ball with hands, not arms, 2 out of 3 trials.
28. Tell child to walk backward, ⬅⚬⚬⚬⚬ toe within 1 inch of heel. Tester may demonstrate. Child must walk 4 consecutive steps, 2 out of 3 trials.

DATE AND BEHAVIORAL OBSERVATIONS (how child feels at time of test, relation to tester, attention span, verbal behavior, self-confidence, etc,):

Figure C-2, cont'd

C, Directions for numbered items on testing form.
(**C** from Frankenburg WK and Dobbs JB, University of Colorado Medical Center, 1969.)

A

DENVER ARTICULATION SCREENING EXAM
for children 2 1/2 to 6 years of age

Instructions: Have child repeat each word after
you. Circle the underlined sounds that he pro-
nounces correctly. Total correct sounds is the
Raw Score. Use charts on reverse side to score
results.

NAME

HOSP. NO.

ADDRESS _____

Date: _____ Child's Age: _____ Examiner: _____ Raw Score: _____
Percentile: _____ Intelligibility: _____ Result: _____

1. table   6. zipper   11. sock   16. wagon   21. leaf
2. shirt   7. grapes   12. vacuum   17. gum   22. carrot
3. door   8. flag   13. yarn   18. house
4. trunk   9. thumb   14. mother   19. pencil
5. jumping   10. toothbrush 15. twinkle   20. fish

Intelligibility: (circle one)   1. Easy to understand   3. Not understandable
                                 2. Understandable 1/2   4. Can't evaluate
                                       the time.

Comments:

Date: _____ Child's Age: _____ Examiner: _____ Raw Score _____
Percentile: _____ Intelligibility: _____ Result: _____

1. table   6. zipper   11. sock   16. wagon   21. leaf
2. shirt   7. grapes   12. vacuum   17. gum   22. carrot
3. door   8. flag   13. yarn   18. house
4. trunk   9. thumb   14. mother   19. pencil
5. jumping   10. toothbrush 15. twinkle   20. fish

Intelligibility: (circle one)   1. Easy to understand   3. Not understandable
                                 2. Understandable 1/2   4. Can't evaluate
                                       the time.

Comments:

Date: _____ Child's Age: _____ Examiner: _____ Raw Score_____
Percentile: _____ Intelligibility: _____ Result: _____

1. table   6. zipper   11. sock   16. wagon   21. leaf
2. shirt   7. grapes   12. vacuum   17. gum   22. carrot
3. door   8. flag   13. yarn   18. house
4. trunk   9. thumb   14. mother   19. pencil
5. jumping   10. toothbrush 15. twinkle   20. fish

Intelligibility: (circle one)   1. Easy to understand   3. Not understandable
                                 2. Understandable 1/2   4. Can't evaluate
                                       the time.

Figure C-3

A, Denver Articulation Screening Examination for children 2½ to 6 years of age.
(From Drumwright AF, University of Colorado Medical Center, 1971.)

To score DASE words: Note Raw Score for child's performance. Match raw score line (extreme left of chart) with column representing child's age (to the closest _previous_ age group). Where raw score line and age column meet number in that square denotes percentile rank of child's performance when compared to other children that age. Percentiles above heavy line are ABNORMAL percentiles, below heavy line are NORMAL.

PERCENTILE RANK

Raw Score	2.5 yr.	3.0	3.5	4.0	4.5	5.0	5.5	6 years
2	1							
3	2							
4	5							
5	9							
6	16							
7	23							
8	31	2						
9	37	4	1					
10	42	6	2					
11	48	7	4					
12	54	9	6	1	1			
13	58	12	9	2	3	1	1	
14	62	17	11	5	4	2	2	
15	68	23	15	9	5	3	2	
16	75	31	19	12	5	4	3	
17	79	38	25	15	6	6	4	
18	83	46	31	19	8	7	4	
19	86	51	38	24	10	9	5	1
20	89	58	45	30	12	11	7	3
21	92	65	52	36	15	15	9	4
22	94	72	58	43	18	19	12	5
23	96	77	63	50	22	24	15	7
24	97	82	70	58	29	29	20	15
25	99	87	78	66	36	34	26	17
26	99	91	84	75	46	43	34	24
27		94	89	82	57	54	44	34
28		96	94	88	70	68	59	47
29		98	98	94	84	84	77	68
30		100	100	100	100	100	100	100

To Score intelligibility:

	NORMAL	ABNORMAL
2 1/2 years	Understandable 1/2 the time, or, "easy"	Not Understandable
3 years and older	Easy to understand	Understandable 1/2 time Not understandable

Test Result: 1. NORMAL on Dase and Intelligibility = NORMAL

2. ABNORMAL on Dase and/or Intelligibility = ABNORMAL

* If abnormal on initial screening rescreen within 2 weeks. If abnormal again child should be referred for complete speech evaluation.

Figure C-3, cont'd

B, Percentile rank.

Glossary

abatement Decrease in intensity of a pain or other symptom.

abdominal regions Surface divisions of the abdomen into nine or four sections.

Abdominal zones Surface division of the abdomen into three sections: (1) the epigastric zone above the transpyloric plane, (2) the hypogastric zone below the transtubercular plane, and (3) the umbilical zone situated between the epigastric and hypogastric zones.

abduction Movement away from the axial line (for a limb) or the median plane (for the digits).

abreaction Release of painful emotion through recall or repressed memories, objective of freudian method of psychoanalysis.

abscess Circumscribed collection of necrotic cellular debris, white blood cells, and microorganisms demarcated by inflamed tissue.

abulia Loss or deficiency in ability to make decisions or to act on decisions; may occur in depression (absence of will power).

accommodation Reflex alteration of the refractory power of the lens of the eye during the viewing of objects at varying distance from the retina. The shape of the lens is changed as a result of the degree of contraction of the ciliary muscle. A blurred image on the retina evokes the brainstem reflex, which is mediated through parasympathetic fibers in cranial nerve III (oculomotor). Change in lens shape occurs equally in both eyes. When the focus is on a near object, accommodation is accompanied by convergence of the eyes and constriction of the pupils.

achalasia Failure of smooth muscle of the gastrointestinal tract to relax; particularly significant for the cardiac sphincter. The condition results from congenital absence of parasympathetic elements of Auerbach's plexus.

achondroplasia Disturbance in cartilage development.

acini Small, saclike dilatations found in various glands.

acromegaly Chronic disease caused by hypersecretion of growth hormone; characterized by overgrowth of the small parts.

acrophobia Abnormal fear of heights.

active range of motion Purposeful joint movement performed by the client without assistance from the examiner.

acute Severe symptoms, usually of rapid onset and of short duration.

adaptation The reduction of pupillary diameter size (constriction) to increased ambient light level and the widening of pupillary size to decreased ambient light level.

adduction Movement toward the axial line (for a limb) or the median plane (for the digits).

adenoid Resembling a gland; hypertrophy of the adenoid tissue situated in the pharynx; sometimes called pharyngeal tonsil.

adenoma Tumor consisting of glandular cells.

adhesion A fibrotic band or structure that joins two surfaces that are normally separated.

adiposis Excessive accumulation of adipose (lipoid) tissue; obesity or corpulence; fatty infiltration of an organ or tissue.

affect Emotional range attached to ideas, outwardly manifested. *Appropriate affect:* emotional tone in harmony with the accompanying idea, thought, or verbalization. *Blunted affect:* a disturbance manifested by a severe reduction in the intensity of affect. *Flat affect:* absence or near absence of any signs of affective expression. *Inappropriate affect:* incongruence between the emotional feeling tone and the idea, thought, or speech accompanying it. *Labile affect:* rapid changes in emotion feeling tone, unrelated to external stimuli.

affective disorders A specific group of psychiatric diagnoses, characterized by mood disturbances on a continuum of depression to mania; unknown as mood disorders in the *DSM-III-R.*

afferent Conduction toward the center or controlling structure; i.e., the afferent nerve conducts impulses to the central nervous system, and the dendrite conducts impulses to the neuronal body.

afterload The load against which a muscle contracts. When used in reference to the heart, afterload is approximately the arterial pressure. An increase in afterload reduces the stroke volume.

ageusia Loss of the sensation of taste or the ability to discriminate sweet, sour, salty, and bitter tastes.

aggression Forceful verbal or physical action that is the motor counterpart of the affect of anger, rage, or hostility.

agitation Restlessness; inability to concentrate or remain motionless.

agnosia Inability to discriminate sensory stimuli. *Acoustic or auditory agnosia:* impaired ability to recognize familiar sounds. *Tactile agnosia:* impaired ability to recognize familiar objects by touch or feel. *Visual agnosia:* impaired ability to recognize familiar objects by sight. *Somatagnosia:* disturbance in recognition of body parts.

agonist (1) Prime mover; a muscle opposed in action by another muscle, the antagonist, i.e., the flexor of the arm (the biceps) and the extensor of the arm (the triceps). (2) A neurotransmitter, hormone, immune complex, or drug that competes for receptors and produces similar (same direction) effects as the substance normal to those receptors.

agoraphobia Marked fear of public places.

akinesia Delay or slowness in beginning and carrying through voluntary motor movements and sudden or unexpected stops in motion. Akinesia is a sign of extrapyramidal disease and is often seen in clients with Parkinson's disease.

akinesthesia Inability to sense movement.

alienation Inability to identify with family, peer group, society, or culture; associated with schizophrenia.

alopecia Loss of hair to baldness.

Alzheimer's disease Progressive condition of atrophy of the brain and degeneration of the neurons that usually occurs in persons over 40 years of age. Histologic changes include the presence of neurofibrillary tangles and extraneuronal senile plaques containing amyloid. The electroencephalogram alpha rhythm is reduced. Behavioral changes may progress from mild cognitive defects to dementia.

amaurosis Blindness without perceptible disease of the visual structures.

ambivalence The coexistence of two opposing impulses or feelings directed toward the same person or object at the same time.

amnestic syndrome Short- and long-term impairment of memory as a result of a specific organic factor.

amyotonia Lack of tone of the musculature of the body.

amyotrophy Wasting or atrophy of muscle tissue.

analgesia Loss of sensation; used particularly to denote relief of pain without loss of consciousness.

anarthria Loss of articulation.

anesthesia Loss of sensation.

aneurysm Dilatation of an artery.

angina pectoris Pain—substernal or radiating to the left arm, neck, or jaw; frequently correlated with myocardial ischemia.

angioma Benign tumor consisting of blood vessels or lymphatic vessels.

anisocoria Unequal dilatation of the pupils.

ankylosis Rigidity and consolidation of a joint.

anonychia Complete absence of the nail.

anorexia Loss of appetite.

anosmia Inability to smell.

anosognosia Lack of insight or loss of ability to recognize one's disease.

antrum Cavity or chamber.

anuria Absence of excretion of urine.

anxiety Motor tension, autonomic hyperactivity, apprehension, or hyperattentiveness.

anxiety disorders Patterns of symptoms and behaviors in which anxiety is either the primary disturbance or a secondary problem that is recognized when the primary symptoms are removed.

anxiety syndrome Anxiety of at least 1 month's duration.

apathy Lack of interest and blunting of affect in conditions that would normally stimulate interest or elicit feeling.

aphakia Absence of the lens of the eye; may be congenital or a result of surgery.

aphasia Dysfunction or loss of the ability to express thoughts by speech, writing, symbols, or signs. *Fluent aphasia:* ability to produce words but with frequent errors in the appropriate choice of words or in the creation of words. *Nonfluent aphasia:* inability to produce words, either in spoken or written form.

aphonia Inability to produce laryngeal voice sounds.

aplasia Failure of cellular formation or development of an organ or tissue or the cellular products from an organ or tissue, as an impairment in blood formation.

apnea Cessation of breathing in the end expiratory position.

apneustic breathing Respiration characterized by a sustained inspiratory phase interrupted by brief expirations.

apraxia Impairment of the ability to carry out purposeful movement (although muscle and sensory apparatus are intact), as an inability to draw or construct forms of two or three dimensions.

aqueous humor Fluid secreted in the ciliary body and found in the anterior and posterior chambers of the eye.

arcus senilis Gray to white opaque ring surrounding the cornea, generally seen in individuals older than 50 years of age, caused by lipoid position.

arrhythmia Any deviation from the normal pace of the heart.

arterial pressure The force exerted by the blood against the arterial walls. Blood pressure is measured in millimeters of mercury above sea level. The contraction of the heart results in a pulsatile ejection of the blood, resulting in variation of the pressure from a systolic peak of about 120 mm Hg at maximum left ventricular stroke output and a minimum *diastolic pressure* of about 80 mm Hg. The *pulse pressure* is equal to the difference between systolic and diastolic pressure. Mean arterial pressure (MAP) may be calculated by the following formula:

$$MAP = \text{Diastolic pressure} + \frac{\text{Pulse pressure}}{3}$$

arteriosclerosis Hardening (sclerosis) and thickening of the walls of arterioles.

arthritis Inflammation of a joint.

arthropathy General term for disease in a joint.

ascites The accumulation of free fluid within the abdominal cavity.

astereognosis Loss of the ability to recognize familiar objects through the sense of touch.

asterixis Liver flap, flapping tremor, or wrist flapping as a result of a sudden relaxation of wrist extensors; appears in hepatic failure with the occurrence of metabolic encephalopathy.

asthenia Weakness; loss of strength or energy.

asthma Proxysmal dyspnea (wheezing) resulting from obstruction of the bronchi or spasm of smooth muscle.

astigmatism Irregularity of the spherical curve of the cornea such that light rays cannot be focused in a point on the retina. Astigmatism is corrected with contact lenses or eyeglasses ground to compensate for the defect.

astrocytoma Tumor composed of astrocytes. Astrocytoma is the most common tumor of the central nervous system.

asystole Cardiac standstill or arrest.

ataxia Impairment of coordination of muscular activity.

atelectasis Incomplete expansion of a lung compromised since birth; collapse of the adult lung.

atheroma Necrosis of a fibrous plaque of the arterial wall with degenerated lipid, seen in atherosclerosis.

atherosclerosis Type of arteriosclerosis characterized by deposits (atheromas) of cholesterol, lipoid material, and lipophages in the walls of large arteries and arterioles.

athetosis Slow, sustained, involuntary, large-amplitude muscle movements that are sinous, writhing, or squirming.

atony Without normal tone or resistance to stretching.

atopy Predisposition to allergy.

atresia Congenital absence or closure of a tubular structure or orifice.

atrioventricular block Impairment of impulse conduction from the atria to the ventricles. Abbreviated AV block.

atrophy Wasting; decrease in the size of a cell, tissue, organ, or body part.

auditory ossicles A series of three small bones (malleus, incus, stapes) that extend across the middle ear.

aura Premonitory sensation, generally applied to sensations preceding epileptiform convulsions.

auscultation Examination made by listening, usually through the stethoscope.

autistic thinking Thoughts, ideas, or desires derived from internal, private stimuli or drives, often incongruent with reality. Most often applied to persons with schizophrenia.

autism Behavioral lack of responsiveness to other persons and defects in language skills; develops within the first 30 months of age.

autotopagnosia Inability to recognize different body parts.

azotemia Elevated serum concentration of nonprotein nitrogen substances, primarily urea.

Babinski's sign Reflex elicited by tactile stimulation of the lateral aspect of the sole and manifested by dorsiflexion and fanning of the toes. This sign is found in upper motor neuron (pyramidal tract) lesions. The sign is normal in infants less than 18 months of age.

Baker's cyst Swelling in the popliteal space resulting from herniation of the synovial membrane of the knee.

balanitis Inflammation of the glans penis.

ballismus Sudden flailing movements of the limbs; *hemiballismus* is the term for the condition affecting only one side of the body.

ballottement A palpation technique used to assess a floating object; fluid-filled tissue is pushed toward the examining hand so that the object will float against the examining fingers.

baragnosis Inability to perceive differences in weight pressure.

basophilia An abornormal increase in the basophilic leukocytosis.

Battle's sign Bluish discoloration along the course of the posterior auricular artery, with ecchymosis first appearing near the tip of the mastoid process; associated with basal skull fracture.

behavior Any observable, recordable, and measurable move, response, or act (verbal or nonverbal) of an individual.

bigeminy Ventricular bigeminy is a pattern of arrhythmia consisting of coupled ventricular beats; alternating QRS complexes are ventricular premature depolarizations.

bipolar disorder An affective or mood disorder characterized by periods of mania alternating with periods of depression, with normal mood intervals in between.

Bitot's spots White or light gray areas of keratinized epithelium on the conjunctiva seen in clients with vitamin A deficiency.

blepharospasm Tonic spasm of the orbicularis oculi muscle.

blind spot The site of penetration of the optic nerve in the retina in which no light-sensitive receptors are found.

blister Vesicle; localized collection of fluid in the epidermis that separates and raises the horny upper layers.

blocking or thought deprivation Sudden pause in the train of thought caused by unconscious emotional conflict.

borborygmus Audible bowel sounds, generally caused by gas propulsion through the intestine.

bradycardia Slower than normal heart rate (<50 beats per minute).

bronchiectasis Chronic dilatation of one or more bronchi.

bronchitis Inflammation of one or more bronchi; condition may be chronic or acute.

bronchophony The sound of the voice as heard with abnormally increased clarity and intensity through the stethoscope over the lung parenchyma.

bronchovesicular Breath sounds from bronchial tubes and alveoli.

bruit Murmur (blowing sound) heard over peripheral vessels.

buccal Pertaining to the cheek.

bullous Characterized by vesicles (blisters) usually 2 cm or more in diameter.

bursa Sac or saclike cavity filled with fluid and located in sites where friction would otherwise develop, as in a joint or over a bony prominence.

bursitis Inflammation of a bursa.

cacosmia Offensive hallucinations of smell.

cachexia Marked malnutrition.

calcinosis Abnormal deposition of calcium salts as nodules in muscles, tendons, and skin.

calculus Stone, abnormal concretion of chemicals, especially in the renal and biliary systems.

callus (1) Localized thickening of the horny layer of the epidermis resulting from hyperplasia. (2) Formation of cartilage and bone at a fracture site.

calor Localized increase in temperature; heat; classic sign of inflammation.

caries Decay of the calcified protein of teeth.

carpal tunnel syndrome Entrapment of the median nerve in the carpal tunnel resulting in paresthesias, pain, and muscle weakness.

caruncle Small elevation of tissue.

cataract Opacity of the lens of the eye or its capsule.

catatonic behavior Motor anomalies not accompanied by organic disease.

catatonic excitement Purposeless excited movement without apparent stimuli.

catatonic negativism Resistance to movement to both verbal instruction and physical attempts to move.

catatonic posturing Voluntary assumption of a bizarre or inappropriate posture; may be maintained for a long period.

catatonic rigidity Rigid posture despite physical efforts to be moved.

catatonic stupor Decreased response to environment; client may appear to be unaware of environment.

catatonic waxy flexibility Body posture and limbs remain in positions in which placed; limbs feel like pliable wax to the examiner.

cephalocaudal direction Starting at the client's head and progressing down to the toes.

cerumen Earwax, produced by apocrine glands within the ear canal.

chalazion Sebaceous cyst on the eyelid formed by distention of a meibomian gland with secretion.

cholangitis Inflammation of the bile ducts.

cholelithiasis Presence of calculi in the bile ducts or gall bladder.

cholesteatoma Cystlike mass common to the middle ear and mastoid region characterized by outer layer of stratified squamous epithelium filled with desquamating debris, including cholesterol; generally associated with chronic infection.

chorea Rapid, brief, involuntary, asymmetric movements worsened by emotional stress; they improve or disappear during sleep.

chorionic Pertaining to the chorion, a fetal membrane composed of trophoblast that forms the fetal portion of the placenta.

chronic obstructive pulmonary disease General term for disease involving airway obstruction, such as chronic bronchitis, emphysema, or asthma. Abbreviated COPD.

Chvostek's sign Spasm of the facial muscle evoked by tapping branches of the facial nerve; may be caused by hypocalcemia or hypomagnesemia.

circadian pattern A cyclic pattern or period of 24 hours.

circumduction A circular movement.

circumstantiality Interruption in the stream of thought caused by excessive associations of an idea reaching the conscious level. Circumstantiality is characterized by digression and extraneous thinking, which serve to avoid emotionally charged areas.

cirrhosis Disease characterized by destruction of liver parenchyma. The liver is characterized by fibrous tissue and yellow-tan nodules.

clanging Speech in which sounds govern word choice; may consist of rhyming or punning; most often observed in schizophrenics and manic individuals.

cleft palate Developmental defect or failure to fuse of the soft palate, hard palate, and the lip. This is the most common developmental defect of the head and neck.

clonus Rapid rhythmic alteration between contraction and relaxation of muscles, induced by stretching the muscle; may result in alternate flexion and extension

closed-ended questions Questions that generally elicit a "yes" or "no" response. Useful in gathering factual data.

clubbing Proliferation of soft tissue of terminal phalanges, generally associated with relative hypoxia of peripheral tissues, loss of the angle between the skin and nail base, and sponginess of the nail base.

coarctation A tightening or compression of the walls of a vessel, producing a narrowed lumen.

cognitive Pertaining to mental processes of knowing, thinking, learning, and judging.

colic Acute abdominal pain associated with smooth muscle contraction of the gastrointestinal tract.

colitis Inflammation of the colon.

coma Deep unconsciousness from which the individual cannot be aroused, even by painful stimuli. *Comatose:* the condition of being affected by coma.

comedo Papule; hyperkeratotic thickening of the duct of a sebaceous gland with retention of sebum, associated with acne.

complex Emotionally charged attitudes and ideas that are unconscious and influence the individual's behavior, such as an Oedipus complex.

compulsion Uncontrollable impulse to perform an act or ritual repeatedly; may be in response to an obsession (unwilled, persistent thought), as in obsessive-compulsive disorder. The act or ritual serves to decrease anxiety. Examples of rituals are handwashing, cleaning, and checking.

conductive hearing loss Diminished ability to hear due to vibrations' inability to travel to or through the inner ear.

condyloma Hyperkeratotic exophytic lesions of stratified squamous epithelium; these develop as small, elevated, soft nodules that enlarge and coalesce to become cauliflowerlike excrescences.

confabulation Fabrication of facts or events in response to questions about situations that are not recalled because of memory impairment.

confrontation A process in which the client is told something about himself or herself by the provider. Most commonly used to clarify an inconsistency.

congenital Present at birth.

consensual Reflex reaction in one pupil mimicking that occurring in the other, which is being stimulated.

consolidation Process in which liquid or solid replacement of lung parenchyma as exudate from an inflammatory condition is amassed.

constipation Infrequent or difficult evacuation of feces; often associated with drying and hardening of the stool.

contralateral On the opposite side.

contour Surface outline or shape of the part being described.

contusion Bruise.

conversion Coordinated medial movement of the eyes in fixing on a near object.

conversion disorder Loss of or alteration in physical functioning suggesting a physical disorder. The symptom allows the individual to avoid some activity that is perceived as noxious or to get support from the environment that otherwise might not be possible. The symptom can be related in time to a psychological conflict or need.

convulsion Series of involuntary muscle contractions.

Cooper's ligaments Suspensory ligaments of the breast.

corneal limbus The edge of the cornea where it meets the sclera.

cor pulmonale Disease of the heart as a result of pulmonary disease; right heart hypertrophy and right ventricular failure resulting from pulmonary hypertension.

cramp Involuntary, painful skeletal muscle contraction.

crepitation, crepitus A dry, crackling sound in (1) the lung, when air passes through abnormally accumulated moisture; (2) the joints, when dry synovial surfaces rub together; and (3) the skin, when air is present subdermally.

cretinism Disease caused by congenital lack of thyroid hormone; characterized by retarded physical and mental development, deafness, dystrophy of bones and soft tissue, and abnormally low concentrations of thyroid hormones.

crisis Sudden change in the course of a disease.

Crohn's disease Inflammatory process that involves the full thickness of the bowel wall and may be associated with mucosal ulcers and cyst abscesses. Bowel obstruction and fistula formation are common complications.

Cullen's sign Bluish coloration in the umbilical region associated with stress accompanying extensive burn injuries.

Curling's ulcer Ulcer of the fundus and body of the stomach associated with stress accompanying extensive burn injuries.

cyanosis Dusky blue color imparted to skin when the hemoglobin saturation is less than 75% to 85% or PaO$_2$ is less than 50 mm Hg.

cyclothymic disorder Periods with some depressive and manic behavior over 2 years but not of sufficient severity or duration to be defined as major depressive or manic episodes; individual may have normal behavior between episodes.

cyst Collection of fluid surrounded by a membrane.

cystocele Herniation of the urinary bladder into the anterior vaginal wall.

dacryadenitis Inflammation of a lacrimal gland.

dacryocystitis Inflammation of the lacrimal sac.

decidua The endometrium during pregnancy that is shed in the postpartum period.

decomposition of movement The performance of normally fluent movements in several parts.

déjà vu A sensation of familiarity with a person, place, or activity during a first encounter; a feeling of "having been there before."

delirium Clouded state of consciousness; reduction in clarity of awareness of environment accompanied by a reduced capacity to shift, focus, and sustain attention to environmental stimuli.

delusion A false belief, improbable in nature; not influenced by contrary experience nor related to the client's cultural and educational background.

dementia Loss of cognitive abilities of sufficient magnitude to interfere with social or occupational functioning; memory impairment and impairment of abstract thinking or impaired judgment or other disturbance of high cortical function.

denial Avoidance of disagreeable realities or threats by ignoring or refusing to recognize them. An unconscious defense mechanism that may be adaptive.

depersonalization Loss of the sense of personal reality or identity; withdrawal and isolation result from disappointments or unbearable sufferings that make one a witness to personal experiences rather than a participant.

depigmentation Loss of pigment, usually of melanin.

depression Term used to define (1) a mood, (2) a syndrome, and (3) an illness. The mood of depression is described as dejection and lowering of functional activity; it is a normal experience that may be incurred in response to frustration and loss. The syndrome of depression includes a depressed mood in combination with one or more of the following symptoms: inability to concentrate, anorexia, weight loss, and suicidal ideas. The illness of depression is characterized by the syndrome of depression but lasts longer. Functional impairment may include inability to carry on daily activities, particularly work.

derealization Feelings that the world around one is not real; generally associated with depersonalization.

dereistic thinking Illogical thought processes.

dermographia Abnormal skin sensitivity, so that firm stroking with a dull instrument or light scratching results in a wheal surrounded by a red flare; may be caused by allergy.

desquamation Scaling, shedding of epithelial tissue.

dextrocardia A rare condition in which the position of the heart is reversed and lies on the right side of the chest.

Diagnostic Statistical Manual-III-R, 1987. A taxonomy of mental disorders by the American Psychiatric Association. Abbreviated *DSM-III-R*.

diarrhea Increased frequency and liquid content of fecal evacuation.

diastasis recti abdominis Separation of the rectus muscles of the abdominal wall; may occur in pregnancy.

dicrotic pulse Presence of two sphygmographic or polygraphic evaluations to one beat of the pulse.

diopter Refractive power of a lens with a focal distance of 1 m; a unit of measure of refractive power.

diplopia Double vision; perception of two images for a single object.

direct auscultation (immediate) The listening to body sounds by the unassisted ear.

disease Abnormality of structure or function that has a single pathogenic mechanism and a predictable course.

disorientation Lack of awareness as to time, place, or person.

diverticulitis Usually refers to inflammation of colonic diverticula.

diverticulum Pouch or sac created by herniation of mucosal lining of a hollow organ (bladder or gastrointestinal tract) through a defect in the muscular wall.

dorsiflexion A backward bending.

dullness Decreased resonance on percussion.

dwarf An abnormally small person.

dysarthria Difficulty in articulating single sounds or phonemes of speech. Individual letters: *f, r, g;* labials—sounds produced with the lips: *b, m, v* (cranial nerve [CN] VII); gutterals—sounds produced in the throat (CN X); linguals—sounds produced with the tongue; *l, t, n* (CN XII).

dysbasia Difficulty in walking, especially from neurologic causes.

dyschezia Difficulty in passing stool; pain associated with defecation.

dyscoria Congenital abnormality in the shape of the pupil.

dysdiadochokinesia Impairment in the ability to stop a movement and to institute the opposite movement, such as pronation to supination.

dysesthesia Impairment of any sensation, particularly of touch.

dysgeusia Impairment or perversion of the sense of taste.

dyskinesia Difficulty of movement.

dyslexia Disturbance in understanding the written word; difficulty in reading.

dysmenorrhea Painful menstruation.

dysmetria An impairment in the ability to stop a movement.

dyspareunia Difficult or painful sexual intercourse in women.

dyspepsia Impairment of the ability to digest food; especially, discomfort after eating a meal.

dysphagia Difficult or painful swallowing.

dysphasia Disturbance in speech evidenced by lack of coordination and failure to express words in proper order.

dysphonia puberum Difficulty in controlling laryngeal speech sounds that occurs as the larynx enlarges in puberty.

dysphoria Restlessness, agitation, malaise.

dysplasia Disorder in the size, shape, or organization of adult cells.

dyspnea Difficult or labored respiration. *Paroxysmal nocturnal dyspnea:* respiratory distress related to posture, especially noted when reclining at night.

dysprosody Difficulty in speech in which inflection, pronunciation, pitch, and rhythm are impaired.

dyssynergia Inability to perform movements smoothly, or an impairment in muscle coordination.

dystrophy Disorder in which muscle wasting, i.e., atrophy, occurs.

dysuria Difficulty or painful urination.

ecchymosis A flat, round or irregular, blue or purplish lesion of the skin or mucous membranes resulting from intradermal or submucous hemorrhage.

echolalia Repetition by a client of words addressed to him or her; may also be the echo of the client's own thoughts; generally a sign of schizophrenia and organic mental disorders.

ectopic Abnormally located.

ectropion Eversion, or turning outward, of an edge, as of the eyelid.

eczema Superficial inflammatory process of the epidermis associated with redness, itching, weeping, and crusting; of multiple cause.

edema Abnormal increase in the quantity of interstitial fluid.

efferent Carrying from the center to the periphery.

egophony Voice sound of a nasal (telephonelike or bleating) quality, heard through the stethoscope; often defined by asking the client to say "ee," which sounds like "ay."

ejection sounds High-pitched, clicking sounds produced by the forceful opening of a diseased aortic or pulmonic valve heard soon after the first heart sound (S).

elation Elevation of mood, emotional excitement; may be temporary response to fortuitous event in a normal individual. Elation is the characteristic mood of mania and is also observed in some schizophrenics.

embolism Sudden obstruction of an artery by a clot or other foreign substance.

emotion A complex feeling state with psychic, somatic, and behavioral components that is related to affect and mood.

emphysema Refers to entrapment of air within tissue either interstitial or pulmonary. *Pulmonary emphysema:* also called chronic obstructive pulmonary disease (COPD); results from permanent dilatation or enlargement of the passages peripheral to the terminal bronchiole, which causes *increased resistance to airflow. Interstitial emphysema:* the presence of air in the subcutaneous tissue mediastinum or connective tissue of the lung resulting from air leakage through a damaged portion of the respiratory passages or alveoli; may result in swelling of tissue or a distinctive crackling sound called crepitation.

empyema Collection of purulent exudate in a body cavity or hollow organ.

encephalitis Inflammation of the cerebrum, cerebellum, or brainstem.

endometriosis Presence of endometrial stroma and glands in ectopic locations such as the ovaries, pelvic peritoneum, or colon.

encephalopathy A general designation for any cerebral disorder.

encopresis Repeated voluntary or involuntary defecation of normal or near-normal feces into inappropriate places.

enophthalmos Recession of the globe of the eye into the orbit.

enteritis Inflammation of the small intestine.

enterocele Herniation of intestinal contents.

entropion Inversion, or tuning inward of an edge, as of the eyelid.

enuresis Involuntary urination during sleep.

epilepsy Paroxysmal disturbances in brain function characterized by loss of consciousness, motor or sensory impairment, and disturbance of emotions or thought processes.

epiphora Abnormal tearing of the eyes.

epispadias Congenital anomaly in which the urethra opens on the dorsum of the penis.

epistaxis Bleeding or hemorrhage from the nose.

epulis Tumor of the gingiva.

equilibrium The ongoing process of maintaining the orientation and position of the body in relationship to the ground and in space.

erectile tissue Tissue that can become rigid and elevated.

eructation Act of belching or bringing up gas (air) from the stomach.

erythema Dilatation of capillaries, resulting in redness of the skin.

esophagitis Inflammation of the esophagus; may be caused by gastric reflux, corrosive chemicals, or infectious agents.

euphoria A false sense of elation or well-being; pathologic elevation of mood. Most notable in clients experiencing the manic phase of bipolar disorder.

eustachian tube The cartilaginous and bony passage between the nasopharynx and the middle ear that allows equalization of air pressure between the inner ear and the external environment.

eversion A turning outward or inside out.

exanthem General eruption of the skin accompanied by fever.

exophthalmos (proptosis) Abnormal protrusion of the globe of the eye.

extension The straightening of a limb so that the joint angle is increased.

external rotation The turning of a body part away from the central axis or midline of the body.

exteroceptive Stimuli originating outside the body received by end organs such as the eye.

extinction Loss of touch perception on one side of the body.

extrasystole Premature contraction.

extravasation Escape of blood or infused substance in extravascular tissue.

facies Term used to indicate the expression of the facial structures or the surface of a structure. *Adenoid f.:* open mouth, dull expression. *Elfin f.:* short, upturned nose, wide mouth, widely spaced eyes, full cheeks; associated with hypercalcemia and mental retardation. *F. hepatica:* sallow complexion, yellow conjunctiva. *F. hippocratic:* pinched expression of face, sunken eyes, hollow cheeks and temples, lax lips, and leaden complexion; associated with debilitating illness. *Leontine f.:* deep folds, lionlike pattern. *Marshall Hall's f.:* disproportion of forehead to head seen in hydrocephalus. *Parkinson's f.:* masklike; infrequent blinking.

facilitation An approach that stimulates the client to continue talking. Examples are use of silence or saying "yes, go on."

faint Temporary loss of consciousness may result from generalized lack of oxygen or glucose to the brain; may be associated with stress.

fasciculation Rapid, fine, twitching movements resulting from contraction of a fasciculus (bundle of muscle fibers) served by one anterior horn cell; usually does not cause movement of a joint.

febrile Characterized by fever.

festination Involuntary tendency to accelerate the speed of walking; occurs in paralysis agitans.

fever Pyrexia; elevation of the body temperature above normal for a given individual.

fiberoptics Transmission of an image along flexible bundles of coated glass or plastic fiber having special optical properties.

fibrillation Fine, continuous twitching caused by contraction of a single muscle or group of fibers.

fist percussion Striking the body with the lateral aspect of the hand to elicit pain or tenderness.

flaccid Relaxed, without tone, flabby.

flatulence Excessive amount of gas in the gastrointestinal tract.

flexion The bending of a joint so that the joint angle is decreased.

flight of ideas Nearly continuous flow of rapid speech with abrupt changes from topic to topic. Flight of ideas is most frequently observed in organic mental disorders, schizophrenia, and psychotic disorders and as a reaction to stress.

fremitus Palpable vibration.

friction rub A crackling, grating sound, heard through the stethoscope when two inflamed, roughened surfaces rub together.

FUO Abbreviation for fever of unknown origin.

fusiform Spindle or cigar shaped.

gait The manner of progression in walking. *Ataxic gait:* foot raised high with sole striking down suddenly.

gallop rhythm Heart rate characterized by three sounds in the presence of tachycardia.

gangrene Necrosis of body tissue associated with ischemia.

gastritis Inflammation of the mucosa of the stomach.

gingivitis Inflammation of the papillary and marginal gingiva.

glabrous Smooth, free of hair.

glaucoma Diseases resulting in increased intraocular pressure. *Angle closure glaucoma:* blockage of the overflow channels for aqueous humor by the iris; results in an acute increase in pressure and pain. *Open angle glaucoma (simple or chonic glaucoma):* degeneration of the outflow channel, trabecular network on Schlemm's canal.

glomus jugulare Globus tympanicum tumor; tumor of the jugular bulb in the floor of the middle ear; may result in hearing loss, sense of fullness, and tinnitus; often seen as a bulging, reddish purple mass through the tympanic membrane.

glossitis Inflammation of the tongue.

goiter Increase in size of the thyroid gland.

goniometer An instrument used to measure joint angles.

gout Disease caused by deposition of crystals of monosodium urate; characterized by a disorder in purine metabolism and associated with exacerbations of arthritis of a single joint.

graphesthesia The ability to identify letters or numbers inscribed with a blunt object on the palm of the hand, back, or other areas.

Grey Turner's sign Bruising of the flank skin.

guilt Painful feeling caused by having transgressed personal or social ethical standards.

gumma Neoplasm composed of soft, gummy tissue resembling granulation tissue; may occur in clients having tertiary syphilis or tuberculosis.

gynecomastia Hypertrophy of breast tissue in a male subject.

habitus Body type, characteristic of the form of the body. *Asthenic:* slender body type, narrow thorax, internal organ at lower position than other body types. *Hypersthenic:* large, thick body type, with broad deep thorax; body organs in a higher position than other body types. *Hyposthenic:* intermediate body type.

hallucination Perception for which no external stimuli can be ascertained; an endogenous experience in an individual whose sensorium is clear. *Simple hallucination:* simple perception, such as seeing light. *Complex hallucination:* more detailed experience, such as seeing a figure or person.

health history A comprehensive body of information obtained from the client and other select sources. It includes information on the client as a whole, the health/illness status past and present, social and phsyical environment, and past interactions with the health care systems.

Heberden's nodes and nodules Small, hard nodules of the terminal interphalangeal joints associated with osteoarthritis.

helix The superior and posterior free margin of the ear.

hemangioma Benign tumor made up of blood vessels; may be capillary or cavernous.

hemarthrosis Hemorrhage into a joint.

hematemesis Vomitus containing blood.

hematoma Localized collection of blood resulting from rupture of a blood vessel.

hematuria Presence of blood in the urine.

hemiballismus Involuntary, coarse, unilateral movements of limbs.

hemiplegia Paralysis involving one side of the body, generally an arm or a leg and sometimes the face, usually resulting from an abnormality of the corticospinal tract of the contralateral side.

hemolytic Pertaining to the release of hemoglobin from red blood cells.

hemophilia Genetic predisposition to bleed more than normal because of a deficiency of the clotting factors.

hemoptysis Spitting or coughing up of blood from the respiratory tract.

hemorrhoid Dilatation of a part of the venous hemorrhoidal plexus in the mucosal membrane of the rectum. Dilatation may occur as a result of increased hydrostatic pressure in the venous system, as in pregnancy, resulting from disease causing portal hypertension and straining at stool. *Internal* *hemorrhoid:* varicosity of superior or middle hemorrhoidal veins below the anal mucosa; may result in bleeding.

External hemorrhoids: varicosity of the inferior hemorrhoidal vein under the anal skin; may cause pain and swelling around the anal sphincter, as well as itching and bleeding.

hernia Abnormal protrusion of an organ or tissue through an opening. *Incarcerated hernia:* protrusion of abdominal contents through a weakness in the abdominal wall, so that the contents cannot be returned to the abdominal cavity. *Inguinal hernia: direct*—protrusion of abdominal contents through a weakness in the abdominal musculature, region of Hesselbach's triangle; *indirect*—protrusion through an internal inguinal ring hernia descending beside the spermatic cord. *Scrotal hernia:* protrusion (generally indirect) of abdominal contents into the scrotal sac. *Strangulated hernia:* hernia in which the blood supply to the protruded tissue is obstructed.

herpes Any inflammatory skin disease caused by herpesvirus (a large group of intranuclear double-stranded DNA viruses capable of establishing a latent infection many years after a primary infection). *Cytomegalovirus:* causes cytomegalic inclusion disease. *Epstein-Barr virus:* causes infectious mononucleosis. *Herpes simplex type 1:* causes fever blister and keratoconjunctivitis. *Herpes simplex type 2:* causes venereal disease. *Herpes zoster:* causes shingles. *Varicella:* causes chickenpox.

hirsutism Excessive hairiness, especially in females.

Holistic Pertaining to totality or the whole (holistic care).

Homan's sign On dorsiflexing the foot, pain is elicited in the calf of the leg; a sign of deep vein thrombosis.

hordeolum Inflammation of a sebaceous gland of the eyelid; sty.

hyaline Glasslike, as of casts in the urine.

hydrocele Circumscribed collection of fluid, particularly in the scrotum.

hydrocephalus Distenion of the cerebral ventricular system from excessive production of cerebrospinal fluid or obstruction of the outflow channels.

hygroma Cystic space, bursa, or sac distended with fluid.

hyperactivity (hyperkinesis) Restless, aggressive, often destructive activity. Prominent in manic states.

hyperesthesia Abnormally increased sensitiviy of the skin or another sense organ.

hyperpigmentation An excess of pigment in tissue.

hyperplasia Cellular overgrowth.

hyperpnea Increase in the depth of respiration with or without an increase in rate.

hyperpyrexia Marked elevation of temperature, usually above 105.8° F (41° C).

hyperreflexia Increased amplitude of muscle contraction to evoked reflex.

hypersplenism Enlargement of the spleen associated with a reduction in red blood cells.

hypertension Persistent elevation of blood pressure.

hyperthermia Abnormally elevated body temperature.

hypertonia Increased resistance of muscle tissue to passive stretching.

hypertrichosis Excessive hairiness, especially in females.

hypertrophy Increase in size of a tissue or organ.

hyperventilation Increase in rate and depth of respiration.

hyphema Blood in the anterior chamber of the eye.

hypochondriasis Unrealistic interpretation of physical signs or sensations as abnormal; preoccupation with the fear or belief of having a serious disease.

hypochromic Abnormally decreased color; used to describe anemias in which the amount of hemoglobin in red blood cells is deficient.

hypoesthesia Abnormally decreased sensitivity of the skin or another sense organ.

hypoglossal Below the tongue.

hypomania A clinical syndrome that is similar to but less severe than that demonstrated in a full-blown manic episode.

hypopyon Purulent material in the anterior chamber of the eye.

hyposmia Partial loss of the sense of smell.

hypospadias A developmental anomaly in which the urethra opens on the underside of the penis.

hysteria Described in Kaplan and Sadock, 1985, as two types. *Conversion disorder:* characterized by bodily symptoms resembling those of physical disease. *Dissociative type:* manifested by such conditions as somnambulism, various forms of amnesia and fugue states, and multiple personality disorder. Anxiety plays a role in each type.

icteric Jaundiced.

illusion Perception based on actual external stimulus with misinterpretation or distortion of the event.

immediate auscultation The use of a sound-augmentation device to detect body sounds.

immediate percussion Using the finger or hand to strike the body to evaluate the sound waves produced.

impetigo Skin infection caused by staphylococcal or streptococcal organisms. The typical lesion is an eroded, ruptured vesicle covered by an amber crust.

incontinence Failure of control of excretory functions.

infarction Obstruction of circulation followed by ischemic necrosis.

inflammation Localized protective condition associated with vascular dilatation, exudation of plasma, and leukocytes. Clinical signs include redness, swelling, pain, heat, and limitation of function.

inspection Visual evaluation of the body incorporating the senses of sight, smell, and hearing.

intellectualization A defense mechanism that consists of ruminating about philosophical or theoretical ideas or engaging in scholarly activities that serves to constrain instinctual drives. Intellectualization constitutes an interruption of the stream of thought.

internal rotation The turning of the body part toward the central axis or midline of the body.

inversion A turning inward.

ipsilateral On the same side.

iritis Inflammation of the iris.

jargon A word or word group commonly used and understood within one profession but seldom used or understood by those outside the profession.

jaundice Accumulation of bilirubin to serum concentration greater than 2 mg/dl; produces yellow-green to bronze color of skin, accompanied by itching.

Jolly test Recurrent stimulation of motor muscles. A positive response includes increasingly weaker muscle contraction, associated with myasthenia gravis.

keratitis Inflammation of the cornea.

keloid Scar formation due to a dense overgrowth of fibrous tissue, usually raised and thickened.

kinesthetic sensation The sensation facilitated by the proprioceptive receptors in the muscles, tendons, and joints.

koilonychia Spoon-shaped nail surface with thin nail, frequently associated with iron deficiency anemia.

Koplik's spots Small white spots on the buccal mucosa that appear in the prodromal stage of measles.

Korotkoff sounds Turbulent sounds heard when auscultating the blood pressure.

kraurosis vulvae Atrophic condition of the vulva with edema of the surface dermis with underlying inflammation.

Kussmaul respiration Rapid and deep respiratory cycles resulting from stimulation of the medullary respiratory center in metabolic acidosis, associated with pH less than 7.2 in diabetic ketoacidosis.

kwashiorkor Protein-calorie malnutrition; generalized pitting edema, ascites, inhibition of growth, skin rash, ulcers, anorexia, diarrhea, liver enlargement.

kyphoscoliosis Deformity of the spine characterized by curvature in lateral (scoliosis) and anteroposterior (kyphosis) planes.

kyphosis Increased posterior convexity of the spine (humpback).

labile Readily altered, unstable.

labyrinth An intricate communicating passageway, such as the bony and membranous labyrinths in the inner ear.

lamella Small sheet or leaf.

lassitude Feeling of weakness or exhaustion.

lethargy Condition of drowsiness.

leukopenia Abnormal diminution of leukocytes.

leukoplakia A disease appearing as white, thickened patches on mucous membranes.

leukorrhea White discharge from the vagina.

lineae albicantes (striae) Atrophic line or streak that differs in texture and color from the surrounding skin due to disrupted elastic fibers of the reticular layer of the cutis.

linea nigra Pigmentation of the linea alba, the tendinous median line on the anterior abdominal wall, during pregnancy.

lipofuscin Brown, granular pigment found in the lysosomes, nerve cells, muscle, heart, and liver in elderly persons.

lithium An element or salt used in the treatment and prevention of manic episodes and other cyclic disorders.

looseness of associations Flow or stream of thought that is vague, unfocused, and illogical. Notable in clients with schizophrenia.

lordosis. Anterior concavity of the lumbar spine (swayback, saddle back).

luxation Dislocation.

lymphadenitis Inflammation of one or more lymph nodes.

lymphadenopathy Disease of the lymph nodes.

lymphadenosis Hypertrophy or proliferation of lymphatic tissue.

lymphedema Edema caused by accumulation of lymph; may result from pathologic condition of lymph ducts or nodes.

lymphoma Neoplastic disorder of lymphatic tissue.

lysis Gradual return to normal following a disease; generally refers to a fever.

macula Small spot on the skin that differs in color from the surrounding tissue and is not elevated.

malaise Feeling of general discomfort or uneasiness.

malignant Tending to become progressively worse and life threatening, especially a disease or tumor.

malingering Simulation of illness.

manic episode Period of behavior characterized by predominantly elevated, expansive, or irritable mood with a duration of at least 1 week. Behaviors that may accompany the elated feeling are increase in activity, restlessness, talkativeness, flight of ideas, feeling that thoughts are racing, grandiosity, decreased sleep time, short attention span, buying sprees, sexual indiscretion, and inappropriate laughing, joking, or punning.

marasmus Malnutrition caused by inadequate intake of all nutrients; atrophy of muscles, growth retardation.

master two-step tests Clinical exercise stress test in which subject repeatedly climbs and descends a two-step stair with 9-in risers for 1½ minutes. Test is meant to reveal subclinical coronary artery disease.

mastication The act of chewing.

mastoid process Bony prominence found posterior to the lower part of the auricle.

mastitis Inflammation of breast tissue.

McBurney's point Approximately 2 in above the right anterosuperior iliac spine on a line between the umbilicus and the spine.

meatus A passage or opening, especially at the external portion of the canal.

mediate percussion The middle finger of one hand strikes the middle finger of the other hand to emit a sound or vibration.

meibomian glands Saebaceous glands found in the tarsal plates of the eyelid.

melanocyte A cell that produces melanin.

melanoma Malignant neoplasm of melanocytes.

melasma Circumscribed hyperpigmentation of the skin, especially the forehead, cheeks, chin, and lips in the presence of normal levels of melanocyte-stimulating hormone (MSH). The "mask of pregnancy" is thought to be a result of progesterone effects.

melena Dark-colored stools that may be black or tarry stained with partially digested blood.

menorrhagia Excessive menstruation.

mental disorder "A clinically significant behavioral or psychological syndrome or pattern . . . typically associated with a painful symptom . . . or impairment, in one or more important areas of functioning" (*DSM-III-R,* 1987).

mental retardation Lack of intelligence to a degree that interferes with social and occupational performance.

mental status examination A record of current findings that include the description of a client's appearance, behavior, motor activity, speech, alertness, mood, cognition, intelligence, reactions, views, and attitudes.

metaplasia Change of cell type as in the presence of squamous cells in the respiratory tract of chronic smokers, replacing columnar epithelium.

metrorrhagia Irregular uterine bleeding.

microcephaly Head circumference measuring less than three standard deviations below the mean for age and sex.

micrognathia Underdevelopment of the jaw.

migraine Paroxysmal headache, frequently unilateral.

milieu The therapeutic environment.

miosis Abnormal contractions of the pupils.

mitral regurgitation Backward flow of blood from the left ventricle to left atrium associated with incompetent mitral valve caused by congenital defects, mitral calcification, papillary muscle rupture, ventricular aneurysm, or bacterial endocarditis. Early in the disease, fatigue and exertional dyspnea may occur, and failure of the right side of the heart may occur with progression of the disease. Auscultation signs include a holosystolic murmur and S_3 gallop. The heart is enlarged.

mitral stenosis Fibrosis and thickening of the cusps of the mitral valve with narrowing of the aperture between the left atrium and ventricle, which is usually seen in the aftermath of rheumatic heart disease. Auscultation reveals accentuated S_1. After the second sound, S_2, an opening snap is heard.

mitral valve prolapse Eversion of the valve cusps of the mitral valve during ventricular systole. Severity is related to the amount of regurgitation or auscultation. A midsystolic click is heard.

Montgomery's glands Small, sebaceous glands located on the areola.

mood disorder A diagnostic category in the *DSM-III-R* that includes the listing of affective disorders.

morning sickness Nausea and vomiting during the fifth or sixth week of pregnancy to the fourteenth to sixteenth week. The cause is unknown.

mumps Viral infection involving the parotid gland.

murmur Blowing sound caused by turbulence of blood flow, heard through the stethoscope over the heart or the great vessels.

Murphy's sign A maneuver done during deep palpation in the approximate location of the gallbladder. On deep inspiration, the liver descends, bringing the gallbladder in contact with the examiner's hand. Pain will be elicited in the presence of cholecystitis.

mydriasis Extreme dilatation of the pupil resulting from paralysis of the oculomotor muscles or the effect of a drug.

myoclonus Jerking movement of one or more limbs or the trunk caused by muscle contractions.

myopathy Disease of the muscles.

myxedema Hypothyroidism. Hypometabolism is present, and nonpitting edema results from the presence of hydrated mucopolysaccharides in connective tissue.

myringitis Inflammation of the tympanic membrane usually resulting from infection.

nabothian follicles Cystlike formations of the mucosa of the uterine cervix resulting from an accumulation of retained secretion in occluded glands.

NANDA Abbreviation for the North American Nursing Diagnosis Association.

narcissistic Extreme self-centeredness and self-absorption (narcissistic personality disorder).

nausea Feeling that emesis is impending.

neologism Newly coined word; meaningless word often uttered by a psychotic client.

nephritis Inflammation of the kidney.

nephrocalcinosis Condition in which there is precipitation of calcium salts in the tubules and parenchyma of the kidney.

nephrolithiasis Condition of renal calculi.

neuralgia Pain associated with the course of a nerve.

neurosis Psychiatric term for an emotional problem thought to be related to unresolved conflict; differs from a psychosis in that hallucinations, delusions, and illusions generally do not occur.

neurotransmitter A chemical found in the nervous system (e.g., norepinephrine, serotonin, dopamine) that facilitates the transmission of the nerve impulses across synapses between neurons. Implicated in affective and schizophrenic disorders.

nevus Well-demarcated malformation of the skin, such as an area of pigmentation or a mole.

night blindness Slow adjustment from bright to dim light.

nociceptive Painful response of reflex evoked by a noxious stimulus.

nocturia Excessive urination at night.

non-verbal communication The process in which information is passed from one individual to another without speaking but by body movements. This may be conscious or unconscious.

nuchal Pertaining to the nape of the neck.

nullipara Woman who has not given birth to a viable offspring.

nursing diagnosis A statement that describes a client's health state, or response to illness, treatable by nurses.

nystagmus Involuntary, rhythmic motion of the eye; may be horizontal, vertical, rotary, or mixed.

obsession Persistent, upsetting preoccupation with an idea that morbidly dominates the mind.

obsessive-compulsive disorder Recurrent obsessions (thoughts) that are ego-dystonic (invasive to the ego) alternating with compulsions (behaviors). Both are unwilled and painful.

obstipation Severe constipation.

oligomenorrhea Decreased frequency of menstruation with an interval of 38 to 90 days.

oligospermia Less than 20 million spermatozoa per milliliter of semen.

oliguria Abnormally decreased urine secretion (<400 ml/24 hours).

omphalocele Congenital umbilical hernia.

onychia Inflammation of the matrix of the nail.

onycholysis Distal separation of the nails from the nail bed.

open-ended statement A statement that elicits further exploration of the client's problem by encouraging communication. Can also be in the form of a question.

opisthotonos Hyperextension of the neck and marked flexion of hips and legs.

organic brain syndromes Clusters of psychological or behavioral abnormalities or symptoms that tend to occur together; the etiology is unknown.

organic mental disorders A class of disorders of mental functioning caused by permanent brain damage or temporary brain dysfunction. Etiology is known and may be primary (originating in the brain) or secondary to systemic disease. Cognition, emotions, and motivation are affected.

orientation Conscious awareness of person, place, and time.

orifice An opening.

orthopnea Dyspnea relieved by sitting upright.

orthostatic (postural) hypotension Lowering blood pressure that occurs on rising to an erect position.

otalgia Earache.

Paget's disease Condition characterized by excoriating or scaling lesion of the nipple, extending from an intraductal carcinoma of the breast.

palpate Examination conducted by feeling or touching the object to be evaluated.

palpebra Eyelid.

palpitation Subjective awareness of the pulsations of the heart and arteries.

papilledema Edema of the optic papilla.

papule Elevated lesion of the skin with a diameter less than 5 mm.

paranoia Oversuspiciousness. May lead to persecutory delusions or projectile behavior patterns.

paraesthesia Abnormal or perverted sensation; may include burning, itching, pain, or the feeling of electric shock.

paresis Slight or incomplete paralysis; weakness.

parkinsonism symptoms Masked facies, muscle rigidity, and shuffling gait; common in clients taking neuroleptic drugs; extrapyramindal symptoms are related to dopamine blockade.

paronychia Inflammation and infection of the folds of tissue surrounding a fingernail.

parosmia Perversion of the sense of smell; olfactory hallucinations.

passive-aggressive personality disorder Resistance to demands for adequate performance in occupational or social settings. Resistance may take the form of "forgetfulness," intentional inefficiency, stubbornness, dawdling, or procrastination.

passive range of motion Joint movement of the client that the examiner produces.

pediculosis Infestation with lice.

perception Awareness of objects and relations that follows stimulation of peripheral sense organs.

percussion Examination conducted by listening to reverberation of tissue after striking the surface with short, sharp blows.

peristalsis Wave of contraction moving along a muscular tube, particularly the gastrointestinal tract.

peritonitis Inflammation of the peritoneum.

personality disorder Exaggerated, pathologic behavior patterns, destructive to the individual and others.

petechiae Very small, flat, purple-to-red skin or mucous membrane lesions caused by submucous or intradermal hemorrhage.

phimosis Difficulty in retraction of the foreskin of the penis.

phobia Persistent and exaggerated fear of a particular object or situation.

phoria Mild weakness of the extraocular muscle(s). *Esophoria:* inward deviation of the eye(s). *Exophoria:* outward deviation of the eye(s).

photalgia Painful sensation in eye following exposure to light.

photophobia Abnormal intolerance of light.

pica Repeated consumption of nonnutritive substance for at least 1 month.

pinguecula Thickened, yellowish area of the cornea, a common degenerative condition.

pinna The projecting part of the external ear; the auricle.

pityriasis Skin disease characterized by the formation of fine, branny scales. *P. alba:* chronic patchy scaling and hypopigmentation of facial skin. *P. rosea:* acure inflammatory disease with oval, tan eruptions of scales in skin cleavage lines. *P. rubra polans:* chronic inflammatory skin condition with pink scales, macules, and papules.

plantar flexion a forward bending.

plantar wart Infection with human wart virus characterized by a wart on the sole of the foot.

-plegia Complete paralysis. *Diplegia:* paralysis of both upper or lower limbs. *Hemiplegia:* paralysis of one side of the body. *Paraplegia:* paralysis of both legs and the lower part of the body. *Quadraplegia:* paralysis of all four limbs.

plethora Pertaining to a red, florid complexion.

pleural effusion Fluid of any kind in the pleural cavity.

pleurisy Pain accompanying pleural inflammation.

polycythemia Abnormal increase in the number of red blood cells.

polydipsia Excessive thirst.

polymenorrhea Abnormally frequent menstruation.

polyphagia Excessive ingestion of food.

polyuria Increased urinary excretion.

Poupart's ligament The inguinal ligament; the fibrous band that runs from the anterior superior iliac spine to the pubic spine.

prepuce Foreskin.

presbycusis Sensorineural hearing loss that develops as a part of the aging process.

presbyopia Reduced capacity of the lens of the eye to accommodate, which develops with advancing age.

preseveration An interruption in the stream of though characterized by multiple repetitions of a word or phrase.

pressure of speech Voluble speech that is difficult to interpret.

preterm infant An infant born before 37 weeks' gestation.

priapism Prolonged erection of the penis.

proctitis Inflammation of the rectal mucosa.

proctoscopy Examination of the rectum with a short cylindric instrument called a proctoscope.

prodromal Sign or symptom indicating the onset of a disease.

progeria Manifestation of aging occurring in childhood.

prognathism Protrusion of the jaw.

prognosis Expected outcome of a pathological condition.

projection Unconscious defense mechanism in which a person attributes, to another person, undesirable thoughts, feelings, and impulses. Anxiety is decreased as feelings are externalized.

pronation (1) Assumption of the prone position; (2) turning the forearm so the palm is posterior; or (3) eversion and abduction of the foot.

proprioceptive sensation Muscle and joint sensations of position in space.

prostatitis Acute or chronic inflammation of the prostate gland, generally in conjunction with cystitis and urethritis. Symptoms: low back and perineal pain, fever, urinary frequency, and dysuria.

pruritus Itching.

psoriasis Papulosquamous dermatosis; characteristic lesion is bright red macule, papule, or plaque covered with silver scales.

psychoanalytic Referring to the structures of the mind, such as the id, ego, and superego, as described by Freud.

psychasthenia Neurosis characterized by depersonalization, delusions, fear, and feelings of inadequacy.

psychogenic amnesia Sudden inability to recall important personal information that cannot be explained by normal forgetfulness.

psychosis Psychiatric term for a mental disorder associated with thought disorders, pathologic perception (delusions, hallucinations), or extremes of affect.

pterygium Abnormal triangular thickening of the bulbar conjunctiva on the cornea, with the apex toward the pupil.

ptosis Drooping of the eyelid.

pulse Palpable rhythmic expansion of the artery.

purpura Small hemorrhage, less than 1 cm in diameter.

pulsus alternans A pulse that alternates strong and weak pulsations with a regular rhythm.

pulse deficit When the peripheral pulse count is less than the ventricular rate taken at the apex of the heart.

pulse pressure The difference between the systolic and diastolic blood pressure.

pustule Elevation of skin containing purulent exudate filled with neutrophils.

pyemia General septicemia marked by fever, chills, and abscesses.

pyorrhea Purulent inflammation of the gums.

pyrexia Fever; elevation of the body temperature above normal for a given individual.

pyrosis Heartburn.

pyuria Presence of pus in the urine.

quinsy Peritonsillar abscess.

rale Discrete, noncontinuous sound resembling fine crackling, radio static, or hairs being rubbed together, heard through the stethoscope; generally produced by air bubbling through an exudate.

rationalization A defense mechanism by which irrational or unacceptable behavior, motives, or feelings are logically justified or made tolerable, by plausible means.

rectocele Herniation of the rectum into the vagina.

regurgitation Reversal of the flow of a substance through a vessel, such as blood flow in the wrong direction or the return of food to the mouth without vomiting.

retinal exudates *Cotton wool exudates:* white, opaque areas seen in the retina in ophthalmoscopic examination; *white, soft, fluffy exudates:* microinfarctions of the retinal nerve that represent swollen axon cylinders, referred to as cytoid bodies. *Soft exudates:* occur in hypertension, collagen vascular disease, and diabetes mellitus. *Hard exudates:* true exudates that are yellowish and in faint clusters or dense masses. These exudates are composed of serum lipids and fat-laden macrophages. Hard exudates occur primarily in diabetes mellitus and severe hypertension.

retraction Condition of being drawn back.

rhinorrhea Excessive, thin nasal secretion.

rhonchus Wheezing or snoring sound produced by airflow across a partially constricted air passage. *Sibilant rhonchus:* wheeze produced in a small air passage. *Sonorous rhonchus:* wheeze produced in a large air passage.

rigor Common term for shivering accompanying a chill or for muscle rigidity accompanying depletion of adenosine triphosphate, as in death (rigor mortis).

salpingitis Inflammation of the fallopian tubes as a result of infection. Leukorrhea, adnexal tenderness, abdominal pain, and fever may be present.

schizophrenic disorder Condition characterized by delusions, hallucinations, or incoherence with flat or inappropriate affect or disorganized behavior. Behavior has deteriorated from a previous level of functioning with regard to work, social relations, or self-care. *Disorganized schizophrenia:* a type of schizophrenia in which there is frequent incoherence, inappropriate affect, but no delusions. *Catatonic schizophrenia:* a type of schizophrenia characterized by any of the following: (1) catatonic stupor reduction in reactivity to environment, spontaneous movements, and mutism; (2) catatonic negativism (resistance to instructions or movement); (3) catatonic rigidity (maintenance of rigid posture even against attempts to move the client); (4) catatonic excitement (excited motor activity not influenced by external stimuli); (5) catatonic posturing (inappropriate or bizarre posturing). *Paranoid schizophrenia:* a type of schizophrenia characterized by persecutory delusions, grandiose delusions, delusional jealousy, or hallucinations with persecutory or grandiose content.

sciatica Pain, weakness, or paresthesias associated with the course of the sciatic nerve; posterior aspect of the thigh, posterolateral and anterolateral aspects of the leg into the foot.

scoliosis Lateral deviation of the spine.

scotoma An islandlike blind gap in the visual field.

sebaceous Pertaining to or secreting sebum, an oily secretion composed of fat and epithelial debris.

sebaceous cyst Retention of the fatty secretion of the sebaceous gland.

sensorineural hearing loss Diminished ability to hear due to the inability of the acoustic nerve transmit nervous impulses from the middle ear to the brain.

sentinel node Also called Virchow's node; enlarged supraclavicular node that may indicate abdominal carcinoma.

sign Objective evidence of disease that is perceptible to the examiner.

simian crease Single transverse crease on the palm; found in 70% of those who have Down's syndrome.

sinus A hollow in a bone or other tissue.

sleep terror (pavor nocturnus) Repeated experience of abrupt awakening from sleep in a state of anxiety or panic, generally occurring in stages 3 and 4 and in the time place of 30 to 200 minutes after the onset of sleep.

somatic Pertaining to the body.

somatization The conversion of mental states or experiences into bodily symptoms; associated with anxiety.

somesthesia Sensation of touch-pressure, temperature, pain, and joint position.

somnambulism (sleepwalking) Sleep disorder characterized by repeated acts of rising from bed during sleep and walking for a few minutes to a half hour, generally occurring in stages 3 and 4 and in the time phase of 30 to 200 minutes after the onset of sleep.

sordes Materia alba; undigested food bacteria encrusting the lips and teeth.

spasm Involuntary sudden contraction of a muscle or a group of muscles accompanied by pain and interference with function.

spastic Rigid; characterized by muscle spasm.

speculum A device made of two narrow blades or a hollow tube, used to assist in opening a body cavity.

steatorrhea Abnormal increase of fat in the feces.

stereognosis Discrimination of objects by the sense of touch.

stereotypy Interruption in the stream of thought consisting of persistent repetition of a word or phrase.

sthenic Sturdy or strong; active.

stomatitis Inflammation of the mouth.

strabismus Disparity in the anteroposterior axes of the eyes; the optic axes cannot be direct to the same object because of lack of muscular coordination.

stress incontinence Involuntary urination incurred on straining, coughing, or lifting.

stressor A stimulus perceived by the individual or the organism as challenging, threatening, or damaging.

striae gravidarum Atrophic, pinkish or purplish scarlike lesions observed on the breasts, thighs, abdomen, and buttocks during pregnancy; lesions later become silvery white.

stridor Harsh, high-pitched respiratory sound heard in clients with respiratory obstruction.

stupor Decreased responsiveness; partial unconsciousness.

succussion Procedure involving shaking an individual to demonstrate fluid in a hollow cavity.

suicidal ideation A verbalized thought that indicates a person's desire toward self-harm or self-destruction.

supine Lying on the back.

symmetry Similar in size, shape, and position to the body part on the opposite side.

symptom A client's subjective perception of an alteration of bodily or mental function from basal conditions; change perceived by the individual.

syncope Fainting; temporary unconsciousness.

syndrome Recognized pattern of signs and symptoms.

tachycardia Rapid heart rate ($\geq$100 beats per minute). *Atrial flutter:* rapid, regular, uniform atrial contraction caused by AV block; ventricular rhythm varies with the degree of AV block. *Atrial tachycardia:* arrhythmia caused by the atria; rapid, regular beat of the entire heart. *Ventricular tachycardia:* arrhythmia caused by the ventricles; rapid, relatively regular heartbeat.

tachypnea Rapid respiratory rate.

telangiectasis Localized group of dilated capillaries.

tenesmus Uncomfortable straining; particularly, unsuccessful attempts at defecation or urination.

term infant Infant born between 37 and 41 weeks' gestation.

thrill Palpable murmur; vibration accompanying turbulence in the heart or the great vessels.

thought disorder Thinking characterized by loosened associations, neologisms, and illogical constructs and conclusions.

thrush A fungal infection of the oral mucus membranes that appears as white adherent patches.

tic Sudden, short contractions of a muscle or group of muscles, always causing movement of affected part.

tinnitus Sensation of noise in the ear caused by abnormal stimulation of the auditory apparatus or its afferent pathways; may be described as ringing, buzzing, swishing, roaring, blowing, or whistling.

tophus Deposits of monosodium urate, seen in gout.

torticollis Contraction of the sternocleidomastoid muscle that results in forward flexion of the head and rotation of the chin away from the affected side.

transient ischemic attack Occlusion of central nervous system vessel resulting in a focal neurologic disturbance. Abbreviated TIA.

tremor Involuntary, somewhat rhythmic, oscillatory quivering of muscles, caused by alternate contraction of opposing groups of muscles. *Cerebellar tremor:* occurs during intentional movement, becoming more pronounced near end of the movement; associated with lesions of the dentate nucleus. *Coarse tremor:* slow rate and large amplitude movements. *Essential (familial) tremor:* begins usually around age 50 with fine tremors of the hands; aggravated by intentional movement; commonly affects head, jaws, lips, or voice. *Fine tremor:* rapid (10 to 20 oscillations per second) and low amplitude movements, usually in the fingers and hands. *Moderate tremor:* medium rate and medium amplitude movements. *Passive tremor:* present at rest, may improve during intentional movement; for example, pill-rolling tremor or Parkinson's disease. *Physiologic tremor:* experienced by healthy people in fatigue, cold, and stress. *Toxic tremor:* caused by endogenous (thyrotoxicosis, uremia) or exogenous toxins (alcohol, drugs).

trimester A period of 13 weeks.

trophoblast The peripheral cells of the blastocyst that attach the fertilized ovum to the uterine wall and become the placenta and the membranes.

tropia Permanent deviation of the axis of an eye.

Trousseau's sign Elicitation of carpopedal spasm by compression of the upper arm with a tourniquet or blood pressure cuff. The sign is associated with hypocalcemic tetany.

turgor The normal resilience of the skin.

two-point discrimination The ability to sense the simultaneous stimulation of two areas of skin.

tympanic membrane (eardrum) A membranous structure separating the external ear from the middle ear.

tympany Drumlike note produced by percussion, generally over a gas-filled region.

ulcer Indentation of the surface of tissue or an organ resulting from the sloughing of necrotic, inflamed tissue.

ulnar deviation Turning the wrist away from the midline of the body.

undulant Wavelike variations, particularly as in fever and diurnal circadian fluctuations.

urticaria Rash characterized by wheals.

uveitis Inflammation of the middle, pigmented layer and vascular coat of the eye; iris, ciliary body, and choroid.

valgus Angulation of an extremity toward the midline. *Genu valgum:* condition in which knees are abnormally close together, knock-knee.

varicocele Distention of the veins of the spermatic cord.

varicose Dilated, particularly a vein.

varus Angulation of an extremity away from the midline. *Genu varum:* condition in which knees are abnormally separated; bowleg.

verbigeration (polyphasia) Repetition of meaningless words or phrases.

verruca Lobulated elevation of the epidermis thought to be caused by papillomavirus.

vertigo Illusion of movement, with imagined rotation of one's self (subjective vertigo) or of one's surroundings (objective vertigo).

vesicle Blister, elevation caused by separation of the epidermis by serous fluid or pus.

Virchow's node See sentinel node.

vital or cardinal signs Indicators of bodily function such as blood pressure, temperature, pulse, and respiration.

vitiligo Skin affliction characterized by patches of depigmented skin caused by destruction of melanocytes associated with autoimmune disorders.

whispered pectoriloquy Increased resonance of the whispered voice as heard through the stethoscope.

xerostomia Dryness of the mouth resulting from decreased production of saliva.

xiphisternum Xiphoid process of the sternum.

Index

An italicized page number indicates an illustration; *l* following a page number refers to a legend; *t* following a page number refers to a table.

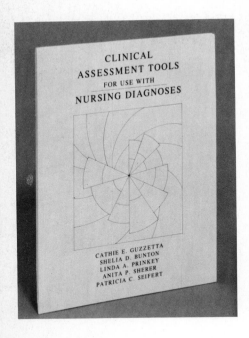
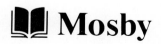